PLASTIC AND RECONSTRUCTIVE SURGERY

PLASTIC AND RECONSTRUCTIVE SURGERY

HANS MAY, *M.D., F.A.C.S.*

THIRD EDITION

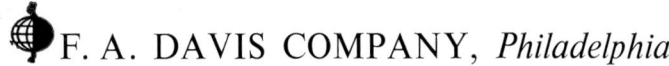 F. A. DAVIS COMPANY, *Philadelphia*

Manufactured in the United States of America

Library of Congress Catalog Card Number 74-103537

ISBN 0-8036-5960-1

TO THE MAIMED
THAT THE ANGUISH
FROM THEIR AFFLICTIONS
BE ALLEVIATED IS THE
EVER-GRATIFYING REWARD
OF OUR PROFESSION'S
HUMBLE EFFORTS

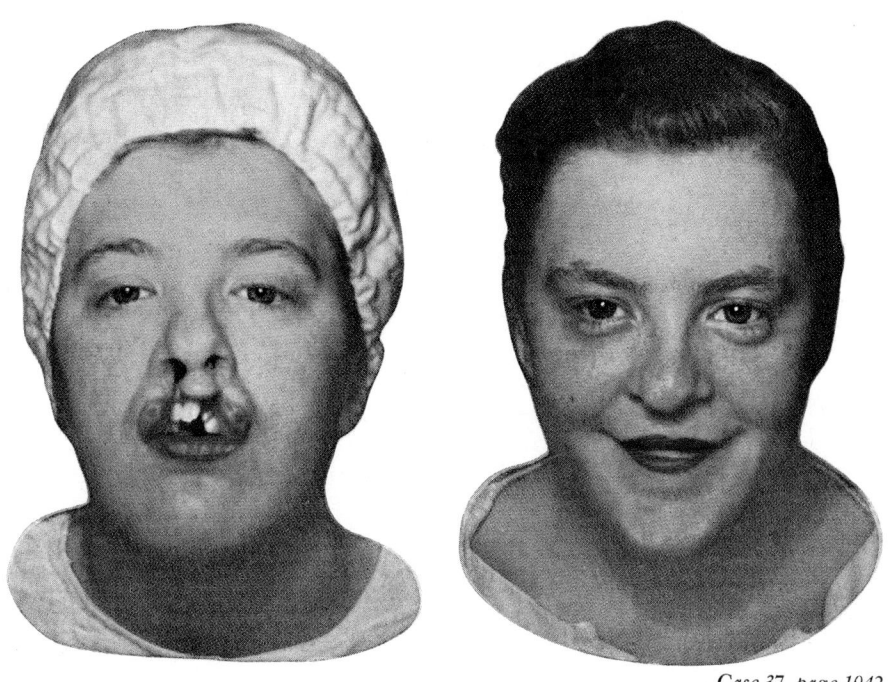

Case 37, page 1042

PREFACE

Twelve years have passed since the publication of the last edition of this book. These were times of peace and times of war; an ugly war is still being waged. Said the Romans, "Mars is the teacher of many things." Indeed he taught plastic surgery a great deal, particularly during the two World Wars. In the present Viet Nam conflict, however, the tables have been turned insofar as it is the civilian-gained knowledge of plastic surgery that can be given back to war surgery. This is the result of vast advances made in this field of surgery during the immediate past, bringing about changes not so much in principle but in refinement and depth. We have obtained a more profound insight into the regenerative processes of tissues and have acquired a keener perception and better control of the forces which encourage or inhibit them. This in turn has influenced the entire field of tissue transplantation and induced organ transplantation. A better understanding of the healing process of a wound and of the physiological and hormonal responses which influence it has aided the treatment of wounds, including the burn wounds. Technical advances have refined numerous reconstructive procedures and new methods have been added. Some will stand the test of time. Some will not, as everything in nature is subject to never-ending changes.

All of this has brought about a sharper definition of plastic surgery, a specialty which is a branch of surgery; as such it must remain, i.e., it must remain attached to the main trunk, lest the branch will wither.

The new revision of the text gave the author a chance for much "pruning" and the opportunity to change, reorganize, and expand. Eliminated or greatly reduced are those chapters which according to experience belong to other branches of surgery, such as the orthopedic and vascular specialties. Expansions or replacements were made in practically every chapter of the book. Treatment and methods, however, that have proved to be constantly efficient have been retained. Some techniques have been mentioned with which the author has no experience but which have proved successful in qualified hands, thus offering the reader convenient access to recent references in these areas.

In spite of expansion, the volume of the book has increased little because of the extensive "pruning." It was not difficult to join the old and the new portions of the text, but the sharper definition of the field of plastic surgery suggested the change of title for the book.

The new revision has maintained essentially the organization of former editions, which is outlined in the preface to the previous edition. The last section of the book, illustrative cases and their histories, has been retained and expanded because of its teaching value. Gathering photographs and detailed case descriptions at the end of the book rather than interspersing them within the main text has satisfied the requirements of practicality.

This revision—the third edition of the book—gives the author the opportunity to acknowledge his debt of gratitude to those who have contributed to it. The drawings were by the celebrated medical illustrators Mr. and Mrs. Wm. B. McNett and Mrs. Dorothy Robinson. The photography throughout was the work of Mr. E. Richard Deats. Dr. David M. Davis contributed the section on congenital malformation of the urethra in the male, Chapter 18, Dr. Michael A. Manko the section on antimicrobial therapy, Chapter 3, and Dr. Thals Bowen the various sections on anesthesiology.

I wish to express my appreciation and gratitude to my secretary, Miss Marian E. Esterly, who is responsible for the painstaking task of transcription of the manuscript.

I am indebted to those authors who graciously permitted reproduction of their illustrations, and last, but not least, to the F. A. Davis Company and its staff for the work involved in publishing the book.

Hans May, M.D.
Christiansted, St. Croix
U. S. Virgin Islands

PREFACE to the Second Edition

TEN YEARS have elapsed since the publication of the first edition of this book—a relatively short span of time, and yet a decade of rapid and profound changes in medicine and surgery effecting improvements and refinement in the art and science of plastic and reconstructive surgery. The experience gained in World War II stimulated the use and evaluation of new techniques in civilian practice, and paved the way for further advances that later were subjected to reevaluation in the Korean conflict. The greater quiescence of recent years has provided an opportunity to digest the vast information offered by the dynamic years of the immediate past.

Plastic surgery is firmly established as a separate branch of surgery, the formative branch of surgery, as the term "plastic"—popularized by E. Zeis through his two scholarly works of 1838 and 1863 —aptly signifies. Specialization is the present trend of medicine— justifiably so. If the tree is to grow it must branch. Overspecialization, however, is apt to lead to segregation, a fact that is being more and more appreciated. It impairs the versatility of the specialist, and he is likely to see only the conditions related to his specialty rather than the patient as a whole. Only through application of the basic principles of general surgery to every surgical specialty can the welfare of the patient be furthered. This book is presented, therefore, with the hope that it may be of practical value and theoretical interest not only to the specialist of plastic and reconstructive surgery but to the general surgeon as well.

The book has five divisions: one on general principles, three on regional features, and one dealing with clinical examples. Division One contains general technique, grafting of tissue, transplantation of flaps, and treatment of burns, wounds, and scars. Divisions Two to Four demonstrate the various reconstructive principles in the different parts of the body: head and neck, trunk extremities other than hand and foot, and hand and foot. Reconstructive surgery deals mainly with the closure of defects and reconstruction in malformations; hence it was considered logical and practical to carry this theme throughout the discussions on regional procedures. Thus, these chapters have been subdivided, whenever possible, under the headings: Defects, Deformities (or Dysfunctions). The last section of the book, Division Five, presents illustrative cases and their histories; formerly arranged on a trial basis, it has proved a worthy adjunct to the text. It has satisfied the requirements of practicality, and therefore in this second edition has been retained and expanded.

This second edition has been largely rewritten. Treatment and methods that have proved consistently to be efficient have been retained. Others have been modified. In addition, the continental literature that was inaccessible during World War II has been studied for values requiring alteration or expansion of the first edition text.

The book has been greatly enlarged to include new information and many recent advances, particularly in the field of tissue transplantation, the treatment of wounds and burns, and the use of the antibiotics. The sections dealing with reconstructive surgery of the face and of the extremities, particularly of the hand, have been expanded greatly. Reference has been made to some techniques with which the author has had no experience but which have proved successful in qualified hands.

This second edition gives the author the opportunity to acknowledge his debt of gratitude to those who have stimulated his efforts through their constructive criticism and affirmation.

It is a particular pleasure to acknowledge the practical values that others have contributed to this book. For those activities, and for the cordial and sympathetic attitudes that accompanied them, I am deeply grateful. The drawings were made by the celebrated medical illustrators, Mr. and Mrs. William B. McNett. Mrs. McNett made many from actual operations. The photography throughout was the work of Mr. E. Richard Deats. Dr. David M. Davis contributed the section on congenital malformations of the urethra in the male, Chapter XVIII, and Dr. Harrison F. Flippin, the section on antimicrobial therapy, Chapter III.

I wish to express my appreciation and gratitude to my secretary, Miss Marian E. Esterly, who is responsible for the painstaking task of transcription of the manuscript and the preparation of the index, and to Mr. Wendell H. Grenman and Mrs. Florence W. Brehm for editing the text.

I am indebted to those authors who so graciously permitted reproduction of their illustrations; and last, but not least, to the F. A. Davis Company and their editorial staff for the excellent work in publishing the book.

HANS MAY, M.D.

CONTENTS

CONTENTS

DIVISION TWO. THE HEAD AND NECK

CONTENTS

DIVISION THREE. THE TRUNK

DIVISION FOUR. THE EXTREMITIES

CONTENTS

CONTENTS

DIVISION FIVE. ILLUSTRATIVE CASES

DIVISION ONE
GENERAL PRINCIPLES

PREOPERATIVE PREPARATION, INSTRUMENTS, SUTURES AND INCISIONS

1

PREOPERATIVE PREPARATION

A PATIENT undergoing a plastic surgical operation requires the same careful preoperative examination and preparation as any other surgical patient. In most instances, the operation is one of election, allowing time for study, physical examination, and laboratory work. The patient's general condition should be judged from the standpoint of risk. Detrimental factors, such as respiratory infection, local infection, anemia, hypoproteinemia, and dehydration, should be overcome first. (For details, the reader should refer to specific subjects in the Index.) The local condition will influence the preparation and the selection of the proper operative method. Many patients require careful preoperative planning and imagination on the part of the surgeon. Close cooperation with other medical departments is often indispensable.

In some lesions, the making of casts and moulages is requisite for a correct outlay of the operative plan. Prostheses and dentures to be employed permanently can usually be prepared or made before the operation. For this, cooperation with the dental surgeon is necessary.

The operating field itself is prepared in various ways: The patient receives a bath the day before operation, and the field is shaved well beyond its boundaries. Even hairless skin should be shaved to remove loose scales of epidermis. (Eyebrows, however, and skin to be transplanted to the face of a woman or to line cavities should never be shaved.) There are two methods to prepare the skin for the operation, physical and chemical.

GENERAL PRINCIPLES

Physical Preparation of Skin

The physical preparation of the skin is done by one of the personnel whose hands are aseptically prepared. It consists of gently scrubbing the skin with green (alkaline) soap and warm sterile water for ten minutes. The soapy solution is frequently rinsed off with sterile water. This procedure causes loosing of the epidermis and dissolving of the greasy sebaceous matter of the skin, removing detritus and organisms. The skin is now dried with a towel to remove any loose epidermis; then ether is applied to dissolve remaining fatty material. Finally, the entire field is washed with 70 per cent alcohol, which dehydrates the skin and is somewhat antiseptic. Some surgeons prefer this method as a routine skin preparation; some use it for certain operations or regions. It is chosen by the majority of operators for all skin-graft operations, since chemical antiseptics may harm the cells of the graft.

Efforts have been made to make the surgical scrub more effective and less time consuming. The synthetic diphenol G-11 (hexachlorophene), incorporated into a bland soap, has been found to produce a marked "degerming" of the skin, much more so than soap alone (Traub et al., Duke et al., Blank et al., and others). Moreover, a highly significant reduction of the permanent bacterial flora may be maintained by scrubbing every other day with this germicide; that is, cumulative action contributes to its effectiveness. A popular G-11 compound is pHisoderm G-11. This is a water-miscible emulsion containing entsufon, lanolin, cholesterols, petrolatum, and 3 per cent hexachlorophene. It is widely used not only for aseptic preparation of the surgeon's hands and arms but also for preoperative preparation of the operative field.

Chemical Preparation of Skin

The second method of preparing the skin is by chemical antiseptics. Application of an alcoholic solution of 3 per cent iodine results in satisfactory disinfection. To prevent irritation of the skin, the solution should be removed immediately by washing the area with a solution of from 70 to 95 per cent alcohol. Another satisfactory antiseptic solution is Arnold's:

Ethyl alcohol	600.0
Acetone	200.0
Mercuric chloride	1.0
Hydrochloric acid	10.0
Chrysoidin	2.0
Distilled water ....q.s. ad	1000.0

4

This solution is not irritating, and is therefore highly recommended. Of other skin antiseptics, picric acid, merbromin (mercurochrome), and merthiolate may be mentioned. Particularly sensitive places, such as the scrotum and the perineal region, are disinfected with an aqueous solution of acriflavine (1:1000). Mucous membranes of the mouth, for instance, are prepared by frequently brushing the teeth and applying a 3 per cent solution of hydrogen dioxide or sodium perborate. Chemical antiseptics do not influence the organisms in the mucous secretion, and may harm the tissues.

INSTRUMENTS, SUTURE MATERIALS, AND SUTURES

Instruments

The instruments needed for an average operation are: knives (the size of the knife blade to be determined by the particular type of operation), scissors (medium-sized and small, curved and straight), hemostats (ordinary size and mosquito type), retractors (with blunt or sharp hooks), forceps (plain and toothed), needles (curved and straight, with and without cutting edge), and a needle-holder. Special types of operations may require special types of instruments.

Instruments are sterilized either by heat or by chemical antiseptics. Since the former is more effective, it should be used whenever possible. Fine cutting instruments, however, should not be subjected to heat sterilization, since heat affects their cutting edges. They are placed in a solution of formaldehyde and alcohol for twelve hours:

Solution of formaldehyde   85
Alcohol   800
Distilled water . . . . .q.s. ad 1000

Suture and Ligature Material

These are classified as absorbable if they are digested by the tissues during wound healing, and nonabsorbable if they become encapsulated.

Catgut: Catgut is the common material for absorbable sutures. Plain, or untreated, catgut is digested more quickly than chromic catgut which has been subjected to certain tanning processes and hence has acquired more resistance to the absorbing power of the tissue fluids. The difficulty with catgut is the local reaction which may arise from the tissues during digestion and absorption. This may lead to delayed healing and even breakdown of the tissues. Furthermore, absolute sterilization of catgut without impairment of its tensile strength is not possible.

Silk: Silk is a frequently used nonabsorbable material (Kocher, Halsted, Whipple, Shambaugh, Mason). It can be autoclaved or boiled. It comes braided or twisted and white or dyed black. The great tensile strength of silk and its pliability allow the use of very fine strands. Silk

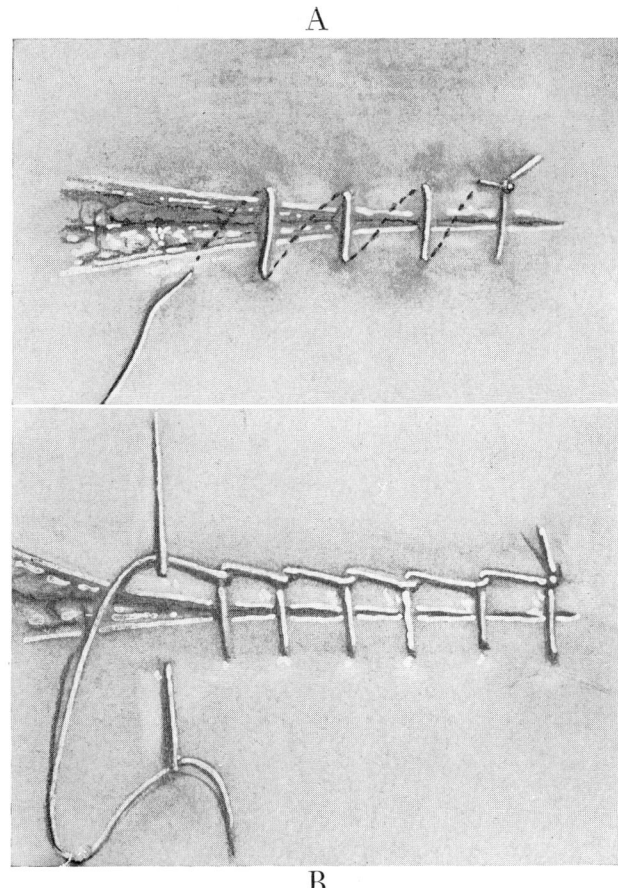

Fig. 1. Continuous suture. *A:* Simple continuous running stitch. *B:* Continuous single-locked stitch.

sutures become encapsulated if used subcutaneously and are not irritating. If embedded in infected tissue, however, organisms may be harbored in interstices, and the suture may become a source of infection until it sloughs out or is surgically removed. To lessen capillarity and increase smoothness, the silk may be drawn through wax or paraffin. This, however, makes the knot more slippery.

SILKWORM GUT: Silkworm gut is unspun silk. It does not consist of fibers, and is smooth and strong; it is principally used for suturing the skin. Dermal suture, a so-called "artificial silkworm gut," is likewise used as a skin suture; it is more flexible than silkworm gut.

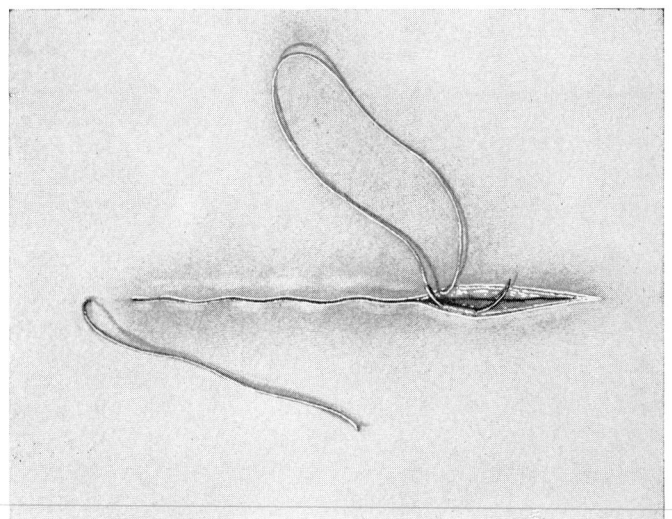

Fig. 2. Cutaneous mattress suture (Halsted), used for closure of straight incisions to avoid stitch marks. A fine curved needle, threaded with fine silk or wire (atraumatic needle, if available), is engaged 1 cm. (⅜ inch) from wound angle and brought out at wound angle. Needle is now passed horizontally through derma on one side and through derma of opposite side until entire wound is closed. At opposite wound angle, needle is brought out 1 cm. (⅜ inch) away from angle.

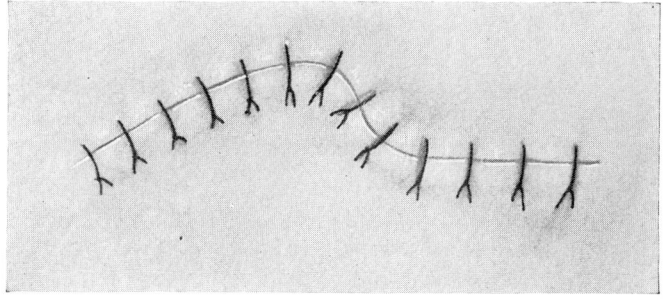

Fig. 3. Interrupted sutures. Stitches lie rectangular to edges of wound.

GENERAL PRINCIPLES

Nylon: Nylon multifilament, a synthetic substitute for silk, has become the most frequently used nonabsorbable suture material. It appears to be stronger than silk (Nichols, Aries, Melick). It is less irritating when used as a skin suture, but seems to be an exciter of tissue reaction when it is placed within tissue; investigators, however, differ

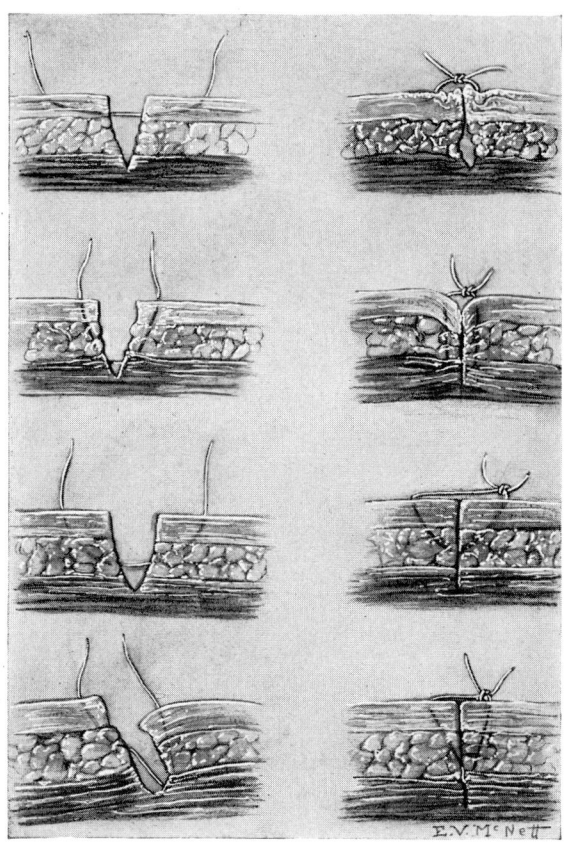

Fig. 4. Various interrupted sutures, passed correctly and incorrectly. *First row:* Suture not passed deeply enough, resulting in dead space beneath and uneven coaptation of skin edges. *Second row:* Suture penetrating too deeply, causing dimpling of wound edges. *Third row:* Suture passed correctly at a distance equal to half the distance from wound edges on each side of wound. *Fourth row:* Uneven wound edges, suture including more tissue on retracted than on elevated side.

as to the amount of tissue reaction (LeVeen and Barberia, Postlethwait et al., Schauble, Dillon, Mager). It can be boiled several times without loss of its original strength.

Cotton: Cotton has come into vogue as suture material and for ligatures (Meade and Ochsner, Thorek, Pannett, Word and Brock). It

8

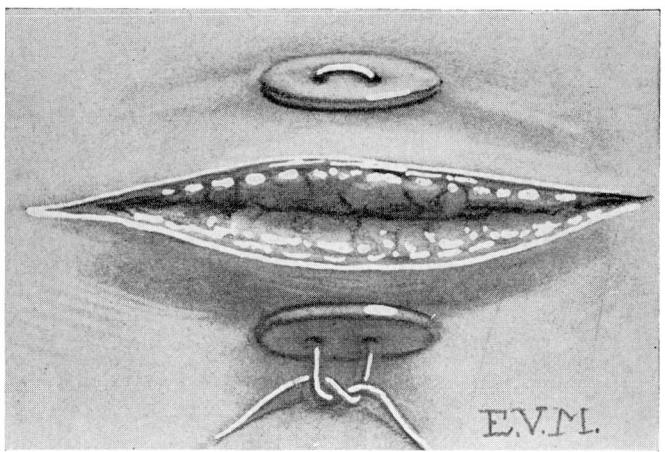

Fig. 5. Relaxation suture tied over metal plate for relief of tension. Buttons, rubber tubing, or rolls of gauze may also be used.

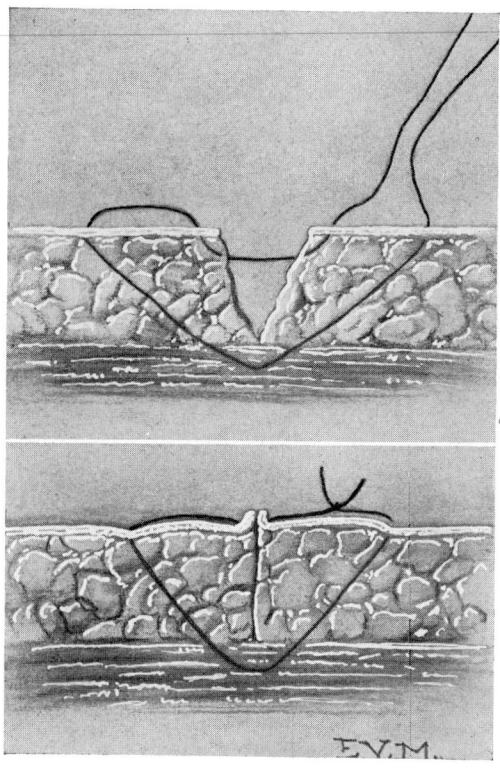

Fig. 6. On-end mattress suture for broad apposition and eversion of wound edges.

9

causes less cellular exudation, but has less tensile strength than silk; it is less capillary, and shows much less tendency to tissue ingrowth, and is, therefore, less likely than silk to cause sinuses in the presence of infection. It is inexpensive, and can be easily sterilized.

Wire: Wire is used by some surgeons routinely, by some only occasionally, as suture and ligature material. It comes in different calibers. The rustless steel wire (an alloy of steel, nickel, and chromium) is smooth, strong, pliable, and noncorrosive, and hence does not irritate the tissue (Babcock). Tantalum wire seems to have the same qualities. Ivy recommends brass wire for interdental use to immobilize the jaws and keep the teeth in occlusion; this kind of wire freely lends itself to such work.

Sutures

Sutures are continuous or interrupted. (Tauber's small monograph on this subject is very descriptive.) A *continuous* suture is a running stitch which approximates the wound edges and is tied only at the beginning and the end. The advantage is that it can be applied quickly;

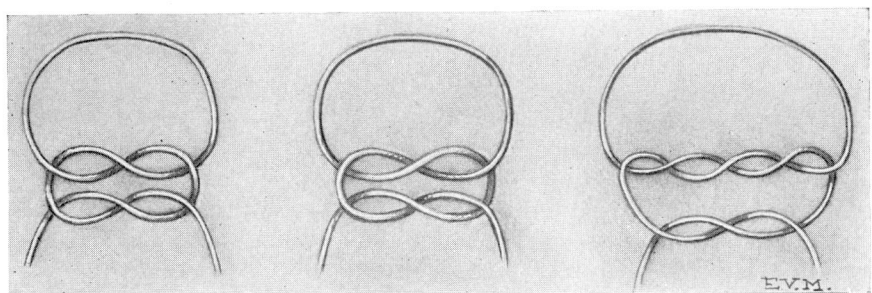

Fig. 7. Knots. *Left to right:* "Granny knot" (not to be used), reef or square knot, surgical knot.

the disadvantages are that it may hold the wound edges under uneven tension, and if it tears it may cause spreading of the entire wound. The continuous suture should not be used in surgery of the face. Various types of continuous suture are depicted in Figure 1. Halsted's cutaneous mattress suture (Fig. 2) is of value in avoiding stitch marks (Case 19, p. 1018). It can be used only for closure of straight incisions. In long incisions, it should be used in sections.

The *interrupted* suture is the more important. The stitches should lie rectangular to the wound edges (Fig. 3). The needle is passed through the skin a few millimeters from the wound edges and then

10

through the subcutaneous tissue. The depth of the suture depends upon its width. If the suture is not passed deeply enough through the tissue, a dead space may be left beneath, resulting in an uneven adaptation of the skin edges, with overlapping or underlapping (Fig. 4, upper row).

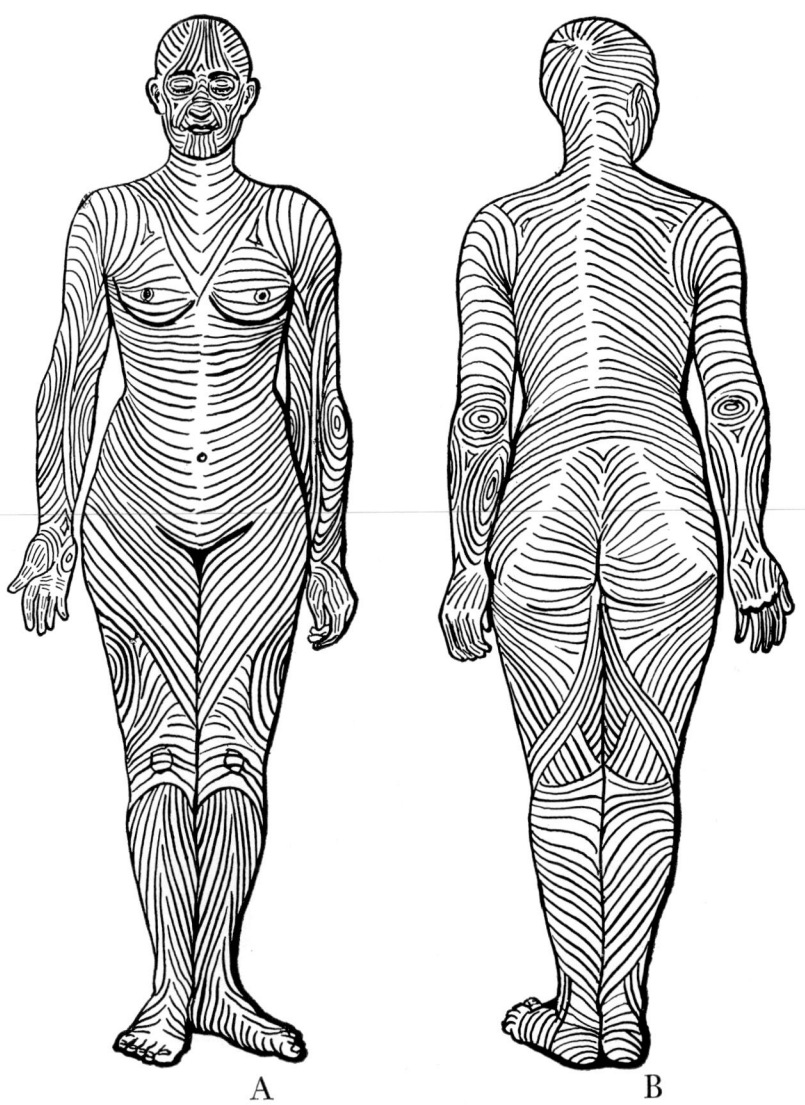

A   B

Fig. 8. Langer's lines of cleavage of skin.

If the suture penetrates too deeply, it may cause dimpling of the wound edges (Fig. 4, second row). As a rule, sutures should penetrate to a distance equal to half the distance from the wound edges on each side

11

of the wound (Fig. 4, third row). If, however, the wound edges are lying uneven to each other, the suture must include more tissue on the retracted side than on the elevated side, to correct the displacement (Fig. 4, fourth row). If the wound edges are under tension, relaxation sutures should be used (Fig. 5). The on-end mattress suture is useful in those cases in which broad apposition and eversion of the wound edges are needed (Fig. 6). It may be used alternately with ordinary sutures.

Knots: In tying sutures and ligatures, too many loops should be avoided. The simple knot forms the basis of practically all knots. It consists of one twist. The reef or square knot is the one most often used in surgery. It consists of a simple twist in one direction and another twist

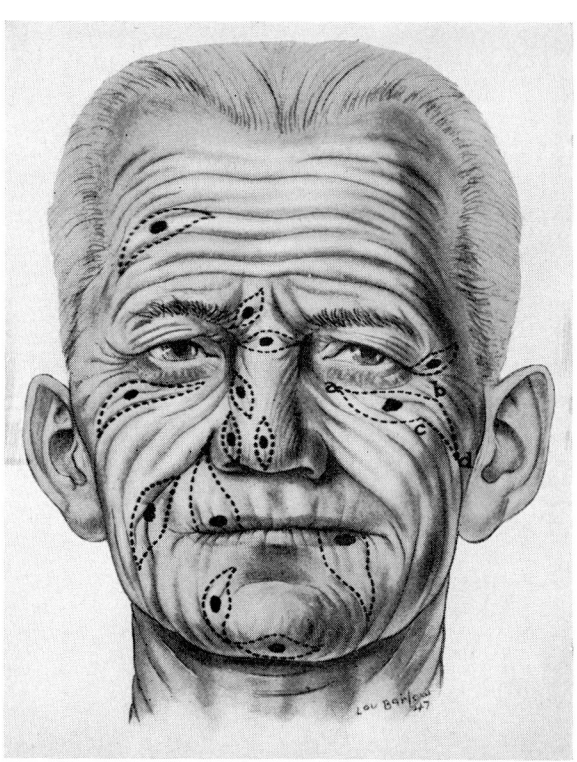

Fig. 9. Skin incisions laid perpendicular to the action of the underlying muscles come to lie within the folds of the adherent facial skin which form at right angles to the action of the underlying muscles. (Kraissl, C. J.: Plast. Reconstr. Surg.)

in the opposite direction. It has less tendency to become untied than a granny knot, which should not be used. The surgeon's knot consists of a double twist in the first part and a single twist in the second. The double twist is used to cause friction and thus prevent slipping of the suture or ligature while the second knot is being tied (Fig. 7). Hayes Martin has written a descriptive article on this subject.

12

INCISIONS

In elective incisions, the incision should, if possible, be placed along the lines of cleavage of the skin to obtain fine-line scars. Langer was the first to point out the advantage of this, and devised lines representing the elastic lines of the skin (Fig. 8). Incisions along these would heal with fine scars. The explanation was twofold: (1) A scar parallel to the lines would be inconspicuous because it resembled a line. This explanation holds. (2) Pull on the wound edges would be avoided owing to the parallel directions of Langer's lines and the muscles. Actually, however, as Rubin, Kraissl, Borges and Alexander, Courtiss et al., and Fongo et al. have observed, the muscle pull tends to separate the wound edges, thus widening the scar.

Facial wrinkles are the result of contracture of the underlying muscles of facial expression. They lie at right angles to the direction of pull. As Kraissl and Conway point out, it is evident that the wrinkles are caused by the shortening of the muscle without corresponding shortening of the skin. Therefore, the skin adapts itself to this irregular mechanism by forming folds that are at right angles to the action of the underlying muscles. In some regions, several muscles act in unison to produce facial expression, with the result that the skin wrinkles are in a curved line (nasolabial fold).

Kraissl offers a revised pattern for making elective incisions on the body surface (Fig. 9). Where the underlying muscles are attached to the skin, as in the face, the incisions are perpendicular to the muscular action. Where there is no attachment to the skin, the incisions are perpendicular to the direction of excursion of the skin produced by normal muscle pull (Blocker). Even with free grafts, particularly when placed on the face or near the joints, the incision should be made in such a manner that the marginal scars are in proper lines; in a contracture of the neck, for example, the relaxation incisions are so placed that the scars will lie horizontally, not vertically. When using a full-thickness graft, the surgeon should attempt to place the skin in its new position with respect to the lines it occupied in its donor site.

ANESTHESIA

Various types of anesthetics and anesthesia are discussed on pages 200, 607, 707.

BIBLIOGRAPHY

ARIES, L. J.: *Experimental studies with synthetic fiber (nylon) as a buried suture.* Surgery, 9:51, 1941.

BABCOCK, W. W.: *Catgut allergy, with note on use of alloy steel wire for sutures and ligatures.* Amer. J. Surg., 27:67, 1935.

BLANK, I. H., COOLIDGE, M. H., SOUTTER, L., and RODKEY, G. V.: *A study of the surgical scrub.* Surg. Gynec. Obstet., 91:577, 1950.

BLOCKER, T. G., HENDRIX, J. H., Jr., HERRMANN, G. C., and HALL, E.: *Application of techniques of reconstructive surgery to certain problems in general surgery.* Ann. Surg., 129:777, 1949.

BORGES, A. F., and ALEXANDER, J. E.: *Relaxed skin tension lines, Z-plasties on scars. Fusiform excision of lesions.* Brit. J. Plast. Surg., 15:242, 1962.

BROWN, J. B., BYARS, L. T., McDOWELL, F., and FRYER, M. P.: *Plastic surgery routine for surgical house staffs.* Plast. Reconstr. Surg., 3:385, 1948.

CANZONETH, A. J. and DALLEY, M. D.: *Bacteriologic survey of scrub technique with special emphasis on pHisoderm with 3 per cent hexachlorophene.* Ann. Surg., 135:228, 1952.

COURTISS, E. H., LONGACRE, J. J., de STEFANO, G. A., BRIZIO, L., and HOLMSTRAND, K.: *The placement of elective skin incisions.* Plast. Reconstr. Surg., 31:31, 1963.

DULL, J. A., ZINTEL, H. A., ELLIS, H. L., and NICHOLS, A.: *An evaluation of pHisoderm G-11 and a liquid soap containing G-11 when used as the preoperative scrub.* Surg. Gynec. Obstet. 91:100, 1950.

FONGO, A., FERRARIS, E., and BOCCA, M.: *Tension lines and skin creases.* Minerva Chir., Torino, 21:627, 1966.

GUEDEL, A. E.: *Inhalation Anesthesia: A Fundamental Guide.* The Macmillan Company, New York, 1951.

HALSTED, W. S.: *The employment of fine silk in preference to catgut and the advantages of transfixing tissues and vessels in controlling hemorrhage.* JAMA, 60:1119, 1913.

KOCHER, T.: *Eine einfache Methode zur Erzielung sicherer Asepsis.* Cor. Bl. f. schweiz. Aerzte, 18:3, 1888.

KRAISSL, C. J.: *The selection of appropriate lines for elective surgical incisions.* Plast. Reconstr. Surg., 8:1, 1951.

KRAISSL, C. J., and CONWAY, H.: *Excision of small tumors of the skin of the face with special reference to the wrinkle lines.* Surgery, 25:592, 1949.

MADSON, E. T.: *An experimental and clinical evaluation of surgical suture materials—II.* Surg. Gynec. Obstet., 97:439, 1953.

MARTIN, H.: *Knot tying in surgery.* Surg. Gynec. Obstet., 115:236, 1962.

MASON, J. M.: *The use of silk sutures and ligatures in clean wounds.* Int. Clin., 1:231, 1938.

PREOPERATIVE PREPARATION

MEADE, W. H., and OCHSNER, A.: *Relative value of catgut, silk, linen and cotton as suture materials.* Surgery, 7:485, 1940.

MELENEY, F. L.: *Treatise on Surgical Infections.* Oxford Univ. Press, New York, 1948.

MELICK, D. W.: *Nylon suture.* Ann. Surg., 115:475, 1942.

NICHOLS, H. M., and DIAK, A. W.: *An experimental study of nylon as a suture material.* West. J. Surg., 48:42, 1940.

PANNETT, C. A.: *A plea for wartime use of cotton ligatures.* Lancet, 242:755, 1942.

POSTLETHWAIT, R. W., SCHAUBLE, J. F., DILLON, M. L., MOYER, J.: *Wound healing. An evaluation of surgical suture material.* Surg. Gynec. Obstet., 108:555, 1959.

PRICE, P. B.: *Stress, strain and sutures.* Ann. Surg., 128:408, 1948.

PRICE, P. B.: *Present day methods of disinfecting the skin: Survey of disinfectants and techniques currently employed in the hospitals of the U. S. and Canada.* Arch. Surg., 61:583, 1950.

RUBIN, L. R.: *Langer's lines and facial scars.* Plast. Reconstr. Surg., 3:147, 1948.

SHAMBAUGH, P.: *Postoperative wound complications. A clinical study with special reference to the use of silk.* Surg. Gynec. Obstet., 64:765, 1937.

TAUBER, R.: *Simplified Knot and Suture Technique.* W. B. Saunders, Philadelphia, 1955.

TAYLOR, F. W.: *Surgical knots and sutures.* Surgery, 5:498, 1939.

THOREK, P., GRADMAN, R., and GLAESS, A.: *Additional experience with spool cotton as a suture material.* Amer. J. Surg., 59:68, 1942.

WHIPPLE, A. O.: *The use of silk in the repair of clean wounds.* Ann. Surg., 98: 662, 1933.
The choice and use of ligature and suture material in the repair of clean wounds. Surg. Gynec. Obstet., 39:109, 1939.

WORD, B., and BROCK, C. E.: *Cotton suture material.* Amer. J. Surg., 63:371, 1944.

15

SHIFTING OF TISSUE, FREE TISSUE GRAFTING, TRANSFER OF FLAPS

2

PLASTIC and reconstructive surgery is concerned mainly with closure of defects, either of the soft tissues or of the framework of the body, and with the reconstruction of malformations, including reestablishment of function and improvement of appearance, with resulting relief of psychological handicaps. The ways by which these two problems can be solved consist chiefly in tissue shifting, free tissue transplantation, and transfer of pedicle flaps.

SHIFTING OF TISSUE FOR CLOSURE OF SURFACE DEFECTS

Shifting of skin and subcutaneous tissue is performed for the purpose of closing certain surface defects. The principle involved in tissue shifting consists of the mobilization of the tissue adjacent to the defect by thoroughly undermining it and sliding it into the defect. Its use is, of course, limited to smaller defects and only to those in which the skin surrounding the defect is freely movable. Sometimes additional incisions (relaxation incisions) are necessary to facilitate the mobility of the undermined tissue. In this respect, the method encroaches on some of the flap methods in which the flap is taken from the immediate neighborhood (French method). The incisions, if possible, should be placed in the direction of the lines of cleavage of the skin (Figs. 8, 9). If the incisions are placed within these elastic lines, the tension of the surrounding tissue does not draw upon the edges of the skin. Hence, the incised wound edges fall naturally together, thus placing the wound under minimal tension and stress.

A

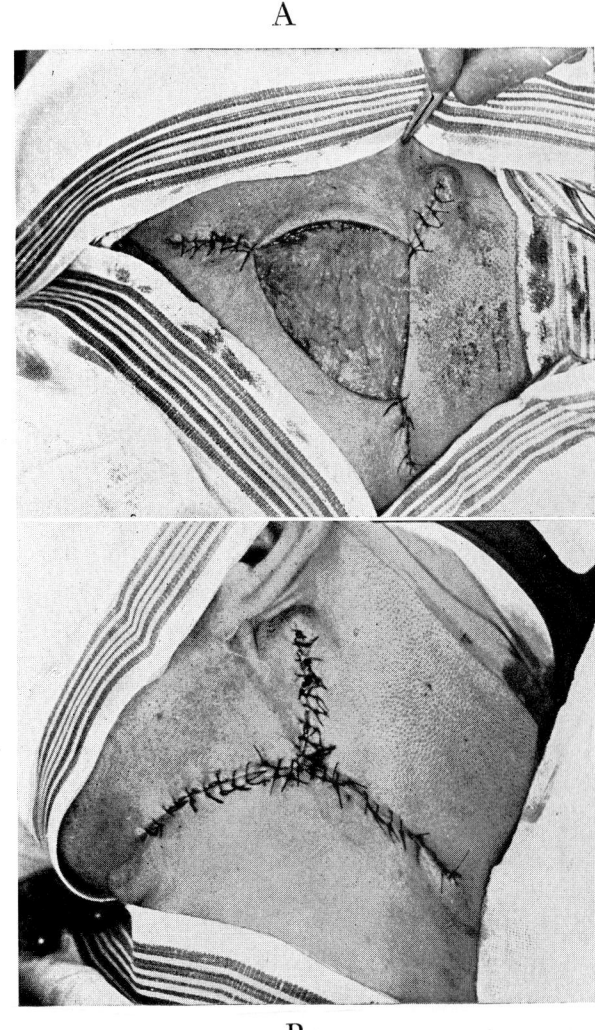

B

Fig. 10. *A:* Closure of triangular defect of neck after excision of flat scar by starting with closure of corners. *B:* Triangular defect changed into Y form.

The simplest form of tissue shifting is the closure of an elliptical defect by mobilization and approximation of the defect edges until a linear suture can be made. Triangular and square defects may be closed by starting with closure of the corners (a method already mentioned by Celsus) whereby the triangle is changed into a Y (Fig. 10) and the square defect into a double Y (Fig. 11).

If additional incisions are necessary to facilitate the mobilization of the tissue, one must be sure that the skin surrounding the defect is freely movable and that a secondary defect can be avoided or, if unavoidable,

A

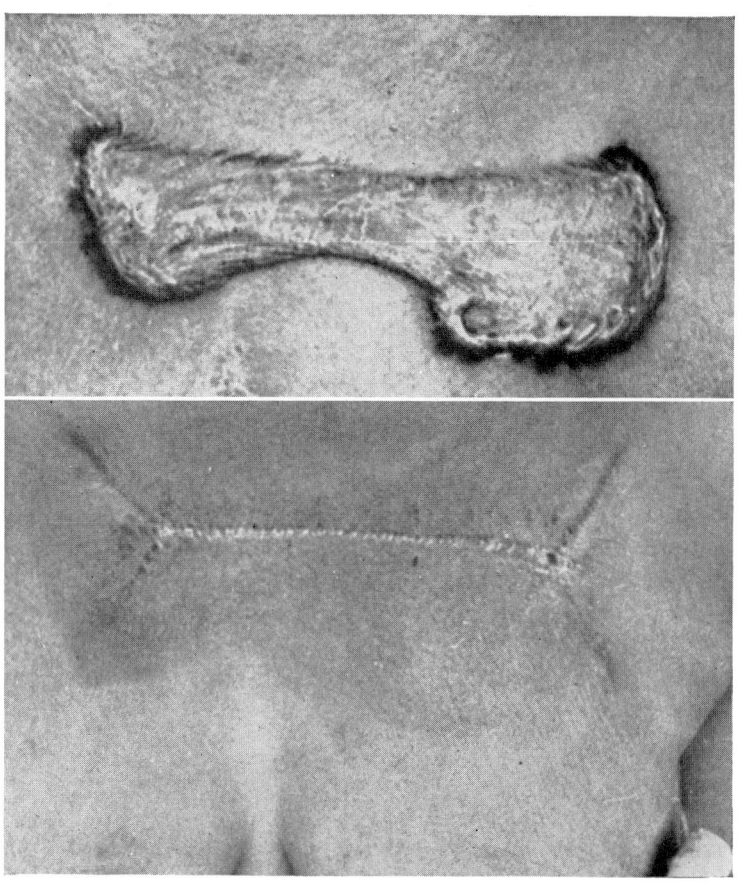

B

Fig. 11. *A:* Large keloid scar of chest. *B:* Resulting defect after excision of scar was square; closed by starting with closure of corners, changing square defect into double Y.

can be closed. A typical example is the closure of a triangular defect necessitating additional incisions (Fig. 12, *a*). One point of the triangle becomes the point of rotation. The side of the triangle op-

19

posite this point is lengthened unilaterally or bilaterally, and the adjoining tissue is mobilized and shifted into the defect. This method becomes more effective if vertical incisions are added to the first incisions, thus covering the triangular defect with one or two square flaps (Dieffenbach, 1834) (Fig. 12, *b*). However, in this method there is a secondary defect which one must be certain can be closed. Its closure may be facilitated by leading the incisions from the corners of the triangle, not horizontally, but obliquely upward (Fig. 12, *c*), so that the outer angles of the secondary defect are less than right angles and thus can be easily closed (von Szymanowski, 1858) (Case 26, p. 1027).

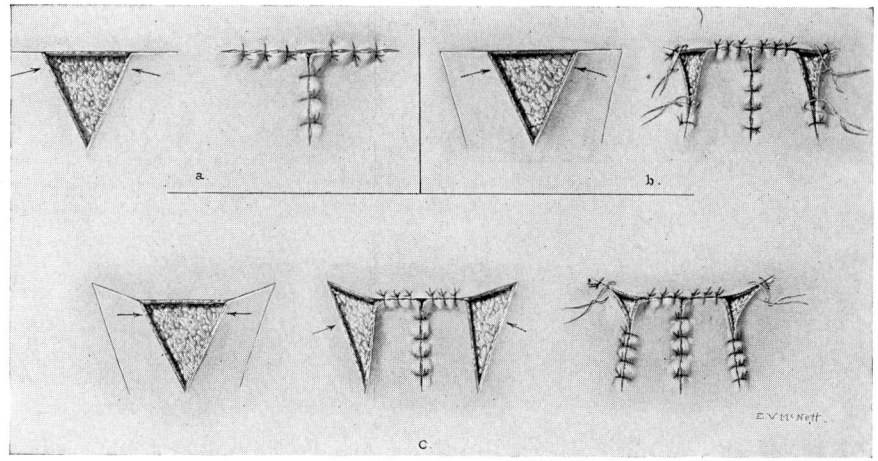

Fig. 12. Triangular defect closed (*a*) by lengthening one side of triangle unilaterally or bilaterally and rotating mobilized tissue into defect; (*b*) by adding vertical incisions to first incision, thus closing defect with two square flaps.. *c*: Facilitating closure of secondary defect by leading horizontal incisions obliquely upward, making outer angles of secondary defects less than a right angle.

Another way of closing triangular defects is that of Burow. The principle of this method consists of sacrificing one or two triangles of tissue in the neighborhood of the tissue to be shifted, where there is surplus of skin, thus facilitating the tissue sliding (Fig. 13, second and third rows) (Cases 27, 28, pp. 1028, 1030).

Closure of a round defect with interchanging triangular flaps is demonstrated in Figure 14.

It is almost impossible to describe all methods which have been devised to facilitate tissue shifting. Those which are still in vogue and which have been found helpful by the author are illustrated in Figures 13, 14.

FREE TISSUE GRAFTING

The history of tissue grafting is ages old; its scientific basis, however, is of recent origin. Ollier's work on transplantation of bone (1858), Reverdin's (1869) and Thiersch's (1874) on epidermis transplantation, and Wolfe's (1875) and Krause's (1893) on cutis transplantation lifted the veil of mysticism and placed this field of surgery upon scientific ground. In spite of numerous contributions, however, many essential questions remained unanswered.

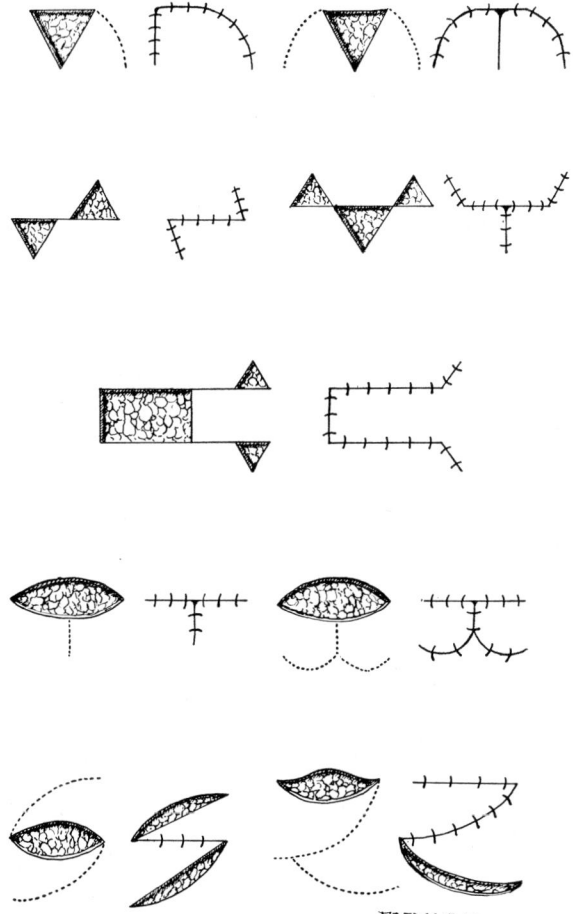

E.V.M⸌Nett.

Fig. 13. Methods of tissue shifting.

GENERAL PRINCIPLES

Bone & Liver

Regeneration of Tissue

Investigation in tissue transplantation received an impetus after the discovery of the tremendous regenerative forces arising from the host tissue. The question of what causes and stimulates regeneration is answered: The loss of tissue and the resulting wound. The wound attracts hyperemia and unleashes the innate force of any tissue for restitution. This is the start of growth and regeneration. Depending upon location, size, and depth of the defect, the healing process of the wound will result in a *restitutio ad integrum* or in a scar. The latter is considered an inferior replacement of the defect. Transplantation of tissue is performed to produce a similar replacement of the lost tissue or to replace an already formed scar.

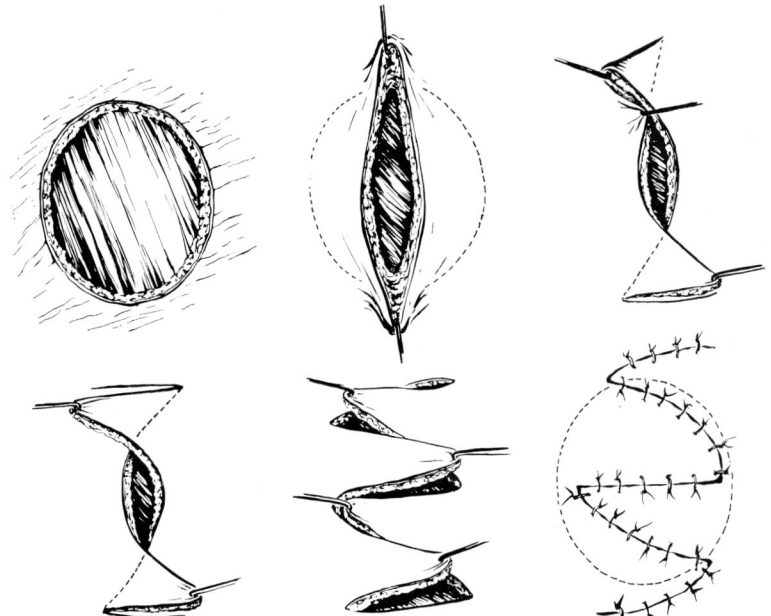

Fig. 14.   Closure of a round defect with interchanging triangular flaps.

The literature on the regeneration of free tissue grafts and the biology of tissue transplantations is voluminous. The world literature has been covered by Lexer's monumental work and by the monographs of Neuhof and R. M. May, and more recently by the stimulating Volume II of Peer and co-workers and the monograph of Purrel and Monak. A recently founded journal called *Transplantation* attempts to keep abreast of the vast accumulation in this field. A detailed description of the whole subject of tissue regeneration would be far beyond the scope of this book.

22

SHIFTING OF TISSUE

Only a few general remarks about the regeneration of autogenous human tissue grafts will be made; as to conclusions concerning the behavior of host tissue and homogenous grafts the reader is referred to page 40.

The fate of some tissue grafts appears to depend upon the type of host with which the grafts are in contact. Peer and co-workers studied the behavior of human tissue grafts (1) when grafts were in contact with unlike tissue, and (2) when they were in contact with like tissue. They came to the conclusion that most of the tissue grafts (skin, cartilage, fat, etc.) tend to survive whether they have been transplanted upon unlike tissue (skin upon fat or fascia, etc., cartilage within soft tissue, etc.) or in contact with like tissue. Bone, muscle, and nerve grafts, however, are exceptions. Bone grafts in contact with unlike tissue are replaced by the host fibrous tissue (except the septal bone graft, which is a so-called "membranous" bone); in contact with living bone, bone grafts regenerate. Muscle grafts always degenerate, whether the graft is in contact with unlike tissue or with muscle. In nerve grafts, Schwann cells disappear when in contact with unlike tissue; when in contact with living nerve, nerve grafts survive. The axons and myelin sheaths, however, degenerate; some become replaced later by ingrowth from the host nerve. All grafts are kept alive initially by the exudation of plasma from the host tissue. This plasma, however, acts rather to prevent desiccation, at least for all but the centrally located cells, than to provide nourishment and oxygen. Peer obtained successful takes of autogenous skin grafts after wrapping them in a rubber sheet to prevent desiccation and keeping them in an incubator at body temperature for four days; those stored longer failed to take. This simple experiment demonstrated that the cells in the skin graft will survive at body temperature without nourishment for four days when the cells are merely prevented from becoming desiccated.

The vascular system in free grafts usually survives. Hence, the ingrowing vessels form a direct anastomosis between the severed vessels of the graft. Enderlen was able to see capillaries—injected with methylene blue —in a transplanted skin graft two days after transplantation. Savenero-Rosselli found red blood corpuscles in the capillaries of the periphery of a transplanted skin graft twenty-four to thirty-six hours after the transplantation. Experiments conducted by the author to study the vascularization of bone grafts demonstrate this vividly (Figs. 29, 30).

In the transplantation of tissue, the operator starts with the preparation of the host tissue, with the stimulation and liberation of the regenerative forces of the graft bed. No regeneration will go out from a scar or from an infection. Therefore, an infection—if any—has to be overcome first. In case of scarring, all atrophic and cicatricial tissue must be removed until sound wound conditions are created. Only under such

23

conditions can the graft be kept alive and regenerated. This alone would not lead to a successful transplantation were it not for the functional stimulus or for the functional adaptation of the graft, which finally causes it to become an organic unit with the host tissue (Roux, Carrel, and Guthrie). So, for instance, the transplanted vein to fill a defect in an artery gradually hypertrophies. A bone graft becomes either thinner or thicker according to the functional demand.

Types of Transplantations

We distinguish autogenous, homogenous, and heterogenous transplantations according to whether the transplant was taken from the same person, from another person, or from a different species. The greatest possibilities for survival and regeneration of a transplant are obtained by autogenous transplantation. The chances of regeneration are much less in homogenous transplantation. In heterogenous transplantations most transplants undergo rapid necrosis and absorption or encapsulation.

SKIN GRAFTING

History

Skin grafting is a development of the nineteenth century. Reverdin (1869) was the first to place skin grafting upon a scientific basis. He took small pieces of epidermis from a patient's right arm and transplanted them to a granulating surface on the left arm. The epidermal islands took and grew and gradually united. Reverdin's observations received great attention. Lawson (1871), Ollier (1872), and Thiersch (1874), stimulated by Reverdin's findings, experimented with larger epidermal grafts, and are responsible for the introduction of this widely used method. (Thiersch's original article is translated into English by H. and L. May, Plast. Reconstr. Surg., 41:365, 1968.) Wolfe (1875) went one step further; he used skin grafts consisting of the entire thickness of the skin. However, the credit for popularizing the use of large full-thickness grafts goes undoubtedly to Krause, who in 1893 reported the successful use of more than one hundred such grafts. (Krause's original article is translated by H. and L. May, Plast. Reconstr. Surg., 41:573, 1968.) In 1914 J. S. Davis introduced the "small deep graft," which was based on Reverdin's idea, but instead of consisting of the superficial layer of skin it included the full thickness of the skin at its center, tapering off toward the periphery.

The real development of skin grafting, however, started after World War I, and resulted mainly from vast experience and improvement in

24

technique. Gillies, Lexer, Davis, Blair, Brown, and Padgett were foremost among others in developing new techniques and increasing immensely the percentage of good results. To J. B. Brown we are indebted for perfecting the technique of skin grafting to such a degree that it has become the method of choice in many instances where a flap formerly was considered indicated. Zoltán gives a vivid account of the development of skin grafting in his recent book.

Choice of Graft

The two most widely used grafts are the large split graft, consisting of partial thickness of the skin, and the large full-thickness graft. The split graft, as originally used by Ollier and Thiersch, was cut thin,

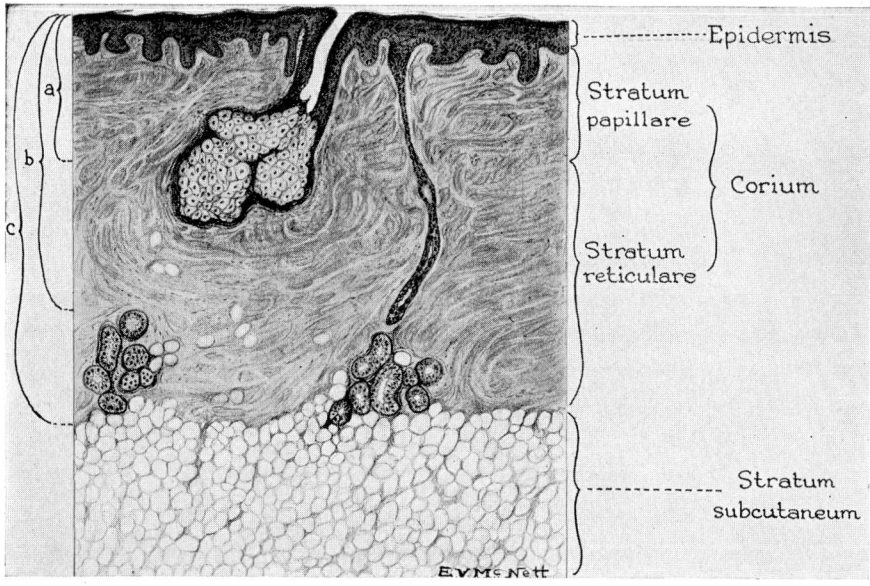

Fig. 15. Section of normal skin. *a:* Thickness of thin split graft; *b:* of thick split graft; *c:* of full-thickness graft.

and consisted only of the epidermal layer of the skin with a small portion of dermis (Figs. 15, 16); these grafts are too thin for use on surfaces where firm coverage is required. Hence, the graft should be cut thicker and should consist of from one half to three quarters of the thickness of the skin (Fig. 16, *c*). The full-thickness graft consists of the full thickness of the skin without any subcutaneous tissue (Fig. 16, *d*).

As to when a split graft is indicated and when a full-thickness graft, it must be said that the question occurs only when the host area is

GENERAL PRINCIPLES

"clean." The full-thickness graft will not take on an infected area, no matter how harmless the infection. Therefore, on granulating surfaces only one type of skin graft comes into consideration, and that is the split graft. But if the host area is "clean," then the question of split or full-thickness graft arises.

In short, it may be said that on all surfaces where the cosmetic effect is not important and on surfaces that will resist subsequent contraction or on which allowance can be made for contraction, split grafts should be used. The split graft is more easily obtained and applied, it takes more readily, and the aftercare is less difficult. Furthermore, the donor area heals more quickly and better because the epithelium regenerates from the hair follicles and sebaceous glands and covers the donor area completely. Its drawback lies in the fact that it changes color, owing to

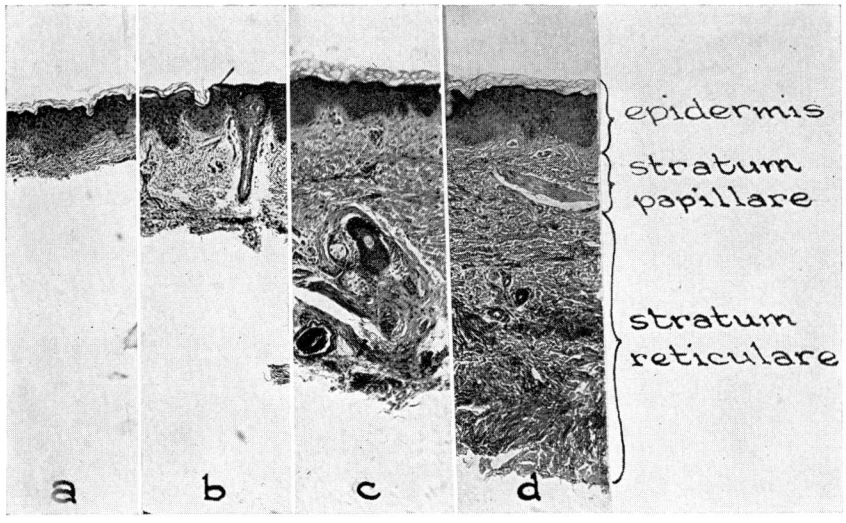

Fig. 16. Photomicrograph showing various thicknesses of skin grafts. *a:* Original Thiersch graft. *b:* Thin split graft (0.010 inch thickness). *c:* Thick split graft (0.022 inch thickness). *d:* Full-thickness graft.

pigmentation, and does not resist subsequent contraction. The work of Byars, Brown and associates, and Conway in matching the color of skin grafts by tattooing appears to be very useful. Brownish discolored grafts can be made lighter by superficial surgical abrasion (p. 191) (Mir y Mir).

The full-thickness graft changes color also, but not so much as the thinner graft. Furthermore, the full-thickness graft prevents recontraction to a certain degree. Secondary contraction does not take place

26

so much in the graft itself as in the underlying host tissue. The thicker the graft, the less is the amount of subsequent shrinkage. Hence, in regions in which the cosmetic effect is of importance or which are exposed to pressure, and in which optimum relaxation is required, the full-thickness graft should be used.

There may be exceptions to this generalization. To obtain a complete "take" of the full-thickness graft, aside from the exercise of careful technique and asepsis, the graft should be in intimate contact with the graft bed. The base upon which the full-thickness graft is placed should be firm and even, so that an adequate pressure dressing can be applied. Complete immobilization is also essential. Therefore, in regions in which a firm, even pressure and immobilization cannot be accomplished, the full-thickness graft is not likely to be successful. In those places (such as the cheek, neck, and axilla, with their irregular contours), a thick split graft is preferable, this graft consisting of 70 to 90 per cent of the thickness of the skin.

Regeneration of Skin Grafts

The regeneration of a free skin graft depends—like that of any other graft—upon the rapid establishment of its interrupted blood supply. In the first twenty-four hours, the vessels of the host tissue dilate; plasma, which preserves the viability of the graft, escapes and fills the spaces between graft and host, and the plasma gradually changes into fibrin. Hence, the graft becomes anchored to the host tissue. After about one to two days, delicate vessels grow from the host tissue into the graft (Thiersch, Garré, Davis and Traut, Enderlen, Savenero-Rosselli, Converse and Rappaport); after the third day, the graft itself takes active part in the regenerative process by marked proliferation of its epithelium. Between the fifth and tenth days after the operation, depending upon the size and thickness of the graft, organic union becomes complete after reestablishment of the interrupted circulation of the graft and development of a subcutaneous connective tissue, which anchors the graft firmly to the host. In addition to proliferative changes, some degenerative changes in the epithelial and endothelial cells and in the elastic fibers, with later regeneration, take place. Subsequent changes, such as change of color and contraction, may occur. Nerves begin to grow into the graft from the surrounding tissues about the third week; however, complete innervation may not occur for several months (Kredel and Evans, Davis and Kitlowski, L. Davis, McCarrol, Fitzgerald, Martin, and Paletta). A very fine description of the regenerative and histiogenic occurrences which lead to an organic unit of graft and host tissue has been published by F. Andina.

GENERAL PRINCIPLES

Condition of Patient

The patient's general condition has much bearing upon the outcome of a skin graft operation. If the patient is in good health, the chances of "take" are much higher than in an anemic, chronically ill, dehydrated person.

Anemia and hypoproteinemia delay wound healing (see Chap. 3). Any disturbance of the fluid balance may affect normal metabolism. No patient should be skin grafted unless the hemoglobin level is well above 60 per cent and the serum protein level above 6.5 gm. per 100 cc. Transfusions of blood and a high-protein diet are the chief remedies for correction of secondary anemia and hypoproteinemia. In some cases, severe burns, for instance, with large denuded areas, the hemoglobin and protein levels may remain low in spite of countermeasures. Under those circumstances, life or death may depend upon covering the raw surfaces; hence, one may be forced to proceed with skin grafting, and even resort to homogenous grafts (p. 40) in spite of the risk. Fluid intake and output should be well balanced. A high-caloric diet is important. Hermansdorfer's suggestion of an acid (salt-free) diet is a good one, but difficult to prepare individually. Vitamin deficiency must be watched for. Vitamin C is essential to wound healing; a deficiency leaves the connective-tissue cells in a state of immaturity. Other vitamins, such as A, B, and D, are also essential to wound healing. Hence, a high-vitamin, high-protein diet with an additional sufficient amount of ascorbic acid, administration of iron, and heliotherapy stimulate general and local health (pp. 137-165).

Preoperative Preparation of Donor Area

The donor area is shaved (with the exception of areas from which grafts are taken to be transplanted to a woman's face or to line cavities); preoperatively, it is washed with pHisoderm G-11 (p. 4), and covered with a sterile sheet. No chemical antiseptic skin preparation should be used, in order to avoid damage of the graft cells.

Preoperative Preparation of Host Area

The host area is prepared in a similar way, unless the surface is granulating. If it is, the chances of "take" of a skin graft depend upon the type of graft used and the condition of the granulations. Large skin (split) grafts will take only on pinkish, flat, healthy-looking granulations. If the granulations are hypertrophic or chronically infected or sluggish, the condition should be improved by general and local measures before skin grafting is attempted.

SHIFTING OF TISSUE

Hypertrophic Granulations: Hypertrophic granulations are exuberant, boggy, and edematous, and overhang the wound edges. To reduce their size and to change them into flat granulations, several measures may be tried: (1) Daily application of silver nitrate with a caustic stick or in 10 per cent solution, followed by application of gauze soaked in Dakin's solution, then a layer of cotton or mechanic's cotton waste and a firm pressure dressing, which eliminates dead spaces and avoids venous and lymph stasis (see Chap. 4). An extremity should be immobilized and elevated; (2) Trimming the exuberant granulations with scissors, followed by application of 10 per cent solution of silver nitrate and a pressure dressing; (3) Daily baths and exposure to ultraviolet rays.

Infected Granulations: These granulations are gray and covered with fibrin, and discharge a purulent exudate. Under such conditions, a daily saline bath is essential. For patients with large infected areas, a daily tub bath, comfortably warm with 5 per cent salt, may be lifesaving. The surrounding skin should be cleansed with soap and water. Daily débridement of dead tissue is necessary. The area is covered with dressings soaked in Dakin's solution, which is added at regular intervals. In profuse discharge, the dressings should be changed daily at frequent intervals according to the description on page 164. Cultures should be taken from the infected area and the proper antibiotic treatment administered (pp. 137-142). If necrotizing processes are present, sprinkling of the area with crystal sugar (which need not be sterile) may be given a trial. The sugar, owing to its hygroscopic properties, causes a profuse exudation and hence an elimination of fibrinous membranes and necrotic tissue. If the granulations have a tendency to bleed, application of zinc peroxide is recommended (Altemeier and Carter). If the discharge lessens, the wet dressings are alternated with ointment, such as cod-liver oil, scarlet red, or mercury ointments, or with balsam of Peru. Heliotherapy may be of value. Twenty-four hours before the operation, isotonic saline dressings are applied, which are moistened at regular intervals.

The Pseudomonas aeruginosa (Bacillus pyocyaneus), harmless to wound healing, is a definite handicap in skin grafting. Grafts do not take well or do not take at all in its presence. The difficulties in eradicating it from the tissues are well recognized. If there is a mixed infection, chemotherapy should be undertaken. The author has found that in combating other germs and checking their growth a marked reduction of the pseudomonas infection could be noticed. Local therapy consists of application of 3 per cent acetic acid solution. The dressings should be kept moist constantly and changed daily. In stubborn cases, 3 per cent acetic acid solution and Dakin's solution are applied alternately at three-hour intervals for forty-eight hours. Sulfamylon has been recently claimed to be the

29

substance most effective against pyocyaneus infections. Muir, Owen and Murphy use a sulfamylon acetate cream applied first by spreading on large gauze squares (8-ply) and then laying these directly on the burned surface. No absorption dressing was used. The dressings were changed every other day except after grafting, when they were left undisturbed for five to seven days. (See also p. 161).

Sluggish Granulations: In sluggish granulations, the response to the wound stimuli is lacking, hence the healing process has to be induced. This may be done by touching the granulations with a caustic stick and applying various stimulating substances, such as Dakin's solution, mercury ointment, and cod-liver oil ointment. If the circulation is at fault, as in old leg ulcers, it should be improved if possible. If an old ulcerative area is surrounded by dense cicatricial tissue, the entire surface, including the granulating area, should be excised to the firm fibrous-tissue base, and this base should be covered immediately with a skin graft.

Time for Grafting Granulations: When are granulations ready to be skin grafted? To determine this, the macroscopic appearance of the granulations is of more importance than a bacterial count. Granulations are ready if they are bright red, small, or at least not too exuberant, and free from purulent discharge. All antiseptic solutions are replaced the day before the operation by isotonic saline dressings, which are moistened at regular intervals.

SPLIT SKIN GRAFTS

Preparation of Recipient Area

The operation starts with the preparation of the recipient, or host, area, which is changed into a clean wound. In case of a granulating area, the granulations are not touched if they are flat. If the granulations are hypertrophic, they are sliced down—not scraped—with a sharp, long knife (transplantation knife) to a yellow, well-vascularized layer, which constitutes the base of the granulations. The next step is thorough hemostasis. Spurting vessels should be ligated. The oozing is controlled by pressing hot wet compresses upon the wound. The heat accelerates coagulation of the blood. If this procedure does not control the oozing, one may try the following: The wound is left open so that the blood has a chance to clot, while a piece of wet gauze, pressed against one edge of the wound, absorbs the blood. When the blood commences to become serous, the wet blood-soaked gauze is pressed firmly upon the wound to promote adherence of the clots. Application of a solution of 1:1000 epinephrine may be the last resort.

30

SHIFTING OF TISSUE

Removal of Graft

The ordinary donor areas are the thighs or upper arms, preferably the hairless inner parts of these extremities, or the back, abdomen, or chest may also be used. The skin of the donor area is moistened with isotonic saline solution, and then stretched between two boards to obtain an even, flat surface (Fig. 17). A common mistake is to press the boards into the

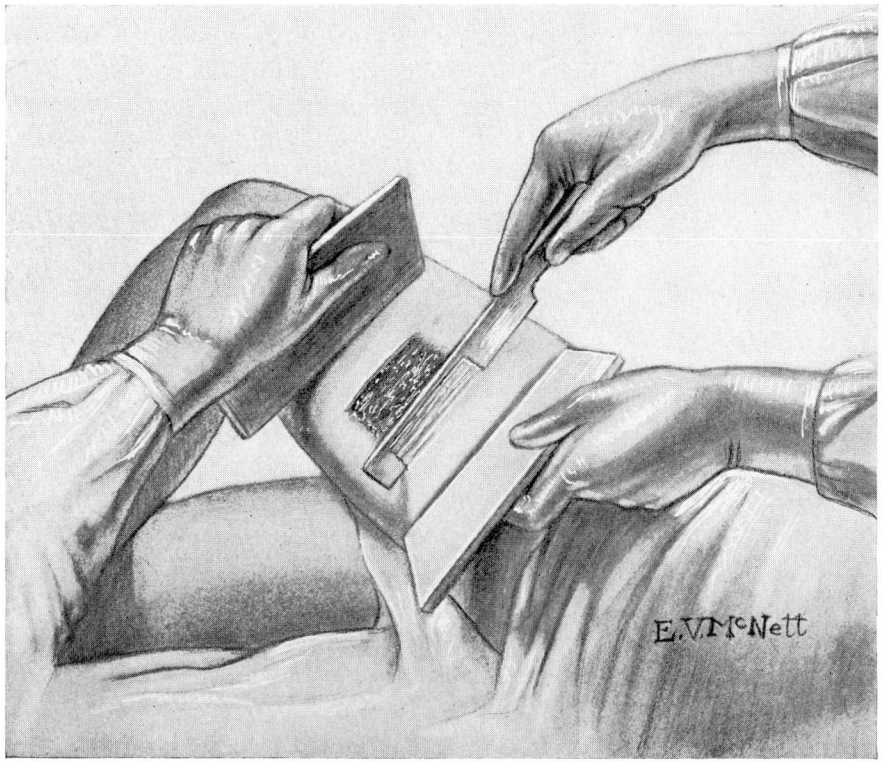

Fig. 17. Technique of cutting split graft with skin graft knife. Skin is stretched between two boards. One board is held by assistant. Second board is pulled by operator immediately in advance of knife.

flesh rather than to pull and stretch the skin flat; the result is an uneven surface. The right board is held by an assistant, the left by the operator. The former board is held firmly in place; the latter is pulled immediately in advance of the knife. The graft is now cut with a long, broad-bladed, sharp knife. Blair-Brown's skin graft knife is a very good one. Marcks added an attachment to the Blair-Brown knife which allows calibration of the skin graft, and thus assures equal thickness of the graft. The knife is placed flat on the skin, and with a rapid forward and backward motion

31

the knife penetrates the skin and splits it (Fig. 17). (For examples of skin grafting, see Cases 107, 108, pp. 1132, 1134.)

Use of Suction Cups: The boards may be replaced by suction cups (Blair-Brown). These are hollow brass boxes with the under side open for suction on the skin. Within the opening, there is a series of transverse bars which prevent the skin from being drawn bodily up into the box. The ends are corrugated for gripping, and are 2.5 cm. (1 inch) square. A tube leads from the top of the box, and is attached to a noncollapsible rubber tube connected to a strong suction machine. There is a valve on top of the box for adjustment of the suction. The suction usually is one half an atmosphere of negative pressure. These boxes come in three different lengths. Before the suction cups are placed on the donor area,

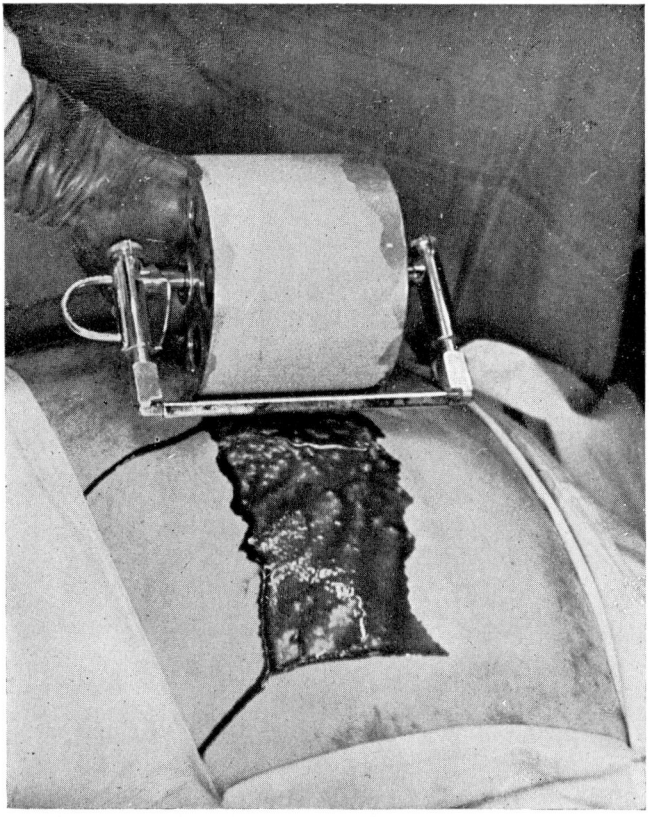

Fig. 18. Technique of cutting skin graft from back with dermatome (Padgett-Hood). Drum and donor area are painted with rubber cement. Drum handle is held in left hand, handle of knife holder in right hand. Drum is placed on area to be cut and knife worked from side to side while drum is turned so as to lift skin slightly.

the skin is greased with a thin film of petrolatum. The boxes are then placed on the skin, neither pressing nor raising the skin; the box in the operator's hand is drawn immediately in advance of the knife. This technique, as developed and used by Blair and Brown, provides an improved means for obtaining grafts of uniform thickness. Another improvement is Barker's Vacu-Tome, a combination of suction cup and movable skin graft knife, which can be adjusted to any thickness of the graft.

Use of Padgett-Hood Dermatome: The best assurance for obtaining a skin graft of uniform thickness is offered by the Padgett-Hood skin graft mechanism, called the "dermatome" (Figs. 18 and 19). The dermatome consists principally of a drum with a movable knife adjustable to any given distance from the drum. A fine film of rubber cement is painted on the drum and on the skin of the donor area. After the cement is allowed to dry slightly, the drum handle is taken in the left hand and the handle of the knife holder in the right hand. Now the drum is placed on the surface to be cut, and is permitted to remain for a few seconds to allow it to adhere. The knife is worked from side to side by making quick, rather short strokes of the knife holder. The drum is turned in such a fashion that it lifts the skin slightly, but not too much (Fig. 18). With this

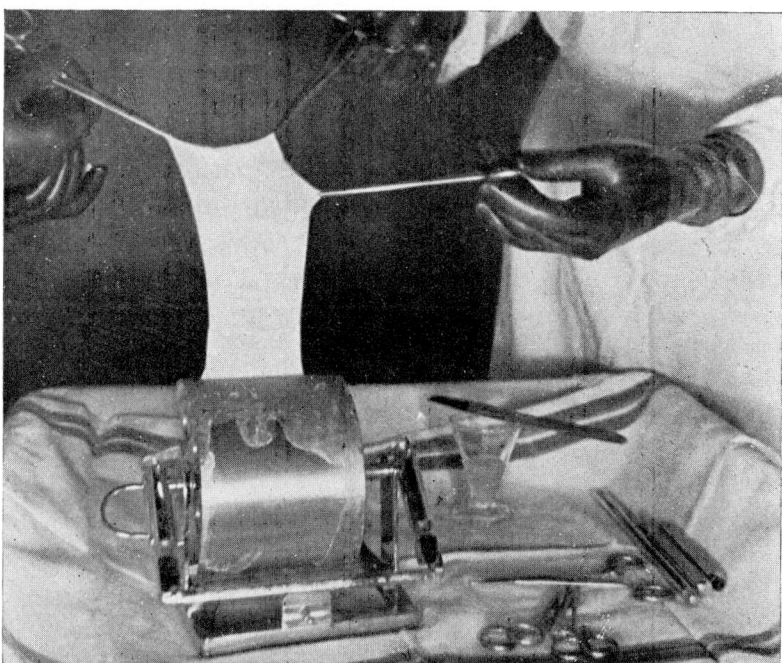

Fig. 19. Skin graft is removed from drum by grasping it with hemostats at extreme points and pulling it from drum.

33

mechanism, it is possible to remove a sheet of skin as large as the drum, or 10 by 20 cm. ($3^{15}/_{16}$ by $7^{7}/_{8}$ inches), or smaller, and to cut it absolutely uniform in thickness; furthermore, the thickness can be varied by turning a calibrating mechanism which varies the distance of the knife from the drum.

INDICATIONS FOR VARYING THICKNESS: Padgett indicates the varying thickness as follows: In an adult when the main indication is one of resurfacing a granulating area, usually the graft is cut from 0.010 to 0.014 of an inch thick. When a clean raw surface is to be covered and the indication is one in which appearance is a prime factor or it is essential to have minimal contracture, the grafts are cut from 0.022 to 0.028 of an inch. It is found that at this thickness sufficient subepithelial elements remain in the base for early regeneration. These, however, are only general rules. The thickness of the skin varies in different persons and in various places of the body surface. For instance, a fairly thick-split skin graft removed from the lateral surface of the thigh may leave a sufficient layer of derma behind while on the median side cutting the same thickness may expose the subcutaneous fat tissue. Hence, it is advisable to check the thickness of the graft according to the thickness of the skin of the donor area. This can readily be done as follows: If at the selected donor site the subcutaneous fat lobules "peep" through the derma when cutting is started the graft can be considered of thick-split thickness for this area. If the fat lobules are not visible at all the graft is of thin-split thickness. The knife may be reset at any stage of the cutting process for readjustment.

REMOVAL OF GRAFT FROM DRUM: The graft is removed by grasping it with hemostats at extreme points and pulling it from the drum (Fig. 19). It should be kept from folding, since the rubber cement may glue the adherent surfaces together. To prevent this, the epithelial side of the graft is rubbed gently with a piece of gauze soaked in the patient's blood (Greely, personal communication, Hirshowitz).

BACKING FOR GRAFT: To prevent the graft from folding and from shrinking, the use of backing material has been advised. Webster uses pliofilm; Green, Levenson, and Lund use nylon backing for dermatome grafts. The author has found the nylon cloth very satisfactory. The drum of the dermatome is coated with cement. A fine-gauge nylon cloth is cut the size of the drum and cemented to the drum as smoothly as possible. A new coat of cement is now applied to the nylon and to the donor site, and the graft is cut as already described. The graft, with its backing, is removed from the drum with hemostats and placed on the host area. Since the backing prevents the graft from shrinking, it may not be necessary to hold the graft in place with sutures. In many cases, however, the graft must be sutured accurately to the wound edges, and this can easily be performed through the nylon backing and the graft. The nylon backing should be removed at the time of the change of the first dressing, but only if it can easily be peeled off. The nylon cloth can be sterilized as easily as any other textile. Backing of a skin graft, as advantageous as it is, should be avoided, however, when the host area is irregular (chin-neck-line, axilla, for example), since the backing material does not yield as readily as the skin.

Reese Dermatome: This is constructed on the same principle as the Padgett dermatome. In addition, it provides a mechanism by which the backing material (dermatape) can be applied. It is very accurate; but if the operator, while cutting the graft, finds its thickness not proper, he must remove the dermatome from the donor area for adjustment.

Electrodermatome: Introduced by Brown, this ingenious mechanism is motor driven and uses an oscillating knife. The knife can be set with a calibrating scale to obtain any graft thickness, and cuts rapidly. It is not necessary to use adhesives to lift the skin. The length of the graft is limited only by the donor area. The availability of donor areas is limited, however; such areas as the abdomen, for example, cannot well be used because of their softness. Furthermore, backing of the graft is not possible. A recent innovation is the Padgett-Hood electrodermatome. This is latched directly to the motor, which serves as the handle.

Schuchardt Dermatome: This is a very useful device, and requires no adhesive, suction, or electricity. Owing to its weight, it adheres to the skin. The graft is cut by side-to-side strokes of a knife blade, which, by means of a knife handle, is attached to the dermatome. The blade can be set by thumbscrews at any distance from the frame.

Transfer of Graft

The skin graft, after it is cut, is transferred to the wound and spread over it. It is not good practice to overlap the graft with the edges of the defect; most of the overlapping tissue would become necrotic and slough. Parts of the overlap, however, would regenerate, thus causing an irregular hypertrophic scar. The graft should be trimmed so that it fits perfectly into the defect. The graft is fastened to the wound edges with continuous or interrupted silk sutures, and also, if necessary, to the base of the graft bed with basting stitches. A few stab holes may be cut in the graft with a pointed knife to allow exudate and air to escape (Case 111, p. 1138). In grafts transplanted to the face and neck, these holes should be omitted. On granulating areas where there has been no evidence of infection, antibiotics should be administered pre- and post-operatively nevertheless.

GENERAL PRINCIPLES

Dressing of Grafted Area

Obviously, much of the success of skin grafting depends upon the proper dressing. The graft must be kept in close contact with the graft bed. This is done by exercising proper pressure. Too much pressure, however, is apt to damage the graft. Furthermore, the grafted area should be immobilized if possible. Before the pressure dressing is applied, a roll of gauze soaked in isotonic saline solution is rolled over the graft to press out air bubbles and blood; the graft is covered smoothly with one or two layers of bismuth tribromophenate (xeroform) gauze (bismuth tribromophenate, 3.0; paraffin, 1.0; white wax, 1.0; petrolatum, 95.0) or scarlet-red gauze. In large areas, rolls of gauze, wrapped around the extremity, for instance, are more convenient than single layers. An ordinary 3- or 4-inch bandage, in which the ointment is incorporated, fulfills this purpose well. Several layers of gauze soaked in isotonic saline solution follow. They should be cut so that the first layer covers only the graft, the second and third ones each being somewhat larger. Then follows the medium which will transmit an even pressure. This may be a thick layer of sterile cotton or mechanic's white cotton waste (J. B. Brown). For a small area, one may also use a sterile marine sponge or rubber sponge. The entire dressing is then placed under firm pressure with gauze bandages followed by elastic bandages. If one is dealing with an extremity, it is immobilized and elevated.

Exposure and Natural Fixation

The first such method was devised by Sano. It consisted of a physiological adhesive medium prepared of two solutions which, when brought together, develop a fibrinous adhesive coagulum simulating, in intensified forms, the normal adhesive process occurring in wounds. The grafted area remained exposed. The disadvantage was the time necessary to prepare the solution.

To obviate such delay, a fibrin-fixation method has been worked out (Tidrick and Warner, Young and Favata, Cronkite, Deaver and Rosner), which in this author's experience does not provide as firm adhesive qualities as does Sano's method. The raw side of the graft is saturated with human plasma (plasma from the plasma bank can be used). The recipient area is flooded with a thrombin solution.* The fibrinogen of the plasma-flooded graft, if brought in contact with the thrombin on the recipient area, clots almost instantly. The graft should not be moved after once applied, to prevent breaking up of the clots. A light moist dressing is applied to protect the graft.

---

* Thrombin topical (Parke, Davis and Company).

SHIFTING OF TISSUE

The author occasionally (when there is much oozing from the wound) uses a modified technique of the fibrin-fixation method by injecting thrombol† (a local thromboplastin). This is a suspension of all blood-clotting principles extracted from fresh brain tissue of the calf. To prevent moving of the graft after application of the thrombol, the following procedure is employed: The graft is sutured in place and just before application of the pressure dressing the required amount of thrombol is injected between graft and host area; the pressure dressing is applied immediately. Thus, the method is used not so much to dispense with suturing as to promote quick adhesion of the graft and control oozing.

Out of these methods grew the recommendation to apply grafts without use of any special solution, depending upon the clotting mechanism of the wound plasma alone (Cannon, Gullick, Freeman, Sherman, Larson et al., Klingenström, Nordzell and Nylen). The grafted areas are left exposed; they must be carefully protected from mechanical interference. For this reason the technique has its limitations.

Care of Donor Area

The donor area is dressed with bismuth tribromophenate (xeroform) gauze or other ointment and covered with dressing pads. The author highly recommends rayon also, which has been introduced by Neal Owens. It has a sufficiently close weave to block ingrowth of capillaries into the fabric, permits adequate drainage, has a low coefficient of friction, and permits easy sterilization. It works even better if it is coated with a thin layer of a bland ointment. There are numerous similar products now available. Artz recommends the exposure treatment (p. 163).

After-Treatment

On clean wounds, the dressing may remain in place for eight to ten days, unless there is evidence of infection. On granulating wounds, it should not remain longer than five to seven days. It is then changed; the sutures are removed. Any slough is trimmed away immediately with scissors. The dressings from now on consist of moist (saline) gauze until the graft has healed (two or three weeks). It is then protected with ointment dressings, and may be massaged daily with cocoa butter or cold cream.

Occasionally a so-called seroma may form beneath the graft (Littlewood). If the graft remains alive it is clear that it is surviving by the plasmatic nutrition from the seroma long enough to receive a vascular

---

† Merck, Sharp and Dohme.

37

supply not from its base but from the adjacent graft, which has become adherent. It is necessary to aspirate the serum immediately, excising a small part of the graft for drainage, followed by basting stitches and by a pressure dressing before the dermal undersurface of the graft becomes epithelized.

The dressing of the donor area is allowed to remain in place until it comes off by itself, i.e., after the donor area has been reepithelized. If the graft has been cut thin, the donor area may heal in one week and—if necessary—be ready in two weeks for furnishing another graft (Fig. 20). If the graft has been cut thick, several weeks may elapse before

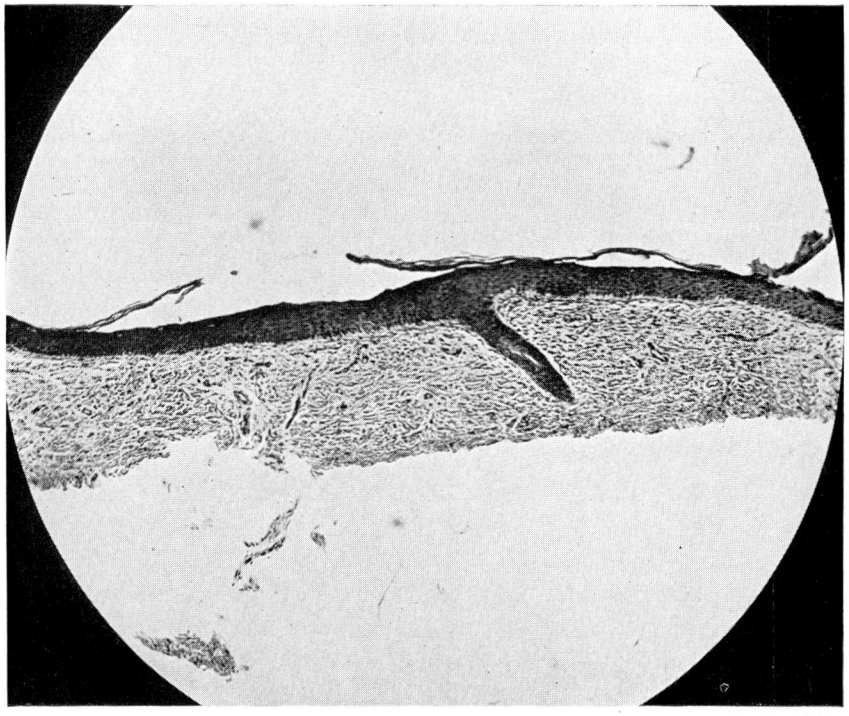

Fig. 20. Photomicrograph of split graft taken from a donor area used twice before.

reepithelization occurs. (See Cases 107, 108, pp. 1132, 1134.) To accelerate epithelization of donor areas from which a thick graft has been taken, application of a Thiersch graft is recommended. This usually involves burying dermal appendages such as hair follicles, sebaceous and sweat glands. Although this is routinely followed by formation of microscopic epidermoid cysts, the vast majority undergo dissolution within one year (Thompson).

SHIFTING OF TISSUE

MESH SKIN GRAFTS

On large granulating surfaces, after extensive burns for instance, autogenous skin coverage may be contraindicated due to lack of donor areas and debilitation of the patient, and homogeneous grafts (p. 40) may not be available. In such cases the technique of Tanner and co-workers in applying expanded autogenous mesh skin grafts can be lifesaving (DiVincenti et al.). By this method a small piece of autogenous split skin graft is placed between the leaves of a plastic carrier and passed through the mesh dermatome, and is then expanded three times the original size. Through a recent modification it is possible to expand the donor material up to twelve times its original surface area. The drawback of this method, however, is a certain amount of contracture resulting from scar tissue which develops between the expanded pieces of skin. Hence joint surfaces should not be treated by this procedure alone. They can be covered by mesh skin grafts at first and contractures repaired later. The author prefers this latter way.

SPLIT INLAY AND OUTLAY GRAFTS

This method is used mainly for the resurfacing of those regions which are difficult to reach or in which no pressure dressing can be applied, as in cavities such as the mouth, orbit, and vagina. This method, which was introduced by Esser in 1917, consists of transplantation of split skin grafts wrapped around a mold of dental compound. Esser used this method for relining the obliterated labiogingival sulcus. From an incision below the chin, the graft with stent was buried without opening the oral cavity; the incision was closed; after ten days the mold was removed through an incision in the mouth. Esser called this method "epithelial inlay-grafting." Later, this principle was modified (Waldron, Gillies, and Pickerill) by applying the graft-covered stent directly to the surface to be lined, and was called "epithelial outlay-grafting."

Technique (Case 88, 101, pp. 1102, 1120)

The surface to be grafted, such as an obliterated labiogingival sulcus, is changed into a fresh wound. A piece of dental compound, softened in hot water, is pressed into the cavity, then carefully removed and placed in cold water. A split skin graft is removed from a hairless region (not to be shaved!), and wrapped around the mold with its raw surface outward. The graft edges are sutured together over the mold. Another way of holding the graft on the mold is by means of collodion applied to the stent before wrapping the graft around it. Stent and graft are now inserted, and kept in place either by suturing the wound edges together and thus burying the stent (inlay-grafting), or by passing a suture through one wound edge and the corresponding edge of the graft. The same suture running across the mold engages the opposite graft edge and its corresponding wound edge, and is then tied. Several such sutures may be necessary (Figs. 206, 232, 302).

After-Treatment

Postoperative care consists of keeping the surrounding area clean with mild antiseptic solutions. The sutures are removed after one week, and the mold is lifted out. The grafted area is cleansed by irrigation and gentle swabbing with boric acid solution, and the mold is reinserted for several days or weeks until the graft has firmly healed in place.

HOMOGENOUS SPLIT GRAFTS

Homogenous grafts (grafts taken from another person) will take satisfactorily, but are absorbed in a few weeks unless used in identical twins (Bauer, Brown, and others). There is apparently no relation between the "take" of a homogenous graft and the blood groups (Loeffler). The main stumbling block to date has been the existence of immunological barriers to any type of graft of foreign origin, which cause rejection of the graft by antibodies. The mechanism by which an antibody causes destruction of the grafted cell is still not known. Considerable literature has accumulated and reports of new observations, ideas, and theories are appearing constantly from highly reputable centers around the world, but investigators are far from agreement. Rogers covered the literature to 1953 and Jones in his fine review of this subject to 1965. Progress in transplantation biology with the emphasis and developments of the past ten years is covered with a wealth of information by Russell and Monaco. Reference is also made to Andina's and Peer's work, Jacob et al., and Köhnlein. It is beyond the scope of this book to go into detail on this topic, but the one theory which has influenced all others must be mentioned. This is that of acquired transplantation immunity as first described by Gibson, a Scottish plastic surgeon, and Medawar, an English zoologist (1943). Medawar must be credited with popularizing and clarifying Gibson's hypothesis by a series of valuable experiments in association with Billingham and other investigators. He was among the first to recognize the mechanism of the puzzling "rejection reaction" caused by development of antibodies. Using the work of Medawar and others as a starting point, Burnet of Australia theorized that the rejection reaction is not full-blown, but instead is gradually developed in the fetus and young child. Burnet speculated that if, during the period of immunological development, the human body could be taught to tolerate grafts from selected

40

donors, it would later be able to accept tissue transplants from those same donors. Seizing on Burnet's thesis, Medawar proceeded to confirm it in a series of laboratory tests. He inoculated mouse embryos in the womb with tissue from a different breed of mice and found that the inoculated animals later were able successfully to tolerate grafts from mice of the same breed as the original donors. Thus far, the Burnet-Medawar discovery hailed in their Nobel Prize citation as "a new chapter in experimental biology" has no direct medical use. It does, however, represent a long step closer to the day when homografts of tissues and whole organs will be successful.

The immediate problems to overcome this reaction are to induce the recipient of a homograft to accept the foreign tissue of the donor or to induce the transplant to accept the recipient. This may be done by depressing or inactivating the reticulo-endothelial, lymphoid and bone marrow systems of the recipient, or by rendering the donor tissue incapable of calling forth a reaction on the part of the graft recipient. Most investigators have been concerned with methods of conditioning the recipient to accept the donor tissue, and have paid less attention to inducing the donor tissue to accept the new host. None of the methods is of permanent value as yet. It is hoped that better matching of donor and recipient will be achieved on a genetic basis through tissue typing as recommended by Converse and Rappaport. Billingham and Barker have discussed recent developments in transplantation immunology.

Although the detailed workings of the immune mechanism are still imperfectly understood, the main outlines are clear. The principal components of immunity are the lymphoid cells. They have the genetically built-in ability to identify other cells as "self" (part of the same body) or "not self" (invaders to be destroyed). In the presence of autogenous cells the lymphoid cells remain passive, but if they detect foreign material they manufacture antibodies to contain or attack the invader. These antibodies are in the form of gamma globulin particles. Some remain on the surface of the lymphoid cells and circulate with them; others, free floating, circulate in the bloodstream. Both kinds adhere to cells in the foreign tissues such as grafts. Which type is more important in graft rejection is still debated. What is certain is that together the two types can be devastatingly effective in destroying a graft.

The only practical side in homogenous skin grafting is the initial "take" of the graft. Its application obviously requires donors; this may in certain cases hamper its practicability. Dogo utilized stored cadaver skin grafts successfully in a few cases, and this may well prove practical, as demonstrated by the establishment of a skin bank for postmortem homografts by Brown and his associates, Burwell, Trier and others.

41

GENERAL PRINCIPLES

Homogenous grafts should be applied only when it is thought that the patient cannot stand a long operative procedure and is steadily slipping owing to debilitation and pain and when there is no sign of subcutaneous epithelization. It may then be lifesaving to apply large sheets of split homogenous grafts. Homogenous grafts take almost as well as autogenous grafts, become vascularized (Converse and Rappaport, etc.), and survive for three to six weeks. During this period, the patient is given a respite from pain and dressings. His general condition picks up, and there is a stimulus to his own epithelization so that complete healing may even occur after absorption of the graft or additional autogenous grafts may be employed (Case 107, p. 1132).

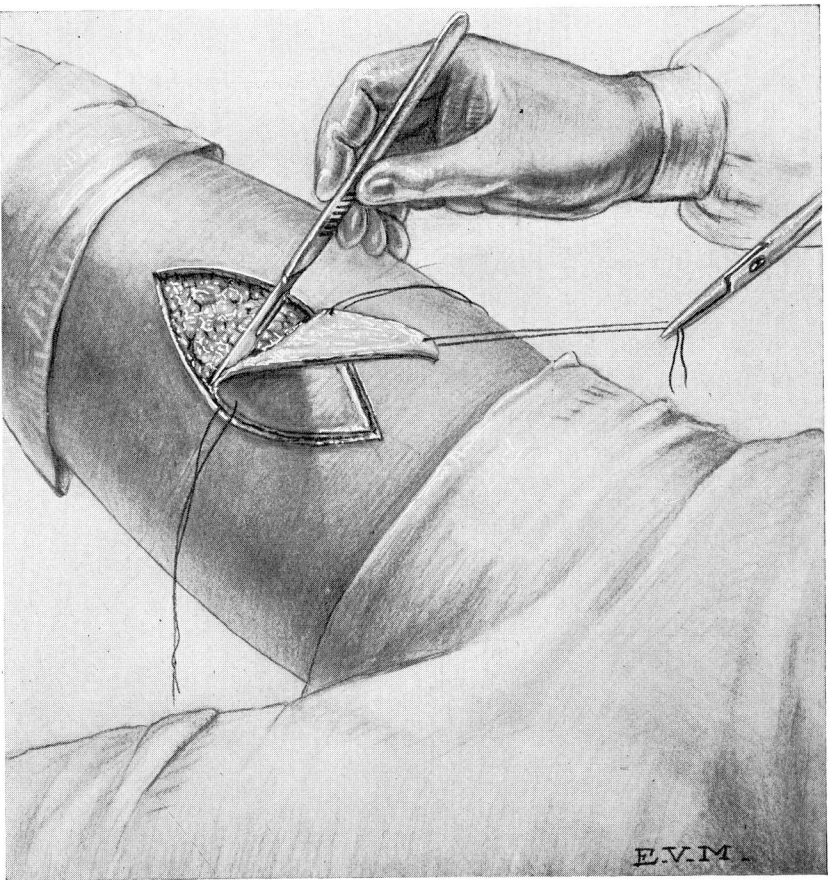

Fig. 21. Removal of full-thickness graft from median surface of thigh. Graft is outlined with incision which penetrates whole thickness of skin, but not subcutaneous fat tissue. Silk sutures, passed through extreme corners of graft, are used for traction. Skin is separated from subcutaneous fat tissue. No fat tissue should remain on graft.

SHIFTING OF TISSUE

FULL-THICKNESS GRAFTS

Technique

In transplanting grafts consisting of the full thickness of the skin, asepsis, thorough hemostasis, and very gentle handling of the graft are of utmost importance. The host area is changed into a clean wound. Then follows thorough hemostasis, in much the same way as already described (p. 30). The next step is to cut a pattern of the host area. Tinfoil, rubberdam, or chamois may be used for this purpose. The simplest procedure is to press a piece of linen upon the wound. Upon its removal, one will find the bloodstained outline of the wound on the material. This is cut out with scissors, and is transferred to the donor area.

The bloodstained side of the pattern is laid upon the skin of the donor area. With a small sharp knife, the outline of the pattern is circumscribed on the skin of the donor area. The incision, after removal of the pattern, is deepened, and includes the whole thickness of the skin. A fine silk suture is passed through each corner of one side of the graft. Under steady traction on these sutures, the skin is separated from the subcutaneous fat tissue. No fat tissue is allowed to remain on the graft (Fig. 21). Another method of cutting the graft is to remove it with some fat tissue attached. The fat tissue is trimmed away with scissors after the graft is removed. The graft is now laid upon the wound in correct position. The traction sutures are used to anchor the graft to the host area. With fine silk sutures, the remainder of the graft is fastened to the wound edges.

Dressing of Grafted and Donor Areas

A firm pressure dressing, similar to that used in split grafts, is applied; if possible, the grafted area is immobilized by proper splinting. The donor area is closed by sliding the wound edges together after undermining the adjacent skin: in case of a large defect, the defect is covered with a split graft, which is kept under proper pressure.

After-Treatment

If there is no evidence of infection, the pressure dressing is allowed to remain in place for eight to ten days. It is then changed, and the sutures are removed. In some cases, blisters may develop on some parts of the graft; they should be opened and trimmed if infected but left closed if they contain clear fluid. The graft is covered with moist (saline) gauze, and another pressure dressing is applied for a period of about three to five days. After the graft has healed, it should be protected from mechanical injury for at least three or four weeks with ointments and dressings, and massaged daily with cocoa butter or cold cream.

GENERAL PRINCIPLES

SMALL DEEP SKIN GRAFTS

These grafts were devised by J. S. Davis in 1914. They are small cones of skin, consisting of the full thickness of the skin in the center, gradually tapering off toward the periphery. They take on many areas (chronic ulcers, for example) where other types of grafts fail. Their simplicity of application and ready "take" are advantages; but the hobnail appearance of the host area, the pitted appearance of the donor areas, the longer healing time, and the tendency to contraction are drawbacks that

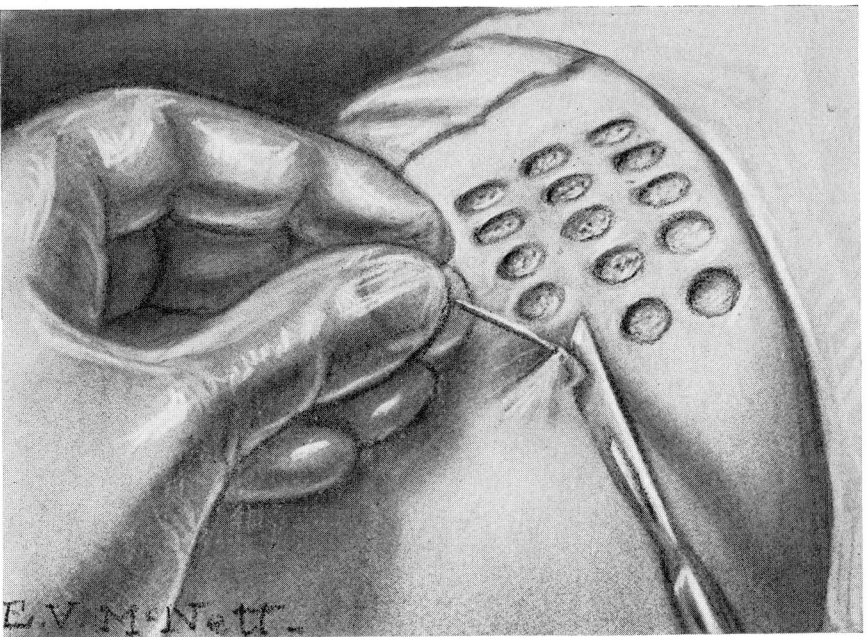

Fig. 22.   Removal of small deep grafts. Straight needle held in artery clamp engages bit of epidermis which is raised to form a small cone. Base of cone is cut through while depressing blade of knife.

make them practical only if necessity demands. These grafts may be used on granulations or on clean wounds. The preparation of these surfaces is the same as described previously (p. 30).

Technique

A straight needle held in an artery clamp is engaged in a bit of epidermis, which is raised to form a little cone. The base of this cone is cut through, after the blade of the knife is depressed (Fig. 22). The graft should be from 0.2 to 0.5 cm. ($\frac{3}{32}$ to $\frac{7}{32}$ inch) in diameter. The graft engaged by the needle is transferred to the host area. The grafts should be placed in rows close to each other.

SHIFTING OF TISSUE

Dressing

The grafted area is covered with a piece of wide-meshed paraffin gauze over which a single thickness of bismuth tribromophenate (xeroform) gauze is placed, followed by a pressure dressing. The grafted part should be immobilized. The donor area is dressed with bismuth tribromophenate gauze.

After-Treatment

If the grafts have been placed on a granulating wound, the original dressing should be changed after four days. If placed on a fresh wound, the dressing is changed after one week. The after-treatment consists in moist (saline) dressings followed by application of some bland ointment; when dealing with granulations which become exuberant, Dakin's solution may be used after one week. The grafted area should be protected from injury for several weeks.

DERMAL GRAFTS

This type of graft consists of the full thickness of the skin minus its epidermal layer (hence the term "dermal" graft; the term "cutis" graft should be avoided since under "cutis" all layers of the skin are understood). The graft is implanted into the body tissues to fill certain defects such as incisional hernias, dural defects, and defects of certain tendons, or to build up depressions in such regions as the face and head (Case 16, p. 1014). It is proved that it heals better and more quickly than other grafts (such as fascia and fat) used for similar purposes, and according to Rehn it adapts itself readily to functional requirements through functional metaplasia (Swenson). Loewe (1913) was the first to use this type of graft. Rehn (1914), however, deserves the credit for popularizing it. The literature upon this subject has been extensively reviewed by Cannaday. The objection that cysts form from the buried glandular structures is apparently not true. Peer and Paddock examined dermal grafts from seven days to one year after implantation, and found disappearance of sebaceous glands and hair follicles and degenerative changes in the sweat glands. This has been recently confirmed by Thompson.

Mair takes the entire thickness of the skin (cutis) to bury as a graft —a method used mainly in repair of hernias. From his rather large series of cases and those of others (Zaveta et al., Marsden), it becomes evident that, in spite of the buried epithelial layer, inclusion cysts do not form. If large buried grafts must be used, the full-thickness skin graft is of no advantage, since the donor area would need another split graft for closure.

45

GENERAL PRINCIPLES

Technique (Cases 16, 18, pp. 1014, 1017)

The graft is obtained in one of two ways: (1) A thin layer of epidermis is sliced off and then the required size of the dermal graft, cut like a full-thickness graft. The resulting defect of the donor area is covered with the removed epidermis. (2) The skin is removed with the dermatome (drum-type dermatome) as thick as possible. The skin remains on the drum while the knife handle is reset. The graft is now split so that only a thin layer of dermis is left behind on the drum which can be utilized to cover the donor area.

Concerning transfer, fixation, and postoperative treatment of dermal grafts, the reader is referred to pages 610 and Case 105, page 1030.

MUCOUS-MEMBRANE GRAFTS

Free transplantation of mucous membrane is not so widely used as that of the skin, owing to lack of material. Large mucous-membrane defects are preferably replaced by skin than by mucous-membrane grafts. The latter's chief use lies in replacing conjunctival lining of eyelids and eye sockets. The chief sources are the lips and cheeks. The lower lip is turned outward and downward, and held in this position with hooks or traction sutures. The graft is sliced off with a razor knife, in the same fashion as a split graft is cut. If the graft is taken from the cheeks, it is cut like a full-thickness graft. For transfer and after-treatment see page 35.

FAT-TISSUE GRAFTS

Transplantation of fat tissue, first attempted by Neuber (1893), attracted attention when Czerny (1895) reported his celebrated case of an actress in whom cystic tissue of the left breast was removed and replaced by a lipoma from the patient's lumbar region. The breast remained well formed, and the lipoma did not grow. The real impetus to this work, however, was given by Lexer and his associates. From experimental and clinical observations he states that about one third of the fat transplant survives; the other two thirds undergoes degeneration in the form of cyst formations. These cysts are due to fat necrosis. The degenerating fat cells coalesce and form cysts. The cysts are invaded by round cells, which absorb the fat globules. Some of the round cells may change into embryonal fat cells, and there may be an actual regeneration of fat. The surviving fat tissue may become atrophic, but does not change character, as the author can confirm.

Further evidence that a portion of fat cells survives was given by Peer in a series of experimental fat grafts in humans. If the fat graft is transplanted together with the overlying dermis, i.e., skin minus the epi-

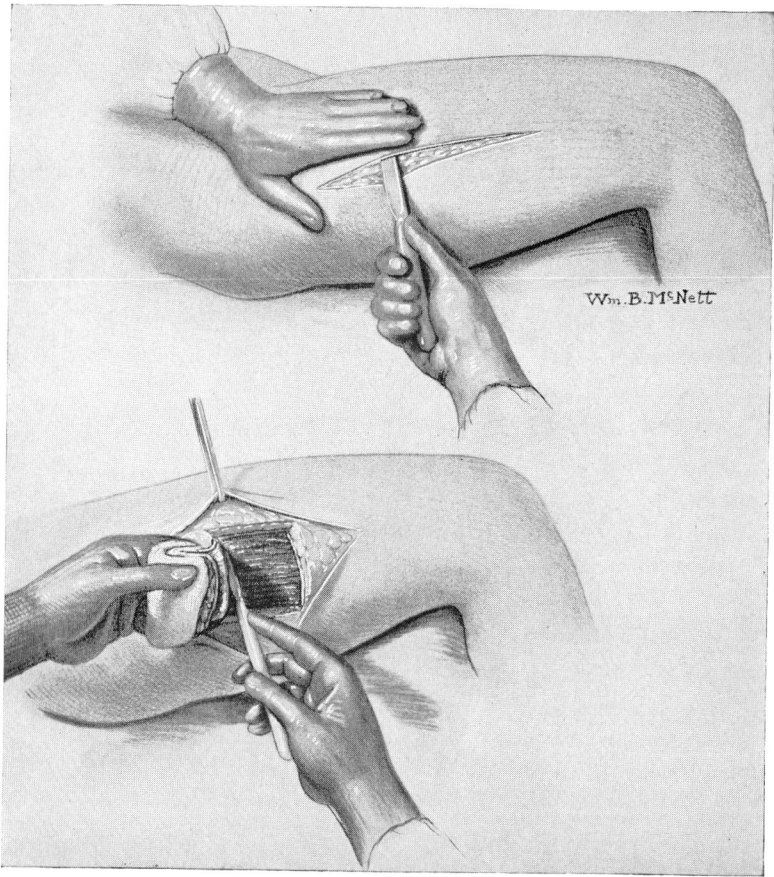

Fig. 23. Removal of fat-tissue graft from lateroposterior surface of thigh. Skin is severed from subcutaneous fat tissue with amputation knife. Fat-tissue graft is removed with underlying fascia lata.

thelial layer (p. 45), even greater parts of the graft seem to survive. The reasons for this are not clear. It is hardly conceivable that proliferating capillaries from the host tissue could invade the dermis and several inches of fat tissue in time to ensure the survival of the graft. Watson, after experimental and clinical experience, came to the conclusion that the dermal element of the composite fat graft, when placed in intimate contact

47

with a competent host tissue, might exert a stronger vaso-inductive effect than fat alone. The larger the surface area of dermis in relation to the mass of fat tissue, the greater the chances of survival. A survival of the dermal part of the graft is of primary importance. Hence, precautions must be taken to bring about an early fusion and vascularization of this part of the graft by establishing a close contact of graft and host tissue, i.e., avoidance of hematomas, application of pressure dressings. Yet, in spite of all safeguards, the regeneration of a fat graft remains unreliable.

Fat-tissue grafts are used to fill surface depressions, to smooth contours, to obliterate dead spaces, and to prevent adhesions. The graft should be taken two thirds larger than required to counteract degeneration and shrinkage. Peer advises having the patient on a fat-free diet before the operation. Derma (p. 45) left in contact with the fat graft seems to limit shrinkage. Sawhney, Bajerjee and Chakravarti, however, believe that whatever bulk persists is mainly the intact unchanged dermis, and the cicatrization of the fat graft.

The graft may be taken from the abdomen, from the lateroposterior surface of the thigh, or from the gluteal folds. If a fat graft plus derma is taken the epidermis is removed with the dermatome. The derma and fat tissue are then cut en bloc and transplanted. The dermal part of the composite graft should be placed upon an even part of the wound cavity. It may also be practical to cut a composite full-thickness skin and fat graft en bloc and remove the epidermis subsequently.

FASCIA GRAFTS

Transplantation of fascia was introduced by Kirschner (1909). It has received widespread acceptance in bridging hernial gaps, in reconstructing facial and other muscular palsies and tendon defects, and in closing defects in such regions as the trachea, esophagus, and diaphragm; it is also used in arthroplasties to prevent ankylosis, and serves as living suture material. Fascia is easily obtainable. It is extremely resistant to infection, and adapts itself readily to the mechanical requirements of the surroundings—factors which make fascia an excellent material for transplantation.

Technique

The best source of fascia grafts is the fascia lata. The simplest way of removing strips of fascia is with a fascia stripper (Fig. 24). Hip and knee are bent, and the extremity is rotated inward. From a small transverse incision at the lateral surface of the thigh above the knee joint, the fascia lata is exposed. With a pair of long-handled dissecting scissors the fat tissue is dissected away from the fascia lata for a distance corresponding to the length of the graft. A small strip of fascia of desired size is outlined with the knife; it is fed through the opening of the stripper, and then grasped with a hemostat and held taut. The stripper is now moved upward, cutting and separating a strip of fascia of desired length. If the stripper is provided with a cutting mechanism, the upper end of the graft is cut; otherwise, it is separated with the knife from a separate small incision. Graft and stripper are removed through the lower incision. If several strips are needed, the graft may be divided or other grafts obtained from the same incisions. Herniation of muscles after this pro-

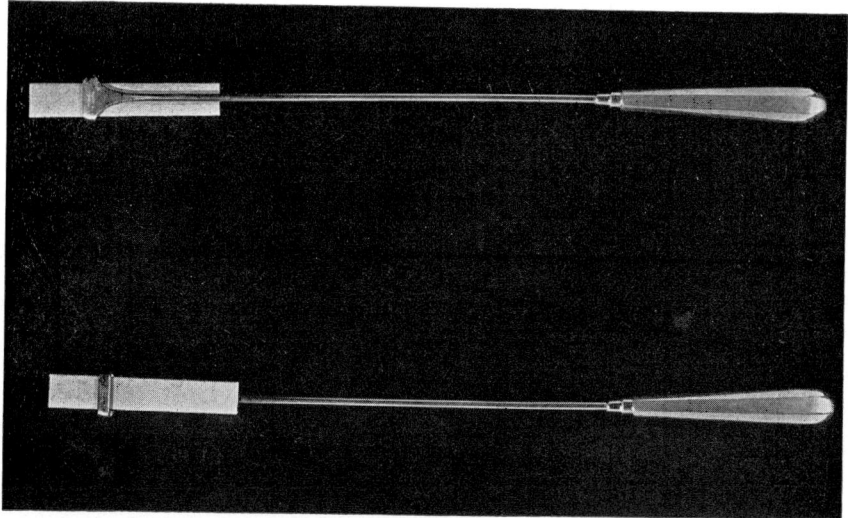

Fig. 24. Fascia stripper, consisting of long handle and transverse slit at end through which fascia strip is passed.

cedure has not been observed by the author. If broad pieces of fascia need to be removed, the fascia must be exposed from a longitudinal incision through skin and fat tissue along the lateral surface of the thigh. The desired piece of fascia is freed from the overlying fat tissue, and then removed with the scalpel. Traction sutures at extreme points of the graft facilitate removal and the marking of boundaries.

STRIATED-MUSCLE GRAFTS

Free transplantation of striated muscle proves to be of little clinical value except for hemostatic purposes in rare instances.

TENDON GRAFTS

Tendon grafts are mainly used to replace tendon defects or diseased tendons. It is an established fact that, in selected cases under the proper operative and postoperative care, a tendon graft regenerates and functions. If the defect is due to infection, one ought to delay the operation for three months. Antibiotics should be administered two days preoperatively and continued for at least four days postoperatively.

For the bridging of tendon defects, various autogenous or homogenous tissues, such as fascia, cutis, tendon, and even heterogenous material (p. 872), have been recommended. Among the pioneers of this work are Kirschner, Bier, Lexer, E. Rehn, Lange, Bunnell, Koch, Mason, Mayer, and Iselin. According to the present consensus, autogenous tendon tissue is favored as graft material (May). The graft sources are the palmaris longus, the long extensor tendons of the second to the fourth toes (the tendon of the fifth toe should not be used since it has only one extensor), the long tendon of the plantaris muscle, and—under certain circumstances to be mentioned later—the flexor digitorum sublimis tendon.

Importance of Paratenon

In all tendon grafting, aside from the regeneration of the tendon tissue, the role of the gliding tissue is of interest and importance. This tissue, called "paratenon," is a loose, fatty meshwork, rich in elastic fibers. The paratenon provides not only the gliding mechanism but also the bulk of the nutrient vessels and nerves of the tendon. The tendon sheath is a closed sac containing fluid. It is found whenever the tendon changes its direction and serves as a fluid buffer to diminish friction at this point. The sheath consists of a parietal and a visceral layer. Both layers are connected with each other by the mesotenon, which carries the nutrient vessels and nerves. Thus, it becomes evident that a tendon graft has little chance to survive and to function unless the gliding tissue of the host area is preserved or, if absent, the gliding tissue is also transplanted. Hence, if the paratenon or the tendon sheath of the graft bed is absent, a paratenon-covered tendon graft must be transplanted. So, for instance, in using one of the long extensor tendons of the toes as a graft, great care should be taken to preserve the loose areolar tissue which surrounds the tendon. It should be not only preserved but firmly held in place with a temporary suture at the extreme end of the graft. The paratenon, like the periosteum of a bone graft, gains quick access to the circulation of the surrounding tissue and is able to reestablish the interrupted blood supply within the tendon graft. That intratendinous vessels do exist is beyond any doubt

(Mayer, Edwards, Brockis). If the paratenon of the graft cannot be preserved, the graft must be taken from other sources as a free graft and wrapped around the tendon graft. The paratendinous tissue differs from ordinary fat tissue. It is a loose areolar fat tissue, which is found over the triceps tendon or directly over the fascia lata or in the interspace between the fascia lata and the muscle fascia. For further details see page 864.

Regeneration of Tendon Graft

Opinions still differ concerning the manner of regeneration of a tendon graft. One group of investigators believes that the graft is replaced by fibrous tissue which is derived from the surrounding tissue. Another group believes in a true or at least a nearly true regeneration of the tendon graft; the graft either survives as a whole (Mason, Shearon, Lindsay and McDougall) or undergoes necrosis but acts as a strut which is replaced by tenoblasts from the stumps of the host (Flynn et al.). The graft is kept alive by reestablishment of its circulation through postoperative adhesions (Peacock). For further consideration of this topic the reader is referred to page 845. All agree that the functional stimulus promotes quicker and better regeneration. Whatever the manner of regeneration, it has been sufficiently proved, experimentally as well as clinically, that a grafted tendon segment, under proper operative and postoperative care, can regain function to transmit the contractile force of its muscle. For technique and after-treatment, the reader is referred to pages 867-876 and to Cases 152-155, pages 1199-1202.

BLOOD-VESSEL GRAFTS

Transplantation of blood vessels became possible only after Carrel and Guthrie at the turn of the century had developed an adequate method of anastomosing vessels; failures, however, were many, chiefly from thrombosis developing at the site of the anastomosis. This problem has been largely overcome by the discovery of anticoagulants. In spite of the feasibility of free transplantation of autogenous and homologous vessel grafts, interest remained lacking until World War II. Since then, the rapid growth of cardiovascular surgery has stimulated interest in vessel grafting.

Vessel grafting is mainly performed to bridge congenital and acquired arterial defects. The graft material is either autogenous (vein), homologous (preserved artery), or heterologous (plastic prosthesis). It is obvious that autogenous material is limited (internal and external jugular, saphenous vein). In a search for a more practical method, the preserved arterial homograft became the chosen graft source. Although Höpfner, Stich, and Carrel at the turn of the century had experimented successfully with such a graft, followed by Klotz, Permar, and Guthrie in 1923, the credit for reintroducing the homologous arterial graft goes to Peirce (working in Gross's laboratory) and Gross. They were followed by a host of enthusiastic researchers, such as Swan and co-workers, Hufnagel, Deterling and co-workers, Debakey and co-workers, McCune and co-workers, Sauvage et al., Kremer of Germany, and Bellman and Gothman of Sweden. A fine review of this topic is presented by Lehr and Blakemore.

The problems of processing, sterilizing and preserving tissue grafts stimulated the search for a prosthetic graft. Such heterogenous grafts in form of a plastic prosthesis made of nylon (Vinyon "N") were introduced by Voorhees, Blakemore, and their co-workers. It is only natural that foreign material was accepted hesitantly at first, but, to judge from numerous recent reports (Poth, Johnson, Edwards, Deterling et al., Wesolowski et al., Harrison et al., and others), it is being used more and more. Edwards published an engagingly written little monograph on this subject, and Eufinger and Vollmar, both of Germany, have also written on the subject. The great advantage is that the material is readily available and inexpensive and that the implants can be tailored to fit the vessels of the host. The immediate results appear to be good; however, the ultimate value must be decided after long-term clinical observations, which are now available. In spite of many disadvantages, such as leakage through the fabric and thrombosis at the site of the anastomosis, plastic prostheses are still widely used. Most attention was focused on the woven plastics. While the ideal prosthesis is still to be found, the knitted dacron prosthesis appears to be satisfactory in most instances (Debakey et al.), and teflon has also many things in its favor. The ultimate fate of the prosthesis is that it becomes encased by hyalinizing fibrous tissue.

Autogenous grafts of blood vessels have the great advantage of remaining alive for a long time. Sooner or later, however, they are replaced by nonspecific fibrous tissue, whereupon the different layers of the transplant become less and less marked. Aneurysmal dilatation of the venous graft, as one might expect, does not occur, and the graft gradually assumes the width of the host artery. Lexer's brilliant and often-quoted case is a vivid example. He extirpated the sac of an arterial aneurysm of the right arteria iliaca externa and arteria femoralis, and bridged the 16-cm. defect with a vessel graft taken from the vena saphena. Five years later, the grafted vessel was still functioning and pulsating and had assumed the width of the artery.

Many successful cases of autograft vein transplants have been described since that time (Murray and others). There is general agreement that autografts (veins) are more desirable than homografts and should be used in bridging peripheral arteries. They are either reversed or the valves are excised, after the vein has been turned inside-out (G. Johnson). However, when dealing with larger arteries, particularly with the aorta, autografts of proper size are not available; hence one must resort to arterial homografts or heterologous material.

The fate of an arterial homograft is of interest. It was first described by Carrel and later in detail by Klotz, Permar, and Guthrie in 1923: (1) rapid degeneration of the intima within forty-eight hours and regeneration of endothelial cells by growth inward from both ends of the graft; (2) gradual replacement of muscle cells of the media by collagen fibers but persistence of elastic fibers for many months; (3) surrounding of the grafted segment by a layer of granulation tissue, replacing degenerated cells with connective tissue. Swan, Gross, Peirce, Halpert, Debakey et al., and others confirmed these findings and came to the conclusion that all cellular layers in the graft are destroyed by host reaction, that the elastic tissue of the media, however, persists for several years, and hence that the host builds a new blood vessel on the scaffold of the elastic tissue of the graft. McCune and co-workers studied the nutrition of blood-vessel grafts. They could demonstrate that practically all of the circulation reaching the graft walls is derived from surrounding structures and to a small extent from the anastomosis of the graft ends. No vessels could be demonstrated entering the graft walls from the lumina. Nevertheless, in cellophane-wrapped grafts the histological appearance of the layers immediately surrounding the lumen was more normal than that of the outer media and adventitia, indicating presumably that some nutrition filters through the endothelium from the lumen to supply the internal and medial coats. It therefore seems important in the employment of arterial grafts that, to promote vascularization, the transplants be surrounded by as much vascular tissue as possible.

A major problem relating to the clinical use of arterial homografts is that of availability and storage. According to Swan, the grafts must be obtained sterile from young persons, from two to thirty-five years of age, previously in good health, whose death is sudden or from a relatively acute cause. The vessels must be obtained within six hours postmortem. The problem of storage is equally important. It has been clearly demonstrated by Gross and his group (Peirce) that viably preserved vessel grafts are more reliable and give better functional results than nonviable vessel segments. They behave for a while like autogenous grafts. Hence, viably preserved grafts should be used. Two methods of storage are available: cold preservation and lyophilization. The latter has the merit of simplicity, but has not gained popularity, mainly owing to lack of large-scale evaluation. Deep freezing (Hufnagel, Deterling, Swan), as well as quick deep freezing (R. B. Brown, Kremer) in a nutrient solution as medium and storage of the graft, has been shown to be successful; however, storing grafts in a stoppered bottle containing a balanced salt solution and 10 per cent plasma or serum at 4° C. is simpler, and accomplishes the same aim for periods up to about forty-five days (Peirce). Swan and Sauvage and Harkins believe that Ringer solution is equally efficient. This subject is broadly discussed by Lehr and Blakemore, Hughes and Bowers.

Technique

Swan summarizes the details of the operation as follows: Suture anastomosis is best suited for insertion of the graft. This may be done by temporarily controlling blood flow proximally and distally with non-crushing arterial clamps, such as Poth's serrated clamps during the anastomosis; or if preservation of blood flow during the procedure is essential—for example, in the carotid artery—the technique of minimal interruption over temporarily placed polyethylene tubes may be employed. All the niceties of technique of vascular suture must be meticulously observed—strict asepsis, avoidance of tissue injury by trauma or desiccation, careful stripping of the adventitia, careful placement of small atraumatic sutures, and careful wound closure without dead space or necrosis. In addition, the employment of a graft of proper size is of paramount importance. The lumen of the graft, when distended by the blood pressure, must match as exactly as possible the lumen of the recipient vessel, thus forming a vessel in continuity of uniform or tapering caliber.

If these precautions are observed, concludes Swan, anticoagulant drugs need not be used unless blood flow has been interrupted for more than an hour. If interruption has been prolonged, thrombosis of the distal artery may occur, and heparin should be used to limit the spread of these distal thromboses.

Linton and Menendez maintain that the end-to-end anastomosis, in many instances, causes a slight stenosis with a chance of subsequent thrombosis. To counteract this, they recommend the end-to-side anastomosis (Figs. 25, 26), modified after the original technique of Kunlin of Paris. With this type of anastomosis, there is a widening at both the end of the graft and host artery itself, thus reducing the chance of stenosis and secondary thrombosis. They also recommend, while preparing the graft, rinsing it frequently with an 0.01 per cent solution of heparin, soaking it in this solution before it is actually inserted, and injecting about 20 cc. of the same solution into the stumps of the host arteries distal to the distal occluding clamp and proximal to the proximal clamp.

If an autogenous vein graft is used, the same meticulous care must be observed: A tourniquet should be used if possible; if it is contraindicated or impossible, the vessel stumps are closed with noncrushing arterial clamps, such as Poth's serrated clamps, which are applied a few centimeters above the wound edges. The vena saphena, cephalia or vena jugularis externa is used as a graft; or if the corresponding vein of the artery to be grafted must be tied, a section of this vein should be transplanted. The graft should be handled with the greatest care. It should be transplanted in the direction opposite to the blood stream to overcome the valvular mechanism. The graft should not run through a dead space.

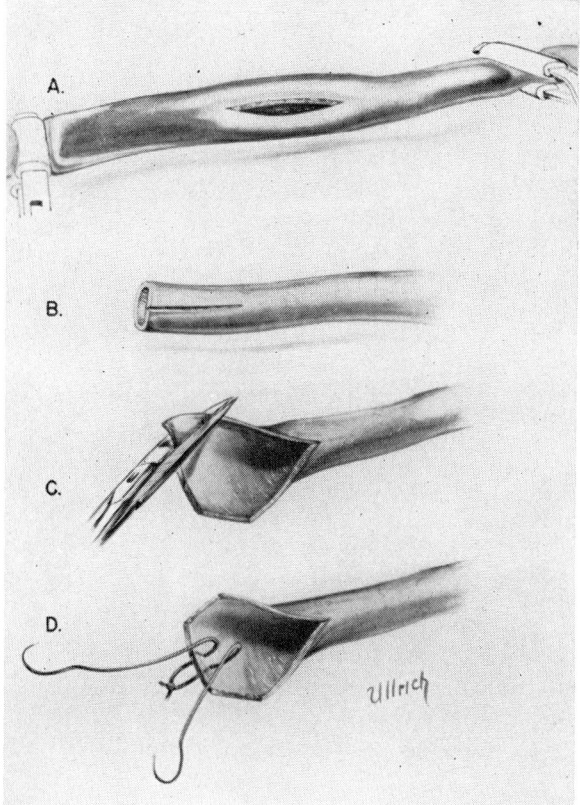

Fig. 25. An artist's drawings to demonstrate the end-to-side technique of an arterial anastomosis. (A) A longitudinal incision is made in a section of the host artery isolated between two bulldog clamps. For most arteries it is two to three times as long as the diameter of the vessel. (B) A longitudinal slit is made in the cleanly divided end of the homograft, approximately equal in length to the incision in the host artery. (C) The corners of the square-ended arterial flap are trimmed. (D) The anastomosis is commenced with two mattress sutures, using two arterial sutures tied together or a double-needled arterial suture. These are placed in the center of the arterial flap, and also at the apex of the incision in the graft. The former is shown; note that the needles have gone through the graft wall from outside to inside. (Linton, R. R. and Menendez, C. V.: Ann. Surg.)

GENERAL PRINCIPLES

Carrel's suture technique is used (Fig. 27). If the grafted vein has a much smaller lumen than the artery, an everting mattress suture (Dorrance) is preferable to a simple overhand stitch (Fig. 27 lower row). It secures a better adaptation of the lumina, a better hold of the tissues, and consequently a better approximation of the intima. The end-to-side anastomosis (Figs. 25, 26) may prove still better. The extremity should be elevated to heart level or to a slightly dependent position (see p. 764). After the wounds are sutured, immobilization is carried out on a molded plaster cast or wooden splint. The first dressing should not be changed for about two weeks if possible. The patient may be permitted to walk after three weeks.

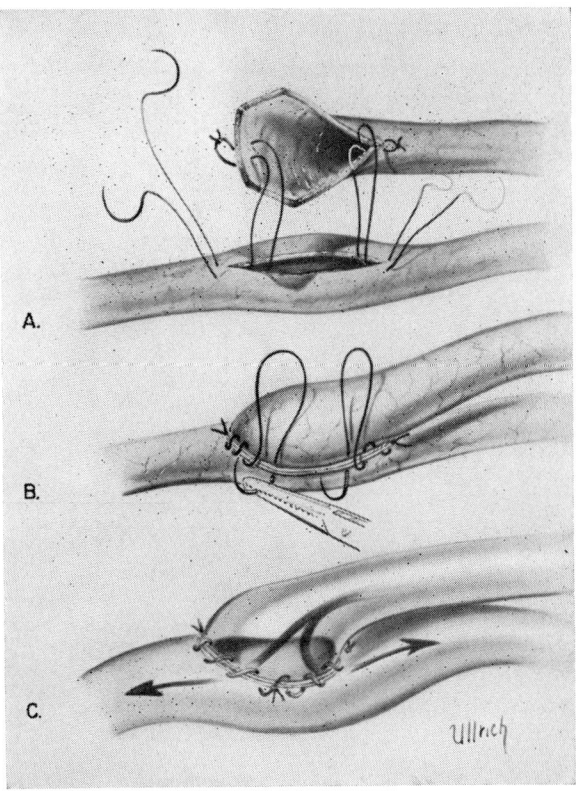

Fig. 26. The end-to-side technique (continued). (A) The two mattress sutures have been placed. Note that the needles have gone through the host artery from inside to outside, to prevent loosening and fragmenting the atheromatous intima. (B) The mattress sutures are tied, then commencing at each end they are used to continue the anastomosis with a simple running over-and-over type of stitch. This everts the edges to give an intima-to-intima approximation, and it is also hemostatic. (C) To complete the anastomosis the two ends of each are tied together where they meet in the center of the suture line on each side. As indicated by the arrows, the blood will flow both proximally and distally in the host artery with this type of anastomosis. (Linton, R. R. and Menendez, C. V.: Ann. Surg.)

56

SHIFTING OF TISSUE

Blakemore and Lord introduced a nonsuture method of blood-vessel anastomosis with the aid of vitallium tubes. A suturing apparatus by means of alloyed steel clips has been tested in the Soviet Union and a similar instrument devised by Inokuchi. The suture anastomosis, however, is simpler, and has remained popular.

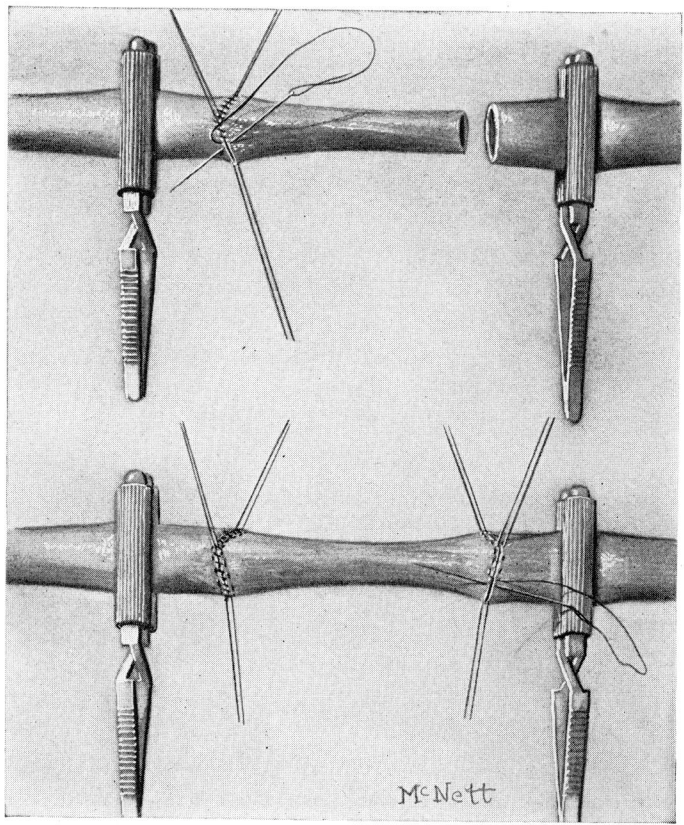

Fig. 27. Section of vein grafted to bridge defect in artery. Arterial stumps are closed with elastic arterial clamps. *Upper row:* Carrel's technique. Three traction sutures are placed at equal distance through entire wall of vessels. If traction is applied, round circumference of vessel becomes triangular, thus facilitating suturing, in which finest arterial silk is used in continuous overhand stitch under eversion of intima. *Lower row:* Dorrance's everting mattress suture, used when grafted vein has much smaller lumen than artery. After completion, a second row of simple sutures (*left*) secures everted edges.

Anticoagulants

Administration of anticoagulants may or may not be necessary, as already pointed out. If necessary, the choice lies between heparin and dicumarol. Heparin was discovered by McLean and finally purified by

57

GENERAL PRINCIPLES

Best, Charles, and Scott; dicumarol was introduced by Link and co-workers. Heparin found in animal tissues is an antiprothrombin and antithrombin as well; it also seems to activate naturally occurring inhibitors of coagulation in the blood. It decreases the coagulability of the blood and hence prolongs the coagulation time. Dicumarol is the active principle in spoiled sweet clover; it acts as a biological antagonist to vitamin K, hence as a suppressor of prothrombin synthesis by the liver, thus lowering the prothrombin level in the plasma. This effect is normally reversible by vitamin K administration. Heparin is administered parenterally, dicumarol orally. Heparin acts immediately upon entering the blood stream, dicumarol after twenty-four to forty-eight hours. The return of the clotting mechanism to normal following discontinuance of the two drugs is rapid with heparin and delayed with dicumarol. Hence, daily prothrombin determinations are necessary when dicumarol is administered, while simply performed clotting-time determinations may be sufficient after heparin administration. Dicumarol is strictly contraindicated in severe liver disease, and should be used with caution or not at all in all conditions where, in the event of bleeding (after recent operation), reversal of its effects may take considerable time. Both drugs may also be used combined (Rhoads and co-workers); here, dicumarol seems to enhance the effect of heparin. An outline of the modern concepts of blood coagulation is collectively presented by Salibi, by Quick and Halse, and by Shapiro and Weiner.

NERVE GRAFTS

Transplantation of nerves was for a long time a discouraging subject, but since Duel and Ballance's (1932) demonstrations of successful nerve transplantation in facial palsies much interest in this subject has been aroused among surgeons. The first thorough information about the degenerative and regenerative processes following nerve transplantation was given by Huber (1895). Many more studies have since been published (Eden, L. Davis and co-workers, Klar, and others), and although more light has been thrown upon this subject, particularly by the experimental work of Sanders, by an extensive clinical research study of Seddon, and by the histological observations of Holmes, agreement is far from complete. If a nerve becomes separated, the peripheral end undergoes degeneration, resulting in atrophy of the axis cylinders. If the nerve continuity can be restored—and even wide gaps may be closed by favorable displacement of the central and peripheral stumps (Babcock, Nigst)—the axis cylinders of the proximal end may grow downward into the peripheral

58

end and regenerate the nerve. If, however, the gap between the severed nerve ends is so wide that direct suture is not possible, a section of another nerve may be transplanted to bridge the defect. This graft undergoes the same degenerative changes as the peripheral end of the severed nerve, but may provide the channels along which the axis cylinders of the central end grow to reach the peripheral end. Whether a graft of a motor or a sensory nerve is used is apparently irrelevant.

Investigators agree that autotransplants are more reliable (see Case 148, p. 1194) than homo- or heterotransplants. The sources of autogenous donor nerves, however, are limited, particularly in bridging large defects of thick nerves. Homogenous nerve grafts are apt to be rejected by the body, as are other homografts (skin, etc.), unless they are conditioned to be accepted (see p. 40). As already pointed out (see p. 41), the ways and means of conditioning the homografts to become accepted by the host tissue are thus far unreliable. Nigst was able to depress the immunological response to the homograft nerve with cortisone, but this did not prevent it altogether. More hopefully, Campbell and Bassett recently reported sensory and motor return after homografting of nerves with defects up to 13.5 cm. in length. They attribute their success to two factors: irradiation of the grafts to condition them to prevent reaction of the host tissue, and the use of "millipore," a porous artificial membrane with which the grafts are surrounded. The pores are so fine (0.45 μ) that no cells can grow through them, hence cicatricial changes around the graft and anatomoses are prevented; yet plasma exchange is not impeded. The graft, like the autograft, acts as a channel for the ingrowth of the axis cylinders of the central end to reach the peripheral end, i.e., the homograft is gradually replaced by autogenous tissue ("creeping substitution"). J. Böhler has had similar results. Lyophilization or deep freezing of the homograft seems to have the same conditioning effect.

The success of nerve grafting depends greatly upon the time that has elapsed since the original nerve injury and upon the skill of the operator. In many cases, nerve grafting must be preceded by replacement of excessive skin scars with pedicled flaps.

Technique

The ends of the severed nerve are exposed by an adequate incision; a tourniquet should not be used, since it may interfere with later regeneration. Thorough hemostasis is of the utmost importance. The dissection of the nerve ends should not be carried too far, and should be as gentle as possible. All scar tissue at the stumps is removed. This is done with a sharp knife by cutting small slices off until normal fibers are exposed. After thorough hemostasis, the wound is covered with gauze soaked in warm isotonic saline solution. (For exposure and handling of the nerve ends, see also p. 749.) The graft is now removed. The aim must always be to implant a graft or a collection of grafts having a total cross section equal, at least, to that of the peripheral stump of the damaged nerve.

Since, according to experimental and clinical experience, sensory nerve grafts are capable of conveying motor responses, it is not necessary to sacrifice a motor nerve to obtain a graft. The nerves which are commonly used as autogenous grafts are the nervus saphenus and the nervus cutaneous surae medialis. The former accompanies the vena saphena magna, and is exposed on the median aspect of the leg on the level of the tuberositas tibiae. The latter accompanies the vena saphena parva, and is found in the midline of the calf beneath the deep fascia in the upper half and superficial to it in the lower half. Other nerves to be considered for autogenous graft material are the superficial radial nerve, between elbow and wrist, and the nervus cutaneus antibrachii. Hanna and Gaisford use the great auricular nerve to replace defects of the facial nerve. The nerve is obtained at the point of exit from the posterior aspect of the sternocleidomastoid muscle and is dissected free as it passes over the lateral and superior portions of this muscle. If the nerve to be bridged has a small caliber, one section of the sensory nerve is used as a graft.

The graft is handled as gently as possible. Neither the recipient nerve nor the graft should be grasped with forceps. The wound should be kept moist constantly. Fine silk and needles are used. The fibers of the graft and recipient nerve are brought into close approximation, and are held in this position by accurate suturing of the epineurium with few interruptions and a continuous suture, care being taken to prevent inversion of the latter.

If the nerve to be bridged has a large caliber, several sections of nerve grafts are taken and sutured together until a cable is formed (Elsberg). Accurate fixation of cable grafts with sutures may be very difficult. To overcome the suture difficulties of a cable graft, the plasma suture is of great value (Tarloff, Young and Medawar, Seddon). Seddon advises the following technique: The field of operation must be dry. The grafts are laid in position and the ends accurately apposed to the cut surface of the stumps. Provided that the grafts have not been moistened with saline, it will be found that they are sufficiently tacky to adhere slightly to the cut surface of the stumps. The operating-room table is then manipulated in such a way as to make the bed of the graft a horizontal lake. Bone wax or fibrin foam may be used (and removed later) to build up any deficiency in the site of the lake so that it will form a convenient receptacle for the plasma. It has not been found convenient to use the plasma-suture molds devised by Tarloff (1944). An assistant then drops the prepared plasma from a fine pipette onto one junction while the surgeon concentrates his attention on the line of suture. He may find it necessary to hold one or more grafts in position with watchmaker's forceps, which can be withdrawn without disturbance after the plasma has clotted. A second batch of plasma is then prepared and used for the distal suture line. In order that the grafts may receive an adequate blood supply from the surrounding tissue, it is probably wise (Tarloff and Epstein) to avoid application of plasma to the grafts throughout their length; in practice this is often difficult. The wound is then closed with avoidance of dead spaces, and the extremity immobilized for four to six weeks. Physiotherapy is then instituted (p. 752).

Rather than transplanting autogenous cablegrafts to bridge defects of large caliber nerves, homogenous nerve grafting can now be resorted to, as recommended some time ago by L. Davis but considered doomed to failure by others. Since Campbell's and Barrett's successful conditioning (see above) and use of the millipore, homografting appears to promise better results.

Technique

The nerve ends are prepared as described above. The gap is filled with an homogenous nerve graft of equivalent length and equal caliber held in contact with the proximal and distal stumps by a continuous epineural suture. The previously lyophilized or frozen grafts preserved at −78° C are procured under aseptic conditions. Graft and anastomoses are shielded with a cylinder of millipore which is made with a millipore membrane. The wrapped-around membrane is held with circular sutures. It is in dry condition, fragile, and when moist tears easily. Hence, it is best placed on a sheath of nylon. It is important that the membrane is not kinked; the course of the nerve should be straight. The extremity should be immobilized for three to four months. The millipore membrane should be removed after six months since it becomes calcified and may then impede proper nourishment of the nerve.

A method of bridging a gap in the median nerve deserves mention: the so-called nerve flap which becomes applicable in combined defects of ulnar and median nerve when the ulnar defect cannot be closed by favorably positioning the nerve. The operation is carried out in two stages (St. Clair Strange, Oakey, personal communication). The first stage consists of anastomosing the proximal stumps of the ulnar and median nerve after proper resection to form a loop. The ulnar nerve is then exposed proximally and at the site of the future section; the distance between anastomosis and section should be somewhat longer than the defect in the median nerve. The central artery, which is visible through the perineurium, is severed to reverse part of the circulation of the ulnar nerve. Six weeks later, in the second stage, the ulnar nerve is severed at the site of the incision and anastomosed with the distal stump of the median nerve.

For the same purpose, i.e., bridging a gap in the median nerve in combined defects of median and ulnar nerve, the author used the proximal end of the ulnar nerve as a free graft to bridge the defect of the median nerve (see Case 148, p. 1194).

Chemical adhesives, supposedly inert synthetic substances—polymers, derived from acrylic acid—have recently been introduced into surgery. The results from "gluing" nerve ends together are thus far inconclusive (Proc. Intern. Symp. on Adhesives in Surgery: Vienna Acad. Med., Vienna, 1968).

CARTILAGE GRAFTS

Transplantation of cartilage has found a widespread acceptance in reconstructive surgery since Mangold introduced it in 1889. (Collective reviews of this subject are presented by Peer and by Sarnat and Laskin.) Cartilage is most satisfactory for filling certain defects in which rigid support is required. Since cartilage is lymph nourished, it survives readily if taken from the same patient, and may become an organic unit with the host tissue. If it is taken from another person, it is apt to die and to become encapsulated like a foreign body. Such a graft may become absorbed gradually. Opinions, however, differ on this subject as well as on the fate of preserved dead cartilage (Gillies, Brown). Peer has reviewed the literature. He also experimented with cartilage preserved in alcohol, and came to the conclusion that the grafts are tolerated by the host tissue as dead foreign bodies for a period of four months, but that after this time definite absorption occurs. O'Connor and Pierce, Kirkham, however, found that dead preserved cartilage may be tolerated by the host tissue for a long time. This has been confirmed by Brown and co-workers, Dingman, Snyder, Rasi, and others, who prefer bank cartilage (preserved human rib cartilage) over autogenous grafts. The author has not used preserved cartilage, since he could always obtain autogenous material. There is also increasing evidence that autogenous cartilage grows in young patients (Dupertuis, Peer).

In using autogenous cartilage grafts, i.e., from the same patient, the ribs are ordinarily the source of supply. The fused portion, from the seventh to the ninth rib on the right side, may be chosen.

62

SHIFTING OF TISSUE

Technique

A longitudinal incision is made over the right costal margin along the middle of the rectus muscle through skin, subcutaneous tissue, and rectus sheath. The rectus muscle is split and retracted. After exposure of the fused cartilaginous portion of the seventh and eighth ribs, the area to be excised is circumscribed with an incision. With a gauge the graft is removed in a fashion similar to that in woodcarving (Fig. 28), care being taken not to injure the pleura.

If larger pieces or the whole thickness of rib cartilage is needed, the rim of the costal margin is exposed and the posterior surface of the ribs is freed by blunt dissection, care being taken not to injure the arteria mammaria interna, pleura, or peritoneum. The desired portion of graft can now be removed with a knife or a pair of strong scissors from the costal margin. One may use Doyen's rib shears and resect a section of rib cartilage similar to resecting a piece of the bony part of the rib. The

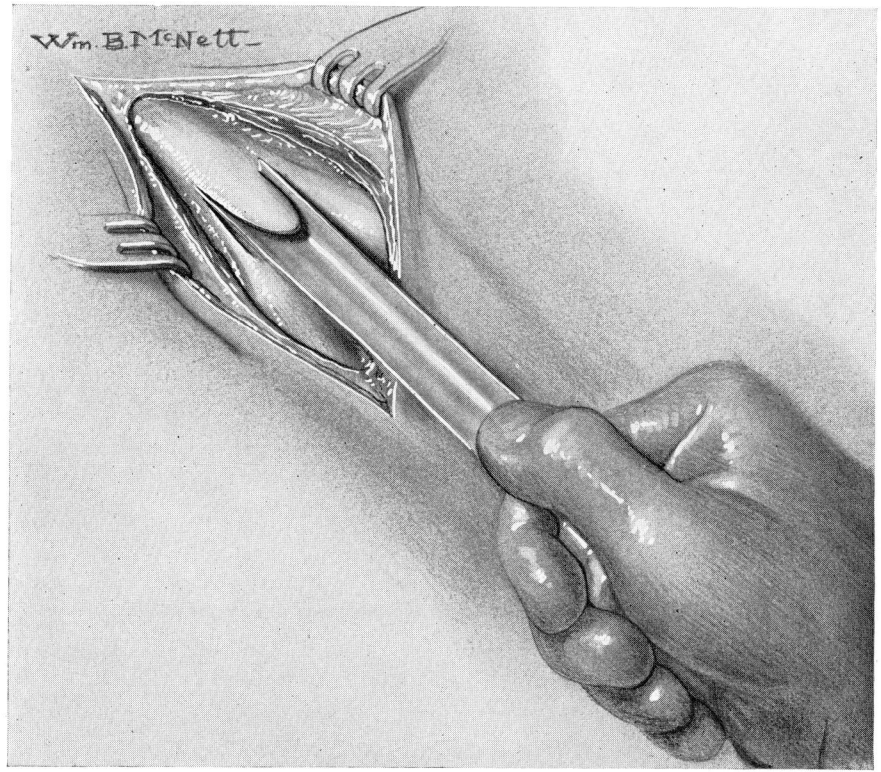

Fig. 28. Removal of cartilage graft. From incision over right costal margin, rectus sheath and muscle are split and retracted. Cartilaginous portion of seventh and eighth rib is exposed and area to be excised is circumscribed with an incision. Graft is removed with a gauge, which is pushed forward with rotary movements.

graft is wrapped in a piece of gauze soaked in warm isotonic saline solution. The donor area is closed after insertion of a drain.

To shape the graft, it is placed on moist gauze and trimmed with a sharp knife to the desired form. If some of the material is left over and a subsequent operation is necessary, it can be stored for further use by inserting it beneath the skin of the abdomen.

For transfer and after-treatment, the reader is referred to special examples (Cases 59, 60, 87, pp. 1070, 1071, 1101).

Gillies noted that if a cartilage graft is carved so that the perichondrium remains along one side only the perichondrium acts as a bowstring, and the graft will curve toward this side. To prevent this he recommended removal of the perichondrium. Yet many grafts continued to warp, as Mowlem and Gibson and Davis could demonstrate. This induced the latter two authors to investigate the cause. They came to the conclusion that in costal cartilage there exists a state of tension; a taut outer layer of cartilage controls the tendency of the main mass to expand. This peripheral layer is the subperichondrial cartilage and not the perichondrium itself. Distortion results from the contraction of the outer layer when the cartilage is carved so that the natural equilibrium is upset. They introduced the "principle of the balanced cross section" in carving a cartilage graft, i.e., to leave in the periphery, the diametrically opposed force equal at all points to balance the cross section as in the use of a complete rib segment or in a graft, in which the layers from two opposite sides have been removed, or from all sides or in which cartilage is removed from the edge only, leaving a D-shaped piece.

Gibson and Davis also call attention to a common misbelief that the ribs forming the costal margin are fused. This, however, is not true in most individuals; the seventh rib articulates with the sternum while the eighth and ninth end freely attached to their neighbors by small interchondral joints at varying distances from the tips. The author is in thorough agreement with this.

Diced Cartilage Grafts

Peer, in repairing defects of the skull and other depressions, used autogenous cartilage grafts cut into many fine squares or cubes. The small grafts are introduced into an exposed depression of the skull, for instance, and gently patted into a rounded contour; the skin of the scalp is sutured over the rounded surface of the cartilage mass. This method has an advantage over the use of large segments of cartilage—the larger grafts, after approximately two months, cause irregularities which may become noticeable and require repair, whereas the diced grafts lend themselves to smoother molding. The small grafts regenerate as well as large grafts. This method is recommended to fill depressions which require firm support, such as of skull, orbital region, and mastoid after extensive mastoidectomy. Limberg of Leningrad injects the diced cartilage into tissue under pressure through a needle of a revolver syringe without tissue dissection. She prefers cadaver costal cartilage preserved by quick refrigeration. Peer also used diced cartilage grafts to form the framework of the auricle in its reconstruction. He made an exact model of the patient's other ear, from which a perforated vitallium mold was made. The mold was filled with diced cartilage grafts and buried beneath the abdominal skin. Connective tissue grew through the perforations. After three months the mold was removed, and the grafts were found bound together in the form of a perfect ear. This method, however, has been largely superseded by other more reliable techniques of forming the cartilaginous framework of an ear (p. 510).

Bank Cartilage (Brown and McDowell)

The material is taken from postmortem examinations in young adults whose blood shows no serological abnormality. The cartilage is removed under sterile technique. Frequent sources are the costal cartilages from the angles of the sixth and seventh ribs. All soft tissue and perichondrium are dissected off.

The cleaned cartilage is placed in a sterile glass jar containing 1:1000 aqueous merthiolate (or 1:1000 merthiolate in isotonic saline solution) and refrigerated at 4° C. for one week with the jar sealed. At the end of this time, a few chips of cartilage are cut off with sterile instruments and cultured. The solution is poured off, replaced with 1:5000 aqueous merthiolate (or 1:5000 merthiolate in isotonic saline solution), and returned to the refrigerator. At the end of the second week, the cartilage is again cultured. If both cultures are negative, the cartilage is ready for use. Cultures are repeated every week, and the cartilage may be used up to one year or possibly longer after removal. If any culture is positive, the whole jar of cartilage is discarded.

Dingman preserves cartilage by irradiation in a cobalt-60 source, so that the cartilage can be stored indefinitely at room temperature. Snyder preserves the grafts in an ethylene oxide gas chamber. Both claim less absorption after transplantation than that evidenced by comparable homografts preserved in merthiosaline.

BONE GRAFTS

Bone grafts are used for healing nonunions, bridging bone defects, and filling other defects in which rigid support is required. The ordinary sources are the anterior surface of the tibia, the crest of the ilium, and, in rarer instances, the median surface of the ilium and a section of the fibula and a rib. Sometimes a sliding bone graft is used, the source of which is the bone from the immediate neighborhood of the defect.

Regenerative Processes

Of all the tissues used for transplantation, none has been more discussed concerning regeneration than bone (May). The consensus is that a bone graft, unlike most other tissue grafts, does not survive after its transplantation; it dies, or at least its osteocytes disappear. The periosteum, however, if the graft transplanted was covered with it, may remain alive. Within a few weeks, vessels grow into the dead graft from the transplanted or host periosteum and from the host bone; these vessels are accompanied by periosteal and endosteal osteoblasts, which transform the dead bone into living bone (Figs. 29, 30). Although the validity of this belief has been questioned ever since Ollier of France first postulated it, it never has been totally disproved (Lexer, Axhausen, Siffert). However, according to recent investigation (Mowlem, Abbott, Ham and Gordon, and others) Ollier's original theory needs modification. It seems that, in a cortical bone graft, the entire graft does not die but parts survive; that in a cancellous graft most of the cells survive if in contact with vascular tissue regardless of whether transplanted on like or unlike tissue, whether transplanted with or without periosteum. Others (Peer et al.) could not verify these latter findings. Another group of investigators (Marchand, Bier, Horwitz, Lacroix) believe that a bone graft is regenerated by immigrating connective tissue cells which undergo differentiation and change into osteoblasts. Recent investigations seem to reconcile both theories. According to Axhausen and others (for reference see Axhausen's most enlightening article), the osteogenetic forces that react first are the specific cells of graft and host bone. Later, however, after about four weeks, a second osteogenetic phase appears which is induced by the unspecific fibrous tissue. Pluripotent mesenchymal cells of the surrounding fibrous tissue change under the influence of resorption of necrotic parts of the graft into osteoblasts and take part in the bone regenerating process. This phase is less intensive than the first and is overshadowed by it. All investigators, however, agree that an autogenous bone graft transplanted on living bone has the best chance of regeneration even if the entire graft should die. (For additional references see articles of May and of Nicoll.) That the bone graft dies and does not become regenerated per se, but from the surrounding osseous regenerative tissue, explains the fact that homogenous and even heterogenous grafting may lead to organic union. Autogenous bone grafts, however, are more reliable and are regenerated more quickly than homogenous grafts (Bürkle de la Camp, Carnesale and Spankus).

A homogenous bone graft has a chance to become regenerated only if it is transplanted upon living bone. When freshly transplanted, some of its cells may survive, but only for a short time. The immediate cellular reaction from the graft bed is considerable, and the ingrowth of vessels and osteogenetic cells from the host bone is sluggish; the process of resorption and transformation of the dead bone into living bone is considerably longer and less complete than in autogenous bone grafts.

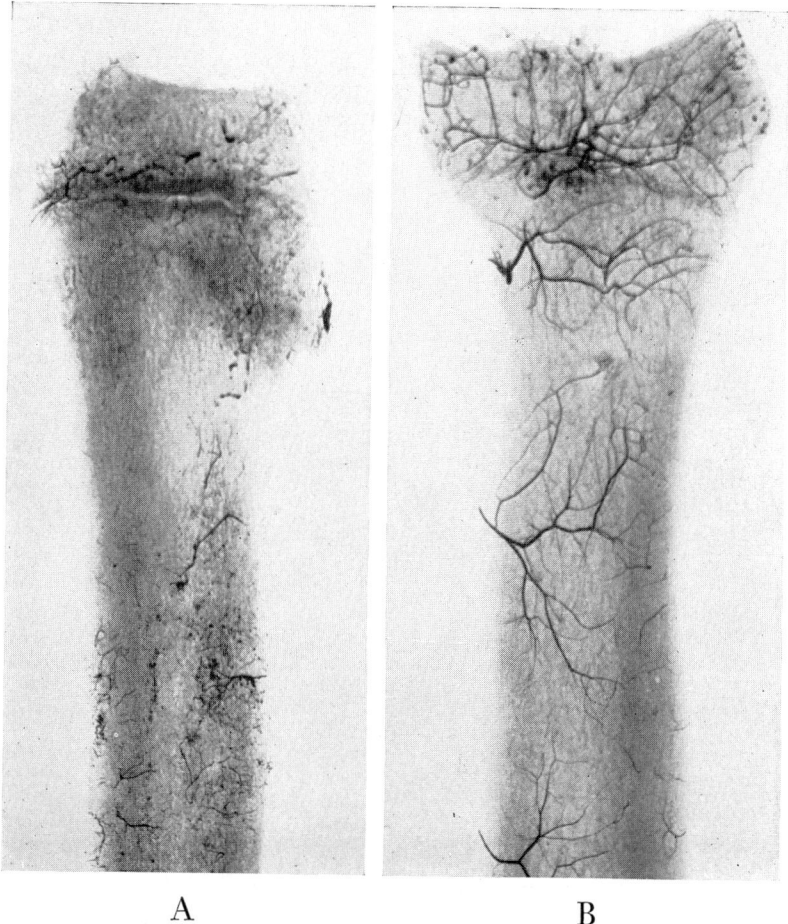

A   B

Fig. 29. Vascularization of bone graft (experimental study by the author in Ann. Surg., 106:441, 1937). *A:* Distal section of reimplanted radius of a dog ten weeks after operation. Vessels have been injected with turpentine-mercury solution through arteria axillaris, periosteum has been removed. Beginning of vascularization and regeneration (compare with Fig. 30). *B:* Another specimen ten months after operation. Complete reestablishment of circulation. Graft is regenerated.

GENERAL PRINCIPLES

There is considerably more reaction and absorption and much less osteogenetic evidence in heterogenous bone grafting. The reason behind the
reaction of the host tissue to a nonautogenous bone graft is that found in
any other homogenous tissue graft—an antibody production (see p. 40).
More fundamental work in this field has been done with skin grafts, and
only recently basic studies of the antigenic components of the bone have

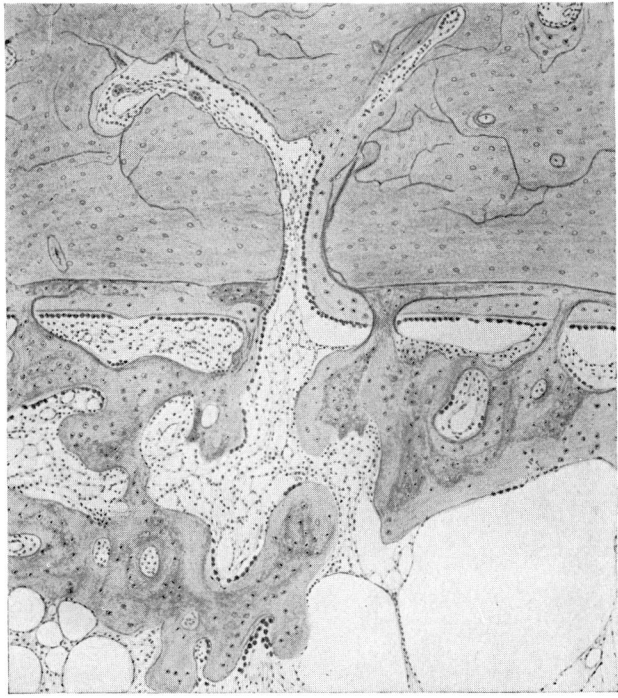

Fig. 30. Histology of bone graft. Section of grafted
bone ten weeks after operation (see Fig. 29, *a*). Cortex
is still dead; lacunae are empty; but trabeculae have been
transformed into living bone tissue by osteoblasts, which,
accompanying the vessels through the haversian canals,
can be seen in their bone-substituting action.

been conducted (Nisbet, Herlap and Zeiss, Burwell and Gowland, Curtis
and Herndon), but to date no practical value has been developed. It is
interesting, however, for practical purposes, that there seems to be no
correlation between osteogenesis and osteocyte survival, which is a little
higher in autografts than in homografts. Indeed, the survival of the osteocytes in a homograft may exacerbate the immunological reaction and
inflammatory response around the graft and so interfere with the repara-

tive osteogenetic activity of the host. This has led to investigation of the practicability of using macerated bone grafts, i.e., grafts from which all antigen causing cells had been destroyed (Orell). The results at first were disappointing, but have been recently improved by better maceration techniques (Maatz, Bauermeister, Bürkle de la Camp).

In conclusion it can safely be stated that the best results in bone grafting may be obtained by using autogenous periosteum- and endosteum-covered grafts; by quick establishment of the interrupted circulation of the graft; and by prolonged complete immobilization (see pp. 780, 781, and Cases 159, 160, 162). The pattern of revascularization of bone grafts has been described in detail, among others, by May and by Stringa, while

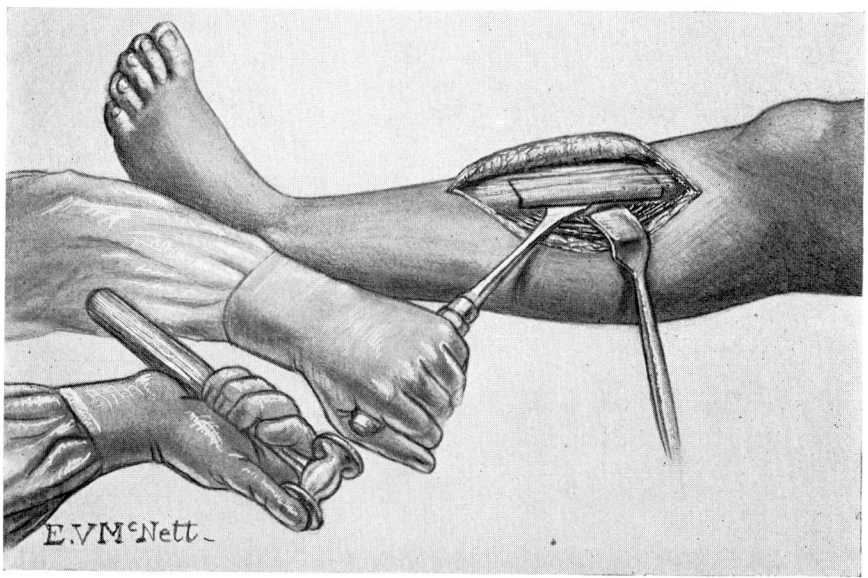

Fig. 31. Removal of bone graft from anterior surface of tibia. Median, proximal, and distal boundaries have been outlined with circular saw. Mobilization of graft is completed from lateral border with chisels.

Trueta in his remarkable investigations described the role of the vessels in relation to osteogenesis of the graft. He confirmed Sr. Arthur Keith's suspicion that the cells which assume a bone-forming role are derived from the endothelium of the capillary system. Hence, the organizer is the osteogenetic vessel from which spring the syncytial frame of cells and the connections on which the bone architecture is established. Thus bone seems to be an organized "soft" tissue of which only part has been made rigid by the deposit of calcium salts.

69

GENERAL PRINCIPLES

Technique

The operation begins with preparation of the host bone. The incision through the skin is curved, so that the subsequent scar will not encroach upon the graft. A tourniquet should not be used. All the bleeding points should be ligated, so that the wound is absolutely dry; otherwise hemorrhage prevents the first adhesions between soft tissue and the periosteum-covered graft. When the bed is exposed, a careful examination for cicatricial tissue is made. It must be completely removed because white, glassy tissue is an obstacle to vascularization. The space in the host bone which receives the graft must be prepared so that the entire surface consists of healthy, bleeding bone and medullary tissue. (For details of the operative procedures, see pp. 778-780.)

Removal of Graft from Tibia: An incision is made along the lateral crest of the tibia. The incision curves mediad, and crosses the anterior surface of the tibia in its lower portion. The skin is separated from the periosteum if the graft is to be transplanted covered with periosteum; otherwise the periosteum is left attached to the skin, and stripped off the bone with a periosteal elevator. The area to be excised is circumscribed with an incision. The graft is excised either with chisels or with a motor-driven saw. The latter has the disadvantage of producing heat; the author uses the saw only to outline the graft, while the actual removal is with chisels and mallet (Fig. 31). The graft is wrapped in saline-soaked gauze for the time being. The donor area is closed. A gauze roll is fitted into the depressed donor area, and a compression dressing is applied. Immobilization may be necessary, depending upon the size of the bone defect.

Removal of Graft from Crest of Ilium: An incision is made along the crest of the ilium commencing just below the spina iliaca, anterior superior. The soft tissues are split on the crest and dissected away from the lateral and median surface of the bone. The graft, consisting of the entire thickness of the crest, is removed with a small (metacarpal) saw or with chisels. During the sawing, the soft tissues are protected by holding them away with wooden boards, similar to those used for stretching the skin to remove split grafts (Fig. 32). A drain is inserted into the wound, which is then closed in layers.

Removal of Graft from Median Surface of Ilium: Grafts from this area were introduced by Pickrell. They are suitable for restoring losses of the skull, depressions of the cheekbone, etc. They are easier to obtain and more adapted in contour and thickness for this particular purpose than grafts from the outer table of the ilium. The median surface of the ilium is exposed from an incision along its crest. The insertions of

70

muscles of the abdominal wall are severed from the superior surface of the chest. They are reflected inwardly, leaving the origins of the muscles arising from the lateral border of the chest undisturbed. Then the musculus iliacus is stripped from the periosteum of the median table. With long, broad retractors, the soft tissues are held mediad. With a V-shaped osteotome, the selected part of the ilium is circumscribed with a groove. The only difficult part is the outlining of the graft in the deep part of the pelvis. I have used for this purpose a motor-driven saw with

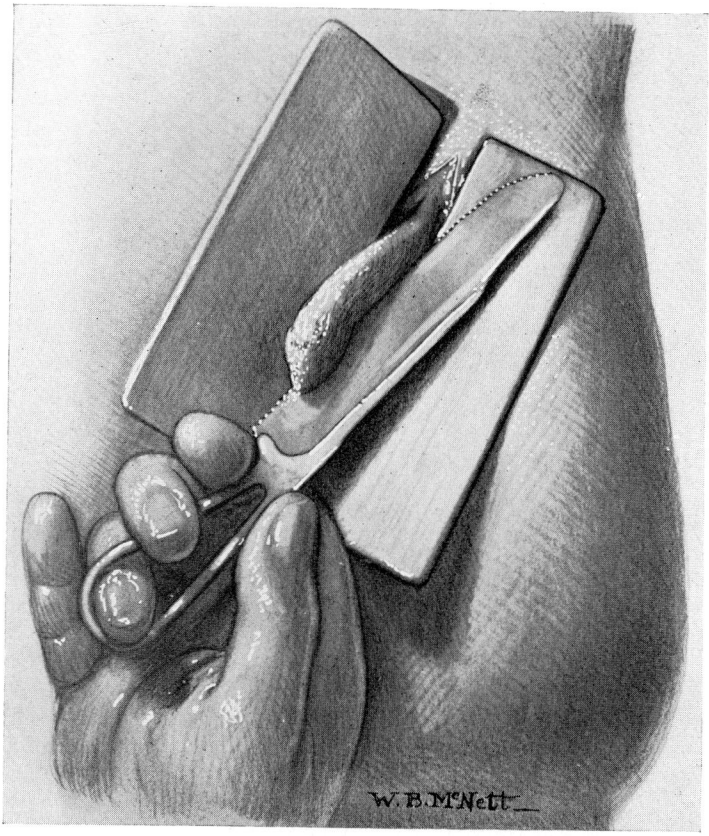

Fig. 32. Removal of bone graft from crest of ilium. From incision along crest, soft tissues are split, dissected from lateral and median surface of bone, and held away with two wooden boards. Graft is removed with hand saw.

a small rotary blade. Oscillating saws, if sufficiently small, would be ideal. The graft is then removed with flat osteotomes, care being taken that the latter do not penetrate too deeply into the pelvic bone. There is considerable oozing from the graft bed, which is temporarily controlled with hot saline compresses. The latter are later replaced with gelfoam. Drains are inserted into the cavity and the wound is closed.

Removal of Graft from Fibula: The fibula is exposed through an incision, as demonstrated in Figures 33 *A, B*. The soft tissues are dissected away from the bone, care being taken not to injure the peroneal artery, which at the median side is in close proximity to the bone. The section of bone to be used is separated either with a costotome or with a Gigli

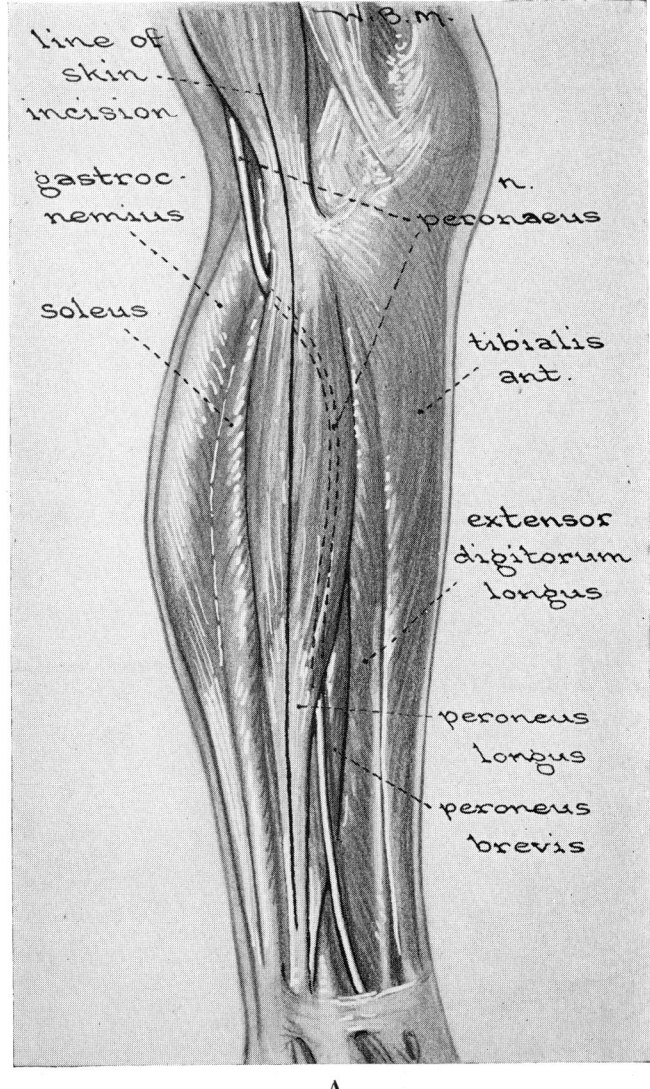

A

Fig. 33. *A:* Approach to fibula (Henry). Skin incision starting 10.2 cm. (4 inches) proximal to head of fibula along biceps tendon, continuing distally over head of fibula toward lateral malleolus.

saw. If the graft is to be used without its periosteum, the latter, together with the soft tissues, is stripped from the bone with Doyen's rib shears similar to those used in rib resection. If the head of the fibula, together with a section of fibula, is to be used, the peroneal nerve must be exposed and carefully held forward while the head of the fibula is detached from its ligaments. The wound is closed after insertion of a drain.

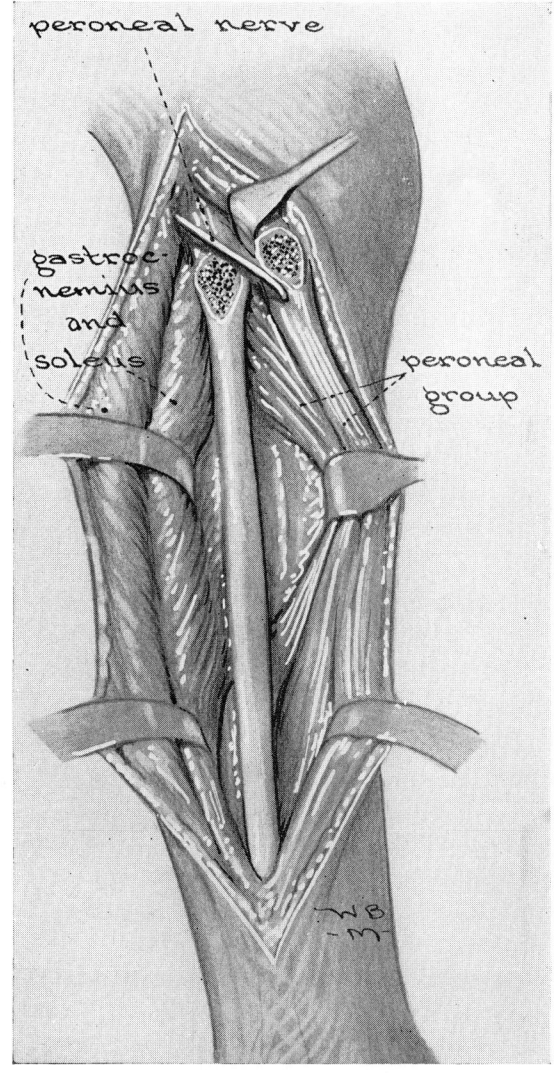

B

Fig. 33. *B:* Exposure of head and shaft of fibula after reflection of peroneal nerve and musculus peroneus longus anteriorly and musculus soleus posteriorly after bony insertion of that portion of the musculus peroneus longus which arises from the lateral surface of the fibula is chiseled off.

GENERAL PRINCIPLES

Removal of Graft from Rib: From an incision along the rib (seventh), the fascia and muscles are split and dissected away from the bone. The lower margin of the rib is freed with a periosteal elevator from all soft tissues, including periosteum, until Doyen's rib shears can be inserted and passed through the rib. The Doyen instrument is pushed forward and backward the proper distance, and the required section of rib is removed with a costotome. Thus, the periosteum of the rib may be left attached to the lateral (outer) surface of the bone but never at its median (inner) surface. The wound is closed in layers.

Removal of Cancellous Bone Chips: Bone chips, consisting of spongiosa bone, regenerate quickly and make a good filling material for dead spaces around a massive graft or in certain kinds of nonunions where the cleft is small, the fragments in good alignment, and the periosteal covering preserved (Matti, Fehr). Spongiosa bone may be available in the tibia after a massive graft has been removed. The spongiosa bone is removed with a medium-sized bone curet. Spongiosa bone may also be obtained from the trochanter region of the femur. The greater trochanter is exposed by a longitudinal incision. A hole is chiseled below its tip and spongiosa bone obtained with the bone curet. The crest of the ilium is the best source. The crest and the inner plate are freed from soft tissue. Below the crest a section of the inner plate of the ilium is removed with the chisel. It consists of a thin cortical layer with cancellous bone attached. If only cancellous bone is needed the cortical part is discarded and more spongiosa can be removed from the defect in the ilium by curettage or with a chisel. The bones are shaved into small pieces, and kept in moist gauze for the time being. The wound is closed in layers after insertion of a drain.

Transfer of Graft: The graft, after it has been made to fit, is transferred to the graft bed and fastened either with stainless steel wires, passed around the bone and graft and twisted, or with vitallium screws which are inserted through holes drilled through graft and host bone (p. 779). The wound is now closed in layers, care being taken that the soft tissues lie closely around the bone. Complete immobilization, including the proximal and distal joint, is necessary.

After-Treatment

The after-treatment is as important as the operation itself, and is carried out according to the course of the regenerative processes, of which three stages can clearly be distinguished: (1) The stage during which the graft is dead. (2) The stage of transformation by substitution of the dead osseous tissue by living tissue. The osseous structure

74

condenses, and the surface becomes smooth. Organic fusion occurs between graft and stump. (3) The stage of functional adaptation in form and increased strength of the graft to its mechanical requirements and surroundings.

From this is derived the important principle of the after-treatment of bone transplantation, i.e., absolute immobilization of the grafted limb during the stage when the graft is dead and being transformed. It is during this stage that the transplant has the least resistance, not only to rough handling but also to minor influences, especially when the latter are ever present. Therefore, fractures or formation of fissures are the consequence of too-early mobilization. If these occur, immobilization must be reapplied immediately. Only after the roentgenogram shows good fusion between stumps and graft can immobilizing dressings be removed and the usual physiotherapy begun.

Bone Bank

The feeling at present among orthopedic surgeons is that a bone bank has a definite place in an institution doing a large amount of elective orthopedic surgery. The reason for the regeneration of homologous bone has been already discussed (p. 66). Bush in this country, Roth and his pupils Betzel and Schilling in Switzerland, and Bürkle de la Camp and Bauermeister in Germany, who are foremost in this field, advise that bank bone (refrigerated homogenous or autogenous bone) should be regarded as a substitute and should not be considered as efficient as the immediate autogenous transplant. Lentz evaluates the usefulness of autogenous, homogenous, and preserved grafts as follows: Any bone graft, even the biologically inferior graft, is a satisfactory transplant as long as it has to supply only a stable framework. Hence, to fill out bone cavities or for use in recent fractures, the homogenous or preserved bone graft should be given priority, since active regenerative participation of the autogenous bone graft is not needed. In other instances—extra-articular arthrodeses, nonunions without actual bone defects—the autogenous bone graft offers the best chance to bring about union, but preserved grafts have been found almost as satisfactory. In all cases, however, in which large bone defects must be bridged and thus part of the graft come to lie within soft tissues, only the autogenous bone graft should be used, since it is biologically superior to any other type. Concerning methods of conservation of bone grafts, the reader is referred to the foregoing references and those of Kawamura, of Carr and Hyatt, and of Bauermeister, and also to the use of denatured macerated bovine bone after Maatz and Bauermeister.

CORNEAL GRAFTS

Attempts to replace opaque or deformed corneas with clear corneal grafts are old. Reisinger (1818), although apparently preceded in the idea by others, is given the credit for having introduced corneal transplantation—or keratoplasty, as he termed it—experimentally. Various authors followed, but results were disappointing until recently. In its March, 1950, issue, the American Journal of Ophthalmology presented an International Symposium on Corneal Surgery, sponsored by the Eye Bank for Sight Restoration, Inc. This brings the status of this fascinating type of surgery up to date. The symposium has been followed by several other publications (Castroviejo, Maumenee, Patan, Thomas, Rycroft et al., and others). Since it is beyond the scope of this book to discuss this special field of surgery, the reader interested in keratoplasty is referred to the publications mentioned.

HETEROGENOUS GRAFTS

Heterogenous grafts are undoubtedly inferior to autogenous grafts since they act as foreign bodies and become encapsulated instead of forming an organic unit with the host tissue. They may at times be superior to homogenous grafts, since they do not cause a rejection reaction resulting in disintegration of the graft, but retain their form and may be tolerated by the host tissue to fulfill their purpose. These two properties are not sufficient to make a heterogenous graft safe for transplantation. Quoting Scales, the "ideal" synthetic prosthesis should (1) not be physically modified by tissue fluids, (2) be chemically inert, (3) not excite an inflammatory or foreign body reaction, (4) be noncarcinogenic, (5) not produce a state of allergy or hypersensitivity, (6) be capable of resisting mechanical strains, (7) be capable of being fabricated in the form required, and (8) be capable of being sterilized. Many synthetic substances have been tried and discarded. Few have proven to be inert and safe. None has ever formed any organic unit with the host tissue. It would not be feasible to go into detail on this subject because of the variety of the materials being used, the discrepancy of opinions, and the many difficulties and challenges still to be overcome. It should be noted, however, that heterogenous grafts have already become an adjunct in reconstructive surgery. The reader is referred to the publications of J. B. Brown and co-workers, Ashley and co-workers, and others. The clinical uses of some of these substances are discussed later in the text.

TRANSPLANTATION OF FLAPS

A flap is a portion of tissue which remains attached by one pedicle (single-pedicle flap) or by two pedicles (double-pedicle flap) to the circulation. Flaps are indicated when skin and subcutaneous tissue need to be replaced. A flap is either simple, consisting of skin and subcutaneous tissue, or compound, consisting of skin, subcutaneous tissue, and bone or cartilage. These flaps may be lined by folding the flap upon itself or by transplanting a skin graft or mucous membrane to that part of the flap which is to replace the lost lining. The viability of every flap depends upon a sufficient arterial and venous circulation, which is supplied through the pedicle. A flap can be taken from the immediate neighborhood of the defect or from distant parts. Flaps taken from the adjoining area have the decided advantage of tissue resemblance and quick healing. Flaps from distant parts may not have this advantage, but—as a rule—have more versatile use.

GENERAL PRINCIPLES

Planning and Mobilization of Flap

There are certain general rules that should be observed in flap transplantation. In selecting the flap, the characteristic features of the skin surrounding the defect should be considered and the donor area chosen to accord in color, texture, and thickness. A flap should be made not longer than twice the width of the pedicle, unless it contains one of the main arteries, whereupon the flap can be made longer and the pedicle narrower. The flap is made one third larger than the defect to counteract immediate and later shrinkage. Normal skin, free of cicatricial tissue, should be selected.

Flap Taken from Immediate Neighborhood: If the flap is to be taken from the immediate neighborhood, the sliding (French method), rotating (Indian method, Carpue), and turnover method are available, and the flap is planned accordingly. The *sliding-flap method* is similar to some of the methods of tissue shifting, and has already been described (p. 17, Fig. 13). The *rotating method* consists of making the flap in such a way that the pedicle borders the defect while the flap itself is some distance from it. To facilitate rotation and lessen the tension in the pedicle, the blind end of the incision should be turned outward (Fig. 34) (Dieffenbach, von Langenbeck) (Cases 1, 44, pp. 988, 1052). In the *turnover method*, the flap is to be hinged around its pedicle to replace a defect of nose or cheek where the skin of the flap is to replace the lining mucous membrane. Covering of the raw outer surface of the flap must be provided for either by skin grafting or by skin sliding (Fig. 78).

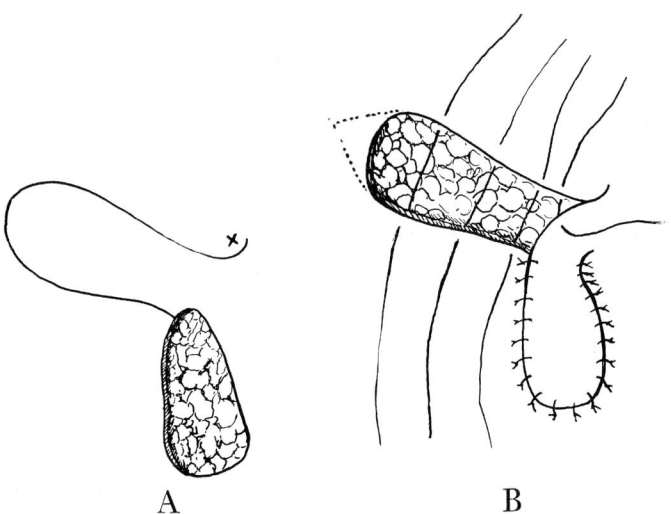

A   B

Fig. 34. *A:* Closure of surface defect by rotating flap taken from immediate neighborhood into defect (Indian method). Pedicle of flap borders defect while flap itself is some distance away from it. To facilitate rotation, blind end of incision (*x*) is turned outward. *B:* Flap is rotated into defect, and donor area is closed by skin sliding.

Flap Taken from Distant Parts: If a flap is to be taken from distant parts (Italian method, Tagliacozzi's method), it should be planned in such a way that it can be transferred by the least number of stages and fastened in a position which will not cause discomfort to the patient.

Pattern Cutting and Outlining: The various flap methods require careful planning and outlining. If possible, the flap should come to lie along the axis of the circulation of the donor area. First, a pattern is made of the defect. The best material for this purpose is chamois, but linen, rubber sheeting, or tinfoil may be used. The pattern is cut one third larger than the defect to make allowance for shrinkage of the flap. The flap is now outlined in reverse to the planned operative steps (Gillies). The method for outlining a tube flap is demonstrated in Figure 40, but is similar for any other type of flap.

In mobilizing the flap, one should cut the flap with equal thickness. This is easy at the scalp and other places where the subcutaneous fat tissue is thin and a firm layer of fascia forms the base. It is difficult in regions with well-developed fat pads.

SHIFTING OF TISSUE

Transfer of Flap

Immediate Transfer: Immediate transfer is understood to mean the mobilization and transplantation of the flap in one stage. It is possible only if the circulation is adequate, that is, if the color of the flap remains normal after the flap is raised. If there is the slightest doubt about the adequacy of the circulation—that is, if the flap becomes cyanotic or pale or its edges are not bleeding—it should be returned to its original site, and transfer should be delayed.

Delayed Transfer: Delayed transfer is understood to mean the mobilization and transplantation of the flap in stages. Mobilization in stages may become necessary to obtain an adequate blood supply. Transplantation in stages may also become necessary because of the distance between the source of the flap and its final site. The following methods of mobilization in stages for developing an adequate blood supply are recommended.

METHOD 1: The flap is raised and returned immediately to its original site (Perthes, Blair) (Case 60, p. 1071). Exact hemostasis is necessary to avoid hematomas beneath the flap. Drains should be avoided if possible. If they are necessary (after mobilization of large flaps), they should be inserted near the base of the pedicle. The author has seen local necrosis where drains were inserted near the periphery. These drains should be attached to an apparatus for continuous suction (McFarlane). The dressing should be free of undue pressure. Moderate pressure, however, is necessary. After the color of the flap has returned to normal and all swelling disappeared (after two or three weeks), the flap is raised again. As a rule, the line of cleavage can easily be found. The flap may be ready for transfer. Should the color of the flap change again, however, transfer should be further delayed.

METHOD 2: Another method of developing an adequate blood supply in the flap consists of raising parts of the flap in successive stages and each time returning the raised parts to the original bed, the stages being ten to fourteen days apart (Case 124, p. 1162).

METHOD 3: Another way of delaying the transfer is by formation of a double-pedicle flap to be converted into a single-pedicle flap. The various stages are described on pages 83-85 for the open double-pedicle flap and on page 87 for the tube flap.

Methods of Transfer: There are two types of transfer: a direct and an indirect. The direct way of transfer is preferred, since it requires fewer stages than the indirect. The *direct* method is possible (1) if a flap by its own length can be transferred to the defect (Fig. 40; Cases 14, 50, pp. 1010, 1060); (2) if the flap and defect can be approximated by favorable posture, whereby the host area is transferred to the flap (Figs. 35, 38) (Cases 120, 122-124, 130-132, pp. 1154, 1158, 1170) or the flap to the host area (Case 13, p. 1008).

GENERAL PRINCIPLES

The *indirect* method of transfer must be chosen whenever defect and flap area cannot be approached directly. It consists of transferring the flap by an intermediate carrier, usually the wrist or forearm (Fig 46) (Case 119, p. 1150), or by successive migration, such as caterpillaring or waltzing.

Fixation and Dressing of Flap

After the flap is transferred and fitted into the defect, it is fastened with sutures, which should not cause tension. Whenever possible, a row of subcutaneous sutures with cotton or catgut should precede the skin sutures. All sutures are interrupted. If a suture causes blanching of the flap edge, it should be loosened or removed.

The dressing should be comfortable and free of undue pressure. Even in places where the dressing is to keep the flap attached to a cavity, like an empty orbit, the pressure should be only moderate. In flaps with long pedicles, the dressing should support the pedicle. The pedicle may be heavy, and may tear the flap from its new position before becoming attached.

Whenever immobilization is needed to hold donor and recipient areas in proper position (flap and defect approximated by favorable posture [Fig. 35]), a plaster cast provides the best fixation. Adhesive strips, as a rule, do not furnish sufficient support. The parts to be immobilized are well padded with layers of cotton. The cast is applied in such a way as to provide sufficient support to keep the flap without tension. Neither the base of the pedicle nor the entire flap should be included in the cast (Fig. 35) (see also Cases 122, 124, 129-130, pp. 1158, 1162, 1168). (For detailed description of arm immobilization and leg immobilization in cross-leg flaps see pp. 720, 808.)

Separation of Pedicle and Final Adjustment of Flap

Unless the flap, together with its pedicle, is to be used for covering the defect, the pedicle must be severed. When a flap can be severed from its pedicle depends entirely upon the extent of surface attachment of flap and host area. Flaps attached only with one edge to the defect will need longer time to gain access to the circulation of the host area than those attached with a broad base. The pedicle may be separated in one stage or in several stages. In either case, however, the circulation must be tested before severance.

Testing Circulation of Flap: A few days before the pedicle is separated, the circulation of the flap should be tested. The circulation, running through the flap in the accustomed way, must be forced to run the reverse way. This is done gradually, and various methods are available.

SHIFTING OF TISSUE

USE OF INTESTINAL CLAMP: With a soft intestinal clamp, the pedicle is compressed daily for several hours. The degree of pressure depends upon the change of color in the flap. To demonstrate the adequacy of the circulation after application of the clamp, the tip of a finger is pressed upon the flap (near the clamp) for a few seconds; this leaves an anemic mark, which—if the circulation is adequate—returns to normal color immediately. If the return to normal color is slow or absent, the pressure

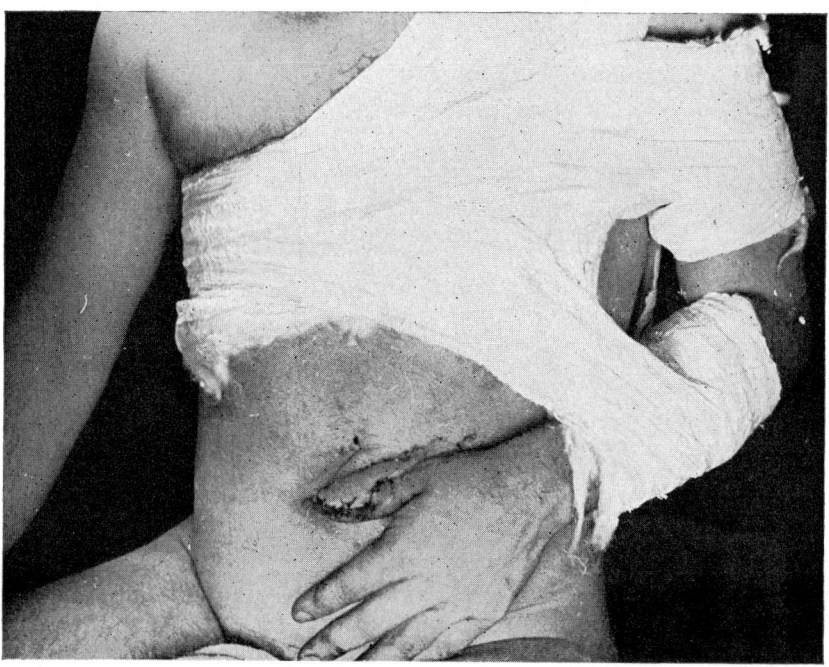

Fig. 35. Abdominal single-pedicle flap covering surface defect of finger. Donor and recipient areas held approximated by plaster cast and figure-of-eight bandage of chest, upper arm, and forearm.

of the clamp must be lessened. When the flap has finally reached a stage where complete interruption of its blood supply by the clamp does not cause change of color, the flap is severed from its pedicle.

USE OF LABORATORY CLAMP: Another method is the application and gradual tightening of an ordinary laboratory clamp, as discussed on pages 84-85. The author prefers this method.

Final Steps: After the flap is severed from its pedicle, the pedicle is returned to its original site and adjusted in place. The flap itself, however, should be left alone for a few days, until all edema has subsided. The granulation of scar tissue of its free edge, as well as of the defect's edge, is then excised and the flap sutured in place.

OPEN PEDICLE FLAPS

The open pedicle flap, as distinguished from the tube flap, can be used whenever a direct approach of flap and defect area can be accomplished, no matter whether the flap is transferred to the defect or the defect to the flap, unless the space between defect area and base of flap is wide. If this is the case, much of the raw undersurface of the flap would come to lie upon normal tissue and constitute a source of drainage, maceration, and infection. In such a case, the flap should be tubed primarily (p. 87), or its pedicle should be tubed after transfer of the flap. The open flap should never be used if the flap must be transferred by a carrier such as the wrist, or if it needs one or more intermediate attachments before reaching the defect.

Open Single-Pedicle Flaps

Two types of single-pedicle flaps are distinguished: one which is made primarily a *single-pedicle* flap; the other a *double-pedicle* flap at first, gradually transformed into a single-pedicle flap.

Primary Single-Pedicle Flap
The rules of formation and transfer of a primary single-pedicle flap are similar to those already mentioned (the reader is referred to pp. 77-79). Mobilization and immediate transfer should be performed only if there is definite assurance of an adequate blood supply within the flap. This is usually the case when the flap is not longer than twice the width of its pedicle, unless it contains one of the major arteries whereupon it can be made longer and the pedicle narrower (Case 1, p. 988). If there is the slightest doubt about the circulation, transfer should be delayed. The most extreme example of a primary single-pedicle flap is the artery, or island, flap devised by Monks, Horsley, and Esser. Monks, in making a new lower eyelid, used a small crescentic piece of scalp which remained attached to the circulation by a long narrow pedicle, consisting of the subcutaneous tissue and the anterior branch of the arteria temporalis and vena temporalis. Near the base of the pedicle the skin was tunneled to the defect, the arterial flap drawn through the tunnel, and the flap sutured in place. The same procedure can be used in other regions where main arteries running in the subcutaneous tissue can be dissected free (p. 475, Converse and Wood-Smith, p. 382, Goumain and Fevrier, p. 382, Barron and Emmett, p. 382, Littler and Tubiana, p. 804).

SHIFTING OF TISSUE

Double-Pedicle Flap Transformed into Single-Pedicle Flap

A double-pedicle flap converted into a single-pedicle flap is constructed for developing adequate circulation in the flap, i.e., when the flap must be made longer than twice the width of its pedicle. The method dates back to Tagliacozzi, who used the double-pedicle flap from the arm to reconstruct noses. According to him, the flap was outlined on the arm, and a longitudinal incision was made on each side, leaving a proximal and a distal pedicle attached. The skin and subcutaneous tissue between the incisions were raised, and a piece of linen was passed between skin and underlying fascia. In another stage the proximal pedicle was severed; thus, the flap was converted into a single-pedicle flap, the flap then being ready to be transplanted.

The advantage of the double-pedicle principle is apparent. Hence, the double-pedicle flap to be converted into a single-pedicle flap has become a popular method of flap transplantation; the passing of linen beneath the flap, however, has been replaced by more aseptic methods, as described below.

Procedure: In this method, the flap is raised, as in the original method of Tagliacozzi, between two parallel incisions, and is left attached at the two pedicles; the flap is thus deprived of all blood supply except for that furnished by the long anastomoses. The pedicle which is to become the peripheral end of the flap is clamped (Fig. 36 and 37 depict types of clamps). If the color of the flap does not change, this pedicle can be severed and the flap transferred immediately. If the color changes, transfer should be delayed to improve the circulation. Drains attached to a continuous suction apparatus should be inserted beneath larger flaps after their return to the flap bed.

The flap is raised again between the parallel incisions after all edema has subsided. To improve the circulation further and to test it, the author has advised the following method: The peripheral pedicle is narrowed by incising it from each side for one third of its distance, leaving the middle third preserved. A laboratory clamp (as depicted in Fig. 36 B for narrow pedicles and in Fig. 37 for broad pedicles) is now attached to the middle third, and all wound edges are sutured together (Broadbent et al. and Oakey modified the ordinary clamp type). On the following day, gradual crushing of the narrowed pedicle is begun by tightening the clamp.

After each tightening, the adequacy of the circulation is tested in the following way: The tip of the finger is pressed upon the flap near the clamp for a few seconds. This leaves an anemic mark, which—if the circulation is adequate—returns to normal immediately. If the return to normal color is slow or absent, the pressure of the clamp is lessened by turning the thumbscrew the reverse way. If the crushing causes pain, a few cubic

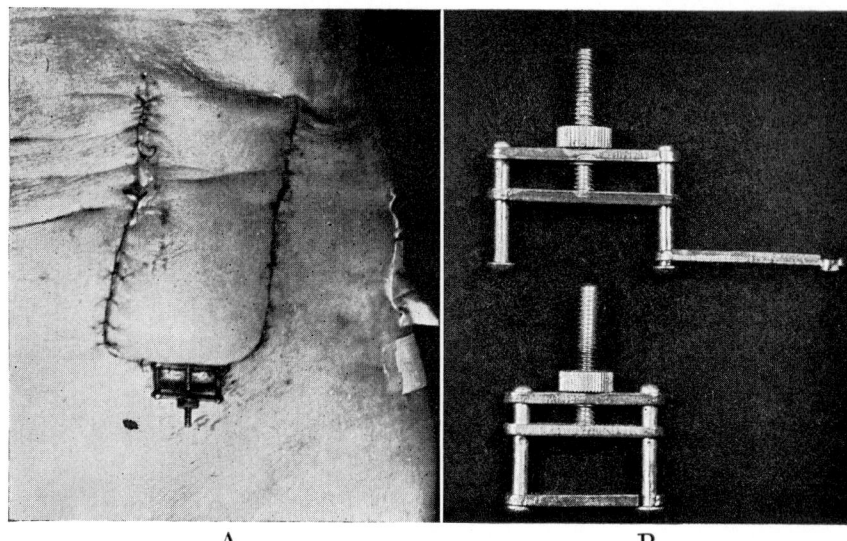

A   B

Fig. 36. *A:* Open double-pedicle flap at abdomen gradually to be converted into single-pedicle flap (see text). Flap was raised between two longitudinal incisions and immediately returned to its original site. Three weeks later, flap was again raised; distal pedicle was incised on each side for one third of its distance, leaving middle third untouched. Laboratory clamp was attached to middle bridge and all wound edges sutured together. Within next few days, blood supply through middle bridge was gradually interrupted by tightening clamp. *B:* Type of laboratory clamp. Closed on all sides with lower crossbar, which is rotatable. (H. May: Surgery.)

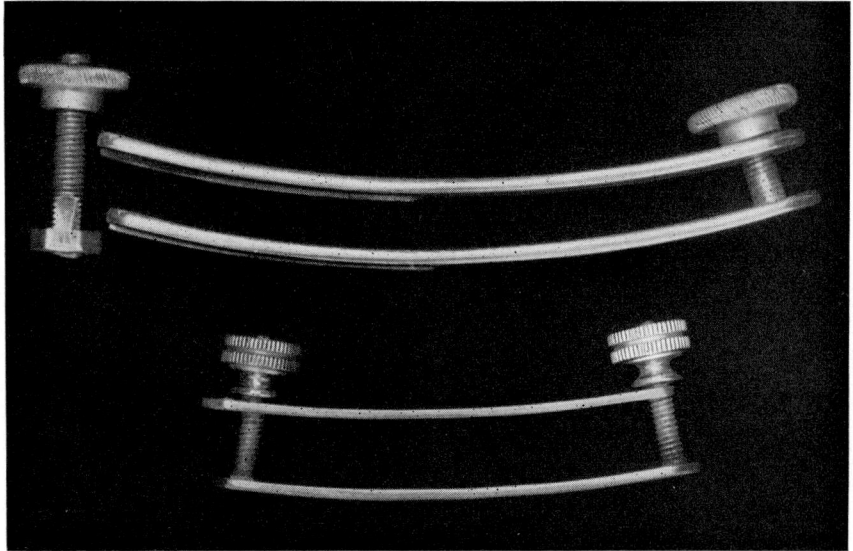

Fig. 37. Clamps for crushing broad pedicles of flaps (compare with Fig. 36*B*).

centimeters of procaine should be injected into the pedicle. Pain can also be avoided by tightening the clamp only slightly but several times daily; this, as a matter of fact, is the recommended procedure. After the pedicle is crushed completely, the clamp can be removed and the flap may be ready for transfer unless the crushing has caused edema. If this is the case, transfer should be delayed until all edema has subsided.

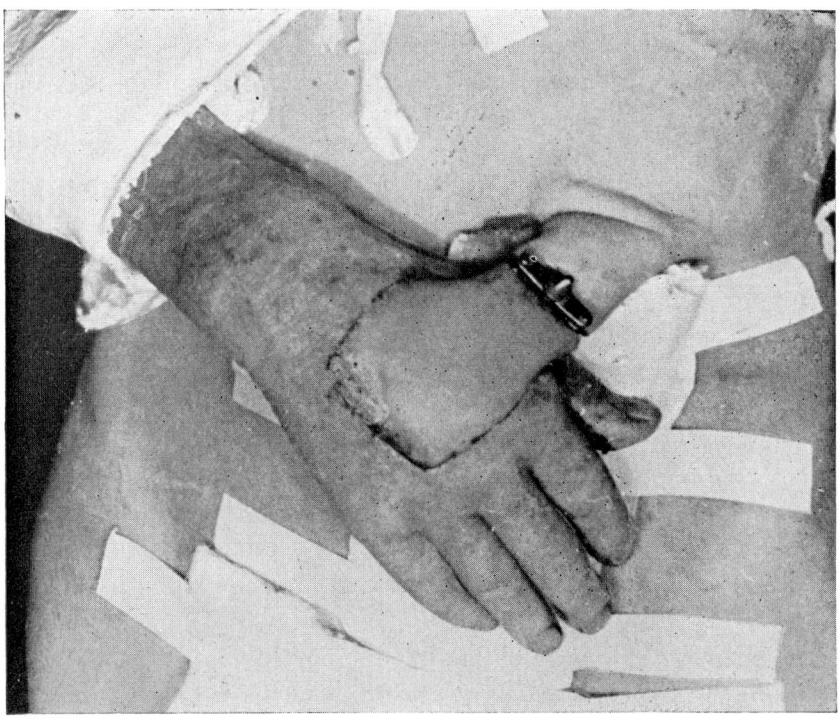

Fig. 38. Separation of pedicle of flap, gradually performed by application and tightening of laboratory clamp.

As a matter of fact, in some instances where the circulation is particularly poor, another raising and returning of the flap—the flap now being a single-pedicle flap—may be advisable (Case 13, p. 1008). In selected cases, one may wish to cover the raw donor area beneath the flap with a skin graft after the second (or the third) time it has been raised (see Case 99, p. 1114) or one may wait with this until the flap is raised for the final transfer (Cases 123, 124, 126, pp. 1160, 1162, 1164).

TRANSFER AND FINAL SEPARATION OF FLAP: For transfer and final separation of the flap from its pedicle, the reader is referred to page 80. As to the method of separation, the author prefers the gradual crushing of the pedicle with a laboratory clamp (Fig. 38). The flap is adjusted in place after a few days.

OPEN DOUBLE-PEDICLE FLAPS

The open double-pedicle flap is used as a pocket, or gauntlet, flap for repair of certain defects of hand or arm (Fig. 39), or as a visor flap, which is a forehead flap pedicled in both temporal regions and brought down to cover defects of face and lips. This flap, being attached by two pedicles, has an excellent blood supply, and hence can be cut thin and transplanted immediately.

Procedure

The flap is raised and, if possible, the flap bed closed immediately by undermining the wound edges and skin sliding. To refer to an example, the injured finger, with its injured dorsum (Fig. 39), is placed beneath the flap of the abdominal wall. The wound edges of the flap are sutured to the wound edges of the defect. The proximal pedicle of the flap is severed and adjusted in place after seven days. The distal pedicle is grad-

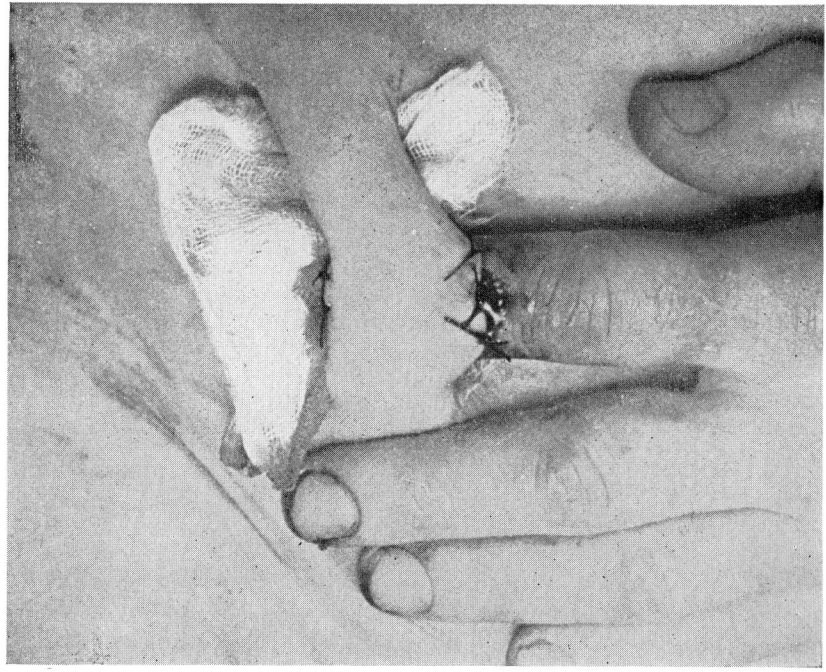

Fig. 39. Open abdominal double-pedicle flap (pocket flap) covering surface defect of dorsum of left index finger.

ually severed after ten days by the laboratory-clamp method (Fig. 38) followed by adjustment of this end of the flap and the raw areas of the abdomen a few days later.

The pocket flap is excellent for small defects (Fig. 39; Cases 127, 131, pp. 1166, 1172). In large defects it has many drawbacks. In large flaps, the tremendous raw surface of the flap bed causes a great deal of drainage, and is a constant source of infection. Primary closure of the donor area by skin shifting or skin grafting has been unsuccessful in the author's hands. Hence, a large pocket flap should rarely be used, but may be indicated for large transverse defects comprising either the entire dorsum or the volar surface of hand or arm (see Case 132, p. 1174). For dorsal defects it is taken from the same or opposite side of the abdomen and lower chest; for volar defects, from the back or, less often, the median side of the thigh of the same side. In all cases in which only a part of the dorsal or volar surface is denuded, a pocket flap is contraindicated, since large parts of the flap—namely, those lying on the uninjured skin of the hand—are not needed. They also add a source of irritation and possible infection to the large raw surface of the donor wound. In those cases, the open single-pedicle flap, as described previously (p. 82), should be chosen in spite of the longer time needed for its preparation and transfer (Case 130, p. 1170).

TUBE FLAPS

The tube flap is a closed-flap method. Hence, danger of infection and of scarring is minimized. It is formed like an open double-pedicle flap at first. It is converted into a closed flap by inverting and suturing the flap edges together. The donor area is closed beneath the flap by skin sliding or skin grafting. This type of flap was devised by Filatow, of Odessa, and Gillies, of London, independently in the same year (1917) (the historical background is well described by Barsky). Gillies, however, deserves the credit for having popularized the method. Schuchardt of Hamburg has published a noteworthy, well-illustrated monograph on this subject.

Indications

A tube flap is indicated whenever the open-pedicle flap is contraindicated (see p. 82); that is, whenever—in using a direct transfer of the flap—defect and base of flap are some distance away from each other, and whenever indirect transfer or successive migration is necessary to convey the flap to the defect.

87

GENERAL PRINCIPLES

Planning and General Principles

As in any other method of flap transplantation, the flap should be carefully planned and outlined. It should be cut so that its long axis comes to lie in the longitudinal direction of the circulation of the donor area. Therefore, as a rule, it would seem inadvisable to extend the flap across the midline of the body, although no harm may result from doing this, as others and the author have found. In long abdominal flaps it is, however, safer to wait for one week before extending the flap across the midline when additional length is required. As a rule, a flap should not

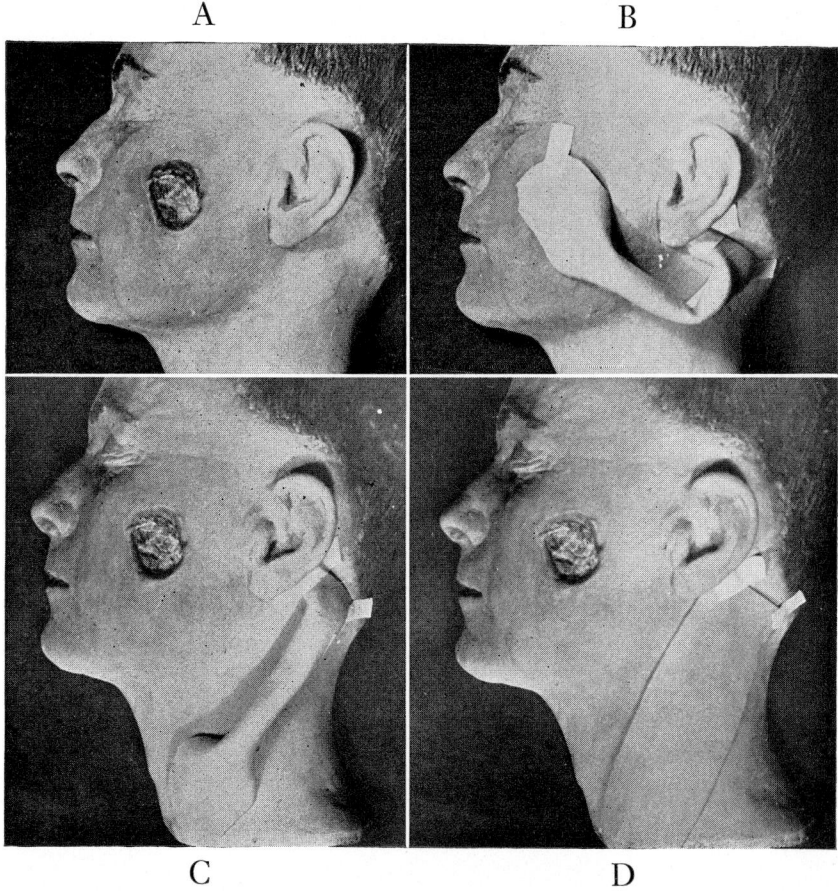

Fig. 40. *A:* Planning a tube flap to be transplanted from left cervical region to left cheek. Method is demonstrated on cast made of patient with cancer of cheek. Various stages are reversed to those of actual transplantation. *B:* Piece of chamois skin is cut and tubed to cover defect and anchored in left mastoid region. *C:* Chamois tube is transferred to left cervical region. *D:* Tube is opened and spread flat.

be more than 20.3 cm. (8 inches) long and from 5 to 6.3 cm. (2 to 2½ inches) wide. In a vascular area and with lean patients, however, flaps can be made longer and narrower. The planning and outlining of the flap is by pattern, and is done best in reverse to the actual operative steps (Gillies), as demonstrated in Figure 40. The flap is outlined along the pattern with an aniline dye. To facilitate later approximation of corresponding flap edges

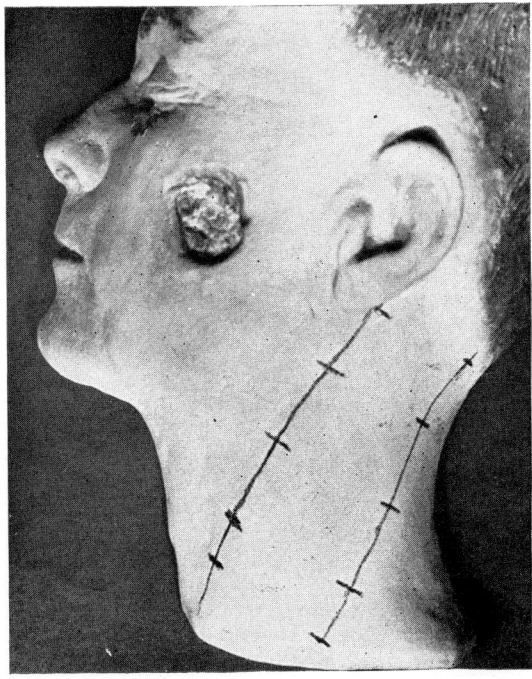

E

Fig. 40. *E:* Width and length of flap is outlined on skin, and cardinal points of approximation of wound and flap edges are marked.

as well as those of the wound edges of the defect, flap and wound edges are marked on each side in equal distance either by scratching the skin or by the intracutaneous injection of a drop of one of the aniline dyes (see Figs. 40 E, 41).

Mobilization of Flap

The skin and subcutaneous tissue are separated with two parallel incisions along the lines previously drawn on the skin (Fig. 41). The depth of the incision depends upon the thickness of tissue needed for covering the defect. As a rule, it reaches the deep fascia, and the flap includes the tissue between the deep fascia and the skin. If a shallow defect is to be covered, less subcutaneous tissue is needed, but it is inadvisable to make the flap too thin. On the other hand, if a thicker flap is needed, the flap should not be made too thick, since it may prevent closure of the tube.

89

GENERAL PRINCIPLES

The skin and subcutaneous tissue are undermined between the two parallel incisions. After thorough hemostasis, the flap is now raised with a strip of gauze.

Closure of Flap Bed

The next step consists of wide undermining of the adjoining donor area to close the bed of the flap. After thorough hemostasis, with the flap held away by means of a strip of gauze, the skin edges of the mobilized

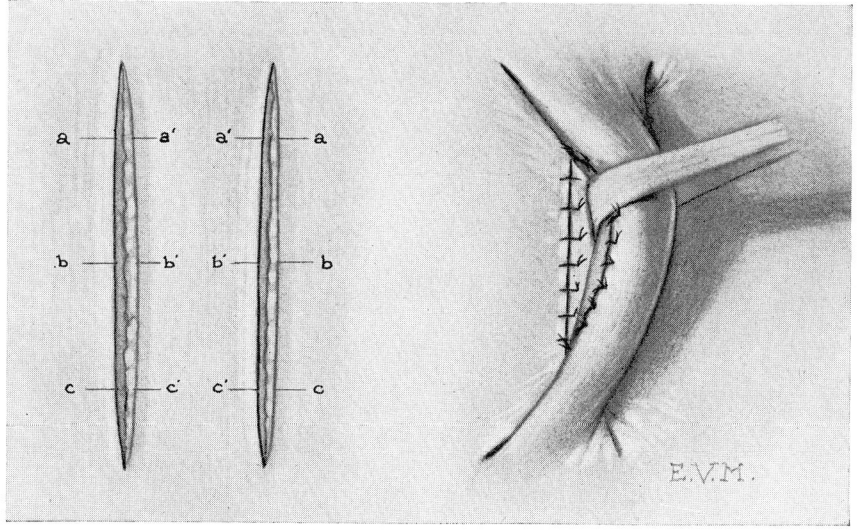

Fig. 41. Construction of tube flap. *Left:* The flap, previously outlined and marked at cardinal points for later approximation of corresponding edges (Fig. 40 E), is incised along its longitudinal edges. Skin and subcutaneous tissue between the two parallel incisions are undermined. *Right:* Flap edges have been inverted and cardinal points (a'-a', b'-b', c'-c') sutured first, followed by closure of remainder of flap. Flap bed has been closed by undermining wound edges adjoining donor area and skin sliding with proper approximation of cardinal points (a-a, b-b, c-c).

area are pulled together beneath the flap and fastened with sutures. First sutures are subcutaneous sutures, followed by skin sutures (on-end mattress sutures) through the marks previously scratched on the skin (Fig. 41). The following sutures (simple interrupted sutures) close the remainder of the wound. If the flap bed cannot be closed by simple skin sliding, the flap bed should be skin grafted.

Formation of Tube

The next step consists of tubing the flap. The skin edges of the flap are inverted and sewn together with simple interrupted silk sutures.

90

The first sutures approximate the marks previously scratched on the skin (Fig. 41). The sutures are placed close to the skin margins. They are left long to facilitate suturing the remainder of the flap edges. There should be no tension along the suture line. If there is tension, too much subcutaneous tissue has been included in the flap, and must be removed with scissors until the flap edges meet with ease.

After the last sutures have been placed, one will notice a triangular raw surface at each end of the flap and likewise at each end of the donor area opposite the raw surfaces of the tube. Gillies closes these areas as

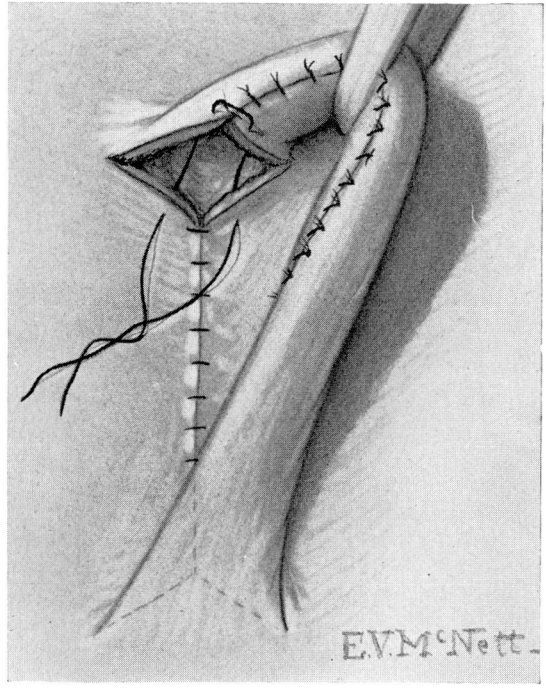

Fig. 42. Closure of triangular raw surface at end of tube flap and flap bed by insertion of mattress suture (Gillies).

demonstrated in Figure 42. To eliminate these small raw areas, Davis and Kitlowski stagger the parallel incisions. The ends of the parallel incisions, instead of being exactly opposite each other, are placed so that at one pedicle end of the proposed flap one of the lines extends from 3 to 4 cm. (1¾₁₆ to 1⅝ inches) or more beyond the point where the flap is to terminate, and conversely at the other pedicle end (Fig. 43).

Dressing and Postoperative Treatment of Flap

Several layers of bismuth tribromophenate (xeroform) gauze are placed beneath the tube on the suture line of the flap bed; the ends of the gauze are cut longitudinally in half to be wrapped around the pedicles of the tube. If the flap bed was skin grafted, a proper pressure dressing must be applied beneath the tube. The dressing, however, should not be so thick as to cause stretching of the overlying flap. Long rolls of gauze

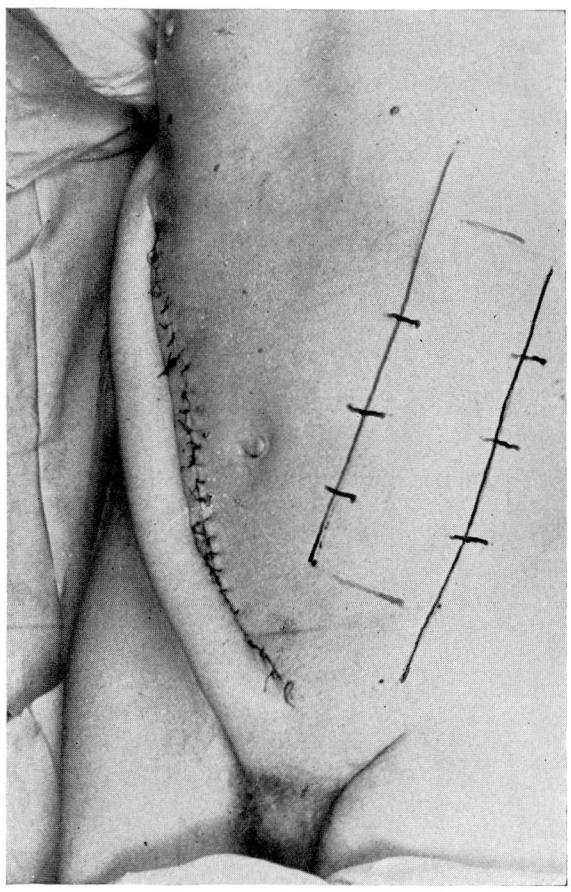

Fig. 43. Demonstration of avoiding raw areas at end of tube flap and flap bed by staggering parallel incisions (Davis and Kitlowski) (compare with Fig. 42). Tube flap on patient's right side had been outlined as depicted on his left side. Ends of parallel incisions are so placed at each pedicle end of proposed flap that one of the lines extends somewhat beyond point where flap is to terminate (Case 119, p. 1150).

somewhat longer and thicker than the flap are now placed along each side of the flap, and held in place with adhesive strips (Fig. 44). A dressing pad is placed over the whole area. The flap should be inspected frequently for possible hematomas or edema, which may interfere with the flap's circulation. If this is the case, the hematoma should be emptied

92

or the edema relieved by removing some of the sutures. The sutures of the flap are usually removed seven or eight days after the operation, as are the simple sutures of the donor area; the on-end mattress sutures of the donor area should remain longer in place.

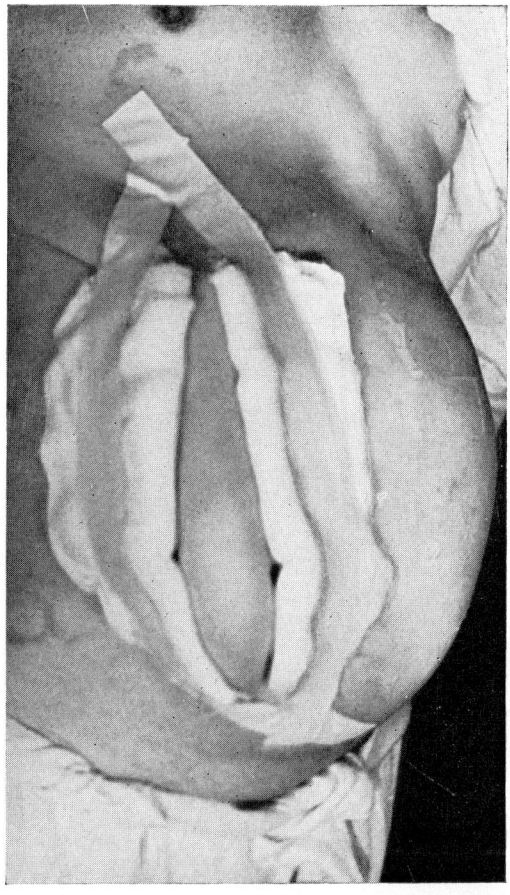

Fig. 44. Dressing of tube flap. Long rolls of gauze, thicker and longer than the flap, are placed along each side of flap and fastened with adhesive strips. A dressing pad is then placed over entire area.

Separation of Pedicle

The next step consists of separating the one pedicle which is to become the peripheral end of the flap. Although German, Finesilver, and Davis, in an experimental study, found the establishment of an adequate blood supply from a single pedicle within seven days, the vascular pattern in a tube flap becomes established much later, according to Braith-

93

waite et al. Hence, the separation of the pedicle, as a rule, should not be performed earlier than three weeks after the operation. In very long flaps, several months may be required before the separation. The blood supply is gradually interrupted by application and gradual tightening of an ordinary laboratory clamp on the pedicle (May) (Fig. 45). Before applying the clamp, it is advisable to incise the skin at this particular site to prevent slipping of the clamp and to lessen the pain and also to inject

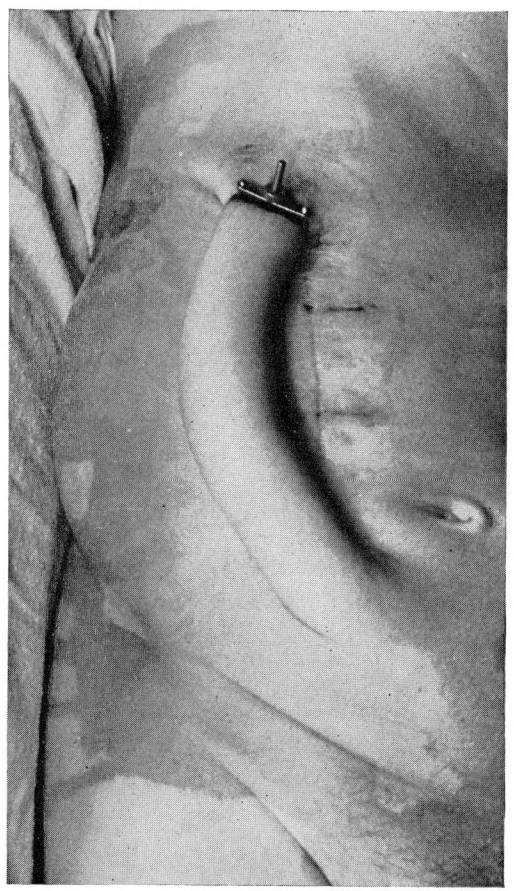

Fig. 45. Separation of proximal pedicle of tube flap by application and gradual tightening of laboratory clamp.

a few cubic centimeters of procaine before each tightening. After each tightening, the circulation is tested as previously described (p. 83). Other clinical, as well as chemical, tests are available (Conway et al. and others). The author, however, has found the clamp method both simple and versatile. Finally, the pedicle is severed, but the flap should not be transplanted immediately. One should wait until all edema has subsided, or until the circulation in the flap has become more adjusted to reversed conditions.

Transfer of Tube Flap

The flap is now ready for transfer. This can be done directly or indirectly.

Direct Transfer: Direct transfer is possible if (1) the flap by its own length can be transferred to the defect (Cases 6, 14, 59, pp. 996, 1010, 1070) or (2) if the flap and defect can be approximated by favorable posture (Case 45, p. 1054). The peripheral end of the flap is then opened along the seam, that is, along the scar where the skin edges were brought together. The cicatricial wound edges, including the scar running to the center of the tube, may need excision. The flap is then unfolded. If it is too thick, some of the fat tissue must be removed; care should be taken not to injure the longitudinal branches of the larger vessels. The flap is now shaped and fitted into the defect. With a few subcutaneous cotton sutures, the base of the flap is anchored to the base of the host tissue. This is the first important step. It is followed by approximation of the edges of flap and defect with subcutaneous cotton sutures and with nylon sutures for the skin. There should be no kinking or tension of the flap. Proper fixation with adhesive strips or plaster of paris may be necessary to avoid tension (Case 45, p. 1054).

Indirect Transfer: Indirect transfer becomes necessary if, owing to long distance between donor and host areas, a direct transfer of the flap is not possible. The flap is transferred by an intermediate carrier, usually the wrist or forearm (Case 119, p. 1150). To avoid too much scarring at the arm, a trapdoor-like flap is formed, which is attached to the tube pedicle (Fig. 46). After establishment of an adequate circulation between intermediate carrier and flap, the other pedicle is severed and the flap transported by way of the arm to the defect. Another way of successive migration is by caterpillaring or waltzing: One pedicle is severed and attached to an area near the other pedicle, or it is swung around toward the defect and implanted; subsequently, the other pedicle is severed and transferred in the same manner until the defect is reached. It is obvious that caterpillaring or waltzing is possible only if the flap is long enough to avoid torsion.

Separation and Adjustment of Flap

Unless the flap, together with its pedicle, is to be used for transplantation, the flap must be separated from its pedicle. Between seven and twenty-one days, depending upon the extent of surface attachment of flap and host area, the flap is gradually severed from its pedicle with the laboratory-clamp technique. The pedicle is now removed from its base with a V-shaped excision and the resulting defect closed by suturing the wound edges together. The suturing of the flap into the defect, however, should be delayed for a few days after adjustment of the flap's reversed circulation. It should be particularly delayed if parts or the entire pedicle are left attached to the flap and are to be used for covering the defect.

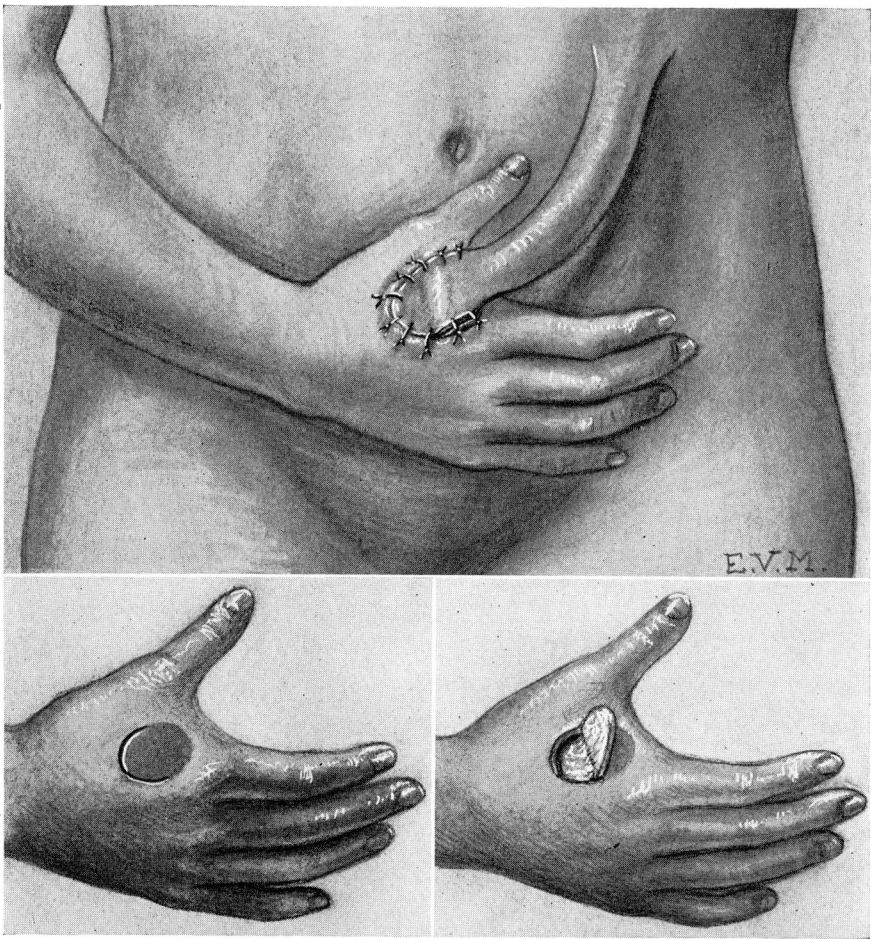

Fig. 46. Successive migration of tube flap by using hand as intermediate carrier. End of pedicle is made oblique. Oblique raw area is pressed upon proposed area of fixation, outlining an oval imprint (*lower row, left*). One half of oval imprint is incised and raised, forming trapdoor-like flap (*lower row, right*). Raw area thus created on hand corresponds in size to that of pedicle. Pedicle is sutured to trapdoor flap and its base. Later, when flap is severed, trapdoor flap is reflected to its original site.

96

In such a case, after a few days or weeks, depending upon the length of the remaining tube, the tube is incised along its scar (seam); the tube is opened and spread out flat to fit into the defect. (For the use of tube flaps, see Cases 45, p. 1054; 116, p. 1146; 119, p. 1150.)

THE PARTLY TUBED FLAP

In this type of flap, the peripheral end—that is, the part of the flap which is to be utilized for covering the defect—remains untubed, and is returned to its original site and sutured in place. After about three weeks

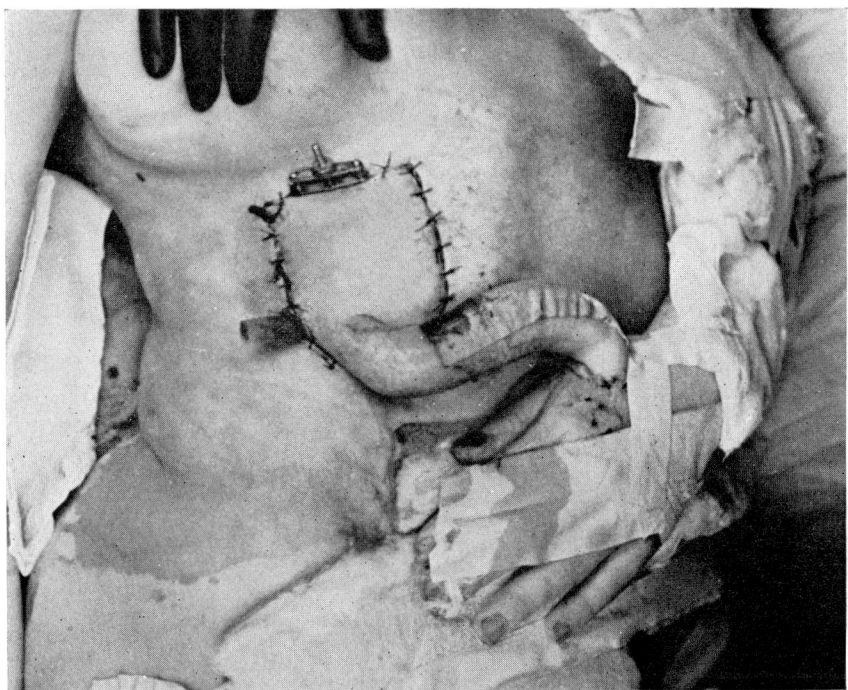

Fig. 47. Partly tubed flap. Peripheral end in stage of gradually being severed. Untubed part has been raised with exception of middle bridge to which laboratory clamp is applied. Raised part has been returned and sutured. Middle bridge is gradually crushed by tightening clamp.

the untubed part is raised again and its peripheral attachment (peripheral pedicle) narrowed from both sides by incisions; a laboratory clamp is attached to the middle bridge (Fig. 47; Case 14, p. 1010). All wound edges are then sutured together. The circulation is now interrupted by gradual tightening of the clamp, as already described. After the middle bridge has been crushed completely, the flap may be ready for transfer after all edema has subsided.

97

GENERAL PRINCIPLES

The advantage of leaving the peripheral pedicle untubed is that it shrinks less than when tubed. It is a well-known fact that the tissues which are included in a tube shrink transversely, so that the full original width cannot be obtained after the tube is spread out flat; furthermore, when a flap has to be lined, it can more easily be folded upon itself, if such is the plan (Case 14, p. 1010). When skin grafts are to be used for lining, the lining can be more conveniently attached to the raw surface of the flap than would be the case if the entire flap were tubed and had to be opened. The skin graft should be applied at the time the untubed part is raised and the laboratory clamp applied. The donor area may be skin grafted at the same time. After the skin-grafted pedicle is sutured back in place, it acts as a pressure dressing.

THE THORACOEPIGASTRIC TUBE FLAP

Blood Supply

The longest and widest flap which can safely be formed is from the thoracoepigastric region, reaching from the axilla to the ligamentum inguinale (Webster) (Figs. 43, 48; Case 119, p. 1150). This region has an abundant blood supply. The largest and longest arteries of the body that course outside the deep fascia to supply the skin and subcutaneous tissue start at each end of this region and approach its middle portion (above: the arteria thoracalis lateralis and suprema; below: the arteria epigastrica superficialis and inferior and arteria circumflexa ilium superficialis). Furthermore, the longest, largest, and most superficial cutaneous veins of all available donor areas are located in the thoracoepigastric region. The course of the vena thoracoepigastrica is visible through the skin in many persons, or can be made visible by washing the area with alcohol.

Procedure

The course of the vena thoracoepigastrica should be marked with one of the aniline dyes. Using this line as the longitudinal center line, the width of the flap as previously determined (8 to 10 cm. [$3\frac{3}{16}$ to $3\frac{15}{16}$ inches] in adults) is marked out on each side of it, as described previously (Fig. 41). The two parallel incisions are then made, and the flap is raised between the superficial and deep layers of the deep fascia. After thorough hemostasis, the tube is formed in the usual way. If there is excess of fat tissue extending beyond the skin edges, it is trimmed away to facilitate closure. The secondary defect is now closed by wide and extensive undermining of the skin, subcutaneous tissue, and superficial layer of the deep fascia on each side of the defect and by suturing first the superficial layer of the deep fascia and then the skin edges, or by skin grafting.

98

SHIFTING OF TISSUE

Dressings and Postoperative Treatment

Dressings and postoperative treatment are the same as previously described (p. 91). The time interval, however, between formation of the tube and separation of one of its pedicles should be much longer than that for flaps of ordinary length (two to three months); the separation should be gradual, by the laboratory-clamp technique.

A

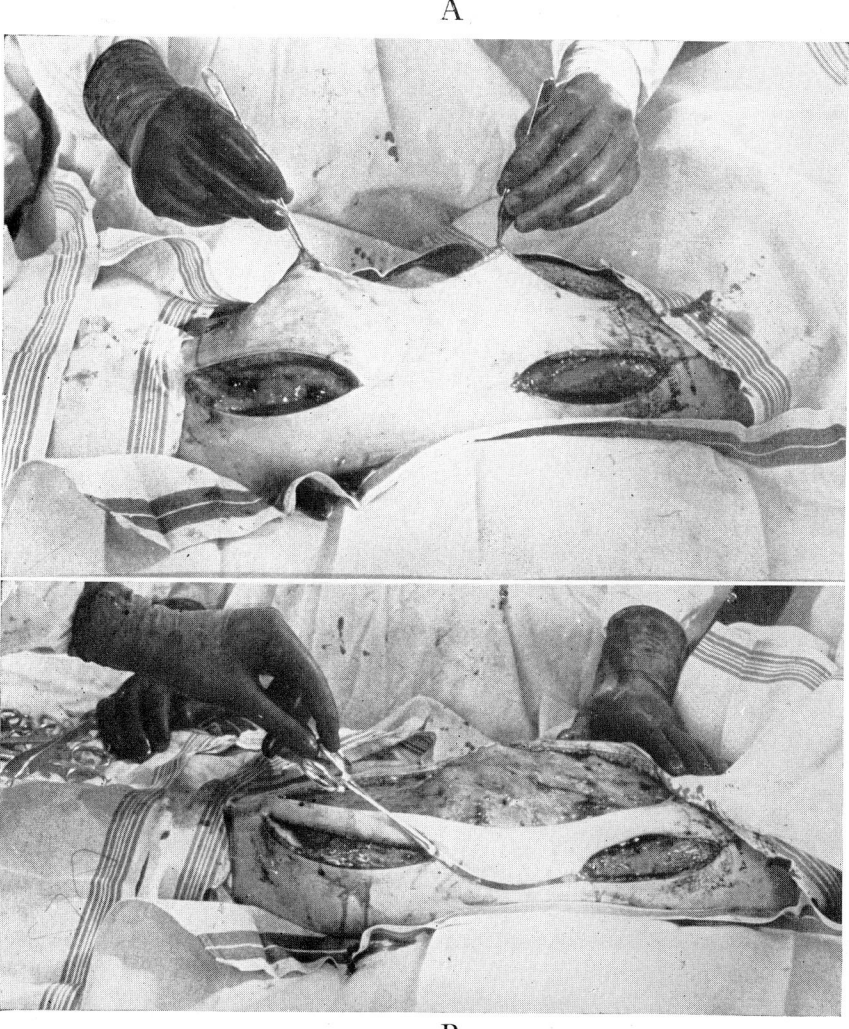

B

Fig. 48: *A:* Method of insuring adequate blood supply in long tube flaps by making one parallel incision of flap (median) uninterrupted and one (lateral) interrupted in its wide portion, thus leaving fairly wide bridge attached to one side of flap. *B:* At end of operation, soft intestinal clamp is applied. If color of flap remains normal, bridge is severed and flap completed; otherwise, bridge is left attached for additional two weeks.

GENERAL PRINCIPLES

Thoracoepigastric Flap in Obesity

If the thoracoepigastric flap is made in an obese patient, it may be necessary to cut through the subcutaneous fat between the skin and the superficial layer of the deep fascia in order to lessen the thickness of the subcutaneous tissue and so make possible the closure of the tube by suturing without excessive pressure. By such a step, the deep arteries and their accompanying veins are cut. Webster advises modifying the procedure under such circumstances by using one of the safety procedures described in the following chapter, preferably the one devised by himself.

Measures for Insuring Adequate Blood Supply in Long Tube Flaps

Generally speaking, a tube flap should not be made longer than from 20 to 30 cm. (7⅞ to 11¹³⁄₁₆ inches). If it is has be made longer, particularly in obese patients, certain measures must be taken to secure an adequate blood supply. There are three possibilities available:

Lengthening in Two Stages: A tube flap of proper secure length is fashioned in the first stage and lengthened to the desired extent in a second stage, from ten to fourteen days later.

Interrupted Tube-Flap Method (DeRiver): The two parallel incisions for the formation of the tube flap are interrupted every 8.8 cm. (3½ inches) by several "jumps" or bridges; these skin bridges are 0.6 cm. (¼ inch) wide. In this way a more abundant blood supply is furnished. After ten to fourteen days, the lateral attachments are separated and sutured together; thus the tube is completed. This method can be modified by the formation of one bridge, but a wider one, left in the middle of the flap on either side.

Unilateral Bridge Attachment (Webster): The principle of this method consists of making one of the parallel incisions of the flap uninterrupted and the other one interrupted in its wide portion, thus leaving a fairly wide bridge attached to one side of the flap (Fig. 48 *A*). After ten to fourteen days, the bridge can be separated and the tube completed. The author (May) found that sometimes the second stage could be undertaken at the end of the first stage; thus, a second operation became unnecessary for the following reason: He had left the flap attached to a unilateral bridge for purposes of safety; a soft intestinal clamp was applied to the bridge (Fig. 48 *B*). If the color of the flap remained normal, the bridge was separated at the end of the operation and the flap completed; otherwise the bridge was left attached for another two weeks.

The unilateral bridge attachment is the preferred method. One of its main advantages is that the tissues on both sides of the defect and on

100

both sides of the flap can be brought together to such an extent that the secondary defect can be closed almost entirely and the tube practically formed in its entire length during the first stage.

BIBLIOGRAPHY

SHIFTING OF TISSUE AND TISSUE GRAFTING

ABBOTT, L. C., SAUNDERS, J. B., and BOST, F. C.: *Arthrodesis of the wrist with the use of grafts of cancellous bone.* J. Bone Joint Surg., 24:883, 1942.

ALLGÖWER, M., BLOCKER, T. G., and ENGLEY, B. W. D.: *Some immunological aspects of auto- and homo-grafts in rabbits, tested by in vivo and in vitro techniques.* Plast. Reconstr. Surg., 9:1, 1952.

ALLGÖWER, M.: *Zur Biologie von Hauthomotransplantaten.* Langenbeck's Archiv für klinische Chirurgie, 279:40, 1954.

ALTEMEIER, W. A., and CARTER, B. N.: *Infected burns with hemorrhage.* Ann. Surg., 115:1118, 1942.

ANDINA, F.: *Grundsätzliches über die freien Hauttransplantationen.* Langenbeck's Archiv für klinische Chirurgie. Deutsche Zeitschrift für Chirurgie, 282:587, 1955.
Die freien Hauttransplantationen einschliesslich der Frage der Homoitransplantation. Ergebnisse d. Chir. u. Orthop., 38:177, 1953.
Annals of the New York Academy of Sciences: Third Tissue Homotransplantation Conference. Vol. 73, Art. 3, pp. 539-868, 1959.
Biologie der Transplantation in Forschung und Klinik. Langenbeck's Archiv für klinische Chirurgie, 292:783, 1959.

ARTZ, C. P., BRONWELL, A. W., and SAKO, Y.: *The exposure treatment of donor sites.* Ann. Surg., 142:248, 1955.

ASHLEY, F. L., BRALEY, S., REES, T. D., TOULIAN, D., and BALLANTYNE, D. L.: *The present status of silicone fluid in soft tissue augmentation.* Plast. Reconstr. Surg., 39:411, 1967.

AXHAUSEN, W.: *The osteogenetic phases of regeneration of bone. A historical and experimental study.* J. Bone Joint Surg., 38A:593, 1956.
Die Bedeutung der Individual—und Artspezifität der Gewebe für die freie Knochenüberpflanzung. Hefte Unfallheilk. H 72, 1962.

BABCOCK, W. W.: *A standard technique for operations on peripheral nerves, with especial reference for the closure of large gaps.* Surg. Gynec. Obstet., 45:364, 1927.

BAETZNER, K.: *Experimentelle Untersuchungen zur homoioplastischen und alloplastischen Aortentransplantation.* Langenbeck's Archiv für klinische Chirurgie. Deutsche Zeitschrift für Chirurgie, 282:647, 1955.

BARNES, R., BACSICH, P., WYBURN, G. M., and KERR, A. S.: *A study of the fate of nerve homografts in man.* Brit. J. Surg., 34:34, 1946.

GENERAL PRINCIPLES

BASSETT, A. L.: *Bibliography of bone transplantation.* Transplantation Bull., 3:103, 1956.

BATEMAN, J. E.: *Plasma silk suture of nerves.* Ann. Surg., 127:457, 1948.

BAUER, G., BOESTROM, H., JORPES, E. and KALINER, S.: *Intramuscular administration of heparin.* Acta Med. Scand., 136:188, 1950.

BAUER, K. H.: *Homotransplantation von Epidermiis bei Eineiigen Zwillingen.* Beitr. z. Klin. Chir., 141:442, 1927.

BAUERMEISTER, A.: *Experimentelle Grundlagen für den Aufbau Einer Neuen Knochenbank.* Berlin, Göttingen and Heidelberg, Springer-Verlag, 1958.
Experimentalle Grundlagen für den Aufbau Einer Neuen Knochenbank. Hefte Unfallheilk. H. 58, 1958.
Zur unterschiedlichen Gewebefreundlichkeit verschiedener Knochentransplantate. Langenbeck's Arch für klin. Chirurgie, 292:828, 1959.

BAXTER, H., ET AL.: *The effect of ACTH on the survival of homografts in man.* Plast. Reconstr. Surg., 7:492, 1951.

BAXTER, H., and ENTIN, M. A.: *Cinical study of the fate of homografts in man. Effect of repeated dosage from the same donor and of refrigeration on these grafts.* Amer. J. Surg., 31:285, 1951.

BAXTER, H., SCHILLER, C., and WHITESIDE, J. H.: *The influence of ACTH on wound healing in man.* Plast. Reconstr. Surg., 7:85, 1951.

BELLMAN, S., and GOTHMAN, B.: *Vascularization of one year old homologous aortic grafts.* Ann. Surg., 139:447, 1954.

BENTLEY, F. H., and HILL, M.: *Nerve grafting.* Brit. J. Surg., 24:368, 1936.

BETZEL, F., and SCHILLING, H.: *Uber die Biologie, Konservierung, und Verpflanzung von Knorpegewebe.* Zentralblatt für Chirurgie, June, 1960.

BIER, A.: *Beobachtungen über Regeneration beim Menschen.* Deutsche med. Wchenschr., 117, No. 29.
Über Knochenregeration, über Pseudarthrosen, und über Knochentransplantate. Arch. für klinische Chirurgie, 127, 1923.

BILLINGHAM, R. E., and BARKER, C. F.: *Recent developments in transplantation immunology, part II.* Plast. Reconstr. Surg., 44:20, 1969.

BILLINGHAM, R. E., and MEDAWAR, P. B.: *"Desensitization" to skin homografts by injections of donor skin extracts.* Ann. Surg., 137:444, 1953.

BILLINGHAM, R. E., BRENT, L., and MEDAWAR, P. B.: *The antigenic stimulus in transplantation immunity.* Nature, 178:514, 1956.

BLAIR, V. P.: *The fullthickness skin graft.* Ann. Surg., 80:298, 1924.
The influence of mechanical pressure on wound healing. Illinois Med. J., 46:249, 1924.

BLAIR, V. P., and BROWN, J. B.: *Use and uses of large split skin grafts of intermediate thickness.* Surg. Gynec. Obstet., 49:82, 1929.

BLAKEMORE, A. H.: *Restorative endoaneurysmorrhaphy by vein graft inlay.* Ann. Surg., 126:841, 1947.

BLAKEMORE, A. H., and VOORHEES, A. B.: *The use of tubes constructed from vinyon "N" cloth in bridging arterial defects—experimental and clinical.* Ann. Surg., 140:324, 1954.

BLAKEMORE, A. H., and LORD, J. W., Jr.: *Nonsuture method of blood-vessel anastomosis with the aid of vitallium tubes.* JAMA, 127:748, 1945.

BLANDFORD, S. E., and GARCIA, F. A.: *Successful homogenous skin graft in a severe burn using an identical twin as donor.* Plast. Reconstr. Surg., 11:31, 1953.

BLOCKER, T. G., and DUKES, C. D.: *Studies on the survival of skin homografts.* Plast. Reconstr. Surg., 10:248, 1952.

BLOCKSMA, R., and BRALEY, S.: *The silicones in plastic surgery.* Plast. Reconstr. Surg., 35:366, 1965.

BÖHLER, J.: *Nervennaht und homoioplastische Nerventransplantation mit Milliporeumscheidung.* Langenbeck's Arch. für klinische Chirurgie, 301:900, 1962.

v. BRANDIS, H. J.: *Die Cutisplastik nach E. Rehn.* Der Chirurg., 14:418, 1951.

BRAUN, W.: *Zur Technik der Hautpfropfung.* Zentralbl. f. Chir., 47:1555, 1920.

BROCKIS, J. G.: *The blood supply of the flexor and extensor tendons of the fingers in man.* J. Bone Joint Surg., 35B:131, 1953.

BROOKS, D. B., HEIPLE, K. G., HERNDON, C. H., and POWELL, A. E.: *Immunological factors in homogenous bone transplantation. IV: The effect of various methods of preparation and irradiation on antigenicity.* J. Bone Joint Surg., 45A:1617, 1963.

BROWN, J. B.: *Homografting of skin: With report of success in identical twins.* Surgery 1:558, 1937.
Preserved and fresh homotransplants of cartilage. Surg. Gynec. Obstet., 70:1079, 1940.

BROWN, J. B., and McDOWELL, F.: *Massive repairs of burns with thick split skin grafts: Emergency dressings with homografts.* Ann. Surg., 115:658, 1942.
Epithelial healing and the transplantation of skin. Ann. Surg., 115:1166, 1942.
Skin Grafting. 3rd Ed. J. B. Lippincott, Philadelphia, 1958.

BROWN, J. B., FRYER, M. P., and ZAYDON, T. J.: *A skin bank for post mortem homografts.* Surg. Gynec. Obstet., 101:401, 1955.

BROWN, J. B., FRYER, M. P., KOLLAS, P., OHLWILER, D. A., and TEMPLETON, J. B.: *Silicone and teflon prostheses, including full jaw substitution: laboratory and clinical studies of etheron.* Ann. Surg., 157:932, 1963.

BROWN, J. B., FRYER, M. P., and OHLWILER, D. A.: *Study and use of synthetic materials, such as silicones and teflon, as subcutaneous prostheses.* Plast. Reconstr. Surg., 26:264, 1960.

BROWN, R. B., HUFNAGEL, G. A., PATE, J. W., and STRONG, W. R.: *Freeze-dried arterial homografts; clinical application.* Surg. Gynec. Obstet., 97:657, 1953.

BUFF, H. U.: *Hautplastiken, Indikation and Technik.* George Thieme, Stuttgart, 1952.

BUNNELL, S.: *Reconstructive surgery of hand.* Surg. Gynec. Obstet., 39:259, 1924. *Surgery of the Hand.* 3rd Ed. J. B. Lippincott, Philadelphia, 1956.

BUNNELL, S., and BOYES, J. H.: *Nerve grafts.* Amer. J. Surg., 54:64, 1939.

GENERAL PRINCIPLES

BÜRKLE-DE LA CAMP, H.: *Knochenkonservierung und Verwendung Konservierten Knochens.* Langenbeck's Archiv für klinische Chirurgie, 279:26, 1954.
Wandlungen und Fortschritte in der Lehre von den Knochenbrüchen. Langenbeck's Archiv für klinische Chirurgie, 276:163, 1953.
Grundzüge der operativen Technik und der Plastischen Chirurgie. Chirurgische Operationslehre Vol. 1. Urban & Schwarzenberg Wien, 1955.
Die Knochenregeneration bei der Transplantation kältekonservierten homoioplastischen Knochens, XVe Cong. Soc. Intern. Chir. S. 1011, 1953.
Knochentransplantation. Extrait du XVIIIe Cong. de la Soc. Internat. de Chir. Munich, 1959.
Knochentransplantation. Verhandlungbericht d. XVIII. Kongr. d. Societe Internationale de Chirurgie. S. 169-203. Imprimerie Medicale et Scientifique, Brussel, 1959.
Plastiken und Transplantationen. Lehrbuch der Chir., Thieme-Verlag, Stuttgart, S. 159-172, 1958.

BÜRKLE-DE LA CAMP, H., and BUDRASS, W.: *Gewebeverpflanzungen in der Unfallchirurgie. Handbuch des gesamtem Unfallheilkunde.* Ferdinand Enke Verlag Stuttgart, Germany, 1963.

BUROW, C. A.: *Beschreibung einer neuen Transplantations—Methode (Methode der seitlichen Dreiecke) zum Wiederersatz verloren-gegangener Teile des Gesichts.* Nauck, Berlin, 1855.

BURWELL, R. G.: *Studies in the transplantation of bone. V: The capacity of fresh and treated homografts of bone to evoke transplantation immunity.* J. Bone Joint Surg., 45B:386, 1963.
Studies in the transplantation of bone. VII. The fresh composite homograft-autograft of cancellous bone. J. Bone Joint Surg., 46B:110, 1964.

BURWELL, R. G., and GOWLAND, G.: *Studies in the transplantation of bone. I. Assessment of antigenicity. Serological studies.* J. Bone Joint Surg., 43B:814, 1961.
Studies in the transplantation of bone. II. The changes occurring in the lymphoid tissue after homografts and autografts of fresh cancellous bone. J. Bone Joint Surg., 43B:820, 1961.

BUSH, L. F., and GARBER, C. Z.: *The bone bank.* JAMA, 137:588, 1948.
The Bone Bank. Monographs on Surgery, 1950, B. N. Carter, Ed. Thos. Nelson & Sons, New York, 1949.

BYARS, L. T.: *Tattooing of free skin grafts and pedicle flaps.* Ann. Surg., 121:644, 1945.

CAMPBELL, C. J., ET AL.: *Experimental study of the fate of bone grafts.* J. Bone Joint Surg., 35A:312, 1953.

CAMPBELL, J. B., and BASSETT, C. A. L.: *Microfilter sheaths in peripheral nerve surgery. A laboratory report and preliminary clinical study.* J. Trauma, 1:139, 1961.

CAMPBELL, H. A., and LINK, K. P.: *Studies on hemorrhage; sweet-clover disease. IV. Isolation and crystallization of hemorrhagic agent.* J. Biol. Chem., 130:31, 1941.

CANNADAY, J. E.: *The use of the cutis graft in the repair of certain types of incisional herniae and other conditions.* Ann. Surg., 115:775, 1942.

CARNESALE, P. L., and SPANKUS, J. L.: *A clinical comparative study of autogenous and homogenous bone grafts.* J. Bone Joint Surg., 41A:887, 1959.

CARR, C. R., and HYATT, G. W.: *Clinical evaluation of freeze-dried bone grafts.* J. Bone Joint Surg., 37A:549, 1955.

SHIFTING OF TISSUE

CARREL, A., and GUTHRIE, F.: *Transplantation biterminale complète d'un segment de veine sur une artère.* Compt. rend. Soc. de biol., 2:412, 1905.

CHANDLER, J. J., and GUSTAVSON, R. G.: *A method of rapid skin graft immobilization.* Surg. Gynec. Obstet., 120:1303, 1965.

CLARKE, S. H. C.: *Formation of inclusion dermoid cysts following whole-thickness skin graft repair of hernia.* Brit. J. Surg., 39:346, 1952.

CONVERSE, J. M.: *Early skin grafting in war wounds of extremities.* Ann. Surg., 115:321, 1942.

CONVERSE, J. M., and DUCHET, G.: *Successful homolous skin grafting in a war burn using an identical twin as donor.* Plast. Reconstr. Surg., 2:342, 1947.

CONVERSE, J. M., and RAPAPORT, F. T.: *The vascularization of skin autografts and homografts.* Ann. Surg., 143:306, 1956.
The development of tissue typing. Plast. Reconstr. Surg., 44:9, 1969.

CONWAY, H., STARK, R. B., and JOSLIN, D.: *Observations on the development of circulation in skin grafts.* Plast. Reconstr. Surg. 12:102, 1953.

CONWAY, H., McKINNEY, P., and CLIMO, M.: *Permanent camoflage of vascular nevi of the face by intradermal injection of insoluble pigments (tattooing): Experience through twenty years with 1022 cases.* Plast. Reconstr. Surg., 40:457, 1967.

COOKE, R. N., ET AL.: *Homologous arterial grafts and autogenous vein grafts used to bridge large arterial defects in man.* Surgery, 33:183, 1953.

CRAFOORD, C., and JORPES, E.: *Heparin as a prophylactic against thrombosis.* JAMA, 131:879, 1946.

CREECH, O., DEBAKEY, M. E., COOLEY, D. A., and SELF, M. M.: *Preparation and use of freeze-dried arterial homografts.* Ann. Surg., 140:35, 1954.

CRONKITE, E. P., DEAVER, J. M., and LOSNER, E. L.: *Experience with use of thrombin with and without soluble cellulose for local hemostasis.* War Med., 5:80, 1944.

CURTISS, P. H., JR., and HERNDON, C. H.: *Immunologic factors in homogenous bone transplantation. I. Serological studies.* Ann. N. Y. Acad. Sci., 59:434, 1955.

CZERNY, V.: *Plastischer Ersatz der Brustdrüse durch ein Lipom.* Verhandl. d. deutsch. Gesellsch. f. Chir., 2:216, 1895.

DALE, A.: *Peripheral vascular grafts. Experimental comparisons of homogenous veins and homogenous arteries and synthetic tubes.* Brit. J. Surg., 156:305, 1959.

DAVIS, J. S.: *Plastic Surgery.* P. Blakiston's Son, Philadelphia, 1919.
The use of small deep skin grafts. JAMA, 63:985, 1914.

DAVIS, J. S., and KITLOWSKI, E. A.: *Regeneration of nerves in skin grafts and skin flaps.* Amer. J. Surg., 24:501, 1934.

DAVIS, J. S., and TRAUT, H. F.: *Plastic Surgery. In Lewis: Practice of Surgery.* W. F. Prior, Hagerstown, 1942, Chap. 8, Vol. 5.

DAVIS, L.: *The return of sensation to transplanted skin.* Surg. Gynec. Obstet., 59:533, 1934.

DAVIS, L., and CLEVELAND, D. A.: *Experimental studies in nerve transplants.* Ann. Surg., 99:271, 1934.

GENERAL PRINCIPLES

DAVIS, L., PERRET, G., HILLER, F., and CARROLL, W.: *Experimental studies of peripheral nerve injuries. III. A study of recovery of function following repair by end to end sutures and nerve grafts.* Surg. Gynec. Obstet., 80:35, 1945.

DEBAKEY, M. E., and COOLEY, D. A.: *Surgical treatment of aneurysm of abdominal aorta by resection and restoration of continuity with homograft.* Surg. Gynec. Obstet., 97:257, 1953.

DEBAKEY, M. E., and SIMEONE, F. A.: *Battle injuries of arteries in World War II; analysis of 2,471 cases.* Ann. Surg., 123:534, 1946.

DEBAKEY, M. E., JORDAN, F. L., ABBOTT, J. P., HALPERT, B., and O'NEAL, R. M.: *The fate of dacron vascular grafts.* Arch. Surg., 89:757, 1964.

DEMUTH, W. E.: *The experimental use of fascia in the repair of large defects of hollow viscera.* Surg. Gynec. Obstet., 96:305, 1953.

DETERLING, R. A., COLEMAN, C. C., Jr., and PARSHLEY, M. S.: *Experimental studies of the frozen homologous aortic graft.* Surgery, 29:319, 1951.

DETERLING, R. A., et al.: *A critical study of present criteria governing selection and use of blood vessel grafts.* Surgery, 33:213, 1953.

DETERLING, R. A., and BHONSLAY, S. B.: *An evaluation of synthetic material and fabrics suitable for blood vessel replacement.* Surgery, 38:71, 1955.

DETERLING, R. A.: *The role of plastics and engineering in vascular surgery.* Arch. Surg., 93:697, 1966.

DIEFFENBACH, J. F.: *Chirurgische Erfahrungen.* Berlin, 1834, Parts 3, 4.

DINGMAN, R. O., and GRABB, W. C.: *Coastal cartilage homografts preserved by irradiation.* Plast. Reconstr. Surg., 28:562, 1961.

DiVINCENTI, G., CURRERI, P. W., and PRUITT, B. A.: *Use of mesh skin autografts in burned patients.* Plast. Reconstr. Surg., 44:464, 1969.

DOGO, G.: *Survival and utilization of cadaver skin.* Plast. Reconstr. Surg., 10:10, 1952.

DORRANCE, G. M.: *An experimental study of suture of arteries with a description of a new suture.* Ann. Surg., (Sept.), 1906.

DOUGLAS, A. S.: *Anticoagulant Therapy.* F. A. Davis Company, Philadelphia, 1962.

DOUGLAS, B.: *The sieve graft: A stable transplant for covering larger skin defects.* Surg. Gynec. Obstet., 50:1018, 1930.

DUEL, A. B., and BALLANCE, C.: *The operative treatment of facial palsy by introduction of nerve grafts into fallopian canal and by other intra-temporal methods.* Arch. Otolaryng., 15:1, 1932.

DUFF, I. F., LINMAN, J. W., and BIRCH, R.: *The administration of heparin.* Surg. Gynec. Obstet., 93:343, 1951.

DUKES, C. D., and BLOCKER, T. G., Jr.: *Studies on the survival of skin homografts. I. Prolongation of life of full thickness grafts by the action of streptokinase-streptodornase.* Ann. Surg., 136:999, 1952.

DUPERTUIS, S. M.: *Growth of young human autogenous cartilage grafts.* Plast. Reconstr. Surg., 5:486, 1950.

SHIFTING OF TISSUE

EASTCOTT, H. G., and HUFNAGEL, C. A.: *The preservation of arterial grafts by freezing.* Surgical Forum, Clinical Congress, Am. Coll. Surgeons 1950, pp. 269, W. B. Saunders, Philadelphia, 1951.

EDEN, R.: *Ueber die freie Nerventransplantation zum Ersatz von Nervendefekten.* Deutsche med. Wchnschr., 45:1239, 1919.
Transplantation der peripheren Nerven. In Lexer: Die freien Transplantationen. Neue Deutsche Ztschr. f. Chir., 26b:537, 1924.

EDGERTON, M. T., and HANSEN, F. C.: *Matching facial color with split thickness skin grafts from adjacent areas.* Plast. Reconstr. Surg., 25:455, 1960.

EDWARDS, W. S.: *Plastic Arterial Grafts.* Charles C Thomas, Springfield, 1957.

ELLISON, E. H., ET AL.: *The effect of ACTH and cortisone on the survival of homologous skin grafts.* Ann. Surg. 134: 495, 1951.

ELSBERG, C. A.: *Technic of nerve suture and nerve grafting.* JAMA, 73:1422, 1919.

ESSER, J. F. S.: *Neue Wege für Chirurgische Plastiken durch Heranziehung der zahnärztlichen Technik.* Beitr. z. klin. Chir., 103:547, 1916.

FITZGERALD, M. J. G., MARTIN, F., and PALETTA, F. X.: *Innervation of skin grafts.* Surg. Gynec. Obstet., 124:808, 1967.

FREEMAN, B. S.; *Immobilization of skin grafts by wide-mesh net. Reintroduction and modification of a valuable method.* Plast. Reconstr. Surg., 27:194, 1961.

FRY, H.: *Cartilage and cartilage grafts: the basic properties of the tissue and the components responsible for them.* Plast. Reconstr. Surg., 40:426, 1967.

GARRÉ, C.: *Uber die histologischen Vorgänge bei der Anheilung der Thierschschen Transplantationen.* Brun's Beitr. z. klin. Chirurg., 4:625, 1888-89.

GEORGIADE, N., PESCHEL, E., and BROWN, I.: *A clinical and experimental investigation of the preservation of skin.* Plast. Reconstr. Surg., 17:267, 1956.

GIBSON, T., and DAVIS, W. B.: *The distortion of autogenous cartilage grafts: its cause and prevention.* Brit. J. Plast. Surg., 10:257, 1958.

GIBSON, T., and MEDAWAR, P. B.: *The fate of skin homografts in man.* J. Anat., 77:299, 1943.

GIBSON, T., DAVIS, W. B., and CURRAN, R. C.: *The long-term survival of cartilage homografts in man.* Brit. J. Plast. Surg., 11:177, 1958.

GILLIES, H. D.: *Plastic Surgery of the Face.* H. Frowde, London, 1920.
Plastic surgery of facial burns. Surg. Gynec. Obstet., 30:121, 1920.

GILLIES, H. D., and MILLARD, D. R.: *The principles and art of plastic surgery.* Little, Brown & Company, Boston and Toronto, 1957.

GINESTET, G., and GINESTET, G.: *Les Lambeaux Cylindriques Dans La Chirurgie Reconstructive.* Expansion Scientifique Francaise, Paris, 1955.

GOHRBANDT, E.: *Homoio-Hetero- und Allo-Plastik.* Langenbeck's Archiv für klinische Chirurgie. 279:14, 1954.

GREEN, R. W., LEVENSON, S. M., and LUND, C. C.: *Nylon backing for dermatome grafts.* New Eng. J. Med., 223:268, 1945.

GENERAL PRINCIPLES

GROSS, R. E.: *Surgical treatment for coarctation of the aorta; experiences from 60 cases.* JAMA, 139:285, 1949.

GROSS, R. E., BILL, A. H., JR., and PEIRCE, E. C.: *Methods for preservation and transplantation of arterial grafts; observations on arterial grafts in dogs; report of transplantation of preserved arterial grafts in nine human cases.* Surg. Gynec. Obstet., 88:689, 1949.

GULLICK, H. D.: *Exposure and natural fixation of split thickness skin grafts.* Arch. Surg., 80:244, 1960.

HAGERTY, R., CALHOON, T. B., LEE, W. H., JR., and CUTTING, J. T.: *Characteristics of fresh human cartilage.* Surg. Gynec. Obstet., 110:3, 1960.
Human cartilage grafts stored in merthiolate. Surg. Gynec. Obstet., 110:229, 1960.

HALPERT, B., DEBAKEY, M. E., JORDAN, G. L., JR., and HENLY, W. S.: *The fate of homografts and prostheses of the human aorta.* Surg. Gynec. Obstet., 111:659, 1960.

HALSE, T.: *Heparin und Heparinode Dicumarol.* S. Hirzel Verlag Zürich, 1950.

HANCE, G., BROWN, J. B., BYARS, L. T., and McDOWELL, F.: *Color matching of skin grafts and flaps with permanent pigment injection.* Surg. Gynec. Obstet., 79:624, 1944.

HANNA, D. C., and GAISFORD, J. C.: *Facial nerve management in tumors and trauma.* Plast. Reconstr. Surg., 35:445, 1965.

HARKINS, H. M.: *Cutis grafts.* Ann. Surg., 122:996, 1945.

HARRISON, J. H.: *A teflon weave for replacing tissue defects.* Surg. Gynec. Obstet., 104:584, 1957.
Synthetic materials as vascular prostheses. II. A comparative study of nylon, dacron, orlon, ivalon sponge, and teflon in large blood vessels with tensile strength studies. Amer. J. Surg., 95:16, 1958.
Synthetic materials as vascular prostheses. III. Longterm studies on grafts of nylon, dacron, orlon, and teflon replacing blood vessels. Surg. Gynec. Obstet., 108:433, 1959.

HENRY, A. K.: *The Hinge Graft.* Williams and Wilkins, Baltimore, 1950.

HERSHEY, F. B., and SPENCER, A. D.: *Autogenous vein grafts for repair of arterial injuries.* Arch. Surg., 86:836, 1963.

HESLOP, B. F., ZEISS, I. M., and NISBET, N. W.: *Studies on transference of bone. I. A comparison of autologous and homologous bone implants with reference to osteocyte survival, osteogenesis and host reaction.* Brit. J. Exp. Path., 41:269, 1960.

HIRSHOWITZ, B.: *Blood as a neutraliser of dermatome cement.* Brit. J. Plast. Surg., 12:82, 1959.

HOLMES, W.: *Histological observations on the repair of nerves by auto-grafts.* Brit. J. Surg., 35:167, 1947.

HORSLEY, J. A., and BIGGER, I. A.: *Operative Surgery.* C. V. Mosby, St. Louis, 1940.

HORWITZ, T.: *Behavior of bone grafts.* Surg. Gynec. Obstet., 89:310, 1949.

HUBER, G. C.: *A study of the operative treatment for loss of nerve substance in peripheral nerves.* J. Morph., 11:629, 1895.

SHIFTING OF TISSUE

HUFNAGEL, C. A.: *The use of rigid and flexible plastic prostheses for arterial replacement.* Surgery, 37:165, 1955.

HUGHES, C. W.: *Traumatic Lesions of Peripheral Vessels.* Charles C Thomas, Springfield, 1961.

INOKUCHI, K.: *A new type of vessel-suturing apparatus.* Arch. Surg., 77:954, 1958.

JACKSON, D.: *A clinical study of the use of skin homografts for burns.* Brit. J. Plast. Surg., 7:26, 1954.

JACOB, S. W., GOWING, D., and DUNPHY, J. E.: *Transplantation of tissues.* Amer. J. Surg., 98:55, 1959.

JOHNSON, G.: *Valve excision in autogenous vein grafts.* Surg. Gynec. Obstet., 123:845, 1966.

JONES, C. J.: *Transplantation and immunity.* Surg. Gynec. Obstet., 120:1317, 1965.

KAWAMURA, B.: *Modern trends in bone grafting.* Sapporo Med. J., 4:381, 1953.

KEEFER, E. B. C., et al.: *The blood vessel bank.* JAMA, 145:888, 1951.

KELLER, W. L.: *Ten years of the tunnel skin graft.* Ann. Surg., 91:924, 1930.

KIRKHAM, H. L. D.: *The use of preserved cartilage in ear reconstruction.* Ann. Surg., 111:896, 1940.

KIRSCHNER, M.: *Ueber freie Sehnen aus Faszientransplantation.* Beitr. z. klin. Chir., 65:472, 1909.
Die praktischen Ergebnisse der freien Faszientransplantation. Arch. für klinische Chirurgie, 92:888, 1910.

KLEMME, R. M., WOOLSEY, R. D., and de REGENDE, N. T.: *Autopsy nerve grafts in peripheral nerve surgery.* JAMA, 123:393, 1943.

KLINGENSTROM, P., NORDZELL, B., and NYLEN, B.: *Open treatment of skin grafts.* Acta Chir. Scand., 129:267, 1965.

KLOTZ, O., PERMOR, H. H., and GUTHRIE, C. C.: *End results in arterial transplants.* Ann. Surg., 78:1923.

KOHNLEIN, H. E.: *Die moglichkeiten der homoio-, hetero-, und allotransplantation bei der behandlungder schwerstverbrannten.* Hefte zur unfallheilkunde, Springer-Verlag, Berlin, 1965.

KRAUSE, F.: *Ueber die Transplantation grosser, ungestielter Hautlappen.* Verhandl. d. deutsch. Gesellsch. f. Chir., 22:46, 1893. Translated by H. and L. May: Plast. Reconstr. Surg., 41:573, 1968.

KREDEL, F. E., and EVANS, J. P.: *Recovery of sensation in denervated pedicle and free skin grafts.* Arch. Neurol. Psychiat., 29:1203, 1933.

KREMER, K.: *Brun's Beitr., 1953, 187:340; Fortschr. Med. ,71:19, 1953.*
Chirurgie der Arterien. Georg Thieme Verlag, Stuttgart, 1959.

KREMER, K., VOLKMANN, E., FRANCKE, D., and SUCHOWSKY, G.: *The problem of transplantation of blood vessels; experimental studies of autoplastic vein transplantation.* Langenbeck's Arch. u. Deut. Zschr., Chir., 277:471, 1953.

LANGE, O.: *Operation an den Weichteilen (Muskeln, Sehnen usw.).* Handb. d. orthop. Chir. Part I.

GENERAL PRINCIPLES

LARSON, D. L., VOGEL, E. H., MITCHELL, E. T., and BUTKIEWICZ, J. V.: *The use of modified exposure in the management of burn wounds.* Surg. Gynec. Obstet., 112:577, 1961.

LAWSON, G.: *On transplantation of portions of skin for closure of large granulating surfaces.* Tr. Clin. Soc. London, 4:49, 1871.

LEHR, H. B., and BLAKEMORE, W. S.: *Arterial Homografts; 84 Cases.* Int. Abstr. Surg., 105:209, 1957.

LENTZ, W.: *Die Grundlagen der Transplantation von Fremdem Knockengewebe.* Georg Thieme, Stuttgart, 1955.

LEXER, E.: *Die freien Transplantationen.* Neue deutsche Chir. Ferd. Enke, 1919, 1924, Stuttgart, Vol. 26a, 26b.
Zwanzig Jahre Transplantationsforschung in der Chirurgie. Arch. für klinische Chirurgie, 138:251, 1925.
Dauerefolg eines Arterienersatzes durch Venenautoplastik nach 5 Jahren. Zentralbl. f. Chir., p. 569, 1917.
Die Verwertung der freien Sehnentransplantation. Verhandl. d. deutsch. Gesellsch. f. Chir., 2:76, 1914. Die freie Transplantation. Internat. Chir.-Kongr., 1914.

LIMBERG, A. A.: *The use of diced cartilage by injection with a needle. Part I. Clinical investigations.* Plast. Reconstr. Surg., 28:523, 1961.

LINTON, R. R., and MENENDEZ, C. V.: *Arterial homografts: A comparison of the results with end to end and end to side vascular anastomosis.* Ann. Surg., 142:568, 1955.

LITTLEWOOD, A. H. M.: *Seroma: An unrecognized cause of failure of split-thickness skin grafts.* Brit. J. Plast. Surg., XIII:42, 1960.

LOEFFLER, C.: *Die auto- und homoplastische Epidermis Implantation.* Deutsche Ztschr. f. Chir., 236:169, 1932.

LOEWE, O.: *Ueber Hautimplantationen an Stelle der freien Faszienplastik.* München med. Wchnschr., 24:1320, 1913.
Ueber Haut-Tiefenplastik. München med. Wchnschr., 51:2125, 1929.

LONGMIRE, W. P., and SMITH, S. W.: *Homologous transplantation of tissues.* Arch. Surg., 62:443, 1951.

LONGMIRE, W. P., STONE, H. B., DANIEL, A. S., and GOOD, C. D.: *Report of clinical experiences with homografts.* Plast. Reconstr. Surg., 2:419, 1947.

MAATZ, R.: *Klinische Erfahrungen mit dem eiweisarmen Tierspan.* Langenbeck's Arch. für klinische Chirurgie, 292:831, 1959.
Der Tierspan in der Knochenbank. Dtsch. Med. J. 8:190, 1957.

MACOMBER, D. W.: *Cancellous iliac bone for depressions of forehead, nose and chin.* Plast. Reconstr. Surg., 3:157, 1949.

MAIR, G. B.: Brit. J. Surg., 32:381, 1945.
Brit. J. Surg., 34:42, 1948.
The Surgery of Abdominal Hernia. E. Arnold & Company, London, 1948.

v. MANGOLD, F.: *Die Einpflanzung von Rippenknorpel in den Kehlkopf zur Heilung schwerer Stenosen und Defekte und Heilung der Sattelnase durch Knorpelübertragung.* Arch. f. klin. Chir., 61:955, 1900.

MARCKS, K. M.: *A modified calibrated skin grafting knife.* Mil. Surgeon, 92:653, 1943.

110

MARRANGONI, A. G., and CECCHINI, L. P.: *Homotransplantation of arterial segments. Preserved by the freeze-drying method.* Ann. Surg., 134:977, 1951.

MARSDEN, C. M.: *Whole skin graft repair of inguinal hernia.* Brit. J. Surg., 35:390, 1948.

MASON, M. L.: *The rate of healing of tendons.* Ann. Surg., 113:424, 1941.

MATTI, H.: *Uber freie Transplantation von Knochenspongiosa.* Arch. Klin. Chir., 168:236.
Uber die Behandlung von Pseudarthrosen mit Spongiosatransplantation. Arch. f. Orthop., 31:218, 1932.

MAUMENEE, A. E.: *Bibliography of corneal transplantation.* Transplantation Bull., 1:107, 1954.
Bibliography of Corneal Transplantation. Transplantation Bull., 2:73, 1955.

MAY, H.: *The regeneration of bone transplants.* Ann. Surg., 106:441, 1937.
Regeneration of joint transplants and intracapsular fragments. Ann. Surg., 116:297, 1942.
Tendon transplantation in the hand. Surg. Gynec. Obstet., 83:631, 1946.
Methods and advances in skin grafting. S. Clin. North America, 1461, Dec., 1947.
Cutis grafts for repair of incisional and recurrent hernias. S. Clin. North America, 517, April, 1948.
Homogenous skin grafts with and without ACTH. Surgery, 3:590, 1952.
Mitteilung über freie Hauttransplantationen. Langenbeck's Archiv für klinische Chirurgie, 273:240, 1952-1953.
Auto- und Homoioplastische freie Hauttransplantation. Langenbeck's Arch. u. Dtsch. Z. Chir. 274:215, 1953.
Untoward effects from skin grafting. JAMA, 173:1347, 1960.

MAY, R. M.: *La Greffe.* Gallimard, Paris, 1952.

MAYER, L.: *Physiological method of tendon transplantation.* Surg. Gynec. Obstet., 33:528, 1921.
Surgery of Tendons. In Lewis: Practice of Surgery. W. F. Prior, Hagerstown, 1943, Vol. 3, Chap. 5.

McCARROL, H. R.: *The regeneration of sensation in transplanted skin.* Ann. Surg., 108:309, 1938.

McCUNE, W. S., THISTLETHWAITE, J. R., KESHUSHIAN, J. M., and BLADES, B.: *The nutrition of blood vessel grafts; an India ink injection study of their vascularization.* Surg. Gynec. Obstet., 94:311, 1952.

McCUNE, W. S., and BLADES, B.: *The viability of long blood vessel grafts.* Ann. Surg., 134:769, 1951.

McGREGOR, I. A.: *The vascularisation of homografts of human skin.* Brit. J. Plast. Surg., 7:331, 1955.

McNICHOL, J. W.: *Experience with a case of simultaneous autograft and homograft in third degree burn with ACTH.* Plast. Reconstr. Surg., 9:437, 1952.

MEDAWAR, P. B.: Bull. War Med. 1:1, 1943.
Behavior and fate of skin autografts and skin homografts in rabbits. J. Anat., 78:176, 1944.
General problems of immunity. In Ciba Foundation Symposium on Preservation and Transplantation of Normal Tissue.

GENERAL PRINCIPLES

The Immunity of Transplantation. The Harvey Lectures. Academic Press, Inc., New York, 1958.

MIR Y MIR, L.: *The problem of pigmentation in the cutaneous graft.* Brit. J. Plast. Surg., 14:303, 1961.

MIUR, I. F. K., OWEN, D., MURPHY, I.: *Sulfamylon acetate in the treatment of Pseudomonas pyocyaneus infection of burns.* Brit. J. Plast. Surg., 12:201, 1969.

MOWLEM, R.: *Bone and cartilage transplants. Their use and behavior.* Brit. J. Surg. 29:182, Oct. 1941.

MURRAY, G.: *Heparin in surgical treatment of blood vessels.* Arch. Surg., 40:307, 1940.
Heparin in thrombosis and blood vessel surgery. Surg. Gynec. Obstet., 72:340, 1941.

NEEDHAM, A. E.: *Regeneration and Wound Healing.* John Wiley and Sons, New York, 1952.

NEUBER: *Fettgewebstransplantation.* Verhandl. d. deutsch. Gesellsch. f. Chir., 1:66, 1893.

NEUHOF, H.: *The Transplantation of Tissues.* D. Appleton & Company, New York, 1923.

NICOLL, E. A.: *The treatment of gaps in long bones by cancellous insert grafts.* J. Bone Joint Surg., 38B:70, 1956.

NIGST, H.: *Freie Nerventransplantationen und Cortison.* Benno Schwabe, Basel, 1959.
Operative Behandlungsmöglichkeiten bei Erkrankungen und Frischen Verletzungen peripherer Nerven. Langenbeck's Arch. für klinische Chirurgie, 301:855, 1962.

NISBET, N. W., HESLOP, B. F., and ZEISS, I. M.: *Studies on transference of bone. III. Manifestations of immunological tolerance to implants of homologous cortical bone in rats.* Brit. J. Exp. Path., 41:443, 1960.

NYHUS, L. M., ET AL.: *Experimental vascular grafts. III. The dimensional changes in short and long length fresh and preserved aortic homografts implanted into the thoracic aorta of growing pigs.* Surg. Gynec. Obstet., 97:81, 1953.

OBELL, S. L.: *Studien über Knochenimplantation und Knochenneubildung. Implantation von "Os purum" sowie Transplantation von "Os Novum."* Acta Chir. Scand. Suppl., 74:31, 1934.

O'CONNOR, G. B.: *Editorial: Establishment of cartilage depots for military and civilian use.* Amer. J. Surg., 58:313, 1942.

O'CONNOR, G. B., and PIERCE, G. W.: *Refrigerated cartilage isografts.* Surg. Gynec. Obstet., 67:796, 1938.

OLLIER, L.: *Recherches expérimental sur les greffes osseueses.* J. de physiol., 3:88, 1860.
Traite expérimental et clinique de la régénération des os. Paris, 1867.
Greffes cutaneous on autoplastiques. Bull. Acad. de med., 1:243, 1872.

OWENS, N.: *Rayon, an ideal surgical dressing for surface wounds.* Surgery, 19:482, 1946.

PADGETT, E. C.: *Calibrated intermediate skin grafts.* Surg. Gynec. Obstet., 69:799, 1939.

SHIFTING OF TISSUE

Skin grafting and the three quarter thickness skin graft for prevention and correction of cicatricial formation. Ann. Surg., 113:1034, 1941.
Skin Grafting. Charles C Thomas, Springfield, 1942.

PATON, R. T.: *Corneal transplantation; a review of 365 operations.* Arch. Ophthal., 52:871, 1954.

PEER, L. A.: *Cartilage grafting.* S. Clin. North America, 24:404, 1944.
Cartilage transplanted beneath the skin of the chest in man; experimental studies with sections of cartilage preserved in alcohol and buried from seven days to fourteen months. Arch. Otolaryng., 27:42, 1938.
Bibliography of cartilage transplantation. Transplantation Bull., 1:104, 1954.
Transplantation of Tissues. Vol. 1. Williams and Wilkins, Baltimore, 1955.
The neglected free fat graft. Amer. J. Surg., 92:40, 1956.
Bibliography of cartilage transplantation. Plast. Reconstr. Surg., 23:438, 1959.
Transplantation of Tissues. Vol. II. Williams and Wilkins, Baltimore, 1959.

PEER, L. A., and PADDOCK, R.: *Histologic studies on the fate of deeply implanted dermal grafts; observations on sections of implants buried from one month to one year.* Arch. Surg., 34:268, 1937.

PEER, L. A., and WALKER, J. C.: *The behavior of autogenous human tissue grafts.* Plast. Reconstr. Surg., 7:73, 1951.
The behavior of autogenous human tissue grafts. Plast. Reconstr. Surg., 7:6, 1951.

PEER, L. A., WALIA, I. S., and PULLEN, R. J.: *Behavior of a first, second, and third crop of skin homografts from the same donor.* Plast. Reconstr. Surg., 26:161, 1960.

PEER, L. A., WALIA, I. S., and BERNHARD, W. G.: *Further studies on the growth of rabbit ear cartilage grafts.* Brit. J. Plast. Surg., 19:105, 1966.

PEIRCE, E. C.: *The use of viably preserved tissue for homologous arterial grafts.* Ann. Surg., 136:228, 1952.

PEIRCE, E. C., GROSS, R. E., BILL, A. H., Jr., and MERRILL, K., Jr.: *Tissue-culture evaluation of the viability of blood vessels stored by refrigeration.* Ann. Surg., 129:333, 1949.

PFEIFFER, D. B., and FLETCHER, D. S.: *Heparin and dicumarol, collective review.* Surg. Gynec. Obstet., 78:109 (Int. Abstr.), 1944.

PICK, J. F.: *Surgery of Repair.* J. B. Lippincott, Philadelphia, 1949.

PICKERILL, H. P.: *Intra-oral skin grafting; the establishment of the buccal sulcus.* Proc. Roy. Soc. Med., 12; Sect. Odont., 17, 1918, 1919.
Note on cranial autoplasty. Brit. J. Surg., 35:204, 1947.

POTH, E. J., JOHNSON, J. K., and CHILDERS, J. H.: *The use of plastic fabrics as arterial prosthesis.* Ann. Surg., 142:624, 1955.

POTTS, W.: *A new clamp for surgical division of the patent ductus.* Quart. Bull. Northwestern Univ. Med. School, 22:321, 1948.

QUICK, A. J.: *The physiology and pathology of hemostasis.* Lea and Febiger, Philadelphia, 1951.

RANDALL, P., McDOWELL, E., and BROWN, J. B.: *The effects of ACTH and cortisone on experimental skin homografts.* p. 475 Surgical Forum Amer. Coll. Surgeons. W. B. Saunders, Philadelphia, 1952.
An experimental method for the study of skin homografts. p. 455 Surgical Forum Amer. Coll. Surgeons, W. B. Saunders, Philadelphia, 1952.

GENERAL PRINCIPLES

RANDALL, P., and LU, M.: *Postmortem homografts as "biological dressings" for extensive burns and denuded areas*. Ann. Surg., 138:618, 1953.

RASI, H. B.: *The fate of preserved human cartilage*. Plast. Reconstr. Surg., 24:24, 1959.

REES, T. D., PLATT, J., and BALLANTYNE, D. L.: *An investigation of cutaneous response to dimethylpolysiloxane (silicone liquid) in animals and humans. A preliminary report*. Plast. Reconstr. Surg., 35: 131, 1965.

REESE, J. D.: *Dermatape: a new method for the management of split skin grafts*. Plast. Reconstr. Surg., 1:98, 1946.

REHN, E.: *Das kutane und subkutane Bindegewebe als plastisches Material*. München. med. Wchnschr., 1:118, 1914.
Die freie funktionelle Kutistransplantation. In Lexer: Neue Deutsche Chir. Ferd. Enke, Stuttgart, 1924, Vol. 26b.

REHRMANN, A.: *Ivalon implantation in der Gerichtschirurgie*. Langenbeck's Arch. n. Dtsch. Ztschr. f. Chir., 292:860, 1959.

REVERDIN, J. L.: *De la greffe epidermique*. Arch. gen. de med., 19:276, 555, 703, 1872.
Greffe epidermique. Bull. Soc. imp. de chir. de Paris, 10:493, 1869.

RIVAS, C. T., and TUCCILLO, O. J.: *Total Free Graft of Nail and Nail Matrix*. Bolet. y. Tra. de la Soc. Arg. de Cirurjanos., 9:453, 1948 (Abst. Plast. Reconstr. Surg., 4:568, 1949).

ROGERS, B. O.: *Guide and bibliography for research into the skin homograft problem*. Plast. Reconstr. Surg., 7:169, 1951.
Bibliography of skin homotransplantation. Plast. Reconstr. Surg., 22:407, 1958.

ROTH, H.: *Die Konservierung von Knochengewebe für Transplantationen (Monograph on bone grafts)*. Wien, Springer-Verlag, 1952.

ROUX, W.: *Der züchtende Kampf der Teile im Organismus oder die Teilauslese im Organismus (Theorie der funktionellen Anpassung)*. In ges. Abhandl. Vol. II, p. 404, 1881.

RUSSELL, P. S., and MONACO, A. P.: *The Biology of Tissue Transplantation*. Little, Brown & Company, Boston, 1965.

RYCROFT, B. W.: *Corneal Grafts*. Butterworth & Co., London, 1956.

SALIBI, B. S.: *Collective review: The mechanism of blood coagulation; historical review and outline of modern concepts*. Surg. Gynec. Obstet, 95:105, 1952.

SANO, M. E.: *Skin grafting, a new method based on the principles of tissue culture*. Amer. J. Surg., 61:105, 1943.
A coagulum contact method of skin grafting as applied to human grafts. Surg. Gynec. Obstet., 77:510, 1943.

SARNAT, B. G., and LASKIN, D. M.: *Collective review: Cartilage and cartilage implants*. Surg. Gynec. Obstet., 99:521, 1954.

SAUVAGE, L. R., WESOLOWSKI, S. A.: *The healing and fate of arterial grafts*. Surgery, 38:1090, 1955.

SCALES, J. T.: *Discussion on metals and synthetic materials in relation to tissues; tissue reactions to synthetic materials*. Proc. Roy. Soc. Med., 46:647, 1953.

SHIFTING OF TISSUE

SCHMID, M. A: *Die freie Verpflanzung Flachenformiger Hautlappen.* Vortrage aus der Praktischen Chir., Ferdinand Enke Verlag Stuttgart 73, 1965.

SCHUCHARDT, K.: *Die freie Hauttransplantation unter besonderer Berücksichtigung der Verwendung von Epidermis-Kutis-Lappen.* Deutsche Zahn-, Mundunder Kiefer-heilkunde Band 12 (1949) Heft 1-3 Johann Ambrosius Barth, Verlag, Leipzig.

SCOTHORNE, R. J., and McGREGOR, I. A.: *The vascularization of autografts and homografts of rabbit skin.* J. Anat., 8:379, 1953.

SCOTT, W., PETERSON, R. C., and GRANT, S.: *A method of procuring iliac bone by trephine curettage.* J. Bone Joint Surg., 31A:860, 1949.

SEDDON, H. J.: *The use of autogenous grafts for the repair of large gaps in peripheral nerves.* Brit. J. Surg., 35:151, 1948.
Nerve grafting. J. Bone Joint Surg., 45B:447, 1963.

SEEGERS, W. H., and SHARP, E. A.: *Hemostatic Agents.* Charles C Thomas, Springfield, 1948.

v. SEEMEN, H.: *Wege und Grenzen der plastischen und Wiederherstellungschirurgie.* Langenbeck's Archiv für Klinische Chirurgie. Deutsche Zeitschrift für Chirurgie, 282:575, 1955.

SHAPIRO, S., and WEINER, M.: *Coagulation, Thrombosis, and Dicumarol.* Brooklyn Medical Press, 1950.

SHAWHNEY, C. P., BAJERJEE, T. N., CHAKARAVARTI, R. N.: *Behavior of dermal fat transplants.* Brit. J. Plast. Surg., 12:169, 1969.

SHEEHAN, E. J.: *Plasma fixation of skin grafts.* Amer. J. Surg., 65:74, 1944.

SHERMAN, P.: *The open method of skin grafting.* Amer. J. Surg., 94:869, 1957. Reviewed in Plast. Reconstr. Surg., 21:241, 1958.

SMITH, F.: *Pressure bags for skin grafting.* Surg. Gynec. Obstet., 42:99, 1926.
A rational management of skin grafts. Surg. Gynec. Obstet., 42:556, 1926.

SNYDER, C. C., WARDLAW, E., and KELLY, N.: *Gas sterilization of cartilage and bone implants.* Plast. Reconstr. Surg., 28:568, 1961.

STRANGE, F. G. St. C.: *An operation for nerve pedicle grafting.* Brit. J. Surg., 34:423, 1947.

STRINGA, G. A.: *Studies of the vascularization of bone grafts.* J. Bone Joint Surg., 39B:395, 1957.

SWAN, H., MAASKE, C., JOHNSON, M., and GROVER, R. S.: *Arterial homograft—II.* Arch Surg., 61:732, 1950.

SWAN, H., and MORFIT, H. M.: *Arterial homografts—III, use of preserved grafts in treatment of neoplastic disease involving peripheral arteries.* Arch. Surg., 62:767, 1951.

SWAN, H., and JOHNSON, M. E.: *Arterial homografts—I, the fate of preserved aortic grafts in the dog.* Surg. Gynec. Obstet., 90:568, 1950.

SWAN, H.: *Arterial grafts.* Surg. Gynec. Obstet., 94:115, 1952.

SWENSON, S. A.: *Cutis grafts. Clinical and experimental observation.* Arch. Surg., 61:881, 1950.

GENERAL PRINCIPLES

v. SZYMANOWSKI, J.: *Handbuch der operativen Chirurgie.* Deutsche Ausgabe von dem Verfasser und C. W. F. Uhde. F. Vieweg u. Sohn, Braunschweig, 1870.

DeTAKATS, G.: *Vascular Surgery.* W. B. Saunders, Philadelphia, 1959.

TANNER, J. C., VANDEPUT, J. J., and BRADLEY, W. H.: *Two years with mesh skin grafting.* Amer. J. Surg., 111:543, 1966.

TANNER, J. C., PATRICK, C., BRADLEY, W. H., VANDEPUT, J. J.: *Large mesh skin grafts.* Plast. Reconstr. Surg., 44:504, 1969.

TARLOV, I. M.: *The plasma clot sutures of peripheral nerves and nerve roots.* Charles C Thomas, Springfield, 1950.

THIEL, R. (Editor): *Ophthalmologische Operations-lehre. (Methodology for Ophthalmologic Operations.)* Leipzig, Georg Thieme, 1943-1950.

THIERSCH, K.: *Uber die feineren anatomischen Veränderungen bei Aufheilung von Haut auf Granulationen.* Arch. f. klin. Chir., 17:318, 1874. Translated by H. and L. May: Plast. Reconstr. Surg., 41:365, 1968.
Ueber Hautverpflanzung. Verhandl. d. deutsch. Gesellsch. f. Chir., 15:17, 1886.

THOMAS, C. I.: *The Cornea.* Charles C Thomas, Springfield, 1955.

THOMPSON, N.: *A clinical and histological investigation into the fate of epithelial elements buried following the grafting of "shaved" skin surfaces. Based on a study of the healing of split-skin graft donor sites in man.* Brit. J. Plast. Surg., 13:219, 1960.
The subcutaneous dermis graft. Plast. Reconstr. Surg., 26:1, 1960.

TIDRICK, R. T., and WARNER, E. D.: *Fibrin fixation of skin transplants.* Surgery, 15:90, 1944.

TRUETA, J.: *The normal vascular anatomy of the human femoral head during growth.* J. Bone Joint Surg., 39B:358, 1957.
The role of the vessels in osteogenesis. J. Bone Joint Surg., 45B:572, 1963.

TRUETA, J., and CALADIAS, A. X.: *A study of the blood supply of the long bones.* Surg. Gynec. Obstet., 118:485, 1964.

TRUETA, J., and BUHR, A. J.: *The vascular contribution to osteogenesis. V. The vasculature supplying the epiphysial cartilage in rachitic rats.* J. Bone Joint Surg., 45B:402, 1963.

VOLLMAR, J.: *Rekonstruktive Chirurgie der Arterien.* Georg Thieme Verlag, Stuttgart, 1967.

VOORHEES, A. B., JR., JARETZKI, A., and BLAKEMORE, A. H.: *The use of tubes constructed from vinyon-N cloth in bridging arterial defects.* Ann. Surg., 135:332, 1952.

WALDRON, C. W. (Quoted by GILLIES, H. D.): *Plastic Surgery of the Face.* H. Frowde, London, 1920.

WALKER, J., and RHOADS, J. E.: *Effect of dicumarol on susceptibility to action of heparin.* Surgery, 15:859, 1944.

WARREN, R.: *Procedures in Vascular Surgery.* Little, Brown & Company, Boston, 1960.

WATSON, J.: *Some observations on free fat grafts: With reference to their use in mammaplasty.* Brit. J. Plast. Surg., 12:263, 1959.

WEBER, R., CANNON, J. A., and LONGMIRE, W. P.: *Observations on the regrafting of successful homografts in chickens.* Ann. Surg., 139:473, 1954.

WEBSTER, J. P.: *Film-cemented skin grafts.* S. Clin. N. Amer., 24:251, 1944.

WEIS, J.: *Neue Gesichtspunkte auf dem Gebiete der homoioplastischen Gefässtransplantationen an der Aorta.* Langenbeck's Arch. u. Dtsch. Z. Chir., Bd., 275:319, 1953.

WEISMAN, P. A., QUINBY, W. C., WIGHT, A., and CANNON, B.: *The adrenal cortical hormones and homografting. Exploration of a concept.* Ann. Surg., 134:506, 1951.
The failure of adrenal cortical hormones to prolong the survival of homologous skin grafts. Plast. Reconstr. Surg., 8:417, 1951.

WESOLOWSKI, S. A., and DENNIS, C., (Eds.): *Fundamentals of Vascular Grafting.* McGraw-Hill, Inc., New York, 1963.

WHITELAW, M. H.: *Physiologic reaction of ACTH in severe burns.* JAMA, 145: 85, 1951.

WOLFE, J. R.: *A new method of performing plastic operations.* Brit. Med. J., 2:360, 1875.

WOLSTENHOLME, G. E. W., and CAMERON, M. P.: *A Ciba Foundation Symposium: Preservation and Transplantation of Normal Tissues.* Little, Brown & Company, Boston, 1954.

WOODRUFF, M. F. A.: *Transplantation of Tissues and Organs.* Charles C Thomas, Springfield, 1960.

YOUNG, F., and FAVATA, B. V.: *The fixation of skin grafts by thrombin-plasma adhesion.* Surgery, 15:378, 1943.

YOUNG, J. Z., HOLMER, W., and SANDERS, F. K.: *Nerve regeneration, importance of the peripheral stump and the value of nerve grafts.* Lancet, 2:128, 1940.

ZINTEL, H. A.: *Resplitting split-thickness grafts with a dermatome; a method for increasing the yield of limited donor site.* Ann. Surg. 121:1, 1945.

ZOLTÁN, J.: *Die Anwendung des Spalthautlappens in der Chirurgie.* Gustav Fischer Verlag, Jena, 1962.

TRANSPLANTATION OF FLAPS

BARRON, J. N., and EMMETT, A. J. J.: *Subcutaneous pedicle flaps.* Brit. J. Plast. Surg., 18:51, 1965.

BARSKY, A. J.: *Filatov and the tubed pedicle.* Plast. Reconstr. Surg., 24:456, 1959.

BELLMAN, S., and VELANDER, E.: *Vascular transformation in experimental tubed pedicles.* Brit. J. Plast. Surg., 12:1, 1959.

BLAIR, V. P.: *The delayed transfer of long pedicle flaps in plastic surgery.* Surg. Gynec. Obstet., 33:261, 1921.
Reconstruction surgery of the face. Surg. Gynec. Obstet., 34:701, 1922.

BRAITHWAITE, F., and MOORE, F. T.: *Cross-leg flaps.* J. Bone Joint Surg., 31B: 228, 1949.

GENERAL PRINCIPLES

BRAITHWAITE, F., FARMER, F. T., HERBERT, F. I.: *Observations on the vascular channels of tubed pedicles using radioactive sodium III.* Brit. J. Plast. Surg. 4:38, 1951.

BROADBENT, T. R., MASTERS, F. W., and PICKRELL, K. L.: *A new compression clamp to test and occlude the circulation in pedicle flaps.* Plast. Reconstr. Surg., 12:187, 1953.

CANNON, B., ET AL.: *The use of open jump flaps in lower extremity repairs.* Plast. Reconstr. Surg., 2:331, 1947.

CANNON, B., LISCHER, C. E., and BROWN, J. B.: *Open jump flap repairs of the lower extremity.* Surgery, 22:335, 1947.

CARPUE, J. C.: *An Account of Two Successful Operations for Restoring a Lost Nose from the Integuments of the Forehead.* Longman, Hurst, Rees, Orme, and Brown, London, 1816. Plast. Reconstr. Surg., 44:174, 1969.

CONVERSE, J. M., and WOOD-SMITH, D.: *Experiences with the forehead island flap with a subcutaneous pedicle.* Plast. Reconstr. Surg., 31:521, 1963.

CONWAY, H.: *Clinical tests for the evaluation of circulation in tubed pedicles and flaps.* Ann. Surg., 135:52, 1952.

CONWAY, H., STARK, R. B., and DOCKTOR, J. P.: *Vascularization of tubed pedicles.* Plast. Reconstr. Surg., 4:133, 1949.

CONWAY, H., STARK, R. B., and NIETO-CANO, G.: *The arterial vascularization of pedicles.* Plast. Reconstr. Surg., 12:348, 1953.

DAVIS, J. S., and KITLOWSKI, E. A.: *A method of tubed flap formation.* South. Med. J., 29:1169, 1936.

DIEFFENBACH, J. F.: *Mémoire et observations sur la Réstauration du Néz.* J. compl. de se méd., 39:162, 1831.

DOUGLAS, B., and MILLIKAN, G. A.: *The blood circulation in pedicle flaps. Preliminary studies on a photo-electric test for determining its efficiency.* Plast. Reconstr. Surg., 2:348, 1947.

EDWARDS, S.: *Evaluation of the open jump flap for lower extremity soft tissue repair.* Ann. Surg., 128:1131, 1948.

ESSER, J. F. S.: *Island flaps.* New York J. Med., 106:264, 1917.

GERMAN, W., FINESILVER, E. M., and DAVIS, J. S.: *Establishment of circulation in tubed skin flaps.* Arch. Surg., 26:27, 1933.

GILLIES, H. D.: *Plastic Surgery of the Face.* Oxford University Press, London, 1920. *The tubed pedicle in plastic surgery.* New York J. Med., 111:1, 1920. *Experiences with tubed pedicle flaps.* Surg. Gynec. Obstet., 60:291, 1935. *Practical uses of the tubed pedicle flap.* Amer. J. Surg., 43:201, 1939.

GILLIES, H., and MILLARD, D. R.: *Principles and Art of Plastic Surgery.* Little, Brown & Company, Boston and Toronto, 1957.

v. GRAEFE, C. F.: *Rhinoplastic order die Kunst, den Verlust der Nase organisch zu ersetzen.* Berlin, 1818.

GOLDWYN, R. M., LAMB, D. L., and WHITE, W. L.: *An experimental study of large island flaps in dogs.* Plast. Reconstr. Surg., 31:528, 1963.

SHIFTING OF TISSUE

GOUMAIN, A. J. M., and FEVRIER, J. C.: *Plastic repair (Les transplants cutanes "en ilot" ou "island flaps" en chirurgie plastique de la face)*. Ann. Chir. Plast., 10: 174, 1965.

HANCE, B., BROWN, J. B., BYARS, L. T., and McDOWELL, F.: *Color matching of skin grafts and flaps with permanent pigment injection*. Surg. Gynec. Obstet., 79:624, 1944.

HORSLEY, J. S.: *Transplantation of the anterior temporal artery*. JAMA, 64:408, 1915.

HYNES, W., and MacGREGOR, A. G.: *The use of fluorescein in estimating the blood flow in pedicled skin flaps and tubes*. Brit. J. Plast. Surg., 2:4, 1949.

KERNAHAN, D. A., and LITTLEWOOD, A. H. M.: *Experience in the use of arterial flaps about the face*. Plast. Reconstr. Surg., 28:207, 1961.

KOCH, S. L.: *The transplantation of skin and subcutaneous tissue to the hand*. Surg. Gynec. Obstet., 72:157, 1941.

v. LANGENBECK, B.: *Fragmente zur Aufstellung von Grundregeln für die operative Plastik*. Göschens deutsche Klin., 1849, 1850.

LIMBERG, A. A.: *Plasmimetrie und Stereometrie des Hautplastik: Theorie und praxis für Chirurgen*. Gustav Fischer Verlag, Jena, 1967.

MAY, H.: *Closure of defects after cancer surgery*. Clinics, 4:53, 1945.
A simple device to test and to improve the circulation in a pedicle flap. Surgery, 21:582, 1947.

McFARLANE, R. M.: *The use of continuous suction under skin flaps*. Brit. J. Plast. Surg., 11:77, 1958.

MONKS, G. H.: *The restoration of the lower eyelid by a new method*. Boston Med. Surg. J., 139:385, 1898.

NEW, G. B., and ERICH, J. B.: *The Use of Pedicle Flaps of Skin in Plastic Surgery of the Head and Neck*. Charles C Thomas, Springfield, 1950.

PENN, J.: *Zigzag modification of the tube-pedicle flap*. Brit. J. Plast. Surg., 1:110, 1948.

PERTHES, G.: *Lappenvorbereitung in situ. Ein neuer Weg zur Bildung langer plastischer Lappen ohne Gefahr der Nekrose*. Zentralbl. f. Chir., 44:641, 1917.

PICK, J. F.: *Surgery of Repair*, J. B. Lippincott, Philadelphia, 1949.

deRIVER, J. P.: *Jump method or interrupted tube flaps*. JAMA, 87:662, 1926.

SCHUCHARDT, K.: *Der Rundstiellappen in der Wiederherstellungschirurgie des Gesichts–und Kieferbereiches*. Georg Thieme Verlag Leipzig, 1944.
Der Rundstiellappen bei der Gestaltung von Stümpfen der unteren Extremität. Georg Thieme Verlag Leipzag, 1945.

v. SEEMEN, H.: *Wege und Grenzen der Plastischen und Wiederherstellungschirurgie*. Langenbeck's Archiv für klin. Chir. Deut. Zschr. für Chirurgie, 282:575, 1955.

TAGLIACOZZI, G.: *de Curtorum chirurgia per Insitionem*. Venice, 1597.

WEBSTER, J. P.: *Thoracico-epigastric tubed pedicles*. S. Clin. N. Amer., 17:145, 1937. In Christopher: *Textbook of Surgery*. W. B. Saunders, Philadelphia, 1942.

WOUND HEALING
AND TREATMENT 3
OF WOUNDS

A WOUND may be defined as a traumatic separation of the skin, mucous membrane, or surface of an organ. A wound is either simple, if no deeper tissues are involved, or compound, involving such structures as muscles, nerves, tendons, and bones. The form of the wound depends upon its cause. The wound due to cuts has smooth edges, does not show involvement of the surroundings, and bleeds freely. It is linear if the cutting force penetrated vertically; it is flap-like if penetrated obliquely. Wounds due to contusion have irregular edges. These edges are bluish and elevated, and may be undermined, forming pockets. The surroundings of the wound show abrasions and subcutaneous hematomas, and may have insensible areas. Bleeding may be minimal. Wounds due to tear show an irregularity of their edges, as in contused wounds, but less involvement of the surroundings.

The immediate consequences of a wound are local pain and bleeding, and—in extensive deep wounds—general shock, collapse, and anemia.

THE HEALING PROCESS

Before discussing the treatment of wounds it is necessary to speak of the various processes which lead to wound healing, since a rational treatment of wounds ought to further the healing process as well as prevent additional damage and infection.

121

GENERAL PRINCIPLES

Wound healing is a many-faceted conglomerate of biological phenomena which are regulated by complicated biochemical processes. Original studies were done by Cohnheim, Virchow, Marchand, Grawitz, Ziegler, and Maximow, and culminated in a wide-ranging discussion of this topic during the Tenth International Medical Congress in Berlin in 1890. Primary attention was paid then and during the subsequent decades to the morphohistological changes during the healing process; these were masterfully described by Marchand in 1901.

A heated discussion was carried on over the origin of the cell forms participating in the inflammatory reaction. Maximow postulated that blood elements are precursors of the infiltrating round cells capable of changing into fibrous tissue formation, while Marchand, Ziegler, and Grawitz denied such a possibility. Even the advent of tissue culture and transparent chamber technique, histochemistry and electron microscopy has not yet definitely settled this issue. Allgöwer has surveyed the history of the dispute recently and has summarized evidence from his own experiments in favor of a blood-borne progenitor.

During recent decades important advances have been made in the studies of other facets of wound healing, which go hand in hand with our knowledge of the growth and metabolism of connective tissue, its change in response to injury, hormones, metabolic disturbances and disease, and confirm Marchand's definition of wound healing as a reaction of the fibrous tissue. Moreover, it is now possible to distinguish among alterations in the ground substance, in the cellular reaction, and in the formation of collagen. The whole topic has been recently discussed in a symposium on Wound Healing and Tissue Repair, edited by W. Bradford Patterson, as part of the Developmental Biology Conference Series (1958), as well as in a volume edited by Sir Charles Illingworth, and during the 79th Annual Meeting of the Deutschen Gesellschaft für Chirurgie, from which the discussions of Kuhnau and Linder are most notable.

We distinguish healing by primary and secondary intention. A wound heals "per primam" if its edges are healthy and remain in close approximation to each other so that epithelial cells bridge the wound. If, however, the edges are devitalized or separated or become so, the resulting defect has to be first filled and bridged by granulation tissue before it finally becomes a scar. This is healing by "secondary intention." In both cases the morphological and other changes do not differ qualitatively, only quantitatively.

Healing by Primary Intention

Depending upon the extent of the injury, the reaction of the body is local or both local and systemic. The local tissue reaction is in form

122

of an acute inflammation which constitutes not only the first defensive reaction but the initial stage of repair as well. It starts with a dilatation of the vessels and the escape of plasma; the plasma changes into fibrin, which dries and forms a scab, acting only as a protective cover. Under this dry and inactive tissue the true wound exudate develops. This consists of a "fluid" (or gel) coming from tissue spaces and from ruptured blood vessels. This exudate is invaded by certain types of cells which speed the removal of the inciting cause and the devitalized tissue; these are polymorphonuclear leukocytes and histiocytes which by phagocytosis and autolysis remove the necrotic tissue and foreign bodies and organisms (destructive or lag phase of wound repair). Almost simultaneously, capillaries and fibrous tissue cells invade the fibrin. In closely adapted wound edges epithelial cells regenerate from the epidermis and grow over the newly formed fibrous tissue (regenerative phase of wound repair), completing the scar which holds the wound edges firmly together.

However, it seems that the epidermis does not unite at the surface but migrates rapidly toward the depth of the wound (Edwards and Dunphy) under dissolution of the previously formed fibrin clot (Clark and Clark), until it reaches a point of tissue continuity. Here the advancing epidermal sheets from opposite sides meet. The epithelial junction thickens and tends to fill in the defect left by its inverted growth down the dermal wound edges.

Healing by Secondary Intention

In wounds in which a more or less wide defect has to be filled, the healing occurs by secondary intention. The wound exudate which develops beneath the protective scab is invaded by the same phagocytic and autolytic cell types (leukocytes, histiocytes) as in "per primam" healing. The proteolytic ferments also liquefy the scab, which is thrown off after a few days; this is the lag phase of wound repair. As the cellular exudation of acute inflammation subsides, the regenerative phase of the healing process becomes evident. It is dominated by the development of granulation and connective tissues. Each granule contains a capillary loop which is formed from endothelial cells of the peripheral inflamed vessels and is its core; it is covered with phagocytes and fibroblasts. This granulation tissue detaches the necrotic tissue through a process of demarcation until finally the entire wound is covered by it. It forms a protective wall against invasion of organisms and is the main source of the development of the final scar. Simultaneously, epithelial cells grow from the epidermis of the wound borders over the granulations, or from preserved epithelial islands, thus gradually closing the wound.

While the origin of the endothelial derivative of the granulations is known, the source of the proliferating fibroblasts is still widely disputed. This has been discussed in two fine collective reviews by Van Winkle, who believes that several cells of mesodermal origin may, under the proper stimulus, differentiate into functioning fibroblasts. At first they proliferate; in the second stage of their activity collagen fibrils are formed by intracellular synthesis (Jackson) and extracellular deposits. Later the fibrils increase in number and size and form fiber bundles, while the number of fibroblasts decreases. There is no longer active cellular division, but instead there is fiber production, which principally accounts for the tensile strength of the scar. Differentiation sets in later and consists of absorption and/or changing the direction of the abundant fibers and enlarging or increasing the number of the oriented fibers present.

The role the ground substance—the interfibrillary and intercellular cement—plays in the healing process of the wound is not yet well understood. The German histologists, starting with Kölliker, distinguished an amorphous substance or gel and a cement substance in the Grundsubstanz, findings which seem to be supported by modern evidence, including electron microscopy. Histological methods, however, are insufficient to define the nature of these substances. Histochemical staining and direct chemical analysis, electron microscopy, and radioisotope studies are expected to provide new information about the ground substance and its role in the healing process of the wound (Karl Meyer, Jackson, Weiss, Dunphy et al., Gross and many others).

A major factor contributing to wound healing is contraction, a process by which a full-thickness skin defect, i.e., a wound, shrinks in size; this process is distinct from the phenomena of exudation and epithelization. It starts one to two days after injury and may well be a physiochemical process resulting from reorientation and shortening of the collagen network. It is uncertain whether contraction is caused by shrinkage within the granulation tissue (Carrel, Lindquist, Eicholz, Abercrombie, Flint and James, Billingham and Russell), or by marginal activity such as a sphincter-like action of contracting narrow tissue bands (Grillo and co-workers). This topic has been well covered by Van Winkle.

Complications

There are numerous local and systemic factors that can influence the normal process of wound healing, such as disturbances of circulation, infection, disturbance of the electrolyte balance, hypoproteinemia, vitamin deficiency, and, last but not least, "stress." Obviously, elimination of disturbing factors and corrections of the deficiencies accelerate the healing process (see pp. 137, 152). The extent of the damage must also be considered: The greater the amount of tissue necrosis, the longer the time required for phagocytosis and repair. Hence, a properly débrided and excised wound is apt to heal more quickly and with fewer complications than a wound that contains much devitalized tissue. Furthermore, a wound heals most quickly and with fewest complications if it heals by primary intention, i.e., without the formation of granulation tissue. This is the rule in wounds in which the wound edges can be closely coapted, but it can and should also be brought about in extensive surface defects if it is possible to apply a skin graft for immediate coverage, even if the skin graft acts only as temporary measure, as a biological dressing. A more detailed discussion of wound healing beneath skin grafts is found on page 27. If a wound is left to heal by secondary intention—i.e., the development of granulation tissue—there is constant danger of infection, epithelization will be only partial, as already mentioned, and some scar formation is the rule. A scar can become harmful if it contracts or, because of instability, breaks down. Hence, wound healing by secondary intention, useful as it may be in closing the raw surface, can be harmful if it results in infection or in contracting or unstable scars. The latter may be prevented by early coverage of the granulation with skin grafts, or better still by inhibition of growth of granulation tissue through primary closure of the surface defect with a skin graft or pedicled flap, as already emphasized.

TREATMENT OF WOUNDS

In treating traumatic wounds, one must realize two facts: first, a traumatic wound is an emergency; second, a traumatic wound is contaminated. Through the trauma, organisms are carried from the surrounding skin, the cloth, or the medium that produced or contacted the wound, into the wound. These organisms remain along the wound tract and on the necrotic tissue for about six hours (Friedrich). Later, they adapt themselves to the new surroundings and commence to multiply and to penetrate into the deeper tissue and lymph channels, the stage of contamination thus passing over into the stage of infection. Therefore, the first six hours constitute a period of relative safety, and it is desirable to treat a wound within this time. The emergency arises from complications, such as hemorrhage and shock. Wound therapy has two general divisions: emergency treatment and final, or definitive, treatment.

EMERGENCY TREATMENT

Anyone who undertakes the emergency treatment of a wound should be cognizant of the fact that he harms more than helps if he secondarily infects the contaminated wound by touching it with the fingers or by covering it with soiled cloths, or if he uses antiseptics which harm the cells of the tissues more than the organisms they attack.

Control of Hemorrhage

Control of hemorrhage, if present, should be the first step of the emergency treatment. This, as a rule, can be accomplished by placing sterile gauze over the wound and using a *pressure dressing*. If sterile gauze is not at hand, freshly laundered linen may be used instead. If the latter is not available, it is better to leave the wound open than to use soiled linen.

In bleeding that cannot be controlled by the pressure dressing, one may apply direct digital pressure proximal to the wound upon the main artery. The use of a *tourniquet* on an injured extremity, particularly in cases of crush injuries, should possibly be avoided since—according to the findings of Blalock and Duncan—the addition of local ischemia and anemia to trauma results in more deleterious effects than are caused by trauma alone. If some form of constriction is necessary, the temperature and thus the metabolic processes of the distal part should, if possible, be lowered by artificial means (surrounding the extremity with ice) (Allen, Blalock, Brooks, and Duncan).

Posthemorrhage Therapy

These steps consist in preventing or combating shock (p. 156), relief of pain with morphine (in severe pain morphine or demerol is injected intravenously, one half to two thirds of the subcutaneous dose), administration of antibiotics, and immobilization and elevation in case of an injured extremity. The patient should then be sent immediately to a place where the final treatment can be carred out.

FINAL, OR DEFINITIVE, TREATMENT

The final treatment should be carried out as soon as possible, that is, as soon as the patient is admitted, unless he is in shock, which must be treated first (p. 156). The final treatment of the wound consists of either an excision of the wound or débridement of it. Wound excision (von Bergmann, Friedrich, von Gaza, Lexer, Duval, von Seemen, Fuss) is permissible only within the stage of contamination, while débridement—removal of retained débris as recommended by Désault and popularized by Baron Larrey during the Napoleonic Wars—is still permissible during the infected stage. Therefore, wound excision and débridement are not synonymous terms (Hook).

126

WOUND HEALING

The general consensus is that all wounds up to six hours after their inception—and those over six hours up to twelve hours that exhibit no definite evidence of infection—are considered to be in the stage of contamination. There may be exceptions where the stage of contamination is prolonged, particularly if antibiotics have been used during the emergency treatment. Wounds coming under treatment during the stage of contamination are best treated by wound excision. Before any operative treatment is instituted, however, an examination for possible nerve, tendon, bone, and other injury should be carried out.

WOUND EXCISION AND PRIMARY SUTURE

Preoperative Preparation

Wound excision should be performed under the same aseptic precautions as any other aseptic operation. It may be done under local or general anesthesia, according to the circumstances. After the patient is undressed, the emergency dressing is removed and the wound covered with sterile gauze. The surroundings of the wound are now shaved (old blood, dirt, grease, and the like having previously been removed with benzene or ether). The direction of the shave is away from the wound, not toward it. The skin is cleansed with soap and water (Lexer, Koch, and Mason), or pHisoderm (p. 4), the wound itself still remaining protected with sterile gauze. The soapy solution is rinsed away with sterile water. Then follows cleansing with alcohol unless pHisoderm has been used, and the operative field is now draped.

Technique

The operation itself starts with the excision of the skin edges, which should be as economical as possible; a contused wound will require removal of more skin than a cut wound. Knife and forceps are now discarded and gloves changed. The excision of the lining of the entire wound tract follows; retractors should be inserted to open up every tract and sinus. All devitalized tissue, foreign bodies, and loose bone must be removed, the instruments being frequently changed. To expose deeper parts of the wound, longitudinal extension of the wound by incisions may be necessary. Hemorrhage is controlled by ligation of the bleeding vessels; severed tendons and nerves are sutured. If the abdominal cavity is open, the peritoneum should be closed and the abdomen opened for inspection through an incision elsewhere. The wound is then closed. No buried sutures should be used if possible. The skin sutures should be interrupted

127

and not too close to each other, allowing the exudate to escape; this might otherwise accumulate and interfere with primary healing. An aseptic pressure dressing is applied which eliminates dead spaces, counteracts the accumulation of exudates and hematomas, and avoids stasis. In the case of an extremity, the injured part is immobilized by proper splinting or by the use of a closed circular plaster cast without padding; the limb is then elevated. (For regional wound surgery, see following chapters.)

If a wound has resulted in a surface defect, the defect should be closed primarily, either (1) by mobilization of the wound edges and skin sliding, with or without relaxation incisions (local flaps) and strictly avoiding tension on the wound edges, or (2) by means of free skin grafts or distant flaps. If coverage requires a flap rather than a graft, but transfer or construction of the flap must be delayed, the raw surface should be covered temporarily with a skin graft to counteract development of granulation tissue and thus the possibility of infection and cicatrization.

It is well known that wounds in certain regions, such as the face, scalp, and hands, heal primarily in a much higher percentage of cases than those in the inguinal and perineal regions. Hence, in the first class of wounds one may safely perform wound excision and primary closure after the twelfth hour; in the second class of wounds, even within the first six hours, open treatment after proper wound excision, followed by secondary closure, is safer (see p. 130). Wounds from human bites are always badly infected and should not be closed primarily, unless treated very early (Curtin and Greeley, Crikelair and Bates). Dog bites, however, can more often be closed primarily after thorough excision, since they cause less infection. The saying "clean as a hound's tooth," however, may be misleading, and thorough treatment with antibiotics is essential.

After-Treatment

The after-treatment of an excised and primarily sutured wound does not differ from that of any other aseptic wound, except for the routine administration of antibiotics (see p. 137). Sutures should be removed between the fifth and seventh days, in facial wounds before the fifth day. However, if there is any evidence of disturbance of the primary healing process, the dressing should be changed earlier and the wound inspected. It is important to recognize a wound infection before complications arise. The struggle between the defense system of the wound and the remaining organisms starts only a few hours after the injury. A wound infection, in overcoming the defense system, gives rise to local and general symptoms: pain, redness, rise of pulse and temperature, and general malaise.

Immediate support of the defense system by local and general measures is now paramount: removal of some or all sutures, spreading of the wound edges to allow exudate to escape, proper drainage, immobilization, application of local heat—dry or moist. The infective strain of organisms should be isolated, its sensitivity to all available antibiotics determined, and the proper antibiotics administered in sufficient quantity. Frequent blood transfusions may become necessary. If in spite of all local and general support the infection is spreading, a wide incision with thorough drainage may be lifesaving; amputation in a rapidly progressing anaerobic infection may be considered (p. 136).

WOUND EXCISION AND DELAYED PRIMARY CLOSURE

War wounds, with the exception of wounds of the face, skull, hands, chest, abdomen, and large joints, as well as severe compound injuries of the extremities in civilian life, should be treated by the open method, since there is more tissue necrosis than in ordinary wounds. Orr's experience of World War I, Trueta's experience during the Spanish Civil War, and the World War II experience of American, British, and German surgeons (Baily, Bürkle de la Camp, Moorhead, Ravdin, Long, and many others) have settled this question. While the principle of immediate treatment—thorough cleansing and excision of the wound and leaving it open—remains sound, the aftercare of such a wound has changed considerably during these years.

The Carrel-Dakin antiseptic treatment of earlier years consisted of frequent dressing (at least once daily) with antiseptic agents, of which there were many, cleansing the granulations, and contributing in other ways to a disturbance of wound healing and promoting infection instead of combating it.

A remarkable advance in open treatment was the closed plaster-cast method applied to wounds of the extremities by Orr, who was followed by Trueta, Löhr, and others. This method was based on the sound principle of encouraging local defense against infection by support and rest. The plaster is applied directly over the wound, which has been excised and packed with gauze; no padding is used except over prominent parts; the cast is not split; no window is cut; the extremity is elevated. In this way, absolute rest for the wound is assured, edema counteracted, and consequently satisfactory circulation maintained. The cast is changed after two weeks unless there is evidence of infection, and the wound is allowed to heal by secondary intention. The disadvantages are undue prolongation of the healing process, danger of secondary infection, and necrotization and sequestration; the resulting scar tissue may be contracting, adherent, and unstable.

129

All this can be avoided by the so-called "delayed primary suture," i.e., closure of the wound after four to ten days if the wound looks healthy. And so the third phase of the aftercare of open-wound treatment was entered, at first hesitantly during the end of World War II, later enthusiastically during the Korean War (Fisher and others). The antibiotics may be credited with this advance; where local antiseptics failed, they have given safety to early closure of the excised wound.

Technique (Delayed Primary Suture)

The initial treatment consists of thorough cleansing, excision and débridement of the wound, insertion of a drain if necessary, application of a petrolatum-gauze pressure dressing and plaster-cast immobilization in the case of an extremity, elevation of the extremity, and antibiotic administration. Closure of the wound follows in four to ten days, whereby the appearance of the wound, not the length of time, is the governing factor, as Fisher has aptly pointed out, with minimum to moderate drainage and healthy-looking pink granulations. If this is the case, delayed primary suture should be undertaken. If it is possible to approximate the wound edges without much mobilization and tension, the wound margins are excised, together with all granulation tissue, and the wound sutured loosely with interrupted stitches. If tension is expected or one is in doubt, it is wise to use a split skin graft to cover the granulating area. Thus, the immediate purposes of closure of the raw area and control of infection are achieved. If the area requires more stable tissue, a graft replacement with a pedicled flap may be considered later. Immobilization is maintained and antibiotic treatment carried out for at least another ten days.

There have been recent trends to delay not only the primary closure but also the wound excision and débridement. Iselin treats all his compound hand injuries with "urgence avec opération différee" (deferred urgency): the surrounding area is cleansed, severed tissue is removed, hemostasis is undertaken if necessary, and then the wound is dressed. The dressings are changed daily, while the definitive treatment, including reconstructive measurements, is deferred up to three to five days. Iselin reasons that after this time the patient's general condition is improved, infection and edema are combated, the line of demarcation is established, and the patient can be operated on under optimum technical conditions; in an emergency situation this may not be the case. Although these reasons are sound, and others, notably Scharitzer of Germany, have proven the rationality of this treatment based on a large number of cases, most surgeons will hesitate to apply the treatment routinely until more widespread experience is gained with it.

130

WOUND HEALING

Maxillofacial Wounds

Wounds of the face require special consideration. In dealing with facial injuries, one must realize that the ultimate outcome depends heavily upon the initial repair. Except for patients having evidence of cerebral injuries, thorough repair of the wounds should be performed to obtain a minimum of deformity and disfigurement. An accurate preoperative evaluation of the extent of the injury is, of course, necessary. This may include neurological and x-ray examinations. The local treatment starts with preoperative cleansing, which should be performed with soap and water or pHisoderm (p. 4). Dirt-stained or oil-impregnated wounds should be thoroughly cleansed with a scrub brush. It is quite easy to remove foreign bodies at this time, but it may be difficult or impossible after healing has taken place. Since infections in the face are rare and gas gangrene almost unknown, the majority of the wounds can be closed primarily, even if seen eighteen to twenty hours after the accident, unless they are badly contused and soiled. The excision of the wound should be as economical as possible. After change of instruments, inspection should follow for damage to deeper tissues, such as muscles and nerves. A divided Stenson's duct should not be overlooked. It is relatively easy to suture it at this time with an end-to-end suture over a dowel (see p. 214). Later, repair work is difficult.

Fixation: Facial fractures should be treated at this stage. Fixation of fractured jaws is aimed at the restoration of normal occlusion of teeth and the function of mastication. The jaws may be temporarily immobilized by bandaging and interdental wiring. Such appliances if needed and not available immediately can be applied a few hours after the wound is sutured (Chap. 12). Depressed fractures, such as those of the nose, orbit, and zygoma, should be elevated.

Suture: Closure of the wound should be thorough. Buried sutures of fine cotton or catgut may be necessary for approximation of deeper structures to avoid dead spaces. Closure of the skin follows, with fine nylon or silk, preferably with an atraumatic needle. Known points if present (vermilion border, nostrils, rim of eyelids) are approximated first, thus facilitating closure of complicated wounds. In long linear wounds, the first suture is placed in the center, thus dividing the wound in two halves, which are divided again, etc. The sutures should not be placed too close together. Drainage is not necessary, except in bad compound fractures that require dependent drainage.

GENERAL PRINCIPLES

Extensive Loss of Soft Tissue and Bone: If the wound has resulted in an extensive defect of soft tissue and bone, an attempt should be made to close the surface defect with a sliding local flap (p. 17). If this is impossible, the following reconstructive steps, recommended by Ivy, are indicated: (1) Arrest of hemorrhage; counteracting loss of control of tongue and thus danger to respiration by pulling the tongue forward with either a suture or a safety pin and anchoring it to the dressing; débridement of the wound and wound excision if necessary; fixation of bone fragments in approximately normal position by wires or other extraoral appliances (Chap. 12); adjustment of torn tissue flaps; dependent drainage; and systemic administration of antibiotics. (2) Final reduction and fixation of the fragments of the mandible by special splints (such as those made of acrylic resin), affording a clear view of the underlying teeth and gum tissue and providing feeding space. (3) After all wounds look clean and healthy, transplanting a flap to cover the soft-tissue defect (pp. 77 and 87). (4) Three months later, replacement of the bone defect with a bone graft unless there has been infection, in which case one ought to wait six months before transplanting bone, and preoperative and postoperative antibiotic therapy. (5) Provision of artificial dentures to replace lost teeth.

Wounds of Hand

For wounds of the hand, see page 797.

Wounds of Joints

Scott's vast experience with joint injuries in the British Armed Forces of World War II confirmed the teaching of Bartos and Mazo that the period of time within which surgical cleansing of a joint wound is possible is longer than for other wounds. It seems that wounds of synovial membrane and articular cartilage are more resistant to infection than any other wound; consequently, the joint capsule can be closed primarily after proper cleansing of the joint spaces long after wounding and in the presence of gross contamination. The periarticular tissue and skin can also be closed loosely if the patient is treated within a few hours of the injury. Otherwise, it is left open and closed secondarily after a few days (p. 130), although the joint capsule is always closed primarily. The limb is immobilized in a plaster cast, and antibiotics are administered. The synovial membrane, however, acts as a barrier to the transmission of drugs from the bloodstream. Hence, it is advisable to introduce penicillin (about 100,000 units in 3 cc. of sterile water) into the joint after closure. A window is then cut into the cast. If the joint swells postoperatively, it should be aspirated as often as necessary; after each aspiration, penicillin is introduced. If the joint becomes actually infected, aspiration must be replaced by drainage.

Wounds of Bones

Since the advent of antibiotics, treatment of open fractures is aimed at closure of the skin wound at the earliest time compatible with safety, either by primary or delayed primary suture or by secondary suture. A certain standardization has thus evolved, based on the vast experience of such authorities on the subject as Watson-Jones, Bürkle de la Camp, Böhler, Key, Magnuson and Stack, Furlong, and others.

The general principles of the treatment can be merely summarized here. Under general anesthesia, cleansing of the involved region is similar to the method described on page 4. The majority of surgeons prefer to operate without the aid of tourniquet. The wound is excised and débrided with minimal sacrifice of viable tissue. The displaced fragments are reduced as accurately as possible by traction and manipulation. Internal fixation, if not vitally needed, should not be used. A substitute can be provided by two Steinmann pins, one through the proximal and one through the distal fragment away from the wound, as recommended by Moore. They are incorporated in the cast.

The wound is sutured with interrupted sutures if the patient is treated within the first ten to twelve hours after the injury. If, however, there is much destruction and crushing of the soft tissues, the wound is left open. In war injuries, the wound is always left open. If primary suture is precluded by loss of surface tissue, a split skin graft should be applied as a temporary measure at this stage; flaps, however, should not be rotated at this time. The wound is covered with petrolatum gauze and a pressure dressing applied, followed by application of a plaster cast, with immobilization of the joints above and below the fracture; the limb is elevated and antibiotic treatment administered.

In wounds that have been left open, delayed primary suture or, in the case of a surface defect, split skin grafting is performed between five and ten days later, as outlined on page 130, unless infection has intervened. These procedures can be carried out through a large window in the cast. Wounds that have been left open and cannot for any reason be practicably closed by delayed primary suture may be permitted to heal by granulation and closed at the earliest time possible. The wound edges must then be excised, as well as the granulations, and the wound edges sutured together. Since this is not often possible without much undermining and tension, it is advisable to cover the granulations with a split skin graft, which, after healing has taken place, can be replaced by more stable tissue, such as that provided by skin sliding or a rotation flap or flaps from distant parts.

WOUNDS IN STAGE OF INFECTION

General Considerations

Generally speaking, a traumatic wound is considered contaminated during the first six hours, becoming infected during the following six hours, and being infected after twelve hours. If, however, antibiotics have been used during the first six hours, the stage of contamination may be prolonged to twenty-four hours and longer. Ordinarily, however, any wound coming under treatment twelve hours after injury should be considered infected and should not be excised. At that time, the defense mechanism of the wound is being built up against the organisms that have adapted themselves to the new surroundings and become invasive. Hence, any extensive operative procedure would break down rather than support the defense of the wound.

Procedure: Débridement in the original sense of the word (Désault, Larrey)—that is, removal of retained débris—may be safely carried out, but any procedure resulting in breaking down the defense mechanism, as wound excision would do, should be avoided. The wound is gently spread, retained debris is removed, and a piece of gauze (plain or petrolatum) is inserted to the depth of the wound. However, if there is evidence of deep infection, incision for free drainage, with removal of dead tissue, should be carried out. The next step consists of supporting local defense by promoting hyperemia and exudation—immobilization and elevation of the extremity, application of local heat, moist or dry, and administration of antibiotics.

The first dressing of the wound may remain in place for several days; if the wound looks clean and free of infection, delayed primary suture can be carried out (p. 130). Where there had been actual infection, however, but the infection remains controlled, promotion of granulations and demarcation and elimination of necrotic tissue should be the policy of further treatment; this may be achieved by local and general measures. Dakin's solution is beneficial if necrotizing processes are present; scarlet red and mercury ointments stimulate formation of granulations; crystal sugar (need not be sterile) sprinkled over the wound and covered with petrolatum gauze promotes exudation owing to its hygroscopic properties; balsam of Peru is an excellent deodorant; cod-liver oil, owing to its bactericidal properties and its vitamin content, is highly recommended to promote early liquefaction of dead tissue and to stimulate granulation

134

and epithelization. The value of ACTH or cortisone (Alrich et al., Baxter et al. [see also p. 152]) in promoting wound healing has remained doubtful. Closure of the wound with skin sliding, grafts, or flaps should be carried out at the earliest time compatible with safety.

TETANUS

Tetanus, also called lockjaw or trismus, is caused by the anaerobic *Clostridium tetani*; its toxin acts upon the neuromuscular end-organs, causing spasm and rigidity of the voluntary muscles. In mild cases, only a local rigidity of a single muscle group near the wound is present. In the generalized form, a typical clinical picture develops, characterized by trismus, stiffness of the jaw, and risus sardonicus, soon followed by painful clonic spasm of the spinal group of muscles, precipitated by external stimuli. The incidence of the disease has diminished since introduction of immunological methods.

Treatment

Prophylaxis by active immunization with tetanus toxoid has apparently greatly diminished tetanus. Those having had active immunization should have a booster dose of 1 cc. of toxoid in case of wounding. In all patients without a history of active immunization in whom the wound has been caused under circumstances that may have introduced the tetanus bacillus, a prophylactic dose of tetanus antitoxin (5000 international units) should be injected after preliminary skin testing for sensitivity to horse serum. All patients who have a history of sensitivity to sera or previous administration of tetanus antitoxin are given 500 units of human tetanus immune globulin intramuscularly. The dose should be repeated after seven days if the possibility of tetanus is great. The disadvantages of the passive immunization are numerous: its effect is short (seven to ten days); it neutralizes only the toxins which circulate through the bloodstream, not those which have entered the cells; and in spite of all precautions (desensitization) it still causes anaphylactic reactions of more or less severity, even death. Active immunization is free of these dangers, and yet provides for a greater protection than passive immunization. This topic has been thoroughly discussed recently during the 79th Annual Meeting of the Deutschen Gesellschaft für Chirurgie, notably by Bürkle de la Camp, Eckman, Scherer, Tilmann, Greisser et al, and Hills and Sykes. The consensus of opinion is to advocate strongly active immunization; in patients who have no history of active immunization and have a wound which may or may not require injection of tetanus antitoxin serum, it is better to start with active immunization than to use the serum, which provides only imperfect and transient protection and may cause untoward side effects. Serum treatment together with active immunization should be reserved as already mentioned for those wounds which have been caused under circumstances making introduction of the tetanus bacillus highly suspicious. The most important prophylactic step, however, is early excision and débridement of the wound.

Should infection become established, the only hope of cure lies in early diagnosis and prompt treatment. The latter consists mainly of heavy sedation with barbiturates or paraldehyde or continuous infusion of a dilute solution of pentothal sodium; wide excision of the wound; early tracheotomy (strongly recommended by Hills and Sykes); 2000 to 3500 international units per kilogram of body weight of tetanus antitoxin injected intravenously after preliminary testing for sensitivity to horse serum; daily repetition of smaller doses (20,000 units); and infiltration of the wounded region with 10,000 units before excision of the wound. If the skin test is positive, rapid desensitization should be carried out to permit injection of a therapeutic dose. Antibiotic treatment is of no value in combating the tetanus bacillus itself, but may be useful in checking secondary infections.

GAS GANGRENE

Clostridium welchii, together with a great variety of other anaerobic gas-producing clostridii, is the common cause of clostridial myositis, or gas gangrene. The characteristic clinical signs are pain, swelling, crepitation of the tissues surrounding the wound, a dry appearance of the wound, a thin, brown, watery, foul-smelling discharge, moderate fever, high pulse rate, low blood pressure, and evidence of toxemia. Serial roentgenograms, for evidence of gas in the soft tissues, may be of diagnostic value.

As far as treatment is concerned, nothing short of surgery can save the patient's life. Altemeier summarizes the treatment as follows: Radical surgery is required as soon after diagnosis as possible. The operation embraces multiple incision for decompression and drainage of the fascial compartments, excision of the involved muscles, or open amputation, if necessary, followed by adequate immobilization of the affected part. Polyvalent gas-gangrene antitoxin is administered before and after surgery—50,000 units every four to six hours, as indicated, to aid in the control of the toxemia. Penicillin is injected in very large doses, up to 1,000,000 or more units, every three hours before and after surgery to aid in the control of the infection. After its obvious control, the dose of penicillin may be gradually reduced. Other antibiotics should also be

136

administered. Streptomycin or Terramycin may be given in daily intra-venous doses of 2 gm. Topical use of zinc peroxide ointment on wound surfaces after radical surgery is recommended.

A new treatment with hyperbaric oxygen has been developed for gas gangrene. It consists of forcing oxygen into the blood in the expecta-tion of bringing more oxygen to the infected tissues. (The treatment can be given only at those institutions equipped with a hyperbaric chamber.) Good results have been reported, but there are also risks and fatalities (Colwill and Mandsley). Until more experience has been gained, most physicians will continue with the treatment outlined above.

SUPPORTIVE THERAPY

In patients with extensive, complicating, infected wounds, general supportive measures are of great value for stimulating local and general health, such as correcting secondary anemia, hypoproteinemia, or any vitamin deficiency, particularly of vitamin C. Hypoproteinemia results in retarded fibroplastic proliferation and delay of wound healing (Thompson, Ravdin, Rhoads and Frank, Rhoads, Koster, and Kasman, Co Tui). This should be counteracted by transfusions of blood and plasma and a high-protein diet (see p. 165). Vitamin C is essential to wound healing (Arey, Lanman and Ingalls, Hartzell, Winfield and Irvin, Hartzell and Crowley, Bartlett, Jones, and Ryan). Deficiency of vitamin C results in failure of conversion of the precollagen substance of the scar to collagen. Moreover, the proliferating connective-tissue cells remain in a state of immaturity (p. 122). These two factors may delay the healing process of a traumatic wound. Daily doses of from 200 to 300 mg. of ascorbic acid (and even more) are normally given. Administration of iron and exposure to ultraviolet light are also valuable.

ANTIMICROBIAL THERAPY

By Michael A. Manko, M.D.

The physician has been helped in the management of infections since the advent of antibiotics. Fortunately, medical science has continued to produce effective drugs even though organisms continue to develop resistance. Because of the large number of antibiotics available today and the constantly changing pattern of organism resistance, the physician must keep abreast of this dynamic field. Knowledge gained as a student, intern and resident must be updated frequently in order to give the patient the best care possible in the management of his infection.

Penicillin and streptomycin were the first two antibiotics available to the physician, and when used together they do offer a certain broad-spectrum effect. Unfortunately, this combination of drugs is frequently ordered by the physician for prophylaxis and oftentimes also when there is a suspicion that an infection has developed. The indications today for the use of antibiotics for prevention of infection are very few. The use of prophylactic drugs in a rheumatic heart patient undergoing a surgical procedure, and also in a patient having an open heart procedure, is definitely indicated. Aside from these two situations, one must show very strong reasons to justify prophylactic antibiotics. After a surgical procedure, the physician must observe carefully for any early signs of infection. If these are detected, he must try to determine the organism or organisms causing the infection. This can first be accomplished by doing a gram stain on the exudate if it is obtainable. Also, a culture of the specimen can be taken and disc sensitivity studies performed as a means to selecting the proper antibiotic. The physical characteristics of the infection can help to determine the likely etiologic agent, as can a knowledge of the natural course of infection followed by certain organisms. The foregoing is important because if the etiologic agent is known or suspected the physician can prescribe the antibiotic most effective for that particular infection. Thus he avoids the "blind" use of antibiotics which many times are ineffective and sometimes harmful.

Antibiotics have been of great value in the treatment of infections. Because of this, there has been a tendency to forget some of the basic principles of surgery. The treatment of a collection of pus is still incision and drainage. If necessary, antibiotics can be used *with* incision and drainage, but rarely should they replace it. This rule applies to abscesses in any part of the body.

A vast number of antibiotics are available today to the clinician, some of them effective against the gram-positive organisms and some against the gram-negative organisms. Some have a broad-spectrum effect, indicating they are effective against both gram-positive and gram-negative organisms, but there is no antibiotic available today that is effective against all bacteria.

Penicillin is the most effective antibiotic in the treatment of gram-positive infections. There are many staphylococci that produce an enzyme called penicillinase. This enzyme acts to make penicillin inactive and, therefore, the staphylococci that produce it are referred to as penicillin resistant. Because these types of staphylococci are now very common, it is necessary for the physician to determine if his patient has an infection with a staphylococcus that is sensitive or resistant to penicillin. If the staphylococcus is resistant, he must use one of the newer penicillins (methicillin, nafcillin, oxacillin, cloxacillin or dicloxacillin). In the treatment of

138

pneumococcus, streptococcus, clostridium and lactobacillus, penicillin is the drug of choice. In addition, the gram-negative cocci, meningococci, and gonococci are sensitive to this drug, and certain gram-negative rods such as Proteus mirabilis and Escherichia coli can be inhibited or killed by high dosages of penicillin.

Allergy to penicillin is not unusual. If the patient has a definite allergy, it should not be used. The patient must also be considered allergic to the newer penicillins, and these drugs should not be used. Toxicity from the penicillins is uncommon; it is manifested by changes in the central nervous system. It will be seen only if the patient is receiving unusually high doses or if he has advanced renal disease and is getting moderately high doses of the drug.

Streptomycin was introduced for clinical use in 1944 by Waksman. It is effective against gram-positive and gram-negative organisms. When this drug is used alone, organisms quickly develop resistance to it; therefore, it should be used only in combination with other drugs. For example, the combination of penicillin and streptomycin is effective in the treatment of the enterococcus group of streptococci. The combination of streptomycin and chloramphenicol is effective against Klebsiella. Of course, in combination with PAS and/or isoniazid, streptomycin is very active against the tubercle bacillus. This drug is given intramuscularly and can cause renal toxicity when used for prolonged periods.

Erythromycin should be used primarily in the treatment of gram-positive organisms and Mycoplasma. It is not as effective as penicillin in the treatment of gram-positive organisms but is much less likely to cause an allergic reaction. If a patient is allergic to penicillin, there are many times when erythromycin can be an adequate replacement.

The tetracycline group of drugs has broad-spectrum activity, but unfortunately many of the gram-negative organisms have become resistant to it over many years of exposure. However, one of the tetracyclines can be used if disc sensitivity studies suggest effectiveness. These drugs are very good in the treatment of Mycoplasma infections. A tetracycline drug can be used to treat clostridial infections if the patient is allergic to penicillin. At this time the tetracycline group consists of: tetracycline, oxytetracycline, chlortetracycline, demethylchlortetracycline, methacycline, and doxycycline. These drugs are equally effective and it appears that there is no important advantage to using one rather than another. The tetracyclines can at times lead to superinfection with Monilia and can cause severe liver disease if used in high intravenous doses.

Chloramphenicol has become a very controversial drug. It is a broad-spectrum antibiotic and has proven to be successful in the treatment of many infections. Unfortunately this drug has a very serious toxic effect on the bone marrow, with resultant aplasia. There are times when high doses of chloramphenicol will cause bone-marrow suppression; this can be reversed when the drug is stopped, but if aplasia occurs the mortality rate is high. The incidence of aplasia following chloramphenicol administration is rare, but since the consequences are so severe it is best not to use this drug unless specifically indicated.

Lincomycin has a spectrum similar to that of erythromycin. A large number of the penicillin-resistant staphylococci are also sensitive to lincomycin. Therefore, if oral therapy is desired for a patient allergic to penicillin, lincomycin can be used. The drug is also available for parenteral use but other antibiotics, such cephalothin and vancomycin, should be used if parenteral therapy is indicated in a patient allergic to penicillin. There is some evidence to suggest that lincomycin is effective in treating bone infections; however, further studies will have to be made to prove its clinical efficacy in the treatment of osteomyelitis.

Vancomycin is useful in the treatment of gram-positive infections, and especially those caused by staphylococci. If a patient allergic to penicillin has a serious staphylococcal infection, vancomycin would be a very good choice. Nephrotoxicity and ototoxicity may result from prolonged use. The physician should use the drug when indicated, bearing in mind the possible toxicity.

Ampicillin is a semisynthetic penicillin. It is one of the newer penicillins but is not effective against the penicillin-resistant staphylococci. This drug has broad-spectrum effects and is very useful, but some gram-negative organisms resist it. Because of this the physician should determine the sensitivity of the gram-negative organism he is treating before assuming the drug will be effective. Ampicillin has been helpful to the clinician in treating Haemophilus influenzae and salmonella infections. Like the other new penicillins, ampicillin is contraindicated in a patient with a history of allergy to penicillin. When ampicillin is given orally, the physician must be aware that diarrhea may develop.

Cephalothin (Keflin) is a semisynthetic derivative of cephalosporin C. Although the structures of the cephalothin nucleus (7-aminocephalosporanic acid) and the penicillin nucleus (6-aminopenicillanic acid) are quite similar, there are differences in the behavior of these drugs, including resistance of cephalothin to degradation by penicillinase. Therefore, cephalothin is effective in the treatment of the penicillin-resistant staphylococci. Cephalothin also has a broader antimicrobial spectrum. Because of this, there is a tendency to use this drug in situations where the etiologic organism is not known. This approach may be successful, but there is danger in it because some gram-negative organisms are resistant to cephalothin. Early experience with cephalothin suggested a lack of cross-allergenicity with penicillin; this of course permitted use of the drug in people allergic to penicillin. Recently there have been reports of patients being allergic to both cephalothin and penicillin. However, definite cross-allergenicity has not yet been established, and therefore the clinician can use cephalothin in a patient allergic to penicillin. When treating such a patient with cephalothin, the physician should have epinephrine available in case of a severe allergic reaction. Pseudomonas is completely resistant to cephalothin and will commonly occur as a superinfection, especially in urine, in patients receiving treatment with cephalothin. This is a drawback to use of the drug and the physician must look for it in any patient being treated with cephalothin. Toxicity is minimal, although neutropenia has been reported.

Cephaloridine is a new analogue of cephalothin. The spectrum and effectiveness of these antibiotics is about the same. Some penicillin-resistant staphylococci have been reported resistant to cephaloridine. This drug does offer some advantages. It is longer acting and can be given every eight to twelve hours, and the intramuscular injection is relatively painless in comparison to cephalothin.

Kanamycin is very reliable. It is also very toxic. This drug is active against most of the gram-negative organisms except Pseudomonas and some of the indole-positive Proteus organisms (morganii, rettgeri and vulgaris). Many staphylococci are sensitive to kanamycin. Because of its potency, the drug is an excellent choice for early use in gram-negative septicemia. When the causative organism has been identified it is wise to switch to a less toxic antibiotic if the sensitivity studies show that this is possible. Kanamycin can cause nephrotoxicity and ototoxicity and, therefore, careful attention must be given to total dosage and to laboratory tests in order to prevent these complications. Despite the toxicity of the drug, it should not be withheld in conditions where it is needed in the treatment of an infection.

Polymyxin B is a potent antibiotic in the treatment of Pseudomonas and other gram-negative infections. It is not effective against Proteus organisms. This drug can be given intramuscularly but procaine should be added to the injection to lessen the pain. Physicians have at times been reluctant to use the drug because of its nephrotoxicity; however, it should not be avoided for this reason if there is an indication for its usage. Most people with normal renal function can tolerate 2 to 3 mg/kg. per day in divided doses for up to two weeks before showing signs of nephrotoxicity. This is frequently sufficient time to have eradicated an infection. In people with abnormal renal function a reduced dose must be given.

Colistin (Coly-Mycin) was isolated in Japan in 1950 and is a member of the polymyxin group of antibiotics. Therefore, the sensitivity pattern of organisms to it is the same as that to polymyxin B. These antibiotics are heavily concentrated in the urine and are, therefore, effective in urinary-tract infections. At the usual doses, colistin is less toxic than polymyxin B and should be used to treat urinary-tract infections. In treating infections elsewhere in the body, polymyxin B is generally superior to colistin. Pain of intramuscular injection with colistin is minimal.

Sulfonamides are useful drugs in treating uncomplicated urinary-tract infections which are usually caused by E. coli. If there are recurrent infections the organisms become resistant to the sulfonamide.

All of the drugs listed above are valuable agents and have reduced surgical morbidity and mortality. However, the dangers of these drugs are significant and they should not be ordered without careful consideration. Toxicity varies with the individual drug and the physician must be aware of this before he writes an order for an antibiotic. He must also know the total condition of the patient; diseases of different organ systems can affect the choice and also the dosage of drugs. Good surgical technique and the discriminate use of antibiotics will greatly reduce the surgeon's problems with infections.

BIBLIOGRAPHY

ABERCROMBIE, M., FLINT, M. H., and JAMES, D. W.: *Wound contraction in relation to collagen formation in scorbutic guinea pigs.* J. Embryol. Exp. Morph., 4:167, 1956.

ABRAHAM, E. P., CHAIN, E., ET AL.:*Further observations on penicillin.* Lancet, 2:177, 1941.

ADELBERG, A.: *Surgical war experiences.* Brit. Med. J., 2:43, 1940.

ALLEN, F. M.: *Surgical considerations of temperature in ligated limbs.* Amer. J. Surg., 45:459, 1939.

ALLGÖWER, M.: *The Cellular Basis of Wound Repair.* Charles C Thomas, Springfield, 1956.

ALRICH, E. M., CARTER, J. P., and LEHMAN, E. P.: *The effect of ACTH and cortisone on wound healing: An experimental study.* Ann. Surg., 133:783, 1951.

ALTEMEIER, W. A., and FURSTE, W. L.: *Gas gangrene.* Surg. Gynec. Obstet., 84:507, 1947.

AREY, L. B.: *Wound healing.* Physiol. Rev., 16:327, 1936.

BAKER, I. D.: *Sulfonamides in traumatic and infected wounds.* J. Bone Joint Surg., 24:641, 1942.

BARON, H.: *Zur Problematik der Wundheilungsstorungen.* Z. f. Therapie, H. 4 u. 5, S. 201-215 u. 276-283, 1963.

WOUND HEALING

BARTLETT, M. K., JONES, C. M., and RYAN, A. E.: *Vitamin C studies on surgical patients.* Ann. Surg., 111:1, 1940.

BAXTER, H., SCHILLER, C., and WHITESIDE, J. H.: *The influence of ACTH on wound healing in man.* Plast. Reconstr. Surg., 7:85, 1951.

BAYLEY, H.: *Surgery of Modern Warfare.* William & Wilkins, Baltimore, 1942.

v. BERGMANN, E.: *Zur Lehre von der putriden Intoxikation.* Deutsche Ztschr. f. Chir., 1:373, 1872.

BILLINGHAM, R. E., and RUSSELL, P. S.: *Studies on wound healing with special reference to the phenomenon of contracture in experimental wounds in rabbits' skin.* Ann. Surg., 144:961, 1956.

BLALOCK, A.: *Effects of lowering temperature of an injured extremity to which a tourniquet has been applied.* Arch. Surg., 46:167, 1943.

BÖHLER, L.: *Die Technik der Knochenbruchbehandlung.* 13th Ed. Whilhelm Maudrich, Wien, 1951. 5th Engl. Ed. Grune and Stratton, New York, 1956.

BONNIN, N. J., and FENNER, F.: *Local implantation of sulfanilamide for prevention and treatment of gas gangrene in heavily contaminated wounds. Suggested treatment for war wounds.* Med. J. Aust., 1:134, 1941.

BOWERS, W. F., and CASBERG, M. A.: *Surgery of Trauma.* J. B. Lippincott, London, 1953.

v. BRANDIS, H. J.: *Praktische und rechtliche Richtlinien zur passiven Tetanusschutzimpfung.* Die Medizinische Wochenschr., 36:1187, 1954.

BÜRKLE DE LA CAMP, H.: *Der derzeitige Stand der Behandlung der Gelegenheitswunde.* Hefte der Unfallheilkunde, 43:11, 1952.
Probleme der Tetanusprophylaxe. Langenbeck's Arch. f. klin. Chir., 301:427, 1962.
Der derzeitige Stand der Behandlung der Gelegenheitswunde Monatsschrift für Unfallheilkunde, 1968, p. 49.
Schock und erste Hilfe am Unfallsart. Ztbl. Verkehrsmed., Verkehrspsych.
Der heutige Stand der tetanus immunisierung. Therapiewoche, 19:43, 1969.

BÜRKLE DE LA CAMP, H., FISCHER, A. W., ET AL.: *Operative Wundversorgung.* Med. Welt., 15:382, 408, 434, 1941.

BÜRKLE DE LA CAMP, H., and BUDRASS, W.: *Wunde und Wundinfektion. Handbuch der gesamten Unfallheilkunde.* Ferdinand Enke Verlag Stuttgart, 1963.

CARPEL, A., and HARTMAN, A.: *Cicatrization of wounds. I. The relationship between the size of a wound and the rate of its cicatization.* J. Exp. Med., 24:429, 1961.

CARRELL, A.: *The treatment of wounds.* JAMA, 55:2148, 1910.

CHAIN, E., FLOREY, H. W., ET AL.: *Penicillin as a chemotherapeutic agent.* Lancet, 2:226, 1940.

CLARK, E. R., and CLARK, E. L.: *Growth and behavior of epidermis as observed microscopically in observation chambers in ears of rabbits.* Amer. J. Anat., 93:171, 1953.

COLEBROOK, L.: *Sulfanilamide and wound infections.* Brit. Med. J., 2:682, 1940.

COLWILL, M. R., MAUDSLEY, R. H.: *The management of gas gangrene with hyperbaric oxygen therapy.* f. Bone. Joint Surg., 50(B):732, 1968.

GENERAL PRINCIPLES

CONWAY, H.: *Principles of wound healing, with indications for the use of the several types of skin grafts.* S. Clin. N. Amer., 32:419, 1952.

CO TUI: *The value of protein and its chemical components (amino acids) in surgical repair.* Bull. N.Y. Acad. Med., 21:631, 1945.

CO TUI, ET AL.: *Nutritional care of cases of extensive burns.* Ann. Surg., 119:815, 1944.

CRICKELAIR, G. F., and BATES, G. S.: *Human bites of the head and neck.* Amer. J. Surg., 80:645, 1950.

CURTIN, J. W., and GREELEY, P. W.: *Human bites of the face. Early treatment and late reconstructive surgery.* Plast. Reconstr. Surg., 28:394, 1961.

DOMAGK, G.: *Ein Beitrag zur Chemotherapie der bakteriellen Infektionen.* Deutsche med. Wchnschr., 61:250, 1935.

DUBOS, R. J.: *Utilization of selective microbial agents in the study of biological problems.* Bull. N.Y. Acad. Med., 17:405, 1941.

DUNPHY, J. E., and UDUPA, K. N.: *Chemical and histochemical sequences in the normal healing of wounds.* New Eng. J. Med., 253:847, 1955.

DUVAL, P.: *Notes on the treatment of flesh wounds in time of war in the surgical formations of the Army.* Med. Bull., 1:273, 1918.

ECKMANN, L.: *Entwicklung und Erhaltung des Impfschutzes beim Starrkrampf.* Langenbeck's Arch. f. klin. Chir., 301:444, 1962.
Tetanus. Benno Schwabe Co., Basel Stuttgart, 1960.

EDWARDS, L. C., and DUNPHY, J. E.: *Wound healing. I. Injury and normal repair.* New Eng. J. Med., 259:224, 1958.
Wound healing. II. Injury and abnormal repair. New Eng. J. Med., 259:275, 1958.

FEKETY, F. R., NORMAN, P. S., and CLUFF, L. E.: *Treatment of gram negative bacillary infections with colistin.* Ann. Intern. Med., 52:214, 1962.

FINLAND, M., ET AL.: *Some recent observations on staphylococcal infections in relation to antibiotic therapy.* Trans. Assoc. Amer. Physicians 64:343, 1951.

FISHER, D.: *Delayed primary closure of Korean war wounds.* Surg. Gynec. Obstet., 96:696, 1953.

FLEMING, A.: *On the antibacterial action of cultures of a penicillium, with special reference to their use in the isolation of H. influenzae.* Brit. J. Exp. Path., 10:226, 1929.
On the specific antibacterial properties of penicillin and potassium tellurite. J. Path. Bact., 35:831, 1932.
Penicillin—Its Practical Applications. C. V. Mosby, St. Louis, 1950.

FLIPPIN, H. F., and EISENBERG, G. M.: *Antimicrobial Therapy in Medical Practice.* F. A. Davis Company, Philadelphia, 1955.

FLOREY, H. W., ET AL.: *Antibiotics: A Survey of Penicillin, Streptomycin, and Other Antimicrobial Substances from Fungi, Actinomycetes, Bacteria, and Plants.* Vols. 1 & 2. Oxford University Press, New York, 1949.

FRIEDRICH, P. L.: *Die aseptische Versorgung frischer Wunden.* Arch. f. klin. Chir., 57:288, 1898.

FURLONG, R. J., and CLARK, J. M. P.: *Missile wounds involving bone.* Brit. J. Surg. War Surg. *Supplement 2—Wounds of the extremities.* 36:291, 1949.

144

WOUND HEALING

GARDNER, D. L.: *Pathology of the Connective Tissue Disease.* Williams and Wilkins, Baltimore, 1965.

v. GAZA, W.: *Grundriss der Wundversorgung und Wundbehandlung.* F. Springer, Berlin, 1921.

GRIESSER, G., BARCK, J., and MAYER, W.: *Klinische Erfahrungen in der Behandlung des schweren Tetanus mit hohen Antitoxin-dosen.* Langenbeck's Archiv. f. klin. Chir., 301:455, 1962.

GRILLO, H. C., WATTS, G. T., and GROSS, J.: *Studies in wound healing. 1. Contraction and the wound contents.* Ann. Surg., 148:145, 1958.

GROSS, J.: *Wound healing and tissue repair.* See Patterson, W. B.

HALL, F. C.: *The value of antitoxin in the prevention and treatment of malignant edema and gas gangrene.* Ann. Surg., 122:197, 1945.

HARBISON, S. P., and KEY, J. A.: *Local implantation of sulfanilamide and its derivatives in wounds.* Arch. Surg., 49:22, 1942.

HARTWELL, S. W.: *The Mechanisms of Healing in Human Wounds.* Charles C Thomas, Springfield, 1955.

HARTZELL, J. B., WINFIELD, J. M., and IRVIN, J. L.: *Plasma, vitamin C, and serum protein levels in wound disruption.* JAMA, 116:669, 1941.

HARTZELL, J. B., and CROWLEY, R. T.: *Vitamin therapy in the surgical patient.* Amer. J. Surg., 56:288, 1942.

HARVEY, S. C., and HOWES, E. E.: *Effect of high protein diet on the velocity of growth of fibroplasts in the healing wound.* Ann. Surg., 91:641, 1930.

HARVEY, S. C.: *The healing of the wound as a biologic phenomenon.* Surgery, 25:655, 1949.

HELLNER, H.: *Die Chirurgische Wundinfektion und ihre Behandlung.* Der Chirurg, 17:385, 1947.

HENDERSON, J.: *Collective review: A summary of the surgical aspects of certain sulfonamide and antibiotic agents.* Surg. Gynec. Obstet. (Intern. Abstr. Surg.), 83:1, 1946.

HERRMANNSDORFER, A.: *Uber den Einfluss der Nahrung auf die Pufferkapazität des Blutes und der Heilverlauf und Keimgehalt granulierender Wunden.* Deutsche Ztschr. f. Chir., 200:534, 1927.

HILLS, W. J., and SYKES, E. M.: *The treatment of tetanus.* Amer. Surgeon, 25:35, 1959.

HOOK, F. R.: *Panel discussion of the war session of the American College of Surgeons.* Bull. Amer. Coll. Surgeons, 27:114, 1942.

ILLINGWORTH, C.: *Wound Healing.* J. & A. Churchill, Ltd., London, 1966.

ISELIN, M.: *Aufgeschobene Dringlichkeit bei der Wundersorgung.* Arch. f. klin. Chir., 301:91, 1962.

IVY, R. H.: *Symposium on military surgery: Plastic and maxillofacial surgery.* S. Clin. North America, 21:1583, 1941.
Early and late treatment of face and jaws as applied to war injuries. South. Surgeon, 11:366, 1942.

GENERAL PRINCIPLES

KAZANJIAN, V. H.: *Primary care of injuries of the face and jaws.* Surg. Gynec. Obstet., 72:431, 1942.

KEEFER, C. S., and ANDERSON, D. G.: *Penicillin in the Treatment of Infections.* Oxford University Press, New York and London, 1945 .

KEEFER, C. S.: *Antibiotics yesterday and today.* Penn. Med. J., 55:1177, 1952.

KEY, J. A.: *Treatment of compound fractures in this antibiotic age.* JAMA, 146: 1091, 1951.

KLEIN, J. O., and FINLAND, M.: *The new penicillins.* New Eng. J. Med., 269: 1019, 1963.

KOCH, S. L.: *Injuries of the parietes and extremities.* Surg. Gynec. Obstet., 76:1, 1943.
The treatment of lacerated wounds. Surgery, 38:447, 1955.

KOCH, S. L., and MASON, M. L.: *Division of the nerves and tendons of the hand.* Surg. Gynec. Obstet., 56:1, 1933.

KOMER, J. A.: *Penicillin Therapy, Including Tyrothricin and Other Antibiotic Therapy.* Appleton-Century, New York, 1945.

KOSTER, H., and KASMAN, L. P.: *Relation of serum protein to well healed and to disrupted wounds.* Arch. Surg., 45:776, 1942.

KUHNAU, J.: *Biochemie der Wundheilung.* Arch. f. klin. Chir., 301:23, 1962.

LANMAN, T. H., and INGALLS, T. H.: *Vitamin C deficiency and wound healing.* Amer. J. Surg., 105:616, 1937.

LARREY, D. J.: *Mémoires de chirurgie militaire.* Paris, 1812, Vol. 1, p. 50.

LEVENSON, S. M., BIRKHILL, F. R., and WATERMAN, D. F.: *The healing of soft tissue wounds: The effect of anemia and age.* Surgery, 28:905, 1950.

LEXER, E.: *Lehrbuch der allgemeinen Chirurgie.* Ferd. Enke, Stuttgart, 1934.

LEXER-REHN: *Lehrbuch der Allgemeinen Chirurgie.* Ferdinand Enke, Stuttgart, 1952.

LINDNER, J.: *Die Morphologie der Wundheilung.* Arch. f. klin. Chir., 301:39, 1962.

LINDQUIST, G.: *The healing of skin defects. An experimental study on the white rat.* Acta Chir. Scand., 94, Suppl. 107:163, 1946.

LOCKWOOD, J. S.: *Symposium on military surgery, prevention and treatment of infections in traumatic wounds.* S. Clin. N. Amer., 31:1739, 1941.
Definition of objectives and the importance of controls in evaluating the local use of sulfonamides in wounds. Surg. Gynec. Obstet., 79:1, 1944.

LOCKWOOD, J. S., WHITE, W. L., and MURPHY, F. D.: *The use of penicillin in surgical infections.* Ann. Surg., 120:311, 1944.

LÖHR, W.: *Ueber die Lebertransalben Behandlung mit und ohne Gipsverband bei frischen Verletzungen, Verbrennungen und Phlegmonösen Entzündungen.* Zentralb. f. Chir., 61:1686, 1934.
Die Behandlung von frischen und älteren Hand und Fussverletzungen mit dem Lebertrangipsverband. Chirurg., 6:5, 1934.

146

WOUND HEALING

MAGNUSON, P. B., and STACK, J. K.: *Fractures.* 5th Ed. J. B. Lippincott, Philadelphia, 1949.

MARCHAND, F.: *Der Prozess der Wundheilung.* Deutsche Chirurgie. 1901.

MARCKS, K. M.: *Soft tissue repair in injuries about the face and head.* Penn. Med. J., May, 1942.

MAY, H.: *Emergency Surgery.* B. J. Ficarro, Ed. F. A. Davis Company, Philadelphia, 1953.

McDOWELL, F., BROWN, J. B., and FRYER, M. P.: *Surgery of Face, Mouth, and Jaws.* C. V. Mosby, St. Louis, 1954.

MELENEY, F. L.: *The past 50 years in the management of surgical infections.* Surg. Gynec. Obstet., 100:1, 1955.

MELENEY, F. L., JOHNSON, B. A., and TENG, P.: *Further experiences with local and systemic bacitracin in the treatment of various surgical and neurosurgical infections and certain related medical infections.* Surg. Gynec. Obstet., 94:401, 1952.

MEYER, K.: *Wound healing and tissue repair.* See Patterson, W. B.

MOOREHEAD, J. J.: *Surgical experience of Pearl Harbor.* JAMA, 118:712, 1942.
War wounds. Amer. J. Surg., 56:338, 1942.
Clinical Traumatic Surgery. W. B. Saunders, Philadelphia, 1945.

ORDMAN, L. J., and GILLMAN, T.: *Studies in the healing of cutaneous wounds.* Arch. Surg., 93:857, 1966.

ORR, H. W.: *Wounds and Fractures.* Charles C Thomas, Springfield, 1941.

OVERTON, L. M.: *The management of open wounds as exemplified in the present European combat.* Surg. Gynec. Obstet., (Intern. Abstr. Surg.), 75:195, 1942.

PADGETT, E. C.: *Severe injuries of the face and jaws.* Amer. J. Surg., 51:829, 1941.
The late care of severe injuries of the face and jaws. Surg. Gynec. Obstet., 72:437, 1942.
Penicillin in warfare: Special issue of the Brit. J. Surg., Vol. 22, July, 1944.

PATTERSON, W. B.: *Wound Healing and Tissue Repair.* Univ. of Chicago Press, Chicago, 1958.

PULASKI, E. J.: *Surgical Infections: Prophylactic Treatment Antibiotic Therapy.* Charles C Thomas, Springfield, 1954.

RAVDIN, I. S., and LONG, P. H.: *Some observations on the casualties at Pearl Harbor.* U. S. Nav. Med. Bull., 40:353, 1942.

REID, M., and CARTER, B. N.: *The treatment of fresh traumatic wounds.* Ann. Surg., 114:4, 1941.

RHOADS, J. E.: *Protein nutrition in surgical patients.* Surg. Gynec. Obstet., 94:417, 1952.

RHOADS, J. E., and HOWARD, J. M.: *The Chemistry of Trauma.* Charles C Thomas, Springfield, 1963.

SCHARITZER, E.: *Die organisatorische Bedeutung der "aufgeschobenen Dringlichkeit" in der Unfall-Chirurgie.* Hefte zur Unfallheilkunde, 1962.

GENERAL PRINCIPLES

SCHERER, F.: *Zur Tetanus-Simultanimpfung des Frischverletzten.* Langenbeck's Arch. f. klin. Chir., 301:447, 1962.

SCOTT, J. C.: *Early treatment of penetrating wounds of joints.* Brit. J. of Surg. War Surg. Supplement 2—Wounds of the Extremities. 36:291, 1949.

v. SEEMEN, H.: *Wundversorgung und Wundbehandlung.* Ferd. Enke, Stuttgart, 1938.

SPAETH, E. B.: *The immediate and late treatment of the injuries around the orbit.* Surg. Gynec. Obstet., 72:453, 1941.

STAFFORD, E. S., TURNER, T. B., GOLDMAN, L.: *On the permanence of anti-tetanus immunization.* Ann. Surg., 140:563, 1954.

Surgery in World War II: The Physiologic Effects of Wounds. (Prepared by Historical Division, Army Medical Library), Superintendent of Documents, Government Printing Office, Washington, 1952.

TAYLOR, W. I., and NOVAK, M.: *Prophylaxis of tetanus with penicillin-procaine.* Ann. Surg., 133:44, 1951.

THOMPSON, W. D., RAVDIN, I. S., and FRANK, I. L.: *Effect of hypoproteinemia on wound disruption.* Arch. Surg., 36:500, 1938.

THOMPSON, W. D., RAVDIN, I. S., RHOADS, J. E., and FRANK, I. L.: *Use of lyophile plasma in correction of hypoproteinemia and prevention of wound disruption.* Arch. Surg., 36:509, 1938.

TILMAN, O.: *15 jährige Erfahrungen mit der aktiven Immunisierung gegen Wundstarrkrampf.* Langenbeck's Arch. f. klin. Chir., 301:453, 1962.

TRÉFOUEL, F. and MME., NITTI, F., and BOVET, D.: *Activité du p-amino phénylsulfanide de la souris et du lapin.* Compt. rend. Soc. de biol., 120:756, 1935.

TRUETA, J.: *Treatment of War Wounds and Fractures.* Paul B. Hoeber, New York, 1940.
The Principles and Practice of War Surgery. C. V. Mosby, St. Louis, 1943.

TURCK, M., ET AL.: *Cephaloridine.* Ann. Intern. Med., 63:199, 1965.

VAN WINKLE, W., JR.: *The fibroblast in wound healing.* Surg. Gynec. Obstet., Collective Review, 124:369, 1964.
Wound contraction. Surg. Gynec. Obstet., 125:131, 1967.
The tensile strength of wounds and factors that influence it. Surg. Gynec. Obstet., Collective Review, 129:819, 1969.

WAKSMAN, S. A.: *Streptomycin: Nature and Practical Applications.* Williams & Wilkins, Baltimore, 1949.

WALLIS, A. D., and DILWORTH, M. J.: *Odor in the Orr treatment of osteomyelitis and its prevention by lactose.* JAMA, 120:583, 1942.

WATSON-JONES, R.: *Fractures and Joint Injuries.* Vol. 1, 4th Ed. Williams & Wilkins, Baltimore, 1952.

WATTS, G. T., GRILLO, H. C., and GROSS, J.: *Studies in wound healing. II. The role of granulation tissue in contraction.* Ann. Surg., 148:153, 1958.

WEISS, P.: *The compounding of complex macromolecular and cellular units into tissue fabrics.* Proc. Natl. Acad. Sci. U.S.A., 42:819, 1956.
Wound healing and tissue repair. See Patterson, W. B.

TREATMENT OF BURNS 4

Historical Phases in Treatment

The treatment of burns has undergone significant change during the past decades, as the vast volume of literature which has accumulated about this subject vividly attests. Among the most recent publications about the burn disease, as it has been aptly called (Bürkle de la Camp), are the monographs and cumulative treatises of Sevitt, Allgöwer and Siegrist, Artz and Reiss, Artz and Montcrief, Blocker, Rehn and Koslowski, Skoog, Bürkle de la Camp, Crews, Moyer et al., Abramson, Wallace, and Moncrief et al. The monograph by E. R. Crews, already in its second edition, is recommended as a down-to-earth approach to the highly complex subject of the burn disease. Up to 1900, the treatment of burns was more or less local. Although laboratory studies were made and the significance of fluid loss and hemoconcentration (Baraduc, Tappeiner) and changes in the morphology of the blood (Wertheim, Lesser) were known, these important facts were, as a rule, not followed up therapeutically. It is estimated that two thirds of the patients burned died from shock and infection. In the beginning of our century, general treatment started to receive more consideration, and was under the influence of the toxin theory. According to the latter, toxic substances are released from the burned area, causing shock and toxemia (Bardeen, Wilms, Pfeiffer, Dale and associates, Cannon, and Bayliss, Robertson and Boyd). The toxin theory lost importance (although it has been revived nowadays in modified form; see Simonart and associates, Fine et al., von Euler, J. Rehn, Bürkle de la Camp, Allgöwer, and Artz) since Underhill and his associates systematically investigated the role of fluid loss in burns (1921 to 1923). Since that time, treatment has gone through four significant phases. Each phase has added a definite improvement, with a lowering of the mortality rate and the lessening of suffering of the patient.

Theory of Hemoconcentration as Cause of Toxemia: In 1921, Underhill and his co-workers had the opportunity of treating twenty-one persons seriously burned in a theater fire in New Haven. At the same time, they made important investigations of fluid loss and blood concentration following burns. Their investigations led them to the conclusion that the clinical picture of toxemia developing in cases of burns is not due to absorption of a toxic substance derived from burned areas but to hemoconcentration. The blood capillaries become injured from the heat and become permeable; this results in a rapid pouring out of fluid on the burned surface and into the tissues, causing marked general edema of the affected part. The rapid and continued loss of fluid from the blood in cases of burns quickly induces a marked concentration of the blood. The condition of the patient depends on the amount of the concentration. Underhill considered restoration of normal concentration of prime significance. His systematic treatment of burns consisted simply of the forcing of fluid by mouth, rectum, hypodermoclysis, or intravenous infusion. Thus, for the first time the important fact of fluid loss and hemoconcentration, although known before, was systematically followed therapeutically, and the dynamic phase of fluid and electrolyte therapy was entered, not only in the treatment of burns but also in other fields of surgery (Crile, Walters, Coller and Madock, Lockwood and Randall, and more recently by Hamit, Fine, Dillon et al., Seeley et al., Moyer, Sorenson and Sejrsen, and others).

Role of Plasma: Remarkable as was the recognition that hemoconcentration, or hypovolemia (i.e., disproportion between circulating volume and the capacity of the vascular system), was the major factor in causing burn shock and toxemia, the recommended treatment did not hold what it had promised, since the escaping fluid was not merely water. Tappeiner (1881) pointed out that death from burns was due to hemoconcentration from loss of plasma, and he was one of the first to advise the infusion of serous fluids. Later, Bayliss for the same reason recommended intravenous use of 6 per cent gum acacia. It was not, however, until much later that their advice was appreciated; this came about mainly through the investigations of Blalock, McIver, McClure, Harkins, Elman, Scudder, Moon, Lee, Elkinton, Wolff, Rhoads, Black, Hecht and Weese, and Schultz. A fine collective review of this subject has been published by Ravdin and Ravdin.

150

TREATMENT OF BURNS

Normally, fluid is kept from leaking disproportionally through the capillaries by the colloid osmotic pressure of the plasma proteins in differential concentrations on either side of the semipermeable capillary membrane. If, as in burns, the capillaries become injured and permeable plasma or a fluid closely corresponding to plasma escapes from the circulation in abnormal amounts, the osmotic pressure is reduced within the capillaries. If, in such a state, aqueous solutions are injected, as in Underhill's treatment, the plasma proteins become diluted to a concentration that makes it impossible to hold the fluid given either intravenously or by other means into the bloodstream. In other words, in severe burns the more that aqueous solutions are administered, the more that fluid is poured out. What is needed is the replacement of the lost plasma. Weiner, Rowlette, and Elman were among the first to stress the importance of replacing the lost plasma by plasma infusions; they also reintroduced the intravenous use of gum acacia, because of its colloidal properties.

Elkinton, Wolff, and Lee, Cope and co-workers, Hegemann, and others state that the capillary permeability with continued shift of plasma and its proteins to the extravascular spaces in burns lasts from thirty-one to forty hours. During this period, excessive hemoconcentration may be prevented by small, repeated transfusions of plasma or plasma expanders. After the capillaries have regained their impermeability to protein, the deficit of plasma protein may be corrected quantitatively by a large transfusion of plasma or plasma expander.

Role of Red Cells: Until recent years, plasma alone has been considered the proper colloid to replace the loss. Whole-blood transfusions have been considered harmful, since they might increase the cellular constituents of the blood with its high cell concentration. However, it has been demonstrated by Colebrook and associates, Cope, Moore, and associates, Evans and Bigger, Raker and Rovit, Brooks and Dragstedt, Kerr, Bürkle de la Camp and others that a thermal burn causes a deficit of the blood volume due to loss of red cells from actual destruction or from being "sludged" or trapped in large masses in the capillaries in and adjoining the burned area, resulting in an anemia. The actual magnitude of the red-cell loss in burned patients, however, could not be accurately estimated because of technical difficulties of red-cell volume measurement. It was not until the introduction of radioactive isotopes into clinical practice that it became feasible to make accurate measurements by means of preparations of suitably labelled red cells. Muir, who carried out such studies, came to the conclusion that red-cell destruction during the shock period is usually not great. The hour-to-hour changes of hemoglobin or hematocrit are valid guides to estimate the plasma volume unless there is

151

positive evidence of severe red-cell destruction: hematocrit falling, but shock not improving in spite of plasma treatment; hemoglobinemia or hemoglobinuria appearing or recurring some hours after burning (early appearance has not the same significance); long tail in the fragility curve. Hence he advises that whole blood not be given routinely to patients with severe burns at an early stage of the shock period but massive transfusions of bank blood should be given during the second day where in general the hemoglobin or hematocrit of the peripheral blood is a reasonable guide to the red-cell volume. Taplay et al. came to similar conclusions.

Role of Sodium and Potassium: Another recent addition to our knowledge of the burn problem is that of severe sodium deficiency, which in itself may aid in the production of shock (Cope and Moore, Roberts, Fitts, Ravdin, Rhoads, Evans, Blocker, Rehn and Koslowski, Moyer et al., and others). Associated with the rapid drop in serum sodium there is a period of sodium retention, usually lasting several days. Following the period of retention, the kidneys as a rule excrete large amounts of fluid sodium. Hence, contrary to the previous consensus, it is now believed that large quantities of sodium should be given in the early phase of burn treatment. Moyer and his associates go so far as to maintain that burn shock is not primarily aligemic, but is mainly related to extravascular sodium deficiency, and that administration of balanced salt solution alone is highly successful in the treatment. Their thought-provoking work has been published in a recent monograph. In a few of our severely burned patients there appeared to be actual damage to the kidneys themselves, with necrosis of the tubular epithelium, resulting in a discharge of excessive amounts of urine. Therapy must then be concentrated upon balancing the electrolytes.

The role that potassium plays in shock is not well understood (Pearson, Soroff, Arney and Artz). A certain degree of potassium depletion seems to occur, but rather in the terminal stages than in the beginning of shock; since renal control of potassium is not so exacting as that of sodium, losses may continue in the face of severe deficit and require special replacement of this ion.

Role of Hormonal Defense: The role of the adrenal cortex in traumatic shock has increasingly become the focus of attention. Swingle and co-workers, Heuer, Andrews, and others showed that adrenal ablation led to shock; this was subsequently found to be due largely to salt depletion. Intravenous administration of adrenal cortical extract was recommended, but the results were questionable and sometimes even harmful. Further research, however, culminated in Hans J. Selye's startling theory and concept of how stress causes disease through the general adaptation syndrome, an expression of adrenocortical activity in response to a wide variety of pathological states.

152

Selye derived his concept from animal experiments. When an animal was subjected to stress, there was an "alarm reaction," i.e., a quick response of the body to the attack by a nervous defense, which had long been known to physiologists, and by an even more important hormonal defense, which was recognized by Selye. According to his theory, the pituitary gland pours out hormones, which in turn stimulate the adrenal glands to pour out others and thus adapt the body to all kinds of stress. If the stresses continued, the alarm reaction was followed by a period of adaptation, "adaptation syndrome," during which the animal learned to live with its stress. If the strain continued or the defenses were inadequate, the "stage of exhaustion" was reached, with reappearance of signs of the alarm reaction, ending finally in death. Autopsy showed a striking variety of pathological changes, which looked like those in human victims of heart and circulatory disorders, arthritis, kidney damage, and other conditions. Evidently, the breakdown was caused by excessive production of hormones by the pituitary and adrenal glands as an emergency defense against stress. After intensive research, Selye found the somatotropic hormone (STH) of the pituitary and desoxycorticosterone (DCA) of the adrenal cortex responsible for it. It became obvious that if STH and DCA could produce a host of diseases, there must be a mechanism to control them or other hormones to neutralize them, since otherwise the resulting pathological changes would be common. Thus, Selye's work foreshadowed the discovery of ACTH and cortisone.

The general consensus is now that the combat mechanism of the body goes into action in response to assault—in burns, for example—and is initiated by the pituitary, which increases the output of ACTH, the adrenocorticotropic hormone of the hypophysis, which in turn stimulates the adrenal cortex to increased secretion of some twenty-five corticosteroids. Of the latter, cortisone (compound E) and hydrocortisone (compound F) are considered the principal hormones basically needed in the defense against injuries that threaten life. Hence, it seems inviting to administer ACTH and cortisone in the treatment of severe burns, thus supporting the defense system of the body (Rehn and Whitelow, Adams and associates, and others).

This subject, however, is quite controversial, since deleterious effects have been reported after such treatment (Evans and Butterfield, Derber and Hegemann). It is also theoretically conceivable that under severe shock the pituitary and adrenal glands are in a condition of maximal stress; further stimulation may be compared to whipping a tired horse, thus inviting rather than preventing a breakdown. On the other hand, it must be admitted that the adrenal response may not be maximal and further adrenal stimulation might be crucial in helping the patient over the critical period. At present, we have no way of evaluating the adrenal cortical reserves. Hence, if strengthening of the hormonal defense is considered replacement therapy with hydrocortisone is safer than whipping with ACTH. Further studies on eosinopenia after secretion of corticotropin (Rud) may become helpful in estimating the strength of the hormonal defense system. All hormones have definitely proved to be ineffective in reducing the abnormal capillary permeability in recent burns (Cope, Raker). More successful treatment is to be expected when more is known of the hormonal basis of shock. In this respect Hardy's publication is enlightening.

Classification of Burns

Thermal burns are usually classified according to penetration. The *first-degree* burn, combustio erythematosa, is characterized by erythema of the skin from enlargement of the dermal vessels due to paralysis of their nerves. The *second-degree* burn, combustio bullosa, is characterized by formation of blisters between the epidermis and the corium. Crews justifiably subdivides this category into superficial and deep second-degree burns. In *third-degree* burns, combustio escharotica, the entire epidermis is destroyed. The eschar is hard and insensitive, brownish or black; the vessels are thrombosed; and the surrounding parts exhibit burns of first and second degree.

Clinical Picture

The clinical picture of a burn depends mainly upon the extent of the involved area. Minor burns cause only local reaction; extensive burns (Verbrennungskrankheit, or burn disease, as it is aptly called in German by Bürkle de la Camp), however, cause general reaction, which may run through the following stages: primary shock, secondary shock, acute toxemia, septic toxemia, healing, or death.

Shock: Shock, in general, is divided into primary and secondary shock. *Primary* shock is the collapse that follows the trauma immediately, and is probably due to pain and to various other reflexes and psychological factors; it is usually not of serious consequence. *Secondary*, or traumatic or hypovolemic, shock is the circulatory collapse that follows one hour after the injury, and is characterized by pallor, cyanosis of lips, cheeks, and extremities, cold, moist, sweaty skin, rapid, shallow respiration, poor pulse volume, collapsed peripheral veins (central venous pressure monitoring, p. 159, may be a valuable aid), restlessness, nausea, vomiting, falling blood pressure, subnormal temperature, increased hematocrit readings, and leukocytosis. In burns, as in other trauma, primary and secondary shock may merge imperceptibly. Comprehensive discussions of this vast subject have been presented recently by Eufinger and by Allgöwer and

154

TREATMENT OF BURNS

Siegrist, Moyer and Butcher, Hamit, and Fine. According to Allgöwer and Siegrist, the following evaluation of signs and symptoms of shock patients is helpful in determining the degree of shock and grouping the cases and recognizing and treating the dangerously ill ones:

(1) Imminent Shock: a. Cold, normotonic tachycardia (cold extremities, pulse 100 to 120, blood pressure over 100 mm. Hg). As a rule such patients have not lost more than 30 per cent of their blood volume. Transfusions are recommended. There is no immediate danger of death, but close watch is necessary since the blood pressure may be deceptively high on account of pain.

b. Cold hypotonic bradycardia (cold extremities, pulse under 100, blood pressure under 100 mm. Hg). Patient feels faint due to vagus stimuli; the vessels of the skin enlarge without increase of the pulse volume.

(2) True Shock: Cold hypotonic tachycardia (cold extremities, sweaty skin, pulse over 100, blood pressure under 100 mm. Hg, most often 80 mm. Hg or lower, cessation of urine secretion). As a rule, such patients have lost more than 30 per cent of their blood volume. If the blood pressure decreases below 70 mm. Hg and the pulse accelerates above 140, life of the patient is in danger. The patient feels nauseated, thirsty, and restless.

Toxemia: The well-known syndrome of toxemia follows extensive burns within the first three or four days, if the patient survives the secondary shock. There is no agreement on the nature of toxemia. The fact that it can occur or persist after the capillaries have regained their impermeability would exclude hemoconcentration as the sole cause; absorption of toxic substances (see p. 149) and infection may also play a role. Vomiting is the first evidence of beginning toxemia. It is soon followed by a typical syndrome characterized by mental and physical disturbances. The patient becomes restless, complains of thirst and pain, and at times is delirious; he is unable to retain food; temperature rises and remains high; and the condition soon assumes a septic character. Pulse and respiration are fast. The tongue is dry; the blood pressure may remain normal. Leukocytes are markedly increased (25,000 and more). The urine is scanty and concentrated; albumin and acetone may appear. Hemoconcentration with a rapid increase in the hematocrit readings, although present early, may reach its peak at the onset of the toxic stage. Blood chlorides and plasma proteins are reduced, blood sugar and nitrogen elevated. This picture of toxemia may last from one to two weeks. Then, if the patient survives, his mental and most of his physical disturbances clear up. However, there may remain an elevated temperature and pulse, marked leukocytosis, and evidence of secondary anemia and hypoproteinemia until the greater part of the raw surfaces has healed.

GENERAL PRINCIPLES

Infection, as already mentioned, is partly responsible for the toxemia syndrome, but toxemia may recur later, days or weeks after the symptoms of acute toxemia have disappeared. The symptoms and findings of septic toxemia (Wilson) resemble those of any other surgical septicemia. The prognosis is grave; fatal signs are apathy and semiconsciousness. Blood pressure drops; the pulse becomes thready and the respiration accelerated and shallow; vomiting, diarrhea, clonicity, coma, collapse, and a marked rise in temperature precede the fatal issue.

TREATMENT OF EXTENSIVE BURNS

The treatment of extensive burns can be divided into immediate and late treatment. The *immediate* treatment consists of combating shock, toxemia, and infection. The *late* treatment consists of combating malnutrition, covering the raw surfaces with skin grafts, and rehabilitation.

IMMEDIATE TREATMENT

Management of Burn Shock

Almost every patient with extensive burns exhibits some evidence of shock, which must be treated before proceeding with local treatment. Everything must be done to combat shock, and everything must be avoided that would increase it. Pain is relieved with morphine or demerol intravenously (one half to two thirds of the subcutaneous dose). The clothes are removed with the least disturbance to the patient. It is now imperative to estimate and chart the extent of the burned area and the patient's weight. The extent of the burned area is estimated according to a modified Berkow chart (Fig. 49). A rough estimate is also the rule of nine which, according to Knaysi, Crikelair, and Cosman, was first used by Pulaski and Tennison: head-neck is estimated at 9 per cent; each arm, 9 per cent; anterior trunk, 18 per cent; posterior trunk, 18 per cent; each leg, 18 per cent; genitalia, 1 per cent. To estimate the extent of smaller burn areas, Allgöwer recommends the palm of the hand as guide; it constitutes roughly 1 per cent of the body surface. The time that has elapsed since the onset of the burn is recorded. The burned area is wrapped in sterile sheets, the foot of the bed or stretcher is elevated, and the patient is wrapped in blankets and kept comfortably warm without overheating. Inhalation of oxygen may be of value, particularly in respiratory-tract burns, which have been revealed as the principal killer of burned patients (Phillips

156

and Cope). Such burns must be recognized early so that fluid and electrolyte administration is limited to the minimum effective to prevent pulmonary edema. A tracheotomy may be greatly beneficial and therefore should be performed early. The patient is observed for any physical sign of shock (see pp. 154-155). Thirst is often an outstanding sign, as are quickening of the pulse and reduced pulse volume, cold extremities, and collapsed veins.

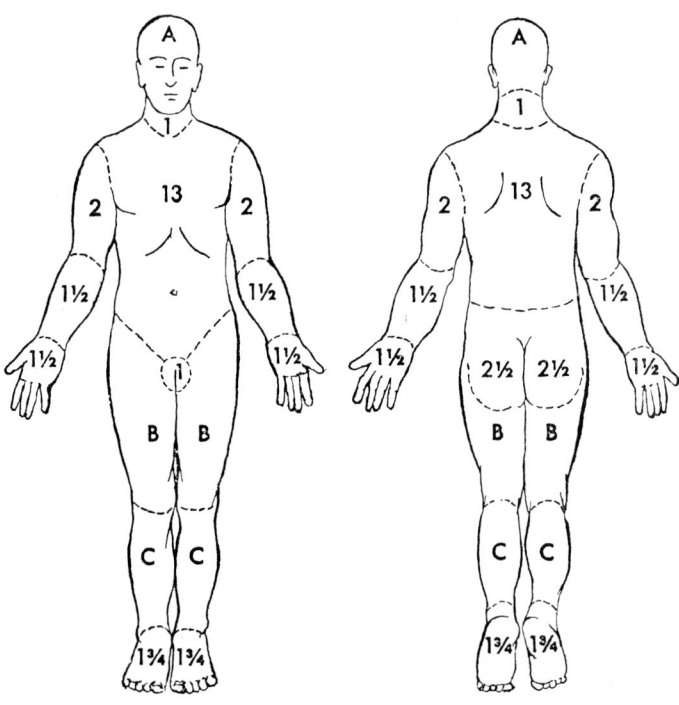

Relative Percentage of Areas Affected by Growth

	Age in Years					
	0	1	5	10	15	ADULT
A — ½ of head	9½	8½	6½	5½	4½	3½
B — ½ of one thigh	2¾	3¼	4	4¼	4½	4¾
C — ½ of one leg	2½	2½	2¾	3	3¼	3½

Total Per Cent Burned _____ 2°+ _____ 3°= _____

Fig. 49. Estimation of body surface expressed in percentage.

157

GENERAL PRINCIPLES

Restoration of Fluids: While the foregoing procedures and observations are carried out, the most important measure to combat shock is undertaken: the replacement of fluid losses and the restoration of blood volume by continuous intravenous infusion of colloids (including blood) and electrolyte solution. As already mentioned, Moyer and associates, who have enthusiastic followers (Dillon et al., Sorenson and Sejrsen, Shirer, and others), do not use colloids at all. From studies of well-conducted burn clinics in the United States and abroad, it is now possible to relate the extent of the burned surface to the volume of fluid loss, which is proportionate. The volume of fluid infused intravenously must correspond to the patient's requirements. There are many formulas for the administration of proper amounts of fluids during the shock phase. The hourly urinary output is one of the most important guides to proper fluid and salt therapy, although it is limited by insensible and, in burns, highly variable loss of fluid from lungs, normal skin, and burned surfaces (Hardy et al., Moncrief, and Moyer). Insertion of an indwelling catheter in the urinary bladder is advised; the bladder is emptied, and the hourly urinary output is from then on recorded. Next, a small polyethylene tube is inserted in one of the ankle veins or in any other available vein to provide blood samples for typing, cross-matching, and hemoglobin and hematocrit estimations; the latter two determinations should be repeated every six hours for the first forty-eight hours. In extensive burns, a suitable colloid solution (plasma, plasma expander, whole blood) and electrolyte solutions are given at once and administered rapidly enough to secure a urinary output of 25 to 50 cc. during the first hour.

Following the lead of the Germans (Hecht and Weese, Schulz), who developed the synthetic colloid polyvinylpyrrolidone (PVP), this and other plasma expanders, chiefly dextran, have been found as effective and safe as pooled plasma. This subject has been critically reviewed by Gropper et al., Ravdin, and Gruber and Siegrist. Evans, whose formula has been widely adopted here and abroad, determines the quantity of colloid solutions to be given during the first twenty-four hours (from time of burn, not from time of fluid start) by multiplying the patient's weight in kilograms by the percentage of body surface involved in second- and third-degree burns. One word of warning is in order: Do not overestimate the area; to overestimate is the tendency. The Evans formula uses saline as electrolyte replacement and uses the same quantity of colloid replacement —blood, plasma, or dextran. The Brooke Army Hospital formula advocates lactated Ringer's solution as the electrolyte replacement and gives this in greater quantities than the Evans formula. It also uses colloids usually in the form of plasma or dextran and in lesser quantity than the Evans formula. Hence, the Brooke formula is a compromise between the Evans

158

formula and Moyer's advocation not to use colloids at all. The author has switched from the Evans formula to the Brooke formula.

BROOKE FORMULA

Fluids During First 24 Hours

a. Colloid (blood, plasma or dextran)—Wt. in kg. $\times$ % burn $\times$ 0.5 cc.
b. Electrolytes (lactated Ringer's solution)—Wt. in kg. $\times$ % burn $\times$ 1.5 cc.
c. Water Requirement (5% dextrose in water)

Adults—   Children—
    2,000 cc.   1 yr.—80 cc. per kg.
                                   5 yrs.—60 cc. per kg.
                                   8 yrs.—40 cc. per kg.

Calculate more than 50 per cent burn as 50 per cent. Little or no colloid is required in second-degree burns. Most third-degree burns do best when colloid in above formula is minimized.

Half of this amount is given within the first eight hours and the remainder within the next sixteen hours. For the second twenty-four hours, only one half of the colloid and half of the lactated Ringer's solution of the first twenty-four hours is administered, plus 2000 cc. of 5 per cent dextrose in water.

This formula, however, should not be followed blindly. In extensive burns, for example, in which the hemoglobin level is more than 19 gm. per 100 cc. and the urinary output is low, more whole blood than plasma is needed; the required colloid solution should then be made up of two parts of whole blood to one of plasma. Less than the estimated amount of fluid should be given to children, older people, those having respiratory-tract burns, and those with over 40 per cent body-surface burns, to prevent pulmonary edema. Each patient must be closely watched. The urinary output and hemoglobin and hematocrit determinations serve as important guides, but are not the only ones used in fluid therapy, since they can mislead. For instance, the hematocrit level may remain normal throughout the shock phase if cells and plasma are lost at the same rate.

Clinical signs and symptoms, such as thirst, rapid pulse, reduced pulse volume, cold extremities, and collapsed veins, have at least as much value as laboratory findings. Monitoring of central venous pressure may be a valuable aid during the initial rapid infusion stage. The cannula should be inserted through the external jugular vein into the vena cava. In general, after the first forty-eight hours, if a good urinary output and a hemoglobin level below 19 gm. are maintained, it is no longer necessary

159

to administer intravenous colloid and electrolyte solutions; by that time every patient takes adequate amounts of fluid and food by mouth. Occasionally, gastric dilatation must be watched for; this may simulate return of shock, with signs of peripheral circulatory collapse and declining urinary output, in spite of adequate fluid intake. A Levin tube should then be passed for gastric suction.

It may be deemed advisable to strengthen the hormonal system. The pros and cons of such therapy have been discussed on page 153.

Admission Order

The following is a routine admission order for the management of a severely burned patient before local treatment. This is a modification of Blocker's admission order. (1) Emergency sedation if required. (2) Typing and cross-matching of blood; draw blood for complete blood count and hematocrit; repeat in twelve hours. (3) Oxygen if required; inspect for respiratory-tract burns. (4) Intravenous colloid, electrolyte and glucose therapy, according to formula (p. 159). (5) No food by mouth for twenty-four hours except by special order. (6) Temperature, pulse, respiration, and blood pressure every two hours for eight hours, then every four hours. (7) Skin test for tetanus antitoxin; administer 1500 units or, if patient has had tetanus toxoid, give 1 cc. booster dose. (8) Insert retention catheter and record hourly volume of urine (25 cc. per hour minimal satisfactory output) for twenty-four hours, then by eight-hour periods; immediate urinalysis; repeat in twelve hours. (9) Record intake and output of fluids on proper form; record emesis volume. Record intake separately for forced feeding. (10) Routine bacteriological culture. (11) Penicillin, 300,000 units parenterally every twenty-four hours. (12) Photograph patient. (13) Record history and physical examination for medicolegal records. (14) Local treatment.

TREATMENT OF THE BURN WOUND

Only after shock treatment is initiated and the patient's general condition stabilized should treatment of the burn wound be undertaken (see Case 108, p. 1134). The treatment of the burn wound is ever changing. What was enthusiastically used in the 1920s, i.e., eschar-forming substances as tannic acid, triple dye, etc., was condemned in the 1930s when the closed pressure dressing treatment became popular. In the 1940s the latter had to give way in popularity to the exposure treatment. Both treatments have been challenged recently by a host of other innovations. Moyer's 0.5 per cent silver nitrate treatment applied continuously with compress is supposed to be bacteriostatic and does not interfere with epidermal proliferation. Electrolytes, however, must be carefully checked to avoid imbalance from sodium chloride depletion. Monafo apparently can prevent such imbalance by using colloidal silver complex instead. Dominguez and associates have put the silver nitrate method to test by treating one hundred burn patients by exposure and one hundred patients with 0.5 per cent aqueous silver nitrate solution. This revealed that the latter did not improve the hospital course nor the mortality but it resulted in a qualitative change in the bacterial flora of the burn wound. From the Brooke Army Hospital Moncrief and associates found a significant lowering of the mortality rate by using Sulfamylon in a water-dispersable base. This is singularly significant since the Brooke Army Hospital probably has the most active burn center in the world. The Sulfamylon supposedly permeates the eschar and diffuses into the subeschar areas; thus it is effective even in the presence of subeschar bacterial invasion while silver nitrate is not. Aluminum powder is used by Lindsay as topical treatment, silicone immersion by Weeder, Brooks and Stephen. It is beyond the scope of this book to go into details of the various treatments of the burn wound, but the two standard treatments which have thus far stood the test of time will be described—those of pressure dressing and exposure.

The advantages of the *pressure dressing*, which according to Blair was first advocated by White (1762) and later by Baynton (1797), are elimination of dead spaces, control of oozing, limitation of venostasis and lymphostasis, and reduction in the flow of plastic material into the wound This method was popularized in the treatment of burns by Allen and Koch in 1942. The dressing consists of covering the wound with gauze, which is impregnated with a bland ointment, followed by application of a heavily padded pressure dressing. The *exposure treatment*, which has been reintroduced by Wallace of Britain, followed by Blocker and Pulaski, and Artz et al. in this country, consists of exposing the burn wound to the air, thus permitting the exudate to dry (within two or three days), to form a hard crust that serves as a natural, occlusive, protective cover for the wound; in deep burns, the dead skin itself forms the occlusive eschar. Hence, as Artz points out, exposure is not an "open method" of treatment because the wound is not left open for invasion of bacteria (except by faulty application of the method), but becomes closed by natural covering.

There are protagonists for each method. The purpose of each is to produce a dry wound, free from infection, and comfortable to the patient. The exposure treatment seems to be preferred at the present time. However, it appears to be far from ideal, and should not be used exclusively. Its success depends much on the rate and effectiveness of drying of the burn wound by exposure to air. Encircling burns of the limbs and trunk, which would require the utmost care to obtain a dry wound, are as a rule better treated by the closed method. Burns of the hand should also be treated by the closed method, which permits immobilization in the position of function and minimizes edema formation, both important factors to counteract dysfunction (see p. 799). It must be pointed out that aftercare of the burn wound requires much more attention in the exposure treatment than in the closed method. On the other hand, in disasters the exposure treatment is the method of choice, since it requires little immediate care and no dressings.

Technique of Pressure Dressing

The patient is placed on an operating table, which is covered with a sterile sheet. The operating-room personnel is prepared as for any other aseptic operation. Oil or grease, if it had been used as a first-aid treatment, is removed with ether. The area around the burn—not the burn itself —is gently washed with soap and water; if, however, the burn wound is dirty, it should be gently sponged with saline solution. Blisters should not be opened; the unopened blister is a fine dressing and provides protection for the new epithelium growing beneath it, as Moyer aptly points out. The entire area is then flushed with copious amounts of warm isotonic saline solution and dried. The injured surface is now smoothly covered with a few layers of fine-meshed sterile gauze, impregnated with petrolatum. Over this are laid a half dozen layers of flat, dry gauze and a mass of gauze fluff, and over the fluff a layer of cotton or mechanic's waste to provide, under the retaining bandage, a resilient covering that produces an even pressure over the injured extremity or the burned surface without causing constriction. An elastic bandage is then applied. Burned limbs are immobilized with splints and elevated. This dressing remains for ten days unless there is evidence of infection. It is changed under sodium pentothal anesthesia. In third-degree burns, sloughs, which start to separate around the tenth day, are excised, and moist dressings with saline solution are applied, followed perhaps later by Dakin's solution to hasten elimination of sloughs and by 3 per cent acetic acid solution dressings in case of Bacillus pyocyaneus infection (see p. 29 for discussion on combating this organism). The dressings are changed every day and all loose slough excised. If the wound becomes infected, the dressings are changed several times daily (see p. 164). Excision of all slough should be completed, necessarily under anesthesia, between the second and third week so that skin grafts can be applied as early as possible (see p. 166). Enzymatic and chemical débridement of slough is still in the experimental stage although hopeful advances in this direction are being made (Connell et al.).

TREATMENT OF BURNS

Technique of Exposure Treatment

The initial cleansing is similar to that described in the foregoing paragraph. The patient is then placed in bed on a sterile sheet, and the burned areas are exposed to the air; burned extremities are elevated. The spraying of powder, such as collodion (Bürkle de la Camp), over the burned area to facilitate quick drying has been recommended. The burned surface should not be in contact with the bedclothes or with other parts of the body. In body burns the sheets are kept away with the aid of a cradle. Electric light bulbs or heat lamps are strongly contraindicated. In circumferential burns of the lower extremities, in which ankles and feet are almost always spared, elevation and exposure may be achieved by placing the feet over folded blankets; a wooden board should be placed beneath the mattress under the buttocks. A Kirschner wire extension (the wire drilled through calcaneus and beneath the tibial tubercle) may be more suitable. In burns of the arms, elevation may be by means of a sling around the wrist, the sling being fastened to an intravenous pole, or by Kirschner wire extension. In spite of these measures encircling burns may be difficult to expose adequately; therefore, they are as a rule better treated by pressure dressings. In some very extensive circumferential burns, however, exposure is indicated to facilitate the total care of the patient. The patient should be placed on a rotating frame (of the Stryker type) and turned at two-hour intervals, thereby permitting the formation of an adequate eschar. The wound usually dries within two to four days to form crusts over partial-thickness burns and eschar over full-thickness burns. The coagulum should now be inspected daily for cracks. Loose parts around the cracks are trimmed; Blocker covers these areas with a single-layer gauze dressing, moistened with saline solution. In spreading infections, crusts and eschars should be excised and moist dressings applied. The exposure treatment ends in partial-thickness burns when complete healing has occurred, and in full-thickness burns when autolysis is evident beneath the eschar. This occurs within the second week. All loose eschar is excised and the burned area is covered with moist dressings (see above). Raw surfaces or granulating areas should never be exposed. If some of the slough has not separated by the end of the third week, all of it should be excised under light anesthesia and the area prepared for skin grafting. Skin grafts should be applied as early as possible, as a rule between the twentieth and thirtieth postburn days (see page 166).

Complications of the Burn Wound

In third-degree circumferential burns of the extremities the eschar at times contracts to such a degree as to cause circulatory disturbances.

Swelling of the uninvolved parts distal to the eschar is the first sign. If this occurs one must act promptly to ward off necrosis of the limb (White and Kaplan). Immediate decompression by means of multiple longitudinal relaxation incisions through the entire length and thickness of the eschar down to the muscles frequently results in return of the circulation and salvage of the limb. When a finger is entirely surrounded by an eschar, prophylactic lateral relaxation incisions are advisable to prevent necrosis of parts or the whole of the finger.

Treatment of the Infected Burn Wound: If a burn wound becomes infected, the treatment as outlined above as a rule will be sufficient to combat the infection. But in some cases the infection is or has become so stubborn that it resists every attempt at treatment—whether antimicrobial, local, or general; grafts fail to take or may take initially but gradually slough away; the donor areas may not heal and also become infected; the patient becomes progressively worse and may die unless the infection is overcome. In cases like these the frequent change of dressings as outlined by Dingman can be lifesaving; as a matter of fact, this therapy should be instituted as soon as an infection of the burn wound is recognized. Dingman advocates this so-called semiopen method as the initial treatment of burns. The frequent daily changing of dressings, however, can be strenuous on the patient no matter how carefully it is conducted; hence, we reserve it only for the infected cases. The treatment is carried out by the nursing staff. Fine-meshed Red Cross gauze moistened with isotonic saline solution is applied to the wound; sterile diapers are laid over the gauze. The patient is laid on a rotating frame if the wound is circumferential, and the dressings are removed with each rotation of the frame. The interval between dressing changes is three to four hours. No changes are made during the night. The dressings are saturated with saline solution one-half hour before removal. Narcotics may be required for the first change in the morning or even later for the subsequent changes. It is important that this treatment is carried out with great care by an understanding nurse. In one of our patients, a 14-year-old boy whose burn had occurred four months previously and who was moribund from uncontrollable infection, the treatment controlled the infection in one week; within six weeks all raw areas were closed with skin grafts although formerly grafts had failed to take in spite of all other therapeutic measures.

Antimicrobial Therapy

It is essential that tetanus antitoxin or a booster dose of tetanus toxoid be injected upon admission of the patient. Antibiotic or chemotherapy is also started immediately (for details see p. 137). Perineal, gluteal, and thigh burns may be partially protected from bacteria-laden feces by giving Sulfasuxidine (p. 142). In spite of potent antimicrobial agents, however, chronic infection of the burn wound is unfortunately often the case, and cross-infection of burn wounds when large numbers of burned patients are involved is frequent. Colebrook's, Ollstein's et al. layout of a burn center, complicated as it may appear, deserves much attention if wound infection and cross-infection are to be reduced.

LATE TREATMENT

Further measures must be directed toward improving the patient's general condition, resurfacing the raw area in third-degree burns, and rehabilitating the patient.

Nutritional Measures

To maintain a good nutritional state and to prevent or counteract secondary anemia, frequent blood transfusions and administration of vitamins, particularly vitamin B complex and vitamin C, and iron in a high-caloric diet, are necessary (see p. 137). Blocker and associates regard the blood loss in severe burns as equivalent to a massive hemorrhage; hence,

HIGH-PROTEIN MIXTURE FOR ORAL FEEDING (LUND)

	Carbo-hydrate	Protein	Fat	Calories
Skim milk (3 liters)	150	110	6	1094
Skim-milk powder (300 gm.)	117	90	6	828
Amigen powder (100 gm.)	0	75	0	600
Valentine's liver extract (30 cc.) ...	0	2	0	8
Salt (15 gm.)	0	0	0	0
Total	267	277	12	2530

HIGH-PROTEIN MIXTURE FOR TUBE FEEDING

	Carbo-hydrate	Protein	Fat	Calories
Skim milk (3 liters)	150	110	6	1094
Skim-milk powder (200 gm.)	78	60	6	598
Amigen powder (200 gm.)	0	150	0	600
Valentine's liver extract (30 cc.) ...	0	2	0	8
Brewer's yeast powder (30 gm.) ...	12	14	1	113
Salt (15 gm.)	0	0	0	0
Total	240	336	13	2413

hemoglobin replacement must have priority over all other types of protein. Other reparative processes require additional caloric and nitrogen intakes. They emphasize that a severely burned patient should be supplied with protein and additional foodstuffs far in excess of normal intake to combat the negative nitrogen balance after the first week of injury. In this author's experience, Lund's recommended diet has been found to meet the nutritional requirements of the severely burned patient. This mixture makes up a large part of the food necessary for twenty-four hours, and should be given in 8-ounce portions every two hours, day and night. Meat and carbohydrate food may be given immediately after at least three liquid feedings. Blocker prescribes routinely 3 to 4 gm. of potassium chloride, enteric-coated, beginning about the fourth or fifth day, if urinary output is adequate. When the patient cannot or will not take this diet, tube feeding may be indicated, and such a mixture may have powdered yeast and more amigen added because palatability is no factor.

Skin Grafting

Another important factor that adds markedly to the improvement of the patient's general physical as well as mental condition is the early closure of raw surfaces with skin grafts. This becomes necessary in third-degree burns, but may also be required in deep second-degree burns. The earlier this is done, the shorter will be the period of debilitation and the more surely will contractures be avoided or counteracted. The raw areas, however, must first be prepared for skin grafting. For details, the reader is referred to page 28, and in preceding chapters to pages 33 and 35. Split skin grafts of medium thickness are used and are rapidly taken with an electric dermatome in long strips. They are spread out in full length over the raw area. If skin is plentiful, they are placed adjacent to each other; otherwise, raw areas of various widths are left between them. Mesh skin autografts (p. 39) and homogeneous grafts (p. 40) may also be considered. With patients on rotating frames, the grafted areas remain exposed and the patients are not rotated for four days. The open treatment of skin grafts is also preferred in other suitable cases. Otherwise a pressure dressing is applied.

Rehabilitation

With a severe burn, and its prolonged treatment, the surgeon may be preoccupied with the physical aspect of the case and be slow in picking up the emotional problem. In the case of a child, it is not only the child that suffers but also the parents, particularly the mother. The child-parent interrelationship of feelings and behavior causes a many-faceted psychological problem which must be dealt with at an early stage (the reader is referred to Woodward and Jackson's excellent article). In the adult the psychological problems vary in degree. They are lessened if the patient has confidence in his surgeon from the start; no matter how many other attendants he has, the patient should feel that there is only one surgeon in charge of his case, and that he can rely upon him then and in the future. If this intimate contact is maintained—and it should be in spite of the fact that the surgeon's patience may be greatly taxed at times by the poor morale and complaints of the patient—psychotherapy may not become necessary. This does not exclude the importance of daily visits from various staff members. When dressings are changed, pain should be avoided by sedation or by the use of light intravenous or inhalation anesthesia. When skin grafting is required, the patient should be given a general outline of the plan, and the expected results should be discussed. Early ambulation, if possible, is important. The services of the physiotherapist may then be sought. Finally, the occupational therapist must join as an important link in the long chain of efforts to solve the many-faceted problems in equipping the patient for his new future.

Electrical Burns and their Treatment

Electrical burns are rarer than others and differ from ordinary heat burns in many respects. Hence they merit separate discussion.

An electrical burn occurs either from direct contact with an electrical current or from an electric flash without contact with a current. The injury occurs only when the body is interposed between two conductors, completing the electric circuit. A whole series of electrical burns can occur if the current is transmitted through several bodies which are joined by contact points (Sturmer). The body itself becomes a conductor through which the current seeks the path of least resistance. Blood vessels and nerves are the least resistant, hence the frequency of vascular and nerve damage after electrical burns; more resistance is offered by muscle, tendon, fat, skin and bone. Although bone is the only tissue with a greater resistance than skin, it is often injured when the current enters through the skull (Case 9); the large surface of the skull and the vascular diploe decrease its resistance (Kragh and Erich). Skin is highly resistant to electric current but may not withstand its force. This depends upon numerous factors involving the type and condition of the skin, the state of the body, and the voltage, amperage and type of current. After the current has penetrated the skin it passes rapidly through the body; it becomes collected again at the point of exit. Hence, the points of entrance and exit receive the maximum effect.

GENERAL PRINCIPLES

As the current passes through the body electric energy is transformed into heat. The latter is highest at the points of entrance and exit, causing full-thickness burns of the skin, the so-called current markings (Jellinek). The dead skin appears gray, becomes depressed, and the edges become erythematous; the lesion is cold and painless. Other immediate effects of the injury may be tetanic muscle contractures, unconsciousness, and occasionally ventricular fibrillation.

If the patient survives the initial effect of the injury, the burned area may look harmless and its extent is often underestimated (Gaby, Lewis, Dale). As days pass, the affected skin becomes black and edematous, yet the real extent of the damage to the deeper tissues may not become apparent until the time of demarcation. The daily increasing extent of the necrosis may then be surprising. This has given rise to the assumption that the necrosis is progressing. Muir and Davies deny that such a phenomenon exists, at least not as a direct and inevitable result of the electrical injury. Muir emphasizes that one must distinguish between two types of necrosis: a local necrosis, in which thrombosis of the main vessels is uncommon, and a necrosis due to vascular thrombosis, i.e., an ischemic gangrene. A local necrosis is characteristic in domestic supply burns. The necrosis may have considerable depth but does not extend beyond the range of damage. If left alone it becomes gradually demarcated and after the dead tissue has been eliminated healing occurs. Healing, however, will be delayed if bacterial infection has intervened. Tissue which is viable, but the viability of which has been depressed by the specific action of the electric current, becomes further damaged by the infection and breaks down; thus a progressive necrosis is started indirectly. The second type of necrosis, which is an ischemic gangrene due to thrombosis of the main vessels, is caused by high-tension injuries where the current passes readily through the body along the paths of least resistance, i.e., the blood vessels. Vascular thrombosis dominates the clinical picture. The extent of the damage may not initially be obvious but later becomes so. Hence, one may gain the impression of a progressing necrosis, which is not true since the parts involved show circulatory embarrassment from the beginning.

Treatment

Treatment is divided into emergency treatment and definitive treatment. Emergency treatment may be carried out immediately in cases in which the general system is damaged, as after high-voltage injuries. The most important emergency treatment is artificial respiration and, in cases of ventricular fibrillation, cardiac massage, which must be started within a few minutes after injury. In ventricular fibrillation breathing continues

168

but the respiratory rate becomes rapid. The patient usually is pale, not cyanotic. When the respiratory center fails, the patient becomes unconscious, the heart beat continues, the blood pressure falls, the patient becomes cyanotic (Artz). Shock may be also present but is usually less severe than with thermal burns.

The general care of the patient is similar to that in thermal burns, page 156. After the patient's general condition has improved attention is paid to the care of the burned area. Opinions differ as to the proper treatment, and surgeons can be divided into two groups. Most favor waiting and allowing demarcation and elimination of necrotic tissue before attempting reconstruction (Jellinek, Lewis, Dale, Brown and Fryer, Kragh and Erich and others); a smaller group (Muir, Davies) are ardent proponents of early excision and immediate closure of the defect with a flap or skin graft, at least in domestic supply burns. They argue that early excision of the necrotic tissue and immediate closure of the defect will prevent bacterial invasion, which they recognize as the course of progression of the necrosis. Muir prefers the flap over the graft even if no important structures are exposed after excision. He argues that the pedicled flap brings its own blood supply and can more readily survive on a host tissue which is viable but may be weakened in its viability by the specific action of the electric current. This treatment of primary or early excision and immediate closure would be ideal if it were not for the difficulty in determining the extent of the necrosis. (This topic has been discussed amongst others by May.)

Experience of the Birmingham Burn Unit (Davies) showed that bleeding is not a good index of viability on the day of injury; under the tourniquet dead fat appears coagulated or pink compared with the normal yellow, and a dead tendon loses its glistening appearance. By careful attention to this they were able to reduce the number of inadequate excisions, thus tacitly admitting the method is not foolproof. Surgeons who have much less experience in dealing with electrical burns will have much more difficulty in finding the proper level of excision. The staining of viable tissues after injection of disulphine blue after Tempest, used by him in more than two hundred cases and by others (Scharitzer, Schmidt-Tintemann, Böhler and Streli, Goulian and Conway), without any harm to the body appears to offer a more reliable method of determining the line of demarcation. According to age, 5 to 20 cc. of the dye are injected intravenously; within three to five minutes the whole organism becomes blue-green. Tissues deprived of blood circulation remain rose-colored, those with impaired circulation exhibit a various amount of spotting; fine spotting evinces partial necrosis, coarse spotting indicates subtotal destruction of tissues, often followed by total necrosis. The dye is excreted through the kidneys within forty-eight to seventy-two hours. (In the United States this method as well as Goulian and Conway's bromphenol blue staining cannot be used clinically since the Food and Drug Administration has not yet granted permission.)

The majority of surgeons, however, wait until a line of demarcation is established to excise the necrotic tissue (May). This can be done ten to fourteen days after injury. If possible, i.e., if one feels assured of the viability of the host tissue, the defect is closed immediately with a flap or a graft depending upon the condition of the host tissue and the depth of the defect, i.e., whether important structures such as tendons are exposed or need later replacement. If a flap is required and needs several stages for mobilization, its preparation can be started during the waiting period. On the other hand, it may be impossible to estimate the ultimate extent of the defect and therefore the size and length of the flap. Hence, preparation of the flap must be delayed and if possible a skin graft used for temporary closure (Cases 157, p. 1204; 9, p. 1000).

In high-tension burns with thrombosis of the main vessels, spontaneous separation of the slough is extremely slow. It should be hastened by excision of the dead tissue at the end of the third week and temporary skin grafting should be done. Even then it may not be possible to recognize the real depth of the necrosis and the line of demarcation, and subsequent excision may become necessary. In high-tension injuries of the scalp and skull, one must wait until the dead bone has separated as a sequestrum. A sequestrostomy is then performed with immediate closure of the surface defect with a sliding scalp flap, followed by replacement of the necrosed bone with an autogenous bone graft after the flap has healed (Case 9).

In electrical burns of the lips, it is well to wait until a line of demarcation is fully established before excising the necrotic tissue, and even then to wait for reconstruction until the healing process is complete and all induration has subsided (May, Thompson, Juckes, and Farmer, Pitts et al.). In many of these cases the resulting cicatricial deformities and defects can be repaired by sliding or rotation of vermilion-lined, full-thickness lip flaps from the immediate neighborhood. Should the procedure fail, other such flaps may not be available. It could fail if the ultimate size of the defect is not established or edema and induration impair local circulation.

Although it is advisable in most cases of electrical burn to delay excision and reconstruction of the burned area, in small domestic supply burns immediate excision and closure of the defect with a flap or graft may definitely be indicated. Early excision is also favored in electrical burns of the hand (Poticha et al., and Peterson).

170

TREATMENT OF MINOR BURNS

Minor burns may be regarded as burns of less than 5 to 10 per cent of the body surface. In most instances, the patient can be treated while ambulatory, unless the location of the burned area is such as to require hospitalization. Usually, no general treatment except for the relief of pain by administration of a sedative is required. In *first-degree* burns, application of antiseptic and analgesic ointments, such as butesin picrate, is recommended. The latter is an excellent analgesic, but should be used with caution—that is, not repeatedly—since it may cause toxic symptoms. *Second- and third-degree* burns require cleansing of the surrounding area. Blisters are not opened; if they are open, they are excised. Then follows application of an analgesic ointment and a pressure dressing; application of splints may be necessary; ultimate treatment does not differ from that of extensive burns.

BIBLIOGRAPHY

ABRAMSON, D. J.: *The care and treatment of severely burned children.* Surg. Gynec. Obstet., 122:855, 1966.

ADAMS, F. H., BERGLUND, E., BALKIN, S. G., and CHISHOLM, T.: *Pituitary adrenocorticotropic hormone in severely burned children.* JAMA, 146:31, 1951.

AHNEFELD, F. W.: *Erstbehandlung von Berbrennungen im Katastrophenfall.* Monatsschrift für Unfallheilkunde und Versicherungsmedizin, Heft, 71:83, 1962.

ALDRICH, R. H.: *The role of infection with special references to gentian violet.* New Eng. J. Med., 208:299, 1933.
Treatment of burns with a compound of aniline dyes. Maine Med. J., 28:5, 1937.
A critical survey of the treatment of burns. Maine Med. J., 33:21, 1942.

ALLEN, H. S., and KOCH, S. L.: *The treatment of patients with severe burns.* Surg. Gynec. Obstet., 74:914, 1942.

ALLEN, H. S.: *Local treatment of the whole thickness burn surface.* Surg. Clin. N. Amer., Feb., 125, 1948.
Treatment of the burned wound. Based on the experience of 1000 hospital patients. Ann. Surg., 134:566, 1951.

ALLGÖWER, M.: *Vollblut in der Therapie des Verbrennungsschocks.* Langenbeck's Archiv für klinische Chirurgie. Deutsche Zeitschrift für Chirurgie, 282:124, 1955.

ALLGÖWER, M., SIEGRIST, J., ET AL.: *Verbrennungen.* Pathophysiologie, Pathologie, Klinik, Therapie. Springer-Verlag, Berlin, 1957.

171

GENERAL PRINCIPLES

ARTZ, C. P., ED.: *Research in Burns. The Proceedings of the First International Congress on Research in Burns.* Blackwell Scientific Publications, Oxford, 1962.

ARTZ, C. P., and GASTON, B. H.: *A reappraisal of the exposure method in the treatment of burns, donor sites, and skin grafts.* Ann. Surg., 151:939, 1960.

ARTZ, C. P., and MONCRIEF, J. A.: *The Treatment of Burns.* Ed. 2. W. B. Saunders, Philadelphia, 1967.

ARTZ, C. P., REISS, E., DAVIS, J. H., and AMSPACHER, W. H.: *The exposure treatment of burns.* Ann. Surg., 137:456, 1953.

BARADUC, H.: *Des causes de la mort a la suite des brulures superficielles des moyens de l'eviter.* Paris, 1862.

BARDEEN, C. R.: *A review of the pathology of superficial burns, with a contribution to our knowledge of the pathological changes in the organs in cases of rapidly fatal burns.* Johns Hopkins Hosp. Rep., 7:137, 1898.

BAUE, A. E.: *Recent developments in the study and treatment of shock.* Surg. Gynec. Obstet., 127:849, 1968.

BAXTER, H., SCHILLER, C., and WHITESIDE, J. H.: *The influence of ACTH on wound healing in man.* Plast. Reconstr. Surg., 7:85, 1951.

BAYLISS, W. M.: *Methods of Raising a Low Arterial Pressure.* Proc. Prog. Soc. Med. Series B, 89:38–1915–1916.

BAYNTON, T.: *Descriptive Account of a New Method to Treat Old Ulcers of the Leg.* Bristol, 1797.

BEARD, J. W., and BLALOCK, A.: *Experimental shock: Composition of fluid that escapes from bloodstream after mild trauma to extremity, after trauma to intestines and after burns.* Arch. Surg., 22:617, 1931.

BERKOW, S. G.: *A method of estimating the extensiveness of lesions (burns and scalds), based on surface area proportions.* Arch. Surg., 8:138, 1924.

BERNHARD, W. G., ET AL.: *Functional and anatomic effect of polyvinylpyrrolidone.* Ann. Surg., 139:397, 1954.

BETTMAN, A. G.: *Tannic acid-silver nitrate in burns.* Surg. Gynec., 62:458, 1936. *The rationale of the tannic acid-silver nitrate treatment in burns.* JAMA, 108:1490, 1937.

BLACK, A. K.: *Treatment of burn shock with plasma and serum.* Brit. Med. J., 2:693, 1940.

BLAIR, V. P.: *Influence of mechanical pressure on wound healing.* Illinois Med. J., 46:249, 1924.

BLALOCK, A., and MASON, M. F.: *Principles of Surgical Care: Shock and Other Problems.* C. V. Mosby, St. Louis, 1940.
Blood and blood substitutes in the treatment and prevention of shock: with particular reference to their use in wartime. Ann. Surg., 113:657, 1941.

BLOCKER, T. G.: *Newer conception of treatment of extensive burns.* Surgery, 29:154, 1951.

BLOCKER, T. G., JR., BLOCKER, V., LEWIS, S. R., and SNYDER, C. C.: *An approach to the problem of burn sepsis with the use of open-air therapy.* Ann. Surg., 134:574, 1951.

172

TREATMENT OF BURNS

Experiences with the exposure method of burn therapy. Plast. Reconstr. Surg., 8:87, 1951.

BLOCKER, T. G., ET AL.: *Nutrition studies in the severely burned.* Ann. Surg., 141:589, 1955.

BLOCKER, T. G., LEWIS, S. R., GRANT, D. A., BLOCKER, V., and BENNETT, J. E.: *Experiences in the management of the burn wound.* Plast. Reconstr. Surg., 26:579, 1960.

BÖHLER, J.: *Die allgemeine und örtliche Behandlung schwerer Verbrennungen.* Langenbeck's Archiv für klinische Chirurgie. Deutsche Zeitschrift für Chirurgie, 282:116, 1955.

BÖHLER, J., and STRELI, R.: *Differentialdiagnose drittgradiger Verbrennungen durch intravenöse Vitalfärbung.* Langenbeck's Arch f. klin. Chir., 297:504, 1961.

BOWE, J. J.: *Primary excision in third degree burns.* Plast. Reconstr. Surg., 25:240, 1960.

BOWERS, W. F.: *Surgery of Trauma.* J. B. Lippincott, Philadelphia, 1953.

BRAITHWAITE, F.: *Plasma and blood transfusions in the treatment of burned patients.* Brit. J. Plast. Surg., 2:95, 1949.

BRENTANO, L., MOYER, C. A., GROVENS, D. L., and MONAFO, W. W., JR.: *Bacteriology of large human burns treated with silver nitrate.* Arch. Surg., 93:456, 1966.

BROOKS, F., DRAGSTEDT, L. R., WARNER, L., and KNISELY, M. H.: *Sludged blood following severe thermal burns.* Arch. Surg., 61:387, 1950.

BROOKS, R., FITTS, WM., and RAVDIN, I. S.: *Treatment of thermal burns. A 10 year progress report.* Amer. J. Surg., 85:364, 1954.

BROWN, J. B., and McDOWELL, F.: *Skin Grafting.* 2nd Ed. J. B. Lippincott, Philadelphia, 1949.

BROWN, J. B., and FRYER, M. P.: *Repair of industrial electrical burns.* Plast. Reconstr. Surg., 18:177, 1956.

BULL, J. P., and SQUIRE, J. R.: *Study of mortality in a burns unit.* Amer. J. Surg., 130:160, 1949.

BUNYAN, J.: *The treatment of burns and wounds by the envelope method.* Brit. Med. J., 2:1, 1941.

BÜRKLE DE LA CAMP, H.: *Die allgemeine und örtliche Behandlung der Verbrennungskrankheit.* Deutsches Med. J., 4:203, 1957.
Die Verbrennungskrankheit. Monatsschrift für Unfallheilkunde und Versicherungsmedizin, Heft, 71:20, 1962.
Die Verbrennungskrankheiten. Koblenz, Verlag Gasschutz und Luftschutz, 1956.
Betrachtungen zur örtlichen Behandlung der Verbrennungschäden. Langenbeck's Arch. f. klin. Chir., 311, 1965.

CANNON, B.: *Procedure in rehabilitation of the severely burned.* Ann. Surg., 117:903, 1943.

CANNON, B., and COPE, O.: *Rate of epithelial regeneration. A clinical method of measurement and the effect of various agents recommended in the treatment of burns.* Ann. Surg., 117:85, 1943.

173

GENERAL PRINCIPLES

CANNON, W. B.: *Traumatic Shock.* D. Appleton Company, New York, 1923.

CLARKSON, P., and EVANS, A. J.: *The Treatment of Burns.* The Med. Press, 232: Dec. 8, 1954.

CLOWES, G. H. A., Jr., LUND, C. C., and LEVENSON, S. M.: *Surface treatment of burns: Comparison of results of tannic acid-silver nitrate, triple dye or boric ointment as surface treatments in 150 cases.* Ann. Surg., 118:761, 1943.

COAKLEY, W. A., SHAPIRO, R. N., and ROBERTSON, G. W.: *The management of severe burns.* Plast. Reconstr. Surg., 3:667, 1948.

COLEBROOK, L.: *A New Approach to the Treatment of Burns and Scalds.* Fine Technical Publications, London, 1950.

CONNELL, J. F., DEL GUERCIO, L. R. M., and ROUSSELOT, L. M.: *Debrecinclinical experiences with a new proteolytic enzyme in surgical wounds.* Surg. Gynec. Obstet., 108:93, 1959.

CONVERSE, J. M.: *Early skin grafting in war wounds of extremities.* Ann. Surg., 115:321, 1942.

CONVERSE, J. M., and ROBB-SMITH, A. H. T.: *The healing of surface cutaneous wounds: Its analogy with the healing of superficial burns.* Ann. Surg., 120: 873, 1944.

COOPER, N., MATSUURA, Y., MURNER, E. S., and LEE, W. H., Jr.: *Analysis of pathologic mechanisms in pulmonary surfactant destruction following thermal burn.* Amer. Surgeon, 33:882, 1967.

COPE, O.: *The treatment of surface burns.* Ann. Surg., 6:885, 1943.

COPE, O., GRAHAM, J. B., MOORE, F. D., and BALL, M.: *The nature of the shift of plasma protein to the extravascular space following thermal trauma.* Ann. Surg., 128:1041, 1948.

CREWS, E. R.: *A Practical Manual for the Treatment of Burns.* Ed. 2. Charles C Thomas, Springfield, 1967.

CRILE, G. W.: *Therapeutic value of water.* Surg. Gynec. Obstet., 34:277, 1922.

CURTIS, R. M., and ROSE, I. W.: *New technique for local treatment of burns.* JAMA, 147:741, 1951.

DALE, H. H., and RICHARDS, A. N.: *The vasodilator action of histamine and of some other substance.* J. Physiol., 52:110, 1918.

DALE, H. H., and LAIDLAW, P. P.: *Histamine shock.* J. Physiol., 52:355, 1919.

DALE, R. H.: *Electrical accidents: A discussion with illustrative cases.* Brit. J. Plast. Surg., 7:44, 1954.

DAVIDSON, E. C.: *Tannic acid in the treatment of burns.* Surg. Gynec. Obstet., 41:202, 1925.
The prevention of toxemia of burns, treatment by tannic acid solution. Amer. J. Surg., 40:114, 1926.

DAVIES, M. R.: *Burns caused by electricity: A review of seventy cases.* Brit. J. Plast. Surg., 11:288, 1959.

DERBER, V. G.: *Untoward Reaction of Cortisone and ACTH.* Charles C Thomas, Springfield.

TREATMENT OF BURNS

DILLON, J., LYNCH, L. H., MYERS, R., and BUTCHER, H. R.: *The treatment of hemorrhagic shock.* Surg. Gynec. Obstet., 122:967, 1966.

DINGMAN, R. O., and FELLER, I.: *Semi-open method in the management of the burn wound.* Plast. Reconstr. Surg., 26:535, 1960.

DOMINGUEZ, O., BAINS, J. W., LYNCH, J. B., and LEWIS, S. R.: *Treatment of burns with silver nitrate versus exposure method: Analysis of 200 patients.* Plast. Reconstr. Surg., 40:489, 1967.

ELKINTON, J. R., WOLFF, W. A., and LEE, W. E.: *Plasma transfusion in the treatment of the fluid shift in severe burns.* Ann. Surg., 112:150, 1940.

ELMAN, R.: *The therapeutic significance of plasma protein replacement in severe burns.* JAMA, 116:213, 1941.

EPPINGER, H., KAUNITZ, H., and POPPER, H.: *Die seröse Entzündung: Eine Permeabilitäts Pathologie.* J. Springer, Berlin, 1934.

EUFINGER, H.: *Schock und Kollaps.* Langenbeck's Arch. f. klin. Chir., 301:128, 1962.

von EULER, U. S.: *Schock, Pathogenese und Therapie.* Springer-Verlag, Berlin, 1962.

EVANS, A. J.: *The early treatment of burns at a regional plastic center (review of 100 cases treated by exposure).* Brit. J. Plast. Surg., 5:263, 1953.

EVANS, E. I.: *The early management of severely burned patient.* Surg. Gynec. Obstet., 94:273, 1952.

EVANS, E. I., and BIGGER, I. A.: *The rationale of whole blood therapy in severe burns.* Ann. Surg., 122:693, 1945.

EVANS, E. I., and BUTTERFIELD, W. J. H.: *The stress responses in the severely burned. An interim report.* Ann. Surg., 134:588, 1951.

EVANS, E. I., ET AL.: *Fluid and electrolyte requirements in severe burns.* Ann. Surg., 135:804, 1952.

FINE, J.: *Current status of the problem of traumatic shock.* Surg. Gynec. Obstet., 120:537, 1965.
The Bacterial Factor in Traumatic Shock. Charles C Thomas, Springfield, 1954.

FINTON, W. L.: *Electrical injuries.* J. Mich. Med. Soc., 29:775, 1930.

GABY, R. E.: *Electrical burns and electrical shock.* Canad. Med. Assoc. J., 17:1343, 1927.

GOULIAN, D., JR., and CONWAY, H.: *Dye differentiation of injured tissues in burn injury.* Surg. Gynec. Obstet., 121:3, 1965.

GOWER, W. E.: *Treatment of fresh burns with scarlet red bandage and moist sulfanilamide dressings.* J. Iowa Med. Soc., 31:234, 1941.

GROPPER, A. L., RAISZ, I. G., and AMSPACHER, W. H.: *Plasma expanders.* Surg. Gynec. Obstet., 95:521, 1952.

GRUBER, U. F., and SIEGRIST, J.: *Der Volumeneffekt verschiedener Plasmaersatzstoffe.* Langenbeck's Arch. f. klin. Chir., 301:128, 1962.

GURD, F. B., and ACKMAN, D.: *Technique in Trauma.* J. B. Lippincott, Philadelphia, 1944.

GENERAL PRINCIPLES

GURD, F. B., ACKMAN, D., GERRIE, J. W., and PRITCHARD, J. E.: *A practical concept for the treatment of major and minor burns.* Ann. Surg., 116:641, 1942.

HAINZL, H.: *Verbrennung grosser Hautgebiete.* Monatsschrift für Unfallheilkunde und Versicherungsmedizin, Heft, 71:60, 1962.

HAMILTON, J. E.: *A comparative study of local burn treatments.* Amer. J. Surg., 58:350, 1942.

HAMIT, H. F.: *Current trends of therapy and research in shock.* Surg. Gynec. Obstet., 120:835, 1965.

HARDIN, R. C.: *Cod liver oil therapy of wounds and burns.* South. Surgeon, 10:301, 1941.

HARDY, E. J., LOVELACE, J. R., NEELY, W. A., and WILSON, F. C.: *Thermal burns in man. IV. Body weight changes during therapy.* Surgery, 38:685, 1955.

HARDY, J. D.: *Surgical Physiology of the Adrenal Cortex.* Charles C Thomas, Springfield, 1955.

HARKINS, H. W.: *Recent advances in the study and management of traumatic shock.* Surgery, 9:231, 447, 607, 1941.
The Treatment of Burns. Charles C Thomas, Springfield, 1942.
The treatment of burns in wartime. JAMA, 119:385, 1942.
The local treatment of thermal burns. Ann. Surg., 115:1140, 1942.

HARTENBACH, W.: *Erfahrungen bei der Behandlung schwerster Verbrennungen.* Monatsschrift für Unfallheilkunde und Versicherungsmedizin, Heft, 71:68, 1962.

HAYASAKA, H., and HOWARD, J. M.: *Septic Shock—Experimental and Clinical Studies.* Charles C Thomas, Springfield, 1964.

HAYNES, B. W., MARTIN, M. M., and PURNELL, O. J.: *Fluid colloid and electrolyte requirements in severe burns.* Ann. Surg., 142:674, 1955.

HECHT, G., and WEESE, H.: *Blutflüssigkeitersatz Münch.* Med. Wschr., 90:11, 1943.

HEGEMANN, G.: *Die Behandlung der Verbrennungskrankheit.* Langenbeck's Archiv für klinische Chirurgie. Deutsche Zeitschrift für Chirurgie, 282:80, 1955.

HEUER, G. J., and ANDRUS, W. D.: *The effect of adrenal cortical extract in controlling shock following the injection of aqueous extracts of closed intestinal loops.* Ann. Surg., 100:734, 1934.

HEYMANN, J.: *Status of Treatment of Burns—Gel Preparation.* Beitr. zur Klinischen Chirurgie, 184:451, 1952.

HIRSCHFELD, J. W.: *A comparison of the effects of straining agents and of vaseline gauze on fresh wounds of man.* Surg. Gynec. Obstet., 76:556, 1943.

JACKSON, D., TOPLEY, E., CASON, J. S., and LOWBURY, E. J. L.: *Primary excision and grafting of large burns.* Ann. Surg., 152:167, 1960.

JELLINEK, S.: *Der Elektrische Unfall.* Ed. 3. Franz Deuticke, Leipzig, 1931.
The pathological changes produced in those rendered unconscious by electric shock and the treatment of such cases. Arch. Radiol. Electroth., 27:316, 1923.

JENNY, F.: *Der Electrische Unfall.* Hans Huber, Bern, 1945.

KAPLAN, I.: *Experimental study of circumferential burns.* Plast. Reconstr. Surg., 31:205, 1963.

TREATMENT OF BURNS

KAPLAN, I., and WHITE, W. L.: *Incisional decompression of circumferential burns.* Plast. Reconstr. Surg., 28:609, 1961.

KERN, R. A.: *The present knowledge on the clinical use of ACTH and cortisone.* Penn. Med. J., 55:1184, 1952.

KNAYSI, G. H., CRIKELAIR, G. F., and COSMAN, B.: *The rule of nines: its history and accuracy.* Plast. Reconstr. Surg., 41:560, 1968.

KOCH, S. L.: *The use of compression as a surgical principle in the treatment of injuries.* Quart. Bull., Northwestern Univ. School, 17:257, 1943.

KRAGH, L. V., and ERICH, J. B.: *Treatment of severe electrical injuries.* Amer. J. Surg., 101:419, 1961.

KYLE, M. J., and WALLACE, A. B.: *Fluid replacement in burnt children.* Brit. J. Plast. Surg., 3:194, 1950.

LARSON, D. L., VOGEL, E. H., MITCHELL, E. T., and BUTKIEWICZ, J. V.: *The use of modified exposure in the management of burn wounds.* Surg. Gynec. Obstet., 112:577, 1961.

LEE, W. E., ELKINTON, J. R., and WOLFF, W. A.: *The management of shock and toxemia in severe burns.* Penn. Med. J., 44:1114, 1941.

LEE, W. E., WOLFF, W. A., ET AL.: *Recent trends in the therapy of burns.* Ann. Surg., 115:1131, 1942.

LESSER, L.: *Ueber die Todesursachen nach Verbrennungen.* Virchows Arch. f. path. Anat., 79:248, 1880.

LEWIS, G. K.: *Burns from electricity.* Ann. Surg., 131:80, 1950.

LEWIS, S. R., GOOLISHIAN, H. A., WOLF, C. W., LYNCH, J. B., and BLOCKER, T. G.: *Psychological studies in burn patients.* Plast. Reconstr. Surg., 31:323, 1963.

LINDBERG, R. B., MONCRIEF, J. A., SWITZER, W. E., ORDER, S. E., and MILLS, W., JR.: *The successful control of burn wound sepsis.* J. Trauma, 5:601, 1965.

LOB, A.: *Mechanische, thermische und elektrische Verletzungen.* Handbuch der gesamten Unfallheilkunde. Ferdinand Enke Verlag, Stuttgart, 1963.

LÖHR, W.: *Die Behandlung grosser, flächenhafter Verbrennungen 1. 2. and 3. Grades mit Lebertran.* Chirurg., 6:263, 1934.
Behandlung von Brandwunden mit Lebertransalbe. Arch. f. klin Chir., 195:203, 1939.

LOOKWOOD, J. S., and RANDALL, H. T.: *The place of electrolyte studies in surgical patients.* Bull. N. Y. Acad. Med., 25:228, 1949.

LUND, C. C.: *The protein nutrition of surgical patients.* Surg. Gynec. Obstet., 83:259, 1946.

LUSTGARTEN, S.: *Zur Theory der primären Todesursache bei Verbrennungen.* Wien. klin Wchnschr., 4:528, 1891.

MADDICK, W. G., and COLLER, F. A.: *Water balance in surgery.* JAMA, 108:1, 1937.

MAGNUSON, P. B., and STACK, J. K.: *Fractures.* 5th Ed. J. B. Lippincott, Philadelphia, 1949.

GENERAL PRINCIPLES

MAHONEY, E. B., KINGSLEY, H. D., and HOWLAND, J. W.: *The therapeutic value of preserved blood plasma.* Ann. Surg., 113:969, 1941.

MASON, M. L.: *Local treatment of the burned area.* Surg. Gynec. Obstet., 72:250, 1941.

MATTER, P., CHAMBLER, K., BAILEY, B., LEWIS, S. R., BLOCKER, T. G., and BLOCKER, V.: *Experimental studies with reference to antigen-antibody phenomena following severe extensive burns.* Ann. Surg., 157:725, 1963.

MAY, H.: *Treatment of burns.* Symposium, Amer. J. Surg., 63:34, 1944.
Electrical burns and their treatment. Transact. of 3rd Intern. Congr. of Plast. Surg., Washington, 1964.

McCLURE, R. D.: *The treatment of the patient with severe burns.* JAMA, 113: 1808, 1939.

MINOT, A. S., and BLALOCK, A.: *Plasma loss in severe dehydration, shock and other conditions as affected by therapy.* Ann. Surg., 112:557, 1940.

MONAFO, W. W., and MOYER, C. A.: *Effectiveness of dilute silver nitrate in treatment of major burns.* Arch. Surg., 91:200, 1965.

MONCRIEF, J. A.: *Complications of burns.* Ann. Surg., 147:443, 1958.
Infection in the early post-burn period. Surg. Gynec. Obstet., 123:837, 1966.

MONCRIEF, J. A., LINDBERG, R. B., SWITZER, W. E., and PRUITT, B. A., Jr.: *The use of a topical sulfonamide in the control of burn wound sepsis.* J. Trauma, 6:407, 1966.

MOON, V. H.: *The dynamics of shock and its clinical implications.* Surg. Gynec. Obstet. (Intern. Abstr. Surg.), 79:1, 1944.
Shock and Related Capillary Phenomena. Oxford University Press, New York, 1938.

MOORE, F. D., PEACOCK, W. C., BLAKELY, E., and COPE, O.: *The anemia of thermal burns.* Amer. J. Surg., 124:811, 1946.

MOYER, C. A.: *Fluid and electrolyte therapy in burns.* Symposium on Burns, National Research Council, Washington, 1951.

MOYER, C. A., BRENTANO, L., GRAVENS, D. L., MARGRAF, H. W., and MONAFO, W. W.: *Treatment of large human burns with 0.5% silver nitrate solution.* Arch. Surg., 90:812, 1965.

MOYER, C. A., and BUTCHER, H. R., Jr.: *Burns, Shock, and Plasma Volume Regulation.* C. V. Mosby, St. Louis, 1967.

MOYER, C. A., MARGRAF, H. W., and MONAFO, W. W.: *Burn shock and extravascular sodium deficiency; treatment with Ringer's solution with lactate.* Arch. Surg., 90:799, 1965.

MUIR, I. F. K.: *Red-cell destruction in burns.* Brit. J. Plast. Surg., 14:273, 1961.
The treatment of electrical burns. Brit. J. Plast. Surg., 10:292, 1958.

MUIR, I. F. K., and BARCLAY, T. L.: *Burns and Their Treatment.* Year Book Medical Publishers, Inc., Chicago, 1962.

OCHSNER, E. W. A., ET AL.: *A new preparation for the study of experimental shock from massive wounds.* Surgery, 43:703, 708, 721, 730, 740, 747, 1958.

178

TREATMENT OF BURNS

OLLSTEIN, R. N., SYMONDS, F. C., CRIKELAIR, G. F., CORLISS, S.: *Creation of a burn center.* Plast. Reconstr. Surg., 43:260, 1969.

OWENS, N., GORNEY, M., and HUGHES, R. W.: *Recent trends in the management of burns. A review.* Plast. Reconstr. Surg., 16:480, 1955.

PACK, G. T., and DAVIS, A. H.: *Burns: Types, Pathology, Management.* J. B. Lippincott, Philadelphia, 1930.

PEARSON, E., SOROFF, H. S., ARNEY, G. K., and ARTZ, C. P.: *An estimation of the potassium requirements for equilibrium in burned patients.* Surg. Gynec. Obstet., 112:263, 1961.

PENBERTHY, G. C., and WELLER, C. N.: *Treatment of burns.* Amer. J. Surg., 46:468, 1939.
Treatment of burns. Surg. Gynec. Obstet., 74:428, 1942.

PETERSON, R. A.: *Electrical burns of the hand.* J. Bone Joint Surg., 48A:407, 1966.

PFEIFFER, H.: *Experimentelle Beiträge zur Aetiologie des primären Verbrennungstodes.* Virchows Arch. f. path. Anat., 180:367, 1905.

PHILLIPS, A. W., and COPE, O.: *Burn therapy. II. The revelation of respiratory tract damage as a principal killer of the burned patient.* Ann. Surg., 155:1, 1962.
Burn therapy. III. Beware the facial burn. Ann. Surg., 156:759, 1962.

PICKRELL, K. L.: *A new treatment for burns—preliminary report.* Bull. Johns Hopkins Hosp., 69:217, 1941.

PITTS, U., PICKRELL, K., QUINN, G., MASSENGILL, R.: *Electrical burns of lip and mouth in infants and children.* Plast. Reconstr. Surg., 44:471, 1969.

POTICHA, ST.M., BELLE, F. H., and MEHIR, W. H.: *Electrical injuries with special reference to the hand.* Arch. Surg., 85:852, 1962.

PRICE, W., and WOOD, M.: *Silver nitrate burn dressing; treatment of 70 burned patients.* Amer. J. Surg., 112:674, 1966.

PULASKI, E. J., ET AL.: *Exposure (open) treatment of burns.* U. S. Armed Forces Med. J., 2:769, 1951.

RAKER, J. W., and ROVIT, R. L.: *The acute red blood cell destruction following severe thermal trauma in dogs; based on the use of radioactive chromate tagged red blood cells.* Surg. Gynec. Obstet., 98:169, 1953.

RAKER, J. W., WRIGHT, A., MICHEL, A. J. D., and COPE, O.: *A clinical and experimental evaluation of the influence of ACTH on the need for fluid therapy of the burned patient.* Ann. Surg., 134:614, 1951.

RANDALL, P., and LU, M.: *Postmortem homografts as "biological dressings" for extensive burns and denuded areas.* Ann. Surg., 138:618, 1953.

RAVDIN, I. S., and RAVDIN, R. G.: *Collective review: Shock, fluids, and electrolytes, 1905–1955.* Surg. Gynec. Obstet., 100:101, 1955.

RAVDIN, I. S.: *Plasma expanders.* JAMA, 150:10, 1952.

REHN, J., and WHITELAW, M. J.: *Die Verbrennungsbehandlung mit ACTH und Cortisone.* Langenbeck's Arch. u. Dtsch. Z. f. Chir., Bd. 274, S. 175-189, 1953.

GENERAL PRINCIPLES

REHN, J.: *Entgiftung der sogenannten Verbrennungstoxine.* Monatsschrift für Unfallheilkunde und Versicherungsmedizin, Heft., 71:38, 1962.
Neuere Ergebnisse der Schockforschung und ihre therapeutischen Schlussfolgerungen. Langenbeck's Arch. f. klin. Chir., 301:109, 1962.

REHN, J., and KOSLOWSKI, L.: *Praktikum der Verbrennungskrankheit.* Ferdinand Enke Verlag, Stuttgart, 1960.

REISS, E., and ARTZ, C. P.: *Current status of research in treatment of burns.* Mil. Surgeon, 114:187, 1954.

RHOADS, J. E., WOLFF, W. A., and LEE, W. E.: *The use of adrenal cortical extract in the treatment of traumatic shock of burns.* Ann. Surg., 113:955, 1941.

RHOADS, J. E., WOLFF, W. A., SALTONSTALL, A., and LEE, W. E.: *Further experiences with adrenal cortical extract in the treatment of burn shock.* Ann. Surg., 118:982, 1943.

RHOADS, J. E.: *Protein nutrition in surgical patients.* Fed. Proc., 11:659, 1952.

RHOADS, J. E., and HOWARD, J. M.: *The Chemistry of Trauma.* Charles C Thomas, Springfield, 1963.

ROBERTSON, B., and BOYD, G. L.: *Toxemia of severe superficial burns.* J. Lab. Clin. Med., 9:1, 1923.

SCHARITZER, E.: *Die organisatorische Bedentung der "aufgeschobenen Dringlichkeit" in der Unfall Chirurgie.* Hefte zur Unfallheilkunde, 1962.

SCHMIDT, M. A.: *Die Grundsätze der plastischen Deckung grosser Verbrennungsdefekte.* Hefte zur Unfallheilkunde 71:46, 1962.

SCHMIDT-TINTEMANN, U.: *Erfahrungen mit der disulphine blue-injektion.* Fortschritte der Kiefer- und Gesichts-Chirurgie band IX:29, 1964.
Zur örtlichen Behandlung der Verbrennungskrankheit. Monatsschrift für Unfallheilkunde und Versicherungsmedizin, Heft 71:78, 1962.

SCHULTZ, E.: *Bluttransfusson und Blutersatzflüssigkeit* Deutsche Med. Wschr., 67:779, 1941.

SCUDDER, J.: *Shock: Blood Studies as a Guide to Therapy.* J. B. Lippincott, Philadelphia, 1940.

SEELEY, S. F.: *Progress in the treatment of shock: An historical perspective.* Plast. Reconstr. Surg., 40:299, 1967.

SELYE, H.: *The general adaptation syndrome and the diseases of adaptation.* J. Clin. Endocr., 6:117, 1946.
The Physiology and Pathology of Exposure to Stress. Montreal, Acta Endocrinologica Inc., 1950.
The Stress of Life. McGraw-Hill, New York, 1956.

SELYE, H., and HEUSER, G.: *Fourth Annual Report on Stress.* Montreal, Acta, Inc., 1954.

SEVITT, S.: *Burns, Pathology, and Therapeutic Applications.* London, 1957.

SHIRER, T.: *Care of the Traumatic Patient.* McGraw-Hill, New York, 1966.

SILER, V. E., and REID, M. R.: *Clinical and experimental studies with the Koch method of treatment of heat burns.* Ann. Surg., 115:1106, 1942.

TREATMENT OF BURNS

SIMONART, M. A.: Sem. Hop. Paris, 34:377, 1958.

SKOOG, T.: *The Surgical Treatment of Burns*. F. A. Davis Company, Philadelphia, 1963.

SORENSEN, B., and SEJRSEN, P.: *Saline solutions in the treatment of burn shock*. Acta Chir. Scand., 129:239, 1965.

SPIETSCHKA, T.: *Ueber Verbrennungen und Verbrennungstod*. Arch. f. Dermat. u. Syph., 103:41, 1910.

STEIN, F. E., WRIGHT, L. T., and PRIGOT, A.: *Streptokinase-streptodornase in the local treatment of burns*. Harlem Hosp. Bull., 5:134, 1953.

STÖR, O.: *Die Verbrennungskrankheit und ihre Behandlung*. Vortr. der Prakt Chirurgie. H. 35. Stuttgart, Ferd. Enke, 1952.

STURMER, F. C.: *Electrical burns*. Ann. Surg., 154:120, 1961.

STRUMIA, M. M., WAGNER, J. A., and MONAGHAN, J. F.: *The intravenous use of serum and plasma, fresh and preserved*. Ann. Surg., 111:623, 1940.

SWINGLE, W. W., PARKINS, W. M., ET AL.: *A study of the circulatory failure of adrenal insufficiency and analogous shocklike conditions*. Amer. J. Physiol., 123:659, 1938.

TAPPEINER: *Ueber Veränderungen des Blutes und der Muskeln nach ausgedehnten Hautverbrennungen*. Zentralbl. f. d. med. Wiss., 19:385, 401, 1881.

TAYLOR, P. H., PUGSLEY, L. Q., and VOGEL, E. H., JR.: *The intriguing electrical burn*. J. Trauma, 2:309, 1962.

TEMPEST, M. N.: *A new technique in the clinical assessment of burns*. Chir. Praxir, 2:265, 1961.

THOMPSON, W. D., RAVDIN, I. S., ET AL.: *Use of lyophile plasma in correction of hypoproteinemia and prevention of wound disruption*. Arch. Surg., 36:509, 1938.

THOMSON, H. G., JUCKES, A. W., and FARMER, A. W.: *Electric burns to the mouth in children*. Plast. Reconstr. Surg., 35:466, 1965.

TOPLEY, E., JACKSON, M. G., CASON, J. S., and DAVIES, J. W. L.: *Assessment of red-cell loss in the first two days after severe burns*. Ann. Surg., 155:581, 1962.

TRUSLER, H. M., GLANZ, S., and BAUER, T. B.: *Use of pituitary adrenocorticotropic hormone (ACTH) in treatment of extensive burns*. Plast. Reconstr. Surg., 9:478, 1952.

UGLAND, O. M.: *Electric burns. A clinical and experimental study with special reference to peripheral nerve injury*. Scand. J. Plast. Reconstr. Surg., Suppl. 2, 1967.

ULLOA, M. G., and STEVENS, E.: *Human Burns*. Latin American Bibliographical Archives, Mexico, 1961.

UNDERHILL, F. P.: *Changes in blood concentration with special referrence to the treatment of external superficial burns*. Ann. Surg., 86:840, 1927.

UNDERHILL, F. P., CARRINGTON, G. L., ET AL.: *Blood concentration changes in extensive superficial burns, and their significance for systemic treatment*. Arch. Intern. Med., 32:31, 1923.

GENERAL PRINCIPLES

UNDERHILL, F. P., KAPSINOW, R., and FISK, M. E.: *Studies on the mechanism of water exchange in the animal organism.* Amer. J. Physiol., 95:302, 315, 325, 334, 339, 1930.

UNDERHILL, F. P., and FISK, M. E.: *Studies on the mechanism of wtaer exchange in the animal organisms.* Amer. J. Physiol., 95:330, 348, 364, 1930.

WALLACE, A. B.: *The exposure treatment of burns.* Lancet, 250:500, 1951. *Burns—past, present, and future.* Plast. Reconstr. Surg., 37:385, 1966.

WALLACE, A. B., and WILKINSON, A. W., Eds.: *Research in Burns. Transactions of the Second International Congress on Research in Burns.* E. & S. Livingstone Ltd., Edinburgh, 1966.

WEEDER, R. S., BROOKS, H. W., and BOYER, A. S.: *Silicone immersion in the care of burns.* Plast. Reconstr. Surg., 39:256, 1967.

WERTHEIM, G.: Wien. med. Presse, 8:1237, 1867. Wien. med. Wchnschr., 18:826, 1868.

WHITE, C. S., and WEINSTEIN, J. J.: *Blood Derivatives and Substitutes.* Williams & Wilkins, Baltimore, 1949.

WILDE, N. J.: *A comparison of silver nitrate treatment with other techniques in the treatment of burns.* Plast. Reconstr. Surg., 40:271, 1967.

WILDE, N. J., and DERRY, G.: *Enzymatic débridement of burns.* Plast. Reconstr. Surg., 12:131, 1953.

WILMS, M.: *Studien zur Pathology der Verbrennungen. Die Ursache des Todes nach ausgedehnter Hautverbrennung.* Mitt. a. d. Grenzgeb. d. Med. u. Chir., 8:393, 1901.

WILSON, W. C., MacGREGOR, A. R., and STEWART, C. P.: *The clinical course and pathology of burns and scalds under modern methods of treatment.* Brit. J. Surg., 25:826, 1938.

WOLFF, W. A., ELKINTON, J. R., and RHOADS, J. E.: *Liver damage and dextrose tolerance in severe burns.* Ann. Surg., 112:158, 1940.

WOLFF, W. A., and LEE, W. E.: *A simple method for estimating plasma protein deficit after severe burns.* Ann. Surg., 115:1125, 1942.

WOMACK, N. A.: *On Burns.* Charles C Thomas, Springfield, 1952.

WOODWARD, J., and JACKSON, D.: *Emotional reactions in burned children and their mothers.* Brit. J. Plast. Surg., 13:316, 1961.

OPERATIVE
CORRECTION   **5**
OF SCARS

Scars usually follow the destruction of tissue resulting from trauma, burns, operation, or disease. Their appearance, their painfulness, or their contraction may cause mental or physical handicaps. Before operative correction is undertaken, the tissue which formed the scar must have reached a state of quiescence, recognizable by the pale color and softness of the cicatrix. Massage and radiation may aid in accelerating the process.

    In discussing the plastic repair of scars, it is important to distinguish between simple and extensive scars. Both types can be smooth, hypertrophic, depressed, or contracted.

SIMPLE SCARS

Simple Smooth or Hypertrophic Scars

    The simple scar, whether smooth or hypertrophic, is not always easy to correct. It is outlined by an incision, which penetrates at either side of the scar to the subcutaneous tissue, but not deeper. The subcutaneous tissue is kept intact to act as a base upon which the wound edges should be approximated (Fig. 50). With a sharp knife, the scar is excised. The wound edges are mobilized and separated from the subcutaneous tissue in a circumference of about 1 cm. (⅜ inch). Exact hemostasis is the next step. If possible, ligatures should be avoided and the bleeding controlled by pressure with hot, moist compresses. If ligatures are unavoidable, they should be made with the finest silk or cotton. The sutures of the wound edges are interrupted, and should be with fine nylon or silk, on a fine, curved cutting-edge atraumatic needle. The wound edges are not grasped with forceps but merely elevated by one prong to facilitate the penetration of the needle. If the wound edges are thick, interrupted subcutaneous sutures with fine cotton should precede the skin sutures.

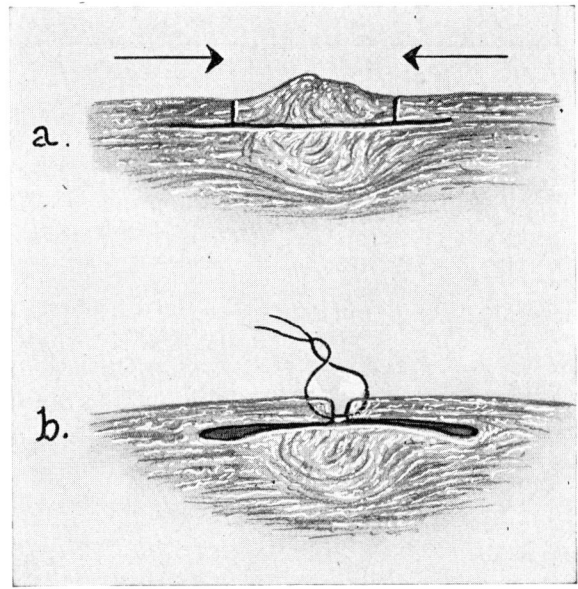

Fig. 50. Correction of simple smooth or hypertrophic scar. Incision outlines scar and penetrates on each side of scar into subcutaneous tissue, but not deeper. Subcutaneous tissue is kept intact to act as base on which mobilized wound edges are approximated.

The sutures are led so that the knot comes to lie toward the base of the scar (Fig. 51). If the wound edges are not under tension and are straight, Halsted's subcuticular wire suture is of value (Fig. 2) (Case 19, p. 1018). The wound is covered with xeroform ointment (see p. 36). The sutures are removed between the third and fifth day after the operation.

Simple Depressed Scars

If the simple scar is depressed, the technique for correction differs. The incision outlines the scar and penetrates at either side to the base of the retracted area, but not farther. The scar is now excised as previously described. From the deep corners of the defect, a bilateral incision is carried obliquely downward and outward, leaving the base of the scar intact to act as a buttress (Fig. 51). The adjoining tissue thus mobilized is approximated upon this buttress, and transfixed with interrupted subcutaneous fine cotton sutures and skin sutures or a subcuticular running wire suture (Case 19, p. 1018). The stitch of the subcutaneous suture is led so that the knot comes to lie toward the base of the scar.

Simple Contracted Scars

If the simple scar is contracted, the entire scar tissue, including the base, must be excised until the whole defect thus created consists of

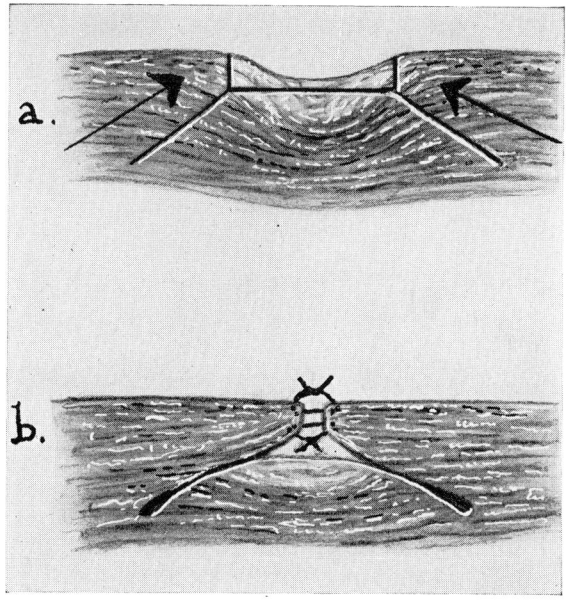

Fig. 51. Correction of simple depressed scar. Scar is excised to base of retracted area. From deep corners of defect, bilateral incision is carried obliquely downward and outward, leaving base of scar intact to act as buttress. Mobilized wound edges are approximated upon this buttress.

normal tissue. One ordinarily succeeds now in releasing the contracture unless it has been of long standing. Usually some sort of tissue shifting, rarely skin grafting, is necessary to close the defect.

In cases where the contracture is due to a binding web, the Z type of relaxation incision with exchanging flaps is the operation of choice. The object of this operation is to interrupt and displace the binding web by the formation and transposition of two triangular flaps, which are placed so that their outlines form a Z. The central line of the Z is laid along the most prominent portion of the web, and the arms of the Z are marked out on opposite sides of the central line. The two triangular flaps thus outlined are mobilized. The contracture is now reduced as far as possible, and the two flaps are transposed (Fig. 52). If the binding web is long, several Zs may be formed and their flaps transposed, as demonstrated in Case 109, page 1135.

The Z-plastic procedure can be applied in many other ways (Dingman). A good example is the breakup of congenital webs of the neck with the multiple Z-operation (see p. 599), and of contracting scars in the hand by the same technique, as already practiced by Morestin. This principle is used currently in the treatment of certain types of

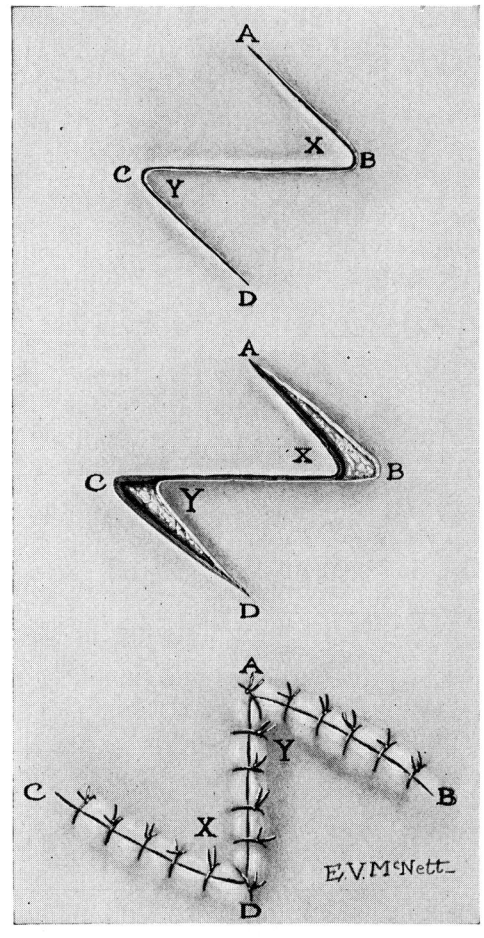

Fig. 52. Z-operation for contracted scars due to binding webs. Central line of Z is laid upon most prominent portion of web; arms of Z marked out on opposite sides of central line in 45-degree angles. Points *A* and *D* should lie in vertical projection of center of *C* and *B*. Thus, two triangular flaps are outlined, which are mobilized and exchanged. Object is to interrupt and displace binding web (note different direction of central line and increased distance between *C* and *D*). (After J. S. Davis: Penn. Med. J.)

186

OPERATIVE CORRECTION OF SCARS

Dupuytren's contracture (see p. 824). The multiple Z-plasty is also of great value in overcoming amniotic furrows of the extremities, as suggested by Stevenson (Farmer, Blackfield and Hauser), and in correcting constricting bands which involve the fingers more frequently than the extremities. They are of various degrees, ranging from superficial furrows to deep grooves and actual amputations. The central line of the Z comes to lie upon the constricting band while the arms are made on the opposite sides. As a rule, several such Zs are necessary. In some cases, particularly those with lymphedema, a several-stage operation (with intervals from one to several months apart) is advisable (Case 138, p. 1180).

The multiple Z principle can be applied in other ways. It is a well-known fact that scars running parallel to the elastic lines of the skin are as a rule less conspicuous than those running against them; the latter are broader and depressed. The elastic or skin-tension lines (or relaxed skin-tension lines, as Borges calls them) run perpendicular to the general direction of contraction of the muscles underlying the skin (see p. 13). They are often, but not always, similar to the wrinkle lines. Scars running perpendicular to the lines of skin tension, if conspicuous, can be improved by Z-plasties (Mir-Chyand Ju). This technique has been much advanced by Borges and Alexander, who describe various situations in detail. In scars running obliquely to the relaxed skin-tension lines, the directions and angles of the limbs of the Zs are important. The simple rule is "Have the limbs follow the relaxed skin-tension lines." The same principle can be used for semicircular or circular or U-shaped scars.

Covarrubias, whom Borges and Marino follow, went one step further. He changed the linear scar after its excision into a zig-zag scar by excision of consecutive small triangular pieces of skin from both skin wound edges, into which fit the small triangular flaps of the opposite side left after the excision (Fig. 53; Case 20, p. 1019). The excisions must be lined out carefully so that the triangular flaps of the one side fit into the triangular defect of the other side. Borges advises that each triangle should have a base of approximately 6 mm., a height of about 6½ mm., and an angle of 50 degrees, except the two at the ends which are 65 degrees. The small skin flaps are mobilized, but not beyond their base, advanced, and each tip is sutured into the angle of the corresponding defect. The author recommends this method highly. Penn achieves a similar result through consecutive small diamond-shaped excisions of the scar. By shifting one side or the other slightly, the wound edges will interdigitate. He removes the sutures after forty-eight hours and applies transparent tape across them. The cross tape, which does not need to be sterilized, should remain in place for two weeks.

Extensive Smooth Scars

Extensive smooth scars are in the same plane as the skin. Ordinarily, they do not cause any trouble, since they do not contract. They tend to become annoying, however, if they are situated in such exposed regions as the face or neck. In these cases, repair work may be requested. If the

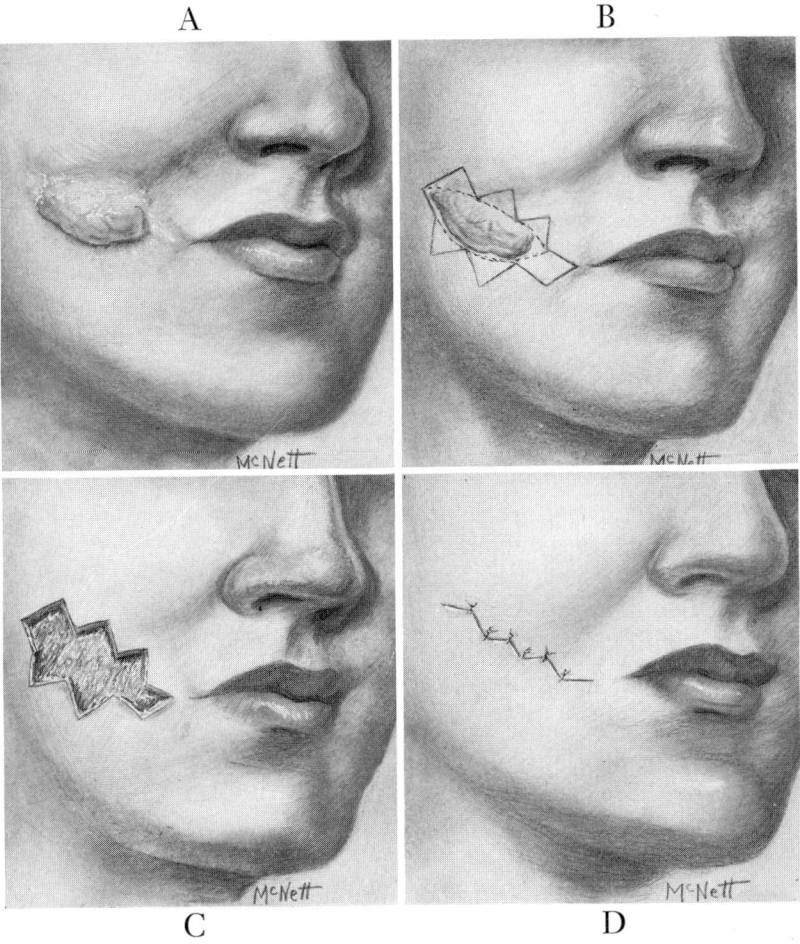

Fig. 53. *A:* Hypertrophic "antitension-line" scar crossing nasolabial fold (compare with Case 20). *B:* Multiple W-plasty for release of tension after excision of the scar. Line of excision marked with dotted lines. The Ws are drawn above and below the lines of excision; note their arrangement at either end of the scar. *C:* Scar and triangles have been excised. The triangular flaps are undermined to the level of their bases. *D:* The wound edges are closed by interdigitation of the various triangular flaps; the tip of each flap is sutured to the triangular notch of the opposing side.

188

scar is not too extensive, is elliptical, and the surrounding skin is freely movable, the scar is treated as if it were simple and smooth. It is excised down to the subcutaneous tissue, but not farther. The wound edges are mobilized subcutaneously and approximated until a linear suture can be established. If the defect left after excision of the scar is triangular (Fig. 10) or rectangular (Fig. 11) and the surrounding skin is freely movable, plastic closure can be achieved by starting with closure of the corners. If undue tension in the sutures is to be anticipated, a multiple-stage procedure is advisable, by which the scar is only partly excised and sutured (Morestin, Sistrunck, Smith). During the intervals—the intervals being three months—the skin is allowed to stretch until all parts of the scar are removed.

If the scar is too large to permit closure of the defect by simple tissue mobilization or tissue sliding, covering the defect by a full-thickness skin graft or thick split graft may be advisable.

Extensive Hypertrophic and Keloid Scars (Cases 5, 22, pp. 995, 1021)

The hypertrophic scar passes through a series of phases. During the healing stage, it becomes raised and looks red. Gradually, however, it fades out and recedes in prominence until it is on a level with the skin. Should, however, the scar maintain its prominence or become thickened and, as often occurs, be accompanied by itching, it then has developed into a keloid. Until recently, we did not know the cause of the keloid (the literature up to 1942 had been well reviewed by Garb and Stone, and more recently by Cosman, Crikelair, Gaulin and Lattes, and Maurer). More light, however, has been thrown upon the subject by Mowlem, and by Gluckmann in collaboration with Fell and Levitt, who investigated the cause of scar hypertrophy. It seems that if hair follicles, sebaceous glands, and their remnants become buried within the scar, the keratin liberated from these structures causes an extreme tissue reaction. The latter can be avoided or at least lessened if the scar is irradiated for the purpose of damaging the buried hair follicles and glands. However, true keloid scars are still a problem. It is a well-known fact that even after a complete excision of a keloid it may recur after a few weeks, whether the defect is sutured primarily, covered by a skin graft, left to granulate, or electrocoagulated. Local injections of the enzyme hyaluronidase, either alone (Cornbleet) or with corticotropin (ACTH) (Conway and Stark), appear to have questionable effect upon reduction of the keloid, although they seem to relieve itching and pain. The most efficient treatment remains radiation by x-ray or radium, preferably after excision of the scar. According to Ketchum et al., Griffith, and Murray, injection of triamcinolone acetonide (Kenalog) into the scar at three-week intervals after

189

surgical excision has proven effective. The author does not agree entirely. If the keloid extends over an area where the skin is freely movable, one may attempt excision of the entire area. The excision is carried out in the confines of the lesion, leaving a narrow margin of keloid at its injunction with normal skin and subcutaneous tissue. The skin surrounding the defect is mobilized and approximated until a linear suture can be established. Radiation is applied postoperatively, as soon as the wound has healed. If the scar, in spite of excision and radiation, develops again into a keloid, the second is many times smaller than the first (Fig. 11).

Extensive Irregular Scars (Hypertrophic or Atrophic)

These scars are often the result of burns or other trauma. If feasible they are excised and replaced preferably with a full-thickness or thick split skin graft; a flap may be required for replacement of scars which are unstable and adherent to underlying bone or poorly vascularized tissues. There are, however, unstable scars which allow removal of a thin surface layer either with a skin-graft knife or by dermabrasion (see p. 191), without exposure of the underlying bone or other deep tissues to which they adhere. The raw surface, which as a rule is freely bleeding from capillary oozing, can now be covered with a thick split skin graft as Webster and co-workers and Hynes have recommended. In this way the unstable scar acquires a thick layer of dermis and becomes less vulnerable. This method is applicable also for previously skin-grafted areas which remain still unstable (overgrafting after Webster). In irregular hypertrophic burn scars of the face, Serafries recommends application of the same method, i.e., deep dermabrasion until the surface is smooth and resurfacing of the raw area with a thick split skin graft.

Extensive Depressed Scars

If an extensive scar is retracted or depressed, the technique of correction differs from that used in simple depressed scars. In the majority of cases, the involved area is too large to allow an approximation of the neighboring subcutaneous tissue to fill the defect. Hence, the repair work involves grafting with fat, derma, bone, or cartilage to restore the normal surface contours. The scar is excised down to its base. The skin surrounding the defect is mobilized; then, after careful hemostasis, a properly shaped graft of dermis fat, dermis, bone, or cartilage is transplanted into the defect before the skin is closed over it (Case 12, p. 1006; Case 18, p. 1017). If simple mobilization of the skin does not suffice to close the defect over the graft, additional incisions must be made to allow more liberal shifting or rotation of skin. In such cases, however, secondary defects may be left, and one must be sure that they can be closed (see Chap. 2). In extreme cases, transplantation of skin by pedicle flaps is the last resort.

Extensive Contracted Scars

Correction of extensive contracted scars is one of the most difficult problems in plastic surgery. Such scars are usually caused by destruction of the deeper parts of the surface tissue, and most frequently appear at the flexor surface of the extremities or at the junction of limb and trunk. In some cases much can be done to avoid them to a greater or less degree by proper immobilization of the affected limb during the healing stage. Before any operative correction is undertaken, one should wait until the scar tissue has reached its final stage, although waiting too long may cause ankylosis and shortening of tendons and ligaments. Active and passive motion exercises of the affected limb and radiation during the waiting time are advisable. The objects of treatment are to remove the scar, to replace it by normal tissue, and to restore function. For technique, the reader is referred to pages 723, 810 and Cases 3, page 992; 111-115, page 1138.

Surgical Abrasion

In 1947, P. C. Iverson of Philadelphia introduced surgical abrasion, which he had devised for treatment of land-mine tattoos during World War II. This ingenious novelty was immediately received with great enthusiasm; its field of application was soon widened, and abrasion became a useful adjunct in the surgical treatment of scars. It was taken up by other branches of medicine, mainly by dermatologists (Kurtin, Burk and others), and used for treatment of all sorts of superficial skin lesions, such as acne pits, pigmentations, birthmarks, and superficial hemangiomas. It was only a matter of time until the increasing number of failures or actual damage from indiscriminate use of the method dampened the original enthusiasm. However, these drawbacks should not distract from the real benefits that surgical abrasion brought.

Its principle consists of removal of the superficial layers of the skin by means of emery paper, a motor-driven emery cylinder, or a wire brush. It is essential that a deep layer of the skin remain behind and intact from which, through regeneration of epithelium, the raw surface becomes epithelialized, as in the healing process of a donor area from which a split skin graft has been removed. The more superficial the abrasion, the quicker and better is the resurfacing. Hence, in lesions of the skin that practically penetrate the entire thickness, such as birthmarks and " professional" tattoos, abrasion may cause irreparable damage. In the treatment of acne scars, it may or may not be of benefit, depending upon the

191

depth of the craters. Patients have varying degrees of pitting. In patients with a preponderance of superficial, well-defined craters, the abrasive treatment is rewarding even in the presence of a few deep pits, which can be excised and sutured during the same procedure. When deep craters are preponderant, the procedure, even by multiple abrasion, is not of benefit; the same is true in patients who present only an indefinite and poorly defined irregularity. If patients have received previous x-ray therapy of the involved area, abrasion may cause actual damage by producing hypertrophic scars.

The greatest benefit derived from surgical abrasion is in the treatment of traumatic tattoos, dirt-stained and certain other scars, and brownish-discolored skin grafts. It may also be of benefit in removing common freckles.

In the treatment of land-mine tattoos during World War II, Iverson observed that after abrasion had been carried to the limits of safety there remained a variable number of small, isolated, deeply embedded deposits, which were excised. The resulting scars from suturing these minute elliptical incisions were rarely visible, while those incised through intact skin without abrasion developed visible scars. Hence, it seems that after abrasion the resulting scar becomes covered with a continuous smooth layer of regenerating epidermis. It is evident that there are limits, and that best results can be hoped for in the repair of narrow scars, for which this treatment is highly recommended. With a fine-grit abrasive, a superficial denudation of the scar and adjacent epithelium is produced before the scar is excised; the wound edges are sutured in the usual way and covered with a strip of rayon (p. 37). The sutures are removed on the fourth postoperative day by cutting the covering strip of rayon over the suture line only. The remainder of the dressing remains in place until it peels off on its own accord.

Technique for Extensive Abrasion (Case 21, p. 1020): The procedure is carried out under general anesthesia or local infiltration anesthesia (1 per cent procaine with epinephrine, 5 to 10 drops per ounce for hemostatic purposes) or by the use of the ethyl chloride spray (Kurtin, Burk). Ordinary waterproof emery paper of various grit (available in any hardware store), cut in strips equal to the width and circumference of a 3-inch bandage and wrapped around the bandage, is used for the abrasive. Smaller pieces may be cut to wrap around a Freer perichondral elevator or curved hemostat to reach crevices or treat narrow areas. Recently, motor-driven (1200 revolutions per minute) sanding cylinders (Iverson) or wire brushes of various widths (Kurtin, Burk) have been recommended. After the surface is surgically prepared, it is abraded vigorously. Capillary oozing can be decreased by applying compresses soaked in epinephrine

192

solution. It is safe to carry abrasion, if necessary, to the point where sub-cutaneous tissue gradually makes its first appearance in pinpoint elevations of fat through the abraded corium. Isolated areas, more deeply embedded and requiring removal, should be excised rather than abraded; the wound edges are sutured. At the end of the procedure, the raw surface is rinsed with copious amounts of warm saline solution to prevent emery particles from becoming buried under the regenerating epithelium. The raw surface is then covered with strips of rayon soaked in epinephrine solution. No other dressings are required. The rayon strips become adherent in a few minutes. They are left in place until they peel off, usually after eight to twelve days.

The erythema of the new skin gradually fades in eight to ten weeks. If a second-stage abrasion of the same area is required, it should not be carried out before this time. Within this time, a small percentage of patients may develop small, white, pinpoint milia, which are prob-ably caused by new epithelium over some of the sebaceous glands. They rupture spontaneously or can be evacuated after puncturing with a sterile needle.

In removal of gunpowder tattoos, the particles or some of the particles may be deeply embedded so that they must be excised as men-tioned above in the course of dermabrasion. Veith recommends another less traumatizing method. He introduces a 23-gauge needle into the skin, approximately 1 mm. to the side of the pigmented particle. The needle is placed so that the angle between it and the involved skin surface is approximately 5 degrees, and thrust into the dermis underlying the pig-mented particle. The needle being kept approximately parallel to the skin surface, the point is elevated. The tattooed skin is thereby raised much in the manner that tissue is presented for the obtaining of a pinch graft. A No. 11 scalpel blade is then used to shave off very thin layers of epidermis, then dermis, until the pigmented area is removed.

BIBLIOGRAPHY

BAER, T. W.: *Abrasive planing of the skin.* Penn. Med. J., 58:573, 1955.

BLACKFIELD, H. M., and HAUSER, D. P.: *Congenital constricting bands of the extremities.* Plast. Reconstr. Surg., 8:101, 1951.

BLAIR, V. P.: *The deep scar.* Surg. Gynec. Obstet., 40:439, 1925.

BORGES, A. F.: *Improvement of antitension-lines scar by the "W-Plastic" opera-tion.* Brit. J. Plast. Surg., 12:29, 1959.

193

GENERAL PRINCIPLES

BORGES, A. F., and ALEXANDER, J. E.: *Relaxed skin tension lines, Z-plasties on scars, and fusion excision of lesions.* Brit. J. Plast. Surg., 15:242, 1962.

BURK, J. W.: *Wire Brush Surgery in the Treatment of Certain Cosmetic Defects and Diseases of the Skin.* Charles C Thomas, Springfield, 1956.

CONWAY, H., and STARK, R. B.: *Corticotropin (ACTH) in treatment of keloids.* Arch. Surg., 64:47, 1952.

CONWAY, H., GILLETTE, R., SMITH, J. W., and FINDLEY, A.: *Differential diagnosis of keloids and hypertrophic scars by tissue culture technique with notes on therapy of keloids by surgical excision and Decadron.* Plast. Reconstr. Surg., 25:117, 1960.

CORNBLEET, T. H.: *Treatment of keloids with hyaluronidase.* JAMA, 154:1161, 1954.

DAVIS, J. S.: *Use of relaxation incisions when dealing with scars.* Penn. Med. J., 41:565, 1938.
Present evaluation of the merits of the Z-plastic operation. Plast. Reconstr. Surg., 1:26, 1946.

DAVIS, J. S., and KITLOWSKI, E. A.: *Theory and practical use of the Z incision for the relief of scar contractures.* Ann. Surg., 109:1001, 1939.

DINGMAN, R. O.: *Some applications of the Z-plastic procedure.* Plast. Reconstr. Surg., 16:246, 1955.

FARMER, A. W.: *Congenital elephantiasis associated with constrictions by anomalous bands.* J. Bone Joint Surg., 308:606, 1948.

GARB, J., and STONE, M. J.: *Keloids: Review of the literature and a report of eighty cases,* Amer. J. Surg., 58:315, 1942.

GLUCKMANN, A.: *Local factors in the histogenesis of hypertrophic scars.* Brit. J. Plast. Surg., 4:88, 1951.

GRIFFITH, B. H.: *The treatment of keloids with triamcinolone acetonide.* Plast. Reconstr. Surg., 38:202, 1966.

HYNES, W.: *The treatment of scars by shaving and skin graft.* Brit. J. Plast. Surg., 10:1, 1957.

IVERSON, P. C.: *Surgical removal of traumatic tattoos of the face.* Plast. Reconstr. Surg., 2:427, 1947.

JU, D. M.: *The physical basis of scar contraction.* Plast. Reconstr. Surg., 7:343, 1951.

KETCHUM, L. D., SMITH, J., ROBINSON, D. W., and MASTERS, F. W.: *The treatment of hypertrophic scar, keloid and scar contracture by triamcinolone acetonide.* Plast. Reconstr. Surg., 38:209, 1966.

KOCH, S. L.: *The treatment of lacerated wounds.* Surgery, 38:447, 1955.

KROMAYER, T.: *Kosmetische Resultate bei Anwendung des Stanzverfahrens.* Dermat. Wchnschr. 101:1306, 1935.
Rotationsinstrumente; ein neues technisches Verfahren in der dermatologischen Kleinchirurgie. Dermat. Ztschr. Berlin, 12:26, 1965.

KURTIN, A.: *Corrective surgical planing of skin.* Arch. Derm. Syph., 68:389, 1953.

OPERATIVE CORRECTION OF SCARS

LEVITT, W. M.: *Radiotherapy in the prevention and treatment of hypertrophic scars.* Brit. J. Plast. Surg., 4:104, 1951.

LEWIS, J. R.: *The Surgery of Scars.* McGraw-Hill, Inc., New York, 1963.

MARINO, H.: *The levelling effect of Z-plasties on lineal scars of the face.* Brit. J. Plast. Surg., 12:34, 1959.

MAURER, G.: *Das Keloid.* Langenbeck's Arch f. klin. Chir., 309:14, 1965.

MAY, H.: *The correction of scars.* Amer. J. Surg., 50:754, 1940.
Correction of cicatricial contractures of axilla, elbow joint and knee. Surg. Clin. N. Amer., p. 1229, October, 1943.
Narben Karrekturen im Gesicht, Fortrchr. d. Kiefer u. Gesichtr Chir. Georg Thieme Verlag, Stuttgart, Vol. VII, 1961.

MORESTIN, H.: *La réduction graduelle des difformités tégumentaires.* Bull. et mém. Soc. d. chirurgiens de Paris, 41:1233, 1915.
Cicatrice très étendue du crâne réduite par des excisions successives. Bull. et mém. Soc. d. chirurgiens de Paris, 42:2052, 1916.

MOWLEM, R.: *Hypertrophic scars.* Brit. J. Plast. Surg., 4:113, 1951.

MURRAY, R. D.: *Kenalog and the treatment of hypertrophied scars and keloids in Negroes and whites.* Plast. Reconstr. Surg., 31:275, 1963.

PENN, J.: *The removal of "cross-hatch" scars.* Plast. Reconstr. Surg., 25:73, 1960.

REID, M., and CARTER, B. N.: *The treatment of fresh traumatic wounds.* Ann. Surg., 114:4, 1941.

SERAFINI, G.: *Treatment of burn scars of the face by dermabrasion and skin grafts.* Brit. J. Plast. Surg., 15:308, 1962.

SMITH, F.: *A Manual of Plastic and Maxillofacial Surgery.* Military Surgical Manuals, National Research Council. W. B. Saunders, Philadelphia, 1942.
Multiple excision and Z-plastics in surface reconstruction. Plast. Reconstr. Surg., 1:170, 1946.

STEVENSON, T. W.: *Release of circular constriction scar by Z-flaps.* Plast. Reconstr. Surg., 1:39, 1946.

TRUSSLER, H. N. GLANZ, S., and BAUER, T.: *Reconstruction of burn scars.* Arch. Surg., 66:496, 1953.

VEITH, F. J.: *A technique for the removal of gunpowder tattoos.* Arch. Surg., 84:45, 1962.

WEBSTER, L. V.: *Dermal overgrafting of leg.* J. Bone Joint Surg., 40A:796, 1958.

DIVISION TWO
THE HEAD AND NECK

INTRODUCTORY ASPECTS OF HEAD AND NECK

6

THE individual appearance or expression of the face and head of a person results mainly from the conformation of the framework of the head and its surrounding soft parts. In numerous places where the framework is covered only by skin and subcutaneous tissue, the framework alone dominates the characteristic features, such as at the ridge of the nose, at the rim of the orbit, and at the zygomatic arch. In other places, where skin and framework are separated by muscles, the muscles not only are additional factors in causing the characteristic features but also provide mimic and other functions, such as the opening and closing of mouth and eyes.

GENERAL CONSIDERATIONS

The aim of any reconstructive operation must be the restoration of form and function. While in some parts of the body restoration of function is the major issue, in exposed parts—particularly in the face—restoration of form is of equal importance. Any external part of the body appears misformed if it differs in shape and proportion from normal appearance. The transition from normal to abnormal form may be either slight or very noticeable. Particularly in the face, any slight deviation from the normal characteristics of a race may become noticeable, making the patient feel self-conscious and causing considerable mental distress. The feeling of having an abnormal appearance is usually reflected in the face, causing a change of the physiognomy, which is under psychic influence. For certain types of patients, disfigurement of the face is more feared than death. These patients become depressed; they seek seclusion and develop a hatred of normal-looking people. It is questionable whether or not some patients will benefit from correction of their deformities. In extensive deformities, particularly those accompanied by functional handicaps (congenital or traumatic), surgical correction probably will be physically and emotionally beneficial; there are, however, some patients—particularly those with profound personality handicaps—for whom not even the finest surgical results can overcome their complexes. When dealing with purely cosmetic cases, the plastic surgeon is aware that he often operates within surgery's twilight zone—past the point of obvious physical need. Hence, he is inclined to weigh his would-be patient's motives and for advice he may turn to a psychiatrist. Unfortunately, not many plastic surgeons have routine psychiatric help available for all of their cosmetic cases, as do the members of the Plastic Department at Johns Hopkins Hospital in Baltimore. This group has done an outstanding job (Edgerton, Jacobson and Meyer).

The various reconstructive procedures for correction of facial deformities or defects can be divided into certain groups: (1) cheeks, temples, forehead, skull regions, (2) lips, (3) nose, (4) lids, and (5) ears. However, it is only natural—particularly if dealing with large defects—that some of the reparative problems cannot be forced into ordinary classifications. Hence, if a surgeon is accustomed to working according to prescribed methods, he is apt to become disappointed. Imagination and artistry must go hand in hand with skill and knowledge to lead to the final result, the success of which can be judged only by a consideration of the gravity of the case, that is, in the light of comparison.

ANESTHESIA IN SURGERY OF HEAD AND NECK

In anesthesia for surgery of head and neck, the patient's emotional and physical condition, the surgeon's requirements, and the anesthetist's ability all contribute to the choosing of the anesthetic method and agent. It can seldom be said that one method or agent is the anesthetic of choice;

there is much variation from person to person and from place to place, with good results.

Ether, which alone or in combination with gases was formerly the most frequently used anesthetic, is becoming less and less popular. Its aftereffects, slow induction and emergence, and explosiveness have contributed to its decline. With ether, the open-drop masks, mouth hooks, and nasopharyngeal airways have largely been abandoned and replaced by endotracheal tube inhalations. Though newer agents, in contrast to ether, depress respiration, they have been steadily replacing it as knowledge of their safe use is acquired. In general they produce smoother inductions and emergences, are nonexplosive, and have fewer aftereffects than ether. The newer general anesthetic agents are intravenous sodium pentothal for induction, followed by gas anesthesia with either nitrous oxide or halothane. Of the local anesthetic agents, Xylocaine and Carbocaine are more frequently used than Novocain.

The chief source of difficulty in head and neck surgery is obstruction of the airway; this complication should be constantly guarded against. The endotracheal tube has become the rule, with few exceptions, for good airway control. Since good control may be lost after the patient is unconscious, tracheal intubation while he is awake is much safer. A topical anesthesia is usually applied to the larynx just before intubation. The endotracheal tube is left in place until the patient regains his own airway control. Short-acting agents are helpful in obtaining smooth and safe emergence. When there is an incision in the mouth with some resultant ooze of blood at the end of the operation, it is wise to allow a good cough reflex to be regained before endotracheal extubation is begun.

For details on these various methods of anesthesia, the reader is referred to standard texts on anesthesiology.

BIBLIOGRAPHY

CLEMENT, F. W.: *Nitrous-Oxide-Oxygen Anesthesia.* Lea and Febiger, Philadelphia, 1951.

DAGLIOTTI, A. M.: *Anesthesia: Narcosis, Local, Regional, Spinal.* S. B. Debour, Chicago, 1937.

DRIPPS, R. D., ECKENHOFF, J. E., and VANDAM, L. D.: *Introduction to Anesthesia: The Principles of Safe Practice.* W. B. Saunders, Philadelphia, 1957.

GILLESPIE, N. A.: *Endotracheal Anesthesia.* University of Wisconsin Press, Madison, 1948.

THE HEAD AND NECK

GUEDEL, A. E.: *Inhalation Anesthesia, a Fundamental Guide*. The Macmillan Company, New York, 1937.
Inhalation Anesthesia. 2nd Ed. The Macmillan Company, New York, 1951.

HALE, D. E.: *Anesthesiology*. F. A. Davis Company, Philadelphia, 1954.

LABAT, G.: *Regional Anesthesia, Its Technic and Clinical Application*. W. B. Saunders, Philadelphia, 1928.

LEIGH, M., DIGBY, M., and BELTON, M. K.: *Pediatric Anesthesia*. The Macmillan Company, New York, 1949.

LUNDY, J. S.: *Clinical Anesthesia: A Manual of Clinical Anesthesia*. W. B. Saunders, Philadelphia, 1943.

MINNITT, R. J., and GILLIES, J.: *Textbook of Anesthetics*. Williams and Wilkins, Baltimore, 1948.

MOORE, D. C.: *Regional Block: A Handbook for Use in the Clinical Practice of Medicine and Surgery*. Charles C Thomas, Springfield, 1953.

PITKIN, G. P.: *Conduction Anesthesia*. J. B. Lippincott, Philadelphia, 1950.

WYLIE, W. D., and CHURCHILL-DAVIDSON, H. C.: *A Practice of Anesthesia*. Year Book Medical Publishers, Inc., 1966.

THE CHEEK,
TEMPLE, FOREHEAD, AND   7
SKULL REGIONS

REPARATIVE surgery of the cheek, temple, forehead, and skull regions is divided into (1) *the closure of defects* and (2) *the correction of deformities.*

DEFECTS

A defect in these regions may be simple or complicated. It may involve the surface structures only or deeper structures including the framework. A defect may be caused by the surgeon himself or may already be present. In the former case, the surgeon is, to some extent, at liberty to give the defect the shape he wants and may thus often facilitate its closure (see discussion of Langer's lines, p. 13, and Fig. 9). In defects already present he is confronted with a predetermined problem.

DEFECTS INVOLVING SKIN ONLY

There are certain defects which involve the skin alone, without the subcutaneous tissue. These defects may be due to trauma, excision of scars, or excision of skin tumors. There are two ways of closing these defects: by *skin shifting* or by *skin grafting.*

Skin Shifting
Skin shifting should be employed, as a rule, only in small defects, since it involves wide subcutaneous undermining of the skin (separation

of the skin from its nourishing base), and hence offers the possibility of necrosis or of secondary deformity. In some cases, this can be avoided by utilizing a several-stage procedure, such as described on page 189. The mole or scar, for instance, is partly removed and the defect closed by skin sliding. After the skin has stretched—that is, after three months—one or more similar procedures are performed.

Skin Grafting

For larger defects, skin grafting is the method of choice (Cases 3, 6, 22, pp. 992, 996, 1021).

Indications for the various types of grafts have been outlined on page 25. One important point, however, should be stressed: simple coverage is not enough. The graft should also match, in color and texture, the skin of the face. Hence, selection of the proper donor area is of importance. The graft which best matches the skin of the face is found, for small defects, behind the ear and supraclavicular region. Even large grafts can be taken from the base of the neck and the supra- and infraclavicular regions with the drum-type dermatome, as Edgerton and Hansen have demonstrated. When the clavicle is prominent and the clavicular fossa deep, the cutting of the skin graft may be greatly facilitated by injecting saline solution into the subcutaneous tissue (Barker).

In skin defects caused by burns with roentgen rays, one word of caution may be said concerning skin grafting: a free graft will take only on healthy well-vascularized tissue. Some x-ray burns may involve deeper structures, causing dense avascular scar formation of the subcutaneous tissue. Such tissue is a contraindication to free grafting; transplantation of a flap should instead be considered.

DEFECTS OF SKIN AND SUBCUTANEOUS TISSUE

Tissue Shifting and Flaps from Immediate Neighborhood

If a defect involves skin and subcutaneous tissue, free skin grafting, as a rule, is not considered, since skin and subcutaneous tissue need to be replaced. Such a defect is covered either by tissue shifting or by a pedicle flap. Tissue shifting (Figs. 12-14, Case 7, p. 997) has the great advantages of tissue resemblance and quick healing. The same is true with flaps taken from the immediate neighborhood. The secondary defect resulting from transfer of the flap may be placed in hidden areas (Cases 1, 4, 8, pp. 988, 994, 998). Seldom will it be feasible and practical to use Esser's cheek rotation principle, as demonstrated in Figure 54. The distinct disadvantage is the large secondary defect, which should be closed by "tugging" the wound edges at strategic points.

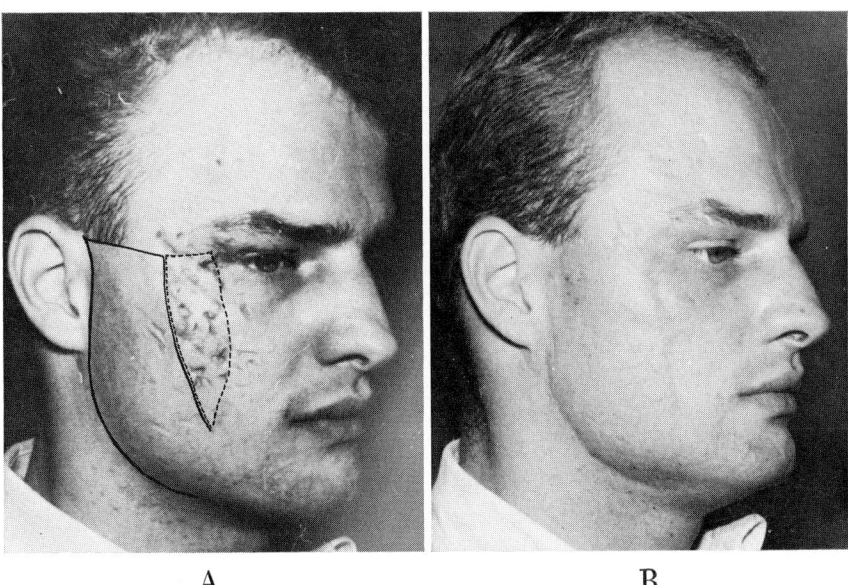

A   B

Fig. 54. Esser's cheek rotation method. *A:* This patient was thrown out of an automobile and his face hit a telegraph pole. He sustained numerous crater-like scars of the face. The area to be excised is marked out in dotted lines. The area of the cheek to be rotated into the defect is marked out with solid lines (note narrow pedicle containing the facial artery). This is not an ordinary pedicle flap, however. The area to be rotated is undermined widely in the periphery, but not mobilized as freely as a flap; it is then shifted into the defect. The secondary defects are closed by tugging and suturing the wound edges. *B:* Four years after the operation and after repair of remaining scars.

Flaps from Distant Parts

Next in choice is a flap from a distant part of the body. Available is the forehead flap or one of the tube flaps. The forehead flap (also the sickle flap, p. 393, and scalping flap, p. 402), best matching cheek color and texture, should in males be used only if necessary; it leaves scars and a denuded area, which in spite of skin grafting may be disfiguring. In females, however, it is the flap of choice if the patient is willing to alter her hair style (Case 49, p. 1059). Large scalp flaps can also be used to cover large defects of the forehead. They are depilated after several weeks by dissecting the hairbearing part of the flap away and covering the raw surface with a split skin graft, preferably taken from the neck clavicular region (Wang, Macomber and Sullivan).

Of the tubed flaps, the vertical or horizontal (mastoid to mastoid) cervical flap is perhaps the simplest, since it can be transplanted directly; secondly, if the flap is planned so that the skin of the clavicular region becomes the peripheral end of the flap, it will match the skin of the cheeks

205

well. Next in choice is a flap from the upper arm (Case 13, p. 1008). Flaps from other regions provide more skin but do not so well match the skin of the cheeks and also necessitate successive migration by the use of intermediate host areas. Where the flap comes to lie on the naked bone of the skull, the external table of this bone should be removed and the medullary spaces exposed to facilitate adherence of the flap's raw surface to the base of the defect.

Flaps or Split Grafts for Scalp and Periosteum

Defects of the scalp which do not include the periosteum are best covered with thick split grafts. The periosteum is an excellent base for the growth of free grafts. The most extensive avulsions of the scalp are incurred by female factory workers whose hair is caught in conveyor belts, rolls, and other machinery (Case 11, p. 1004). If the general condition of the patient is satisfactory, the raw areas should be covered immediately by split-thickness grafts. Quoting Robinson, attempts to replace the avulsed scalp in its original form have invariably failed. Very recently, however, a successful replacement of the avulsed scalp is reported by Lu, who attributes his success to an early operation (within $1\frac{1}{2}$ hours after the accident), prevention of drying of the inside scalp and exposed skull, avoidance of irritation in the preparation of the scalp, and strictly atraumatic technique. Neglect in those areas may be the reason for O'Conner and Hankins' experiences. Hankins prepared the avulsed scalp by shaving all hair and scrubbing both sides vigorously with a stiff brush and green soap, then rinsing with saline solution. The vessels were flushed with heparin solution; the avulsed scalp was replaced; the temporal vessels were anastomosed (a questionable procedure). The replacement of the scalp proved successful in that the base of the scalp took. After twenty days the leathery necrotic outer layer could be removed in toto, uncovering healthy granulating tissue which was immediately covered with skin grafts. Osborne reports success in the application of split grafts from the shaved and aseptically prepared avulsed scalp with the dermatome, using Zintel's resplit technique (p. 170).

Defects which include the periosteum, exposing the naked bone, are best covered with flaps taken from the preserved parts of the scalp. Before one resorts to this method in large defects, however, a more conservative method may be given a trial: removal of the outer table of the skull with a chisel to expose the medullary spaces and to promote the growth of granulations, followed by transplantation of a split graft. This procedure has been successful in one of the author's cases, and is also highly recommended by Kazanjian and Webster. It may not even be necessary to wait

until granulations have formed but instead to transplant the grafts immediately upon the medullary space (Case 10, p. 1002), as is done after saucer-
ization of other bones. If this does not succeed, the flap method should be
used. The flap should be planned to contain one of the larger arteries
(temporal, frontal); because of the abundant blood supply of scalp flaps
they can be transferred immediately. Care should be taken that the
periosteum of the donor area is not included in the flap but left behind
upon the bone. The periosteum is an excellent base for a skin graft.
Hence, after transfer of the flap, the raw area of the flap bed can be
covered with a split graft immediately, which invariably takes well (Cases
1, 4, 9, pp. 988, 994, 1000). Orticochea makes use of four flaps to close
the scalp defect as well as flap beds. If a sliding flap cannot be used—the
defect may be too large—a tube flap from the abdomen migrated via the
forearm should then be selected (Bagozzi).

Hair-bearing punch grafts may be used for bald areas (Orentreich,
Cronin, and Strough).

DEFECTS OF SKIN AND MUSCLE

Defects of this type are best covered with pedicle flaps to which
a sufficient amount of fat tissue is attached. (For defects of *muscles*, see
under Deformities, p. 228.)

DEFECTS OF FULL THICKNESS OF CHEEKS

Defects involving the entire thickness of the cheeks require replacement of skin plus lining. There are numerous possible ways to do this,
and many methods have been described; only a few of them are worthwhile from the cosmetic standpoint. All those methods which employ
local flaps in such a way that they leave disfiguring scars should be
discarded.

Local Flaps

These should be used only for closure of small defects. The principle consists of the formation of a flap from the direct neighborhood of
the defect; its pedicle is sutured to the bordering mucosa to obtain
maximal blood supply at its base. Later, the flap is turned over to replace
the lining and another flap from the neighborhood is rotated or slid to
cover the raw areas. The defect left by the latter is closed by skin sliding
(F. Smith).

Technique (F. Smith) (see Fig. 78 for comparison): The flap to be utilized as the lining-hinged flap is outlined. It must receive its blood supply from the lining mucosa and the muscles bordering the defect. Consequently, the mucosa on this edge must be undermined and accurately approximated to the skin or the pedicle with fine sutures. This produces a minimal scar and a maximal blood supply. The blood supply may be guaranteed by partially mobilizing the flap and returning it to its original site. The next step (three weeks later) consists, if necessary, of destroying the hair follicles of the lining flap by shaving off (with a skin-graft knife) a layer of epidermis sufficiently thick to destroy them. The raw area is covered with a split skin graft. Two weeks later, the lining flap, with some of the underlying fat tissue, is turned over and sutured to the incised free margins of the mucosa of the defect. The raw surfaces are covered with a flap rotated or slid from the neighborhood; the defect left by the latter is closed by skin sliding. The blood supply of the covering flap may be guaranteed by mobilizing and returning it to its former site during one of the previous stages. The muscle defect, if it results in a depression, may be corrected later by transplantation of a dermal graft.

Flaps from Distant Parts

For larger defects, flaps from distant parts must be chosen (Case 14, p. 1010). These flaps must, of course, be lined, unless other flaps—for instance, large temporal flaps (McGregor and Reid)—can be used for lining. Concerning the source and lining, see page 77.

DEFECTS OF LINING OF CHEEKS

Large defects of the lining mucous membrane due to trauma or infection cause early contractures. These contractures should be released as soon as possible and the defect covered either with a split skin graft, according to the in-lay or on-lay method (p. 39), or with a pedicle flap. Grafts should be used in cases where only the mucosal lining is to be replaced; for deeper defects, a pedicle flap is indicated and most useful (Blair). The pedicle flap should have a hairless skin (cervical or acromiopectoral) flap. The flap is introduced through an incision below the mandible. The incision, commencing at the anterior border of the masseter muscle anterior to the crossing of the arteria maxillaris externa, is led forward and penetrates between cheek and mandible. The flap is sutured in place after removal of all scars and reduction of the contracture. The pedicle is severed after two to three weeks, followed by adjustment of the flap and proper closure of the wound along and below the mandible.

THE CHEEK, TEMPLE, FOREHEAD, AND SKULL

DEFECTS OF SKULL

Defects of the skull may cause deformity as well as functional impairment and symptoms (traumatic epilepsy) (Drevermann, Bürkle de la Camp, Grant and Norcross). Closure of such defects can be achieved with autogenous or heterogenous material. The preferred autogenous material is the bone graft (Lexer, Gulecke, Grant and Norcross, McClintock, Dingman, and others). Of the heterogenous material, vitallium (Geib, Peyton and Hall, Beek), celluloid (Ney), tantalum (Pudenz, Mayfield and Levitch, Gardner, Woodhall and Spurling, Weiford and Gardner, and others), and stainless steel (M. Scott et al.) have been used. Tantalum has gained popularity. The concepts of this subject up to 1950 have been well covered by Reeves in a monograph that also contains an up-to-date collection of references. He prefers tantalum plates. More recently, Dingman strongly advocates autogenous bone plates, Longacre and de Stefano use split rib grafts, and Streli and Nockemann recommend frozen cranial homografts. Autogenous material becomes an organic unit with the host bone; heterogenous material becomes encapsulated. Tantalum, however, appears to induce less tissue reaction than the other foreign materials, but it remains a foreign body and as such may upon injury cause infection, which is the chief source of failure in cranioplasty. This is unlikely when autogenous bone grafts are used, particularly after the bone graft has become incorporated as an organic unit; this outweighs the apparent disadvantage of the greater magnitude of the operation and inhibits epilepsy.

Closure of Skull Defect with Autogenous-Bone Graft

Technique: The covering skin receives first attention. Any broad scar must be replaced, preferably by skin shifting or transfer of a pedicle flap (see p. 77 and Case 9, p. 1000) a few weeks before the main repair work is done. After traumatic injury, it is still believed wise to postpone the closure of the skull defect for three months after primary healing and six months after infection. In preparing the bone-graft bed, it is to be emphasized that (1) cranial periosteum is to be preserved; otherwise, a periosteum-covered graft must be chosen; (2) the preparation of the defect's edges is to be done in such a way that a broad apposition of graft and host bone is possible. The defect is exposed by forming and reflecting a properly shaped scalp flap. The flap should be made larger than the underlying bone defect so that its wound edges do not superimpose upon the edges of the cranial defect. The dura is carefully dissected free. Then the medullary spaces of the bony defect's edges are exposed for at least 1.5 cm. (⅝ inch) by removing the external table, thus preparing a broad, well-vascularized graft bed (Figs. 55, 56). This is done as follows: At a distance of about 1.5 cm. (⅝ inch) from the defect's edges, a shallow groove is carved in the bone with a V-shaped chisel. Then with a flat chisel the external table is removed from the bone edge to the groove.

GRAFT FOR SMALL DEFECT: The removal of the graft follows. Only seldom will the classic method of Müller and König be possible: they shifted a pedicle flap (skin, periosteum, lamina externa) from the neigh-

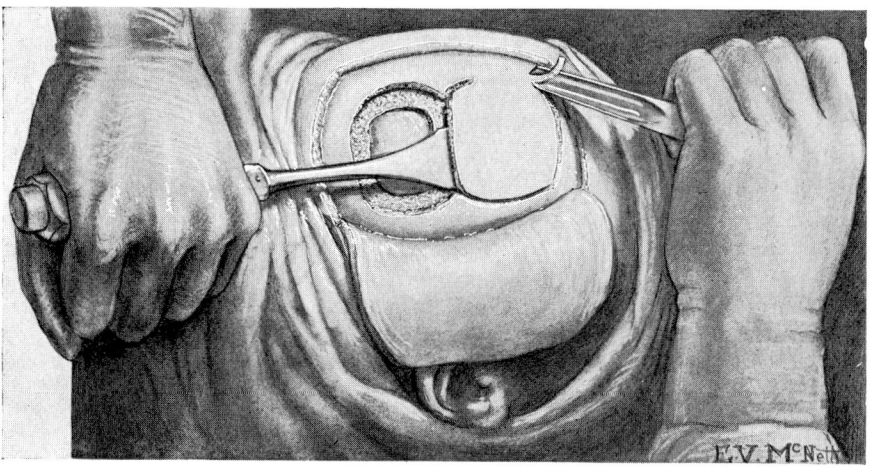

Fig. 55. Closure of medium-sized skull defect with tabula externa graft. Scalp flap reflected. Graft bed prepared by removal of rim of external table around defect edges. Tabula externa graft being removed.

borhood into the defect. But a free lamina-externa graft for defects not larger than 5 by 5 cm. (2 by 2 inches) is the graft of choice (Fig. 55). It is best taken from a thick part of the skull, such as the occipital region. An extension of the incision or a secondary incision for exposure of the occipital region may become necessary. The periosteum should be left attached to the graft if a periosteum-covered graft is needed. A pattern of the defect is made and placed upon the donor area. With a V-shaped chisel, a groove is made around the pattern down to the diploe; with a straight chisel, held almost flat, the graft is removed. The graft is now laid upon the defect and its periosteum sutured to the periosteum of the defect's edges.

GRAFT FOR LARGE DEFECT: For larger defects, the graft should be taken from the ilium or from the anterior surface of the tibia and be about

210

0.5 cm. (³⁄₁₆ inch) thick (Fig. 56), or it should be in the form of split rib grafts (Longacre and de Stefano). The graft from the ilium is given preference. If a periosteum-covered tibial graft is used, it is bent by sawing transversely through the cortex to, but not through, the periosteum. If more than one plate of graft is needed, the defect is covered as outlined in Figure 57. It is important not to place the plates side by side, but to overlap them; this requires shaping of the edges in a staircase-like manner. In this way, the grafts are in broad apposition not only with the defect's

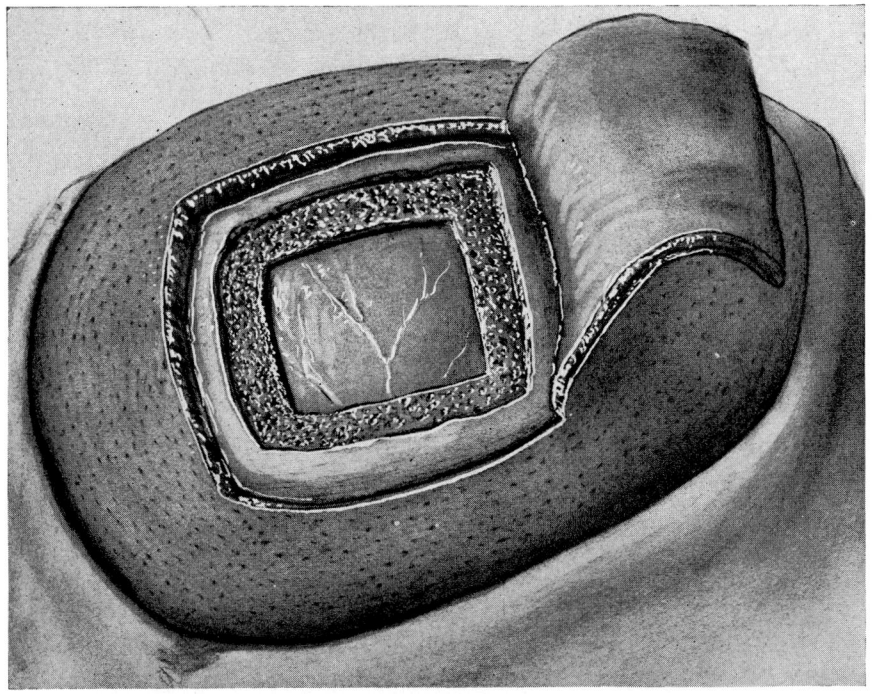

Fig. 56. Closure of large skull defect with autogenous bone graft. Scalp flap for exposure of defect is reflected. Graft bed is prepared by removal of external table around defect edges.

edges but also with each other. They are held in place with long mattress sutures of cotton. If rib grafts are used, alternate entire ribs, e.g. sixth, eighth, and tenth rib, are removed subperiosteally; each rib is split. The grafts are bent and contoured to fit the defect and are placed as scaffold between the edges of the cranial defect to stimulate new bone formation between skull and grafts and between the rib grafts themselves. If ilium grafts are used (see Case 9, p. 1000), they are removed from the inner table of the ilium, as recommended by Pickrell and described on page 70.

211

Coming from the median side of the pelvis, they are naturally curved. The concave side, which comes to lie upon the dura and brain, is smooth and covered with periosteum. As large grafts must be used, it may be necessary to remove the median rim of the crest of the ilium, togther with the median plate. The graft is properly shaped with rongeur and chisels. To obtain additional curvature of the graft, the margins may be bent with pliers and broken in greenstick fashion. The graft is then placed upon the cranial defect's edges and held in place with long mattress sutures of cotton similar to those demonstrated in Figure 57. The skin flap is now replaced and sutured. If there was much oozing, it is wise to insert two fine rubber dam drains at the most dependent points for forty-eight hours.

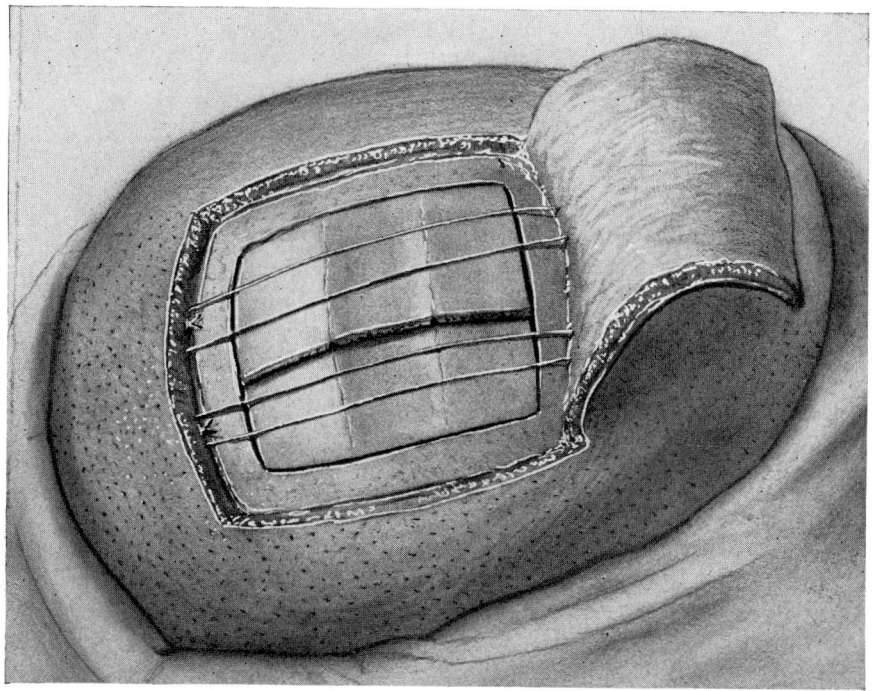

Fig. 57. Two periosteum-covered tibial grafts are placed upon graft bed and held in place with mattress sutures. Grafts have been bent after sawing transversely through cortex in two places to periosteum, but not through it.

After-Treatment: A heavily padded pressure dressing is applied. The dressing is changed after forty-eight hours and a moderately padded dressing applied until removal of the sutures on the eighth postoperative day. The grafted cranial area must be protected by means of well-padded dressings for about three weeks.

THE CHEEK, TEMPLE, FOREHEAD, AND SKULL

Traumatic Epilepsy: Traumatic epilepsy is benefited by cranioplasty alone, as the follow-up studies of Drevermann, Bürkle de la Camp, Grant and others demonstrate (see Case 9, p. 1000). There are, however, opinions to the contrary. Lexer recommended for cases of dural defects replacement of the cicatricial tissue with a fat-tissue graft (Drevermann). The operation is then carried out in two stages: (1) removal of scar from the brain and transplantation of the fat-tissue graft, and (2) closure of the bone defect with bone grafts three months later.

Closure of Skull Defect with Tantalum Plate

Technique: The defect is exposed and the defect's edges prepared as just described. The groove in the outer table encircling the defect, however, is made less wide and less deep. A sheet of tantalum, 0.3 mm. (0.0125 inch) thick, is shaped at the operating table to fit into the prepared groove and to conform with the contours of the skull. The necessary implements are a pair of tin shears, a metal punch, a round-headed hammer, and a concave wooden block (Gardner). The plate is then set upon the prepared bone shelf and held in place with small tantalum screws, drilled through punch holes of the plate into the bone. The skin flap is reflected back and the wound edges sutured.

After-Treatment: A well-padded dressing is worn until the wound has healed. Postoperative fluid collections between scalp and implant may be aspirated or controlled by a pressure dressing.

DEFECTS OF THE DUCTUS PAROTIDEUS (SALIVARY FISTULA)

Injuries to the ductus parotideus may occur in the region of the parotid gland or of the masseter or buccinator muscle. Injury to the buccal and zygomatic branches of the nervus facialis is also likely to be present. If the division of the duct is overlooked or primary repair neglected or unsuccessful, distressing fistulas of the duct may develop and may offer difficulties in successful repair. Hence, it is most desirable to attempt a primary repair, which in clean-cut wounds can be performed up to twelve hours after the accident. Repair of the fine-caliber facial-nerve strands should not be attempted, since it is hardly possible and spontaneous regeneration nearly always occurs. The literature on primary repair of the severed parotid duct has been thoroughly reviewed by Sparkman. From his experience, it becomes evident that a dowel should be inserted into the severed ends only temporarily while the divided ends are being anastomosed, and also that postoperative salivary secretion should be augmented to counteract obstruction rather than suppressed.

Hence, as soon as it is feasible the patient is placed on a regular diet. Oral hygiene with frequent mouthwashes should be maintained pre- and postoperatively.

Technique

Primary Repair: After the usual cleansing and under local anesthesia with 1 per cent procaine, bleeding is controlled and the severed duct ends are exposed. Lacerated oral mucous membrane and muscles are sutured first. A small-caliber urethral catheter is inserted into the distal portion of the duct while the other end of the catheter is cut on a bevel and placed into the proximal portion. The anastomosis of the divided duct ends is now accomplished over the catheter with interrupted everting mattress sutures of fine silk on an atraumatic needle (compare with Fig. 27). The catheter is then withdrawn through the mouth and the wound is closed.

If the laceration of the duct is overlooked or primary repair is unsuccessful, a salivary fistula will usually develop which may be external or internal. Fistulas of smaller branches of the duct in the gland region heal spontaneously; fistulas of the duct proper often do not, and require repair. If the gap between the peripheral and central ends of the duct is not excessive, simple suturing of the two ends after their mobilization over a dowel may be tried, as described previously; the dowel is removed after completion of the anastomosis. In the majority of cases, however, the duct ends cannot be united or the anastomosis would be under tension. In such cases, short-circuiting operations, with rerouting of the central end into the mouth, have been advised but should be reserved only for extreme cases (see below), since this method does away with the valve-like action of the papilla and there is no protection against ascending infection from the mouth. Instead, it is recommended that the two ends be bridged with a dowel, which should remain in place for two to three weeks. The use of a dowel with a lumen (urethral catheter) is not necessary, since most of the saliva passes between dowel and mucous membrane. While the flow of saliva is augmented after anastomosis, it should be slowed when a gap is present. Bailey and Saff describe a simple method of secondary repair.

Secondary Repair: Under local anesthesia, the divided duct is exposed after excision of the former scar. The blunt end of a probe is inserted from the mouth through the papilla into the peripheral end of the duct, and escapes through the wound of the cheek; a strand of cotton (No. 10) or heavy silk is tied as a double loop to the probe, and both are withdrawn through the mouth. The patient is given a few drops of lemon juice to stimulate the salivary flow; this facilitates identification

214

of the proximal end of the severed duct. The two ends of the cotton or silk strand are threaded through a long, curved Mayo needle. The needle is passed backward, with the blunt end first into the proximal duct. With gentle manipulation, the needle is forced through the parotid gland to the skin. A tiny nick is made in the skin, and the thread is carried through. A small square of rubber sheeting is threaded on each end of the thread, and this is followed by application of a lead shot on top of each square to hold the thread snugly in place. The incision is now closed.

After-Treatment

This consists of routine administration of antibiotics, mouthwash, and liquid diet until the initial swelling has subsided; a watery fluid will drain from the wound for about a week. The suture dowel may be removed after the fourteenth postoperative day, provided all the swelling has subsided.

If the papilla of the duct in the mouth is destroyed or obliterated and the central end of the duct is sufficiently long, it can be rerouted into the mouth.

Technique (Langenbeck)

If an external fistula is present, a probe is inserted, and the fistula is circumscribed by an incision, which leaves a small disk of skin attached to the external opening (Delore). From here, the central part of the duct is dissected free for a short distance. A perforation is now made in front of the masseter muscle through the buccinator muscles and the mucous membrane of the mouth. The freed part of the duct is pulled through this opening into the mouth and held in this position by suturing the small disk of skin to the edges of the mucous membrane. The wound is closed in layers. A similar procedure, but without the disk of skin, is possible for internal fistulas.

If the papilla of the duct in the mouth is destroyed or obliterated and the central end of the duct is too short to permit rerouting into the mouth, plastic elongation of the duct becomes necessary.

Technique (Küttner) (Fig. 58)

The central part of the duct is dissected free for a short distance. The incision through skin and subcutaneous tissue and fascia is now led forward beyond the anterior border of the masseter muscle. Through an opening in the buccinator muscles, the mucous membrane is exposed. It is incised so that a tongue-like flap is tubed, by proper suturing, and connected with the central end of the duct after temporary insertion of

215

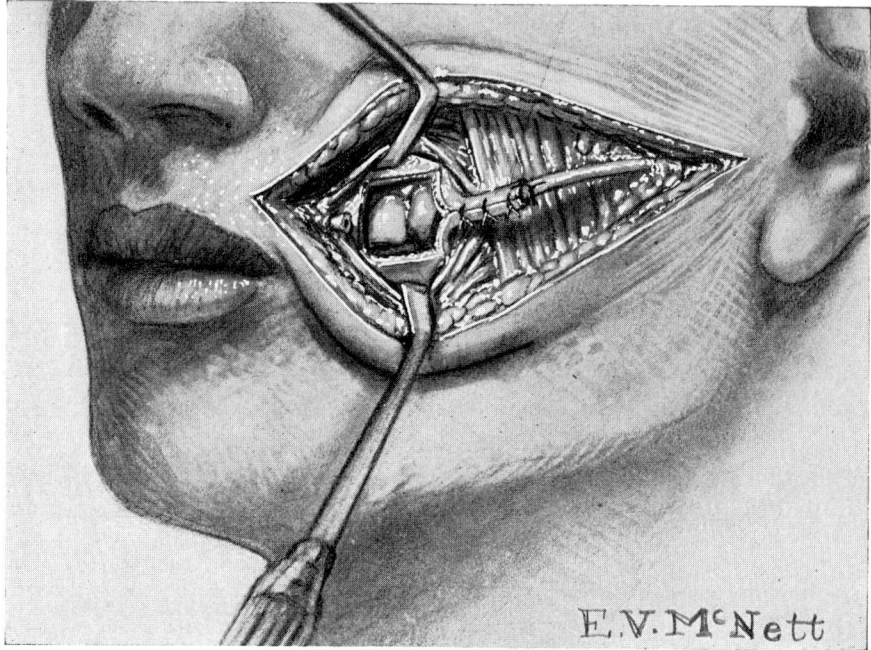

Fig. 58. Repair of defect of Stensen's duct with tubed buccal mucous membrane flap (Küttner). Mucous membrane has been exposed through opening in buccinator muscle.

a urethral catheter as a dowel. Closure of the opening in the mucous membrane is not difficult.

When it was impossible to restore the continuity of the duct and the fistula persisted, Baron followed Morestin's original suggestion and excised the fistula and the surrounding cicatrix, ligated the central part of the Stensen's duct and closed the wound without drainage. He was able to cure five cases of salivary fistulae by this method. Sparkman suggested similar procedures.

DEFORMITIES

PALSY FROM PERIPHERAL LESION OF FACIAL NERVE

A peripheral lesion of the facial nerve can occur with or without interruption of the continuity of the nerve substance. In the absence of nerve interruption, it may be due to cold (toxic neuritis, primary or idiopathic paralysis, Bell's palsy), to inflammation of the surroundings, or to pressure. Comprehensive treatises about this subject have been published by Kottel and by Miehlke.

Complete or incomplete paralysis of one side of the face is the most outspoken symptom. The treatment is either conservative or surgical.

CONSERVATIVE TREATMENT

In all cases where there is no evidence of severance or compression of the nerve, conservative treatment is indicated, at least for several months: daily massage and stimulation with the galvanic current for a few minutes three times weekly. If, however, the faradic response is still absent or does not recur after five or six months, surgery is indicated.

SURGICAL TREATMENT

Surgical treatment is required if the paralysis of the facial nerve appears to be the result of pressure or of severance of the nerve. The presence or absence of response to the faradic current is of diagnostic and locating value. In compression, the loss of response to faradic stimulation distal to the lesion is—as a rule—gradual, while in severance the loss occurs after forty-eight hours. Furthermore, in complete severance, the loss of response distal to the injury is complete; in compression, the loss may be incomplete, particularly if the site of the lesion is in the soft parts and not in the bony canal with its unyielding wall. The operation should be carried out as soon as the diagnosis is made.

Decompression

If the lesion appears to be outside the bony canal—that is, beyond the foramen stylomastoideum—the nerve is exposed at its exit from the foramen, following the posterior belly of the digastric muscle. The nerve is carefully dissected free until one finds the lesion, which may be located posterior to, within, or anterior to the parotid gland. The nerve is now decompressed by removing the compressing cause and slitting the sheath of the nerve to gain further relief from pressure. If the site of the pressure appears to be in the bony canal, the canal is opened by a mastoid operation, during which the descending and horizontal portion of the fallopian aqueduct is defined and opened. The exit of the facial nerve at the foramen stylomastoideum serves as a guide. Such an operation should be performed only by a surgeon competent in this particular field. The pressure is released by removing the compressing cause and slitting the sheath of the nerve.

217

THE HEAD AND NECK

Nerve Suture

If the facial nerve is severed it should be sutured as soon as possible, unless the accident has occurred under septic conditions. It should be remembered that the distal end of the severed nerve ceases to respond to the faradic current only after forty-eight hours. Thus, location of the distal end by use of the faradic current is greatly facilitated during this period. The severed ends are approximated and held accurately together by suturing the nerve sheath with 8-0 black monofilament nylon suture on an atraumatic needle—all principles of microsurgery to be used in this technique—unless the severance is in the bony canal (see following paragraph). Even small gaps may be closed by direct nerve suture, rerouting the nerve along a shorter course (Bunnell). McCabe states that, unless the distal segment is depolarizable with a square wave stimulator inserted percutaneously, repair should be carried out preferably on the twentieth day after injury, or as soon as possible thereafter. The question frequently arising is: how may one determine if it is too late for successful nerve repair? Edgerton points out that electromyography is a valuable tool when used to detect fibrillation action potentials. If the denervated muscle fibers are still contractile, neurorrhaphy may also be useful.

Nerve Grafting

If loss of substance has occurred (due to operation, crushing injury) or is to be anticipated (considerable extent of compression), bridging of the defect with an autogenous nerve graft is indicated (for technique, see p. 59). Such an operation is contraindicated if the paralysis is older than one year. If during parotid gland removal the nerve is resected, it should be immediately bridged with a graft. As graft is used, the greater auricular nerve and the nerves to be bridged are the branches to mouth and eyelids. The same microsurgical technique is used as described in the previous paragraph. The nerve is obtained at point of exit of the posterior aspect of the sternocleidomastoid muscle and is dissected free transversely over the lateral and superior portion of the muscle (Hanna and Gaisford, Nanson, McCabe). A branching pattern of this nerve makes it possible to replace all the important branches of the facial nerve. If the lesion is in the bony canal, the canal is opened as just described and the nerve is followed along its course; after identification of the lesion, the nerve is resected with a sharp knife until normal nerve fasciculi are exposed. The nerve graft is fitted accurately in place; it does not require suturing, since the body fluid, serum, and blood clots anchor the graft in place. Ballance and Duel cover the grafted area with pure gold leaf (22½ carat) for protection, then follow with a piece of gauze soaked in isotonic

218

saline solution. This dressing is left undisturbed for two weeks; from then on it is changed daily. After complete healing, one should massage the paralyzed muscles daily and stimulate them with the galvanic current for a few minutes three times weekly. A return of active function of the muscles may not occur for three to six months after the operation.

Facial-Nerve Anastomosis

Anastomosis of the facial nerve with another healthy motor cranial nerve is seldom employed, and should be performed only by a competent neurosurgeon.

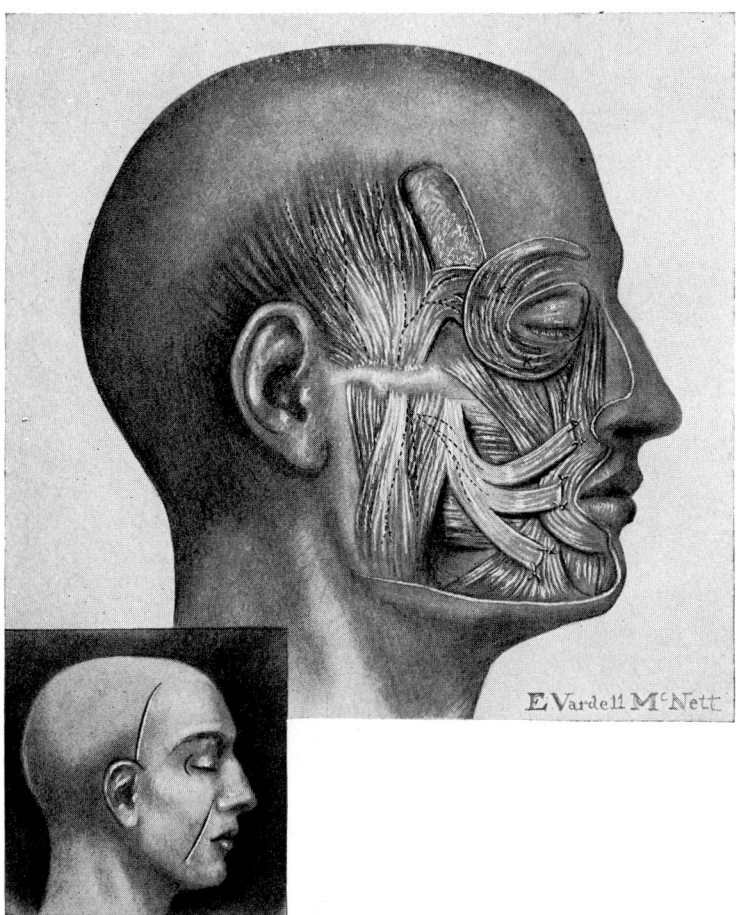

Fig. 59. Operation for dynamic support (muscular neurotization) in facial paralysis (Lexer). From two functioning muscles, musculus temporalis and musculus masseter, muscle flaps are separated and brought in contact with paralyzed muscles. Note that flaps are made parallel to direction of nerve trunk. Insert depicts incisions. (E. Lexer: Die Gesamte Wiederherstellungschirurgie. J. A. Barth, Leipzig.)

219

THE HEAD AND NECK

Suspension of Paralyzed Muscles

The object of the operation is to fix mechanically the sagging tissue of the paralyzed side and to counteract overactivity of the unparalyzed side. This operation is indicated if suturing of nerves or nerve grafting is contraindicated or has failed. Suspension of the muscles is also advisable after nerve anastomosis to prevent overstretching of the paralyzed muscles by their opponents while nerve and muscles are regenerating. The suspension is achieved either by static fixation with lifting and anchoring of the sagging cheek portion to an immobile structure—such as parotid fascia, zygomatic arch with loops of fascia lata, or wire—or by dynamic support either directly through transposition of muscle flaps from adjacent functioning muscles (reanimation) or indirectly by transmission of muscle action from functioning muscles via loops of fascia, etc., to the paralyzed muscle. Everyone who has experience with various types of operations for this problem can attest to the fact that the lasting results are still disappointing in a high percentage of cases (Ragnell, Conway, and others). Starting with the methods which attempt a direct dynamic support, it must be borne in mind that the dynamic support must be also a static support. Muscle implantation operations (Fig. 59) (Lexer, Rosenthal, Sheehan, Neal Owens, Maurer, and others) may fail in this respect since their success depends mainly on regeneration of the paralyzed muscles by so-called "neurotization" (Erlacher).

The author has had opportunity to evaluate some of Lexer's patients in whom functioning muscle flaps had been transplanted. Lexer of Germany, who is credited for being the first (1908) to introduce this principle of reanimation in facial palsy, reported on follow-up examinations of thirty-two patients, of whom ten were markedly improved, twelve moderately improved, and the remainder unimproved. The unimproved cases were mostly among those whose palsy had existed two years or longer before the operation. The author concludes that muscle implantations in markedly sagging palsies do not supply sufficient static support.

The indirect method of dynamic suspension consists generally of inserting loops of fascia lata (1 cm. wide) into the paralyzed orbicularis oris muscle, either directly, after Brown, or through a second loop of fascial slings laid through the paralyzed orbicularis oris, after McLaughlin, and insertion of the fascial strips to the temporal muscle after suspension of the paralyzed side of the face. The failures of these techniques stem from overstretching or teasing of the fascia. To overcome this flaw, stainless steel wires were substituted for fascia (Schuessler and others). However, this method too had numerous failures from the cutting effect of the wire or breakage from metal fatigue (Backdahl and D'Alessio of the Ragnell Clinic). As to the methods of static suspension (Fig. 60), the

220

results are not much better because of the same instability of tissue or material used for suspension as that found in the method of indirect dynamic support.

After a thorough analysis of the failures following various methods of reconstruction of facial paralysis, Ragnell developed a method that would satisfy the following considerations:

1. The entire dynamic force of the temporal muscle supplied by the trigeminus nerve should be utilizable for facial movements on the paralyzed side.

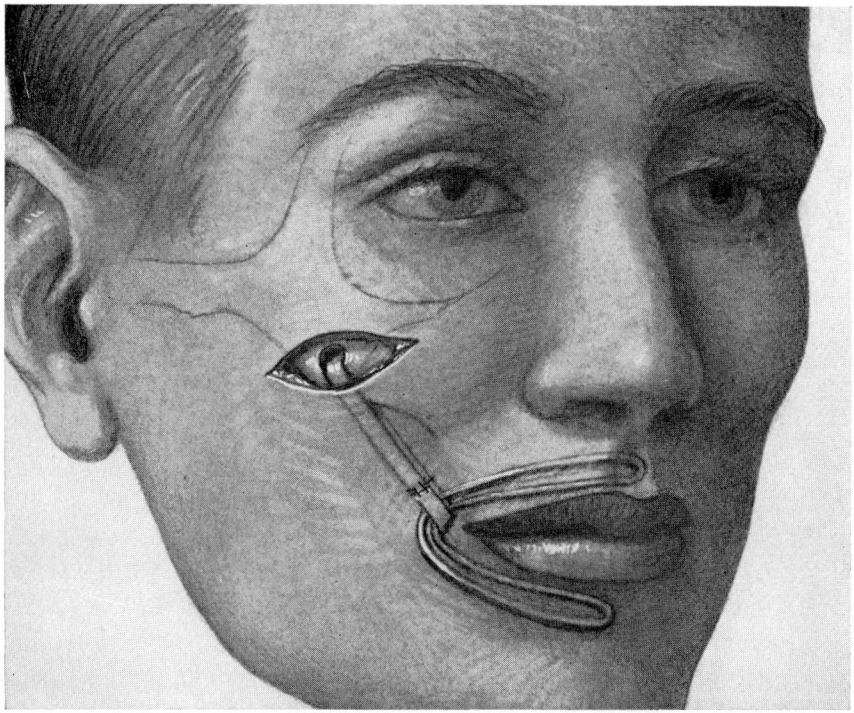

Fig. 60. Static support of paralyzed muscles from facial palsy. From three tiny incisions a double loop of fascia lata strips is laid around the paralyzed muscles of the mouth; a second fascia strip is looped around the first loop and—from a separate incision—drawn through a drill hole of the malar bone. (McLaughlin, C. R.: Plast. Reconstr. Surg.)

2. This force should be transmissible to the orbicularis oris muscle by means of a graft especially suited to the purpose by virtue of satisfactory gliding properties and little tendency to resorption—tendon.

3. The attachment in the orbicularis oris muscle should enable the symmetry of the lips to be restored, while at the same time eliminating secondary gliding as far as possible.

221

4. The movement should proceed from a static position of equilibrium.

5. Active movements should be instituted forthwith in order to prevent immobilization of the dynamic apparatus by fibrous adhesions.

Ragnell's method is a combination of various other techniques; he has added, however, many of his own ideas to give it the stamp of novelty and has proven the value of this method by a long-term follow-up of his patients. The two outstanding new features are the two stages and the combination of static suspension and dynamic action. The author has used Ragnell's technique repeatedly in the past years and endorses its principles wholeheartedly. A few details, however, were modified. For instance, the fascia lata sling which Ragnell devises to encircle the entire mouth has caused in two patients a marked stenosis of the oral orifice; this was due to a technical mistake by the author which, according to Ragnell, can be corrected by excision of the knot on the sound side after healing. In spite of this the stenosis could not be overcome completely. Others had similar experiences (Winkler, Schmidt-Tintemann). Hence, I advise incorporation of the fascial sling into the paralyzed half of the orbicularis oris muscle, with the inclusion of only the median portions of the unparalyzed side. There are a few other minor changes which will be described in the following text.

Technique

First Stage (Case 15, p. 1012): Three tiny verticle incisions are made: one in the upper lip just beyond the philtrum on the sound side, the second one in the lower lip opposite the one in the upper lip, and the third one just lateral to the commissure of the paralyzed side. A strip of fascia lata 0.6 cm. (¼ inch) wide and 18 cm. (7 inches) long is removed with the fascial stripper (see p. 49). With a fascial carrier (Fig. 61) one end of the fascial strip is carried from the lateral incision between the oral mucous membrane—care being taken not to perforate it—and the paralyzed part of the orbicularis oris of the upper lip to escape through the muscle of the sound side and the incision in the upper lip. A similar procedure is carried

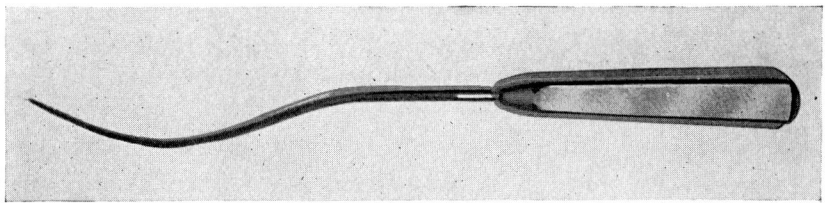

Fig. 61. Fascia-carrier needle used for insertion of fascial strips.

222

out along the lower lip. Each fascial end is then carried back between subcutaneous tissue and orbicularis oris muscle to escape through the lateral incision at the commissure. The loops are tightened to take up the slack of the paralyzed side, but care must be taken to avoid stenosis of the mouth. If dentures are worn, they must be worn during this operation, or, after sterilization, they must be inserted before tightening of the fascial loops. The two loose ends of the fascial strips are then fastened by putting the first part of a surgeon's knot in the slips and clamping them with two mosquito forceps; fixation is firmly effected with three or four fine sutures of black silk put through the loops and tied around them. More for localizing purposes for the second-stage operation than for anything else, the author loosely ties the knotted and unknotted loops together at the lateral wound with heavy black silk. The small wounds are closed and covered with collodion (compare with Figs. 60, 62).

Second Stage: This operation is carried out two months or longer after the first stage. From an incision just within the anterior hairline of the temporal region of the paralyzed side, curving backward to extend along the anterior part of the auricle, the zygoma is exposed. The posterior part of the masseter muscle attachment of the inferior border of the zygomatic arch is divided, thus exposing the coronoid process of the mandible directly below and median to the lower and posterior part of the rim of the zygoma (this rim is much more posterior than one may assume). Wide separation of the jaws (by the anesthetist) facilitates palpation of the coronoid process. With the chin held down, a hole is drilled through the process just below the apex. With an Allis clamp or another suitable clamp, the coronoid process is steadied and held down while it is severed with a nasal saw a little below the hole. With the process still steadied, a wire loop is passed through the hole (the closed end of the loop to be on the lateral side of the process) (Fig. 62), and the sharp-cut edges of the process, attached to the temporal muscle, are smoothed with a rasp. The clamp is then released, and the ends of the wire loop are secured.

Two tendon grafts are taken from the long extensor tendons of the third and fourth toes of the foot. Lately I have used the plantaris tendon as a graft (p. 865). As a rule these tendons fuse proximally beneath the transverse ligament. They are removed with their fused part; the fusion is firmly reinforced with a thin stainless-steel wire to form one long tendon graft. The small scar lateral to the commissure of the mouth is in- or excised, and the fascial loops, which had been inserted in the first stage and had been marked with a heavy black silk thread, are exposed. One end of the tendon graft is passed around the fascial loop, starting anteriorly to escape posteriorly. This end is passed with a fascial carrier (Fig. 61) in a straight line deeply through the fat pad of the cheek posterior

223

to the zygoma to the coronoid process, where it is attached to the closed end of the wire loop and pulled through the hole in the bone (Fig. 62). It is fastened to the coronoid process by pulling the first part of a surgeon's knot in the graft and clamping it with two mosquito forceps. Fixation is firmly effected with three or four medium-sized sutures of black silk put through the ends and tied around them. The other end of the tendon sling is passed through the fat pad of the cheek to the zygoma and looped

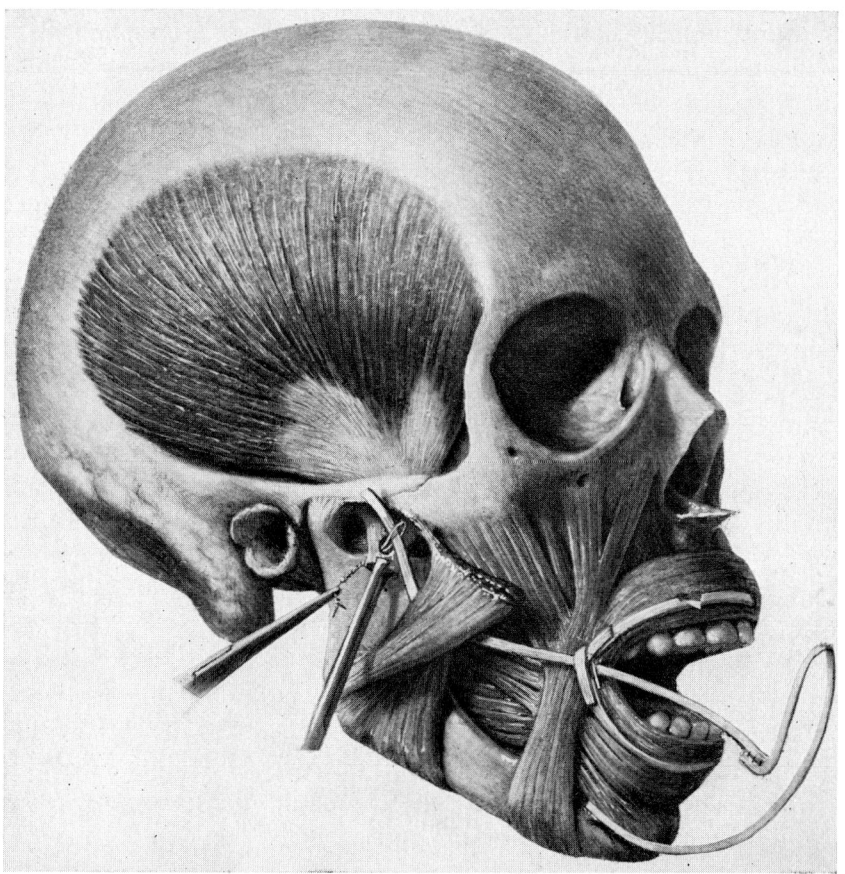

Fig. 62. Two-stage static and dynamic muscle suspension in facial palsy after Ragnell. In the first stage a facial sling was incorporated into the paralyzed half of the orbicularis muscle of the mouth with incorporation of the median portions of the unparalyzed side. This illustration depicts the second stage which is carried out two months later. First the coronoid process, into which a hole has been drilled, is severed from the mandible. Then two tendon grafts, taken from the long entensor tendons of the third and fourth toes, are sutured together at their fused portion. One end is passed around the facial sling and median to it toward the median side of the zygoma. It is pulled through the hole in the severed coronoid process, looped around and fastened to itself. (After A. Ragnell: Plast. Reconstr. Surg.)

224

around it in the following way (Fig. 63): An aneurysm needle is led from the inferior rim of the zygoma along its median surface (the arch of the zygoma is more posterior than one may assume) to escape on its upper rim; the tendon sling is attached to it and withdrawn. This part of the sling is tightened. Before it is tightened completely, one must make sure—and this is important—that the juncture part of the tendon sling where the two tendon grafts have been sutured together has passed the fascial sling at the mouth to prevent locking of the tendon loop at this point. (In using the plantaris tendon, there is no knot.) It is also good to suture

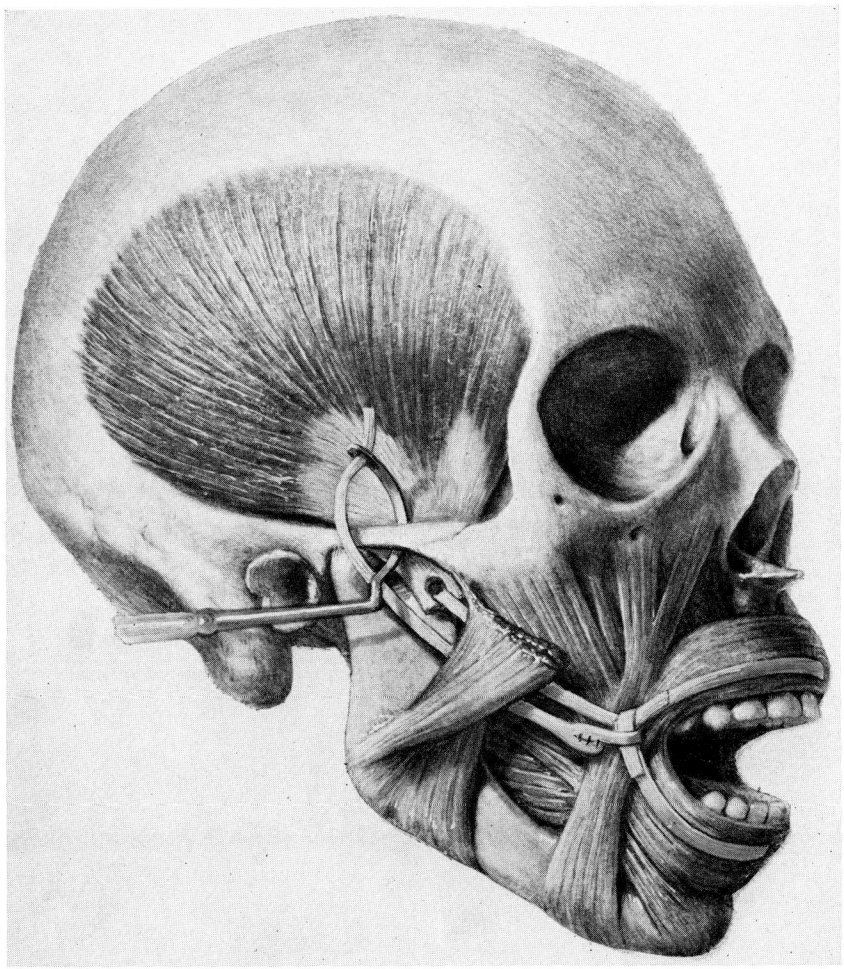

Fig. 63. The other end of the tendon sling is passed through the fat pad of the cheek to the outer side of the zygoma and then looped around its median side. It is then tightened to overcorrect the paralyzed side and sutured to itself. (After A. Ragnell: Plast. Reconstr. Surg.)

the small wound at the mouth at this stage. The tendon loop is then pulled tight around the zygoma to overcorrect the paralyzed side of the face, the first part of a surgeon's knot is put into the tendon loop, and the ends are clamped with two mosquito forceps. Then fixation is firmly effected with three of four silk sutures put through the ends and sutured and tied around them. The lateral skin wound is closed. Before closure, one may consider excising redundant skin or postponing this procedure.

If the eyelids are paralyzed, a lateral tarsorrhaphy (p. 484) is the simplest procedure to lessen the lagophthalmos. This narrows the palpebral fissure, reapplies the lower lid against the eyeball, and relieves the epiphora. Fascial support of the lower lids is seldom satisfactory.

After-Treatment

A firm pressure dressing is applied. Speaking and chewing should be prohibited for one week. The patient should be on a liquid, high-caloric diet, fed through a Jutte tube. The dressing is changed after one week, and the side of the face operated upon is supported for about three weeks with adhesive strips running from the side of the mouth to the temporal region. Later the patient must train his facial movements to separate the functions of chewing and smiling, and he should particularly avoid overactivity of the sound side. This training is best done before a mirror.

Supplementary Procedures for Improvement of Appearance after Operation for Facial Nerve Palsies: The suspension operations improve the appearance of the face and restore some function to the paralyzed side, so that the face is symmetrical as long as it is in repose; however, as soon as the patient smiles broadly, the face is thrown out of balance. Niklison, and subsequently Curtin, and Greeley et al., have reported promising results with excisions of sections (3 cm. wide) of the quadratus labii superior and inferior, zygomaticus, risorius, and triangularis muscles of the unparalyzed side to diminish facial activity on this side without inhibiting it completely.

Another valuable method to improve the appearance of the paralyzed side is removal of redundant skin in front of the ear by means of a partial face-lift operation. Furthermore, I have found excision of an ellipsoidal strip from the nasolabial fold most beneficial; this not only helps to elevate the paralyzed half of the upper lip but the resulting scar creates an image of the nasolabial fold which is usually effaced on this side (Case 15). Care must be taken not to sever the underlying tendon and fascia loops. Thirdly, one may consider elevation of the eyebrow on the paralyzed side by an oval excision of skin from its upper border.

THE CHEEK, TEMPLE, FOREHEAD, AND SKULL

PARALYSIS OF MUSCLES OF CHIN

Paralysis of the depressor muscles of the chin is not infrequent. It occurs particularly after surgery for removal of the cervical lymph nodes or tumors of the parotid region. When the patient is relaxed, the lip appears normal; when he talks, the asymmetry becomes evident by contraction toward the unaffected side. In these cases, fascial suspension and muscle transplantation are not successful. Marino advises neurectomy of the ramus marginalis mandibuli of the opposite side. This is a simple and effective procedure. Before the operation is recommended, however, one should ensure the result by injecting a few cubic centimeters of 2 per cent procaine near the angle of the mandible on the unparalyzed side to block the mandibular nerve. If the reaction is satisfactory it is considered sure evidence for predicting a good result from the operation. However, in two out of three of the author's cases, the postoperative result was a disappointment. This seemed to be a mystery until Dingman and Grabb solved it after thorough study of the surgical anatomy of the mandibular ramus of the facial nerve based on the dissection of one hundred facial halves. In only 21 per cent of the specimens was there a single ramus, while in the remainder there were two or more major branches. There were even peripheral anastomoses between the mandibular and buccal rami in a few specimens. Hence, if procaine is injected, it is possible that in multibranch cases all branches are paralyzed; however, if only one branch is removed by operation, the other branch or branches may take over its function. Therefore the procaine test is of value only if it is negative. If the operation is recommended, the patient must be forewarned of the possibility of failure.

Technique

The operation is performed under general anesthesia. A small incision is made about 1 cm. (³⁄₁₆ inch) behind the angle of the mandible of the unparalyzed side. The ramus marginalis of the facial nerve is located. This may be facilitated by using a cortical stimulator with a bipolar electrode. After the nerve is completely dissected free, the stimulator is applied again to determine exactly the group of muscles supplied by the exposed nerve. This will avoid damage to the buccal branches; it will also ascertain whether there is only one or several branches leading to the depressor muscle of the lower lip. All such branches must be resected to ensure success. Neurectomy is performed. A few millimeters of the nerve are removed to prevent regeneration. The small wound is closed with fine sutures.

227

DEPRESSIONS RESULTING FROM SKELETAL INJURIES OR DESTRUCTION, FACIAL ASYMMETRIES

These are due to fractures or destruction of the skeletal parts. In case of a *fracture*, reduction and retention of the reduced fragments (zygomatic arch, etc.) will correct the deformity in the majority of cases (see p. 565). Depressions resulting from bone *destruction* can be corrected by transplantation of dermal, fat, cartilage, or bone grafts, depending upon the depth and location of the depression. If the depression is the result of an *infection*, the corrective operation should be delayed until at least three months have elapsed after closure of the last fistula, and antibiotics should be administered preoperatively and postoperatively. Any broad scar should be corrected first by skin sliding or by skin flaps, so that the involved area is covered with normal skin. As far as the filling material goes, dermal or derma fat grafts are suitable for shallow depressions (Case 12, p. 1006). For *deeper depressions*, however, particularly those requiring rigid support, bone grafts (Lexer, Kazanjian, Sheehan, and others) or cartilage grafts, solid or diced (Peer) should be chosen (Case 17, p. 1016). Diced cancellous bone grafts from the ilium are also recommended (Mowlem, Macomber). Converse inserts bone grafts through the mouth to overcome depressions of the cheek. The danger of infection seems to be minimal with antibiotics. In *large defects of the skull*, with exposure of brain, bone grafts offer more protection, as already described (p. 209). For reconstruction of depressions and defects after radical operations for *osteomyelitis of the frontal bone*, a two-stage operation as a rule is necessary. Kazanjian and Converse recommend: (1) closing the defect in the soft tissues by skin sliding (preferably from an inverted T-incision above the eyebrows) (see Case 7, p. 997); (2) replacing the absent bone with a tibial graft several months later. Diced cartilage grafts also may be chosen.

Repair of facial asymmetries is discussed on page 355; see also Case 17, page 1016, and following paragraph.

DEPRESSIONS DUE TO DESTRUCTION OR ATROPHY OF SOFT PARTS

These may be local, due to destruction or defects of muscles, for instance, or may involve one whole side of the face. In the latter instance, the deformity is due to atrophy of the soft tissues including skin, subcutaneous tissue, and muscles; in rarer instances, cartilage and bone are involved as well. The cause of hemiatrophy of the face is rather obscure.

THE CHEEK, TEMPLE, FOREHEAD, AND SKULL

Previous injuries may be the causative factors. These alone, however, would not explain the distribution of the atrophy. Archambault and Fromm suggest an involvement of the cervical sympathetic system from infection or trauma with disturbance of the vegetative function, as of the vasomotor, pilomotor, and other such systems. Crikelair et al. substantiated this theory experimentally, but could not reveal any evidence of comparable nerve involvement in their patients. Kazanjian and Sturgis have reviewed the literature on this interesting subject. They divide the therapeutic approach into three phases: (1) investigation of the underlying condition (infection, tumors, congenital cysts of the neck, bony anomalies of the spinal vertebrae and face, vasomotor disorders); (2) treatment of the local manifestations while the disease is in progress; and (3) treatment of the final deformity resulting from this condition.

In the final stage of hemiatrophy, the main object of treatment is filling out the depressions and restoring contours. Free grafts, such as dermal grafts (Case 12) or derma fat grafts, used to be the preferred filling material. The grafts were inserted through small incisions made in inconspicuous areas. In spite of initial success the ultimate results were disappointing owing to absorption of most of the graft, no matter what type of graft was used. Schuchardt (1944, 1960) was the first to recommend the use of the subcutaneous fat part of a tube flap as filling material. He "peeled" the entire cutis from the distal end of the flap, spread the fat, and transplanted it beneath the skin of the cheek. Newmann (1953), apparently unaware of Schuchardt's technique, recommended a similar procedure. He, however, did not remove the entire thickness of the skin but left the derma attached to safeguard the circulation of the flap. This makes the flap rather bulky, which occasionally (as in extensive cases of atrophy), but not usually, may be an advantage.

Technique (Schuchardt)

A lateral lower chest-abdominal tube flap (Fig. 42) is constructed on the same side as the atrophy of the face, so that its cranial pedicle can be later attached to the median side of the upper arm of the same side. After three months the cranial pedicle is gradually severed (p. 93) and attached to the median side of the upper arm. Four weeks later the distal end is gradually severed. The final transfer of the flap, however, should be delayed for at least six weeks to permit maturation of the circulation of the flap. The distal end of the flap, i.e., the part to be buried, is denuded by removal of the entire thickness of the skin and the fat portion of the flap is spread out. An incision is then made through the skin only, either behind or below the angle of the mandible, and the skin of the atrophied portions of the cheek is undermined subcutaneously

229

by blunt dissection with a pair of curved scissors along the superficial fascia. After hemostasis (by packing) the arm is moved toward the cheek with the forearm resting upon the head. Several nylon sutures are passed through the terminal part of the fat flap without tying them; with a long straight needle both ends of each suture are passed through the highest point of the depressed area. The needle is clamped longitudinally within the branches of a hemostat. The tip of the needle should not project. The hemostat is passed through the undermined compartment. When its blunt end has reached the blind end, the hemostat is opened and the needle is pushed through the skin. By pulling on the threads one inserts the fat portion of the flap. The sutures are then tied over small rolls of gauze, and the rim of skin of the tube flap is sutured to the skin edge of the cheek wound. The arm is immobilized with a plaster cast (see p. 80). After four weeks the flap is gradually severed as described on page 93, and after adjustment the skin edges of the cheek and upper arm are closed.

DEFORMITY FROM HYPERTROPHY OF
MASSETER MUSCLE

Benign hypertrophy of the masseter muscle is a rare condition, and is described here only in brief; for details, the reader is referred to publications of Adams, Masters et al., Gelbke, Dencer, and others. This condition, which is a soft, ill-defined, contractile mass within the masseter muscle, may be unilateral or bilateral. It may mimic parotid disease; hence, sialography may be necessary for differential diagnosis. It can be corrected readily, according to Adams' technique, by resection of the medial part of the hypertrophied muscle, together with any abnormal bony spur formation at the angle of the mandible which often accompanies the masseteric hypertrophy.

CORRECTION OF THE AGING FACE
(RHYTIDECTOMY, MELOPLASTY,
FACE LIFT)

This may be necessary for economic, as well as for purely cosmetic and psychic, reasons. Most individuals who desire a "face lift" complain that the wrinkling and sagging of the facial skin gives them a tired and depressed appearance, and this in turn causes a downcast feeling. They expect from a face-lift operation not only a physical improvement but also a psychic "uplift" and consequently a reactivation of their vitality. It is obvious that such miraculous change is not always possible. Unfor-

230

tunately, this type of operation has been commercially exploited by char-latans, well advertised by them as a minor but effective procedure. It should be understood that to be effective the operation becomes a major procedure. It is apparent that the elastic facial skin, under the influence of the mimic muscles, cannot remain smooth after removal of strips of skin alone. Such a procedure is of only temporary success, unless the skin is widely undermined toward the face and upper part of the neck to cause broad adhesions with the underlying inelastic fascia and is firmly anchored to fascia or periosteum. Hence, one must be careful in the selection of the patient. The most satisfactory patients are those with fine skin and well-molded chins; the least satisfactory are those with fleshy skin and recessive chins. The whole procedure must be discussed frankly with the patient from all angles, including the result that can be expected and the possibility of postoperative complications (p. 237).

Among the pioneers of the correction of the aging face are Lexer (1910), Passot (1919), and Joseph (1921). This subject has been more recently discussed by Aufricht, Johnson, McIndoe, Gonzales-Ulloa, Marino, Morel-Fatio, Edgerton et al., and very recently by Baker and Gordon, Spira, Gerow and Hardy, and by Conley in a monograph which is both amusing and interesting.

There are various skin incisions recommended, but none is ideal. All those incisions (beginning with Joseph's original technique) which are made within the temporal scalp region have the obvious advantage of concealing resulting scars. Their disadvantage is that after excision of the redundant skin from the anterior wound edge the temporal hairline will recede; this becomes increasingly true with subsequent operations. Incisions along the temporal hairline do not have this disadvantage but are not so well concealed (Figs. 64 and 65). The author has for many years preferred the latter incisions, including incisions along the posterior hairline, and still uses this technique if more than two rhytidectomies are indicated (Figs. 64, 65). For the majority of cases, however, he has changed his technique according to Aufricht's. Aufricht does not claim originality but modestly states that his technique is a combination of those of other authors, particularly Joseph, Johnson, and McIndoe. He, however, has added many of his own ideas to this operation to give it the stamp of novelty.

Technique (Figs. 66, 67, 68, 69, 70)

The patient is told to have her hair shampooed on the day before admission to the hospital. The operation is performed under local or general anesthesia. (The author prefers general anesthesia.) Prior to the induction of anesthesia, the lines of incisions within the temporal and

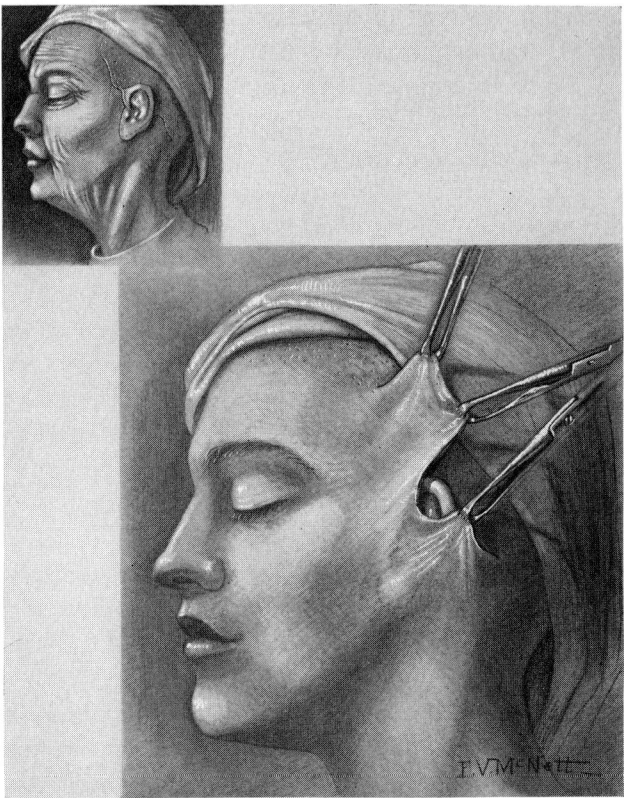

Fig. 64. Correction of facial wrinkles from incisions along the hairlines as outlined in insert. After wide undermining of facial and cervical skin the loose skin is pulled backward over the ear. (For details of technique compare with Figs. 66-70.)

occipital scalp regions are outlined with a dye, and a strip of skin is shaved along those lines. The outline of the temporal scalp incision starts at the hairline above the ear. This point, however, may be influenced by the anterior temporal hair margin. If the latter is receding from the eyebrow, exposing a broad area of skin between temporal hairline and eyebrow, the starting point of the incision is somewhat further posteriorly, and vice versa. The incision proceeds upward and forward from this starting point for about 2 to 2½ inches in an angle of 45 degrees with an imaginary line between the starting point and the eyebrow. (If the hair margin in front of the ear is down and low, the angle may be less, and if higher it may be more than 45 degrees.) The strip of skin to be shaved along and below this line is about 1 to 1½ inches wide. The hairs below the shaved area are curled and bound with a heavy silk thread (Fig. 66).

232

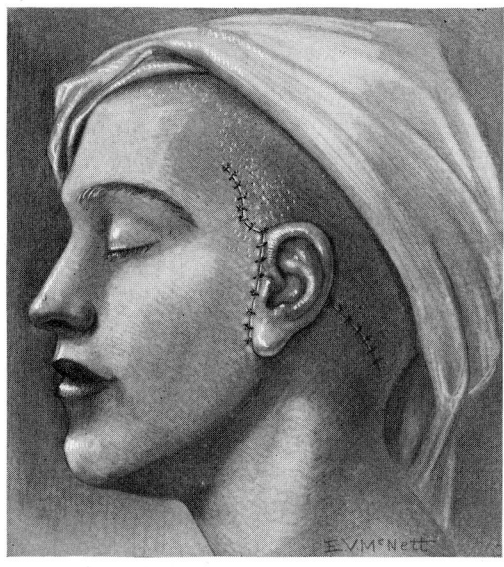

Fig. 65. After proper excision of redundant skin median wound edges are fastened with subcutaneous cotton sutures to fascia of lateral wound edges, followed by closure of skin wound. (For details of technique compare with Figs. 66-70.)

The posterior scalp incision starts in the postauricular fold at the insertion of the upper part of the concha and proceeds backward into the scalp in an angle of about 135 degrees with the future incision along the lower auricular fold. The scalp is shaved along and below this line. The incisions are then marked with scratch marks. The hairs below the shaved areas are curled and bound with a heavy silk thread (Fig. 66). Endotracheal anesthesia is administered. (If local anesthesia is used, it is injected after the patient is draped.) The face is washed with pHisoHex, scalp areas are painted with red Zephiran which is washed off with alcohol, and a head drape is laid just posterior to the shaved areas and sutured to the skin. It is advisable to outline the extent of the undermining of the skin with one of the dyes. Overly extensive undermining may result in hematomas, necrosis of the skin, and injury to the fine branches of the facial nerve. Dissection of the skin in an area of about 5 to 8 cm. in front, below and back of the ear suffices.

The operation starts with the anterior scalp incision and proceeds anteriorly along the hairline and down to the insertion of the helix and continues just in front of the tragus. Between the anterior insertion of the helix and tragus the incision should not be straight but curved posteriorly (almost "dot-like") to avoid later webbing of the scar above the tragus (Fig. 66). The anterior skin portion is undermined, first with the knife and later with curved dissecting scissors. The dissection is carried out rather superficially along the subcutaneous layer of the skin. This reduces bleeding and avoids injury to the nerves. The translucency of the skin is a good

233

guide. At this point I have the overhead light directed against the skin. The most vulnerable branches of the facial nerve are over the zygoma and around the lateral canthus of the eye; injury may result in palsy of the respective half of the fontalis muscle and drooping of the upper eyelid (in two personal experiences the palsies were temporary from instrument pressure on the fine zygomatic nerve branches during dissection). Hence, in the zygomatic and canthal areas dissection must be superficial. In the temporal area, however, undermining is done beneath the temporal fascia to protect the circulation of that part of the skin which will be tightened most. The next step consists of an incision along the oblique posterior scalp line which is continued from its median point at the ear downward along the posterior auricular fold around the ear lobule and in front of the ear to join the anterior incision. The skin is undermined subcutaneously first behind the ear, then in the submental area. In front the skin must be elevated beyond the rim of the fascia parotideomasseterica. Below the ear lobule dissection should also be superficial; if it is too deep, difficulty may be encountered because of tough fascial extensions from the anterior rim of the musculus sternocleidomastoideus to the platysma. If dissection is carried out in this plane, these fascial extensions must be severed, but care must be taken not to injure the posterior auricular nerve in front and the nervus accessorius in back of the musculus sternocleidomasoideus (Fig. 67). Thorough hemostasis follows (many of the smaller vessels can be electrocoagulated). The wound surfaces are flushed with thrombin topical intermittently during the operation.

The most important phase of the operation is the "lifting" of the face. This should be carried out in two separate steps (Aufricht),

--→

Fig. 66. Rhytidectomy (after Aufricht). Incisions are outlined before hair is shaved around the temporal and posterior scalp incisions. The hairs below the shaved areas are curled and bound with a heavy silk thread.

Fig. 67. Dissection of skin of temporal area and 5 to 8 cm. in front, below and back of the ear. The fat pad in front of masseter muscle is implicated and sutured to the fascia parotideomasseterica.

Fig. 68. Two subcutaneous suspension sutures of heavy Dermalon are being passed through the subdermal tissue level with and lateral to the mouth and below the mandible and led through the skin posterior to the upper and posterior oblique incisions. They are tightened over a roll of cotton (see Fig. 70).

Fig. 69. Mobilized skin is pulled upward and backward over the ear and is held temporarily with a mattress suture above and behind the ear.

Fig. 70. The anterior and posterior redundant skin has been excised and wound edges have been sutured. Earlobe is still buried. A short vertical incision through the overlapping skin in level of the buried earlobe for adjustment of the skin around this portion of the ear is marked out (vertical dotted line).

234

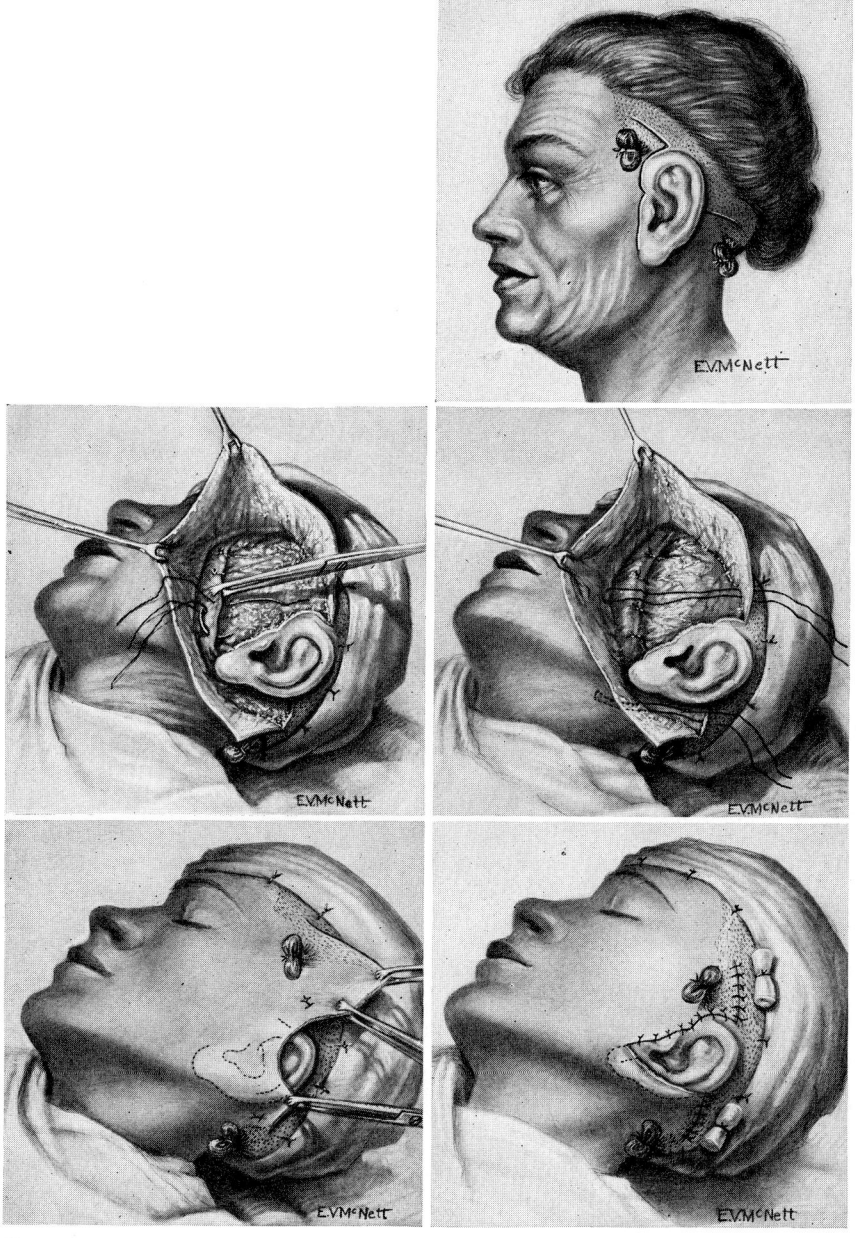

Figs. 66-70.

consisting of, first, "lifting" the fat tissue of the cheek and submental areas and, secondly, tightening the skin. The loosely hanging fat tissue in front of the masseter muscle is implicated and sutured with cotton sutures to the fascia parotideomasseterica, thus effacing the nasolabial fold (Fig. 67). Tightening and excision of the skin follow, first above and in front of the ear, and then in back of it. This sequence is important; if the steps are reversed, an undesirable fullness of the lower posterior portions of the face may result. Before the skin is excised, a subcutaneous suspension suture of heavy Dermalon is passed as a mattress suture through the subcutaneous fat tissue and subdermal tissue in front of the cheek fat pad, and is led through the skin edge posterior to the upper oblique incision near the center of it. It is tightened over a roll of cotton (such as the dentist uses). In some cases a second such suture for suspension of the anterior skin flap may be necessary (Fig. 68).

The lower skin flap is suspended with a similar suture which engages the subcutaneous tissue at the lowest point of mobilization in the chin-neck line and is led out through the skin just posterior to the center of the posterior oblique incision.

The relaxed loose anterior skin flap is then pulled over the posterior oblique wound edge. A temporary mattress suture is placed through the overlapping skin and upper wound edge near its starting point (Fig. 69). The redundant skin is excised along the oblique incision and the wound sutured with interrupted 000 Dermalon sutures. The temporary mattress suture is removed and the redundant skin in front of the upper half of the ear is excised.

The operation is now continued in the posterior scalp region. The relaxed loose posterior skin flap is pulled over the posterior oblique wound edge. A mattress suture is placed through the upper oblique wound edge at or near the hairline and through the overlapping skin (Fig. 69). The redundant skin is excised along the oblique incision and the wound sutured with 000 Dermalon. Some of the redundant skin behind the ear is excised.

The lower half of the ear is still buried beneath the redundant skin. To adjust the skin around this portion of the ear a short vertical incision is made through the overlapping skin in level of the buried ear lobule (Fig. 70). The incision should end in level with the lowest inserting point of the lobule, which can then be pulled out from beneath the redundant skin flap. This is followed by removal of the remaining redundant skin in front and in back of the ear and suture of the posterior and anterior wound edge with 000000 Dermalon.

A drain is inserted through an opening behind the earlobe and

236

above the ear. If the bleeding is profuse, the drain should be a multi-perforated polyethylene tube attached to a continuous suction apparatus.

The wound edges are covered with a gauze strip containing bland ointment. Numerous long strips of dressing gauze are laid around the ear donut-like. A dressing pad is perforated and laid upon this layer, and then a perforated piece of thick rubber sponge (the perforation being as large as the ear). The perforation over the ear is filled with fluffed gauze. A towel is placed over the entire dressing and clamped to the head drape above and below. The patient's head is then turned for operation on the other side, which is carried out in a similar manner. The last step consists of holding the donut-like paddings on the ears with a semielastic head dressing such as Curlex, with figure-of-eight turns around the forehead and neck.

This dressing is changed, and removed together with the drains on the third postoperative day; all sutures but the suspension sutures are removed on the fifth day, and the suspension sutures are removed on the twelfth postoperative day.

Complications, such as hematoma formation, infection, excessive scarring, skin necrosis, salivary fistula, paresthesia of cheeks and earlobes, and motor nerve damage occur, but fortunately seldom. If a massive hematoma develops, it should be evacuated immediately after removal of most of the skin sutures and drained with a catheter attached to a continuous suction apparatus. Smaller hematomata are evacuated through a smaller opening and drained in a similar way. In two cases of salivary fistula, the author kept the patient on a liquid (Metracal) diet, and the fistula closed after a few days. Nerve damage, as a rule, is only temporary, but may take months for recovery, as the author observed in two cases of temporary palsy to the zygomatic branch of the facial nerve which supplies the frontalis muscle. Baker and Gordon have recently discussed this subject. It is imperative that the possibility of such complications is discussed preoperatively with the patient.

With the technique described above, the longitudinal wrinkles in the chin-neck line can be eradicated; however, they are the first ones to recur, a fact which should be pointed out to the patient preoperatively. To remove the redundant cervical skin from an anterior T-incision is not advisable because of the obvious scarring. Spira, Gerow, and Hardy combine the posterior incisions and remove the redundant skin from a posterior cervical T-incision. In a marked deformity, the so-called "turkey gobbler" deformity, which is due to redundancy of skin plus increase of the submandibular fat pad, Adamson, Horton and Crawford demonstrated good results after a transverse incision within the upper neck crease, removal of the fat pad, and vertical plication of the platysma muscle. This operation should be done in a second stage.

THE HEAD AND NECK

Millard, Pigott and Hedo solve the problem of reconstructing a pleasing concave chin-neck line in individuals with a deposit of adipose tissue in the submental area, often combined with an extension laterally beneath the inferior edge of the mandible, by a submandibular lipectomy in combination with the face-lifting procedure. The operation starts with a 3-cm. horizontal incision in a submental crease from which the submental skin is dissected from the fat pad down to the level of the thyroid cartilage with long blunt scissors. Then under direct vision using a No. 5 right-angle nasal retractor and strong overhead lighting, the fat pad is dissected away from the platysma and excised laterally only as far as one can see clearly. The wound is left open for possible later hemostasis. Then, through a routine face-lift incision as described above, the skin is freed from the deeper structures. The undermining is carried well forward until it joins the anterior submental dissection. Under direct vision, the excess fat in the submandibular area is excised with careful consideration of the mandibular branch of the facial nerve. Injury to this nerve can be avoided by keeping the dissection strictly below the inferior border of the mandible and superficial to the platysma at all times. The face-lift procedure is then completed as described above.

If longitudinal forehead (frown) wrinkles and wrinkles around the eyes and on the eyelids are conspicuous, these are corrected in another stage (three weeks later). Correction of eyelid wrinkles is described on page 499.

Correction of frown wrinkles is uncertain, and this should be pointed out to the patient. They may be improved after Pangman and Wallace by making a small incision at the medial end of each eyebrow and elevating the skin from the corrugator muscle. The entire muscle is severed along a line curving upward and medially from the eyebrow incision, but only a segment of muscle in the area between eyebrow and nose is removed. The incisions are sutured with fine nylon and a pressure dressing is applied. Insertion of strips of dermal grafts to elevate the frown wrinkles has not been permanently successful in the author's experience.

Correction of horizontal forehead wrinkles is rarely attempted by the author since the results—as in correction of the vertical wrinkles—are uncertain. Ushida and Marino and Gandolfo appear to have more success with their techniques.

In conclusion, chemical face peeling (Linton, Baker) with a solution of phenol and carried out in conjunction with rhytidectomy should be mentioned. This method is still in the investigative stage and will need much more evaluation before its merits can be judged.

238

BIBLIOGRAPHY

ADAMS, W. M.: *Bilateral hypertrophy of the masseter muscle: An operation for correction.* Brit. J. Plast. Surg., 2:78, 1949.

ADAMSON, J. E., HORTON, C. E., and CRAWFORD, H .H.: *The surgical correction of the "turkey gobbler" deformity.* Plast. Reconstr. Surg., 34:598, 1964.

ANDERSON, R., and BYARS, L. T.: *Surgery of the Parotid Gland.* C. V. Mosby Co., St. Louis, 1965.

ARCHAMBAULT, LaSALLE, and FROMM, N. K.: *Progressive facial hemiatrophy.* Arch. Neurol. Psychiat., 27:529, 1932.

ASCHAN, P. E.: *Muskel- und Sehnentransplantation bei Facialisparese. Forschritte der Kiefer- und Gesichts-Chirurgie,* 2:143, 1956.

ASHLEY, F. L., GRAZER, F. M., MACHIDA, R. C., McCONNELL, D. V., and MORGAN, S. C.: *A modified operation for the correction of facial paralysis.* Plast. Reconstr. Surg., 41:58, 1968.

AUFRICHT, G.: *Chirurgische Korrektur des alternden Gesichts.* Fortschritte der Kiefer- und Gesichts-Chirurgie, Georg Thieme Verlag, Stuttgart, VII:179, 1961.
Surgery for excess skin of the face and neck. In Trans. Int. Soc. of Plast. Surgeons, Second Congress, edited by A. B. Wallace. Williams and Wilkins, Baltimore, 1960. p. 495.

BACKDAHL, M., and D'ALESSIO, E.: *Experience with static reconstruction in cases of facial paralysis.* Plast. Reconstr. Surg., 21:211, 1958.

BAGOZZI, I. C.: *Reparative procedure in large losses of scalp and bone of the skull by serious electrical lesions.* Brit. J. Plast. Surg., 8:49, 1956.

BAILEY, H. A., and SKAFF, V.: *Surgical repair of lacerations and fistulas of the parotid duct.* Ann. Surg., 129:103, 1949.

BAKER, T. J.: *Chemical face peeling and rhytidectomy. A combined approach for facial rejuvenation.* Plast. Reconstr. Surg., 29:199, 1962.

BAKER, T. J., and GORDON, H. L.: *Complications of rhytidectomy.* Plast. Reconstr. Surg., 40:31, 1967.

BALLANCE, C. A., and DUEL, A. B.: *The operative treatment of facial palsy.* Arch. Otolaryng., 15:1, 1932.

BARON, H. C.: *Surgical correction of salivary fistula.* Ann. Surg., 153:545, 1961.

BATTLE, R. J. V.: *A technique for reanimation of the face after paralysis of the seventh nerve.* Brit. J. Plast. Surg., 5:247, 1953.

BECK, C. S.: *Repair of defects in skull by ready-made vitallium plates.* JAMA, 118:798, 799, 1942.

BLAIR, V. P.: *Notes on the operative correction of facial palsy.* South. Med. J., 19:116, 1926.
The surgical restoration of the lining of the mouth. Surg. Gynec. Obstet., 40:165, 1925.
Further observations upon the compensatory use of live tendon strips for facial paralysis. Ann. Surg., 92:694, 1930.

THE HEAD AND NECK

BODECHTEL, G., KRAUTZUN, K. J., and KAZMEIER, F.: *Grundriss der Traumatischen Peripheren Nervenschädigungen.* 2 Erweit, U. Verb. Aufl. Stuttgart: Georg Thieme, 1951.

BOERING, G., and HUFFSTADT, A. J. C.: *The use of derma-fat grafts in the face.* Brit. J. Plast. Surg., 20:172, 1967.

BROWN, J. B.: *The utilization of the temporal muscle and fascia in facial paralysis.* Ann. Surg., 109:1016, 1939.

BROWN, J. B., FRYER, M. P., and ZOGRAFAKIS, G.: *Reanimation in ptosis and in facial paralysis.* Plast. Reconstr. Surg., 41:343, 1968.

BUNNELL, S.: *Suture of the facial nerve within the temporal bone.* Surg. Gynec. Obstet., 45:7, 1927.
Surgical repair of facial nerve. Arch. Otolaryng., 25:253, 1937.

BÜRKLE DE LA CAMP, H.: *Plastische Deckung von Knochenlücken der Schädels (mit Kurzer Bemerkung zur operativen Behandlung der traumatischen Frühepilepnie).* Ztrbl. f. chir., 1938.

CLARKSON, P.: *Reanimation of the face in paralysis of the facial nerve.* Brit. J. Plast. Surg., 5:259, 1953.

COLEMAN, C. C.: *Surgical lesions of the facial nerve: With comments on its anatomy.* Ann. Surg., 119:641, 1944.

COLLIER, J.: *Reanimation of facial paralysis.* Brit. J. Plast. Surg., 5:243, 1953.

CONLEY, J.: *Face-Lift Operation.* Charles C Thomas, Springfield, 1968.

CONVERSE, J. M.: *Restoration of facial contour by bone grafts introduced through the oral cavity.* Plast. Reconstr. Surg., 6:295, 1950.

CONWAY, H.: *Muscle plastic operations for facial paralysis.* Ann. Surg., 147:541, 1958.

CRIKELAIR, G. F., MOSS, M. L., and KHURI, A.: *Facial hemiatrophy.* Plast. Reconstr. Surg., 29:266, 1962.

CRONIN, T. D.: *Use of hair-bearing punch grafts for partial traumatic losses of the scalp.* Plast. Reconstr. Surg., 42:466, 1968.

CURTIN, J. W., GREELEY, P. W., GLEASON, M., and BRAVER, D.: *A supplementary procedure for the improvement of facial nerve paralysis.* Plast. Reconstr. Surg., 26:73, 1960.

DELORE: *Procédé nouveau pour l'operation de la fistule du canal de Stensen.* Bull. gén. de thérap., 77:184, 1869.

DENCER, D.: *Bilateral idiopathic masseteric hypertrophy.* Brit. J. Plast. Surg., 14:149, 1961.

DINGMAN, R. O.: *Iliac bone cranioplasty.* Plast. Reconstr. Surg., 9:130, 1952.

DINGMAN, R. O., and GRABB, W. C.: *Surgical anatomy of the mandibular ramus of the facial nerve based on the dissection of 100 facial halves.* Plast. Reconstr. Surg., 29:266, 1962.

DREVERMANN, P.: *Ueber den Ersatz von Dura und Schädeldefekten, unter besonderer Berücksichtigung der Dauerfolge in der Verhütung und Heilung der traumatischen Epilepsie durch Dura Ersatz mit frei transplantiertem Fettgewebe.* Bruns' Beitr. z. klin. Chir., 127:674, 1922.

240

THE CHEEK, TEMPLE, FOREHEAD, AND SKULL

EDGERTON, M. T.: *Surgical correction of facial paralysis: a plea for better reconstructions.* Ann. Surg., 165:985, 1967.

EDGERTON, M. T., and HANSEN, F. C.: *Matching facial color with split thickness skin grafts from adjacent areas.* Plast. Reconstr. Surg., 25:455, 1960.

EDGERTON, M. T., WEBB, W. L., SLAUGHTER, R., and MEYER, E.: *Surgical results and psychological changes following rhytidectomy.* Plast. Reconstr. Surg., 33:503, 1964.

ERLACHER, PH.: *Ueber die motorischen Nervenendigungen.* Ztschr. f. orthop. Chir., 34:561, 1914.
Direct and muscular neurotization of paralyzed muscles. J. Orthop. Surg., 13:22, 1915.

ESSER, J. F.: *Studies in plastic surgery of the face. Use of skin from the neck to replace face defects. Plastic operations about the mouth. The epidermic inlay.* Ann. Surg., 65:297, 1917.
Rotation der Wangen. F. C. W. Vogel, Verlag Leipzig, 1918.

FREEMAN, B. S.: *Fluorescein as an adjunct in the treatment of radionecrotic ulcers.* Surg. Gynec. Obstet., 89:566, 1949.

FREY, R.: *Die Injektionsbehandlung der Auesseren Speichelfistel.* der Chirurg., 17:401, 1947.

GARDNER, W. J.: *Closure of defects in the skull with tantalum.* Surg. Gynec. Obstet., 80:303, 1945.

GEIB, F. W.: *Vitallium skull plates.* JAMA, 117:8-12, 1941.

GELBKE, H.: *The operative correction of angular face deformity due to hyperplasia of the masseter muscle and prominent angle of the mandible.* Langenbeck's Arch. und Deut. Zschr. Chir. 288:248, 1958.

GILLIES, H. D.: *Hemiatrophy of the face. (unilateral lipodystrophy.) Conditions improved by insertion of fat grafts.* Proc. Roy. Soc. Med., 27:64, 1934.

GONZALEZ-ULLOA, M.: *Facial wrinkles: integral elimination.* Plast. Reconstr. Surg., 29:658, 1962.

GRANT, F. C., and NORCROSS, N. C.: *Repair of cranial defects by cranioplasty.* Ann. Surg., 110:488, 1939.

GROCOTT, J.: *Experiences in cranial bone grafting.* Brit. J. Plast. Surg., 5:51, 1952.

GULECKE, N.: *Ueber das Schicksal bei Schädelplastiken verpflanzter Gewebe.* Bruns' Beitr. z. klin. Chir., 107:503, 1917.

HANKINS, E. A.: *Total scalp avulsions.* Ann. Surg., 158:277, 1963.

HANNA, D. C., and GAISFORD, J. C.: *Facial nerve management in tumors and trauma.* Plast. Reconstr. Surg., 35:445, 1965.

HEINECKE, H.: *Verletzungen und chirurgische Krankheiten der Speicheldrüsen.* Deutsche Ztschr. f. Chir., 33:2, 1913 (Part 2).

HOLLANDER, M. M.: *Rhytidectomy: anatomical, physiological, and surgical considerations.* Plast. Reconstr. Surg., 20:218, 1957.

JAEGER, A.: *Closure of skull defects.* Plast. Reconstr. Surg., 1:69, 1946.

THE HEAD AND NECK

JANVIER, H.: *Traitment Chirurgical De La Paralysie Faciale–Place des Plasties Musclaires Tendlinenses et Cutanees*. Paris: Librairie Arnett. 1952.

JOHNSON, J. B., and HADLEY, R. C.: *The Aging Face*. In Reconstructive Plastic Surgery, J. M. Converse, ed. W. B. Saunders, Philadelphia, 1964.

JOSEPH, J.: *Plastic operation on protruding cheek*. Deutsch. Med. Wschr., 47:287, 1921.

KAZANJIAN, V. H.: *Reconstruction after radical operation for osteomyelitis of the frontal bone*. Surg. Gynec. Obstet., 79:397, 1944.
Repair of partial losses of the scalp. Plast. Reconstr. Surg., 12:325, 1953.

KAZANJIAN, V. H., and CONVERSE, J. M.: *Reconstruction after radical operation for osteomyelitis of the frontal bone*. Arch. Otolaryng., 31:94, 1940.
The Surgical Treatment of Facial Injuries. Williams and Wilkins, Baltimore, 1949.

KAZANJIAN, V. H., and STURGIS, S. H.: *Surgical treatment of hemiatrophy of the face*. JAMA, 115:348, 1940.

KAZANJIAN, V. H., and WEBSTER, R. C.: *The treatment of extensive losses of the scalp*. Plast. Reconstr. Surg., 1:360, 1946.

KÖNIG, F.: *Der knöcherne Ersatz grosser Schädeldefekte*. Zentralbl. f. Chir., 17:467, 1890.

KÜTTNER: *Plastik des Ductus Parotideus aus der Mundschleimhaut*. München. med. Wchnschr. 1906, p. 100.

LANGENBECK, C. F. M.: *Behandlung der Speichelfistel*. Bibliot. f. Chir., 2:686, 1808.

LEWIS, S. R., BLOCKER, T. G., and EADE, G. G.: *Problems of scalp reconstruction*. Plast. Reconstr. Surg., 20:133, 1957.

LEXER, E.: *Die Gesamte Wiederherstellungschirurgie*. J. A. Barth, Leipzig, 1931, Vols. 1 and 2.
Zur Gesichtsplastik. Langenbeck's Arch. f. klin. Chir., 92:749, 1910.

LEXER, E., and EDEN, R.: *Ueber die chirurgische Behandlung der peripheren Facialislähmnung*. Beitr. z. klin. Chir., 73:116, 1911.

LINDEMANN and LORENZ: *Zur chirurgisch-plastischen Deckung der Weichteildefekte des Gesichtes*. Urban-und Schwarzenberg, Berlin-München, 1949.

LITTON, C.: *Chemical face lifting*. Plast. Reconstr. Surg., 29:371, 1962.

LONGACRE, J. J., and deSTEFANO, G. A.: *Further observations of the behavior of autogenous split-rib grafts in reconstruction of extensive defects of the cranium and face*. Plast. Reconstr. Surg., 20:281, 1957.
Reconstruction of extensive defects of the skull with split rib grafts. Plast. Reconstr. Surg., 19:186, 1957.

LONGACRE, J. J., deSTEFANO, G.A., and HOLMSTRAND, K.: *The early versus the late reconstruction of congenital hypoplasias of the facial skeleton and skull*. Plast. Reconstr. Surg., 27:489, 1961.

LU, M. N.: *Successful replacement of avulsed scalp*. Plast. Reconstr. Surg., 43:231, 1970.

MACOMBER, D. W.: *Cancellous iliac bone depressions of forehead, nose and chin*. Plast. Reconstr. Surg., 4:157, 1949.

THE CHEEK, TEMPLE, FOREHEAD, AND SKULL

MACOMBER, W. B., SHEPARD, R. A., and CROFUT, V. E.: *Mandibular bone grafts.* Plast. Reconstr. Surg., 3:570, 1948.

MARINO, H.: *Paralysis of the muscles of the chin; surgical treatment.* Surg. Gynec Obstet., 96:433, 1953.
Paralysis des N. facialis. Forschritte der Kiefer- und Gesichts-Chirurgie, 2:184, 1956.

MARINO, H., and GANDOLFO, E.: *Treatment of forehead wrinkles.* Prensa Med. Argent., 51:1368, 1964.

MASTERS, F., GEORGIADE, N., and PICKERILL, H. P.: *The surgical treatment of benign masseteric hypertrophy.* Plast. Reconstr. Surg., 15:215, 1955.

MATTHEWS, C. N.: *Reanimation of facial palsy.* Brit. J. Plast. Surg., 5:253, 1953.

MAURER, G.: *Die operative Behandlung der Fascialislähmung.* Langenbeck's Archiv für Klinische Chirurgie. Deutsche Zeitschrift für Chirurgie., 282:637, 1955.

MAY, H.: *Transplantation and regeneration of tissue.* Penn. Med. J., 45:130, 1941.
Closure of defects after cancer surgery. Clinics, Vol. 55, June, 1945.
Gesichtsplastiken nach Krebsbehandlung. Langenbeck's Arch. f. Chir., 289:501, 1958.

MAYFIELD, F. H., and LEVITCH, L. A.: *Repair of cranial defects with tantalum.* Amer. J. Surg., 67:319-322, 1945.

McCABE, B. F.: *Facial nerve grafting.* Plast. Reconstr. Surg., 45:70, 1970.

McCLINTOCK, H. G., and DINGMAN, R. O.: *The repair of cranial defects with iliac bone.* Surgery, 30:955, 1951.

McGREGOR, I. A., and REID, W. H.: *The use of the temporal flap in the primary repair of full thickness defects of the cheek.* Plast. Reconstr. Surg., 38:1, 1960.

McLAUGHLIN, C. R.: *Surgical support in permanent facial paralysis.* Plast. Reconstr. Surg., 11:302, 1953.

MIEHLKE, A.: *Die Chirurgie des Nervus Facialis.* Urban und Schwarzenborg, Munchen, 1960, p. 208.

MILLARD, D. R., PIGOTT, R. W., and HEDO, A.: *Submandibular lipectomy.* Plast. Reconstr. Surg., 41:513, 1968.

MOREL-FATIO, D.: *Cosmetic Surgery of the Face.* In Modren Trends in Plastic Surgery, T. Gibson, ed. Shoe String Press, Hamden, Conn., 1964, p. 216.

MOREL-FATIO, D., and LALARDRIE, J. P.: *The eyelid spring (Le ressort palpebral).* Neurochirurgie, Paris, 11:303, 1965.

MÜLLER, W.: *Zur Frage der temporären Schädelresektion an Stelle der Trepanation.* Zentralbl. f. Chir., 17:65, 1890.

NANSON, E. M.: *The surgery of the deep lobe of the parotid salivary gland.* Surg. Gynec. Obstet., 122:811, 1966.

NEUMANN, C. G.: *The use of large buried pedicled flaps of dermis and fat; clinical and pathological evaluation in the treatment of progressive facial hemiatrophy.* Plast. Reconstr. Surg., 11:315, 1953.

NEY, K. W.: *The repair of cranial defects with celluloid.* Amer. J. Surg., 44:394-399, 1939.

THE HEAD AND NECK

NICOLADONI: *Ueber Fisteln des ductus Stensonianus.* Verhandl. d. deutsch. Gesellsch. f. Chir., 25:81, 1896.

NIKLISON, J.: *Contribution to the subject of facial paralysis.* Plast. Reconstr. Surg., 17:276, 1956.

NÖCKEMANN, P. F.: *Comparison of autologous and homologous bone grafts for cranioplasty (Allgemeinchirurgische Probleme bei der Schaedelachplastik).* Langenbeck's Arch f. klin. Chir., 297:12, 1961.

OPPENHEIM, H., and WING, M.: *Benign hypertrophy of masseter muscle.* Arch. Otolaryng., 70:207, 1959.

ORTICOCHEA, M.: *Four flap scalp reconstruction technique.* Brit. J. Plast. Surg. 20:159, 1967.

OSBORNE, M. P.: *Complete scalp avulsion. Rational treatment.* Ann. Surg., 132:198, 1950.

OWENS, N.: *Preliminary report on the development of neuromuscular junctions in cases of facial paralysis followed by masseter muscle transplantations.* Plast. Reconstr. Surg., 6:345, 1950.

PASSOT, R.: *Surgical correction of wrinkles.* Bull. Acad. Med. Paris, 82:12, 1919.

PEER, L. A.: *Types of buried grafts used to repair deep depressions in the skull.* JAMA, 115:357-360, 1940.

PEYTON, W. T., and HALL, H. B.: *The repair of a cranial defect with a vitallium plate.* Surgery, 10:711, 1941.

PICKERILL, H. P.: *Note on cranial autoplasty.* Brit. J. Surg. 35:204, 1947.

PUDENZ, R. H.: *The repair of cranial defects with tantalum, an experimental study.* JAMA, 121:478, 1943.

RAGNELL, A.: *A method for dynamic reconstruction in cases of facial paralysis.* Plast. Reconstr. Surg., 21:214, 1958.
Experience with dynamic and static reconstruction in cases of facial paralysis. Scand. Plastic Reconstr. Surg., 41:343, 1968.

REEVES, D. L.: *Cranioplasty.* Charles C Thomas, Springfield, 1950.

ROBINSON, F.: *Complete avulsion of the scalp.* Brit. J. Plast. Surg., 5:37, 1952.

ROSENTHAL (Quoted by Lexer): *Die geramte Wiederherstellungschirurgie.* J. A. Barth, Leipzig, 1931.

ROSENTHAL, W.: *Die muskuläre Neurotisation.* Forschritte der Kiefer und Gesichts-Chirurgie., 2:139, 1956.

SCHMIDT-TINTEMANN, U.: *Behanlungsverfahren und-Ergebnisse bei der peripheren Facialislähmung.* Langenbeck's Arch. f. klin. Chir., 298:951, 1961.
Die Gesichtsspannung. Langenbeck's Arch. f. klin. Chir. 309:83, 1965.

SCHUCHARDT, K.: *Fortschritte der Kiefer- und Gesichts-Chirurgie Vol. 7.* Georg Thieme Verlag, Stuttgart, 1961.
Der Rundstiellappen in der Wiederherstellungschirurgie des Gesichts-Kieferbereiches. Georg Thieme Verlag, Leipzig, 1944, p. 37.

SCOTT, M., WYCIS, H., and MURTAGH, F.: *Long-term evaluation of stainless steel cranioplasty.* Surg. Gynec. Obstet., 115:453, 1962.

244

THE CHEEK, TEMPLE, FOREHEAD, AND SKULL

SEELEY, R. C.: *Maxillo-facial injuries. Reconstructive surgery of the dehiscent parotid duct and dehiscent peripheral facial nerve.* Amer. J. Surg., 73:551, 1947.

SHEEHAN, J. E.: *A Manual of Reparative Plastic Surgery.* Paul B. Hoeber, New York, 1938.
The use of iliac bone in facial and cranial repair. Amer. J. Surg., 52:55, 1941.

SISTRUNK, W. E.: *Plastic surgery, removal of scars by stages; open operation for extensive laceration of anal sphincter; kondoleon operation for elephantiasis.* Ann. Surg., 85:185, 1927.

SMITH, F.: *Manual of Standard Practice of Plastic and Maxillofacial Surgery; Military Surgical Manuals.* National Research Council, W. B. Saunders, Philadelphia, 1942.
Plastic and Reconstructive Surgery; A Manual of Management. W. B. Saunders, Philadelphia, 1950.

SPARKMAN, R. S.: *Primary repair of severed parotid duct.* Ann. Surg., 129:652, 1949.
Lacerations of the parotid duct. Ibid., 131:743, 1950.

SPIRA, M., GEROW, F. J., and HARDY, S. B.: *Cervicofacial rhytidectomy.* Plast. Reconstr. Surg., 40:551, 1967.

STEINDLER, A.: *The method of direct neurotization of paralyzed muscles.* Amer. J. Orthop. Surg., 13:33, 1915.

STOUGH, D. B., III: *Punch scalp autografts for bald spots.* Plast. Reconstr. Surg., 42:450, 1968.

STRAITH, C. L., and McEVITT, W. G.: *Total avulsion of the scalp.* Occup. Med., 1:451, 1946.

STRELLI, R.: *The use of deep-frozen cranial bone homografts in the repair of defects of the skull.* Brit. J. Plast. Surg., 12:200, 1959.

UCHIDA, J.: *A method of frontal rhytidectomy.* Plast. Reconstr. Surg., 35:218, 1965.

WAKELEY, C.: *Surgery of Salivary Glands.* Ann. Roy. Coll. Surgeons England, 3:289, 1948.

WEIFORD, E. C., and GARDNER, W. J.: *Tantalum cranioplasty; review of 106 cases in civilian practice.* J. Neurosurg., 6:13, 1949.

WHALEN, W. P.: *Avulsion of the scalp.* Plast. Reconstr. Surg., 19:225, 1957.

WHITE, J. C.: *Late complications following cranioplasty with alloplastic plates.* Ann. Surg., 128:743, 1948.

WINKLER, E.: *Uber die chirurgische Behandlung der Fazialisparese* Zentral. Bl. Chir., 79-2093, 1954.
Erfahrungen mit der chirurgischen Behandlung der Facialisparese etc. Langenbeck's Arch. f. klin. Chir. 298:955, 1961.

WOODHALL, B., and SPURLING, R. G.: *Tantalum cranioplasty for war wounds of the skull,* Ann. Surg., 121:649, 1945.

WOOLF, J. I., and WALKER, A. E.: *Cranioplasty.* Surg. Gynec. Obstet., (Int. Abstr.), 81:1, 1945.

ZINTEL, H.: *Resplitting split thickness grafts with a dermatome; a method for increasing the yield of limited donor site.* Ann. Surg., 121:1, 1945.

245

THE LIPS, CHIN, AND PALATE

8

WOUNDS OF LIPS

WOUNDS of the lips are treated like wounds elsewhere. Unless the wound is grossly infected, however, it should be sutured primarily, regardless of the lapse of time. Excision of the ragged wound edges should be made as sparingly as possible. Whenever the full thickness of the lip, including the vermilion border, is severed, accurate suturing of the different layers is of the utmost importance. The first suture to be placed is through the mucocutaneous junction of the vermilion border. Traction on this suture causes the other structures to fall in line. Mucous membrane and muscle layer are sutured from the buccal side with an on-end mattress suture of 00000 chromic catgut through both layers; skin and vermilion borders are closed with silk or nylon. No dressing is required. The skin sutures are removed on the third day, the mucous-membrane-muscle sutures on the eighth day.

DEFECTS OF VERMILION BORDER OF LIPS

These defects may include the partial or total length of the vermilion border, as well as varying widths of it. If narrow strips are to be replaced, an adjacent mucosal flap, consisting of the entire oral length of

247

the lower lip down to the gingival sulcus, should be mobilized and shifted forward to reach the external wound edge (see Spira and Hardy, Bakamjian). For larger defects, flaps from the opposing lip should be used. Langenbeck's often-quoted method, as a rule, does not give the satisfactory cosmetic results which the classic illustrations make one believe. There are various more reliable methods available, among them a recent innovation consisting of the use of lingual flaps (Bakamjian, McGregor), with which the author has no experience.

Closure of Narrow Defects of the Vermilion Ridge

Under local anesthesia the vermilion border ridge is excised (for removal of leukoplakia or superficial squamous cell carcinoma). The depth of the excision stops at the level of the orbiculari oris muscle. A flap of adjacent oral mucous membrane is now formed by extending the incision from the lateral wound edges of the vermilion defect to the gingivolabial sulcus. The rectangular mucous-membrane flap should be thick enough to include the mucous glands. The latter, however, should be excised from the peripheral end of the flap, i.e., from that part of the flap which is to form the new vermilion border. (In one of the author's cases these glands hypertrophied on the vermilion border, with much mucous discharge, and had to be removed.) The flap is pulled outward over the defect and sutured with 00000 chromic catgut. Moist dressings, frequently changed, are applied for twenty-four hours. The author has used this method to replace the entire length of the vermilion border of the lower lip in leukoplakia cases and has never encountered an inversion of the lip.

Closure of Broad Defects of Middle Section of Vermilion Border (Gillies-Lexer)

The principle of this method is the formation of a mucous-membrane flap from the buccal side of the opposing lip; the flap has its free border at the gingivolabial sulcus, and is pedicled at the vermilion border. The flap is hinged, and is sutured into the defect; immobilization can be achieved with a Barton bandage. The pedicle of the flap is severed after fourteen days, and pedicle and remainder of flap are adjusted in place.

Closure of Vermilion-Border Defects at and Adjacent to Angle of Mouth

These defects are closed with sliding mucous-membrane flaps (see above) or mucous-membrane flaps taken from the mucous membrane of the opposing lip; they are pedicled and hinged in a way similar to that just described. The form of the flap, however, must be triangular, and the tip

248

of the triangle is at the commissure of the mouth, while the base is the median border of the flap. The after-treatment is the same as that described for the foregoing method. Another method may also be applicable, namely, the first-stage method after Joseph (p. 73).

Closure of Deep Defects of Entire Length of Vermilion Border (Af Schultén)

The principle is the formation and transplantation of a double-pedicle mucous-membrane-muscle flap from the opposing lip. It is important that the flap and its two pedicles, which are situated near the angle of the mouth, be thick enough to prevent necrosis (Figs. 71, 72).

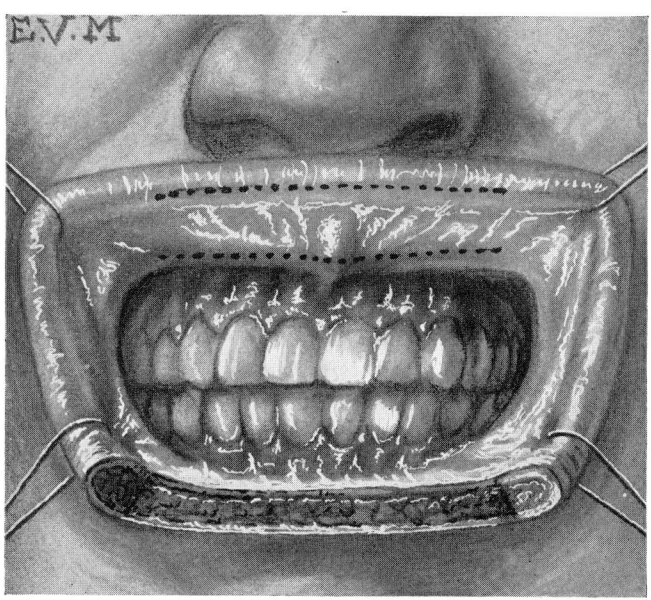

Fig. 71. Closure of defect of entire length of vermilion border of lower lip with double-pedicle mucous-membrane muscle flap from upper lip (Af Schultén). Upper and lower lip are everted with traction sutures.

1. A traction suture is passed through the lip near each commissure. The lip is now put under tension and turned outward.

2. An incision is made from one angle of the mouth to the other within the vermilion border in such a way that it bisects the vermilion border. The incision should be made about 1 to 1.5 cm. (⅜ to ⅝ inch) behind and proximal to the first one within the mucous membrane of the lip. Both incisions meet in a right angle within the muscle layer of the lip. Thus, a bridge flap of vermilion border, mucous membrane, and muscle is formed.

249

3. The flap is now rotated into the defect of the other lip. To facilitate rotation, the proximal incision can be lengthened toward the angle of the mouth, care being taken not to make the pedicle too thin or too narrow. The posterior, or mucous-membrane, edge of the flap is sutured to the skin edge of the defect, and the anterior, or vermilion-border, edge

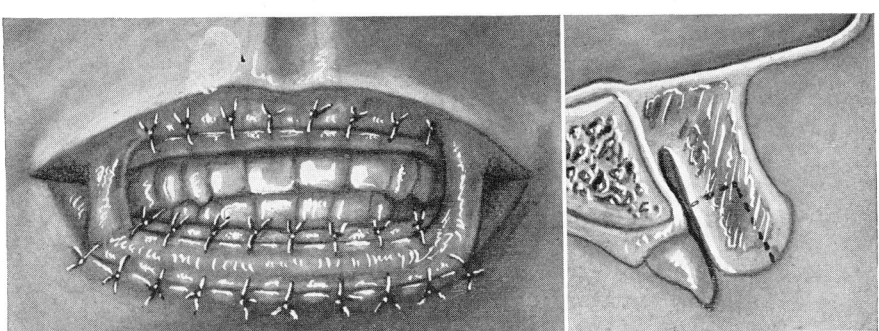

Fig. 72. Bridge flap of upper lip, with pedicles near commissures of mouth, is rotated into defect of lower lip. Secondary defect of upper lip is closed. Insert shows depths and shape of bridge flap on transverse section.

is sutured to the mucous-membrane edge of the defect. Thus, the flap is rotated about 90 degrees.

4. The secondary defect of the donor area is closed by simple suturing. Immobilization is achieved by a Barton bandage.

5. Separation of the pedicles and final adjustment are performed on the fourteenth day.

Method of Joseph: This is a two-stage operation covering one half of the vermilion-border defect at a time. Example: closure of a vermilion-border defect of the upper lip (Fig. 73).

STAGE 1: The edges of the right half of the defect are pared; then one forms a single-pedicle flap from the posterior surface of the left side of the lower lip. The peripheral end of the flap is near the commissure of the mouth, the pedicle near the middle of the lip. The flap is now raised and turned over in such a way that the peripheral end of the flap can be sutured into the lateral corner of the defect. Adjustment of the remainder of the flap and closure of the donor side follow. The pedicle is severed fourteen days later.

STAGE 2: Three weeks after the first operation, the same procedure is performed on the opposite side.

FULL-THICKNESS DEFECTS OF LIPS

VERTICAL DEFECTS

Small Vertical Defects

Small vertical defects can be closed by suturing the wound edges together. To achieve such a simple closure, the defect is given the shape of a wedge, the base of the wedge lying toward the vermilion border, the tip of it toward the chin. Mucous membrane, muscles, and skin are sutured separately, care being taken to bring the vermilion-border edges in exact alignment. Alternately, mucous membrane and muscles are su-

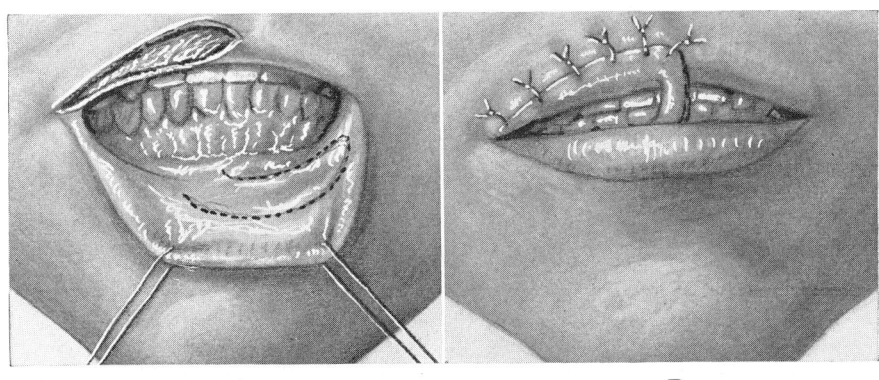

A   B

Fig. 73. *A:* Reconstruction of vermilion border of upper lip in two stages with flaps from buccal side of lower lip (Joseph). Flap for right half of defect is outlined on left side of lower lip. *B:* Flap is hinged into defect. After separation of pedicle, same procedure is carried out on opposite side.

tured together with an on-end mattress suture tied at the mucous-membrane side; the skin is sutured separately. After closure of the defect, the upper lip should not protrude much; if it does, the wound should be opened and the defect closed by one of the procedures described later.

Vertical Defects Not Larger than Half the Width of the Lip

These defects are best closed according to a method first described by Estlander (1872). The principle of the method consists in formation and rotation of a full-thickness flap from the opposing lip into the defect. The flap is pedicled at one side of the vermilion border which contains the coronary artery. The latter must be preserved since it is the only nutrient

251

artery. Estlander's original operation was devised for closure of triangular defects of the lower lip near the commissure of the mouth (Fig. 74). The flap, consisting of the full thickness of upper lip and cheek, was rotated into the defect in such a way that the pedicle formed the new angle of the mouth. This operation has been modified in many ways since. Abbé used the same principle for closure of defects of the upper lip (Case 24, p.

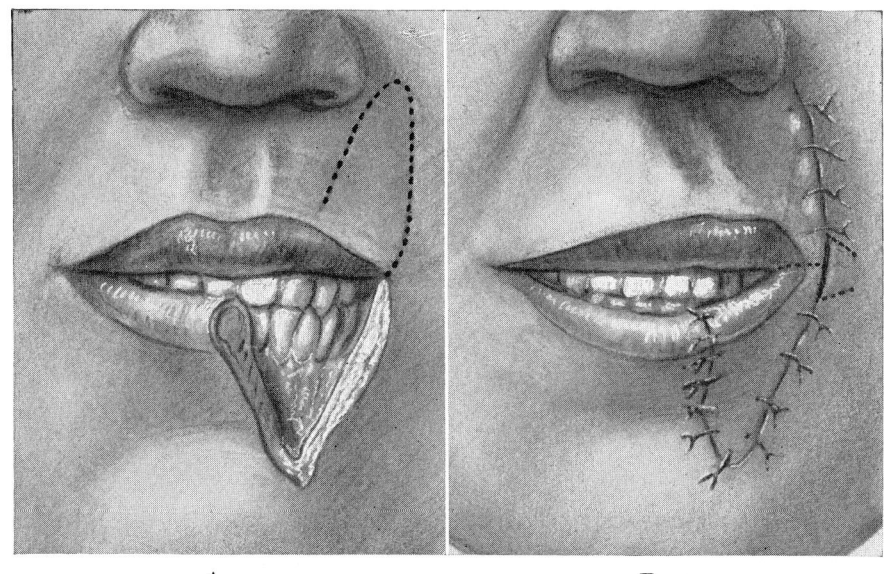

A   B

Fig. 74. *A:* Closure of triangular defect of lower lip with flap from upper lip in defects not larger than one half the width of lip. Defect includes lower border of left angle of mouth. To close defect, a vermilion-border lined flap is rotated from upper lip and nasolabial region. Pedicle of flap containing the coronary artery is to replace the commissures of mouth. Flap should be made one half as wide as defect to shorten upper and lower lip proportionately. (H. May: Ann. Surg.) *B:* Flap is rotated into defect. Secondary defect is closed by suturing wound edges together.

1024). He also demonstrated that the method is useful for defects not including the commissure. In such a case, the pedicle of the flap crosses the mouth and has to be separated later (Fig. 76; Case 23, p. 1022). Other modifications include those of Buck, Brown, Padgett, Cannon, and Smith.

Technique (Estlander): Some of the different ways in which Estlander's principle can be used are outlined in Figures 74 to 77 (see also Cases 23, 24, pp. 1022, 1024). Only a few important points for achieving a closure of the defect and a satisfactory cosmetic result need be emphasized. The defect is made triangular. The incisions are outlined with one of the aniline dyes. The shape of the flap is now outlined opposite the defect within the nasolabial region. The length (height) of the flap should be equal to that of the defect; the width of the flap should be only half that of the defect, in order to shorten upper and lower lip proportionately. In the majority of cases, the pedicle of the flap lies at its median side, and consists of the vermilion-border thickness of the lip. The pedicle should be made narrow to facilitate rotation, but great care must be taken not to injure the coronary artery which runs within the vermilion. One may be guided as to the level of the coronary artery by comparison with the other side of the flap, where the artery has already been severed and ligated.

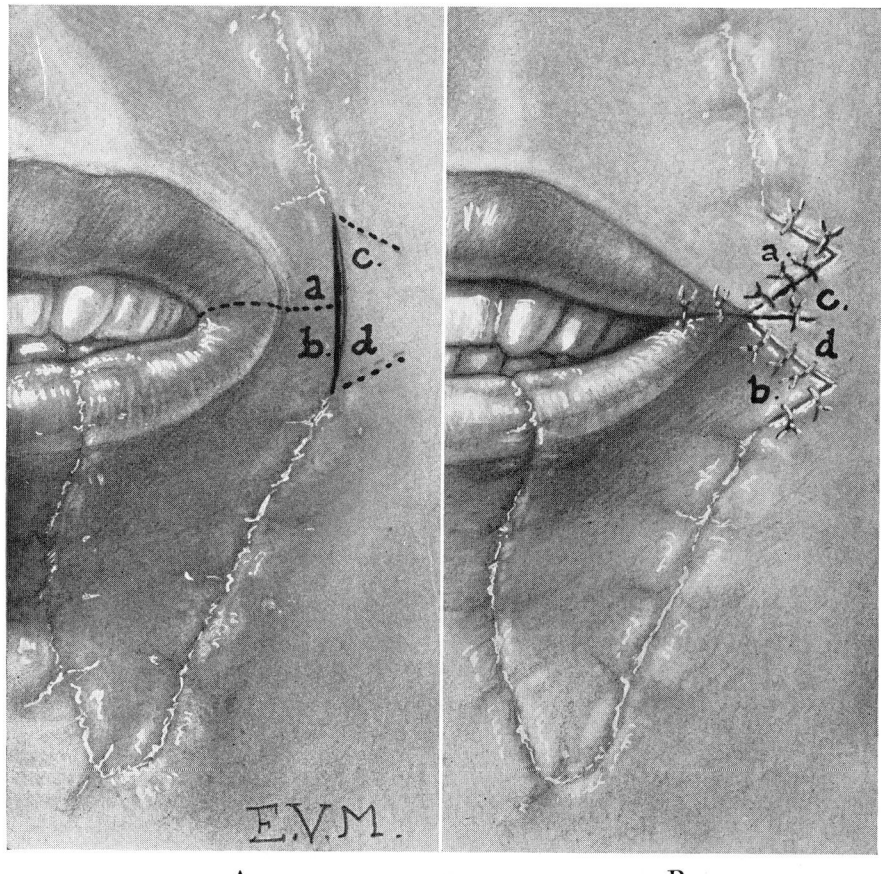

A   B

Fig. 75. Reconstruction of commissure of mouth in cases where pedicle of flap (see Fig. 74) forms new angle of mouth. Vertical shortness is overcome by switching triangular flaps (double Z-operation; compare with Fig. 52). Flap *a* is exchanged with flap *c*, flap *b* with flap *d*. Thus, not only is the oral orifice widened but a more natural commissure of the mouth is achieved. (H. May: Ann. Surg.)

253

After the flap is formed, the secondary defect is closed in layers as far as possible. The flap is now rotated into the defect. Mucous membrane, muscles, and skin are sutured separately. The side toward the pedicle and the corresponding side of the defect should be sutured first. Accurate approximation of the vermilion border of the flap and the edge of the defect is necessary. This may sometimes be difficult owing to difference

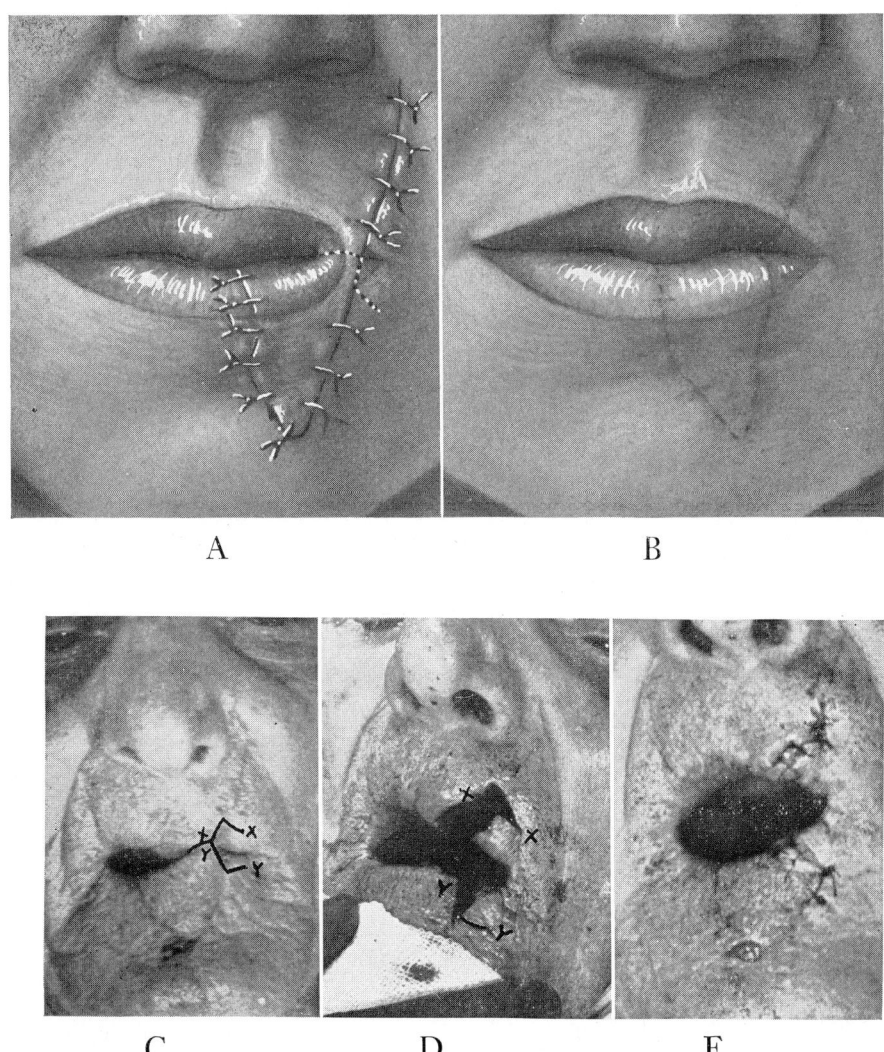

A   B

C   D   E

Fig. 76. In defects not including commissure, method of Fig. 74 is applicable; pedicle of flap, however, crosses mouth and must be severed. After severance, flap and pedicle are adjusted in place with Z-type incisions as outlined in *A* and *C*, *D* and *E*.

in width, but then at least the mucocutaneous borders should be brought in alignment.

After-Treatment: After the application of a dry dressing, a Barton bandage may be used for one week and the patient fed a liquid diet.

OVERCOMING VERTICAL SHORTNESS: In those cases in which the angle of the mouth was included in the defect and the pedicle of the flap forms the new commissure, some vertical shortness is caused. This consequently

A   B

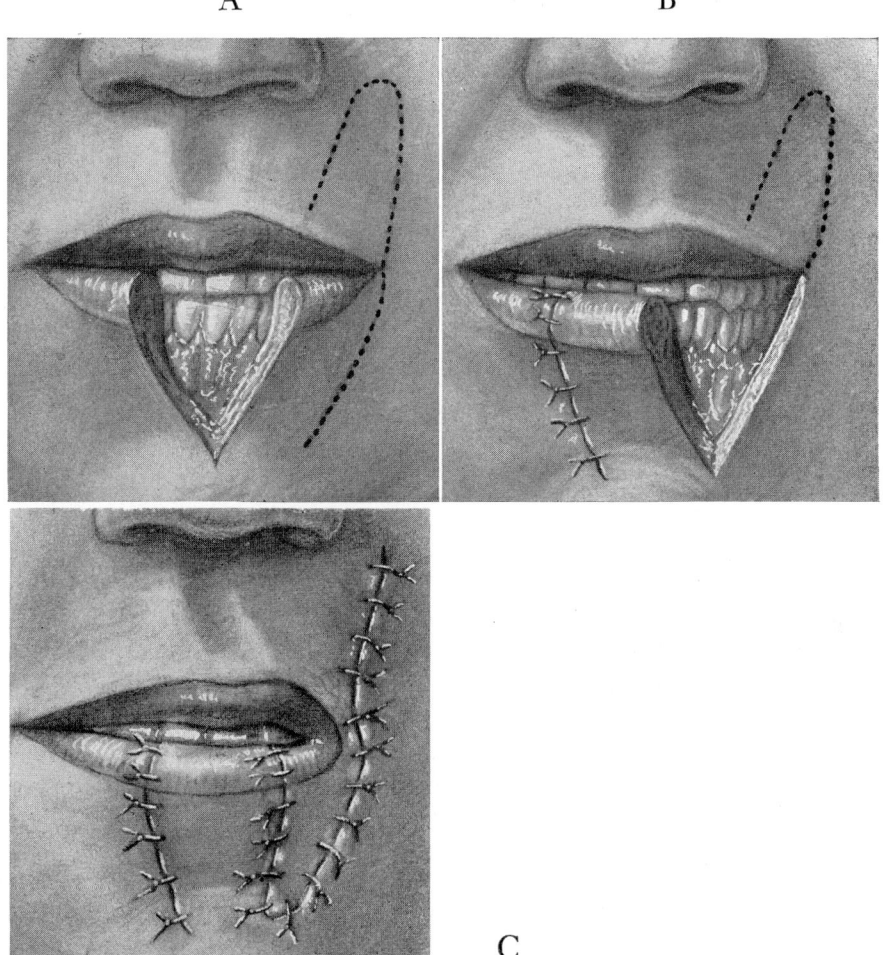

C

Fig. 77. *A:* Triangular defect in middle portion of lower lip. To make possible the method shown in Fig. 74, defect must be transferred laterally. This is achieved by closure of center defect with square flap. Outlines of this flap and flap of upper lip are illustrated. *B:* Square flap for closure of center defect is rotated into defect. This creates similar defect in lateral portion of lip. *C:* Flap from upper lip is rotated into lateral defect. Secondary defect of nasolabial region is closed (Buck). (H. May: Ann. Surg.)

prevents the patient from opening the mouth fully. To overcome the handicap, the author recommends a procedure (to be performed three weeks after the first operation) as outlined in Figure 75. The principle is based on the switching of triangular flaps, as in Z-operations. Thus not only is the oral orifice widened but a more natural commissure achieved (Case 24, p. 1024).

CROSSING OF MOUTH BY PEDICLE: If the pedicle of the flap crosses the mouth, it must be severed (Fig. 76; Case 23, p. 1022). This is done after four weeks. After it is severed, it is adjusted into its original place, followed by adjustment of vermilion borders of flap and defect. To facilitate adjustment, the author uses a Z-type incision, as demonstrated in Figure 76.

Defects in Middle of Lower Lip

For defects in the middle of the lower lip, the procedure depicted in Figure 77 is recommended. The commissure of the mouth can be reconstructed according to the method shown in Figure 75.

HORIZONTAL DEFECTS

These defects may involve partial or full length of the lips. Depending upon the size of the defect, flaps from the immediate neighborhood or from distant parts can be transplanted. There are a number of procedures described which recommend the use of full-thickness cheek flaps. The literature on this subject has been reviewed by Pierce and O'Connor. Some of the procedures have never been practiced, and some of them give such poor cosmetic and functional results that they should be abandoned, not only from surgical practice but also from textbooks. Brun's operation is still highly recommended in some textbooks. This method was tried by the author, but the result was far from that which the classic illustrations would lead one to expect. There are a few excellent procedures available, however, which make use of flaps from the immediate neighborhood, consisting of skin and subcutaneous tissue only, and these are recommended whenever they are possible.

Transplantation of Local Flaps

Technique (F. Smith) (Case 31, p. 1035): This reconstruction is completed in four stages, with proper intervening periods of time (Fig. 78).

STAGE 1. COMPLETE DÉBRIDEMENT AND PREPARATION (IMMEDIATE): The management of the borders of the defect must anticipate reconstruction of the lip. Flaps for a lining to replace the lost mucosa, for the outer skin covering, and for the vermilion margin must be so planned that ample material enjoying an adequate blood supply is available.

The blood supply of the lining flap, which will be reflected from the skin adjacent to the angle of the mouth, must come from the buccal mucosa and the muscle bordering the defect. Consequently, the mucosa on this edge must be undermined and accurately approximated to the skin with fine, closely placed nylon sutures. This produces a minimum of scar and a maximal blood supply. This blood supply is usually adequate, but it can be guaranteed by outlining, partially undercutting, and again approximating this skin flap at this stage (Fig. 78, *a*).

A   B

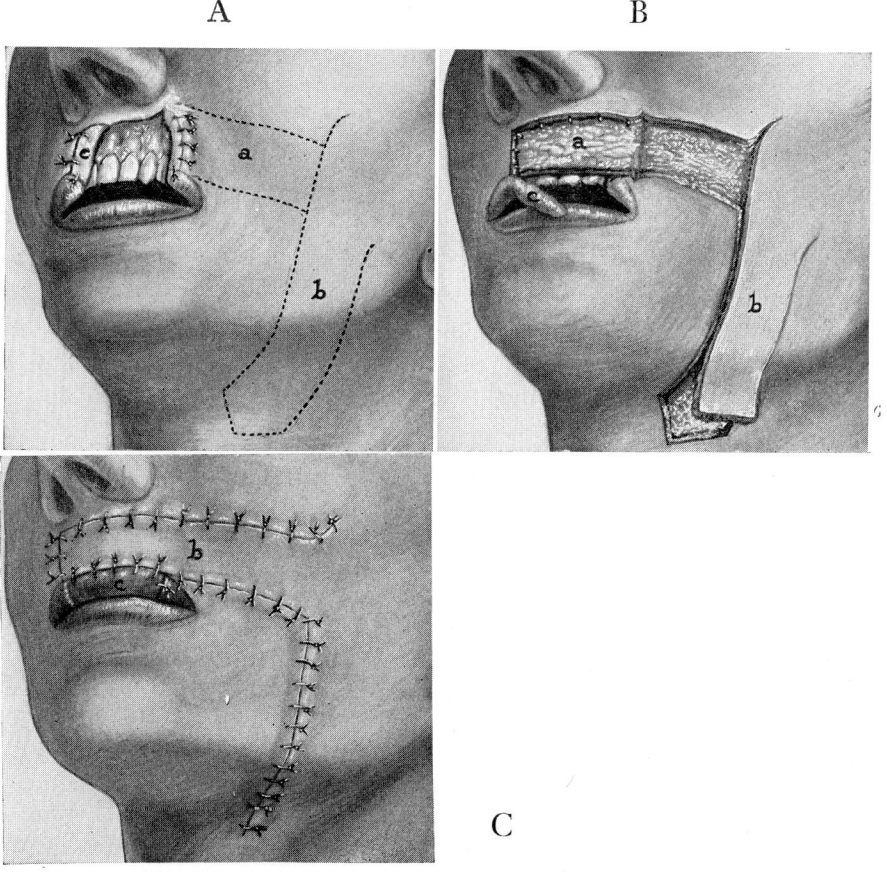

C

Fig. 78.   *A:* Subtotal loss of upper lip replaced with flaps from immediate neighborhood. Method of managing skin and mucous membrane on margins of defect; outline of lining flap, *a*, and covering flap, *b*, for the reconstruction. (F. Smith: Manual of Standard Practice of Plastic and Maxillofacial Surgery. W. B. Saunders.) *B:* Lining flap in situ, *a*; covering flap, *b*; and mucocutaneous margin flap, *c*, dissected. *C:* Skin-covering flap rotated and sutured in position, *b*; mucocutaneous-border flap sutured in position, *c*; skin defect in face and neck closed and sutured.

257

The covering flap (Fig. 78, *b*) is outlined next. It can be raised and sutured in its original location at this time if the blood supply is questionable. The blood supply, however, is usually excellent.

It is sometimes advisable to utilize flaps from both sides of the mouth in the construction of an entire lip. When this method is followed, a long covering flap and a shorter lining flap should be cut on one side and the reverse procedure practiced on the opposite side. This will place the junction line of the covering flaps at a different place from that of the union of the lining flaps and will prevent a depressed, adherent scar line.

The mucosa bordering the edge of the remnant of the lip is similarly undercut and sutured. This mucosa will be utilized to form the vermilion border of the reconstructed portion of the lip (Fig. 78, *A, B, C*). (This, however, is not necessary if the vermilion border is replaced by the Gillies-Lexer or Af Schultén method; see p. 248.) The remaining skin bordering the defect—chin or face and nose—is undercut and accurately approximated to the mucosal remnant along the buccal sulcus.

STAGE 2. PREPARATION OF LINING: The purpose of this is to destroy hair follicles. The operation is performed three weeks after Stage 1.

The hair-bearing derma of Flap *a* (Fig. 78, *A*) is excised like a full-thickness graft; one must be sure that all hair roots are removed. After thorough hemostasis by sponge pressure, the surface is covered with a thick, split skin graft from a hairless region of the arm or leg (donor area not to be shaved). The graft is covered with a strip of bismuth tribromophenate (xeroform) gauze and mechanic's waste; pressure is applied by tying the skin sutures, which have been left long, over the mechanic's waste.

STAGE 3. RECONSTRUCTION: This is performed two weeks following Stage 2.

The mucous membrane on the edge of the remnant of lip is removed between two parallel incisions 1 cm. (⅜ inch) apart. (This step can be eliminated if the vermilion border is replaced by the Gillies-Lexer or Af Schultén methods; see p. 248). One incision is carried down its line of union with the skin, and the other through the mucosa on the posterior surface of the lip. The blood supply of the remnant is provided by the mucosa on the free margin of the lip and a broad portion of mucosa posteriorly. Flap *c*, formed by the maneuvers just described, is held on a sharp hook; it will form the vermilion border of the reconstructed lip (Fig. 78, *B*).

The skin flap, *a* (in Fig. 78, *A, B*), carrying underlying fat, is turned from the face on a hinge and sutured to the incised margin of the mucosa

258

on the posterior surface of the remnant of lip and along the superior border of the defect.

The covering flap, *b*, is incised and elevated with the underlying fat (Fig. 78, *B*). The skin of the face on each side of the defect, resulting from elevation of the covering flap, *b*, is freely undercut and approximated with nylon sutures. Approximation of these skin edges adds two thirds of the width of the flap to its length. This covering flap, *b* (Fig. 78, *B*, *C*), is rotated 90 degrees to cover the lip and the defect left by reflection of the lining flap, *a* (Fig. 78, *B*). The opposing skin edges are sutured with nylon.

The anterior edge of the mucosal flap, *c* (Fig. 78, *B*, *C*), is sutured to the free edge of the covering flap with nylon. Its posterior edge is sutured to the lining flap.

The suture lines about the mouth are painted with collodion and left exposed; the wound at the neck is dressed.

STAGE 4. CORRECTIONS: The procedures are performed from thirty to sixty days after Stage 3.

The teat created by the rotation of the covering flap, *b* (Fig. 78, *C*), is adjusted by removal of excess skin. This should not be done sooner than the twelfth day because of possible damage to the blood supply of the transplanted flap prior to this time. Any other cosmetic defects are corrected at this period.

The same principle can be used for some of the larger defects of the lower lip excluding the chin. The covering flaps will then, of course, be extended well below the mandible toward the neck. In large defects this method may be performed bilaterally. The vermilion border, however, must then be furnished from the sound lip (see p. 248) or by means of two buccal mucous-membrane flaps (see foregoing discussion, Fig. 73).

Technique (Dieffenbach-Webster) (Fig. 79): Jerome P. Webster called attention to a method of upper-lip reconstruction which was devised by Dieffenbach over a century ago but which had been mentioned only sporadically in the literature and much less used. It consists of a crescentic perialar cheek excision in preparation for advancement of a lip flap. It can be used unilaterally or bilaterally; it also can be used in conjunction with other methods, such as the Estlander-Abbé flap from the lower lip, and for closure of defects as well as for correction of certain deformities of the upper lip, such as cicatricial changes.

An incision is made in the alar fold along the base of the ala of the nose down to the periosteum. It can if necessary be carried up above the ala along the nose. This incision follows the ala on the base of the nostril to the defect. The lip and cheek are then retracted upward, and the

259

mucosa is incised along the upper labiogingival sulcus. The muscles are stripped away from the attachment to the maxilla; this dissection is carried up to the infraorbital foramen. This procedure allows the cheek to be brought medially, and in this advanced position the mucous membrane is closed with interrupted sutures along the labiogingival sulcus. The flap is then drawn forward and tentatively held in position by temporary

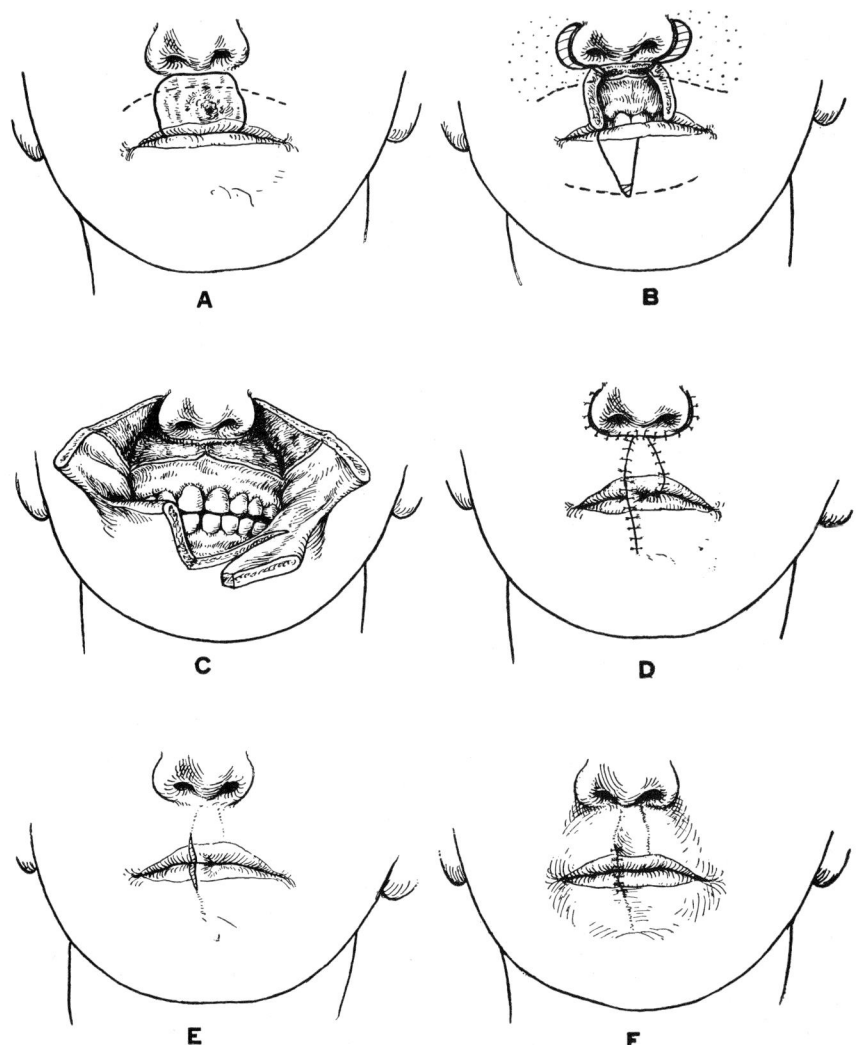

Fig. 79. Crescentic perialar cheek excision in preparation for advancement of upper lip flaps. *A:* Condition before excision of basal cell epithelioma of upper lip. *B:* Condition following excision of tumor, bilateral excision of perialar cheek crescents and undermining of both cheeks. Upon drawing the wound edges together lip was found to be too tight. Hence an Estlander-Abbé flap from lower lip is added, *B* to *F.* (J. P. Webster: Plast. Reconstr. Surg.)

260

sutures. A crescentic portion of perialar cheek tissue is excised so that the skin edges of the cheek incision fit those of the ala without distortion. The cheek flap is anchored at the ala by heavy buried sutures, either to the periosteum or to the fibrous tissue of the ala, so that the pull of the cheek will not displace the nostril. The lip is sutured in layers, with due attention to satisfactory lip formation, length, and protrusion, and with no discrepancy of skin junction at the vermilion border. A similar procedure is performed on the other side.

If it is found, with the trial suture of the flap in position, that the upper lip is too tight and that the lower lip protrudes with a possible narrowing of the mouth, the lip sutures may be cut and the defect closed by an Estlander-Abbé flap from the lower lip (see Fig. 79, B to F). The bridge between the lips is severed at a secondary operation.

There is another adaptation of the Dieffenbach principle. Of the four tissue layers that make up the lip, the mucous-membrane lining and the vermilion borders are the more elastic ones. Hence, after mobilization of the horizontal flaps it may be possible to unite the oral mucous membrane and the vermilion borders, but one may not be able to close the muscles and the skin. If such a situation is likely to arise, it may be good to have a distant flap previously prepared (a tube flap, for instance; see below) for coverage of the remaining defect, or to close the defect temporarily with a skin graft.

Transplantation of Distant Flaps

Whenever the defect is of such a size that flaps from the immediate neighborhood cannot be used without leaving secondary deformities, flaps from distant parts of the body must be transplanted. Available flaps are the acromiopectoral, arm, and cervical—the forehead flaps only in exceptional cases. These flaps have to be lined unless local flaps can be hinged or turned over to replace the lining of the lips; the previously mentioned method for lining (see above) can also be used. Schuchard describes the construction and use of such flaps in his well-illustrated monograph.

Tube Flap Lined with Split Graft: If a tube flap is to be lined, the peripheral part is left untubed and lined with a free skin graft, as described on page 98. It must, however, be pointed out that flaps lined with free skin grafts tend to buckle from shrinkage of the graft. Hence, the method of lining described below is preferable, although it may be more complicated.

When the flap is ready to be transferred, the edges of the defect are split so that free skin and mucous-membrane edges are available. The flap is now transferred to the defect and sutured in place—the lining to the mucous-membrane edges, the skin to the skin edges of the defect. An immobilizing dressing may be necessary. The remaining raw area of the donor site, from which the flap was raised, is skin grafted. After two to three weeks, the flap is gradually severed from its pedicle and adjusted in place. Four weeks later, the vermilion border is replaced from the opposing lip (see p. 248). In the case of an upper lip, a new philtrum can be formed by subcutaneous excision of a section of tissue after the flap has healed in place; this may be achieved by subcutaneously introducing the scalpel from the middle of the vermilion border to the septum or by making an incision in that region and excising a flat section of subcutaneous tissue.

Tube Flap Lined by Folding Peripheral End Over (Compare with Figs. 83, 84, 85 and Case 14, p. 1010): In constructing the tube flap, its peripheral part is left untubed and returned to its original site. After four to six weeks, the untubed part is mobilized again and the peripheral pedicle gradually severed, as described on page 97.

After all edema has subsided in the untubed flap, this part is again elevated with the exception of a small bilateral bridge, which is left unsevered near the transition of the untubed into the tubed part. The purpose of this is to hold the flap in place until it is ready for its transplantation into the defect. The raw surface of the elevated untubed part is thinned by trimming away some of the fat tissue; it is then folded upon itself and sutured together. The raw surface of the donor area is skin grafted. After two weeks, the small skin bridges are severed and the flap elevated and transferred into the defect. The following procedures differ somewhat for lower and upper lips.

LOWER LIP: The edges of the defect are split until free skin and free mucous-membrane edges are obtained. The flap is now sutured in place; the part which is folded over is sutured to the mucous-membrane edges, the other part to the skin edges; an immobilizing dressing may be necessary. After two to three weeks, the flap is gradually severed from its pedicle and adjusted in place. After three weeks, the folded skin edge of the flap, now forming the free edge of the flap, is split and covered with a mucous-membrane flap from the sound lip (see p. 248), thus replacing the vermilion border.

UPPER LIP: The defect's edges are split as described; the folded skin edge of the flap is incised so that this part of the flap can be sutured to the proximal, or upper, wound edge of the defect—the folded part to the mucous membrane, the outer part to the skin edges. Adjustment of the remaining parts follows; the subsequent steps are similar to those previously described.

262

DEFECTS OF LOWER LIP AND CHIN WITHOUT LOSS OF BONE

Transplantation of Local Flaps

For closure of defects not larger than three quarters of the width of the lip and centrally located, Burow's and Bernard's methods are recommended (Fig. 80; Cases 27, 28, pp. 1028, 1030) (compare also with Fig. 13).

Technique (Burow): This method is used only if the defect is triangular. Flaps are shifted from the immediate neighborhood into the defect after sacrificing two triangles of tissue in the nasolabial region (Fig. 80).

EXCISION OF LIP AND CHIN: The lower lip and soft parts of the chin are excised in a heart-shaped, rather than wedge-shaped, piece (Dieffenbach). This results later in a more normal-looking profile, with a dimple in the center of the chin.

EXCISION OF NASOLABIAL REGION: The next step consists of excision of additional triangles in the nasolabial region. They are marked out first with one of the aniline dyes. The base of the triangle, instead of lying

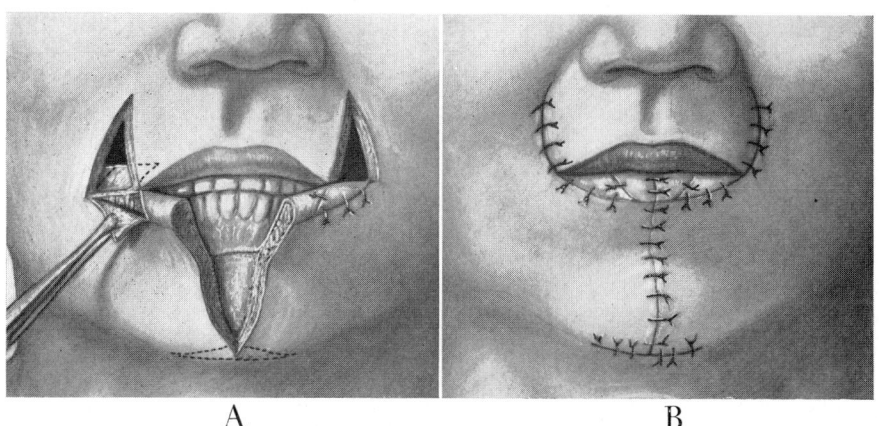

A   B

Fig. 80. *A:* Burow's method of closure of triangular defects of lower lip and chin when defect is not larger than three quarters the width of lip. Closure of defect by shifting tissue from immediate neighborhood into defect after sacrificing two triangles of tissue in nasolabial region. Excision of triangles should consist of skin and muscle only. Incision of mucous-membrane flap of triangular defect is outlined. Turned outward, the mucous-membrane flaps lengthen vermilion border. A small triangle of skin near corner of mouth must be removed for adjustment of mucous-membrane flap. Horizontal incision and excision of skin triangles below chin may facilitate shifting of main flaps and avoid pointing of chin. (H. May: Ann. Surg.) *B:* After closure of primary and secondary defects.

263

in line with the vermilion border of the lower lip, is slightly slanting laterally and upward and equals in length half the width of the defect. The median side of the triangle follows or parallels the nasolabial fold so that after closure of the defects the suture line comes to lie within or parallel to the nasolabial fold. The height of the triangle varies according to the length of its base. Of these triangles, only skin and muscles are excised. The mucous membrane is separated as outlined in Figure 80, *A*. If turned outward, it will lengthen the vermilion border. The purpose for shaping the small mucous-membrane flaps, as outlined in Figure 80, *A*, is twofold: to provide (1) a gradual tapering off of the new vermilion border at the outer angles which are to form the new angle of the mouth, and (2) a more satisfactory adjustment of the mucous-membrane flap to the gradually disappearing original vermilion border. As a rule, a small triangle of skin needs to be removed at the angle of the mouth to make room for the tip of the mucous-membrane flaps (New and Figi). The flaps are now turned outward and sutured in place. The lateral part, however, where the new vermilion border tapers off, may be too broad, owing to thickness of the cheek tissues; it should be thinned somewhat by excision of a wedge of subcutaneous and muscle tissue.

MOBILIZATION OF CHEEK FLAPS: With an incision along the lower gingivobuccal sulcus, the mucous membrane is severed as far back as the last molar. A rim of mucous membrane should be left attached to the gingival side to facilitate later suturing. Then follows separation of the lateral cheek flaps from the outer surface of the horizontal rami of the mandible with the knife and with the aid of a periosteal elevator, care being taken not to injure the alveolar nerve bundle where it escapes from the foramen mentale. The dissection should be carried back to the anterior border of the masseter muscle; if mobility of the flap is not sufficient, the masseter muscle may be separated from its insertion, care being taken not to injure the arteria maxillaris externa.

CLOSURE OF DEFECTS: The mobilized flaps are now pulled forward and anchored in this position to the gums by suturing the mucous membrane in the gingivobuccal sulcus. Each suture should be placed obliquely so that it advances the flap forward. The last suture should attach the mucous membrane of both sides in the midline of the mandible. Closure of the triangles in layers follows, starting with the mucosal side. The next step is connecting the lateral edge of the new vermilion border to that of the upper lip, then the vertical connection of both flaps in the midline in layers. Some adjustment may be necessary at the bottom of the incision to avoid pointing of the chin (Fig. 80, *B*). A drain is inserted in the lower corner of the vertical wound.

VARIATIONS: In defects less than half the length of the lip, and particularly off-center defects, only one triangle needs to be sacrificed (the triangle does not need to be as wide as the defect) and the cheek of the affected side mobilized. One may be tempted to mobilize the other cheek also to facilitate closure, but this may result in a deviation of the mouth, as the author has once experienced. For other variations, see page 269. If dissection of the cervical glands is necessary, it should be performed in a second stage.

Technique (Bernard): This operation is similar to Burow's, with the exception that the defect is made square instead of triangular. Martin improved the technique by modification. Figure 81 demonstrates the vari-

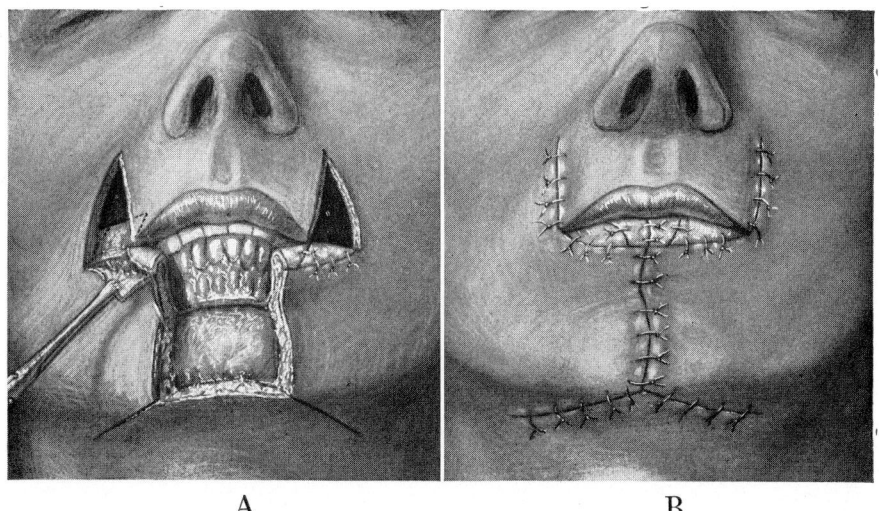

A   B

Fig. 81.   Bernard's method, modified by Martin, in closing square defects of lower lip and chin when defect is not larger than three quarters of lip. Method similar to that of Fig. 80.

ous steps. Freeman and R. Webster and co-workers have worked out other modifications of the method, with which the author has had no experience.

Technique (Dieffenbach) (Modification after Adelmann, Syzmanowski, May): For closure of defects of the entire lower lip and chin without loss of bone, a lined flap from a distant part of the body will be the method of choice in a number of cases, particularly for square, irregularly shaped defects. If, however, the defect can be made triangular, transplantation of composite flaps from the immediate neighborhood may still be possible. The writer recommends Dieffenbach's operation in such a case. This method has been frequently criticized as being mutilating and ex-

265

tensive. The operation is extensive, but, correctly performed, it is not mutilating. The writer has endeavored to improve the technique by slightly modifying it. From cosmetic, functional, and economic standpoints, it is by far superior to distant flap transplantations. The advantages are: excision of the diseased part and closure of the defect in one sitting, thus short hospitalization; replacement of lost structures by similar structures, thus restoring original function and appearance (Fig. 82; compare also with Fig. 12) (Cases 26, 29, 30, 32, pp. 1027, 1032, 1034, 1036).

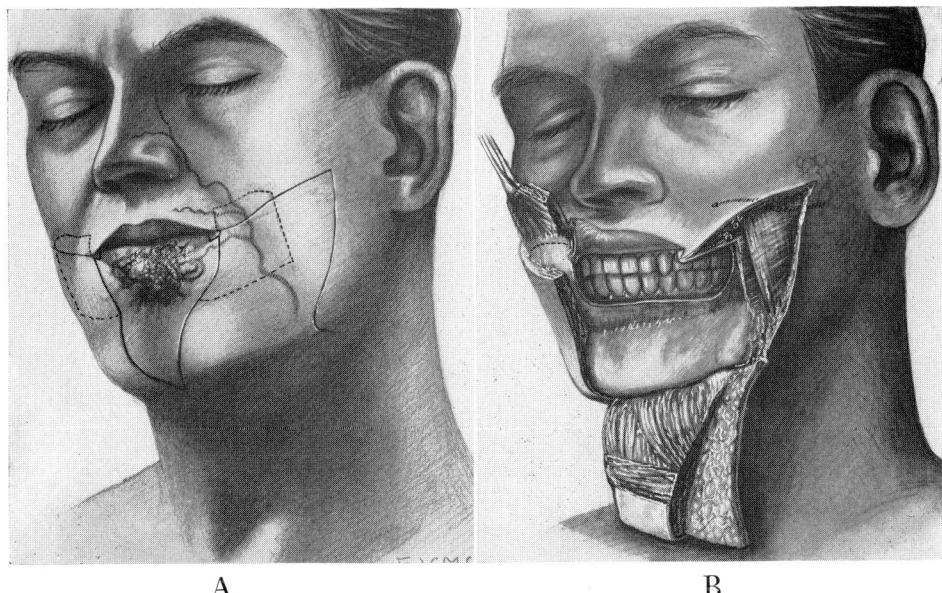

A   B

Fig. 82. *A:* Modified Dieffenbach method for closure of large defects of lower lip and chin. Heart-shaped excision of lower lip and chin is outlined, as well as two square flaps which are to cover defect. Two small flaps at angle of mouth are preserved. Inside incisions for mobilization of flaps from mandible and from anterior border of masseter muscles are outlined by dotted lines, also small mucous-membrane flaps for formation of vermilion border. *B:* Left flap is mobilized. Small mucous-membrane flap is sutured to outer edges of main flap. Right mucous-membrane for formation of vermilion border is being freed. (H. May: Surg. Gynec. Obstet.)

The principle is based upon the creation of a triangular defect, which is closed by shifting two square flaps around one point of rotation from the immediate neighborhood into the defect (Figs. 12, 82). The incisions are outlined with one of the aniline dyes. Before the anesthesia is administered, the patient is requested to contract his masseter muscle; its anterior border is marked out at its upper and lower insertion

266

with a drop of methylene blue injected percutaneously. Before operation, the orifice of Stensen's duct is also marked with a drop of dye.

EXCISION OF LIP AND CHIN: The tumor, together with the soft parts of the entire chin, is excised in a heart-shaped, rather than a wedge-shaped, piece (Dieffenbach). This results later in a more normal-looking profile, with a dimple in the center of the chin. If possible, the excision should not include the entire vermilion border at the commissure of the mouth. The reconstruction of a labial commissure involves another problem.

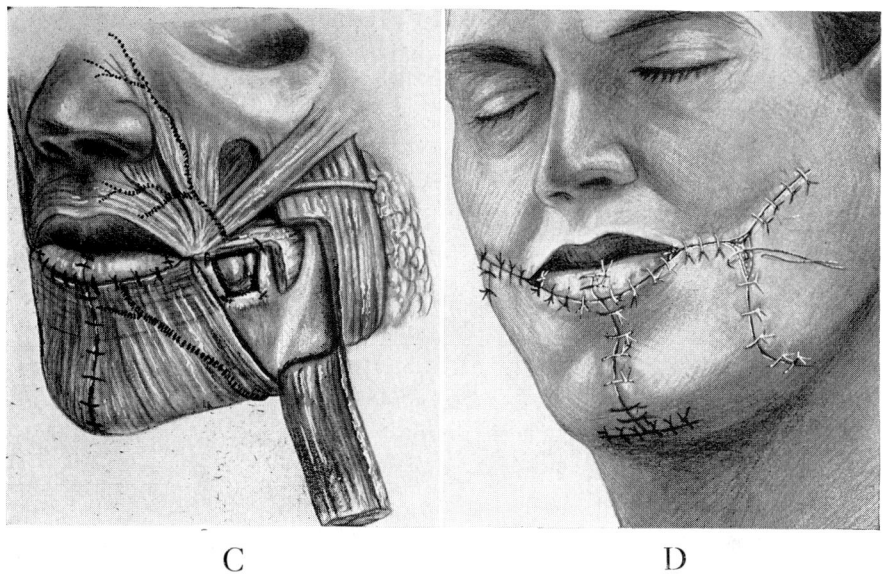

C   D

Fig. 82. *C:* Closure of triangular muscle and mucous-membrane defect in front of masseter muscle by mobilization of mucous membrane as far as possible and transplantation of flap consisting of lower anterior half of masseter muscle. (Mobilization of flap is exaggerated in drawing for demonstration purposes.) *D:* Original and secondary defects are closed. Horizontal incision and excision of skin triangularly below chin may facilitate shifting of main flaps and avoid pointing of chin (see Fig. 80).

In these cases, a very small flap of the vermilion at either side of the mouth is left as outlined in Figure 82, *A, B.* Also, if resection of the mandible is not required, a rim of mucous membrane should be left attached to the gingival side of the sulcus to facilitate later suturing. The incisions on each side meet each other at a point below the center part of the mandible. This point becomes the point of rotation around which two square flaps are turned from the immediate neighborhood.

OUTLINES OF FLAPS AND FORMATION OF VERMILION BORDER: For forming the left flap—likewise the right—the following incisions are made

THE HEAD AND NECK

(Fig. 82, *A*). From the left commissure, an incision is carried obliquely upward to about 3.8 cm. (1½ inches) in front of the tragus of the ear. It is imperative that this incision be made obliquely, *not* horizontally. From there the incision is carried downward at an angle less than a right angle, ending below the mandible.

The next step is the formation of the left half of the vermilion border. From the angle of the mouth to the anterior border of the masseter muscle, the incision includes skin and muscles, while the mucous membrane is dissected free from the upper wound edge for about 1 cm. (⅜ inch). In this way, the external maxillary artery is encountered and ligated. Posterior and more superficial to the external maxillary artery, the facial vein is found, and is also ligated and separated. Still more posterior and above is Stensen's duct; care must be taken not to injure it. The mucous membrane is now separated 1 cm. (⅜ inch) above the main flap, tapering off in its lateral half (Fig. 82, *A* and *B* right side). This tiny mucous-membrane flap is now turned outward to form the left half of the vermilion border (Fig. 82, *B*). The lateral third of this new lip, owing to the thickness of the subcutaneous and muscle tissue, is broader than the median parts; this results in protrusion instead of gradual disappearance of the lateral part of the vermilion border. It can be avoided by excising some of the subcutaneous and muscle tissue of the lateral third of the new lip and trimming the mucous membrane accordingly.

MOBILIZATION OF FLAP: The entire flap is now mobilized (Fig. 82, *B*). Its lateral half is mobilized by outside incisions consisting of skin only. Its median half is mobilized by inside incisions, comprising the entire thickness of the cheek. The incisions for the lateral half penetrate not deeper than to the fascia parotideomasseterica, from which the lateral half of the flap is separated. The incisions for the median half begin with separation of the mucous membrane along the lower gingivobuccal sulcus. A rim of mucous membrane should be left attached to the gingival side to facilitate later suturing. The incision should reach from the defect to the anterior border of the masseter muscle, including only the mucous membrane. The other inside incision, leading vertically upward, connects this latter point with the outer edge of the newly formed vermilion border. This incision penetrates the mucous membrane and the muscles. The entire flap is now turned downward and, by blunt dissection, separated from the mandible until the submandibular spaces are exposed—an important step, since the flap will not be flexible enough unless it is separated entirely from the mandible. As a rule, the alveolar nerve bundle must be severed at the foramen mentale; the resulting loss of sensitivity around the chin is only temporary. Great care, however, should be taken not to injure the arteria maxillaris externa. The right flap is formed and mobilized similarly.

268

CLOSURE OF DEFECTS: Both flaps, which have surprising mobility, are shifted toward the midline into the defect. This creates a secondary mucous-membrane and muscle defect in front of the masseter muscle, as well as a secondary skin defect at the origin of the lateral half of the flap. To close the muscle and mucous-membrane defect, the author advises the following precedure: By retracting the free edge of the masseter and buccinator muscles backward (Fig. 82, *B*) the oral mucous membrane is widely mobilized so that it can be pulled forward. This may be facilitated by a posterior relaxation incision and an incision along the lower gingivo-buccal sulcus. The muscle defect is closed with a flap of the masseter muscle, consisting of its anterior lower half, which is separated from the underlying buccinator muscle and shifted anteriorly into the muscle defect (Fig. 82, *C*); or a vertical relaxation incision may be made through the middle of the masseter muscle and the anterior half of the muscle shifted forward. The closure of all defects is carried out in the following order: Connection of the lateral edge of the new vermilion border to form the commissure of the mouth; suturing of the mucous membrane of the flap to the gingival mucous membrane; closure of the posterior mucous-membrane defect as far as possible by mobilization of the posterior mucous membrane; connection of both flaps to each other in a three-layer suture; shifting forward of the masseter flap to fill the defect; suturing of the lateral half of the main flap to the skin edges. This should be done without causing undue tension to the flap. The remainder of the secondary triangular defect lateral to the flap is closed by starting with closure of the lateral corner. This is easily accomplished since the outer angle has been made smaller than a right angle (Szymanowski) (Fig. 82, *D*). A drain is inserted in the lateral lower wound angles. Some adjustment may be necessary below the chin to avoid pointing (Fig. 82, *D*).

After-Treatment: The patient is fed by a Jutte tube inserted through the nose. Blood transfusions and antibiotics are necessary. After three days, he is fed by mouth, his diet being liquid and high caloric. The buccal wounds are cleansed with boric acid solution after each feeding. Drains are removed after two days, the sutures after five days (Case 26, p. 1027).

Variations and Combinations: The same operation can be performed unilaterally for unilateral lesions. In extensive unilateral tumors, particularly those extending into the cheek, a unilateral Dieffenbach operation can be performed on the affected side and a Burow operation on the other side (Case 30, p. 1034). If in the unilateral lesion the tumor has grown around the commissure into the upper lip, a unilateral Dieffenbach operation is performed, with excision of a Burow triangle at the upper lip (Case 29, p. 1032). If the tumor involves the entire lower lip and part of the upper lip, a bilateral Dieffenbach operation is performed, with excision of a sufficiently wide triangle of the affected part of the upper lip (Case 32, p. 1036).

Additional Procedures: If the mandible is involved, it can be resected at the same sitting and splinted temporarily with an intramedullary wire (see p. 557). Sometimes it is possible to leave a rim of the lower edge of the mandible behind; this part of the bone now acts as a splint. Dissection of the cervical lymph glands if indicated, however, should be carried out in the second stage, since this procedure necessitates resection of the external maxillary vessels. This would consequently endanger the circulation of the cheek flap if carried out primarily. Günther and Spissl's experience seems

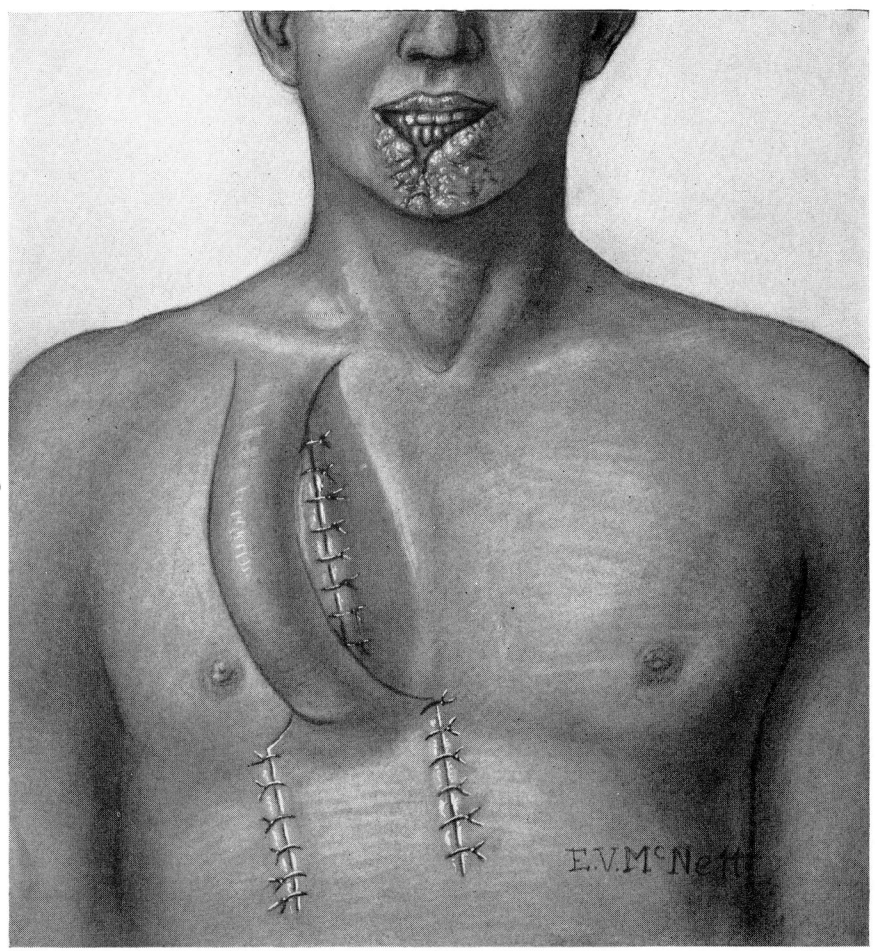

Fig. 83. Large defect of lower lip and chin to be closed with tube flap from right pectoral region. Peripheral end of flap is left untubed.

270

however to differ in this respect. If bone grafts are needed to replace defects of the horseshoe-shaped section of the mandible, they should be inserted three months later.

Transplantation of Distant Flaps

    Use of Lined Flap: In very large defects in which flaps from the neighborhood are not applicable, a flap from a distant part must be used. If possible, the acromiopectoral or chest region should be the donor site. The lined open-flap method or the tube-flap method is applicable (for

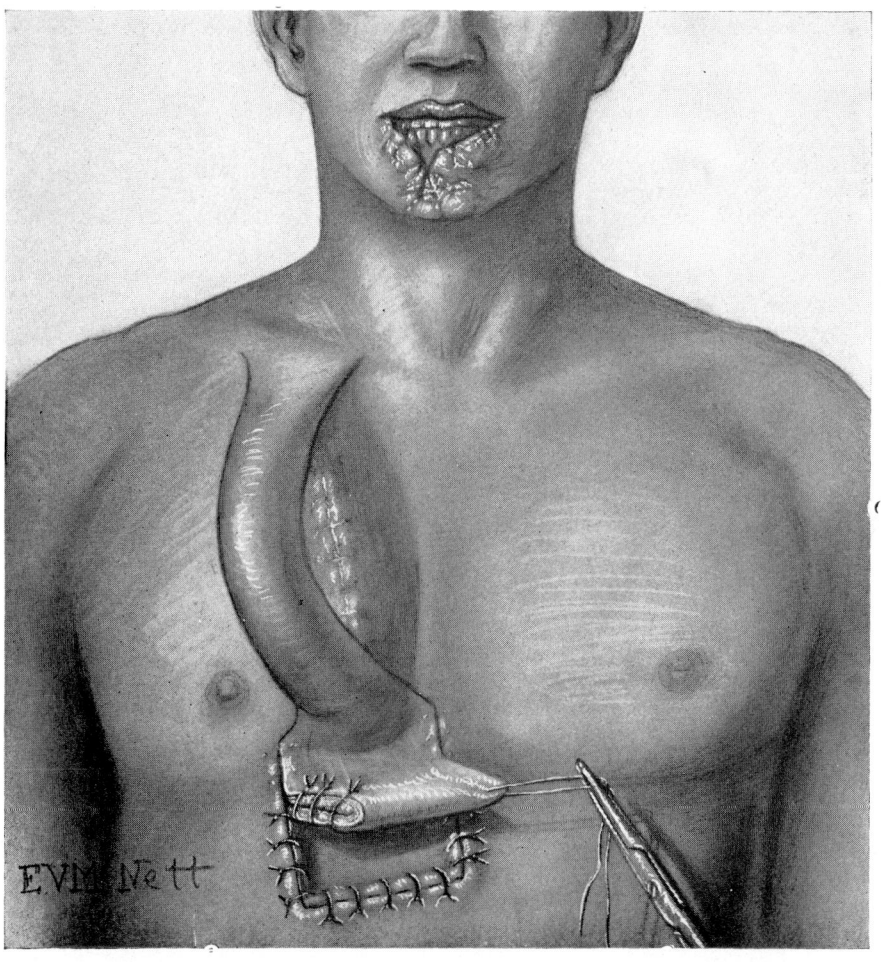

Fig. 84. Two or three months later, flap is lined by folding peripheral end over. Note that untubed part is raised with exception of bilateral small bridge near transition of untubed part into tubed part, to hold flap in place. Raw surface of flap bed is skin grafted.

271

lining of flaps, see p. 98; compare also with Case 14, p. 1010). If the latter is used, the distal pedicle is left untubed; the length of this part should be carefully planned and measured. If it is to provide the lining by folding the distal end over, the untubed part has to be made longer than it would be if skin grafting were to provide the lining. The different steps necessary for transplantation of a lined tube flap to cover lip and chin are outlined in Figures 83, 84, 85. The vermilion border is replaced from the opposing lip (Figs. 71, 72, 73).

Reconstruction in Extensive Injuries

Extensive Loss of Soft Tissues and Bone in War Injuries: If the soft-tissue defect cannot be closed by the use of local flaps, as after exten-

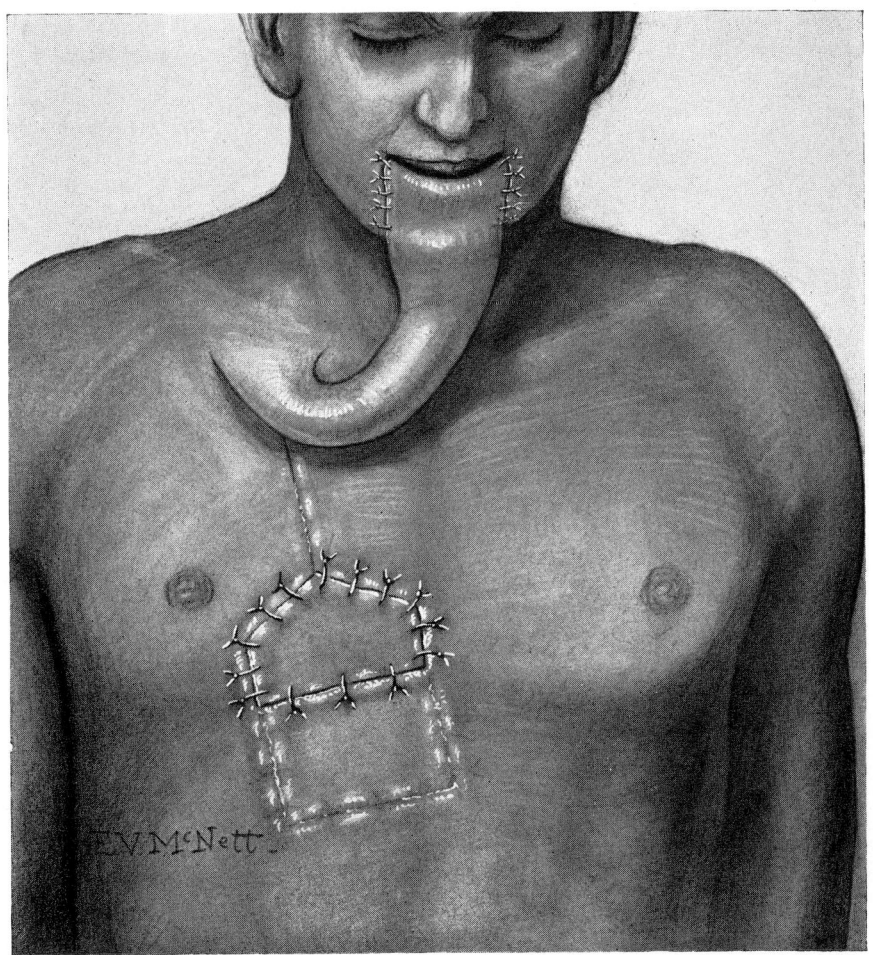

Fig. 85. Flap is sutured into defect.

272

sive war or other injuries, the necessary reconstructive steps are as follows (Ivy):

1. Arrest of hemorrhage, counteraction of loss of control of tongue and thus danger to respiration by pulling the tongue forward (either with a suture or large safety pin, anchored to the dressing); débridement of the wound and wound excision if necessary; fixation of bone fragments in approximately normal position by wires or other (extraoral) appliances; adjustment of torn tissue flaps; dependent drainage; antibiotics.

2. Final reduction and fixation of the fragments of the mandible by special splints (such as made of acrylic resin, affording a clear view of the underlying teeth and gum tissues and providing feeding space).

3. After all wounds look clean and healthy, transplantation of a lined flap to cover the soft-tissue defect.

4. Three months later, replacement of the bone defect by bone transplantation unless there has been infection, in which case one ought to wait three months before transplanting bone (and to provide preoperative and postoperative administration of antibiotics).

5. Provision of artificial dentures to replace lost teeth.

As far as choice of flaps is concerned, the open acromiopectoral flap is best suited (for construction of open flaps, see p. 83). Local flaps, if available, are utilized to replace the missing lining. These flaps may be taken from the cervical region with the base at the tongue and hinged upward. Smith's principle to improve the circulation at the base of the flap may be advisable (p. 257). If local flaps for lining are not available, the pectoral flap is constructed so that the peripheral pedicle is folded over. This principle and the way of transfer are similar to those described on page 271 (Case 14, p. 1010). Schuchardt and more recently Kazanjian and Converse have described many useful flap transplantations in their well-illustrated monographs.

DEFECTS OF COMMISSURE OF MOUTH AND PARTS OF ADJACENT CHEEK

If the defect includes only one half of the commissure of the mouth (the corner part of either the upper or the lower lip) and parts of the adjacent cheek and if the defect can be made triangular, Estlander's method is the operation of choice. Case 24, page 1024, is a typical example. Before rotating the vermilion-bordered triangular flap into the defect, the defect is made smaller by starting with closure of the lateral corner of the triangle. Now the triangular flap is formed from the sound lip opposite the defect (for technique, see p. 74), and rotated into the defect.

THE HEAD AND NECK

The closure of the secondary defect follows. In a second stage, the pedicle of the flap is severed and adjusted as outlined in Figure 75.

If the defect includes the entire commissure of the mouth together with larger parts of the cheek, the Dieffenbach or Burow method for closure of the defect may be applicable (see p. 269; Cases 25, 29, pp. 1026, 1032) or the Estlander method in conjunction with a lined or unlined tube-flap. For reconstruction of the oral commissure in transverse facial clefts, see page 357. See also page 360, reconstruction of cicatricial contractures of oral commissure and cheek.

CLEFTS OF LIP AND PALATE

Congenital clefts of the face and palate are caused by lack of fusion of the various processes that form the face and its bony structures. For better understanding of the problem, a short discussion of the developmental errors that lead to facial clefts and at times to concomitant deformities (see also p. 355, Transverse Clefts) is essential.

The face and neck develop from the branchial arches which appear on the ventral-lateral surface of the embryonic head during the fourth week of gestation. There are five branchial arches, each containing a cartilaginous core, a blood vessel, and appropriate muscles and nerves. The arches are separated by four ectodermal grooves. At the same level as these external grooves, the entoderm of the pharynx pushes aside the mesenchyme and bulges outward to become the pharyngeal pouches. The ectoderm of each groove and the entoderm of its complementary pouch meet and unite to form thin plates which rarely rupture (Arey). The clefts close off between the sixth and the eighth week. Imperfect closure leads to the formation of branchial cysts or fistulae.

The development of the face is closely related with the formation of the first and, to a lesser degree, with the second pair of branchial arches; the face develops between the fifth and eighth week of gestation. In early fetal life the oral and nasal fossae form one continuous chamber between head and pericardium, the so-called stomodeum or primitive mouth. The latter soon changes and becomes bounded by several prominences above, below, and at the sides. Above projects the frontonasal process which is formed by the prominence of the forebrain. The lower boundary is formed by the mandibular processes which grow forward to meet in the midline, forming the lower jaw and chin and thus representing the first pair of visceral arches (Fig. 86). The mandibular arches presently bifurcate, and out of this bifurcation develop the maxillary processes which form the lateral boundary.

274

THE LIPS, CHIN, AND PALATE

As it grows downward, the frontonasal process becomes divided by two oval depressions, the olfactory pits, which form the first rudiments of the nose. They divide the lower part of the frontonasal process into one median process and two lateral nasal processes. The median nasal process fuses with the maxillary processes to form the upper jaw. Each lateral nasal process joins the maxillary process of the same side to form the sides and wings of the nose (Fig. 87). At the same time, the upper portion of the original frontonasal process becomes the forehead. Its downward con-

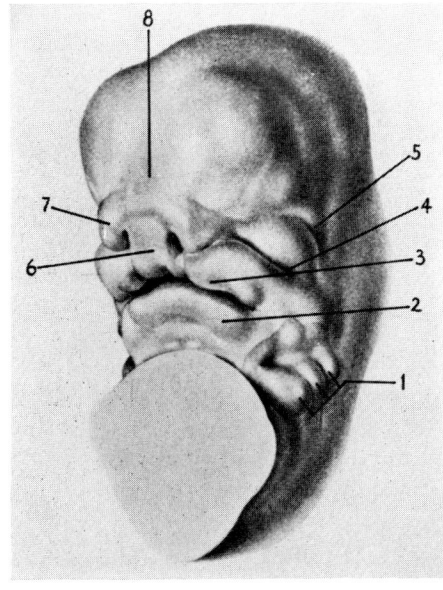

Fig. 86. Embryo 14 mm. long. *1:* Anlage of the auricle. *2:* Mandible, first visceral arch. *3:* Maxillary process. *4:* Nasolacrimal groove. *5:* Eye. *6:* Median nasal (or frontal) process. *7:* Lateral nasal process. *8:* Triangular area. (From G. L. Streeter; Carnegie Contr. Embryol. Carnegie Inst. Washington, 14:111, 1922.)

tinuation, the so-called triangular area (His), elevates slowly into the bridge and the apex of the nose (Figs. 86, 87).

The median nasal process develops a globular process (Merkel) at each lateral angle; both fuse and form the prelabium or philtrum of the lip, the columella and nasal septum, the premaxilla and anterior palate. The lateral nasal processes form the lateral nasal walls, the nasal alae, and the adjoining cheek regions. The maxillary processes, aside from becoming the major parts of the upper jaws, form the greater part of the cheeks, the lateral part of the upper lip and the palate (Fig. 87).

The lips are originally not separated from the alveolar parts of the jaws. They split away from the gum regions in the seventh week (Arey). The original lateral extent of the opening of the mouth is at the point of bifurcation of the maxillary and mandibular processes (Figs. 86 and 87). The parotid glands develop near these original angles of the

275

mouth; later, they grow backward toward the ear, while the parotid duct opening is left behind in this area (Fig. 87). Later, this broad mouth slit is reduced markedly in its lateral extent by progressive fusion of the lips and by the development of the muscles of mastication and of facial expression. The latter are derived from the second branchial arch. In this way the cheeks are established and the lips become pursed.

According to His, the auricle traces its origin to six branchial hillocks on the mandibular (first branchial arch) and hyoid (second branchial arch) bars adjacent to the first branchial cleft (Fig. 86). Streeter, however, considers these hillocks incidental rather than fundamental to the devel-

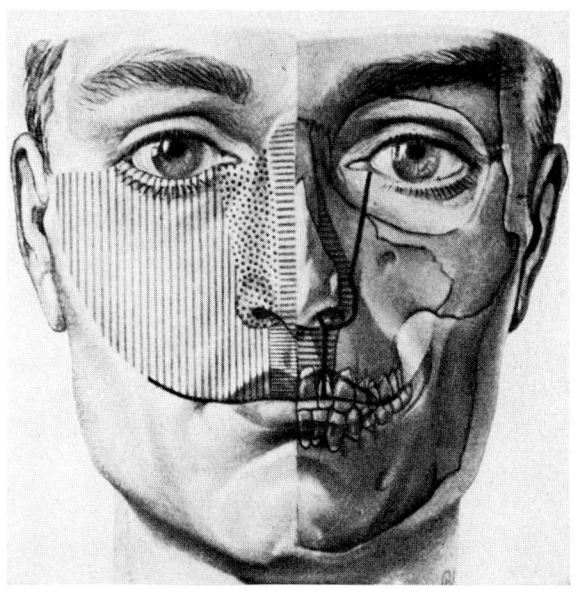

Fig. 87. Sketch demonstrating participation of various facial processes in formation of face. (From F. Merkel in Die Anatomie des Menschen, 2nd ed., edited by E. Kalius, J. F. Bergmann, 1927.) The parts of the *right* side of the face are designated (after His) as follows: *broad horizontal bars*, triangular area (downward continuation of the original frontonasal process forming bridge and apex of nose); *narrow bars*, area of median nasal process (premaxilla, columella, nasal septum, philtrum, os incisivum); *vertical bars*, area of maxillary process; *dotted area*, lateral nasal process (lateral nasal wall, ala, adjoining cheek regions). The *horizontal line* extending from the oral commissure into the cheek marks the original lateral extent of the opening of the mouth. At its lateral point is the Anlage of the parotid gland in the embryonic stage, further the parotid duct opening. The *left* side of the face (facial bones inserted) is marked as follows: *horizontal bars*, premaxilla; *black line*, approximate direction of clefts which result from lack of fusion of various facial processes (compare with right side). The *upper part* of this line indicates an oblique cleft between lateral nasal and maxillary process. The *middle part* indicates a cleft between the lower parts of the lateral nasal and the median nasal process. The *lower part* demonstrates the site of a lip cleft. An alveolar cleft would extend between premaxilla and maxillary process where the fissure between bisects the lateral incisor.

276

opment of the auricle. The consensus of opinion appears to be that the tissue for helix and tragus is furnished by the first (mandibular) branchial arch and for the anthelix, antetragus, earlobe, and concha by the second (hyoid) arch.

The middle ear (external auditory canal, Eustachian tube, and part of the tympanic membranes) represents a drawn-out first pharyngeal pouch. The internal ear is derived from a thickened ectodermal plate near the hindbrain.

It is readily understandable that lack of fusion, derangement of fusion, or underdevelopment of the various parts which are to form the face will lead to single or to a variety of clefts or deformities (Fig. 87). Continuation of this discussion is found on page 355 (Transverse Facial Clefts).

Undoubtedly, some of these malformations are inherited, as Fogh-Andersen deduces from an excellent genetic study of his large Danish material. Stiegler and Berry's studies seem to support the belief that the chief etiological basis of clefts and other structural malformations resides in gene transmission. It seems likely that a so-called recessive gene is responsible in most cases; this is, however, by no means always the case. In addition to the inheritance factor a second significant factor has emerged: unfavorable maternal environment during the "critical period" of the first twelve weeks of gestation until the various clefts have fused. Tondury, Oldfield, Stark, Schlegal and others discuss in detail several factors, such as malnutrition, vitamin A in excess or deficiency, and rubella infection, which might contribute to an unfavorable maternal environment.

Much of our original information about developmental errors in this area has come from the teachings of William Roux and the fascinating researches of Hans Spemann and his numerous pupils and followers. Bautzmann has contributed much to this research and has presented an interesting discussion of this topic. The Ciba Foundation and Haring and Lewis present excellent symposia on congenital malformations which bring the reader up to date on the latest thinking on the subject.

Clefts of the lip and palate are very frequent. Clefts of the nose and oblique and transverse clefts of the face are rare, and their structural appearance is not so regular as that in clefts of the lip and palate. Hence, the surgical procedures differ and have to be adapted to each case (see p. 355).

The subject of cleft lip and palate has been pursued in its diverse ramifications in recent monographs by Burian, Gabka, Holdsworth, and Stark, and in reports by Hotz of the First International Symposium on Early Treatment of Cleft Lip and Palate in Bern, by K. Schuchardt of the

THE HEAD AND NECK

Second International Congress in July, 1964, in Hamburg, and by P. Randall at the International Congress in Houston in April, 1969 (in print).

CLASSIFICATION OF CLEFTS

From the embryonic viewpoint, the cleft of lip, alveolar process, and palate must be considered as one unit; from the surgical viewpoint, however, a subdivision is more feasible, since the operative requirements differ with each cleft. Ritchie, impressed by the observation that the condition of the alveolar process has the most important influence in determining the requirements for surgical repair, grouped the cases according to the presence or absence of a cleft in the alveolar process. The underlying embryonic concepts, however, have been recently challenged (Kernahan and Stark, Harkins et al.). It appears that normal fusion begins at the incisive foramen; hence, clefts should be grouped with this foramen, rather than the alveolus, as the line of division. A more precise classification is depicted in Figure 88.

GENERAL CONSIDERATIONS

The object of the operation is the closure of the cleft and, as far as possible, the providing of normal anatomical conditions. In a through-and-through cleft, closure of the entire cleft in one sitting would be too extensive. Hence, the repair work must be divided into two or more stages. The cleft of the lip and the alveolar process is closed first, since it is not only the most visible part of the defect but also, as far as feeding and development of the severed alveolar process are concerned, the most disturbing factor. The cleft of the palate impedes feeding, but not to such a degree that it causes nutritional disorders. Hence, its closure is delayed until it causes a definite handicap to the child, that is, when the child learns to speak.

When the *cleft of the lip* should be closed has been a matter of dispute for a long time. The present consensus is that the baby should be given at least two weeks' time to become adjusted both to his feeding and to life in general. Accordingly, the earliest time to operate is the fourteenth day. In cases where the cleft of the lip is associated with an alveolar-process cleft, it is inadvisable to wait longer than three months. The cleft tends to become wider with each consecutive month, and closure becomes more and more difficult. This concept, however, has been challenged by two recent innovations which have become milestones in the progress of cleft lip and palate surgery: dental orthopedics (orthodontia) and bone grafting of the alveolar cleft. More will be said about these later (see

278

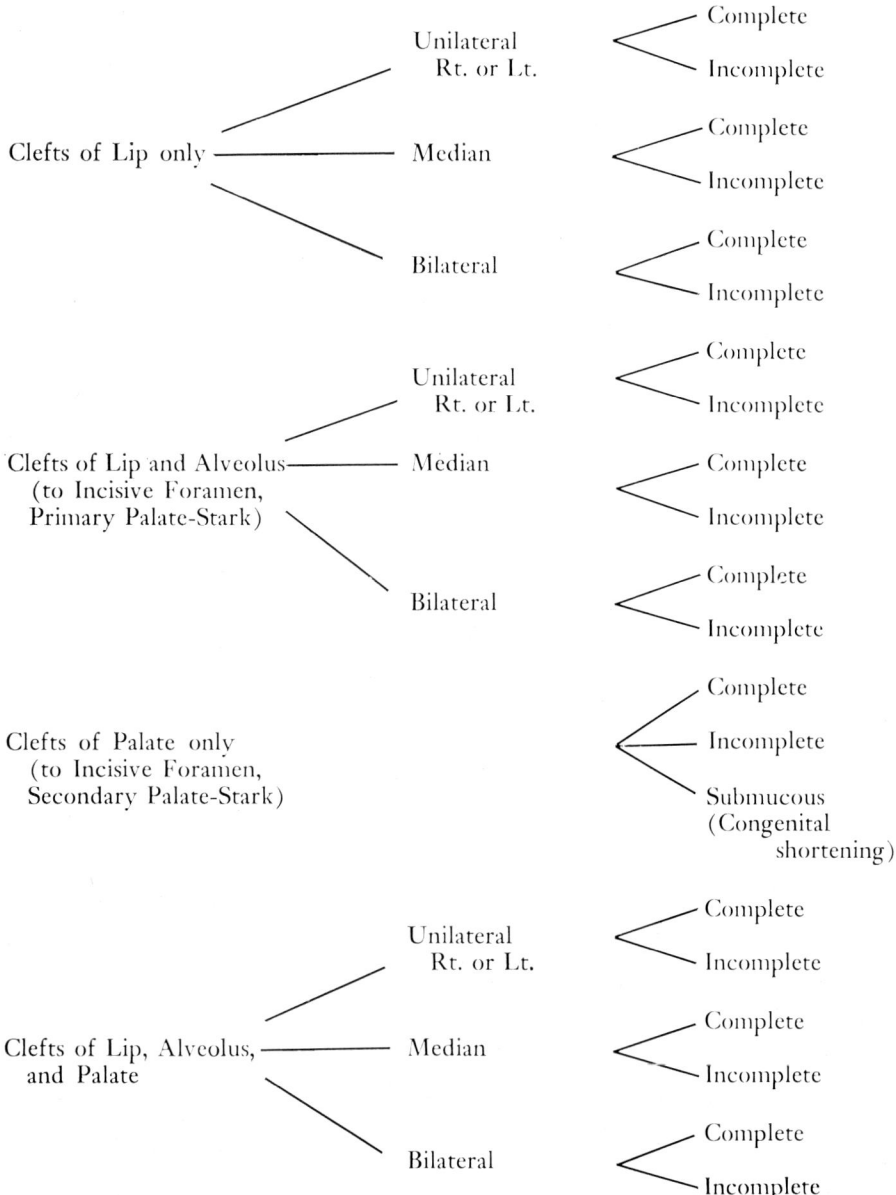

Fig. 88. Classification of cleft lip and cleft palate.

p. 295 and p. 299). The author prefers to repair the cleft lip between the ages of four to six weeks, if the child has regained his birth weight and is healthy. If primary bone grafting is considered (see p. 298), the operation is performed between the ages of three to four months.

As to when the *cleft in the palate* should be closed, controversies have arisen recently. As a result of the extensive and interesting research of Slaughter and Brodie on facial growth, they advise a delay of closure of clefts in the palate until the child is about five years old. According to their findings, the face develops rapidly until about the fifth year. The middle portion of the face develops from the growth centers of the maxilla (frontonasal, zygomaticomaxillary, pterygomaxillary sutures); any disturbance of these growth centers, as may be caused in cleft-palate operations by an impairment of blood supply to the maxilla, might result in failure of the middle portion of the face to move forward at the same rate as the rest of the face. Kazanjian had previously called attention to the development of the maxilla in operated and nonoperated cleft-palate cases. In the nonoperated cases, the separate halves of the palate developed and achieved a harmonious relation to the mandible, even though the cleft in the palate remained. Hence, a reasonable operative delay may result in more normal growth; on the other hand, however, it may cause a permanent speech impediment, since functional development will not occur in an unoperated soft-palate cleft unless it is subjected to normal use. Not all cleft-palate operations with early closure result in interference with maxillary growth, particularly not those for closure of partial clefts, and such interference seems to be directly proportional to the amount of injury to the growth centers and to diminution of blood supply to the parts concerned. Thus, if the delicate tissues are handled with the utmost care, it may be better to operate than to delay the closure beyond the time the child learns to speak, i.e., beyond the second to the third year. Instead of extensive mobilization of oral mucous-membrane flaps, greater use should be made whenever possible of the mucoperiosteal vomer flap (Waldron, Dunn).

The author has seldom seen postoperative retrusion of the maxilla, and is supported in this by Trusler and others, but it does occur. Some of these deformities result, not from disturbance of the maxillary growth centers, but from tightness of the upper lip after lip repair in through-and-through clefts. Bone grafting of the alveolar cleft may be the answer to this problem (p. 295).

Another practical way out of this dilemma is the method of Schwenkendiek of Germany (1951), which is reported by his co-worker Kehl and by Hamelmann based on their experience with nine hundred cases. Unaware of Schwenkendiek's work, Slaughter and Pruzansky published in 1954 a similar procedure based on their experience with two hundred cases. The difference between this method and the usual one is the different sequence of closure of the various clefts. Schwenkendiek closes in through-and-through clefts, the cleft of the soft palate first between the ages of fourteen to sixteen months; the lip cleft is closed earlier. The hard palate is closed between the ages of four to five years. Thus impairment of growth is counteracted by deferring operating near the maxillary growth centers.

Preoperative Preparation

The preoperative preparation should start with an evaluation of the general condition of the child. No operation should be planned unless the child is gaining weight and is in good general health. Close cooperation with the attending pediatrician is absolutely necessary; he will inform the surgeon whether or not the child is ready for the operation. If ready, the child is admitted to the hospital forty-eight hours before the operation. A careful physical examination is made, which includes urinalysis, Wassermann blood test, a complete blood count, and bleeding and clotting time. The latter two should be normal and the hemoglobin above 10 gm. Feeding is given up to six hours, water up to two hours before operation. Atropine (dosage to be determined by the pediatrician) is given one hour before the operation. A blood donor should be on hand if primary bone grafting is considered.

The child is anesthetized with ether and later with ether and oxygen, which is administered intraorally. Some surgeons prefer local anesthesia. An intravenous drip should be employed, for there are two things that an infant cannot tolerate: lack of oxygen and lack of fluids.

CLEFT LIP

Cleft lip, ordinarily called "harelip," is a prealveolar cleft if confined to lip or to lip and nostril. In the majority of cases, however, cleft lip is associated with an alveolar and postalveolar cleft. Innumerable procedures are proposed for closure of the defect. An excellent collective review of the history and technical development of cleft-lip repair has been made by A. D. Davis. The older methods aimed at the closure in primitive fashion, without regard to the cosmetic result. The vermilion border lining the cleft edges was sacrificed and the cleft closed by simply uniting the wound edges. Mirault was the first to utilize the vermilion-border lining, thus improving the appearance of the lip. His method became, more or less, the basic principle for modern procedures.

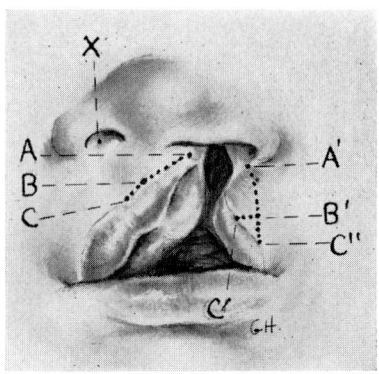

Fig. 89. The triangular flap operation for cleft lip repair. The V-excision is marked out first. c' is on the mucocutaneous junction at the most medial point of good full vermilion. b' is on the line a'-c'' equidistant from c' and c''. The incision is a'-b'-c' saving the mount of lip indicated by the shaded isosceles triangle in the insert drawing. b is on the mucocutaneous junction, the same distance from c that b' is from c'. (J. B. Brown and F. McDowell: Surg. Gynec. Obstet.)

One objection is the straight-line scar, which produces a straight, flat lip in the profile view and may, if contracting, cause a notch in the vermilion border. A normal lip, as seen in profile, bulges forward at and just above the vermilion border. To reproduce this "break," or pout, in cleft-lip repair (it occurs about two thirds or three fourths of the way down the lip), Blair and Brown modified the Mirault operation in such a way that an extra amount of tissue was provided at and above the vermilion border, but the standard flap that was described then was half the length of the lip and too large in some patients. Brown and McDowell overcame this by using a small triangular flap to produce the fullness in only the lower one third or one fourth of the lip (Figs. 89 to 92). This principle

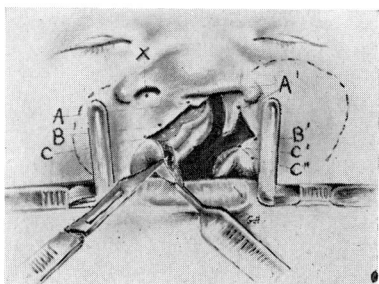

Fig. 90. The lightly incised lines a-b-c and a'-b'-c' are cut completely through the lip with a stab blade, with care to keep knife exactly perpendicular to lip. All angles should be completely opened. The vermilion is inspected and any attached skin removed with a stab blade. The rectangular flap freed from a'-b'-c' must be loose enough to be rotated up 180 degrees into nostril floor. Dotted lines indicate area undermined. (J. B. Brown and F. McDowell: Surg. Gynec. Obstet.)

282

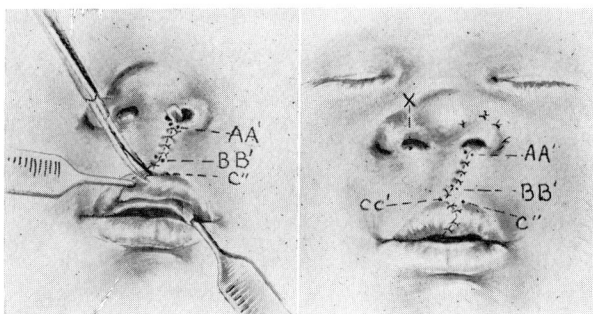

Fig. 91   Fig. 92

Fig. 91. *a* and *a'* are approximated with a deep stitch of white silk or cotton or 000 catgut (knot on the mucosal side) and a surface suture of 000 black silk. *b* and *b'* are approximated with a fine deep white stitch and a black one on the surface. Intervening fine surface sutures are placed and an oblique cut is made in the vermilion flap from *c'*. For the incisions and trimming fine, very sharp scissors are most useful. (J. B. Brown and F. McDowell: Surg. Gynec. Obstet.)

Fig. 92. *c* and *c'* are united and the vermilion flaps are interdigitated in a zigzag fashion, fitting them so that they lie naturally together without any pull or stretching. Suturing is then continued on around the vermilion border and up the inside to the fornix. The little flap in the nostril is trimmed to fit with the one from the opposite side, and they are sutured together to form the floor. A few key mattress sutures are placed through the ala to unite the lining and covering (which were separated during the undermining). (J. B. Brown and F. McDowell: Surg. Gynec. Obstet.)

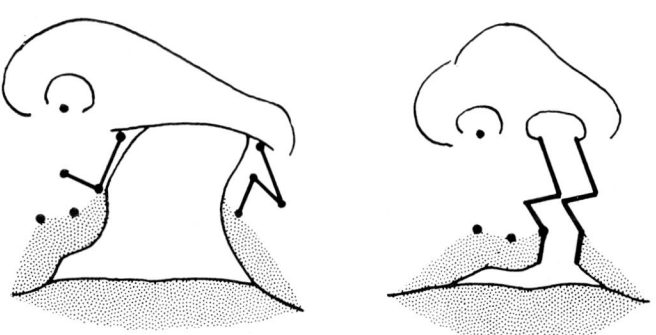

Fig. 93. The triangular flap operation. An incision is made along the medial edge of the cleft to the superior peak of the cupid's bow on the cleft side. The incision then extends at right angles into the philtrum about to the midline or far enough to allow the cupid's bow to come down to a horizontal position. The size of the triangular flap from the lateral side can be determined by subtracting the distance from the base of the columella on the cleft side to the incision made into the philtrum from the vertical height on the noncleft side. (P. Randall: Plast. Reconstr. Surg.)

283

became widely accepted until it was challenged by LeMesurier, who modified the old Hagedorn quadrangular-flap method. He was soon followed by Steffensen, Bauer, Trusler and Glanz, Brauer, May, Gelbke, and others. In this operation, a quadrangular flap is used from the side of the cleft and swung down and over to the median side of it to fit into a notch created in the philtrum (Figs. 95, 105-107). Some of those who now use the quadrangular-flap method after LeMesurier formerly used the triangular-flap method of Mirault, Blair, Brown, and McDowell. According to their experience, the quadrangular method produces consistently better results than any other, that is, it provides adequate fullness of the lower third of the lip; notch formations are counteracted by the change in the direction of the scar to a "stepline."

The Hagedorn-LeMesurier technique, however, has several disadvantages. The main one stems from the necessity for removal of a certain amount of tissue from the lip margin, which results in tightness of the upper half of the lip. The method also requires accurate measurement of the skin incisions, which once made are irrevocable; in case of mistakes, deformities become magnified with the growth of the child. (The author has overcome these disadvantages, as elaborated on p. 286.)

A new feature in cleft lip repair was introduced by Tennison's Z-plasty, in which for the first time the natural cupid's bow was preserved. The latter is normally present on the median side of the cleft, as noted by Cardoso and Marcks and associates. With a simple but effective bent-wire technique Tennison draws the lip markings. He constructs a triangular flap on the lateral side of the cleft which fits into a triangular defect above the cupid's bow on the median side without excising any tissue. This rather simple method was further developed by Skoog, Trauner, Randall, Brauer and others (Fig. 93). The one disadvantage of the Z-plasty principle is that the scars do not come to lie in a normal contour of the lip and thus may remain conspicuous. To overcome this disadvantage, Millard developed a large rotation advancement flap which is brought down on the medial side of the cleft, while the tissues on the lateral side are used to fill a triangular defect resulting from the rotation high up on the median side beneath the columella (Fig. 94). Thus the scar is in a much better position, and very little tissue is discarded. This technique also has the advantage that the incisions are not irrevocable and alterations during the operation are still possible; it is a "cut-as-you-go" technique. This procedure has been enthusiastically endorsed by many surgeons.

The author has seen much merit in the quadrangular-flap method (Hagedorn-LeMesurier) and adopted this principle and incorporated it into the Axhausen technique which he has followed for many years. He has tried to minimize the above-mentioned disadvantages and has achieved with this modification a fullness of the lower one fourth of the lip without sacrificing much skin; in simplifying the design, final determination of length and adjustment of the quadrangular flap are made at the end of the operation so that changes can still be made. This is an important feature.

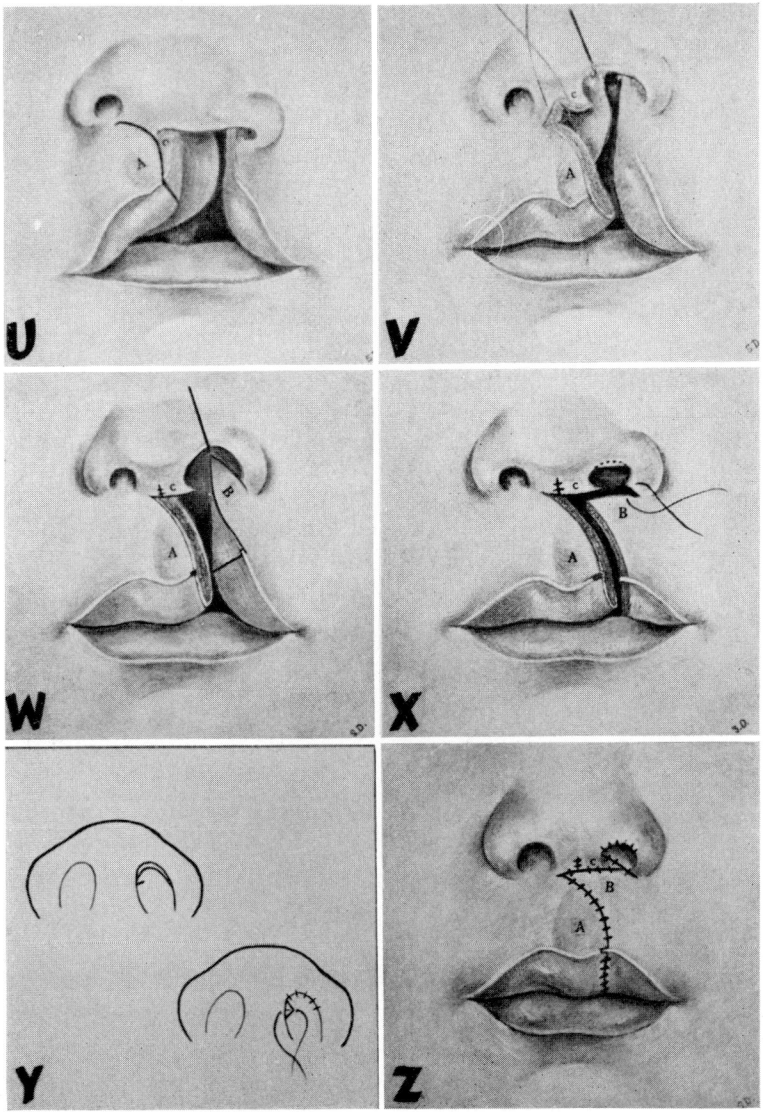

Fig. 94. The rotation-advancement operation of Millard. *A* drops down, *C* shifts up. As *B* moves across into the gap between *A* and *C* it not only pulls the alar base but maintains the correct position of *A* and *C*. A crescent excision of the web across the alar arch is also carried out. (D. R. Millard: Plast. Reconstr. Surg.)

THE HEAD AND NECK

The technique of Axhausen modified after LeMesurier will be described in detail for this most common deformity, the through-and-through cleft (Fig. 95; Cases 34-36, pp. 1039-1041).

Technique (Axhausen-LeMesurier)

The preoperative preparation has been described. The repair is divided into the following stages:

1. Outlining of the lip incisions
2. Formation of the floor of the nostril
3. Correction of the alar displacement
4. Correction of the septal displacement
5. Closure of the lip.

Outlining of Lip Incisions (Figs. 95, 96): Although it is possible without previous designs to create a square notch on the philtrum side and a quadrangular flap on the lateral side to fit into this notch (Figs. 95, 105), it is more accurate to plan the incisions as shown in Figure 96. The

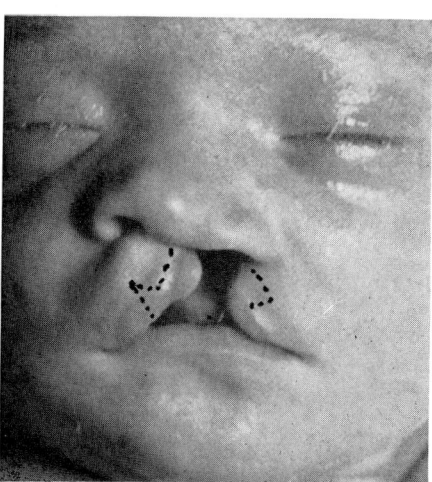

Fig. 95. Outline of square notch on the philtrum side of cleft and quadrangular flap on lateral side to fit into notch (compare with Figs. 96 and 105).

design is made immediately. The actual incisions, however, are made later; that is, any time after Stage 2 and one may wait until Stage 5. Should the markings prove later to be not quite accurate, adjustment is still possible in Stage 5. The markings are made with percutaneous dots by the tip of a hypodermic needle dipped into methylene blue.

286

Point *a* is marked out first. It is located on a level with the base of the columella at the very tip of the median vermilion-border lining (mucocutaneous junction) of the lip cleft. Point *a'* is located at the tip of the lateral vermilion border where it joins the tip of the laterally displaced ala. Points *b* and *b'* are found as follows: The median part of the upper lip is pulled by a finger into correct position; in this way, the cupid bow (juncture of philtrum and mucocutaneous border of the

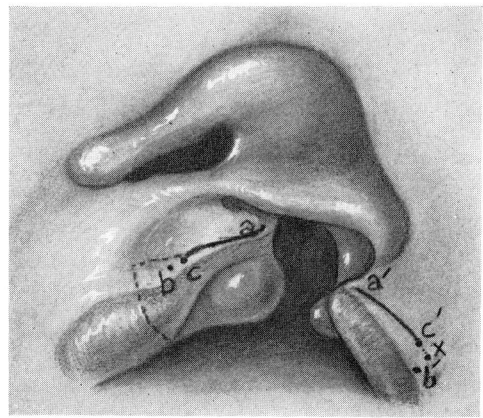

Fig. 96. Outline of lip incisions (Axhausen-Hagedorn-LeMesurier Technique of Cleft Lip Repair): Point *a* is marked out first. It is located in level of the base of the columella at the very tip of the median vermilion border line of the lip cleft. Point *a'* is located at the tip of the lateral vermilion border where the latter joins the tip of the laterally displaced ala. Points *b* and *b'* are found as follows: The median part of the upper lip is pulled with a finger into correct position; in this way the cupid bow becomes visible, at least its point opposite to the cleft. If the corresponding point at the cleft is not visible it is imagined at the vermilion border in the same level as the other point—this is point *b*. Point *b'* is marked on the lateral cleft side and is of equal distance from *a'* as is *b* from *a*; *c* is marked out from 2 or 3 mm. above *b*. To find *c'* a perpendicular is erected on *b'* for about 2 to 3 mm. (equal distance of *b* to *c*). This is point *x*; *c'* is 2 to 3 mm. from *x* toward *a'*. (H. May: Plast. Reconstr. Surg.)

vermilion) becomes visible, at least its point opposite the cleft. If the corresponding point at the cleft is not visible, it is imagined near the vermilion border at the same level as the other point. This is point *b*. Point *b'* is marked out on the lateral cleft side, and is the same distance from *a'* as *b* is from *a*; *c* is marked out 2 or 3 mm. above *b*. *To find c'*, a perpendicular is erected on *b* for 2 or 3 mm. (equal distance of *b* to *c*); this is point *x*; 2 or 3 mm. from *x* toward *a'* is *c'*. Point *c'* is marked out and connected by a slightly laterally curved line with *a'*. Adjustment of these markings for formation of the lateral vermilion-border flap can still be made at the end of the operation (compare with Fig. 105).

Formation of Floor of Nostril (Figs. 97 to 99): Only the anterior part of the floor is reconstructed, that is, no farther back than just behind the alveolar process. It is constructed by using turnover flaps taken from the median and lateral walls of the cleft. Thus, the cleft of the alveolar process is closed but the cleft behind remains open until the palate is repaired, unless the bone grafting method is used (see p. 298).

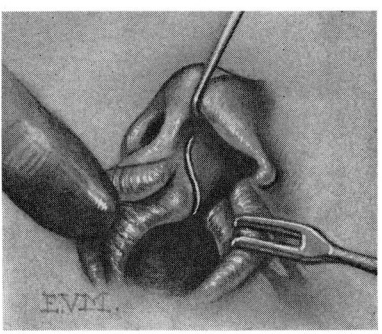

Fig. 97. Formation of the median turnover flap: Incision is made just behind the rim of the columella from its tip to the ridge of the alveolar process. The incision then is curved around the alveolar process and posterior where premaxilla and vomer meet. Under sharp dissection the flap is mobilized. (H. May: Plast. Reconstr. Surg.)

The first step is the formation of a median turnover flap (Fig. 97). With a retractor, the nostril is shifted forward, and an incision is made just behind the rim of the columella, from its tip to the ridge of the alveolar process. The knife is now turned horizontally and the incision curved around the alveolar process, ending posteriorly where premaxilla and vomer meet. The mobilization of the flap is difficult; it should be carried out under sharp dissection, avoiding perforation of the flap and injury to the septal cartilages. The flap should not be extended farther posteriorly than to the groove that is formed by the insertion of the vomer to the premaxilla; otherwise, the flap will tear at this point, and may need replacement by a small turnover flap from the vomer.

The next step is the formation of the lateral turnover flap. This step is combined with an incision along the gingivolabial sulcus and mobilization of the soft tissues of the cheek (Figs. 98, 99). The incision starts at the edge of the alveolar process and is led to the point where alveolar process, tip of ala, and vermilion border meet, and from there upward into the nostril (Fig. 98). The location of this latter part of the incision, the nostril incision, is important: if it is too close to the rim of the nostril, the nostril will be weak and collapse when rotated. If it is too far posteriorly, it will make the nostril too bulky. As a rule, the incision should be made so that it is one quarter anterior to the mucous-membrane skin line and three quarters of the skin lining of the nostril is left in front of the incision.

The lateral turnover flap is now formed by freeing the tissues from the edge of the alveolar process upward, beyond the lower turbinated bone.

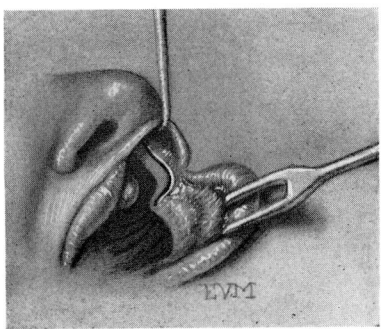

Fig. 98. Formation of lateral turnover flap: This step is combined with an incision along the gingivolabial sulcus and mobilization of soft tissue of the cheek. The incision starts at the edge of the alveolar process and is led to the point where alveolar process, tip of ala, and vermilion border meet, and from there upward into the nostril. The location of this latter part of the incision, the nostril incision, is important. If it is too close to the rim of the nostril the nostril will be weak and collapse when rotated. If it is too far posterior it will make the nostril too bulgy. As a rule, the incision should be made so that it is one fourth anterior to the mucous-membrane skin line, and three fourths of the skin line of the nostril is left in front of the incision. The lateral turnover flap is now formed by freeing the tissues from the edge of the alveolar process and beyond the lower turbinate bone. (H. May: Plast. Reconstr. Surg.)

Median and lateral turnover flaps are now united with sutures of 00000 chromic catgut (Fig. 99). The lower suture is left long for later use.

Correction of Displaced Ala (Figs. 99, 100): For the formation of a well-formed nostril, it is necessary to mobilize the laterally displaced ala and to unite its tips with the columella of the septum at the site of the tuberculum. At this particular place, the recipient site is already prepared; it is the wound which has resulted from turning over the median flap for formation of the floor of the nose (Figs. 97, 99). To facilitate smooth approximation of ala and recipient site, the tip of the ala is mobilized in the form of a small flap which should be made rather too short than too long. There is usually a small portion of skin available median to the tip. This, however, is not sufficient; the flap must

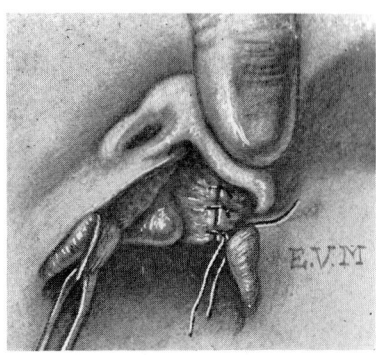

Fig. 99. Median and lateral turnover flaps are united with sutures of 00000 chromic catgut; the lower suture is left long for later use. A small alar flap is cut with a curved pair of scissors along the base of the nostril; it should be rather too short than too long. On the median cleft side a vermilion border flap is cut (from *a* to *c* of Fig. 96). (H. May: Plast. Reconstr. Surg.)

be made longer. Its posterior (inner) edge is already made, resulting from turning over the lateral nostril flap (Fig. 98). Hence, only the anterior (outer) incision needs to be added. It starts at the point where the tip of the ala and lateral vermilion-border lining join each other (Fig. 99), and proceeds upward and laterally along the base of the ala for about 0.5 to 1 cm. ($\frac{3}{16}$ to $\frac{3}{8}$ inch). After the anterior and posterior incisions have been connected, the small alar flap is cut with sharply curved scissors and sutured into the upper wound angle of the columella; the posterior edge is sutured to the median and lateral turnover flap, the anterior edge to the outer wound edge of the columella (Fig. 100). Care should be taken to unite the tip of the ala with the tuberculum of the columella, which is near point *a* of Figure 96. Its location can be facilitated by forming part of the vermilion-border flap (*a-c* of Fig. 96) before adjustment

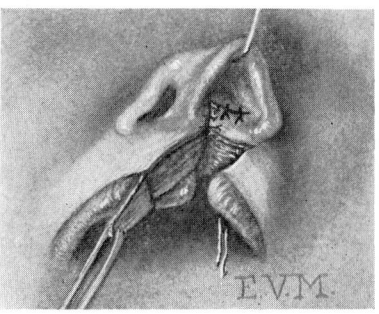

Fig. 100. The alar flap is sutured posteriorly to the turnover flaps and with its tip to the tuberculum of the columella which is near point *a* of Fig. 96. (H. May: Plast. Reconstr. Surg.)

290

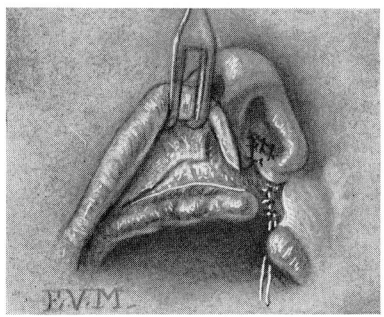

Fig. 101. Correction of the septal displacement: An incision is made along the sulcus, care being taken to leave a rim of the mucosa attached to the gums to facilitate later suturing. The soft tissues are mobilized from the bone until the cartilaginous septum and the floor of the nose is reached. (H. May: Plast. Reconstr. Surg.)

of the ala. After application of an elastic clamp to the lip to reduce bleeding, an incision is made from *a* to *c* just within the skin (Figs. 96, 100). The tip of the vermilion border is grasped, and a whole-thickness vermilion-border flap cut down to point *c* but not farther. The alar flap can then be accurately adjusted as previously described (Fig. 100).

Correction of the displaced ala does not necessarily correct the nasal tip, which as all surgeons admit is one of the most difficult problems of cleft-lip repair. For reasons explained on page 294, the author prefers to replace the alar cartilages in a more natural position. He only frees the skin over the alar tip cartilages subcutaneously with a pair of Mayo scissors to give the underlying cartilages a chance to move into a more elevated position.

Correction of Septal Displacement (Figs. 101, 102): The extramedian displacement of the septum is corrected by advancement of the

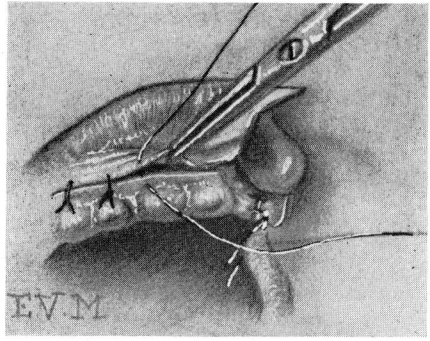

Fig. 102. The mobilized mucosa is now advanced laterally by pulling it with a forceps in that direction and fastening it in this position with catgut sutures. (H. May: Plast. Reconstr. Surg.)

291

mucous membrane along the median gingivolabial sulcus. An incision is made along the sulcus, care being taken to leave a rim of mucosa attached to the gums to facilitate later suturing. The soft tissues are mobilized from the bone until the cartilaginous septum and the floor of the nose are reached. The mobilized mucosa is now advanced laterally by pulling it with a forceps in that direction, and is fastened in this position with catgut sutures.

Formation of Lip (Figs. 104, 105): Prior to the closure of the lip cleft, a vermilion-border flap must be made from each side of the cleft. The median one is already partly formed. It is now extended along the dotted line of Figure 96—i.e., across the philtrum and parallel to the vermilion border—and cut off along the vertical dotted line of Figure 96. The lateral vermilion-border flap is now cut along the line *a'-c'*; however, it is better to stop the incision before reaching *c'* and to estimate the proper length of the flap at the end of the operation. Before the lip is sutured the mucosa along the lateral gingivolabial sulcus is advanced. The cheek is then mobilized from an incision along the lateral gingivolabial sulcus—a rim of mucous membrane should be left attached to the gingival side to facilitate later suturing—and is thoroughly detached from the underlying bone with knife and periosteal elevator up to the foramen infraorbitale, i.e., until the infraorbital nerve is reached (Fig. 103) and advanced mediad along the lateral gingivolabial sulcus (Fig. 104).

SUTURING: The lateral and median wound edges are united in front of the alveolar-process cleft (Fig. 104). The last suture to be inserted is taken from the nostril suture, which has been left long (Figs. 99, 104). One end of this suture is passed through the lateral, the other end through the

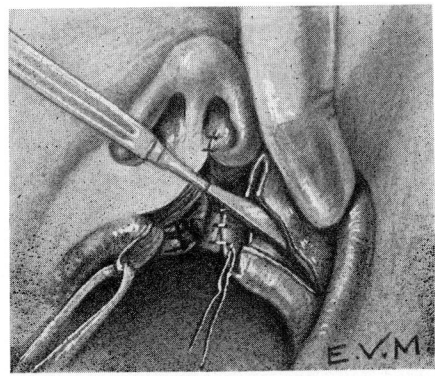

Fig. 103. The cheek is mobilized from incision along the lateral gingivolabial sulcus—a rim of mucous membrane should be left attached to the gingival side to facilitate later suturing—and is thoroughly detached from the underlying bone with knife and periosteal elevator up to the foramen infraorbitale, i.e., until the infra-orbital nerve is reached. (H. May: Plast. Reconstr. Surg.)

292

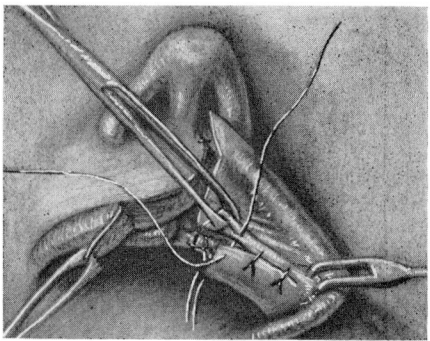

Fig. 104. Median advancement of the lip lateral to the cleft by advancement of the mucosa along the lateral gingivolabial sulcus. The lateral and median wound edges are united in front of the alveolar process with the stitch which had been left long previously (Fig. 99). (H. May: Plast. Reconstr. Surg.)

median, mucosal edge. After the suture is tied, the remaining gap in the alveolar process is closed.

The lip is now formed, and is sutured in three layers. First, the oral mucous membrane is sutured with 00000 chromic catgut; this is followed by suturing of the muscle layer with the same material. The stitches are laid in such a way that they can be tied posteriorly. The skin edges are mobilized from the muscles for a short distance, to prevent inversion, and sutured together with fine nylon. The lowest suture unites point c and point c' of Figure 105. If it is now evident that the two wound edges are of unequal length (the lateral one being the shorter if, in the begin-

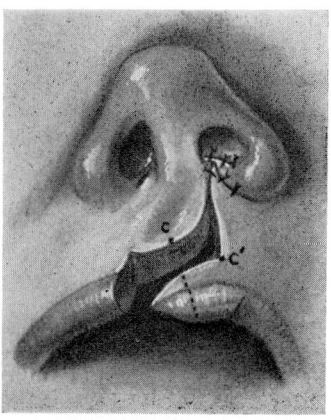

Fig. 105. Closure of the lip: Formation of the square notch on the median side of the vermilion border flap; the lateral side of the vermilion border flap is cut square and is adjusted into the notch on the median side. (Compare with Fig. 96.) (H. May: Plast. Reconstr. Surg.)

293

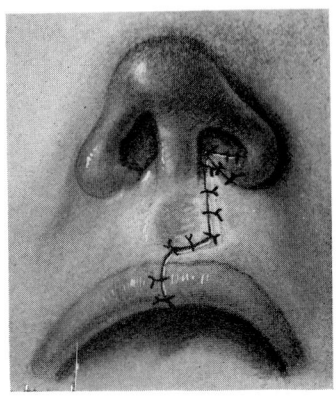

Fig. 106. Wounds are closed in layers. (H. May: Plast. Reconstr. Surg.)

ning, the incision was not completely extended to point c'), it is possible to correct the inequality by merely lengthening the lateral vermilion-border flap. The next step is fitting the lateral vermilion border into the notch of the median side by proper shortening. (For final results, see Figs. 106, 107; Cases 34-36, pp. 1039-1041.)

At the end of the operation, the nostril of the cleft side may not match the other side. No attempt should be made to correct the deformity at this stage, but should be postponed until the child is about five years of age for the following reasons: The pull of the soft tissue after closure of the cleft will in time cause the displaced underlying bony framework to change position, and this in turn will cause a shift of the soft tissues. Any correction of residual deformities around the nose before the anatomy has settled is a waste of time, although others, notably G. B. O'Connor and Gelbke, disagree with this statement (see also p. 316). Fur-

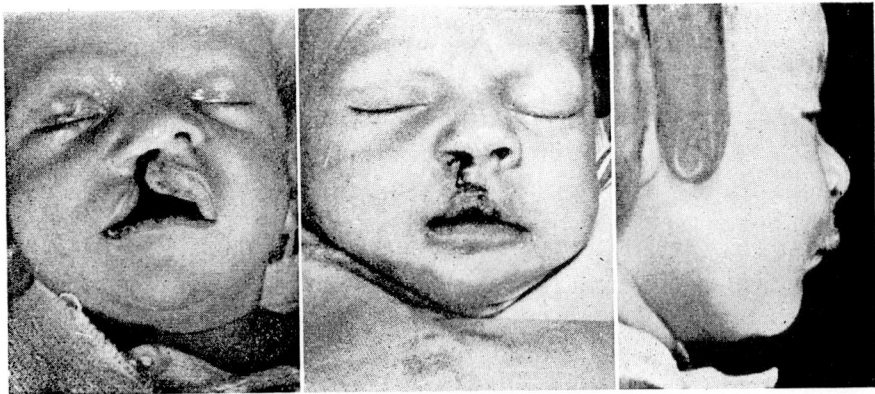

Fig. 107. *A-C:* Patient before and after the Axhausen-Hagedorn-LeMesurier cleft lip operation. Note normal forward bulge of vermilion.

294

ther, should the immediate correction not have been successful, the cartilages may be so damaged from the primary correction that secondary repair is fruitless.

After-Treatment

The lip wound is painted with collodion. A Logan bow is strapped to the cheeks to relieve tension on the suture lines and to protect the lip. As soon as the child is awake, he is fed with a small spoon or a dropper. The elbow joints are immobilized with cardboard cylinders or splints so that the child cannot touch the wound. The skin wound remains exposed. The skin sutures are removed on the fifth postoperative day. The baby can usually be fed with a bottle after the tenth postoperative day, but the holes in the nipple should be enlarged.

INCOMPLETE CLEFT LIP

A technique similar to that described in the foregoing paragraphs is applicable whether the cleft reaches the floor of the nostril or not. In the latter case, the triangular-shaped indented skin above the cleft is excised. The tip of the triangle becomes point *a-a'* of Figure 96, from which the remaining marking points are selected. The technique from then on is practically the same as already described, except that the floor of the nostril is already formed. There is always, however, asymmetry at the nasal entrance, which requires advancement of the vestibular mucosa on the median as well as on the lateral side.

For results, see Case 33, page 1038. For after-treatment, see above.

BRIDGING CLEFTS OF THE ALVEOLAR PROCESS
WITH BONE GRAFTS

In through-and-through clefts (unilateral or bilateral) early closure of the lip cleft is considered advantageous not only from the cosmetic and functional (feeding) point of view but also because normal pressure of the closed lip upon the alveolar process tends to favor approximation of the severed bony arches. This latter advantage, however, is turned into a disadvantage and handicap in unilateral as well as bilateral clefts if the shorter and more posteriorly displaced lateral process fails to meet the anterior one but moves behind it and causes a collapsed arch. It then becomes the task of specially-trained dentists to overcome the malocclusion by orthodontic measures (see p. 299).

THE HEAD AND NECK

To prevent the collapse of the alveolar arch or its recurrence after orthodontic correction, bridging the alveolar cleft with a bone graft, as introduced by German and Swedish surgeons, has become one of the great milestones in the progress of cleft lip and palate surgery. Twenty-eight years ago Axhausen already expressed this thought, but it was E. Schmidt of Stuttgart who in 1952, after extensive preliminary work (from 1944), published his method of inserting bone grafts from the tibia into the alveolar cleft some time after closure of the lip cleft. Independently and unaware of Schmidt's work, B. Johanson and co-workers at Göteborg proceeded along similar lines in 1955. They concentrated mainly upon secondary restoration of the collapsed alveolar arch through orthodontic measures and subsequently filled the alveolar defect with bone grafts (spongiosa chips and cortical grafts from the crest of the ilium). In 1956, Schrudde and Stellmach of Düsseldorf recommended a "primary osteoplasty," i.e., bone grafting (graft from rib) and closure of the lip cleft in one sitting. Schuchardt and Pfeifer of Hamburg (1958) and Rehrmann became convinced of the soundness of the principle of primary bone grafting and applied this method with modifications routinely to all through-and-through cleft cases. Schuchardt and co-workers have thus far treated more than six hundred thirty cases and have followed up most of them (personal communication). From these studies it becomes evident that the method is safe and that the bone graft becomes regenerated. The graft is inserted either at the time of primary repair (Schrudde and Stellmach, E. Schmidt, Schuchardt)—Schuchardt emphasizes that the graft must be solid and wedged between the alveolar processes to keep them separated—or secondarily some time after the soft tissue closure preceded by expansion of the alveolar arches and application of prosthetic appliances (Johanson and co-workers, Skoog, Maisels).

Georgidade, Pickerill and Quinn have recently reviewed the various bone-grafting techniques, and Pickrell, Quinn and Massengill reported on a four-year study of twenty-five cases of primary bone grafting. Very recently Robinson and Wood presented favorable reports on primary bone grafting. The author has only limited experience with this method. There is no question that this procedure is more formidable and time consuming, but it has many advantages as it eliminates tedious preoperative orthodontic treatment. It is also a physiological method insofar as it promotes growth of the alveolar process in the proper direction through pull of the operatively closed obicularis muscle on the lateral segment and pressure on the maxillary segment; it thus creates a normal well-rounded alveolar arch and prevents crowding of the teeth. It is amazing how nature can accomplish this when one realizes that in the vast majority of unilateral cases the lateral alveolar process is posterior to the median one and considerably

296

shorter. Evidently the bone graft not only keeps the alveolar processes separated, thus preventing the arch from collapsing, but also causes a molding effect by stimulating a forward growth of the lateral alveolar process (law of Roux, p. 114). However not all experts agree on this (Pickerill et al.). In bilateral cleft lip and palate cases the bone-graft operation should not usually be performed primarily when the premaxilla is displaced.

Technique (Primary Bone Grafts)

The operation is performed at four months of age. The child receives an intravenous infusion and a small blood transfusion during the operation. The anesthetist must be prepared for positive pressure technique in case the thin pleura is accidentally perforated.

The right side of the chest (axillary line) is prepared for taking a rib bone graft. It is removed subperiosteally in the first stage of the operation from a horizontal incision in the right axillary line. The graft is taken from the seventh or eighth rib and should be somewhat longer than the actual length of the alveolar cleft. Great care should be exercised not to perforate the thin pleura.

The author follows Schuchardt's advice and closes the soft-tissue cleft and the anterior cleft of the palate in the same operation, as Veau and Ivy have practiced. Although this prolongs the procedure somewhat, it facilitates the formation of the pockets for the bone graft. The anterior palatal cleft should be closed first, the lip cleft secondly. This sequence facilitates the formation of the turnover flaps.

On the median side a turnover flap of the vomerine mucoperiosteum is made from an incision along the borderline between the pale palatine and the dark-red vomerine mucosa (Fig. 108 A and compare with Fig. 155 and pp. 336-339). The knife is then turned horizontally and the incision curved around the alveolar process and continued just behind the columella. The entire flap is then mobilized. The vomer flap is elevated with a small periosteal elevator, and the anterior part is mobilized by sharp dissection. Care must be taken that the entire flap is mobilized in continuity. To facilitate this, a few cubic centimeters of adrenalin-saline solution (consult anesthetist before injecting adrenalin) or saline solution alone may be injected submucously before dissection is started. The lateral turnover flap consisting of nasal mucosa on the lateral side of the palatal cleft and nostril (Fig. 108 B, compare also with Fig. 98) is now elevated and median and lateral turnover flaps are sutured together. Two anterior palatal flaps pedicled posteriorly (Fig. 108 A and B) are mobilized subperiosteally and sutured together in the midline.

The width of the alveolar cleft is measured. A groove is cut into the rib graft with a narrow-mouthed rongeur for dove-tailing to embrace

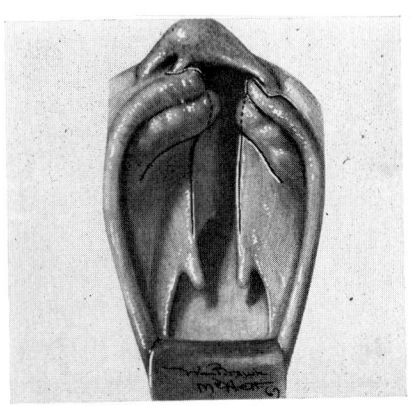

Fig. 108. *A:* Primary bone grafting for bridging of a unilateral alveolar cleft (after Schuchardt) and closure of lip cleft and anterior cleft of palate. Lines of incisions.

the bony edges of the alveolar process. The sharp cut edges are smoothed with a rasp. The periosteum is removed from the edges of the alveolar processes and the graft is pushed into the defect. It should come to lie high above the alveolar ridges beneath the columella (spino nasalis) and the base of the ala. It must be long enough to fit snugly into the defect to keep the alveolar processes well separated. The remainder of the defect is filled out with bone chips. The graft is already covered above by the two turnover flaps forming the floor of the nostril and nose. A flap must now be made to cover the graft from the oral side. Before this is done, the nostril is formed and the vermilion border for closure of the lip is cut as described in detail on pages 292-294, or according to the surgeon's preference of method. The cheek is mobilized from an incision along the upper gingivolabial sulcus as demonstrated in Figure 103 and described on page 292, and a rotation flap after Schuchardt pedicled on the median side (Fig. 108 *B* and *C*) is made wide enough to fill the alveolar cleft and to cover the bone graft. Rehrmann uses a vomer flap to avoid occasional pulling of the upper lip. The author agrees that this may happen with Schuchardt's device in wide

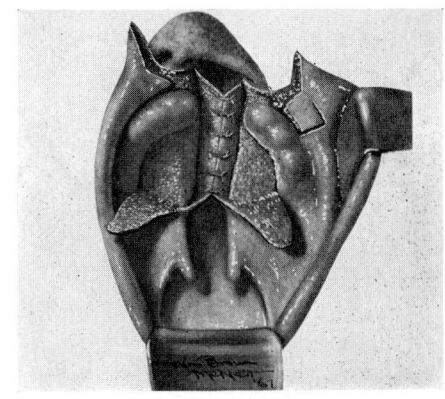

Fig. 108. *B:* Formation of floor of nose with a median vomer and lateral turnover flap; palatal mucoperiosteal flaps are elevated. Rotation flap for anterior closure of alveolar cleft and bone graft is outlined on oral side of cleft side of lip; it is pedicled on median side. Vermilion-border flaps of closure of lip cleft are formed.

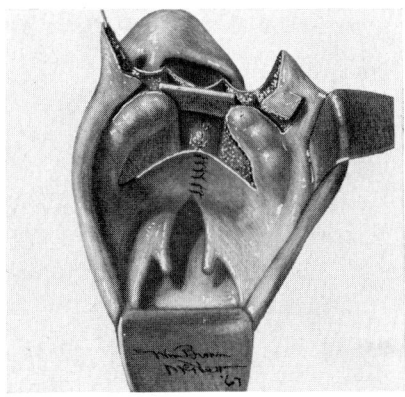

Fig. 108. *C:* Anterior palatal flaps are sutured together. A dovetailed rib bone graft embraces the bony edges of the median and lateral cleft edges above the alveolar ridges. The rotation flap on cleft side of lip is mobilized.

clefts, but it is only temporary. To facilitate the formation of such a flap, the oral mucous membrane of the lateral half of the lip is mobilized submucously within the extent of the outline of the flap; then a vertical incision for formation of the flap and a horizontal one for rotation of the flap are made (Fig. 108 *B*). The lip is advanced mediad along the lateral gingivolabial sulcus as depicted in Figure 104 and described on page 292. The flap is laid into the alveolar cleft and fastened to either the anterior rim of the palatal flaps (Fig. 108 *D*) or, if they are too short, to the turn-over flaps. If the latter is the case, it is good also to fasten the anterior rim of the palatal flaps, with one suture, to the turnover flaps. An incision is made along the gingivolabial sulcus on the median side of the cleft (Figs. 101, 102) and the lip is advanced laterally, followed by suture of the oral mucosal edges of the lip and completion of the closure of the left cleft as described on pages 292-294.

Dental Orthopedic Procedures and Secondary Bone Grafting of the Alveolar Cleft: These procedures, performed some time after the lip cleft is closed, are preferred by numerous surgeons (Ohlson

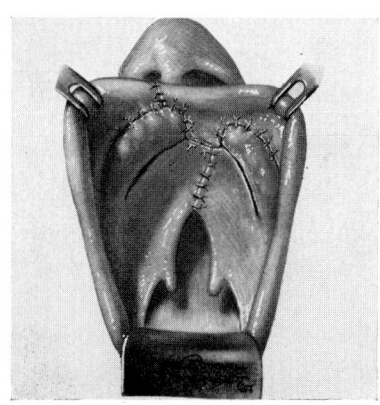

Fig. 108. *D:* The rotation flap is covering the bone graft after advancement of the lip along the gingivolabial sulcus and is sutured to palatal flaps. The median side of the lip is advanced along the median gingivolabial sulcus and the lip cleft closed.

299

and Kling, co-workers of Johanson, who have probably had as much experience in this field as anybody, state that good growth and development are not maintained in all cases of early bone grafting). Since the introduction of dental orthopedic procedures in the treatment of alveolar clefts, a better relationship of the alveolar processes prior to bone grafting can be achieved. This idea was conceived by Mc-Neil of Glasgow (1954), Burston of Liverpool (1958), followed by Nordin and Johanson, Häuple and Schrudde, Rehrmann, E. Schmidt, Shiere and Fisher, Wallace, Matthews, Horton et al., Brauer and Cronin, Harkins, Maisel, and others who have developed this treatment to its present high degree of refinement. The objectives of the treatment are correction of the misalignment of the alveolar processes and their development to a well-balanced normal maxillary arch. The treatment is started within forty-eight hours after birth by application of expansion splints. The bone-grafting operation, together with repair of the lip and anterior palate, is performed four to six months or more after birth, whenever an optional alveolar arch has been obtained. Alternatively, the lip cleft may be closed first (four months) and bone grafting done later. The bone grafting is done by means of a solid graft and bone chips, and orthodontic treatment by means of retention splints is continued for at least six months.

There are many opponents to routine early orthopedics and bone grafting in the alveolar cleft. They maintain that in a large percentage of cases the relationship of the alveolar processes after the cleft lip repair will be satisfactory. In those cases in which it is unsatisfactory, expansion of the alveolar arch and insertion of a bone graft is still possible at the age of five years. This is an argument well to be considered.

TOTAL BILATERAL CLEFT

In total bilateral clefts, the prominence of the premaxilla increases the width of the cleft (Fig. 109), and hence makes closure more difficult. The premaxilla is the anterior part of the embryonic frontonasal process, which as a rule fuses with the lateral maxillary (alveolar) processes to form the upper dental arch (p. 275). In complete bilateral lip clefts, the three processes are separated from each other. The premaxilla with the prelabium sits in front of the vomer, and usually protrudes forward, with or without lateral or upward tilt. Its shape varies. All these factors have considerable bearing upon the proper surgical management of the premaxilla. Hence the primary consideration in the treatment must center around the premaxilla (Barsky). The following three groups of displacement of the premaxilla are considered in relation to surgical repair: (1) premaxilla is aligned with lateral alveolar processes; (2) premaxilla is for-

300

ward displaced but can be aligned with lateral alveolar processes; (3) premaxilla is forward displaced but cannot be aligned with lateral alveolar processes.

Thus, if the premaxilla is already aligned with the lateral alveolar processes nothing needs to be done but closure of the soft-tissue clefts in one stage (for technique see p. 303). If the premaxilla is separated from the alveolar processes and is prominent, the question arises as to how to force it into the space of the maxillae to complete the alveolar arch. (Speaking of an arch is erroneous and unrealistic since, due to missing tissue and marked displacement of the various segments, a normal maxillary arch can hardly ever be achieved.)

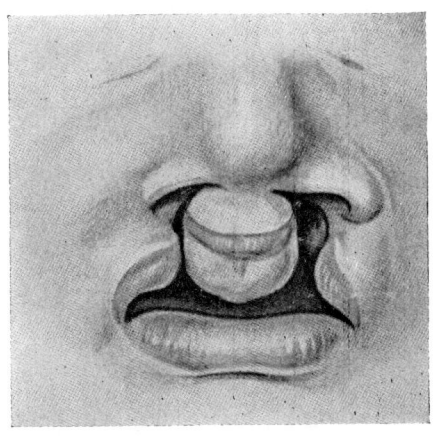

Fig. 109. G. Axhausen: Technik und Ergebnisse der Lippenplastik. G. Thieme, Leipzig.

If the premaxilla is not too prominent and not too badly tilted and the alveolar processes are sufficiently separated, it is advisable to keep the latter expanded by maxillary orthopedics (see following paragraph), instituted forty-eight hours after birth, and to close the soft-tissue clefts in one or two stages four to six weeks after birth (for technique see p. 303). Thus, the premaxilla is gradually pushed backward by the pull of the soft tissue. A bone-grafting operation (see p. 310) will later be required to firmly unite and stabilize the premaxilla to the alveolar processes.

In a third group of cases (Barsky), a very prominent, often tilted and rotated premaxilla is found, in which manual pressure or pressure after closure of the soft tissues—if possible at all—would cause the cartilaginous portion of the nasal septum to buckle and block the nasal airways. Complicated and prolonged orthodontic treatment may be considered and may result in pushing the premaxilla backward and simultaneously keeping the alveolar processes sufficiently spread. The author, however, prefers an operative recession of the premaxilla (for technique see p. 308). This method has had many followers since it was introduced by von Bardelen in 1868, but many have condemned it because of a justified fear of damaging the growth centers of the maxilla, leading to diminished development of the middle face and recession of the upper lip (this may nowadays be avoided; see p. 308). Veau, after reviewing his cases, had second thoughts about this procedure because of harmful effects which became noticeable in late adolescence. His viewpoint is supported by Bauer, Trusler and Tondra, Glove and others, to name recent investigators. Other authors, however, feel that possible harmful effects should not detract from the great benefit operative recession has in cases of extreme forward displacement of the maxilla (Brown, McDowell and Byars, Matthews, Gelbke, Sedfield, Harkins, Cronin, Barsky, Kahn and Simon, Monroe and others).

One important point must nonetheless be stressed: that operative recession of the premaxilla should be performed only if the alveolar processes are—or can be—sufficiently separated to permit wedging of the premaxilla into the maxillary space. If the maxillary processes have already collapsed behind the premaxilla so that prolonged orthodontic treatment must be anticipated, the author advises closing the lip clefts in two stages (starting four to six weeks after birth) without forced recession of the premaxilla unless it is absolutely impossible to close the lip clefts without some recession. One should wait until the child is eighteen months old to close the posterior part of the bilateral cleft of the palate. An attempt should then be made to correct the alveolar collapse with orthodontic measures, which may now be easier to achieve since some of the teeth have erupted, permitting firmer attachment of the expansion plates. If this procedure is successful and the premaxilla can be lodged into the maxillary space, the anterior part of the clefts of the palate can then be closed by elevating two anterior palatal flaps and by utilizing vomer turnover flaps (see p. 339). By bringing down a small turnover flap from the oral side of the lip, which is based at the fissure and laid into it and sutured to the anterior palatal flaps, and by suturing the mucosal flap beds over the hinged flaps, pockets are made into which bone grafts can be inserted subsequently. (For insertion of bone grafts see p. 310.) Splinting must be maintained until the bone graft is organized.

Should it be impossible to overcome the so-called "dog-mouth" appearance resulting from the forward displaced premaxilla, the latter should be removed when the child is about five years of age. This is not as harmful as it sounds, particularly in cases in which the alveolar processes can be spread to some degree to permit dental occlusion of the lateral segments. A removable prosthesis can be applied to the teeth of the lateral upper alveolar processes to maintain the spread of the latter, to replace the front teeth, and to keep the upper lip forward as in a normal profile. Having achieved many good cosmetic and functional results with this treatment, I do not hesitate to recommend it in selected cases. For technique see page 320 and Cases 37, 39, pages 1042, 1045.

As far as the technique of bilateral lip closure in general is concerned, it was mentioned above that if the premaxilla is already aligned with the lateral alveolar processes nothing need be done but closure of the soft tissue in one stage. This, however, is seldom the case. The second group of cases consists of patients in whom the premaxilla is separated but not too prominent and in whom the alveolar processes are sufficiently spread or can be spread by orthodontic means. In those cases, orthodontic treatment to permit the premaxilla to recess between the lateral segments is started forty-eight hours after birth, and the soft-tissue clefts are closed in one or, more often, in two stages, the first (the wider of the two clefts) at four to six weeks of age and the second three to four weeks later.

Technique (*Axhausen*) (Cases 37-39, pp. 1042-1045)

Formation of the floor of the nostril is similar to that described for the unilateral cleft. Here again the posterior border of the median turnover flap should not be extended beyond the insertion of the vomer to the premaxilla.

The various steps for the formation of the floor of the nostril, as well as for the formation of the median vermilion-border flap, are depicted in Figures 110 to 113.

The soft tissues of the cheek are mobilized from an incision along the lateral gingivolabial sulcus, followed by advancement of the mucosa. To unite the lateral vestibular mucosa with the mucosa of the premaxilla requires mobilization of the lower mucosal-wound edge of the premaxilla (Fig. 114). The lateral mucosal flap is advanced and sutured to the

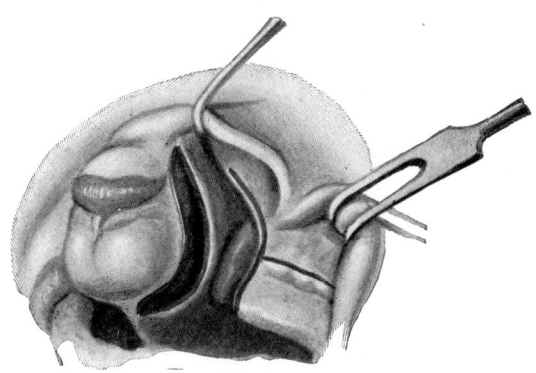

Fig. 110. (Figs. 110-118 are from G. Axhausen: Technik und Ergebnisse der Spaltplastiken. C. Hanser, München.)

303

THE HEAD AND NECK

premaxillary mucosa, thus bridging the cleft between alveolar process and premaxilla in front (Figs 115, 116). It is then sutured to the floor of the nostril (Fig. 117).

Formation of the median vermilion-border flap is shown in Figure 113, of the lateral one in Figure 114. Closure of the lip and adjustment of the vermilion-border flaps are shown in Figure 118.

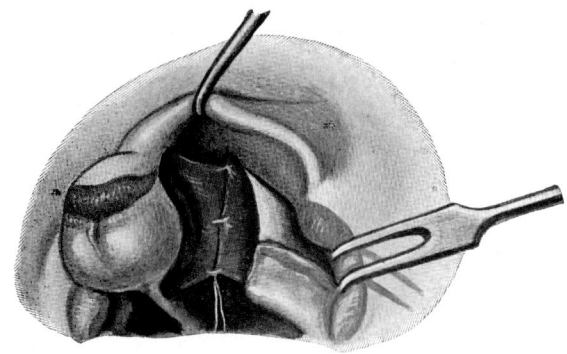

Fig. 111.

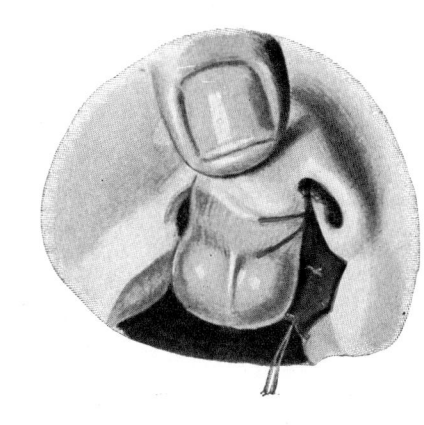

Fig. 112.

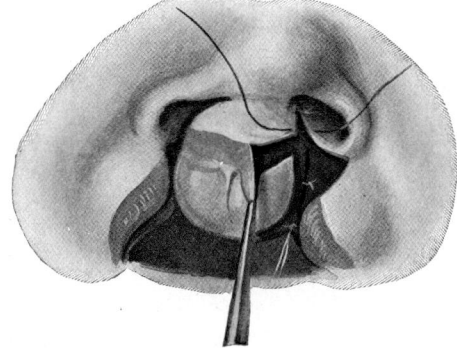

Fig. 113.

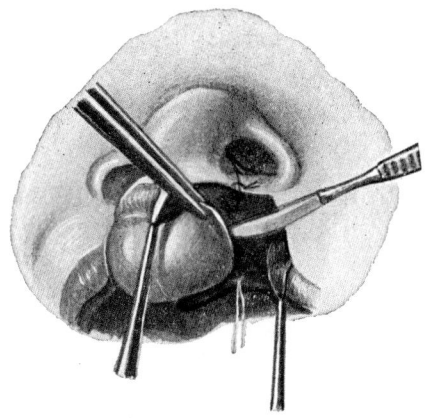

Fig. 114.

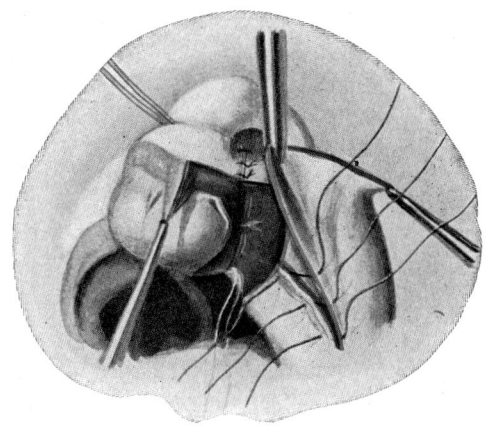

Fig. 115.

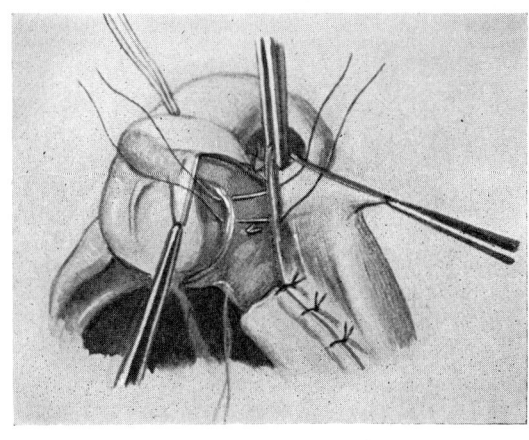

Fig. 116.

The author, however, agrees with J. B. Brown and others that the vermilion of the prelabium should not be included in the vermilion of the reconstructed lip when the vermilion of the prelabium is thin, as in most cases. The procedure tends to result in a double notch or a scant vermilion-border lining in the center of the lip. It is better to make an incision at the mucocutaneous junction all the way around the prelabium and to turn the vermilion of the prelabium backward as a hinge flap, to use it as part of the oral lining of the lip and backing of the center part of the vermilion, as depicted in Figures 119 to 121. (Cases 37-39, pp. 1042-1045).

The second side may be closed in the same operation. If there is too much tension resulting from closure of the first side, however, repair of the second side is postponed for four to six weeks.

As already mentioned, closure of the lip cleft is followed immediately by dental orthopedic treatment until the premaxilla is aligned with the maxillary processes. The premaxilla is then stabilized in this position by bone grafting (see p. 310).

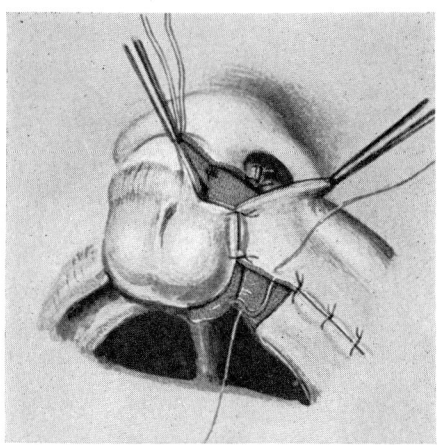

Fig. 117.

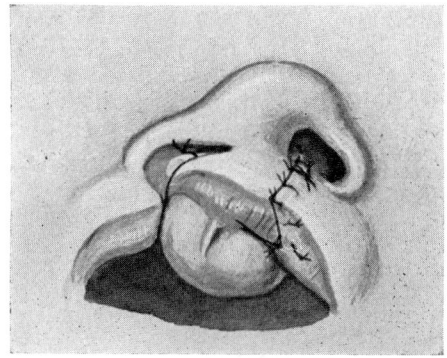

Fig. 118.

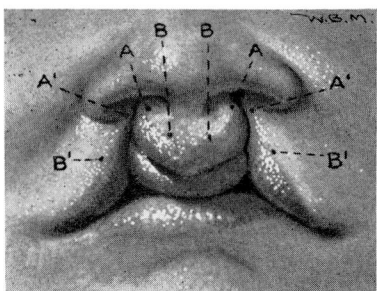

Fig. 119. Closure of bilateral cleft lip—after J. B. Brown and F. McDowell. The narrow vermilion of prelabium is not used for reconstruction of vermilion of prelabium per se, but turned backward to be used as a hinge flap for oral lining and backing the center part of the vermilion. Corresponding points of junction between lip and prelabium are marked out. *A* is marked out on mucocutaneous border of prelabium in level of base of columella. *A'* is located at tip of lateral vermilion border, where it joins the laterally displaced ala. *B* is marked out on lower mucocutaneous border of prelabium perpendicular to lateral border of base of columella. *B'* is of equal distance from *A'* as *A* from *B*.

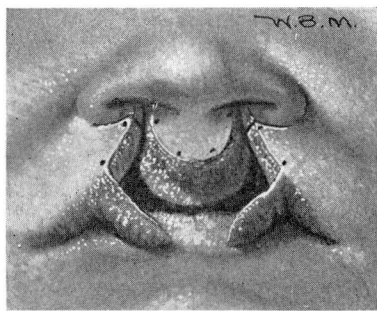

Fig. 120. From an incision at the mucocutaneous junction of the prelabium all the way around the latter vermilion of prelabium is turned backward. Vermilion border flaps of lips are formed. Small relaxation incision at base of ala.

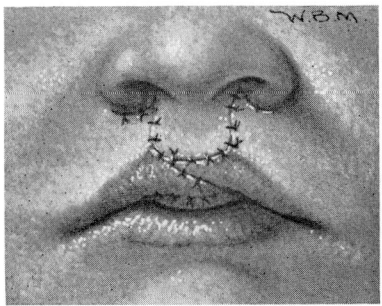

Fig. 121. Formation of lip. Note backing of center part of vermilion by use of hinged vermilion of prelabium.

307

In the third group of cases the premaxilla is so prominent and tilted that orthodontic treatment (prolonged and comprehensive) would have little chance to align the premaxilla with the lateral alveolar processes or, if alignment were possible, a buckling and distortion of the nasal septum with blockage of the nasal passage would result; in these cases a surgical recession of the premaxilla is performed. This is best done by a subperiosteal resection of a square block of vomer as recommended by Brown, McDowell and Byars. By removal of a rectangular piece of bone instead of a wedge-shaped piece, the premaxilla is slid straight backward; this prevents abnormal tilting of the teeth. By adding a submucous horizontal incision through the septal cartilage (Cronin), recession is facilitated. The resection should be done behind the prevomerine groove since the latter, the cartilaginous junction between premaxilla and septum, appears to be the area responsible for the greatest bone growth (Monroe) and hence should not be disturbed. The recessed premaxilla is stabilized with one (Brown et al.) or two (Barsky et al.) Kirschner wires. The lip clefts are closed six weeks later.

Technique (Cronin) (Recession of Premaxilla)

An incision is made through the mucosa over the free border of the vomer starting 1 cm. posterior to the premaxilla. Under subperiosteal dissection the wound edges are elevated from each side of the vomer. The amount of protrusion is measured and 3 to 4 mm. less than this amount of vomer is removed, as a rectangle, with a small sharp chisel.

The mucoperichondrium of both sides of the septal cartilage in front of the defect is undermined; this may be facilitated through a vertical incision through the mucoperichondrium of the anterior edge of the septum. A submucous horizontal incision is then made through the septal cartilage parallel to the inferior edge of the vomer leading from the upper bony wound edge toward the nasal tip (Fig. 122). The premaxilla can now be slid straight back without tilting. The prolabium is lifted up with a hook and a Kirschner wire (0.035-inch) is drilled through the premaxilla (far enough superiorly to avoid injury to the intraosseous teeth buds) and the inferior or thickest portion of the vomer until it escapes on the cut surface. The drill is removed and the excess wire is cut off. The two vomerian fragments are lined up carefully and the Kirschner wire is driven into the posterior portion with a mallet. If stablization is not sufficient, a second diverging Kirschner wire is drilled obliquely through the premaxilla and one of the lateral alveolar processes. The resected piece of vomer is cut into small chips which are packed around the junction of the fragments, and the mucosal incision is sutured. The protruding end of the wire is cut short so that the prolabial tissues can be pulled over it.

Closure of the soft-tissue clefts (possibly in one stage) is postponed for about six weeks. At that time the Kirschner wires are removed.

Stabilization of the premaxilla by bone grafting the alveolar clefts is postponed until a satisfactory alveolar arch has been established by means of orthodontic treatment (see p. 299 and following page).

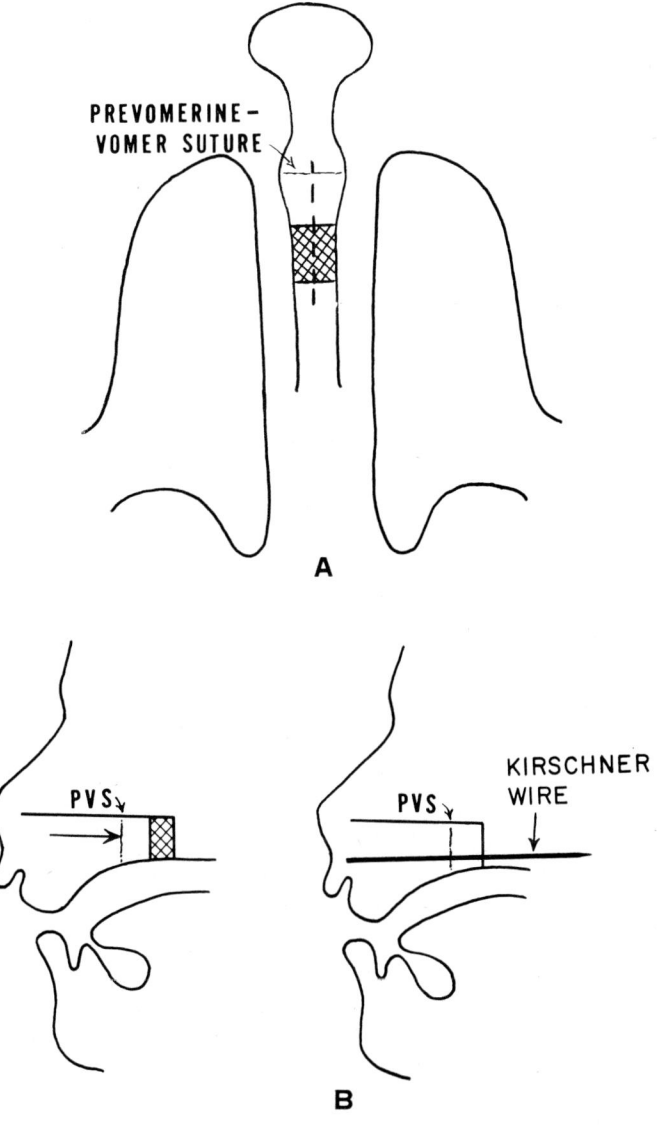

Fig. 122. *A:* Incision of mucosa on inferior border of vomer. *B:* Attention is called to the rectangular shape of the excised vomer and the submucous incision of the cartilage extending toward the tip of the nose. Note the better definition given to tip of nose and columella when premaxilla is set back to a more normal position (Cronin, T. D. J.: Plast. Reconstr. Surg.)

THE HEAD AND NECK

In the most severe group of cases, the alveolar processes have almost or are already closed behind the premaxilla. For these cases no fast rules of management can be established. One may try immediate orthodontic treatment with expansion splints before closure of the lip cleft. This, however, is a prolonged procedure and may unduly delay the lip repair. Another approach is closure of the soft tissue defects, performed first (in two stages), with later expansion of the collapsed alveolar processes. I prefer the second approach and delay the dental orthopedic work until the time of the cleft-palate repair. When the child is eighteen months old, the posterior part of the palate is closed as far front as possible. Then an attempt is made to expand the collapsed alveolar processes and to align the premaxilla. If this is successful, the anterior part of the cleft of the palate is closed and soft-tissue pockets are formed to bridge the alveolar clefts as described on page 302. Bone grafts are subsequently placed into these pockets to stabilize the premaxilla.

The pockets are exposed from an incision along the upper oral sulcus. There is no need to reopen the lip to obtain access to any part of the operative field (Skoog). The incision is carried down to the bone on both sides. The bony margin of the alveolar and premaxillary bone edges are subperiosteally exposed on the labial as well as the palatal sides. Great care must be exercised to prevent tear of the delicate membranes, particularly on the side of the premaxilla. As Skoog points out, even if there seems to be alignment of the visible parts of the median and lateral segments, a defect of several millimeters will be present when the segments are exposed (Fig. 123). This is because the premaxilla bulges, overhanging the vomer and thus concealing the actual cleft. Skoog uses split-rib grafts to fill the pockets and one or two longer pieces wedged across the cleft. The author uses split-rib grafts simply to bridge the cleft and fills the space between the cleft edges with bone chips (Fig. 123). Needless to say, the graft should be taken at the beginning of the operation before the cleft repair to avoid possible infection of the donor area. Both sides are operated on at the same time.

The dental splints must be worn for three months or longer to assure proper immobilization of the various segments during the regeneration of the bone graft. This procedure is also applicable for handling late (after infancy) cases with so-called "floating" maxilla. However, if attempts at expansion of the alveolar processes are unsuccessful or if expansion is insufficient, so that the forward-displaced premaxilla causes a "dog-mouth" deformity, one should not hesitate to remove the anterior portion of the premaxilla and replace it with a dental prosthesis as described on page 320 (Cases 37, 39, pp. 1042, 1045).

310

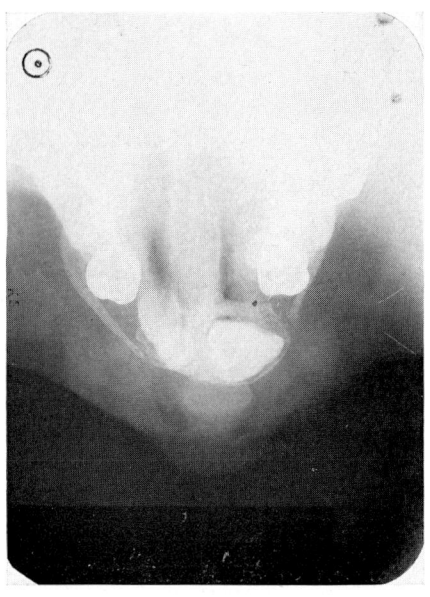

Fig. 123. Bilateral cleft lip and palate. The lateral alveolar processes were found closed behind premaxilla upon examination of this girl soon after birth. Since it would have taken too much time to expand them by orthodontic treatment, the lip clefts were closed first in one stage six weeks after birth. The posterior part of the cleft of the palate (⅔ of the cleft) was closed twenty-two months after birth. At three years of age, expansion of the collapsed alveolar processes by orthodontic expansion splints was started and completed one year later. At that time the front part of the cleft of the palate, which had become very small, was closed and pockets for reception of bone grafts were made between the alveolar clefts (see p. 302). The retention splint was not worn for ten days so as not to disturb the healing process. After this rather short time expansion became necessary to make it fit again. Two months later a bilateral bone graft operation was performed (pp. 310.) The retention splint was not worn for ten days. Three months later the premaxilla was firmly in place by palpation. After six months it was found fused by x-ray examination and the retention splint was discarded. At five years of age the columella of nose was elongated and a philtrum was made with a skin graft (pp. 318). This illustration of an röentgenogram at two years after the bone graft operation shows both clefts consolidated; the left alveolar cleft is filled with the regenerated spongiosa chips, while the bridging cortical bone graft is partially absorbed but clearly visible on the right side.

SECONDARY DEFORMITIES AFTER UNILATERAL CLEFT-LIP REPAIR

These deformities follow dehiscence or faulty primary correction or perhaps are a combination of both. In unilateral cases, the most frequent type exhibits four characteristic deformities which are always present, although varying in degree: (1) downward-displaced nostril, (2) laterally displaced ala, (3) extramedian position of the septum, and (4) a connection between nasal cavity and vestibulum oris (Figs. 124, 125,

311

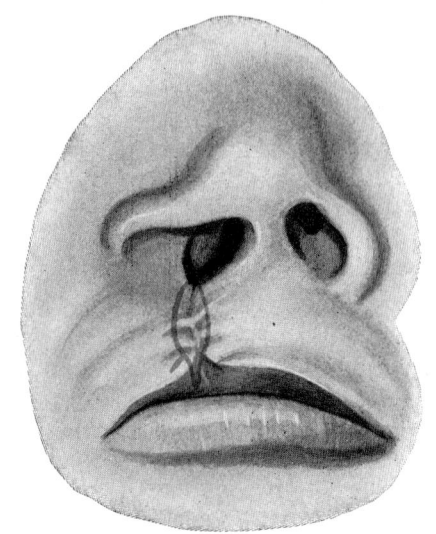

Fig. 124. (Figs. 124-130 are from G. Axhausen: Technik und Ergebnisse der Spaltplastiken. C. Hanser, München.)

131). This frequent type occurs following closure of the lip only, without formation of a nasal floor and without closure of the vestibular cleft. Satisfactory correction is possible only after undoing the former repair and secondary reconstruction.

Technique (Axhausen)

The scar at the lip is excised; a short incision is made along the mucocutaneous junction of the vermilion (Fig. 124). With one branch of a pair of straight scissors inserted through the vestibular hole into the nasal cavity, the remainder of the lip is severed. The result is depicted in Figure 126.

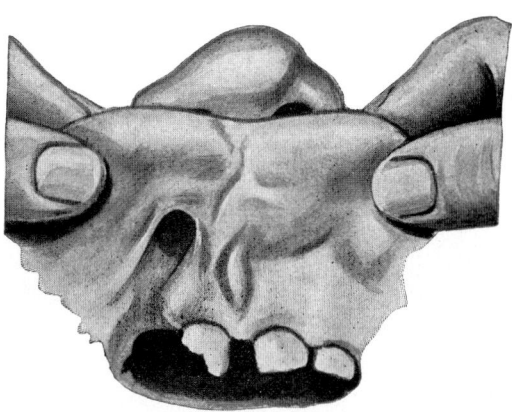

Fig. 125.

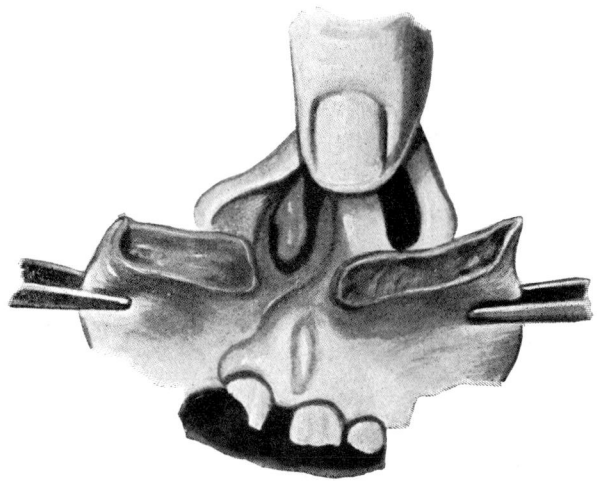

Fig. 126.

Two incisions are made upward from the upper edge of the wound for formation of the floor of the nostril. The median incision is made just posterior to the outer border of the columella and extended upward, almost to the juncture of the ala (Fig. 127). The lateral incision is made on the inside of the ala, in a way similar to that described on page 288. Both incisions are connected with each other just below the original vestibular hole (Fig. 127). Two turnover flaps are formed, as described on page 289, and are sutured together (Fig. 128).

The next step is mobilization of the soft tissues median and lateral to the cleft from incisions along the gingivolabial sulcus and advancement and suturing of the mucosal flaps (Fig. 128). The formation of an alar

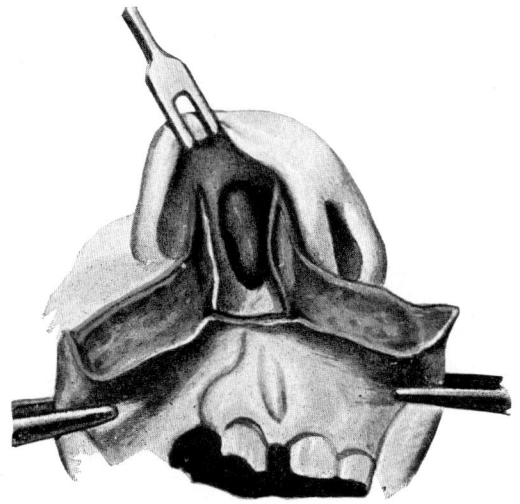

Fig. 127.

313

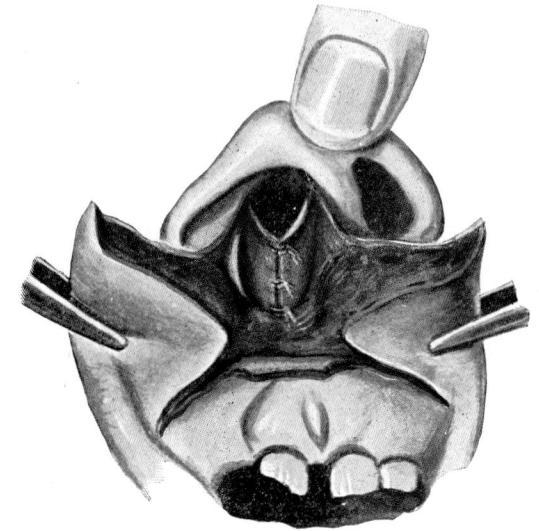

Fig. 128.

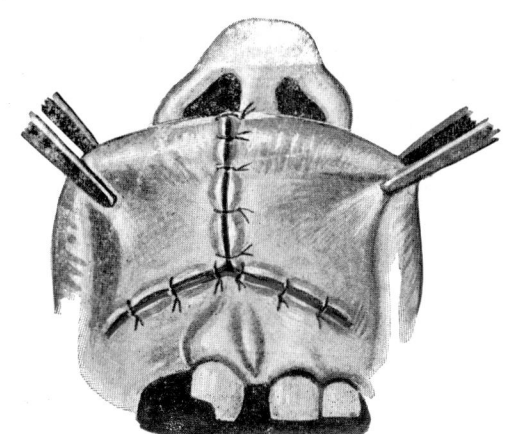

Fig. 129.

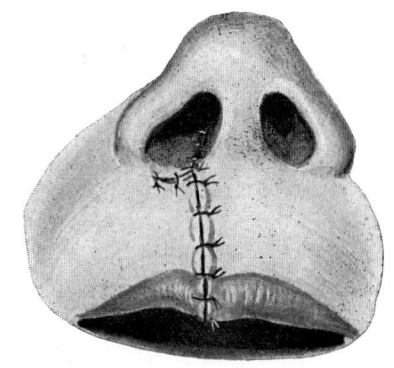

Fig. 130.

flap, as already described (p. 289), follows. The tip of the flap is sutured in the upper corner of the wound behind the columella. The posterior edge of the flap is connected with the turnover flaps, the anterior border with the anterior edge of the wound at the columella.

Two small vermilion-border flaps are made, and the lip is sutured together in layers (Fig. 130).

Since the quadrangular-flap method (after Hagedorn-LeMesurier) has come into vogue (compare with pp. 284, 286), attempts have been made to utilize this method in repair of secondary cleft-lip deformities (Trusler and Glanz, Brauer). Hence, in suitable cases, it is possible to combine the Axhausen technique with the quadrangular-flap method of lip repair (Fig. 131). In the author's experience, this procedure invariably

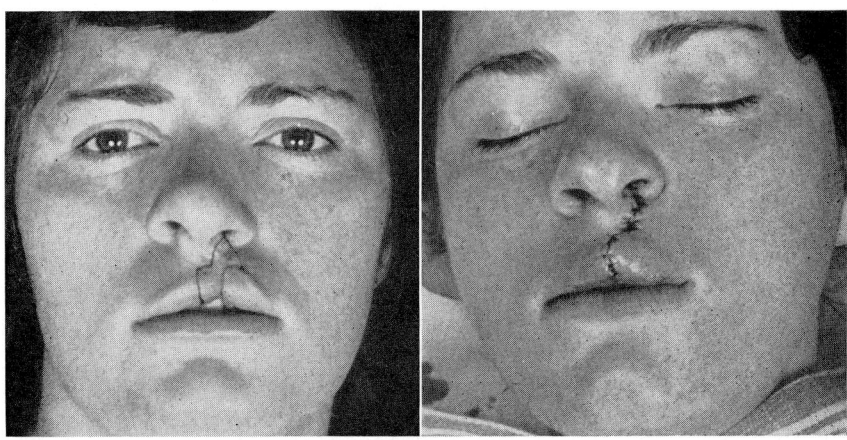

Fig. 131. Repair of secondary cleft lip deformity with quadrangular flap method (compare with Figs. 95, 96, 105, 106). A rectangular lip-vermilion notch on the median side is filled with a quadrangular lip-vermilion flap from the lateral side. The scar above is excised wedge-shaped through full thickness of lip. The apex of the wedge is within the floor of the nostril.

has corrected the deformity of the lip, lengthened the contracted scar and overcome the notch. Marcks and associates put a multiple Z-plasty to good use for this purpose.

If in addition to the soft-tissue deformities the alveolar arch is also deformed through collapse, dental orthopedic work (p. 299) must precede the soft-tissue repair. Johanson and co-workers advocate starting this procedure after age seven to correct the inversion of the front teeth, the median-posterior displacement of the lateral alveolar process and the lateral open bite. After good occlusion of the teeth is obtained, a removable retention plate is made. Bone grafting can now be carried out to fill the

315

alveolar defect (p. 300). The operation requires separation of the lip to facilitate exposure and the formation of suitable mucous-membrane flaps for formation of a pocket between the alveolar processes to receive the bone graft (compare with Figs. 124-130). Johanson uses spongiosa bone chips and one cortical graft from the iliac crest. Rib grafts are also available (p. 298). Secondary deformities of the lip and defects of the hard palate can be corrected in the same sitting. The removable retention plate is fitted in place and worn for about six months; it is then replaced with a permanent denture.

In cases in which some of the foregoing deformities are not marked and in which there is no connection between vestibulum and nasal cavity, correction of the outstanding deformities is done without reopening the cleft.

If the *vermilion-border edges are displaced upon one another*, only a Z-plastic operation is necessary (compare with Fig. 175). A *notch in the lip* is overcome by a diamond-shaped excision of the notching part of the vermilion border and closure of the gap in layers, or, in suitable cases, the technique of Figure 131 has much to be recommended; great care is taken to accomplish exact adaptation of the mucocutaneous juncture of the vermilion. If the *pout of the lip* (the bulge at or above the vermilion border) *is missing* and the lip looks flat, Pickrell et al. advise the subcutaneous insertion of a folded free fascia or dermal graft or a tendon graft (for example, of the musculus palmaris or the musculus peroneus brevis) above the vermilion border.

Lateral Displacement of the Ala. (This is corrected in Z-type fashion and in the opposite way, as depicted in Fig. 203.)

In the majority of cases, the lateral displaced ala is accompanied by flatness of the tip cartilage of the same side so that this half of the nasal tip is lower than the other side and a wide columella ala angle. This may be due to abnormal pull exerted upon the columellar and alar bases by the cleft itself, due to malposition rather than malformation of the nasal structures (Huffman and Lierle, Stenstrom and Oberg), but the possibility of over- and underdevelopment of the involved lower lateral cartilage secondary to the lip repair cannot be excluded. In all cases, the structures are present but in faulty position. In general, the correction must consist of freeing, repositioning, and transfixing the ala tip cartilage. This is generally acknowledged to be a difficult task. Numerous methods are available, but none is ideal. The author is now following Reynold's and Horton's technique and has obtained better results than with previous methods. The main difference here is found in the fixation of the repositioned tip cartilage to the opposite upper lateral cartilage which, being attached to the nasal bone, provides a firm anchorage. In the majority of other techniques, the median crura are sutured together in an attempt to hold the unstable abnormal alar cartilage in position.

The author in following Reynold's and Horton's technique found the Réthi approach convenient; temporary severance of the base of the affected ala and, if necessary, simultaneous correction of its malposition are also advantageous.

Technique: From a bilateral intercartilaginous incision, to which a transfixion incision down to the nasal spine and a Réthi incision are added (p. 422), a wide exposure of the upper and lower-upper cartilaginous structures of both sides is achieved. For a more extensive exposure of the deformed alar cartilage, the rim incision is extended much further than on the other side. The intercartilaginous incision of the affected side is extended down to the base of the ala and from there to the tip of the ala. A short incision is now added on the outside along the base of the ala and, with a sharply curved pair of scissors, the base of the ala is severed. A mattress suture of 0000 chromic catgut is now placed through the heights of the flattened dome of the affected and the upper part of the upper lateral cartilage of the other side. By pulling on the suture it becomes evident whether or not the cartilages and the mucosal lining need to be trimmed. The suture is then tied. The wound edges of the rim incisions are adjusted and sutured. Invariably the laterally displaced base of the ala must be adjusted in Z-type fashion and in the opposite way as depicted in Figure 203. The nostril of the repaired side is packed with a strip of vaselinized gauze for three to four days.

If the ala is very flat, Royster and co-workers use a more formidable method for primary as well as secondary cleft lip repair; the author has no experience with this method, but has seen their good results. They make a midcolumellar incision which is carried over the tip between the upper and lower nasal cartilage as a through incision. Another through incision is made from the freed half of the columella just below the vestibule of floor around the base of the nostril to the upper end of the nasolabial fold. The whole nostril is now rotated clockwise. This requires excision of a small crescent-shaped piece of skin of the dorsum from the affected side for smooth approximation of the wound edges and excision of a small triangular piece of skin lateral to the ala.

SECONDARY DEFORMITIES AFTER BILATERAL CLEFT REPAIR

The most frequent deformities encountered after bilateral cleft lip repair consist of (1) shortness of the columella, (2) "dog-mouth" deformity from the forward displaced premaxilla, and (3) vertical shortness and flatness of the lip.

317

THE HEAD AND NECK

Shortness of the Columella

Numerous suggestions have been made to overcome this deformity (Brown and McDowell, Straith, Matthews, Marcks, Trevaskis and Payne, Musgrave, Skoog, Berkeley, Millard, Converse, Symonds and Crikelair, Schmidt, and others). All are variations of the principle of advancing tissue from the prolabium. The author follows the basic outline of Brown and McDowell's technique, which is depicted in Figure 132. Some modifications, however, are added. One of them is that the operation is performed in two stages. In the first stage, the philtrum flap is outlined and raised, then returned to develop better circulation. After all edema has subsided, which should be in about four weeks, the main operation is performed.

Technique: The philtrum flap, consisting of the skin of the prolabium (no subcutaneous fat tissue is included), is outlined and reaches from the vermilion borderline to the floor of the nose; it includes the little "darts" which will be used later to fill the little "dart" openings at the nasal tip. The flap is raised and after thorough hemostasis is returned to its bed and sutured. After all edema has subsided (four weeks), the flap is raised again with its little "darts." The membranous septum is now incised to sever the columella from the cartilaginous septum, and the prolabium flap and columella are elevated. The nasal tip must then be freed and elevated. This is facilitated by incising the mucosa high up over the septum. This opens up dart-like defects into which the little darts of the prolabium flap are sutured after the dorsum of the nose has been thoroughly mobilized. The prolabium flap is folded together; if it is too wide and makes the new columella too bulky, it should be trimmed; it is shifted from the lip into a position below the septum and held with catgut sutures. It is necessary that the new columella make practically a right angle with the lip; if the prolabium flap is too long it should be shortened. Care must be taken that the lower flap edge is not sutured back down into the lip, producing an ugly web.

Seldom can the raw flap bed be closed as demonstrated in Figure 132 unless the Dieffenbach-Webster cheek-sliding procedure is performed (see p. 259). The latter has the drawback of additional tightening of the upper lip, which may already be tight. In patients where this is not the case, I have found the method very helpful. The crescent excision of skin lateral to the base of the ala—see Figure 79—may not be necessary, since the alae are laterally displaced and their shape will benefit from a more median displacement. Otherwise, a full-thickness skin graft taken from the supraclavicular region is transplanted for closure of the flap bed; this is widened if the scars bordering the prolabium must also be repaired. Before placing the full-thickness graft on the lip, the wound edges of the

318

lip are pulled slightly together with two horizontal mattress sutures of fine chromic catgut. This inevitably raises the wound edges and depresses the center of the raw surface to the degree of a normal philtrum, and facilitates closure of small dart openings at the floor of the nose. The raw area is

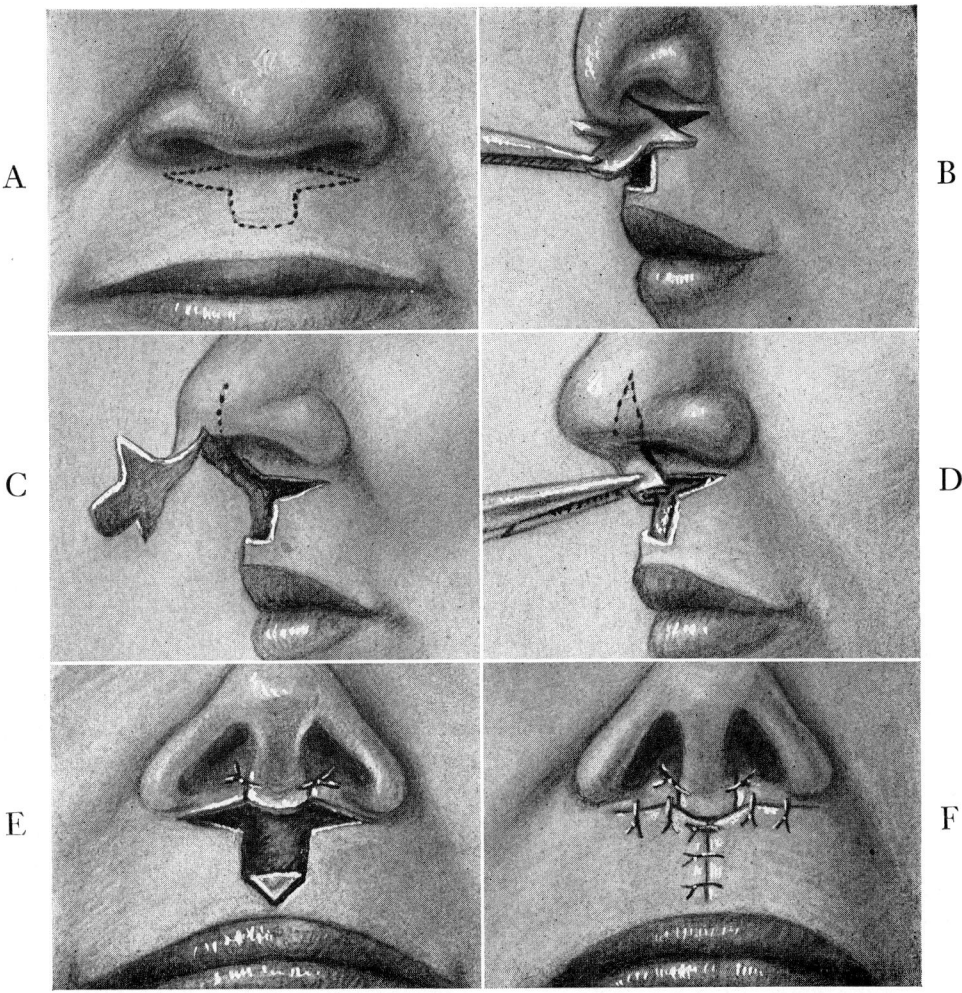

Fig. 132. *A:* Elongation of columella in secondary correction after repair of bilateral cleft. Design of flap to be advanced from upper lip; flap has lateral triangles to fill opening in septum and to allow for shortening of lip. *B:* Flap is raised. *C:* Membranous septum has been severed; area over nasal tip has been freed; incisions are made into mucosa high up over septum. *D:* Flap being sutured in place; lateral triangles of flap are sutured into triangular defect over septum. *E:* Flap in position at right angle to lip. *F:* Lip is closed by shifting it to midline. No sutures should be inserted at base of columella to prevent dragging down the latter. (J. B. Brown and F. McDowell: Ann. Surg.)

319

then covered with the graft, which is sutured in place. The sutures are left long and are tied over the pressure dressing. (For results, see Cases 37, 39, pp. 1042, 1045.)

"Dog-mouth" Deformity

This is due to the forward-displaced premaxilla, which rests upon the medially displaced alveolar processes. In many cases this deformity can be overcome or lessened by orthodontic procedures, which have been outlined in detail on page 299. If the premaxilla can be brought into alignment with the alveolar processes, it must be stabilized in this position with bone grafts (p. 310). If it is impossible to overcome the deformity appreciably by dental orthopedics, one should not hesitate to remove the anterior part of the premaxilla and replace it with a dental prosthesis. This is not as deforming as it sounds. As a matter of fact, I have obtained in numerous cases far better cosmetic and functional results (Cases 37 and 39) than would have been the case with the premaxilla left behind and protruding.

I even recommend partial removal of the premaxilla where dental orthopedics have brought improvement but have not produced an acceptable arch. In these cases, a retention splint containing a frontal dental prosthesis must be worn after partial removal of the premaxilla to prevent the lateral alveolar processes from collapsing.

Technique: In removing the premaxilla, usually before the child goes to school or even earlier, it is essential to leave the posterior shell since this facilitates fitting of the dental prosthesis. The bone of the premaxilla is exposed by submucosal dissection. It is important to make the anterior (gingivolabial) flap as long as possible, including all the anterior mucosa of the premaxillary bone. After excision of the anterior part of the premaxilla, which is done with chisels and bonecutters and includes all dentigenous elements, this flap makes an excellent lining of the anterior gingivolabial sulcus, which is often shallow and can be deepened with this flap; the flap is sutured to the posterior lining of the premaxillary bone. As soon as the wounds have healed, a removable prosthesis should be applied to the upper teeth to replace the front teeth and particularly to keep the upper lip forward as in a normal profile.

If a lengthening of the columella is also planned, excision of the premaxilla, as described in the foregoing paragraph, and the first-stage columella lengthening (raising and returning of the prelabium flap; see previous paragraphs) can be combined.

Loss of Tissue and Flatness of the Lip

If the lip is too tight, a vermilion-border lined flap is rotated from the middle of the lower lip into a center split of the upper lip (Estlander,

Abbé) (see Fig. 76). This may be done with a triangular flap if vertical shortness is no problem. Otherwise, a W-shaped Abbé flap is formed from the central part of the lower lip (Cannon and Converse, Horowitz and Wood-Smith). Vertical increase of the upper lip can be achieved and controlled by the amount of curvature of the edges of the upper lip defect. The W-flap is rotated and sutured into the upper lip defect with each tongue of the W extending into the nasal floor. The lower lip defect is closed, starting with closure of the lower corners. The pedicle is divided after three weeks, followed by adjustment of the vermilion borders according to the method described on page 256. If the alar bases are too wide, they may be narrowed by a modified Z-plasty (the reverse of Fig. 203).

Cleft Palate

For general considerations, time of operation and preoperative treatment, see page 280.

Choice of Operation

The classic operation for closure of a cleft palate is the so-called "von Langenbeck operation." Its principle is the median displacement and approximation of lateral palatine bridge flaps which are pedicled in front and back. Bridge flaps had been used by numerous surgeons preceding Langenbeck (Dieffenbach, 1826; J. M. Warren, 1841; and others); for historical facts the reader should refer to Dorrance's excellent book, *The Operative Story of Cleft Palate*, to Wallace's historical remarks, and to Stark's recent excellent summary in *The Historical Basis for Contemporary Cleft Palate Surgery* and his monograph "Cleft Palate: A Multidiscipline Approach." The first recorded palate sutures by C. von Graefe entitled "The Gaumannaht" (1817, translated in part by H. May and to be published 1970 in Plast. Reconstr. Surg.) is a noteworthy article from the historical point of view. It was Langenbeck (1861) who based the operation on sound principles, thus improving results and popularizing its merits. Operators preceding Langenbeck failed to realize the value of including the periosteum in the flaps. Langenbeck took the courageous step of including it—courageous since, according to the teaching of that time, to deprive a bone of its periosteum must inevitably lead to necrosis of the bone. Including the periosteum in the flaps secured the circulation in them.

In 1931 appeared the monumental work of Veau and his pupil Plessier, which was to break with the principles of the classic operation of Langenbeck. Veau's criticisms of the bridge-flap principle were sound: He criticized it as resulting in a dropping and flattening of the palatal arch, in the creation of a dead space above the flaps, and in cicatricial changes of the flaps with consequent contracture and shortening of the soft palate. Veau considered the principle of the bridge flap as the sole cause of the imperfections. He believed that mobilization and approximation of two lateral bridge flaps inevitably lead to a drop from their levels, particularly so if, for better mobilization, the nasal mucosa at the posterior edge of the hard palate is severed. Hence, the two flaps are hanging free in the oral cavity, anchored only on the anterior and posterior pedicles. This creates a deep wound sac above the flaps, which becomes particularly hazardous since the nasal side of the flaps, deprived of mucosa, is raw and discharging. The stagnation of the wound secretion may lead to infection, endanger the suture line, and bring about cicatricial changes and shortening and thickening of the palatal flaps and muscles.

To eradicate these disadvantages, Veau developed a technique which is based on the following principles: formation and median displacement of single-pedicle flaps (pedicled posteriorly) of the palatine mucoperiosteum, mobilization and suturing of nasal-mucosa flaps, anchoring of the palatine flaps to the nasal mucosa with mattress sutures, and approximation of the separated palatine muscles.

The Veau operation has not remained unchallenged. Its chief adversary became Lexer, for whose conversion Veau devoted much space in his work, but Veau gradually achieved recognition of the principles of his procedure all over the world.

Thus for the first time in cleft-palate repair closure of the raw surface on the nasal side became established as a principle. However, successful closure of the cleft will not lead to normal speech—and this is the primary object of cleft-palate repair—unless a sufficiently long and mobile palate is provided to establish good closure of the pharyngeal isthmus. Thus the two principles of an effective cleft-palate repair are: avoidance of scars and good velopharyngeal closure. The latter is no problem in sufficiently long palates, but becomes one when the palate is short. It can be solved in any of three ways (see p. 342 and Fig. 163): by moving the palate closer to the posterior pharyngeal wall (lengthening the palate), by transferring a pharyngeal pedicle flap to the soft palate, or by a combination of both. While the lengthening of the palate is done more often primarily, the pharyngeal flap method is performed by many surgeons secondarily if speech training was unsuccessful in overcoming impediments such as nasality and denasality.

Other developments have influenced our views on cleft-palate repair, mainly recent research (p. 280) on facial growth (Graber, Slaughter and Brodie, Waldron, Subtelny). Formerly, we were all too much concerned with the technical details of closing the cleft, and neglected or

322

overlooked a most important problem that still remained—the maldevelopment of the maxilla with consequent malocclusion and functional and cosmetic handicaps which often followed the conventional types of cleft-palate repair. The maxilla grows by sutural and surface deposition of bone. The growth is arrested if the blood supply is impaired. This may result if the maxilla is denuded of its periosteum after periosteal elevation, as frequently happens in the surgical repair of cleft palate. To prevent interference with growth, one must either delay closure or avoid extensive mobilization of the palatal flaps that might interfere with growth. In the majority of cases, delayed closure is not advisable, since by far not all cleft-palate operations with early closure result in noninterference with maxillary growth, particularly in the closure of partial posterior clefts; furthermore, delayed closure may cause a permanent speech impediment.

On page 280, I have mentioned that Schweckendiek and his followers in Germany and later Slaughter and Pruzansky in this country tried to overcome this dilemma by closing the cleft in two stages. The velum cleft is closed when the child starts to speak, usually at fourteen to sixteen months of age, while the cleft of the hard palate is repaired three to four years later. By that time the anterior cleft may have become quite small, so that closure becomes simple and atraumatic to the growth centers. This two-stage method is excellent and deserves consideration with an excessively wide cleft (see also p. 339).

In through-and-through clefts, bridging of the alveolar cleft with bone grafts, as described in detail on page 295, counteracts impairment of growth to a large extent.

As already mentioned cleft-palate repair must aim at a good velopharyngeal closure, which in short palates can be achieved by moving the velum backward or the posterior pharyngeal wall forward. More will be said about this later (p. 342), since some of the more extensive methods are carried out much later as a secondary procedure. There are, however, some methods which aim at lengthening the palate during primary repair. This can be achieved only by elongation of the palate on the buccal aspect, namely by dividing the mucoperiosteum on the hard palate, actually creating palatal flaps, and the aponeurosis from the posterior palatal rim. The nasal mucosa, however, must remain intact (as explained on p. 321) to avoid raw surfaces and consequent scarring (compare with Fig. 163). Hence, the extent to which the palate can be lengthened is rather limited. There are numerous surgeons who use this type of palate lengthening routinely during primary repair, whether the palate seems to be sufficiently long or not. The best known procedures are the V-Y repositioning of the mucoperiosteum of the hard palate as devised by Ganzer (1917) and adapted by Veau and Rupps (1922). This method was further advanced to a W-V flap by Halle, Ernst, Moorhead, Wardill and Killner, and his pupils Peet, Osborne and Reidy (the Oxford Group). The amount of retropositioning and thus of lengthening the palate depends, however, upon the degree to which the nasal mucosa can be stretched, and this, in the majority of cases, is limited.

The author practices the modern Langenbeck method as developed by Axhausen, who modified and improved the Langenbeck operation by including modern principles as brought forward by Veau, Halle, Ernst and others. To prevent the Langenbeck bridge flaps from dropping from their levels—which was thought by Veau to be the inevitable imperfection of the classic method—Axhausen introduced two important features: (1) the mucoperiosteal flaps were more thoroughly mobilized, and (2) the nasal mucosa was not severed behind the hard palate but carefully freed from the bony edge after the aponeurosis was separated from the bony plate. The method has found many enthusiastic followers (Schuchardt, Ivy and Curtis, Luhmann, and others).

The Langenbeck-Axhausen operation is described in detail below for a cleft involving the soft and posterior part of the hard palate. Axhausen recommends local anesthesia (the author uses endotracheal anesthesia). A small pillow is placed beneath chest and shoulders to allow a backward bend of neck and head. The mouth is held open with a Lane or other type of spreader; the tongue, if necessary, is grasped with a towel clamp or suture and held forward. A small pharyngeal pack is inserted behind the tongue. The field of operation is kept free of blood with a sucker, which is manipulated by an assistant, who also holds the tongue down with a tongue depressor. To reduce the amount of bleeding, saline-adrenalin solution may be infiltrated beneath the palatine mucosa. (The anesthesiologist should be consulted if adrenalin is used.) Instruments to be used are fine but simple.

CLEFT OF SOFT PALATE AND POSTERIOR PART

OF HARD PALATE

Technique (Langenbeck-Axhausen)

Formation of Lateral Bridge Flaps: The operation starts with the lateral relaxation incision on the left side. Anteriorly, the incision commences somewhat in front of the level of the anterior cleft angle (Fig. 133) and runs along the alveolar process until the posterior edge of the process is reached, where the hamulus behind the alveolus can be felt. The incision, following the same direction slightly more laterally, is continued into the soft palate (Fig. 134) through the palatoglossal arch for about 1.5 to 2.5 cm. (⅝ to 1 3⁄16 inches).

324

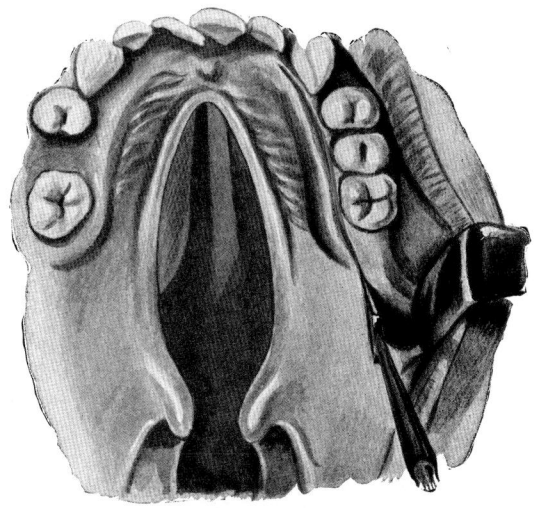

Fig. 133. (Figs. 133-154 are from G. Axhausen: Technik und Ergebnisse der Spaltplastiken. C. Hanser, München.)

With a small periosteal elevator (the Joseph type, Fig. 192), the mucoperiosteum median to the incision is elevated from the bone. The position of the tip of the instrument should be checked with the thumb of the other hand (Fig. 134). The mobilization is extended to the median border of the cleft—but should not perforate the mucosa at this point—and to the posterior edge of the palate. In front of the cleft, undermining is extended beyond the midline and close to the cleft angle (Fig. 135).

Mobilization of Soft Palate: The next step is mobilization of the soft palate. A retractor is inserted into the lateral wound region (Fig. 136) and the wound deepened by spreading a pair of dissecting scissors, until the glistening tendon of the musculus pterygoideus internus is visible

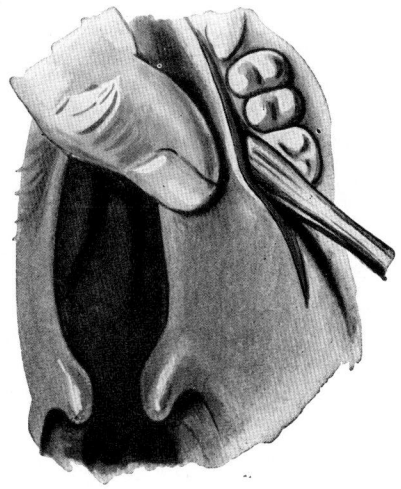

Fig. 134.

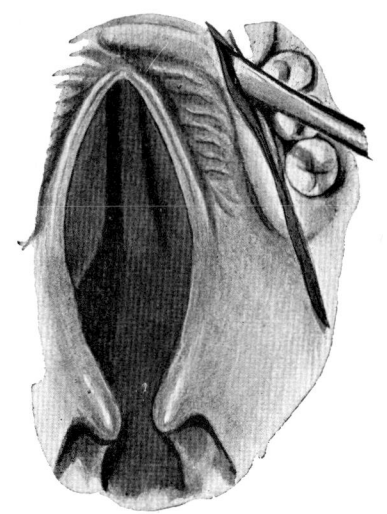

Fig. 135.

(Fig. 136). Sometimes visualization of the tendon may be facilitated by stripping off all the overlying tissue with a piece of gauze. Exposure of the tendon is important, since it is the path along which the mobilization of the soft palate is carried out. To avoid protrusion of the fat pads of the cheek, care should be taken not to penetrate too far laterally. If protrusion occurs, the fat should be retracted and the tendon localized more mediad. Median to the tendon one finds the space which surrounds the pharyngeal organs. This space can easily be opened up beyond the tonsil to the cervical spine, either with an elevator or with the finger. The lateral pharyngeal wall (soft palate, pillars, and tonsil) is displaced

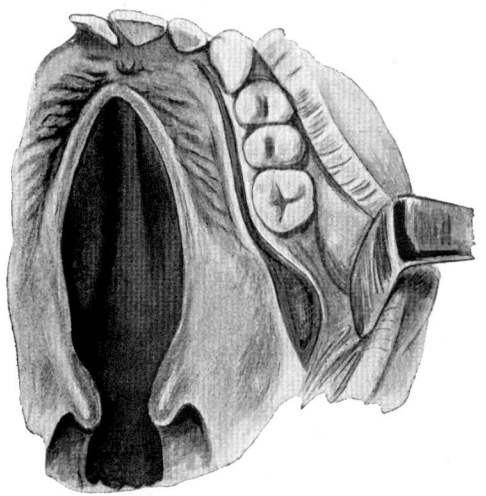

Fig. 136.

326

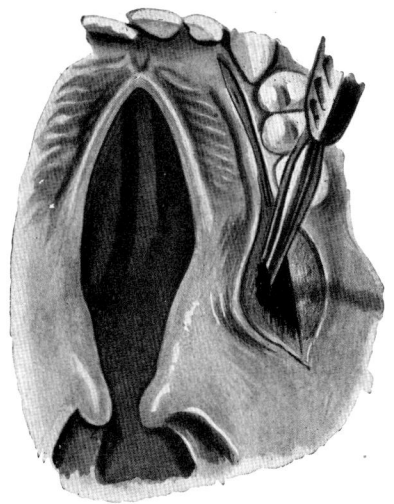

Fig. 137.

mediad (Fig. 137) until it touches the opposite side. The space is temporarily packed with plain gauze.

Middle Portion of Incision: Attention is now paid to the middle part of the incision, where the flap is still firmly attached to the posterior edge of the palatine bone. The flap is severed from the bone, bluntly or under sharp dissection, until the insertion of the pterygoid tendon to the bone is clearly visible. Median to it one finds the hamulus, either close to the tendon or somewhat in front of it. The best way to locate the hamulus is to lead a small elevator along the pterygoid tendon, forward and upward, until the bony insertion is felt. If the instrument is now pushed mediad,

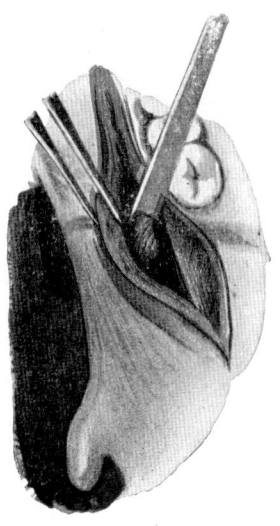

Fig. 138.

327

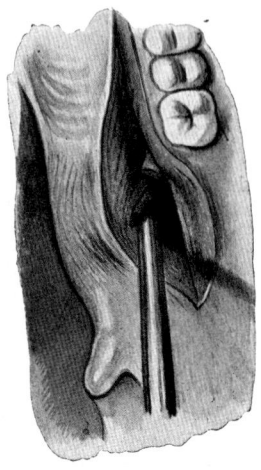

Fig. 139.

the resistance of the hamulus is palpable. After dissection of the hamular process with the elevator, one sees the tensor veli palatini extending obliquely over it into the soft palate. A small chisel is placed in front of the tendon (Fig. 138) and the hamulus severed, thus allowing the tensor tendon to be displaced mediad and relaxing the soft palate (Fig. 139). More relaxation can be achieved if the tensor tendon directly in front of the hamulus is divided as it fans out in the palatal aponeurosis. Median to the hamulus stump is the posterior rim of the hard palate, which is now freed from muscle and fibrous tissue by separating the aponeurosis, which is the common insertion of the palatal muscles, from

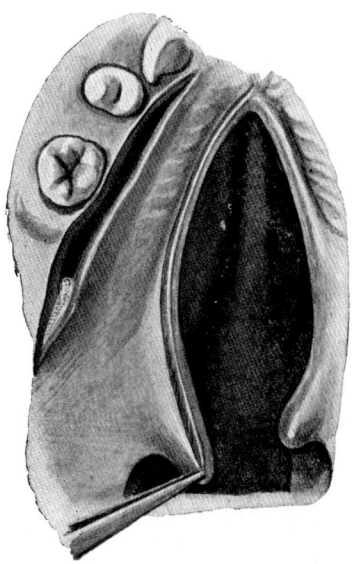

Fig. 140.

328

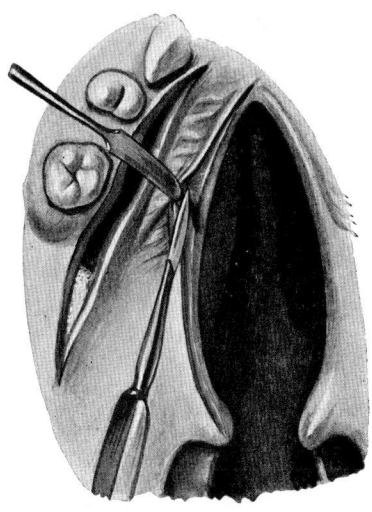

Fig. 141.

the posterior palatal edge. Thus further relaxation of the soft palate is achieved. Care, however, must be taken not to sever the nasal mucosa, for reasons explained on page 321.

As the next step, Axhausen advises ligation and separation of the arteria palatina for better mobilization of the bridge flap. The author has found no advantage in this procedure, since the flap can be stretched sufficiently as described on page 347. Indeed, severance of the arteria palatina may be a disadvantage if additional procedures, such as a pushback operation (p. 344), are required later on.

The same procedure is carried out on the right side.

Preparation of Cleft Margins: The incision is made on the right side, starting just above the cleft angle, and is led parallel to and somewhat

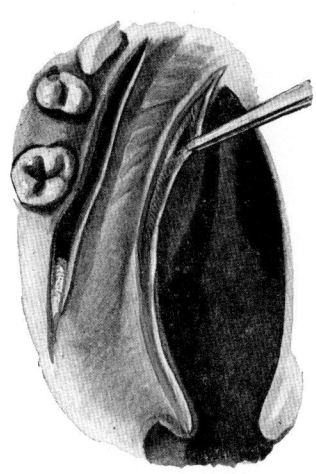

Fig. 142.

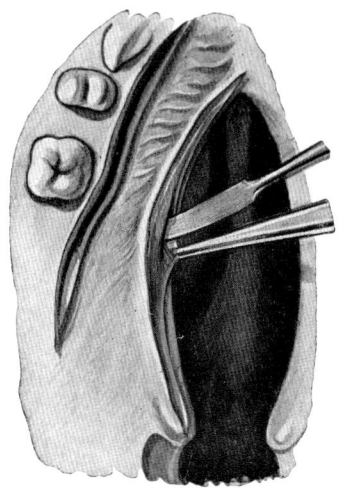

Fig. 143.

away from the cleft margin (Fig. 140). The line of incision is marked
by nature; it is the line where the pale mucosa of the margin joins the
darker mucosa of the palate proper (Fig. 133).

The knife is led along this line upon the bone until the posterior
edge of the hard palate is reached. The uvula is now grasped with a forceps and the margin of the soft-palate cleft incised longitudinally. The
incision starts near the uvula and in front joins the first incision. The
uvular margin is incised in the same way, and the tip is split with a pair
of scissors.

From the marginal incision the mucosa of the hard palate is split
into two layers: nasal mucosa and oral mucosa. Mobilization of the nasal
mucosa is the most difficult part of the procedure. Partly under blunt,

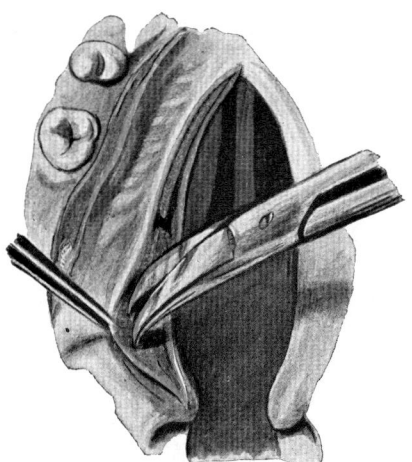

Fig. 144.

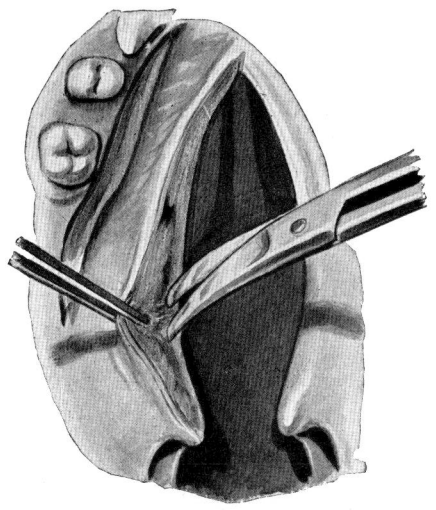

Fig. 145.

partly under sharp dissection, the median wound edge at the margin is severed from the oral surface of the palatine bone until the bony margin itself is reached (Fig. 141). The mucosa is then carefully mobilized from the bony edge. This is best done with the knife, which at all times must remain in contact with the bone. Gradually, the pale-colored edge of the bone becomes visible. The edge of the mucosal wound is grasped with a pair of forceps and pulled into the cleft (Fig. 142), thus permitting visualization of the remaining connecting fibrous bands, which must be severed with the knife. A small curved elevator, such as dentists use for

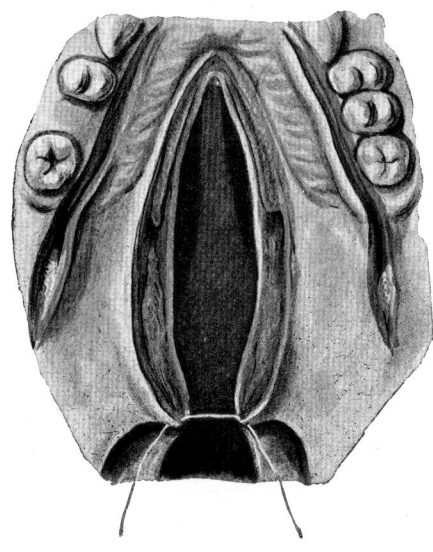

Fig. 146.

331

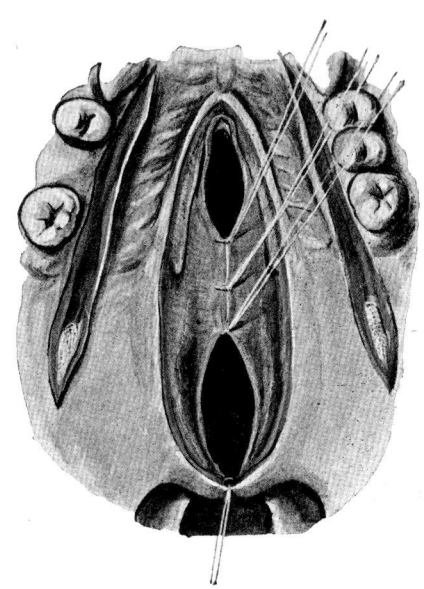

Fig. 147.

filling teeth, can then be led around the bony edge submucously to the nasal side of the bone.

At this point, one may be tempted to push the instrument forward and backward to free the nasal mucosa. This may, however, tear the mucosa, and in this location a rent is apt to enlarge rapidly. Hence the same procedure should be followed as on the oral side and the elevator used only after the connecting fibrous bands have been separated with the knife (Fig. 143). At the posterior edge of the palatine bone, the small bony process (spina nasalis posterior ossis palatini) is reached, from which the insertion of a tiny muscle bundle is severed (Fig. 143). The elevator can now be led around the posterior bony edge.

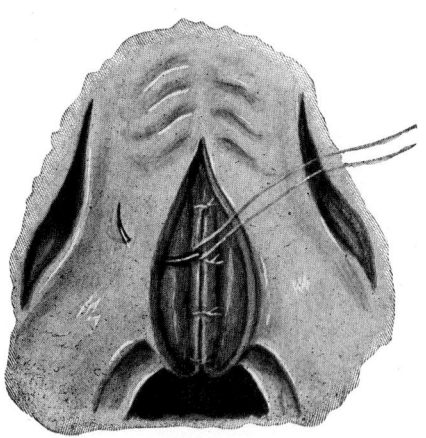

Fig. 148.

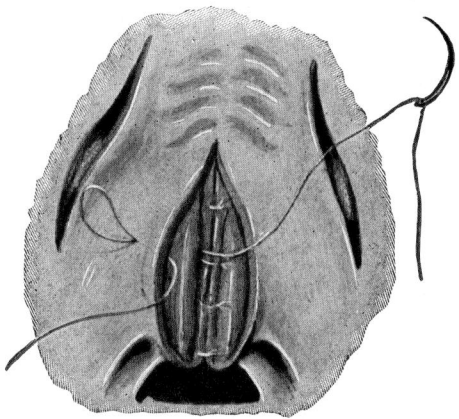

Fig. 149.

Mobilization and formation of the nasal-mucosa flap are now carried out. With the small, curved elevator, the nasal mucosa is elevated from the nasal side of the palatine bone, starting posterior to the bony rim of the palate and gradually working forward until a broad nasal-mucosa flap is formed, which, if pulled mediad, easily reaches the midline.

Preparation of the Cleft Edges of the Soft Palate: From the marginal incision of the soft palate, the latter is split in layers. The oral mucosa is severed from the musculature with knife and scissors (Fig. 144). The uvula itself is dissected in the same way. Muscles and oral mucosa are retracted and the nasal mucosa severed from the muscles (Fig. 145) until the muscle layer is clearly visible as a separate layer, thus permitting a separate suture.

The left side of the palate is prepared in the same way as the right side, in front completing the anterior commissure on the oral as well as

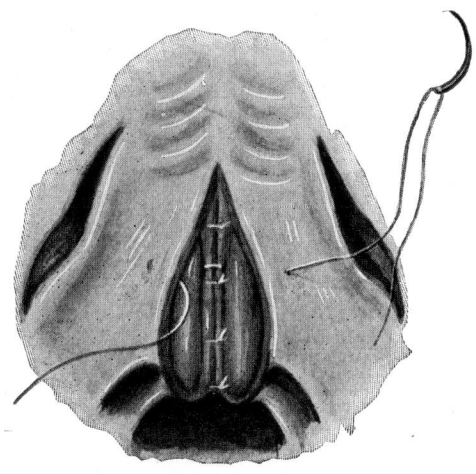

Fig. 150.

333

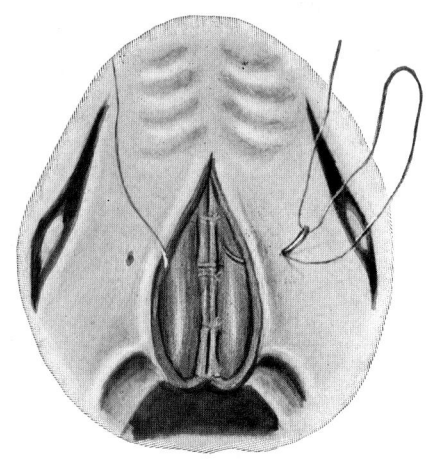

Fig. 151.

on the nasal side. Mobility of the bridge flaps is checked. The importance of adequately freeing the soft tissue from the bone cannot be emphasized too strongly. Both portions of the palate must meet in the midline without any tension.

Suture of Flaps: Approximation of the nasal mucosa is carried out first, and starts with suture of the uvula tip (Fig. 146), followed by sutures of the middle part; 00000 chromic catgut is used, and the sutures are left long for traction (Fig. 147). The remainder of the sutures can be inserted without difficulty.

The muscles of the soft palate are united with two or three sutures of 000 chromic catgut as demonstrated in Figures 148 to 152.

Approximation and suture of the oral bridge flaps now follow. If the assistant pulls the uvula posteriorly by grasping the uvular traction

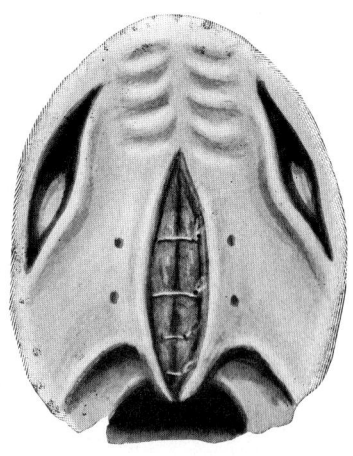

Fig. 152.

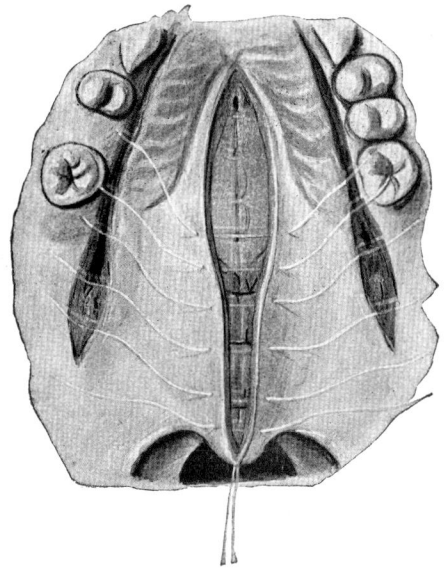

Fig. 153.

suture, approximation is facilitated. The posterior part is sutured first
and then the anterior one (Figs. 153, 154), care being taken that the
wound edges are well adapted.

The temporary packings are removed. Axhausen advises packing
the pharyngeal pockets to keep the soft palate relaxed during the healing
period (dry gauze, Oxycel, is good). We have seen no need for this if
dissection has been thorough.

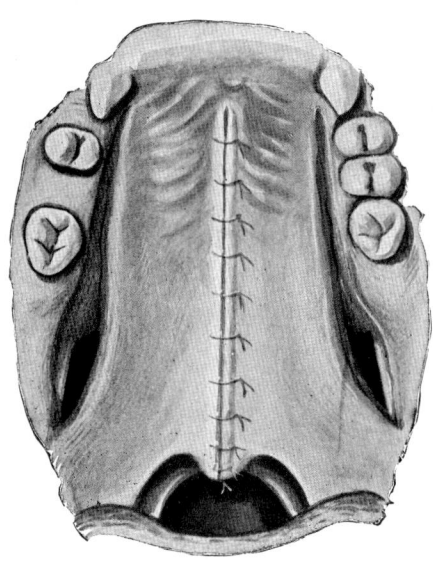

Fig. 154.

335

Axhausen, Wassmund, and Schuchardt now insert a celluloid plate which has been prepared preoperatively. It is fastened to the upper teeth. Its purpose is to hold the palatal flaps snugly against the roof of the palate. This prosthesis is changed frequently for cleansing and replacing a gauze pad which is placed upon the plate. The gauze pad is later replaced by a gutta-percha plug. This support is discarded after four or five weeks. The author has found no need for this prosthetic aftercare; however, in special cases the palatal flaps must be supported. This is done either with the above-described method or with the simpler one described on page 341.

After-Treatment

The patient is placed in bed on his abdomen and given fluids intravenously. Antibiotics do not need to be administered routinely. Sterile water by mouth is given after nausea if the patient is able to swallow. In children the arms are splinted, as described on page 295. After the first twenty-four hours, the patient receives liquid diet including milk, gelatine, ice cream, and the like. The diet is changed to soft foods as soon as the patient can swallow without difficulty (three to four days postoperatively). After the temperature has returned to normal, the patient is allowed to sit up and get out of bed. The patient is discharged eight or ten days after operation.

UNILATERAL CLEFT PALATE

In this form of cleft, the cleft reaches in front between the processus maxillaris on the lateral side and the vomer on the median side. The vomer is attached to the processus palatinus; hence, only one half of the nasal cavity is open. A typical example is the through-and-through cleft-lip-cleft-palate case in which the lip and alveolar clefts have been closed previously, as depicted in Figure 155. Again the improved von Langenbeck operation is performed. At the vomer, however, a flap of mucoperiosteum is made and turned over to the lateral side, where it is attached to the palatal mucosa (Veau). For reasons already mentioned on page 280, the bridge flaps should not be carried too far anteriorly. Shifting a mucoperiosteal flap from the maxilla across and over the vomer flap is rarely necessary and is unwise from the standpoint of future growth (Waldron, Dunn).

Technique

The lateral incisions for formation of the palatine bridge flaps are similar to those described in the foregoing (Figs. 133, 134), but they are not carried as far forward as demonstrated in these figures. Fig-

ure 155 shows their approximate length. The development of the pharyngeal pocket and severance of the hamulus are similar to the steps depicted
in Figures 136 to 139. On the median (closed) side, a turnover flap of the
vomerine mucoperiosteum is now made (Figs. 155, 156). The borderline between the pale palatine and the dark-red vomerine mucosa is clearly
visible. An incision is made along this line, starting in front and connected
in back with the incision along the margin of the soft-palate cleft. The
vomerine mucoperiosteum is elevated. This is not difficult in front, but

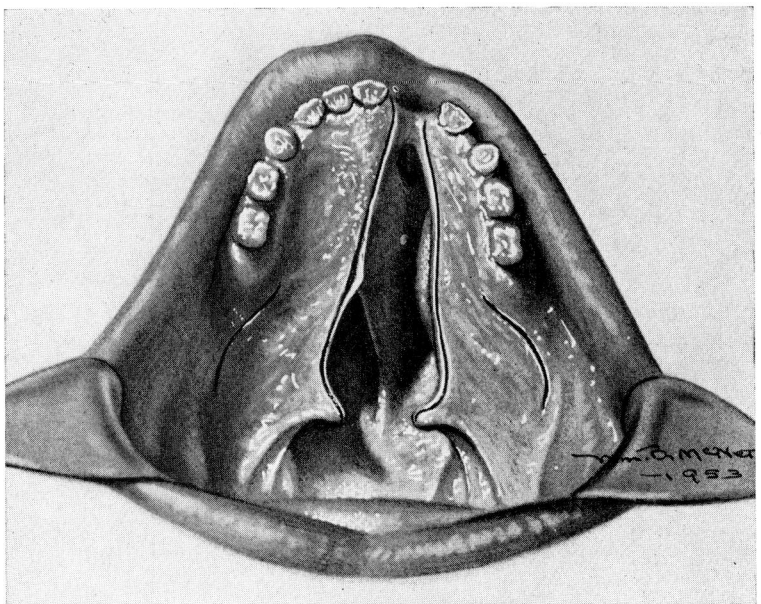

Fig. 155. Closure of unilateral cleft palate with utilization of vomer flap; incisions
are lined out.

at the posterior rim great care should be taken not to sever the vomerine
mucosa from the nasal mucosa of the soft palate. The posterior osseous
connection with the posterior edge of the hard palate is dissected free
with the knife, and the muscular and fascial attachments of the spina nasalis
posterior ossis palatini are severed until the small elevator can be led
around the posterior rim of the hard palate to the nasal side. To obtain
free motility of the vomerine nasal-mucosa flap, the posterior rim of the
vomer must be freed submucously (Fig. 156). The margin of the soft
palate is split in the usual way (compare with Figs. 144, 145).

On the lateral side of the cleft, an incision is made along the rim of
the hard palate, and the mucoperiosteum of the margin is elevated for
about 2 or 3 mm. (Fig. 156). The vomerine mucoperiosteal flap is now

337

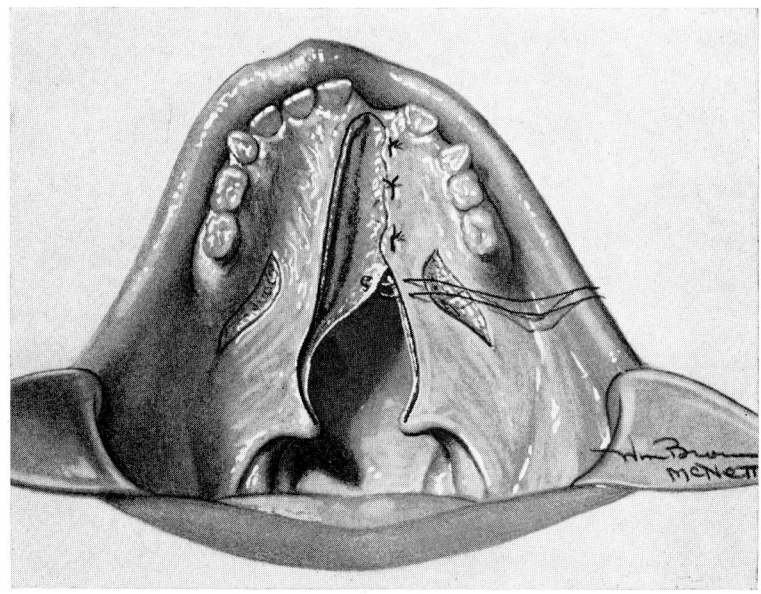

Fig. 156. Closure of unilateral cleft palate with utilization of vomer flap. Vomerine flap turned over to be tucked beneath lateral mucoperiosteal flap with "vest-over-pants" type of mattress sutures.

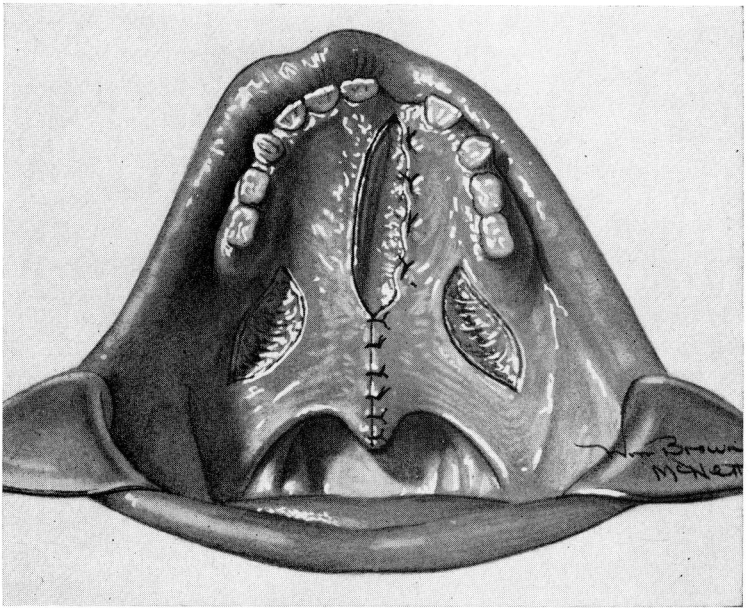

Fig. 157. Closure of unilateral cleft palate with utilization of vomer flap. Remainder of cleft closed as far anteriorly as possible.

338

turned over to the lateral side and sutured beneath the elevated periosteal surface of the lateral mucoperiosteum with three mattress sutures of the "vest-over-pants" type (Fig. 156; see also p. 611). At the posterior rim, the vomerine flap passes gradually over into the nasal mucosa of the soft palate, which is sutured to the other side. The following steps are as described (Fig. 157; compare also with Figs. 146 to 153).

After-Treatment

See page 336.

BILATERAL CLEFTS

The term "bilateral cleft of the palate" may not be quite correct, but it is descriptive. In this type of cleft, there is no connection between the vomer and the palatine process (compare with foregoing paragraph); the oral cavity communicates with either nasal cavity; the vomer hangs free in the middle. To this group belong the extensive postalveolar clefts and the bilateral through-and-through lip-palate clefts. The type of closure of these bilateral clefts depends upon the condition of the vomer, i.e., whether the vomer is fully developed or rudimentary and short. In the former case, closure can be accomplished in one stage, while in the latter case two stages are required. A typical example of closure of the former type (i.e., with fully developed vomer) is the repair of the bilateral cleft of a case of through-and-through lip-palate cleft in which the lip and alveolar clefts have been closed previously (see also p. 303).

Technique (in Cases with Fully Developed Vomer)

The operation is similar to that described for closure of unilateral cleft palates in which much use is made of a vomer flap (see Figs. 155-157), the only change being that the mucous membrane of the vomer—the vomer hangs free in the middle—is split upon the vomerine ridge and a flap of mucoperiosteum is reflected on either side of the vomer and turned over to the lateral sides, tucked beneath, and attached to the palatine mucosa as in the unilateral type and depicted in Figure 156. The vomer bone is left denuded to granulate and heal.

In cases in which the vomer is rudimentary, the operation is divided into two stages. In the first stage, the posterior part of the cleft is closed; in the second stage, the anterior part is closed. This operation requires extensive denudation of the hard palate; this may result in a disturbance of the growth centers if the operation is carried out too early (see p. 280). Hence, it may be advisable to follow Schweckendiek's advice and close the posterior part of the cleft first as far anteriorly as possible, and close

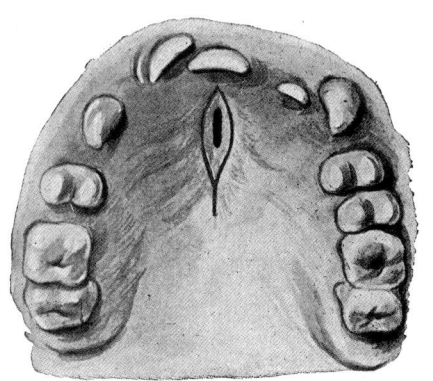

Fig. 158. (Figs. 158-162 are from G. Axhausen: Technik und Ergebnisse der Spaltplastiken. C. Hanser, München.)

the remaining anterior cleft much later, when the child is seven years old (see p. 280).

Technique (in Cases with Underdeveloped Vomer)

Stage 1: The posterior part of the palate is closed as described on page 324; it is emphasized that the palatine arteries should not be severed or ligated but stretched as described on page 347. The cleft is closed as far anteriorly as is possible without causing tension of the flaps.

Stage 2: The anterior hole (often larger and longer than depicted in Fig. 158) is closed after four or five weeks, or later if much dissection of the hard palate is required (see foregoing paragraph). The rim of the hole is circumscribed with an incision which is extended posteriorly for a short distance (Fig. 158). The incision should penetrate deeply but not through the whole thickness of the tissues. A bilateral turnover flap is made and hinged inward (Fig. 159). Two single-pedicle lateral flaps are now made, which are to be shifted mediad (Fig. 160). The undermining

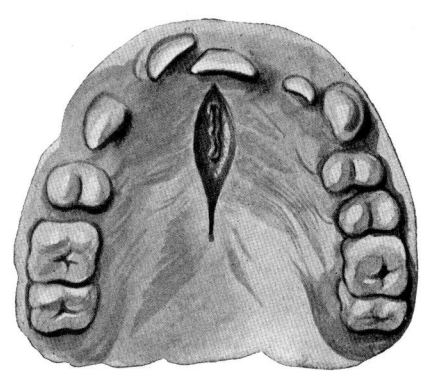

Fig. 159.

340

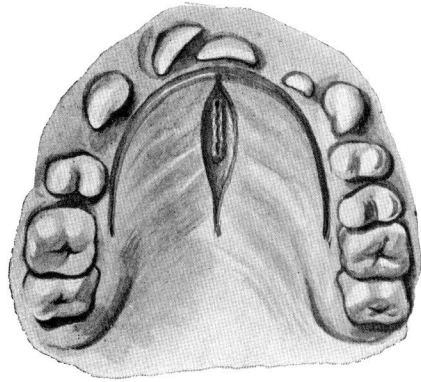

Fig. 160.

for mobilization of the flaps should start from the median side. The oral mucosa is severed from the nasal mucosa until the palatine bone is reached. Mobilization can then be completed from the lateral side; starting from the lateral side may tear the nasal mucosa. The base of the pedicles of the flaps should be level with the posterior point of the median incision. Mobilization, however, should be carried farther back (Fig. 160). To achieve perfect coaptation of both flaps in the midline, it is necessary to split the median wound edge (Fig. 161). After the flaps are sutured together (Fig. 162), they are held in place for one week with a piece of dental compound, which is softened in warm water, molded in place, and fastened with dental wires which cross from one side of the dental arch to the other and are made to pass through the mold while the latter is still soft.

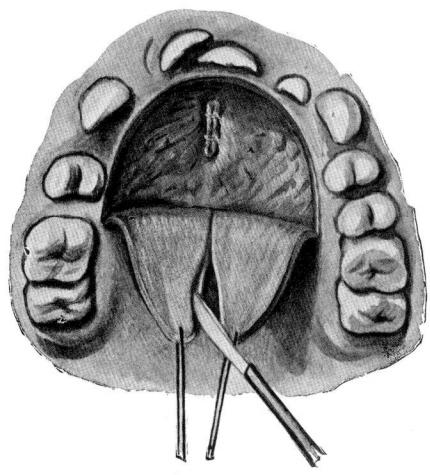

Fig. 161.

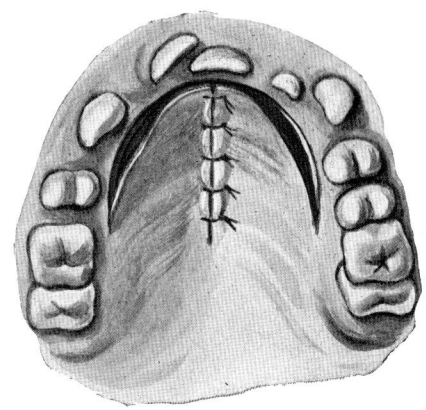

Fig. 162.

CLEFTS ASSOCIATED WITH SHORT PALATE

In this type of cleft, not enough tissue is present to achieve sufficient length of the palate posteriorly. Hence, the nasopharynx cannot be entirely closed by the patient. Such velopharyngeal insufficiency causes a speech defect.

As previously mentioned (p. 323), velopharyngeal closure can be achieved (1) by moving the palate closer to the posterior pharyngeal wall through lengthening the palate, (2) by moving the posterior pharyngeal wall forward (transfer of a pharyngeal flap to the soft palate), or (3) by a combination of these methods. Steffenson presents an excellent review of this topic to 1952.

Palate Lengthening: This can be achieved by elongation of the palate on the buccal aspect as mentioned on page 323; it can be carried out during primary repair. Although in these procedures dividing the mucoperiosteum transversely in front and the aponeurosis in back along the bone plate permit some elongation (see Fig. 163, *B, C*), the intact nasal mucosa limits the amount of elongation considerably. A great degree of palatal lengthening can be achieved through transverse division of the nasal mucosa and aponeurosis. However, a large open area posterior to the bony plate will remain, and development of granulations and of cicatricial contracture of the raw surface would nullify the initial success (Fig. 163 *D*). Hence, closing of this area is a necessary aim which has evoked considerable ingenuity. The earliest method is the so-called "pushback" operation of Dorrance, who skin grafted the raw surface (Figs. 163 *E*, 166). The other methods of palate lengthening can be divided into those in which nasal or vomerine mucosa is utilized for lining (Cronin and Brauer) and those in which palatal mucosa is used (Millard, Edgerton) (Fig. 169).

342

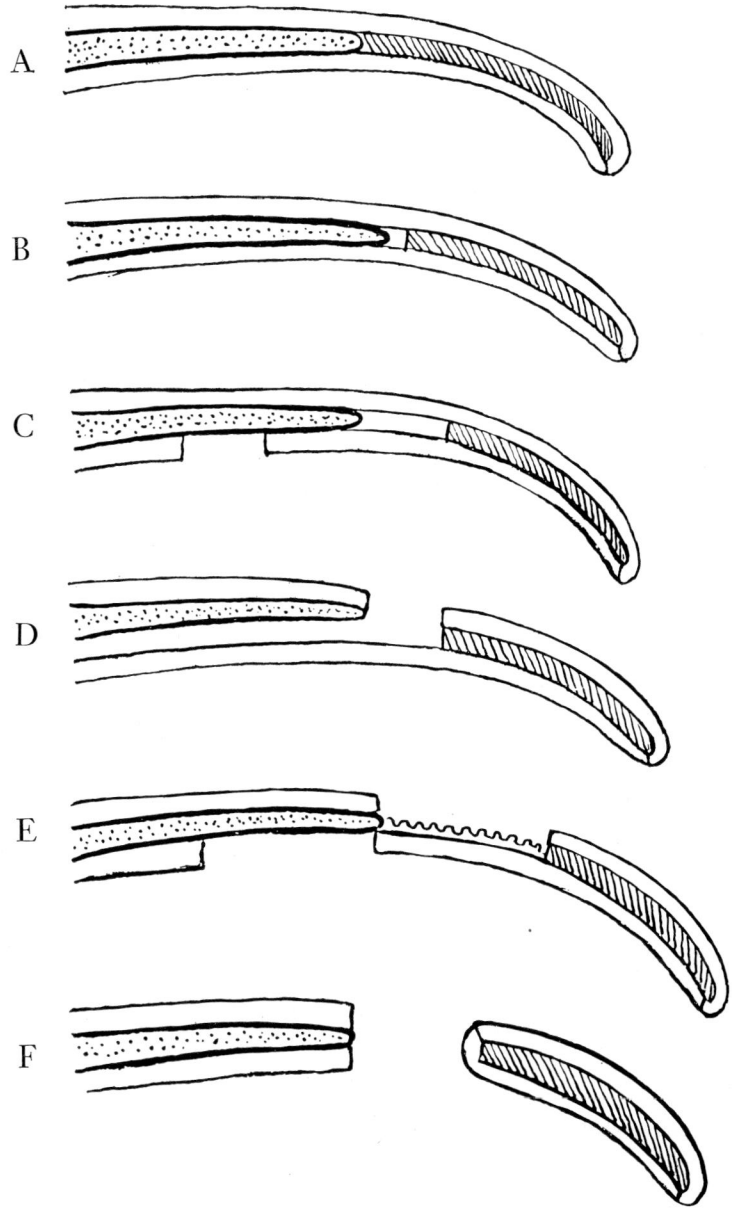

Fig. 163. Palate lengthening procedures. Attention has centered principally on the junction of the hard and soft palates as site for elongation. (Holdsworth, W. B.: Cleft Lip and Palate, 3rd ed., W. Heinemann, 1967.)

THE HEAD AND NECK

The principle of lengthening the palate through division of nasal mucosa dates back to Gillies (1921), who, after severing the nasal and buccal mucosa, inserted a dental prosthesis after Fry to fill the hole (Fig. 163 F). A much more practical method was later devised and popularized by Dorrance under the name "pushback" operation (1925). It consists of freeing almost the entire mucoperiosteum from the hard palate with a horseshoe-shaped incision, dividing the greater palatine vessels, the nasal mucosa, and the aponeurosis from their attachment to the hard palate. Thus the whole palate can be pushed back. Much later (1943), Dorrance became concerned about the resulting raw surface on the nasal side; he advocated skin grafting this surface. J. B. Brown adopted Dorrance's principle, but he did not sever the palatine vessels, and he condemned skin grafts for nasal lining to avoid the foul odor caused by the normal discharge from skin grafts. Although the pushback principle of Dorrance is still favored in certain types of short palates, the closure of the raw surface is achieved in a different and more effective way (p. 347). The pushback operation can be performed primarily in cases with definite shortness of the palate, or more often as a secondary operation where the first operation has resulted in velopharyngeal insufficiency. The operation should not be performed until the patient has reached the age of five since it requires extensive denudation of the hard palate; this may disturb its growth centers if the procedure is performed too early (see p. 322).

Technique (Dorrance's Pushback Operation)

Stage 1: Through an incision along the alveolar arch, a flap of mucoperiosteum is raised from the hard palate (Figs. 164, 165). The posterior palatine vessels are divided and the flap freed from its bed all the way back to the attachment of the palatine aponeurosis (Fig. 165). A split-skin graft is sutured to the raw surface of the flap (Fig. 166). The flap is then returned to its original site and sutured (Fig. 167). Pressure dressing is applied with dental compound, as described on page 341.

Stage 2: From three to ten weeks later—depending upon the color of the flap—the flap is again raised and the palatine aponeurosis and nasal mucosa freed from their connection with the posterior border of the hard palate. The hamular process is divided with a chisel. The relaxation incisions are extended backward around the maxillary tuberosity and over the pterygomandibular fold, freeing the palate from all bony attachments. The entire palate is now pushed back and the anterior portion of the flap sutured with four wire sutures to the fibrous membrane and to the bone at the apex of the defect (Fig. 168). The borders of the cleft are denuded. Interrupted sutures are passed through the nasal mucosa but not tied until the insertion of the intramuscular wire suture around

344

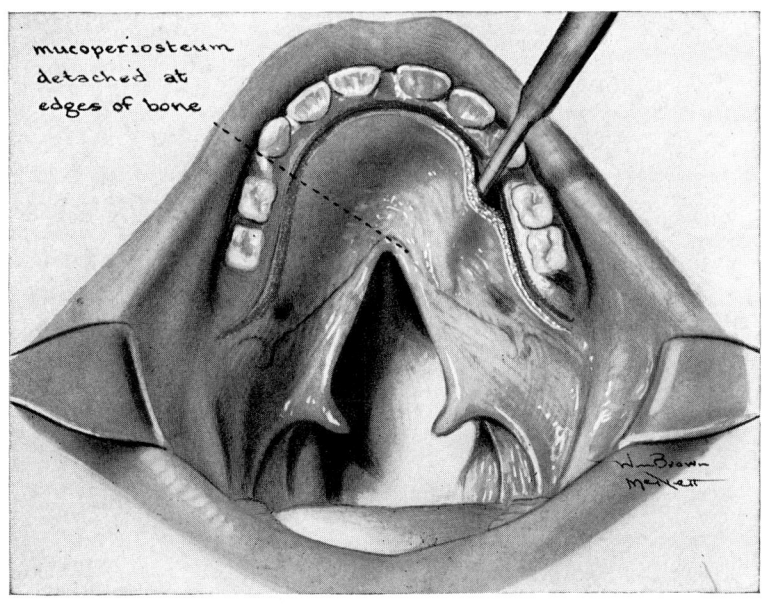

mucoperiosteum
detached at
edges of bone

F i g. 1 6 4.
(Figs. 164-
168 are from
G. M. Dor-
rance and J.
W. Brans-
field: Ann.
Surg.)

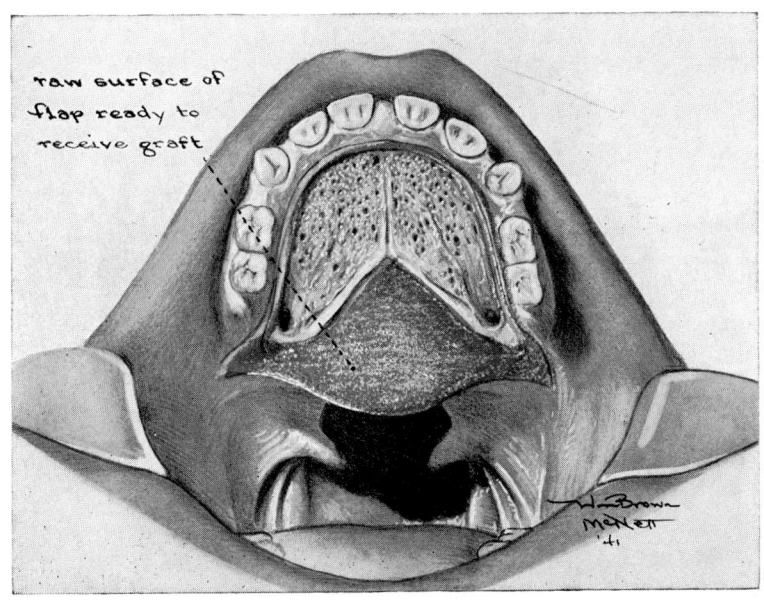

raw surface of
flap ready to
receive graft

Fig. 165.

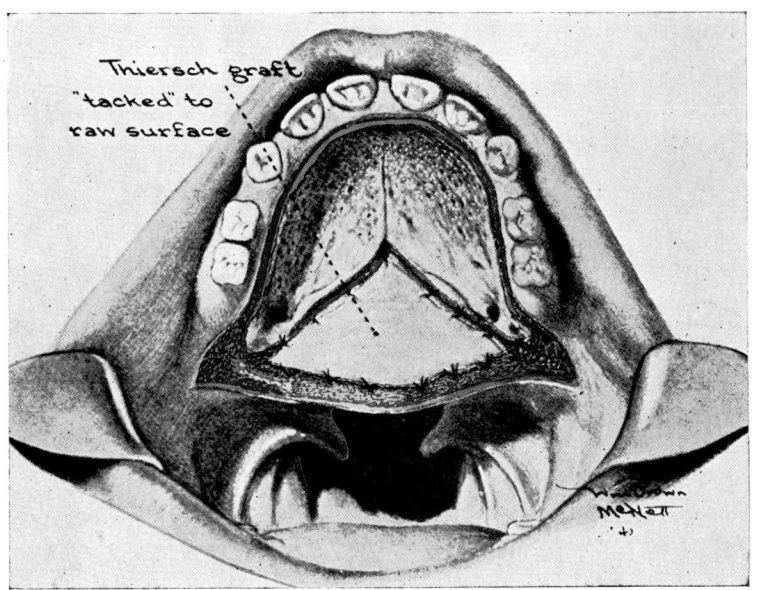

Fig. 166.

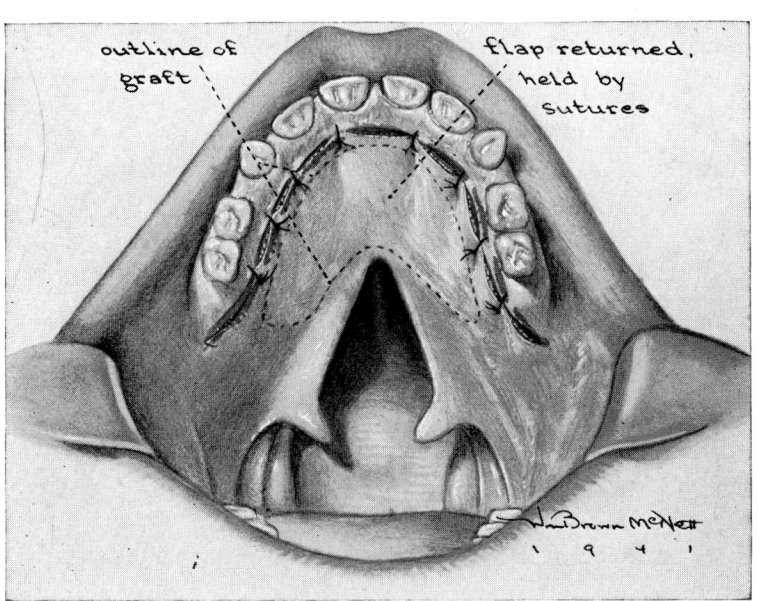

Fig. 167.

the muscles, as in Veau's procedure. The interrupted sutures are then tied, followed by twisting of the wire suture and approximation and suture of the oral mucosa.

This pushback type of palate lengthening has certain disadvantages. Brown's objection to the odor which emanates from the skin graft must be respected. Brown also objects to severing the descending palatine vessels and advocates blunt mobilization of the vessels from the major palatine foramen. Limberg had previously described removal of the bone from around the palatine vessels to gain more vessel length and thus more length for palatal pushback. Edgerton found that by cutting the neurovascular

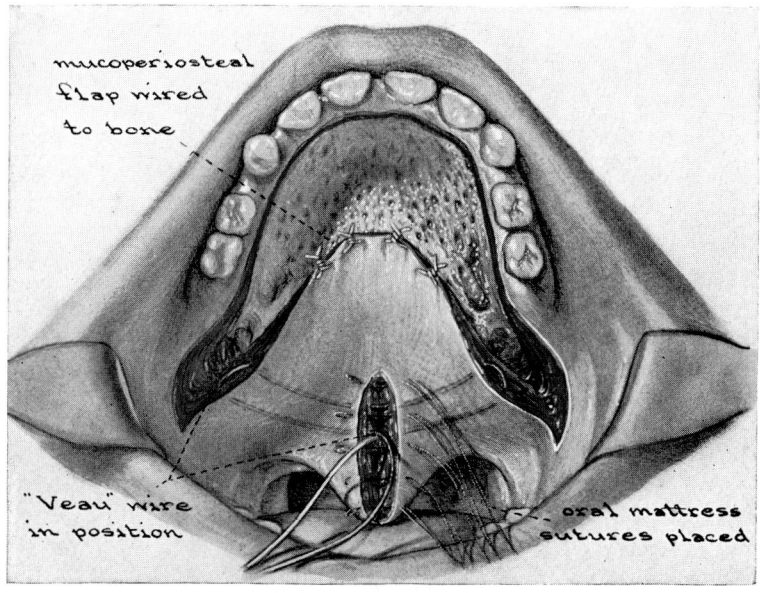

Fig. 168.

bundles free from the undersurface of the palatal mucoperiosteal flap or flaps the same amount of vessel length is gained. Still, the problem of coverage of the raw nasal surface remains. Cronin's method of mobilizing nasal-floor mucosa is said to be technically difficult and bloody. It was Millard who solved this problem by means of transfer of an island flap of mucoperiosteum on the palatine neurovascular bundle of one side. This principle was enthusiastically endorsed by Edgerton; the author also recommends it highly.

Technique (Fig. 169)

A horseshoe-shaped flap of mucoperiosteum is elevated from the hard palate and the major palatine foramina are located. Under sharp dis-

347

section, the neurovascular bundles, containing the palatine artery and vein and two small nerves, are dissected free from the undersurface of the mucoperiosteal flap. On the side of the island flap, the dissection is carried forward to within 1.5 cm. of the tip of the flap. The island flap is then cut, consisting of an ellipse of mucoperiosteum of 2 to 3.5 cm. in size. The aponeurosis and the nasal mucosa at the posterior border of the hard palate are divided. The incisions are prolonged as required behind the maxillary tuberosities and over the pterygomandibular fold so that the hamuli may be broken and the attachments of the soft palate to bone can be completely divided. The island flap is turned over 180 degrees and sutured to the defect edges of the nasal mucosa to supply the missing lining. The whole palate is now pushed back. The half of the palate opposite to the island flap, after sharp dissection of the neurovascular bundle from its undersurface, is moved toward the midline and transposed posteriorly until it overlaps the posterior edge of the bony cleft. Holes are drilled through bony edges and the flap is sutured with wire into its new position.

Millard uses this operation also in primary repair when the palate is short, repairing the soft-palate cleft at the same time. Edgerton uses this technique almost routinely in primary-cleft closure. In unilateral cases, the island flap is taken from the cleft side.

Moving the Posterior Pharyngeal Wall toward the Palate (Velopharyngoplasty): Moving the posterior pharyngeal wall toward the palate can be achieved by mobilization and transfer of a flap from the posterior pharyngeal wall (Passavant, 1862; Schoenborn, 1876; Rosenthal, 1924; Padgett, who introduced this method to this country in 1930; Conway, Stark; Sanvenero-Roselli; Moran; Marino; Dunn; and Skoog). It can also be achieved by suturing the velum into the posterior pharyngeal wall (Trauner).

Through the flap itself, as well as through its pull, the soft palate is lengthened and retrodisplaced without narrowing the nasopharynx to such an extent that it would interfere with breathing or swallowing; yet,

———————————————————————————————➤

Fig. 169. *A:* Incomplete cleft in a short palate. Potential island marked. *B:* Dorrance mucoperiosteal flap turned back with the neurovascular bundles intact. *C:* Nasal attachment to posterior edge of hard palate has been divided completely allowing pushback of palate. One neurovascular bundle is dissected from mucoperiosteal flap to allow cutting off the island flap which has been marked. *D:* neurovascular bundle carrying mucoperiosteal island flap has been turned easily into the nasal lining defect. Chisel ostectomy of posterior bony wall of the greater palatine foramen is being accomplished on opposite side. *E:* Cleft closure and pushback completed. Island flap has supplied the nasal lining of the lengthened soft palate. (D. R. Millard: Plast. Reconstr. Surg.)

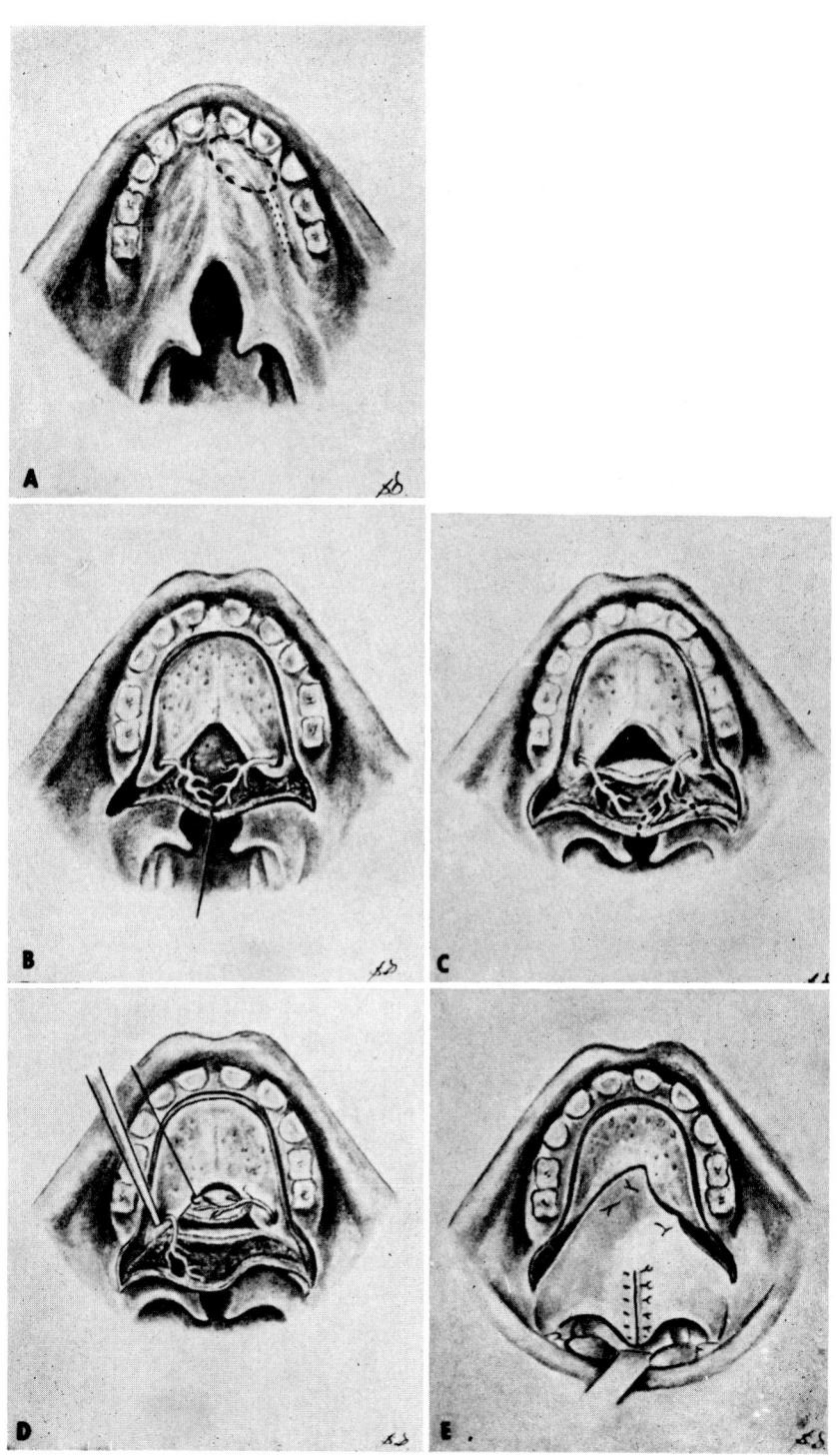

as Rosenthal emphasizes, the flap should not be made too narrow. Moran points out that the pharyngeal-flap operation should be restricted to those secondary palate cases where operative correction has not brought about the desired speech, in spite of vigorous speech training. He suggests that the operation should not be delayed too long; an incompetent palato-pharyngeal sphincter may not respond quickly to thorough training exercises. It is better to achieve early improvement of the sphincter with a flap operation than to have the patient form poor speech habits with objectionable nasality. Moran does not combine the pharyngeal-flap operation with the pushback operation, since he considers it unnecessary in the majority of cases. Conway, Burian, Marino and Segre, however, report better results after the combined operation than after the pharyngeal-flap operation alone. R. Stark warmly advocates this procedure in primary repair. Dibbel et al. even use the flap for resurfacing the raw nasal surface after pushback. Rosenthal, Conway, and Stark pedicle the flap downward; Padgett, Sanvenero-Roselli, and Moran pedicle it upward. Skoog has used both ways and did not notice any significant difference in speech nor any influence on hearing or nasal function. The author has used the downward pedicled flap.

Technique (*Postpharyngeal Flap*)

The operation is performed under local or general anesthesia (endotracheal anesthesia through the mouth). The posterior pharyngeal wall is distended with procaine to facilitate dissection and minimize bleeding. The soft palate is retracted forcibly (Fig. 170). A tongue-shaped flap is outlined at the posterior wall of the pharynx; its free edge is placed as high (cranially) as possible; the pedicle comes to lie downward. It should be at least 2 cm. ($1\frac{3}{16}$ inch) wide. The orifices of the Eustachian tubes should be looked for and avoided. To outline such a flap, the arches of the soft palate must be retracted anteriorly. Traction sutures are placed at the lateral margins of the flap, and incisions are made through the mucosa and superior constrictor pharyngeus muscle. The flap is dissected away from the prevertebral fascia and the donor area at the postpharyngeal wall closed with catgut sutures. Rosenthal emphasizes the importance of this step, since it helps bring about a "mesopharyngoconstrictio" for improvement of phonation. A mucosal flap is now made from the oral surface of the soft palate (Fig. 171). This flap is hinged posteriorly. The pharyngeal flap is now laid upon the raw surfaces of the palate and of the hinge flap and sutured to the wound edges (Fig. 172).

350

Technique (Velopharyngorraphy after Trauner)

In this method, part of the posterior rim of the soft palate is united with the posterior pharyngeal wall so that only two small lateral openings and one median are left to permit nasal breathing and passage of nasal secretion. From an incision along the posterior rim of the soft palate, starting near the tonsillar fossa and crossing the uvula, the velum is split in three layers, as in preparation for closure of clefts of the soft palate. The palate is now pressed against the posterior pharyngeal wall. A curved incision is made through the latter in line with the posterior palate rim. The inci-

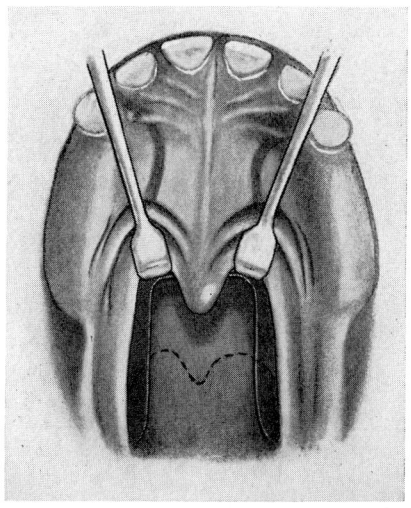

Fig. 170. Conway's technique of transfer of postpharyngeal flap to soft palate. First step in the construction of a posterior pharyngeal flap. The rigid soft palate is retracted forcibly so that the flap will have sufficient length to bridge the gap of the wide-open velopharyngeal aperture. In a typical procedure the flap is 2 cm. wide and 6 cm. long. If the flap is not fashioned from a high enough level, attempts to mobilize a shorter flap by caudal extensions of the two parallel incisions may cause undue tension on the flap when sutured to the soft palate. Mucosa and superior constrictor pharyngeus muscle are included in the flap. The posterior pharyngeal defect is closed by undercutting and suture of the cut margins of muscle and flap so that the sphincteric action of the constrictor muscle is regained. (H. Conway: Plast. Reconstr. Surg.)

sion goes through the mucosa and muscle layer. The lower part of the pharyngeal wound is mobilized and elevated a short distance. If possible, the posterior or nasal mucosa of the soft palate is sutured to the upper pharyngeal wound edge. The main suture, however, is a mattress suture of nylon through the muscles of the velum and pharynx; two such sutures are placed, one on the right and one on the left side. A long, curved

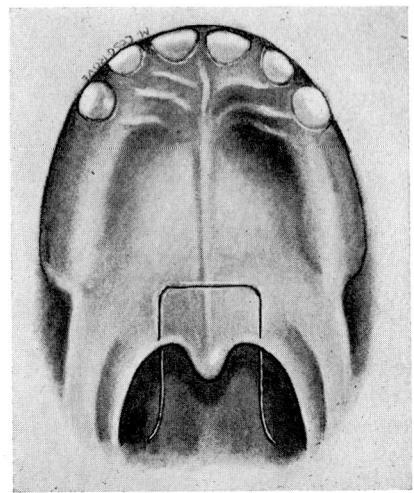

Fig. 171. The lines on the soft palate indicate the incision for attachment of the soft palate. The mucosa thus outlined is rotated posteriorly so that a rectangular raw surface presents on the oral side of the soft palate to which the pharyngeal flap is sutured. (H. Conway: Plast. Reconstr. Surg.)

needle enters the oral mucosa of the velum about 1.5 cm. (⁹⁄₁₆ inch) from the wound edge in front of the tonsillar fossa, penetrates the muscle layer, and escapes near the wound edge of the nasal mucosa. The other end of

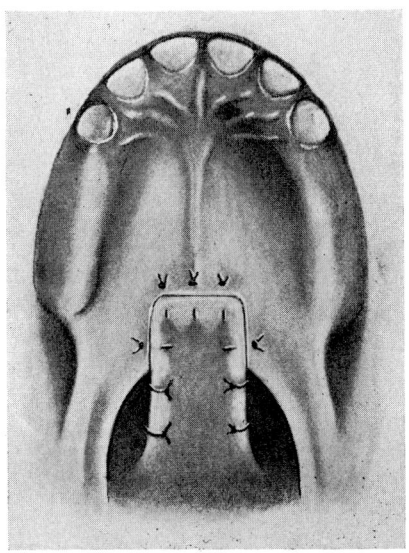

Fig. 172. The posterior pharyngeal flap (based inferiorly) is sutured to the raw area on the oral aspect of the soft palate. (H. Conway: Plast. Reconstr. Surg.)

the thread is laid more mediad and about 1 cm. (⅜ inch) from the wound edge in a similar way. Both ends are now passed behind the muscle layer of the lower pharyngeal wound flap to escape through the pharyngeal mucosa through different exits, which should be about 1.5 cm. (%₁₆ inch) from the wound edge. They are now tied over small, short rubber tubings. Suture of the oral palatal and lower pharyngeal wound edge follows. Trauner originally left a 5-mm. (¼-inch) hole in the middle, but recently has not done so. If the lateral openings are not adequate to permit sufficient drainage of nasal secretion, it is easy to create an opening in the center with a pair of scissors. The nylon sutures are removed on the tenth postoperative day.

Trauner and those who have had experience with this method claim greater improvement of speech following it than with any other. The author endorses it enthusiastically. If the palate is too short, a pushback operation may be performed in the same or a preceding sitting.

SUBMUCOUS CLEFT PALATES

This type of cleft palate is uncommon, but should be recognized if it exists. Gylling and Soivio recently reviewed the literature and paid tribute to the valuable work of Calnan. They, themselves, contributed to the diagnosis and treatment of the cleft. In the German literature Kriens and Wulff discuss this subject in great detail.

Speech impairment (rhinolalia aperta), evident since birth or becoming manifest later, for instance after adenoidectomy, is a common symptom. Hence, in many cases patients are referred because of speech nasality. A common finding is a bifid uvula. Also, upon saying *ah*, the patient may reveal a median thinned portion in the mobile soft palate which widens with palatal movements, revealing the absence of muscles in this area. This can further be ascertained by transillumination (Massengill) and palpitation, which may also reveal a V-shaped defect in the hard palate. X-ray examination according to the method of Calnan may be of value. Speech training should be given a trial in these cases. If it fails, the submucous cleft should be repaired in conjunction with a pushback operation of the type of Millard-Edgerton (p. 347). If this procedure is not entirely successful in achieving marked improvement of speech, a velopharyngoplasty, preferably of the Trauner type (p. 351), should secondarily be added. The author has used the latter procedure without repair of the submucous cleft or pushback operation in two cases of congenital short palate with excellent functional result. The same good experience has been recently recorded on a larger scale by Crickelair, Striker and Casman.

THE HEAD AND NECK

SECONDARY REPAIR OF PALATINE DEFECTS

Small or large holes or defects of the palate following primary repair can be successfully closed surgically in the majority of cases. It is the consensus that obturators, fastened to the dental arch, should be recommended only in exceptional cases, since most patients grow dissatisfied with these appliances. It goes beyond the scope of this book to describe in detail all the various methods which have been recommended for repair. Size and location of the defect vary; consequently, surgical methods differ and have to be adapted to each case. Padgett, in an excellent article, evaluates many of the applicable procedures.

Small fistulas, usually located at the junction of soft and hard palate, may be successfully closed by frequent touching of the area with tincture of cantharides or silver nitrate. *Larger holes* are circumscribed by an incision, the inner wound edges are turned inward (a similar procedure is depicted in Figs. 158, 159), and the defect is covered with a single, posteriorly pedicled flap, which is taken from the immediate neighborhood of the defect. The secondary defect, resulting from shifting the flap, is left to granulate. In defects with *extensive loss of tissue,* in the hard or soft palate or both, flaps from the palate itself are not available. Hence, one must resort to the transfer of buccal mucous-membrane flaps or, if the soft palate is defective, pharyngeal flaps. Occasionally, lined flaps from distant parts of the body are required, such as from the hairless region of the upper arm or neck and chest. Edgerton and Zovikian and others have demonstrated remarkable successes. In patients with large anterior holes and short and even partially cleft soft palates, Struppler performs closure of the cleft with such a flap and a velopharyngorraphy after Trauner. He prepares the flap for closure of the hole in the same sitting (velopharyngorraphy), while closure of the hole with the flap is performed in subsequent sittings.

SPEECH TRAINING AND ORTHODONTIA

Cleft-palate repair has two aims: anatomical restoration and development of normal speech. If the repair has resulted in a well-arched palate and sufficient velopharyngeal closure, the young patient as a rule is able to develop normal speech. In other patients, however, even after good surgical closure, a speech defect may be left, owing to shortness of the palate, or dental malocclusion, or psychological handicaps, and the like. Speech training alone is often not enough, and additional surgery may be required (see pp. 342-353), as well as an effective rehabilitation program.

354

These patients should have the benefit of opinions from various special-
ists, such as the surgeon, orthodontist, otolaryngologist, psychologist, and
speech therapist. Recognition of this fact is leading to the etablishment,
in various parts of this country, of group clinics, which are financed
either privately or publicly, for the rehabilitation of cleft-palate patients.

RARE FACIAL CLEFTS

For reasons explained on page 274 (see also Fig. 87), these clefts are
often associated with other facial deformities. This topic has been recently
discussed by May, Stark and Saunders, Randall and Royster, Fogh-Anderson, Grabb, and Longacre, deStefano and Holmstrand, Khoo Boochai.
The distribution of these deformities varies; what does not vary is maldevelopment of the mandible and of the ear, which is nearly always
present to some degree.

There is good reason for this. After fusion in the midline, the mandibular arches bifurcate and develop the maxillary processes. The lips
split away from the gum region and form the mouth. The original lateral
extent of the mouth is at the point of bifurcation (Fig. 86). Directly behind
this point the auricle develops, derived from the mandibular arch and
also the hyoid arch (second branchial arch) (Fig. 86). Hence, a close
interrelationship in the development of mandible, mouth and ear is apparent. In some of these interrelated deformities the mandibular parts of
the external ear (tragus, crus helicis, and helix) as well as the hyoid parts
(anthelix, lobule and concha) may remain rudimentary and retain their
embryonic proportions in the form of skin and cartilage elevations or tabs.
The external auditory canal may also be absent or only apparent as an
amniotic-like furrow, since it develops from the first branchial groove,
bounded by the first two arches (Fig. 173).

Aside from deformities or underdevelopments of the ear, a host of
other deformities may be present which have been classified under various
names. In 1944, Franceschetti and Zwahlen recognized the common nature
of this complex of deformities and called it dysostosis mandibulo facialis.
They recognized that other writers, such as Treacher Collins (1900),
had already described similar syndromes, but they considered these cases
"abortive." In 1949, Straith and Lewis reported this syndrome for the
first time in American literature under the name Treacher Collins syndrome; they were followed by O'Connor and Conway and others. This
syndrome is now well recognized and includes: lack of development of
lower eyelids, oblique palpebral fissures, notching of rims of outer thirds of
lower lids, deficiency of malar bone and infraorbital ridge, micrognathia,
and ear deformities. These deformities may be bilateral, unilateral, and

355

accompanied by transverse clefts, less often by other clefts and deformities of the extremities.

Recently, subgroups with characteristic deformities have been picked out and classed under such terms as the dysostosis mandibularis which occurs as a rule unilaterally, involves only the lower part of the face (Case 17, p. 1016), and in which transverse clefts are very often present (Case 40, p. 1046). Francois and Haustrate, who discuss this topic thoroughly, suggest collection of all the dysostoses under the term "syndrome of the first arch (mandibular)." All of these dysostoses have one fundamental significance in common: aplasia of the mandible. It would lead too far from the main topic to go into more detail here. The pathogenesis of these congenital defects is ably discussed by recognized authorities in an international symposium edited by J. T. Longacre.

Of all the rare clefts, transverse clefts are most often encountered. They vary in extent, and may range from a mere broadening of the oral commissure (Case 41, p. 1048) to a complete unilateral or bilateral division of the face. Ordinarily, however, they are unilateral and do not extend beyond the anterior border of the masseter muscle (Fig. 173; Case 40, p. 1046). The cleft edges are lined with a vermilion border-like membrane. In some cases, only the median cleft borders are vermilion lined, while the lateral part of the cleft edges are lined with skin. Sometimes at the point where the commissure would normally be there is a step-like elevation beneath the vermilion which is caused by the free edges of the orbicularis oris muscle (Case 42). The direction of the cleft is horizontal or obliquely upward, depending upon the location of the ear. It seems to radiate toward the tragus or its rudiments. With the mouth closed the cleft may or may not close tightly. In short clefts the defect may not even be visible. It shows up as soon as the mouth is opened and particularly upon smiling. The mouth then becomes a macrostoma, not only from the increased width of the aperture, but also from lack of a muscular commissure since the orbicularis muscle is divided and cannot act as a checkrein to prevent lateral displacement. In the more extensive cases another phenomenon becomes apparent. When the child cries, the lower cleft side is drawn downward and backward. There are two reasons for this. Transverse clefts are often part of a mandibular arch syndrome, and hence are frequently accompanied by underdevelopment or partial absence of the mandible and underdevelopment of the mandibular parts of the cheek. This in itself gives the appearance of a downward displacement or deviation of the lower cleft side. The deformity, however, becomes accentuated upon crying or laughing when the powerful triangularis and quadratus labii muscles contract, together with the risorius muscle. Because of the division of the orbicularis oris muscle, a strong oral commissure is absent; these muscles are unopposed and, upon

356

contraction, cause the downward displacement, even in cases in which the mandibular parts of the cheek are normally developed.

Technique of Repair of Transverse Facial Clefts
(Fig. 173; Cases 40-42, pp. 1046-1049)

Hence, the key point in the repair of the cleft must center upon the reconstruction of a muscular commissure, i.e., the closure of the orbicularis ring at the cleft side. This can be done effectively by means of the Estlander method. The principle of this method is the formation and rotation of a full-thickness vermilion-lined flap from one lip into the opposing one. The author suggests that the flap be taken from the lower cleft side; it should contain the free edge and full thickness of the orbicularis muscle. A corresponding defect should then be created on the upper cleft side where the normal commissure would be and the flap rotated into the defect. This not only closes the orbicularis ring but also keeps the sagging lower cleft side "uplifted." The remainder of the cleft edges are denuded of their lining and sutured together in layers. This step, as well as the closure of the secondary defect at the donor site of

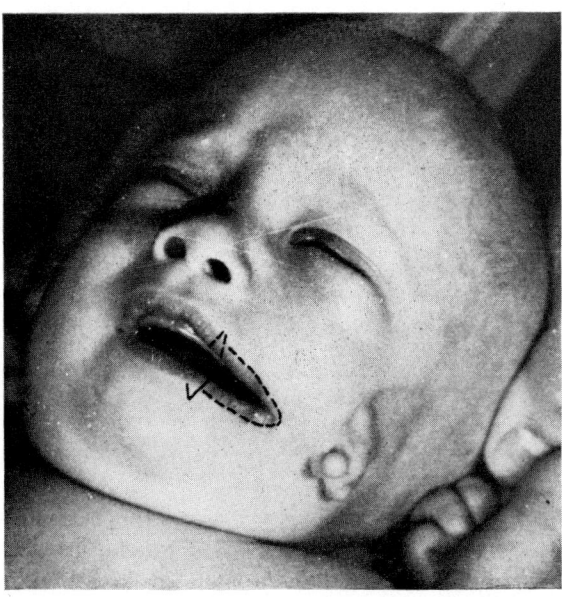

Fig. 173. Transverse facial cleft. Commissure of mouth to be formed by rotation of a small full-thickness, vermilion-border lined flap from lower lip into triangular defect of upper lip. The flap should contain the free edge and full thickness of orbicularis muscle. Flap at lower lip and defect at upper lip are outlined as are the incisions for closure of the cleft. From experience with this case (for end result see p. 1047) I advise using a multiple W-plasty for skin closure (p. 187) instead of a straight line to counteract possibility of subsequent contracture. (H. May: Plast. Reconstr. Surg.)

the flap, should be completed before rotation of the flap. The flap can be made rather small since it need only contain the orbicularis muscle. Hence, it is similar only in principle to the Estlander flap. It is made triangular to facilitate closure of the donor site. It must contain the coronary artery, since this is the main nutrient vessel. Since in wide transverse clefts the resulting transverse scar crosses the elastic lines of the cheek vertically, hypertrophy and contracture of the scar may result (Case 40, p. 1046), which later can be broken up by a multiple Z-plasty. Schuchardt advises the Z-plasty during the primary repair. The author agrees and recommends breaking up the straight line by a multiple W-plasty to counteract the possibility of subsequent contracture (the multiple W-plasty is described on p. 187). The mucous membrane which is redundant can be closed in a straight line.

Early closure of the transverse cleft (six to twelve weeks of age) is desirable. Major correction of concomitant deformities of ears, mandible, and so forth, must be postponed until the child is twelve to fourteen years old. If the mandibular segment is underdeveloped and the malar arch absent, the latter, which also will form a ledge for the mandibular joint, is replaced with a bone graft from the pelvis, inserted from an incision well below the branches of the facial nerve, followed at a later date by replacement of the ascending ramus of the mandible with the fifth metatarsal bone (see p. 555). Should the ramus be present, lengthening of the under developed mandible with a bone graft would suffice (Case 42, p. 1049).

Much rarer than those described above are median clefts of the upper lip and, still rarer, those of the lower lip, sometimes associated with clefts of the mandible and tongue. This topic has been thoroughly described by Gutierrez.

DEFORMITIES

MICROSTOMA

Technique for Cicatricial Microstoma (Dieffenbach; Modified after Lexer)

A triangular-shaped piece of skin and muscle is removed lateral to each side of the microstoma, leaving the mucous membrane intact. The tip of the triangle should come to lie on a level perpendicular with the pupilla. The vermilion border, together with the mucous membrane, is now cut across to a point close to the tip of the triangular defect, leaving a mucous-membrane angle which should be sutured to the tip of the triangular skin defect. This may be facilitated by blunt separation and mobilization of the adjacent mucous membrane of the cheek. The mucous-membrane flaps are now united with the skin edges. There may be some buckling where the vermilion border passes over into the mucous membrane. Removal of a rhomboid piece of the vermilion-border edge will correct the deformity.

Technique (May)

In microstoma following the switching of vermilion-border-lined flaps, a double Z-operation is applicable, as described on page 256.

A

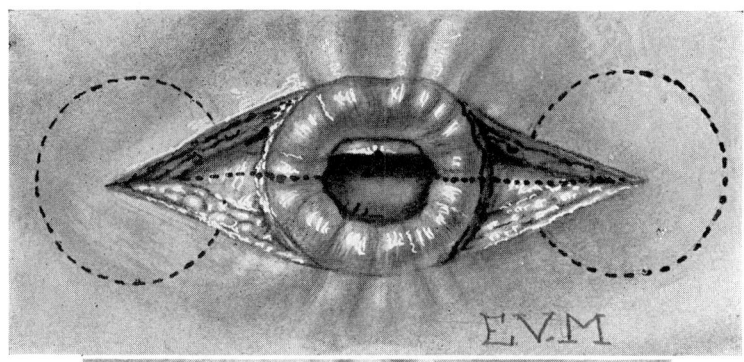

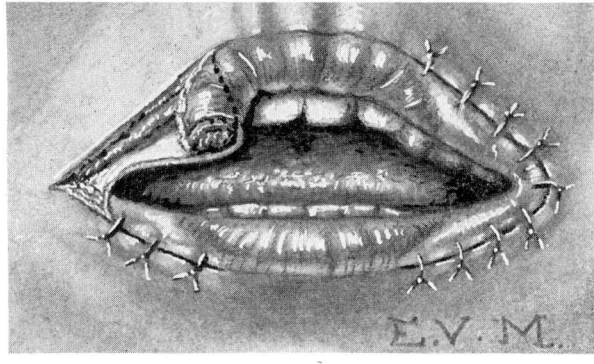

B

Fig. 174. *A:* Repair of cicatricial microstoma (Dieffenbach-Lexer). Removal of triangular pieces of skin and muscles. Dotted lines indicate extent to which surrounding skin is undermined. *B:* Vermilion border and mucous membrane are cut across and sutured to wound edges.

THE HEAD AND NECK

CICATRICIAL ECTROPION OF LIPS

These deformities are, in the majority of cases, due to burns. In cases of the lower lip, the contracture may involve the lip alone or may be due to pull from scars involving chin and neck (Cases 3, 22, 89, pp. 992, 1021, 1103). The correction of the ectropion consists in excision of the entire contracting scar, reduction and overcorrection of the contracture, and application of a thick split graft. The sutures of the graft are left long and tied over mechanic's waste to exert pressure. In those cases, however, in which much of the subcutaneous tissue is destroyed and replaced by scar tissue, a flap should be transplanted after removal of all cicatricial tissue. In selecting the flap site, a flap from the immediate neighborhood may not be available because of extensive cicatricial scarring. The best flap site may be the supraclavicular area, with the flap pedicled on a lateral neck tube.

CICATRICIAL ENTROPION AND RECONSTRUCTION OF OBLITERATED GINGIVOLABIAL SULCUS

The entropion of the lip is due to scar formation at the mucous-membrane side and, as a rule, is combined with cicatricial obliteration of the gingivolabial sulcus. The repair of the latter corrects the deformity of the lip. The reconstruction of the gingivolabial sulcus is done according to the Esser-Waldron technique (see p. 39). With an incision along the obliterated sulcus, the lip is freed from the bone deeper than required so that secondary shrinkage may be counteracted. A mold of dental compound is now prepared, as described on page 39, and a skin graft draped around it with the raw surface outward; after insertion of mold and graft, the margins of the wound are sutured, thus burying the mold. If the margins of the wound cannot be sutured, the mold must be held in place by other means. In the case of a lower lip, this is done with two circumferential wires placed between two teeth around the mandible, as described on page 552. Mold and graft are inserted into the gutter between the wire loops and the wires tightened around them. In the case of an upper lip, sutures are placed around the mold through the upper parts of the lip and tightened at the outside over small rolls of gauze. For postoperative treatment, see page 39.

CICATRICIAL DISPLACEMENT OF ANGLE OF MOUTH

This condition is corrected with the "N" type of incision. The operation starts with a V-like incision circumscribing the angle of the mouth

(Fig. 175). The incision penetrates through the whole thickness of the cheek. In the case of an upward displacement, an incision is made through the cheek, starting from the lower end of the V and running parallel to its upper arm. Thus, two triangular flaps are created which are exchanged with each other in a manner similar to that in the Z-operation (see p. 186). Downward displacements can be repaired by a reversal of the procedure.

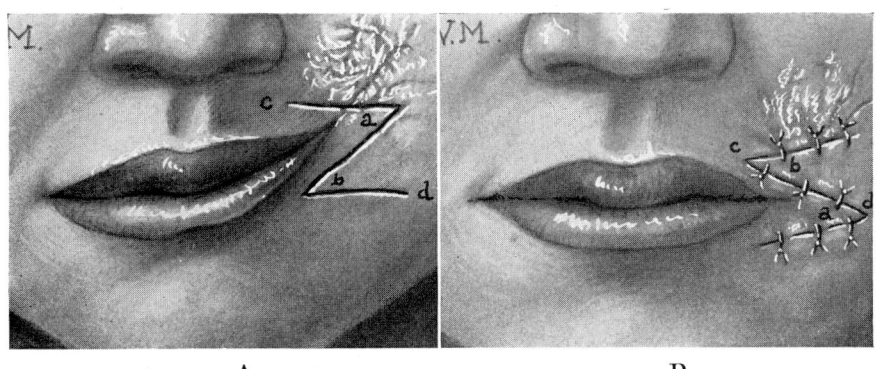

A.   B.

Fig. 175. Repair of cicatricial displacement of angle of mouth by formation of two triangular full-thickness cheek flaps. Their outlines form an N. *B:* Two triangular flaps are exchanged with each other.

If the scars of the adjacent parts of the cheek must also be repaired, they are excised and the defects covered either with a graft (Case 5, p. 995) or a flap preferably taken from the clavicular area on a lateral cervical tube.

HYPERTROPHY OF LIP AND DOUBLE LIP

Simple hypertrophy of the lip becomes particularly noticeable if associated with a hanging lip. The operation for repair of the deformity is simple. With an elliptiform incision, reaching from commissure to commissure along the mucous membrane on the posterior side of the lip, a wedge-shaped piece of tissue of proper thickness is removed and the defect closed by simple suturing. To avoid buckling of the midportion of the lip, additional excision of a vertical wedge-shaped piece of tissue may become necessary, as is done for correction of a double lip (Fig. 176). The latter, usually the upper lip, is due to a groove bisecting the vermilion border, occasionally containing large openings from deep mucoid cysts. Concerning repair of this deformity, Figure 176 is self-explanatory. Cysts, if present, must be removed.

361

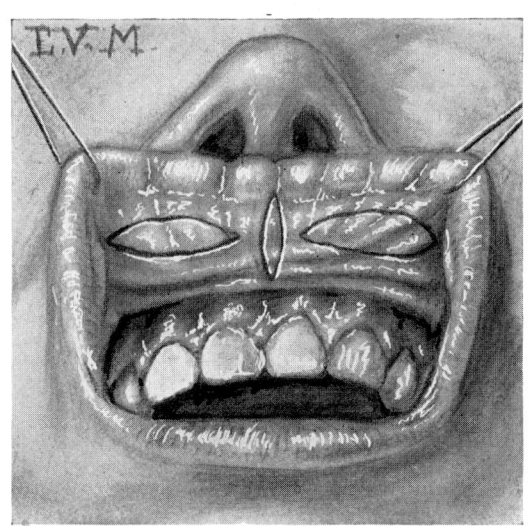

Fig. 176. Correction of double lip. Horizontal excision of ellip-tiform piece of buccal tissue from each side of lip. Excision of vertical piece to avoid buckling of midportion.

SECONDARY DEFORMITIES AFTER REPAIR OF CLEFT LIP

For repair, see page 311.

DEFORMITIES OF CHIN

For reparative surgery of deformities of the chin, see pages 571-584.

BIBLIOGRAPHY

DEFECTS (OTHER THAN CLEFTS) OF LIPS AND CHIN

ABBÉ, C. R.: *A new plastic operation for the relief of deformity due to double harelip.* M. Rec., 53:477, 1898.

AF SCHULTÉN, M. W.: *Eine Methode um Defekte der einen Lippe mit einem brückenformigen Lappen aus der anderen zu decken.* Deutsche Ztschr. f. Chir., 39:97, 1894.

ASHLEY, F. L., SCHWARTZ, A. N., and DRYDEN, M. F.: *A modified technique for creating a lower lingual sulcus.* Plast. Reconstr. Surg., 22:204, 1958.

BAKAMJIAN, V.: *Use of tongue flaps in lower lip reconstruction.* Brit. J. Plast. Surg., 17:76, 1964.

THE LIPS, CHIN, AND PALATE

BERNARD, C.: *Cancer de la lèvre inferieur Operé par un procedé nouveau.* Bull. et mém. Soc.d. chirurgiens de Paris, 3:357, 1853.

BROWN, J. B.: *Switching of vermilion bordered lip flaps.* Surg. Gynec. Obstet., 46:701, 1928.

BUCK, G.: *Contributions to Reparative Surgery.* D. Appleton & Co., New York, 1876.

BUROW, C. A.: *Berschreibung einer neuen Transplantations Methode (Methode der seitlichen Dreiecke) zum Wiederersatz verlorengagangener Teile des Gesichts.* Nauck, Berlin, 1855.

CANNON, B.: *The split vermilion bordered lip flap.* Surg. Gynec. Obstet., 73:95, 1941.
The use of vermilion bordered flaps in surgery about the mouth. Surg. Gynec. Obstet., 74:458, 1942.

DIEFFENBACH, J. F.: *Chirurgische Erfahungen.* Abb. 3: u. 4, Berlin, 1834, p. 101.

ESTLANDER, J. A.: *Eine Methode aus der einen Lippe Substanzverluste der anderen zu ersetzen.* Arch. f. klin. Chir., 14:622, 1872.

FREEMAN, B. S.: *Myoplastic modification of the Bernard cheiloplasty.* Plast. Reconstr. Surg., 21:453, 1958.

GELBKE, H.: *Abbé-plastik, Technik und Möglichkeiten.* Langenbeck's Arch. u. Deutsche Zeitschrift f. Chir., 289:668, 1958.

GILLIES, H. D.: *Plastic Surgery of the Face, Based on Selected Cases of War Injuries of the Face, Including Burns.* H. Frowde, London, 1920.

GILLIES, H. D., and MILLARD, D. A.: *The Principles and Art of Plastic Surgery.* Little, Brown and Co., Boston, Toronto, 1957.

IVY, R.: *Early and Late Treatment of the Face and Jaws as Applied to War Injuries.* South. Surgeon, 11:366, 1942.

JOSEPH, J.: *Nasenplastik und sonstige Gesichtsplastik.* Curt Kabitzch, Leipzig, 1931.

KAZANJIAN, V. H.: *Treatment of Extensive Loss of the Mandible and Its Surrounding Tissues.* J. Oral Surg., 1:30, 1943.

KAZANJIAN, V. H., and CONVERSE, J. M.: *The Surgical Treatment of Facial Injuries.* Williams and Wilkins, Baltimore, 1949, 1959.

LEXER, E.: *Die Gesamte Wiederherstellungs Chirurgie.* J. A. Barth, Leipzig, 1931.

MARINO, H., GANDOLFO, E. A., and RIZZO, M.: *Reconstructive surgery in cancer of the lower lip.* Prensa Med. Argent., 52:973, 1965.

MARTIN, H. E.: *Cheiloplasty for advanced carcinoma of the lip.* Surg. Gynec. Obstet., 54:914, 1932.

MAY, H.: *One-stage operation for closure of large defects of lower lip and chin.* Surg. Gynec. Obstet., 73:236, 1941.
Closure of defects of lips with composite vermilion-border lined flaps. Ann. Surg., 120:214, 1944.
Closure of defects after cancer surgery. Clinics, 4:53, 1945.
Surgical treatment of cancer of lips. J. Plast. Reconstr. Surg. 9:424, 1952.
Gesichtsplastiken nach Krebsbehandlung. Langenbeck's Arch. u. Deutsche Zeitschrift f. Chir., 289:501, 1958.

THE HEAD AND NECK

McGREGOR, I. A.: *The tongue flap in lip surgery*. Brit. J. Plast. Surg., 19:253, 1966.

NEW, G. B., and FIGI, F. A.: *The repair of postoperative defects involving the lips and cheeks secondary to the removal of malignant tumors*. Surg. Gynec. Obstet., 62:182, 1936.

OWENS, N.: *Simplified method of rotating skin and mucous membrane flaps for complete reconstruction of the lower lip*. Surgery, 15:196, 1944.

PADGETT, E. C.: *Cheiloplasty for Cancer of the Lip*. Int. J. Orthodont. 22:939, 1936.

PIERCE, G. W., and O'CONNOR, G. B.: *A new method of reconstruction of the lip*. Arch. Surg., 28:317, 1934.

REINHARDT, W.: *Die Plastische Chirurgie*. Stuttgart, F. Enke, 1953.

SANVENERO-ROSSELLI: Rev. Chir. Struct. (Belg.) 6:413, 1936.

SCHUCHARDT, K.: *in Bier, Braun, Kümmell's Chirurgische Operationslehre*, 7th Edition, Vol. 2. J. A. Barth, Leipzig, 1954.

SCHUCHARDT, K. and WASSMUND, M.: *Fortschritte der Kiefer- und Gesichts-Chirurgie*. A Yearbook, Vol. II. Georg Thieme, Verlag, Stuttgart, 1957.

SMITH, F.: *Reconstructive Surgery of the Head and Neck*. Nelson Loose-Leaf System. Thomas Nelson & Sons, New York.
Manual of Standard Practice of Plastic and Maxillofacial Surgery. Military Surgical Manuals, National Research Council. W. B. Saunders, Philadelphia, 1942.
Plastic and Reconstructive Surgery; a Manual of Management. W. B. Saunders, Philadelphia, 1950.

SMITH, J. W.: *Clinical experiences with vermilion bordered lip flap*. Plast. Reconstr. Surg., 27:527, 1961.

SPIRA, M., and HARDY, S. B.: *Vermilionectomy. Review of cases with variations in technique*. Plast. Reconstr. Surg., 33:39, 1964.

SZYMANOWSKI, J.: *Zur plastischen Chirurgie*. Vrtljschr. f. d. prakb. Heilk., 60:127, 1858.

WEBSTER, J. P.: *Crescentic peri-alar cheek excision for upper lip flap advancement*. Plast. Reconstr. Surg., 16:434, 1955.

WEBSTER, R. C., COFFEY, R. J., and KELLEHER, R. E.: *Total and partial reconstruction of the lower lip with innervated muscle-bearing flaps*. Plast. Reconstr. Surg., 25:360, 1960.

CLEFTS OF LIP AND PALATE

ADAMS, W. M., and ADAMS, L. H.: *The misuse of the prolabium in the repair of bilateral cleft lip*. Plast. Reconstr. Surg., 12:225, 1953.

AREY, L. B.: *Developmental Anatomy*, ed. 5. W. B. Saunders, Philadelphia, 1947.

AXHAUSEN, G.: *Technik und Ergebnisse der Gaumenplastik*. Georg Thieme, Leipzig, 1936.

THE LIPS, CHIN, AND PALATE

Technik und Ergebnisse der Lippenplastik. Georg Thieme, Leipzig, 1941.
Technik und Ergebnisse der Spaltplastiken. Carl Hanser, München, 1952.

BACKDAHL, M., NORDIN, K., NYLEN, B., and STROMBECK, J.: *Bone grafting to the maxillary defect in cleft lip and palate by the method of Backdahl and Nordin. In Transactions of the Third International Congress of Plastic Surgery.* Excerpta Medica Foundation, Amsterdam, 1964, p. 193.

BARSKY, A. J., KAHN, S., and SIMON, B. E.: *Early and late management of the protruding premaxilla.* Plast. Reconstr. Surg., 29:58, 1962.

BATTLE, R. J. V.: *The past, present, and future in the surgery of the cleft palate.* Brit. J. Plast. Surg., 7:217, 1954.

BAUER, T. B., TRUSLER, H. M. and GLANTZ, S: *Repair of unilateral cleft lip.* Plast. Reconstr. Surg., 11:56, 1953.

BAUER, T. B., TRUSLER, H. M., and TONDRA, H. M.: *Changing concepts in the management of bilateral cleft lip deformities.* Plast. Reconstr. Surg., 24:321, 1959.

BAUTZMANN, H.: *Entwicklungsphysiologische Grundlagen zum Verständnis der normalen und abnormalen Entwicklung des Gesichts- und Kauschädels.* Fortschr. der Kiefer- und Gesichts-Chirurgie VI:1, 1960.
Versuche einer Analyse der Induktionsmittel in der Embryonalentwicklung. Gemeinsam mit 3 Aufsätzen von J. Holtfreter, H. Spemann und O. Mangold. Die Naturwissenschaften 20:971, 1932.

BERKELEY, W. T.: *The cleft lip nose.* Plast. Reconstr. Surg., 23:567, 1959.
The concepts of unilateral repair applied to bilateral clefts of lip and nose. Plast. Reconstr. Surg., 27:505, 1961.

BLAIR, V. P., and BROWN, J. B.: *Mirault operation for single harelip.* Surg. Gynec. Obstet., 51:81, 1930.

BRAUER, R. O.: *A consideration of the LeMesurier technic of single harelip repair with a new concept as to its use in incomplete and secondary harelip repair.* Plast. Reconstr. Surg., 11:275, 1953.
Observations and measurements of non-operative setback of premaxilla in double cleft patients. Plast. Reconstr. Surg., 35:145, 1965.
Push-back repair of the cleft palate with nasal mucosal flaps to prevent late contracture; follow-up results of the Cronin procedure. Plast. Reconstr. Surg., 36:529, 1965.

BRAUER, R. O., and CRONIN, T. D.: *Maxillary orthopedics and anterior palate repair with bone grafting.* Cleft Palate J., 1:31, 1964.

BRAUER, R. O., CRONIN, T. D., and REAVES, E. L.: *Early maxillary orthopedics, orthodontia and alveolar bone grafting in complete clefts of the palate.* Plast. Reconstr. Surg., 29:625, 1962.

BRAUER, R. O. and FOERSTER, D. W.: *Another method to lengthen the columella in the double cleft patient.* Plast. Reconstr. Surg., 38:27, 1966.

BROPHY, T. W.: *Cleft Lip and Palate.* P. Blakiston's Son & Co., 1923.

BROWN, G. V.: *The Surgery of Oral and Facial Diseases and Malformations.* Lea & Febiger, Philadelphia, 1938.

THE HEAD AND NECK

BROWN, J. B.: *Elongation of the partially cleft palate.* Amer. J. Orthodont. & Oral Surg., 24:878, 1938.
Elongation of the partially cleft palate. Surg. Gynec. Obstet., 63:768, 1936.
Switching of Vermilion-bordered lip flaps. Surg. Gynec. Obstet., 46:701, 1928.
Double elongations of partially cleft palates and elongations of palates with complete clefts. Surg. Gynec. Obstet., 70:815, 1940.

BROWN, J. B., and McDOWELL, F.: *Secondary repair of cleft lips and their nasal deformities.* Ann. Surg., 114:101, 1941.
Simplified design for repair of single cleft lips. Surg. Gynec. Obstet., 80:12, 1945.
Small triangular flap operation for single cleft lip. Plast. Reconstr. Surg., 5:392, 1950.

BROWN, J. B., McDOWELL, F., BYARS, L. T.: *Double clefts of the lip.* Surg. Gynec. Obstet., 85:20, 1947.

BURIAN, F.: *Surgery of Cleft Lip and Cleft Palate.* Prague—Statni Zdravotnicke Nakladatelstvi, 1955.
Chirurgie der Lippen-und Gaumenspalten. VEB Verlag Volk- und Gesundheit, Berlin, 1963.
Chirurgie roz stepu rtu a patra. Vytvarny Spolupracovnik Juroslav Benda, Praha, 1954.

BURSTON, W. R.: *The early orthodontic treatment of cleft palate conditions.* Dent. Pract. 9:41, 1958.
The pre-surgical orthopedic correction of the maxillary deformity in clefts of both primary and secondary palate. In Transactions of the Second International Congress of the International Society of Plastic Surgeons. Williams and Wilkins, Baltimore, 1960, p. 28.

CALNAN, J.: *Submucous cleft palate.* Brit. J. Plast. Surg., 6:282, 1954.

CARDOSO, A. D.: *New technique for harelip.* Plast. Reconstr. Surg., 10:92, 1952.

COLLINS, E. T.: *Case with symmetrical congenital notches in the outer part of each lower lid and defective development of the malar bones.* Trans. Ophthal. Soc. UK, 20:190, 1900.

CONVERSE, J. M., HOROWITZ, S. L., GUY, C. L., and WOOD-SMITH, D.: *Surgical-orthodontic correction in the bilateral cleft lip.* Cleft Palate J., 1:153, 1964.

CONWAY, H.: *Combined use of the push-back and pharyngeal flap procedures in the management of complicated cases of cleft palate.* Plast. Reconstr. Surg., 7:214, 1951.

CONWAY, H., and STARK, R. B.: *Pharyngeal flap procedure in the management of complicated cases of cleft palate.* Ann. Surg., 142:662, 1955.

CRICKELAIR, G. F., STRIKER, P., and CASMAN, B.: *The surgical treatment of submucous cleft palate.* Plast. Reconstr. Surg., 45:58, 1970.

CRONIN, T. D.: *Management of the bilateral cleft lip with protruding premaxilla.* Amer. J. Surg., 92:810, 1956.
Lengthening the columella by use of skin from nasal floor and alae. Plast. Reconstr. Surg., 21:417, 1958.
Surgery of the double cleft lip and protruding premaxilla. Plast. Reconstr. Surg., 19:389, 1957.

DAVIS, A. D.: *Collective review—management of the wide unilateral cleft lip with nostril deformity.* Plast. Reconstr. Surg., 8:249, 1951.

THE LIPS, CHIN, AND PALATE

DAVIS, W. B.: *Harelip and cleft palate deformities: Some of the types and their operative treatment.* Ann. Surg., 76:133, 1922.
Harelip and cleft palate. Ann. Surg., 87:536, 1928; 88:140, 1929.
Methods preferred in cleft lip and cleft palate repair. J. Int. Coll. Surg., 3:116, 1940.

DENECKE, H. J., and MEYER, R.: *Plastiche Operationen an Kopf und Hals.* Vol. 2. Springer-Verlag, Berlin, 1964.

DIBBELL, D. G., LAUB, D. R., JOBE, R. P., and CHASE, R. A.: *A modification of the combined pushback and pharyngeal flap operation.* Plast. Reconstr. Surg., 36:165, 1965.

DORRANCE, G. M.: *The Operative Story of Cleft Palate.* W. B. Saunders, Philadelphia, 1933.
Lengthening of the soft palate operations. Ann Surg., 82:208, 1925.
Congenital insufficiency of the palate. Arch. Surg., 21:185, 1930.

DORRANCE, G. M., and BRANSFIELD, J. W.: *Cleft palate.* Ann. Surg., 117:1, 1943.

DRILLIEN, C. M., INGRAM, T. T. S., and WILKINSON, E. M.: *The Causes and Natural History of Cleft Lip and Palate.* Williams and Wilkins, Baltimore, 1966.

DUNN, F. S.: *Observations on the pharyngeal flap operation for the improvement of speech in cleft palate patients.* Plast. Reconstr. Surg., 7:530, 1951.
Management of cleft palate cases involving the hard palate. Plast. Reconstr. Surg., 9:108, 1952.

EDGERTON, M. T., Jr.: *Reconstruction of major defects of the palate.* Plast. Reconstr. Surg., 17:105, 1956.
The island flap push-back and the suspensory pharyngeal flap in surgical treatment of the cleft palate patient. Plast. Reconstr. Surg., 36:591, 1965.
Surgical lengthening of the cleft palate by dissection of the neurovascular bundle. Plast. Reconstr. Surg., 29:551, 1962.

ERICH, J. B.: *A technic for correcting a flat nostril in cases of repaired harelip.* Plast. Reconstr. Surg., 12:320, 1953.

ERNST, FRANZ: *Zur Frage der Gaumenplastik.* Centralbl. f. Chir., 52:464, 1925.
Die Gaumenspalten und ihre Behandlung. In KIRSCHNER, M., and NORDMANN, O.: *Die Chirurgie.* Wien, Urban and Schwarzenberg, Berlin and Wien, 1927, Vol. 4, p. 666.
Die Gaumenspalten und ihre chirurgische Behandlung. Fortschr. d. Zahnh., 2:999, 1926.

FEDERSPIEL, M. N.: *Harelip and Cleft Palate.* C. V. Mosby Co., St. Louis, 1927.

FOGH-ANDERSEN, P.: *Incidence of cleft lip and palate: constant or increasing?* Acta Chir. Scand., 122:106, 1961.
Rare clefts of the face. Acta Chir. Scand., 129:281, 1965.
Inheritance of Harelip and Cleft Palate. Nyt. Nordisk Forlag-Arnold Busck, Copenhagen, 1942.
Pharyngeal flap operation in velopharyngeal insufficiency. Acta Chir. Scand., 105:92, 1953.

FOSTER, T. D.: *Maxillary deformities in repaired clefts of the lip and palate.* Brit. J. Plast. Surg., 15:182, 1962.

THE HEAD AND NECK

FRANCESCHETTI, A., and KLEIN, I.: *The mandibulo-facial dysostosis, a new hereditary syndrome.* Acta Ophthal., 27:144, 1949.

FRANCESCHETTI, A., and ZWAHLEN, P.: *Un nouveau syndrome: la dystose mandibulo-faciale.* Bull. schweiz. Akad. Med. Wissensch. 1:60, 1944.

FRANCOIS, J., and HAUSTRATE, L.: *Anomalies colobomateuse anglobe oculaire et syndrome du premier arc.* Ann. ocul. 187:340, 1954.

GABKA, J.: *Hasenscharten und Wolfsrachen, Entstehung und Behandlung,* ed. 2, 1963.

GELBKE, H.: Die Schnittführung nach LeMesurier und andere moderne Gesichtspunkte bei der Operation von Lippenspalten. Bruns' Beiträge zur Klinischen Chirurgie. Band 188, Heft 4 (1954).
Unsere derzeitige Lippenspaltenchirurgie. Langenbeck's Archiv für Klinische Chirurgie. Deutsche Zeitschrift für Chirurgie, 282:616, 1955.
The nostril problem in unilateral harelips and its surgical management. Plast. Reconstr. Surg., 18:65, 1956.

GEORGIADE, N. C., PICKRELL, K. L., and QUINN, G. W.: *Varying concepts in bone grafting of alveolar palatal defects.* Cleft Palate J., 1:43, 1964.

GILLIES, H. D., and FRY, W. K.: *A new principle in the surgical treatment of congenital cleft palate and its mechanical counterpart.* Brit. Med. J., 1:335, 1921.

GLOVER, D. M., and NEWCOMB, M. R.: *Bilateral cleft lip repair and the floating premaxilla.* Plast. Reconstr. Surg., 28:365, 1961.

GRABB, W. C.: *The first and second branchial arch syndrome.* Plast. Reconstr. Surg., 36:485, 1965.

GUNTER, G. D.: *Nasomaxillary cleft.* Plast. Reconstr. Surg., 32:637, 1963.

GÜNTHER, H., and SPISSL, B.: *Rekonstruktion der Unterlippe nach Carcinomentfernung und gleichzeitiger Ausräumung regionärer Lymphknoten.* Chirurgia Plastica et Reconstructiva 3:229, 1967.

GUTIERREZ, H.: *Median cleft lips (fissures labiales medianes).* Ann. Chir. Plast., 10:97, 1965.

HAGEDORN: *Uber Eine Modifikation der Hasenschartenoperation.* Centralb. f. Chir., 11:756, 1884.
Die Operation der Hasenscharte mit Zickzacknaht. Centralb. f. Chir., 19:281, 1892.

HALLE, M.: *Zur Operation der Gaumenplastik.* Berl. klin. Wchnschr., 55:892, 1918.
Gaumensegelplastik. Laryngologische Gesellschaft zu Berlin, January 20, 1922. Reviewed in Zentralbl. f. Hals-, Nasen- u. Ohrenh., 2:148, 1922, 1923.

HAMELMANN, H.: *Zur Operation der Lippen-Kiefer- und Gaumenspalten nach Schweckendiek.* Langenbeck's Arch. f. klin. Chir. 295:890, 1960.

HARING, O. M., and LEWIS, F. J.: *The etiology of congenital developmental anomalies.* Int. Abstr. of Surg., Surg. Gynec. Obstet., 113:1, 1961.

HARKINS, C. S.: *Surgery and prosthesis in the rehabilitation of cleft palate.* Plast. Reconstr. Surg., 7:32, 1951.
Retropositioning of the premaxilla with the aid of an expansion prosthesis. Plast. Reconstr. Surg., 22:67, 1958.

368

THE LIPS, CHIN, AND PALATE

HARKINS, C. S., BERLIN, A., HARDING, R. L., LONGACRE, J. J., and SNODGRASS, R. M.: *A classification of cleft lip and cleft palate.* Plast. Reconstr. Surg., 29:31, 1962.

HÄUPL, K., and SCHRUDDE, J.: *Kieferorthopädische Gesichtspunkte bei der Behandlung von Lippen- Kiefer-Gaumenspalten.* Langenbeck's Arch. f. klin. Chir. 295:900, 1960.

HERFERT, O.: *Two-stage operation for cleft palate.* Brit. J. Plast. Surg., 16:37, 1963.

HIS, W.: *Anatomie menschlicher Embryonen.* Vogel, Leipzig, 1885.

v. HOCHSTETTER, F.: *Entwicklungrgesichichte des äusseren Gehörganges und der Ohrschel des Menschen.* Denkschrift der Akad. der Wissensch., 109:1948.

HOLDSWORTH, W. G.: *Cleft Lip and Palate.* ed. 3. Grune and Stratton, Inc., New York, 1963.

HONIG, C. A.: *The surgical treatment of median fissure of the face.* Semaine hop. Ann. chir. plast., 33:17, 1957.

HORTON, C. E., CRAWFORD, H. H., ADAMSON, J. E., BUXTON, S., COOPER, R., and KANTER, J.: *The prevention of maxillary collapse in congenital lip and palate cases.* Cleft Palate J., 1:25, 1964.

HOTZ, R.: *Transactions of the First and Second International Symposia on Early Treatment of Cleft Lip and Palate.* Berne, 64, 1946.

HUFFMAN, W. C., and LIERLE, D. M.: *Studies of the pathologic anatomy of the unilateral hare-lip nose.* Plast. Reconstr. Surg., 4:225, 1949.

IVY, R. H.: *Clefts of the Lip and Palate.* Surgery of the Mouth and Jaws, Nelson Loose-Leaf Surgery, 2:631, Thomas Nelson & Sons, New York.
Experiences in cleft palate surgery. Ann. Surg., 112:775, 1940.
Modern concept of cleft lip and palate management. Plast. Reconstr. Surg., 9:121, 1952.
Some thoughts on posterior pharyngeal flap surgery in the treatment of cleft palate. Plast. Reconstr. Surg., 26:417, 1960.

IVY, R. H., and CURTIS, L.: *Procedures in cleft palate surgery; experiences with the Veau and Dorrance technique.* Ann. Surg., 100:502, 1934.

JOHANSON, B., and OHLSSON, A.: *Bone grafting and dental orthopaedics in primary and secondary cases of cleft lip and palate.* Acta Chir. Scand., 122:112, 1961.
Die Osteoplastik bei Spathehandlung der Lippen-Kiefer-Gaumenspalten. Langenbeck's Arch. f. klin. Chir., 295:876, 1960.

JOSS, G., and ROULLIARD, L. M.: *A critical evaluation of the rotation-advancement (Millard) method for unilateral cleft lip repair.* Brit. J. Plast. Surg., 15:349, 1962.

KAHN, S., and WINSTEN, J.: *Surgical approaches to the bilateral cleft lip problem.* Brit. J. Plast. Surg., 13:13, 1960.

KAZANJIAN, V. H.: *Secondary deformities of cleft palates.* Plast. Reconstr. Surg., 8:477, 1951.
Congenital absence of the ramus of the mandible. J. Bone Joint Surg., 21:761, 1939.

THE HEAD AND NECK

KAZANJIAN, V. H., and HOLMES, E. G.: *Treatment of median cleft lip associated with bifid nose and hypertelorism.* Plast. Reconstr. Surg., 24:582, 1959.

KEHL, H.: *Zur Operation der Lippen-Kiefer- und Gaumenspalten nach Schweckendiek.* Langenbeck's Arch. f. klin. Chir., 295:893, 1960.

KERNAHAN, D. A., and STARK, R. B.: *Classification of cleft lip and palate.* Plast. Reconstr. Surg., 22:435, 1958.

KITLOWSKI, E. A.: *Preoperative and postoperative care of congenital clefts of the lip and palate.* Ann. Surg., 95:659, 1932.

KLING, A.: In: *Transactions of the First and Second International Symposia on Early Treatment of the Cleft Lip and Palate.* R. Hotz, ed. Huber, Berne, 1964, p. 193.

KOENIG, P.: *Corrective procedures after operations for harelip or cleft jaw and palate (Ueber Korrektureingriffe nach Operationen von Lippen-Kiefer-Gaumenspalten)* Langenbeck's Arch. u. Deut. Ztschr. Chir., 269:435, 1951.

KRIENS, V. O., and WULFF, J.: *Die submuköse Gaumenspalte Ein Beitrag zu Diagnose, Anatomie, Operations und Sprechpädagogischer Behandlung.* Chir. Plast. Reconstr., 6:255, 1969.

LAMONT, E. S.: *Reparative plastic surgery of secondary cleft lip and nasal deformities.* Surg. Gynec. Obstet., 80:422, 1945.

LANGENBECK, B.: *Die Uranoplastik mittels Ablösung des mucoperiostalen Gaumenüberzuges (5 Operations geschichten).* Arch. f. klin. Chir., 2:205, 1862.

LATTES, and FRANTZ, V.: *Absorbable sponge tests.* Ann. Surg., 121:894, 1945.

LeMESURIER, A. B.: *The treatment of complete unilateral harelips.* Surg. Gynec. Obstet., 95:17, 1952.
The quadrilateral Mirault flap operation for hare lip. Plast. Reconstr. Surg., 16:422, 1955.
Harelips and Their Treatment. Williams and Wilkins, Baltimore, 1962.

LEXER, E.: *Gaumenspalten Operationen.* Deutsche Ztschr. f. Chir., 200:109, 1927.
Grundlegende Neuerrungen bei der Operation angeborener Lippen-Kiefer-Gaumenspalten. Zentralbl. f. Chir., 59:2793, 1932.
Die gesamte Wiederherstellungchirurgie. J. A. Barth, Leipzig, 1931.

LIMBERG, A.: *Neue Wege in der radikalen Uranoplastik bei angeborenen Spaltendeformationen: Osteotomia interlaminaris und pterygomaxillaris, resectio marginia foraminis palatini und neue Plättchennaht, Fissura ossea occulta und ihre Behandlung.* Zentralbl. f. Chir., 1745, 1927.

LONGACRE, J. J.: *The surgical management of the first and second branchial arch syndrome.* Brit. J. Plast. Surg., 18:243, 1965.
Craniofacial Anomalies, Pathogenesis and Repair. J. B. Lippincott, Philadelphia, 1968.

LONGACRE, J. J., deSTEFANO, G. A., and HOLMSTRAND, K. E.: *The surgical management of first and second branchial arch syndrome.* Plast. Reconstr. Surg., 31:507, 1963.

LUHMANN, K.: *Die angeborenen Spaltbildungen des Gesichtes.* Johann Ambrosius Barth, Leipzig, 1956.
Der primäre Verschlus von Gaumenspalten. Langenbeck's Arch. f. klin. Chir., 295: 885, 1960.

LYNCH, J. B., LEWIS, S. R., and BLOCKER, T. G., Jr.: *Maxillary bone grafts in cleft palate patients.* Plast. Reconstr. Surg., 37:91, 1966.

MAHLER, L.: *Die Entwicklung der plastischen Chirurgie der Lippen-Kiefer-Gaumenspalten.* Münchener Medizinische Wochenschrift., 27:1385, 1963.
Über Art und Behandlung von 360 Gesichtsspalten, operiert in den Jahren 1935-1942 in der chirurgischen Universitäts-Klinik Frankfurt am Main. Langenbeck's Arch. f. klin. Chir., 206:66, 1944.

MAISELS, D. O.: *The timing of the various operations required for complete alveolar cleft and their influence on facial growth.* Brit. J. Plast. Surg., 20:230, 1967.

MARCKS, K. M., TREVASKIS, A. E., and DACASTA, A.: *Further observation in cleft lip repair.* Plast. Reconstr. Surg., 12:392, 1953.

MARCKS, K. M., TREVASKIS, A. E., and KICOS, J. E.: *Repair of nasal deformities associated with secondary cleft lip defects.* Transactions of International Society of Plastic Surgeons, 1960.

MARCKS, K. M., TREVASKIS, A. E., and PAYNE, N. J.: *Elongation of columella by flap transfer and Z-plasty.* Plast. Reconstr. Surg., 20:466, 1957.

MARINO, H., and SEGRE, R.: *Cleft palate: Pharyngo-staphyline fixation.* Brit. J. Plast. Surg., 3:222, 1950.

MASSENGILL, R., Jr.: *An objective technique for submucous cleft palate detection.* Plast. Reconstr. Surg., 37:355, 1966.

MATTHEWS, D. N.: *The premaxilla in bilateral clefts of the lip and palate.* Brit. J. Plast. Surg., 5:77-86, 1952.

MATTHEWS, D., and GROSSMAN, W.: *A combined orthodontic and surgical approach to the problem of the collapsed maxilla in cases of cleft palate. In Transactions of the Third International Congress of Plastic Surgery.* Excerpta Medica Foundation, Amsterdam, 1964, p. 239.

MAY, H.: *Cleft lip repair after Axhausen.* Plast. Reconstr. Surg., 1:139, 1947.
The Axhausen operation for cleft lip repair modified after the Hagedorn LeMesurier principle. Plast. Reconstr. Surg., 15:15, 1955.
Transverse facial clefts and their repair. Plast. Reconstr. Surg., 29:240, 1962.

MAZAHERI, M., HARDING, R. L., and NANDA, S.: *The effect of surgery on maxillary growth and cleft width.* Plast. Reconstr. Surg., 40:22, 1967.

McDOWELL, F.: *Late results in cleft lip repairs.* Plast. Reconstr. Surg., 38:444, 1966.

McINDOE, A., and REES, T. D.: *Synchronous repair of secondary deformities in cleft lip and nose.* Plast. Reconstr., Surg., 24:150, 1959.

McNEIL, C. K.: *Congenital oral deformities.* Brit. Dent. J., 101:191, 1956.
Oral and Facial Deformity. Isaac Pitman and Sons, Ltd., London, 1954.

MERKEL, F.: *Die Anatomie des Menschen.* ed. 2, Part I, edited by E. Kallius. J. F. Bergmann, Munchen, 1927.
Handbuch der topographischen Anatomie zum Gebrauch für Aerzte, Vol. 1. Vieweg und Sohn, Braunschweig, 1891, p. 341.

MILLARD, D. R.: *Adaptation of the rotation-advancement principle in bilateral cleft lip.* Presented at Inter. Congress of Plastic Surgeons, London, 1959.
Complete unilateral cleft of the lip. Plast. Reconstr. Surg., 25:595, 1960.

THE HEAD AND NECK

A radical rotation in single harelip. Amer. J. Surg., 95:318, 1958.
Refinements in rotation-advancement cleft lip technique. Plast. Reconstr. Surg., 33:26, 1964.
Wide and/or short cleft palate. Plast. Reconstr. Surg., 29:40, 1962.

MILLARD, D. R., and WILLIAMS, S.: *Median lip clefts of the upper lip.* Plast. Reconstr. Surg., 42:4, 1968.

MIRAULT, G.: Malgaigue's f. Chir., 1844, p. 265.

MONROE, C. W.: *Recession of the premaxilla in bilateral cleft lip and palate.* Plast. Reconstr. Surg., 35:512, 1965.
The surgical factors influencing bone growth in the middle third of the upper jaw in cleft palate. Plast. Reconstr. Surg., 24:481, 1959.

MORAN, R. E.: *The pharyngeal flap operation as a speech aid.* Plast. Reconstr. Surg., 7:202, 1951.

NBOO, BOO CHAI: *The transverse facial cleft.* Brit. J. Plast. Surg., 22:119, 1969.

MORLEY, M. E.: *Cleft Palate and Speech.* ed. 6. Williams and Wilkins, Baltimore, 1966.

MUSGRAVE, R. H.: *Surgery of nasal deformities associated with cleft lip.* Plast. Reconstr. Surg., 28:261, 1961.

MUSGRAVE, R. H., and DUPERTIUS, S. M.: *Revision of the unilateral cleft lip nostril.* Plast. Reconstr. Surg., 25:223, 1960.

NEUNER, O.: *A new method for the velopharyngeal operation.* Plast. Reconstr. Surg., 37:111, 1966.

NORDIN, K. E.: *Bone grafting to the alveolar process clefts following orthodontic treatment of secondary cleft palate deformity.* Transactions of the Inter. Soc. of Plastic Surgeons. Williams and Wilkins, Baltimore, 1957, p. 228.
Early jaw orthopaedics in the cleft palate programme with a new orthopaedic surgical procedure. Transactions of the European Orthodontic Society, 1960.

NORDIN, K. E., and JOHANSON, B.: *Freie Knochentransplantation bei Defeten im Alveolarkamm nach kieferorthopädischer Einstellung der Maxilla bei Lippen-Kiefer-Gaumenspalten.* Fortschr. Kiefer und Gesichtschir. 1:168, 1955.

NYLEN, B.: *Surgery of the alveolar cleft.* Plast. Reconstr. Surg., 37:42, 1966.

O'CONNOR, G. B., and CONWAY, M. E.: *Treacher Collins' syndrome (dysostosis mandibulo facialis).* Plast. Reconstr. Surg., 5:419, 1950.

OHLSSON, A.: In: *Early Treatment of Cleft Lip and Palate,* R. Hotz, ed. Huber, Berne, 1964, p. 187.

OLDFIELD, M. C.: *Cleft palate and the mechanism of speech.* Brit. J. Surg., 29:197, 1942.
Modern Trends in harelip and cleft palate surgery. Brit. J. Surg., 37:178, 1949.
Some observations on the cause and treatment of harelip and cleft palate based on treatment of 1041 patients. Brit. J. Surg., 46:311, 1958.

OLDFIELD, M. C., and TATE, G. T.: *Cleft lip and palate: some ideas on prevention and treatment, based on 1166 cases.* Brit. J. Plast. Surg., 17:, 1964.

PADGETT, E. C.: *The repair of cleft palates primarily unsuccessfully operated upon.* Surg. Gynec. Obstet., 63:483, 1936.

372

THE LIPS, CHIN, AND PALATE

PEET, E.: *The Oxford technique of cleft palate repair.* Plast. Reconstr. Surg., 28:282, 1961.

PFEIFER, G., and SCHUCHARDT, K.: *Growth of the nose, upper jaw and teeth after primary osteoplastic completion of the cleft alveolar ridge in patients with cleft lip and palate. In Transactions of the Third International Congress of Plastic Surgery.* Excerpta Medica Foundation, Amsterdam, 1964, p. 282.

PICKRELL, K., MASTERS, F., GEORGIADE, N., and HORTON, C.: *Restoration of lip contour using fascia, tendon and dermal grafts.* Plast. Reconstr. Surg., 14:126, 1954.

PICKRELL, K., QUINN, G., and MASSENGILL, R.: *Primary bone grafting of the maxilla in clefts of the lip and palate: a four year study.* Plast. Reconstr. Surg., 41:438, 1968.

RANDALL, P.: *Congenital deformities. Chap. 1 in Modern Trends in Plastic Surgery,* T. Gibson, ed. Butterworth, Washington, 1964.
The management of cleft lip and cleft palate patients. Amer. J. Med. Sci., 233:204, 1957.
A triangular flap operation for the primary repair of unilateral clefts of the lip. Plast. Reconstr. Surg., 23:331, 1959.

REES, T. D., GUY, C. L., and CONVERSE, J. M.: *Repair of the cleft lip-nose: addendum to the synchronous technique with full-thickness skin grafting of the nasal vestibule.* Plast. Reconstr. Surg., 37:47, 1966.

REHRMANN, A.: *Bone grafting in cleft palate repair: rationale of palatal bone grafting. Chap. 2 in Modern Trends in Plastic Surgery,* T. Gibson, ed. Butterworth, Washington, 1964.
In die chirurgische Behandlung der angelborenen Fehlbildungen. Georg Thieme Verlag, Stuttgart, 1961.
Korrekturoperationen nach Verschluss von Lippenspalten. Langenbeck's Arch. f. klin. Chir., 295:919, 1960.
Neue Aufgaben der Kieferorthopädie in der Rehabilitation der trager von Lippen-Kiefer-Gaumenspalten. Dtsch. Zahnärztl. Z., 17:917, 1962.

REINHARDT, W.: Die Plastische Chirurgie, Stuttgart, F. Enke, 1953.

REYNOLDS, J. R., and HORTON, C. E.: *An alar lift procedure in cleft lip rhinoplasty.* Plast. Reconstr. Surg., 35:377, 1965.

RITCHIE, H. P.: *Congenital Clefts of the Face and Jaw.* In Dean Lewis: *Practice of Surgery.* W. F. Prior Co., Hagerstown, Md., 1930.

ROBERTS, A. C.: *Obturators and Prostheses for Cleft Palate.* E. and S. Livingstone, Edinburgh, 1965.

ROBINSON, F., and WOOD, B.: *Primary bonegrafting in the treatment of cleft lip and palate with special reference to alveolar collapse.* Brit. J. Plast. Surg., 12:336, 1969.

ROGERS, R. O.: *Berry-Treacher Collins Syndrome: a review of 200 cases.* Brit. J. Plast. Surg., 17:109, 1964.

ROSENTHAL, W.: *Erfahrungen auf dem Gebiete der Uranoplastik.* Deutsche. Ztschr. f. Chir., 140:50, 1917.
Pathologie und Therapie der Gaumendefekte. Fortschr. d. Zahnh., 4:1021, 1928; 5:1044, 1929; 6:953, 1930; 7:989, 1931.

THE HEAD AND NECK

Platische Massnahmen zur Erzielung einer deutlichen Sprechweise bei Lippen-, Kiefer-, Gaumenspalten. Langenbeck's Archiv für Klinische Chirurgie. Deutsche Zeitschrift für Chirurgie., 282:631, 1955.

ROUX, W.: *Gesammelte Abhandlungen über Entwicklungsmechanik der Organism,* Vol. II. Engelmann, Leipzig, 1895.

ROYSTER, H. P., and WHITACRE, W. B.: *A technique for primary and secondary nasal reconstruction in the unilateral cleft lip patient.* Int. Col. Plast. Surg., 1963.

SANVENERO-ROSSELLI, G.: Rev. Chir. Struct. (Belg.) 6:413, 1936.
Les Palatoplasties, les Pharyngoplasties et la voix. Paris: S. A. Maloine, 1953.
Die Gaumenplastik unter Verwendung von Pharynxlappen. Langenbeck's Arch. f. klin. Chir., 295:895, 1960.
Malformazioni congenite. Minerva Chir., 13:921, 1958.

SCHLEGEL, D.: *Kritische Beiträge zum Stand der Spaltchirurgie.* Zbl. Chir., 84:1489, 1959.

SCHMID, E.: *Die aufbauende Kieferkammplastik.* Ost. Z. Stomat., 11:51, 1954.
Entwicklung und gegenwärtiger Stand der Knochenplastik in der Spaltchirurgie. Acta Chir. Plast., 9:15, 1967.

SCHMID, E.: *Zur Operationstechnik der Cheilognathopalatoschisis.* Medizinische, 42:1428, 1954.
Die Osteoplastik bei Lippen-Kiefer-Gaumenspalten. Langenbeck's Arch. f. klin. Chir., 295:868, 1960.
Widerherstellungsprobleme im Philtrumbereich der Lippe unter Berücksichtigung der Unterentwicklung des Nasenteges. Dtsch. Zahn-, Mund-und Kieferheilk, 26:397, 1957.

SCHOENBORN: *Ueber eine neue Methode der Staphylorraphie.* Verhandl. d. deutsch. Gesellsch. f. Chir., 4:235, 1875-1876. Arch. f. klin. Chir., 19:527, 1876.

SCHRUDDE, J.: *Die Knochenbildung unter funktionellen Gesichtspunkten.* Dtsch. Zahn-, Mund- und Kieferheilk, 32:3, 1960.

SCHRUDDE, J., and STELLMACH, R.: *Primäre Osteoplastik und Kieferbogenformung bei Lippen-Kiefer-Gaumenspalten.* Zbl. Chir., 15:849, 1958.

SCHUCHARDT, K.: In Bier, Braun, Kümmell's Chirurgische Operationslehre, 7th edition, vol. 2, J. A. Barth, Leipzig, 1954.
Zur Frage des günstigsten Termins für den operativen Verschluss von Gaumenspalten. Dtsch. Zahn- usw. Heilk. 20, H. 9 (1954).
Der derzeitige Stand der Lippen- und Gaumenplastik. Arch. Ohren-usw. Heilk. und Z. Hals-usw. Heilk., 186:517, 1962.
Die Entwicklung der Lippen-, Kiefer- und Gaumenspaltenchirurgie unter besonderer Berücksichtigung ästhetischer und funktioneller Momente. Langenbeck's Arch. f. klin. Chir., 295:850, 1960.
Treatment of patients with clefts of lip, alveolus, and palate. Second Hamburg International Symposium. Georg Thieme Verlag, Stuttgart, 1964.
Zur Technik des Verschlusses der queren Gesichtsspalte. Langenbeck's Arch. f. klin. Chir., 306:119, 1964.
Primary bonegraft in clefts of lip, alveolus and palate. In Modern Trends in Plastic Surgery, T. Gibson, ed., Butterworth, London, 1966.

SCHUCHARDT, K., and PFEIFER, G.: *Erfahrungen über primäre Knochentransplantation.* Langenbeck's Arch. f. klin. Chir., 295:881, 1960.
Die primäre Knochentransplantation beim Verschluss von Lippen-Kiefer-Gaumenspalten. Dtsch. Zahn-, Mund- und Kieferheilk., 37:185, 1962.

SCHUCHARDT, K., and WASSMUND, M.: *Fortschritte der Kiefer–und Gesichts-Chirurgie, A Yearbook, Vol. I.* Georg Thieme, Verlag, Stuttgart, 1956.

SCHWECKENDIEK, H.: *Zur Behandlung der angeborenen Gaumen- und Lippenspalten.* Landarzt, 31:1, 1955.
Zur Frage der Früh- und Spätoperationen der angeborenen Lippen-Kiefer-Gaumenspalten. Laryngol. Rhinolog., 30:51, 1951.

SHIERE, F. R., and FISHER, J. H.: *Neonatal orthopedic correction for cleft lip and palate patients: a preliminary report.* Cleft Palate J., 1:17, 1964.

SKOOG, T.: *A design for the repair of unilateral cleft lips.* Amer. J. Surg., 95:223, 1958.
The management of the bilateral cleft of the primary palate (lip and alveolus). Part I. General considerations and soft tissue repair. Plast. and Reconstr. Surg., 35:34, 1965.
The management of the bilateral cleft of the primary palate (lip and alveolus). Part II. Bone grafting. Plast. Reconstr. Surg., 35:190, 1965.
The pharyngeal flap operation in cleft palate. Brit. J. Plast. Surg., 18:265, 1965.

SLAUGHTER, W. B., and BRODIE, A. G.: *Facial clefts and their surgical management in view of recent research.* Plast. Reconstr. Surg., 4:311, 1939.

SLAUGHTER, W. B., and PRUZANSKY, S.: *The rationale for velar closure as a primary procedure in the repair of cleft palate defects.* Plast. Reconstr. Surg., 13:341, 1954.

SMITH, J. K., HUFFMAN, W. C., LIERLE, D. M., and MOLL, K. L.: *Results of pharyngeal flap surgery in patients with velopharyngeal incompetence.* Plast. Reconstr. Surg., 32:493, 1963.

SPEMANN, H.: *Embryonic Development and Induction.* Yale University Press, New Haven, 1938.

STARK, R. B. (ed.): *Cleft Palate: A Multidiscipline Approach.* Hoeber Medical Division, Harper and Row, New York, 1968.

STARK, R. B.: *The historic basis for contemporary cleft palate surgery.* Proceedings of the Symposium on Orofacial Abnormalities. Wilmington, Del., 1965.
The pathogenesis of harelip and cleft palate. Plast. Reconstr. Surg., 13:20, 1954.
Plastic Surgery. Hoeber Medical Division, Harper and Row, New York, 1962.

STARK, R. B., and SAUNDERS, D. E.: *The first branchial syndrome.* Plast. Reconstr. Surg., 29:229, 1962.

STEFFENSEN, W. H.: *Further experience with the rectangular flap operation for cleft lip repair.* Plast. Reconstr. Surg., 11:49, 1953.
Palate lengthening operations. Plast. Reconstr. Surg., 10:380, 1952.

STELLMACH, R.: *Die funktionskieferorthopädische Behandlung der Kieferdeformitäten bei Lippen-Kiefer-Gaumenspalten im Säuglingalter.* Fortschr. Kieferorthop., 16:247, 1955.
Die Osteoplastik bei Lippen-Kiefer-Gaumenspalten. Langenbeck's Arch. f. klin. Chir., 296:880, 1960.

375

STENSTROM, S. J., and OBERG, T. R. H.: *The nasal deformity in unilateral cleft lip.* Plast. Reconstr. Surg., 28:295, 1961.

STIEGLER, E. J., and BERRY, M. F.: *A new look at the etiology of cleft Palate* Plast. Reconstr. Surg., 21:52, 1958.

STRAITH, C. L.: *Elongation of the nasal columella.* Plast. Reconstr. Surg., 1:79, 1946.

STRAITH, C. L., and LEWIS, J. R.: *Associated congenital defects of the ears, eyelid and malar bones (Treacher Collins' syndrome).* Plast. Reconstr. Surg., 4:204, 1949.

STREAN, L. P., and PEER, L. A.: *Stress as an etiologic factor in the development of cleft palate.* Plast. Reconstr. Surg., 18:1, 1956.

STREETER, G. L.: *The development of the auricle in the human embryo.* Carnegie Contr. Embryol., Carnegie Inst., Washington, 14:111, 1922.

STRUPPLER, V.: *Zum plastischen Verchluss von Gaumenspalten im Erwachsenenalter.* Langenbeck's Archiv für Klinische Chirurgie. Deutsche Zeitschrift für Chirurgie, 282-635, 1955.

SUBTELNY, J. D.: *A review of cleft palate growth studies reported in the last 10 years.* Plast. Reconstr. Surg., 30:56, 1962.

SYMONDS, F. C., and CRIKELAIR, G. F.: *Auricular composite grafts in nasal reconstruction.* Plast. Reconstr. Surg., 37:433, 1966.

TENNISON, C. W.: *The repair of the unilateral cleft lip by the stencil method.* Plast. Reconstr. Surg., 9:115, 1952.

THOMPSON, J. E.: *The simplification of technique in operations for harelip and cleft palate.* Ann. Surg., 74:394, 1921.

TONDURY, G.: *Über die Genese der Lippen-Kiefer-Gaumenspalten.* Fortschr. der Kiefer- und Gesichts-Chirurgie, 1:1, 1955.

TRAUNER, R.: *Über eine neue Methode der Velo- Pharynxplastik bei zu kurzem weichen Gaumen.* Langenbeck's Arch. u. Dtsch. Z. Chir., 374:204, 1953.
A new procedure in velopharyngeal surgery for secondary operations on too short soft palates. Brit. J. Plast. Surg., 8:291, 1956.
Korrekturoperationen bei Lippen-Kiefer-Gaumenspalten. Langenbeck's Arch. f. klin. Chir., 287:744, 1957.
Operationen bei Lippen-Kiefer-Gaumenspalten. Urban and Schwartzenberg, Vienna, 1955.
Der Verschuluss einseitiger Lippenspalten. Langenbeck's Arch. f. klin. Chir., 295:856, 1960.

TRAUNER, R., and TRAUNER, M.: *Results of cleft lip operations.* Plast. Reconstr. Surg., 39:168, 1967.
Results of cleft lip operations. Plast. Reconstr. Surg., 40:209, 1968.

TRUSLER, H. M., and GLANZ, S.: *Secondary repair of unilateral cleft lip deformity.* Plast. Reconstr. Surg., 10:83, 1952.

TRUSLER, H. M., BAUER, T. B., TONDRA, J. M.: *The cleft-lip cleft-palate problem.* Plast. Reconstr. Surg., 16:174, 1955.

THE LIPS, CHIN, AND PALATE

ULLIK, R.: *Die plastische.* Chirurgie des Gesichtes. Wien, 1948.
Uber den operativen Verschluss von durchgehenden LKG-Spalten. Wien. med. Wschr., 1953, Nr., 46, 874.
Verbesserung der Resultate in der Spaltenchirurgie. Langenbeck's Arch. f. klin. Chir., 295:915, 1960.

UNRUH, C. C., and KENYON, W. O.: *Investigation of the properties of cellulose oxidized by nitrogen dioxide.* J. Amer. Chem. Soc., 64:127, 1942.

VAUGHN, H. S.: *Important factors in the treatment of cleft lip and cleft palate.* Ann. Surg., 84:223, 1926.
Congenital Cleft Lip, Cleft Palate and Associated Nasal Deformities. Lea & Febiger, Philadelphia, 1940.

VEAU, V.: Bec-de-Liévre, Masson, Paris, 1938.
Division Palatine. Masson, Paris, 1931.

WALDRON, C. W.: *Management of unilateral clefts of the palate.* Plast. Reconstr. Surg., 5:322, 1950.

WARDILL, W. E. W.: *Cleft palate.* Brit. J. Surg., 16:127, 1928.
The technique of operation for cleft palate. Brit. J. Surg., 25:117, 1937.

WALLACE, A. B.: *Canadian-France-Scottish cooperation: a cleft palate story.* Brit. J. Plast. Surg., 19:1, 1966.
The problem of the premaxilla in bilateral clefts. Brit. J. Plast. Surg., 16:32, 1963.

WANG, M. K. H.: *A modified LeMesurier-Tennison technique in unilateral cleft lip repair.* Plast. Reconstr. Surg., 26:190, 1960.

WARREN, J. M.: *Operations for fissure of the soft and hard palate.* New Eng. R. G. M. & S., 1:538, 1842-1843.
Operation for fissure of the soft and hard palate, with the result of twenty-four cases. Amer. J. Med. Sci., 15:329, 1848.

WASSMUND, M.: *Lehrbuch der praktischen Chirurgie des Mundes und der Kiefer.* Bd. 1, 1935, Bd. 2, 1939.
Praktische Chirurgie des Mundes und der Kiefer: II. J. A. Barth, Leipzig, 1939.

WILDE, N. J.: *Repositioning of the premaxilla and its fixation.* Brit. J. Plast. Surg., 13:28, 1960.

WYNN, S. K.: *Lateral flap cleft lip surgery technique.* Plast. Reconstr. Surg., 26:509, 1960.
Technical clarification of the bone-flap method in surgery for cleft palate. Amer. J. Surg., 98:811, 1959.

THE NOSE AND
INTRANASAL   9
REGIONS

ANATOMY

THE external part of the nose is pyramidal. Its root, located below the glabella, forms with the latter the frontonasal angle. From here the dorsum, or the ridge, of the nose descends downward ending at the tip. The base of the nasal pyramid is represented by the two nostrils. The lateral walls connect the dorsum with the cheeks (Fig. 177). A detailed description of the anatomy of the nose, particularly with reference to plastic surgery, has been presented by Converse, Straatsma, Broadbent and Matthews, and Denecke and Meyer.

The various parts forming the external nose can be divided into framework, covering, and lining. The framework is osseous in its upper half; it is cartilaginous in the lower half. The *osseous framework* (Fig. 177*a*) consists of the two nasal bones which rest upon the anterior processes of the maxilla. At the root of the nose, they articulate with the frontal bone and the perpendicular plate of the ethmoid bone. The *cartilaginous framework* consists of the lateral cartilages and the cartilaginous part of the septum. The upper lateral cartilages (cartilagines nasi laterales) (Fig. 177*b*) are triangular and join the septal cartilage in the midline. The caudal two thirds are separated from the cartilaginous septum by a narrow connective-tissue cleft, while the cephalic third is continuous with the cartilaginous septum (Straatsma and Straatsma): The lower lateral cartilages (alar cartilages—cartilagines alares) (Fig. 177*c*) consist of two parts: a crus laterale, which forms and determines the shape of the ala and nostrils, and a crus mediale, which, with its fellow from the other side, forms the tip of the nose and the mobile part of the septum called the "columella." These alar cartilages are semimobile, since they are attached only loosely to the upper lateral cartilages and the septum. They shape the nasal tip and, through their continuation into the columella, determine the height of the nose. Sometimes there are additional smaller cartilages.

The *nasal septum* is the partition of the nasal fossa, and consists of the crus mediale of the lower lateral cartilages (columella), the cutaneous septum (skin connection between columella and edge of septal cartilage),

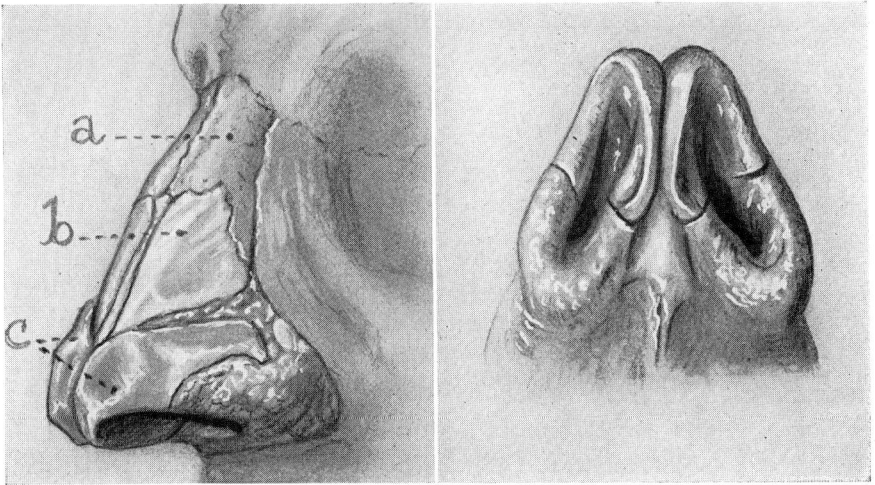

Fig. 177. Anatomy of nose.

the septal cartilage, the perpendicular plate of the ethmoid, and the vomer. The septal cartilage is the most important part of the nasal septum. It is flexible and if distorted, bent, twisted, deviated, or dislocated from its base at the nasal spine or the vomer it may displace the surrounding structures.

The *skin* covering the upper part of the nose is thin and freely movable, while the skin covering the alae and tip is thick and firmly attached to the subcutaneous structures. The *nasal muscles* are insignificant; they belong to the facial muscles, and have some influence in enlarging and narrowing the nares.

The *arteries* are the arteria dorsalis nasi, a terminal branch of the arteria ophthalmica, and branches of the arteria maxillaris externa. The terminal branch of the latter, the arteria angularis, anastomoses with the former. The *veins* empty into the vena facialis anterior; there are also connections with the vena ophthalmica superior. The following

380

sensory *nerves* supply the external nose: the nervus ethmoidalis anterior, the nasal tip and alae; the nervus infraorbitalis, the dorsum and lateral parts; the nervus infratrochlearis, the skin of the root. The nasal cavity is supplied by the nervus olfactorius, the nervus nasopalatinus, and the nervus ethmoidalis anterior.

For esthetic considerations and preoperative planning, see page 405.

DEFECTS

Defects of the nose are quite often composite, requiring the replacement of the missing tissue by similar tissue. The defects may involve only parts of the nose or the entire nose; they may involve the soft tissue or the framework or both.

DEFECTS OF SKIN OF NOSE

Defects of the nasal skin are more often due to removal of tumors than to injuries. These defects are replaced by either skin grafts or flaps, depending upon the depth of the defect. If sufficient soft tissue (subcutaneous tissue, periosteum, perichondrium) is left behind, transplantation of a free skin graft is the best choice. The full-thickness graft taken from behind the ear (compare with Fig. 210) or from the supraclavicular region is preferred, since it best matches the facial skin. In small defects of skin and cartilage, MacFee uses a composite graft of skin and cartilage from the posterior surface of the ear for closure. The auricular donor area is covered with a split skin graft. The author recommends taking the composite graft from the anterior surface of the concha, since skin and cartilage are more firmly attached (see Fig. 184); this, however, depends upon the matching of the curvature. (For other types of grafts, see p. 395.)

Dupertuis, who was preceded by Zeno, reports successful use of free earlobe grafts of skin in closure of skin defects about the nostril and the tip of the nose. He takes the grafts from the straight portion of the lobe between the tail of the helix and the dependent curve. A triangular, wedge-shaped piece of lobe is excised and the resultant defect then closed by laminated approximation of the cut edges. Although he was able to transplant such a graft successfully in correcting full-thickness defects about the nostril and the tip of the nose, he also demonstrated good results from splitting the earlobe graft to accept the cartilaginous edges if the alar cartilage was intact.

THE HEAD AND NECK

If bone and cartilage are exposed or missing, transplantation of a flap becomes necessary.

For closure of defects around the root of the nose, a rhomboid flap from the glabellar region pedicled near one of the canthal regions is highly recommended (Case 2, p. 990). The so-called banner flap (Elliott, compare with Fig. 179) or bilobed flap after Zimany may also be useful. For larger defects, a vertical forehead flap pedicled above the root of the nose is available (Case 44, p. 1052). The island forehead flap may also be available; this is rotated on a subcutaneous pedicle, which contains the frontal vessels, over one of the supratrochlear regions, as described by Converse and Wood-Smith, Heanley, Kubacek, Kernahan and Littlewood, Wilson and Gournain, and Fervier. If the temporal artery is used, the pedicle is based in front of the ear. Denecke and Meyer use the frontal artery and operate in two stages. The flap is circumscribed in the first stage, care being taken to keep the incision superficial where the entrance of the frontal artery is suspected to be. The second stage involves reconstruction of the subcutaneous pedicle containing the frontal artery from an incision along the anatomical course of the artery and transfer of the flap through a subcutaneous tunnel. Barron and Emmett recommend rotation flaps with subcutaneous tissue pedicles. (For other flap sources, see pp. 393, 402.)

DEFECTS OF COLUMELLA

The technique of replacing the columella alone differs from that used in replacement of subtotal or total defects of the nose. For technique of the latter, see Figures 185 and 186.

Numerous methods are available, including the transplantation of free composite grafts from the base of the alae or the helix of the ear for replacement of partial defects. Paletta summarized the literature, and Denecke and Meyer described and profusely illustrated the various methods.

Technique (Lexer) (Fig. 178)

A mucous-membrane flap, about 1.5 cm. (⅝ inch) long and pedicled in the gingivobuccal fold, is tubed and transferred through a slit of the upper lip. The site of the lip perforation is above and close to the base of the pedicle. The peripheral end of the flap is adjusted to conform with the shape of the columellar defect at the nasal tip and sutured into the latter. The secondary defect in the upper lip is either closed or left open. The red color of the mucous-membrane flap becomes paler and less noticeable after a few weeks.

Technique (Smith)

A double-pedicle flap is formed from the same region, as in Lexer's method. The posterior raw surface of the flap is covered with a skin graft. After two weeks, the proximal (superior) pedicle is severed, and the lip is everted and fixed in this position to the cheek with silver wires passed through a lead plate and held with adhesive tape. The flap is turned over, and the peripheral end is sutured into the defect at the nasal tip. After three weeks, the base of the flap is severed from the lip and sutured into the skin of the lip at the point of the columellar attachment.

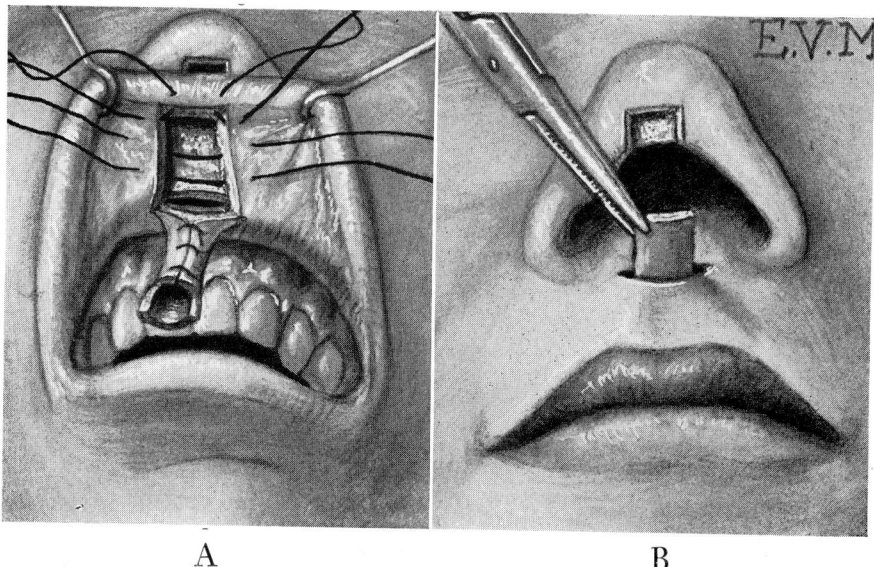

A   B

Fig. 178. *A:* Replacing columella (after Lexer). A mucous-membrane flap, pedicled in the gingivobuccal fold of the upper lip, is tubed. *B:* Flap is transferred through slit of upper lip to be sutured to nasal tip.

To lengthen a congenitally short columella, Pegram divided the columella at the base, advanced it anteriorly, and filled the resulting defect with a composite graft taken from the base of one ala. Apparently closure of the latter defect did not result in asymmetry.

Technique (Savenero-Roselli)

The philtrum is elevated as a bridge-flap; the undersurface is covered with a split skin graft. After the graft has healed in place, the peripheral pedicle of the flap, near the vermilion border, is severed; the flap is hinged upward and sutured to the tip of the nose. The area at the donor site is closed by skin sliding.

383

Lexer and Smith's techniques have not found many followers. The philtrum flap of Savenero-Roselli has only limited use, i.e., in patients with long upper lips in whom the columella is short.

Savenero-Roselli offers another method whereby a lined pedicle flap, pedicled near the nostril, is transferred from the cheek. Schuchardt mobilized the flap, not from the cheek but from an area lateral to the nose; the flap is made narrow and thick, and transferred and sutured to the nasal tip after the graft has healed in place. The resulting scar from closure of the donor area is satisfactory, since it lies along the base of the nose; four weeks after transfer of the flap, it is severed from its pedicle near the nostril and flap and pedicle are adjusted in place.

Champion raises a flap 5 cm. long by 1 cm. wide from the nasolabial fold with its base just below the ala. The raw flap surface is covered with a split skin graft which is wrapped tightly around the flap and sutured to itself for fixation. The flap is then sutured to a trapdoor flap (for comparison see Fig. 46) at the base of the columella. This trapdoor flap is raised to permit later rotation of the main flap to the new columella position. The flap bed is closed. Four weeks later, the flap is severed from its base and sutured to the tip of the nose.

DEFECTS OF TIP OF NOSE

Transplantation of a free skin graft can be successful only in superficial defects which do not involve the framework (see p. 381, particularly Dupertius-Zeno method). In deeper defects, a forehead flap (see p. 392; Case 44, p. 1052) or a flap from the side of the nose, pedicled over the nasomaxillary angle and extending obliquely downward along the nasolabial fold, is used. The arterial island flaps mentioned in the previous chapter (p. 382) may also be considered. In still deeper and extensive defects, particularly those involving parts of the alae and columella, a tube flap, preferably from the lateral cervical region or in women from the upper-neck region across its anterior surface or from the upper arm, should be transplanted. After the flap is severed and sufficient time has elapsed to allow for shrinkage, the tubed part of the flap is opened and adjusted in such a way as to form the upper rim of the nostrils and to replace the uppermost part of the columella (Case 45, p. 1054).

Another good method, originally devised by Schmid and modified by Meyer, is the use of a narrow-bridge flap formed above one of the eyebrows with a wider extension in the temporal area. The bridge pedicle is about 1 cm. wide; it is elevated between the glabella and temporal region. The raw surface is skin grafted and the flap bed is closed; subcutaneous sutures through the upper wound edge and periosteum of the upper orbital rim will prevent displacement of the eyebrow. In the same sitting, a conchal graft from the ear with its convex surface outward (see p. 381) is placed beneath the temporal extension of the flap from an incision close to the hair border. This graft will serve as a support for the nasal tip and the adjacent crural angle. About three weeks later, the temporal skin surrounding the cartilage graft is circumscribed with an incision (the outline of the incision depends upon the shape and size of the defect to be covered, and hence it must be carefully measured) and skin and cartilage are elevated. Care must be taken to leave a 1-cm. bridge of skin untouched between the lateral end of the pedicle and the flap; further, the undersurface of the cartilage graft must not become exposed but should remain covered by a thin layer of soft tissue. The entire raw surface of the flap and flap bed is skin grafted. After three weeks, the entire flap is lifted up and transferred to the defect.

DEFECTS OF ALA

Defects of the ala may comprise parts of the ala, the entire ala, or ala and parts of the nasal tip. It is fully realized that—as far as the various reparative methods are concerned—a division as outlined in the previous sentence is insufficient, since a full-thickness defect, for instance, may be surrounded by cicatricial tissue instead of normal skin. The removal of the scar tissue inevitably increases the size of the defect and, furthermore, forces a change in the reparative plan if the use of some of the surrounding skin is to be used as a lining. Nevertheless, only concrete examples can be quoted, leaving variations to the ingenuity of the operator. In the majority of instances, replacement of the covering and lining is sufficient. In some instances, however, a thin cartilage graft (ear cartilage) is required for support.

Small Defects of Ala Near Nasal Tip

Technique (Denouvilliers-Joseph) (Fig. 179)
A flap is formed consisting of the whole thickness of the entire remainder of the ala. The flap, pedicled at the base of the ala, is rotated downward and its peripheral end sutured to the lateral border of the nasal tip. The secondary defect above the ala is covered with a flap from the lateral wall of the nose. This flap also consists of the full thickness of the nasal wall. The donor area, from which this flap was taken, is closed by simple suturing.

Another method is the free transplantation of a composite graft from the helix of the ear (see Fig. 182; Case 43, p. 1050).

THE HEAD AND NECK

MEDIUM-SIZED DEFECTS OF ALA NEAR NASAL TIP

These defects are best closed by hinging a skin flap from above the defect downward to provide the lining; the entire raw surface is covered with a full-thickness graft from the posterior surface of the ear. The hinge flap should be sufficiently long to permit the peripheral part—after the flap has been turned downward—to be turned over to form the rim of the nostril (F. Smith) (compare with Fig. 78).

Another method is the free transplantation of a composite graft from the helix of the ear (see Fig. 182; Case 43, p. 1050).

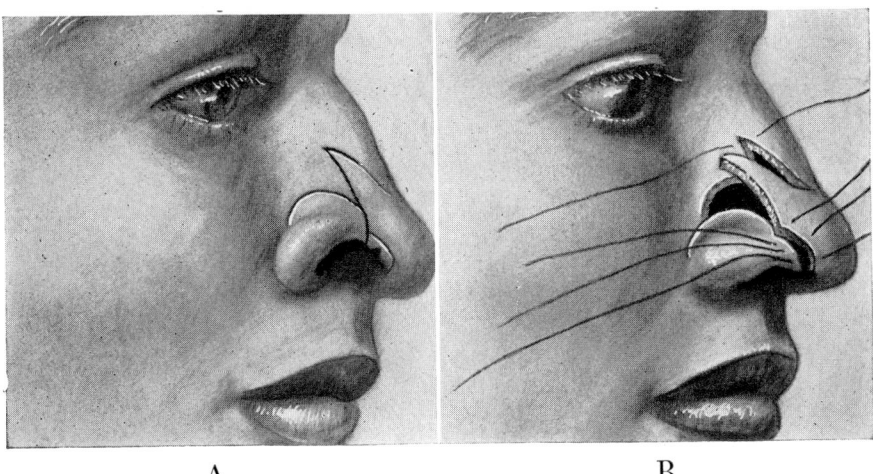

A   B

Fig. 179. *A:* Repair of small defect of ala near nasal tip (Denouvilliers-Joseph). A triangular full-thickness flap of entire remainder of ala is formed and a similarly shaped flap of lateral wall of nose. *B:* Alar flap is moved downward and sutured to prepared place at tip of nose. Flap of lateral wall of nose is rotated into defect above ala. Defect at lateral wall of nose is closed by simple suturing.

SMALL AND MEDIUM-SIZED DEFECTS NEAR BASE OF ALA

The lining of these defects is provided by hinging a flap from the nasolabial region; the covering is provided by a skin graft.

Technique (F. Smith) (Fig. 180)

Stage 1: A flap of sufficient size, with its pedicle near the base of the ala, is outlined in the adjacent nasolabial region. The inferior part of the flap should be made so broad that after the flap is hinged it can be turned over to form the rim of the nostril. The flap is raised and returned to its original site.

386

Stage 2: After two weeks, the flap is again raised and transplanted; if the blood supply is still insufficient, however, the flap should be returned for another two weeks. The edges of the defect are split and the flap sutured to the mucous-membrane lining, with the sutures tied intranasally. The inferior border of the flap is rolled outward to form the rim of the

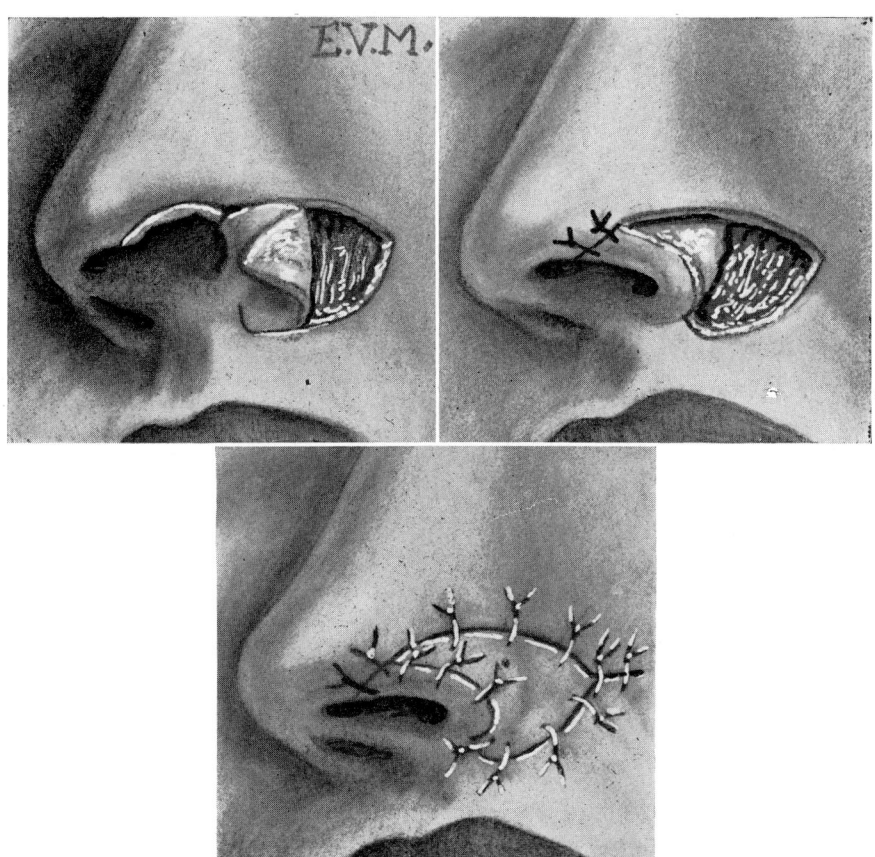

Fig. 180. Repair of smaller and medium-sized defects near base of ala. Lining is provided by hinging flap from nasolabial region. Inferior part of flap should be made so broad that after flap is hinged it can be turned over to form rim of nostril. Covering is provided by skin graft. (F. Smith: Manual of Standard Practice of Plastic and Maxillofacial Surgery. W. B. Saunders.)

nostril. The donor area in the nasolabial region is closed by skin sliding after mobilization of the borders of the wound, unless the area is too large and consequently requires transplantation of a skin graft from the posterior surface of the ear. The raw area of the hinged flap is covered with the same full-thickness graft or with a full-thickness graft from the

387

posterior surface of the other ear. The repaired side of the nose is packed with plain gauze and a pressure dressing is applied to the outside, or the sutures which have been left long are tied over mechanic's waste. This is left in place for ten days.

Variation

Another method is the free transplantation of a composite graft from the helix of the ear (see Fig. 182; Case 43, page 1050) or from the base of the sound nostril (Davis).

DEFECTS OF RIM OF ALA

Technique (*Kazanjian*) (Fig. 181)

The borders of the defect are utilized to form the alar rim. A curved incision is made a few millimeters behind the margin of the defect through the skin and cartilage only; the mucous membrane is carefully separated from the overlying skin and cartilage and part of the nasal bone. A mucous-membrane flap is now cut, as indicated by the shaded area of Figure 181 *B;* the mucous-membrane flap is brought down, together with the alar rim; the defect at the inside of the nose above the mucous-membrane flap is left to granulate, and the skin defect above the alar rim is covered with a full-thickness graft from the posterior surface of the ear. The nose is packed with plain gauze and a proper pressure dressing is applied upon the graft, or the sutures which have been left long are tied over mechanic's waste.

Another method is the free transplantation of a composite graft from the helix of the ear (see Fig. 182; Case 43, p. 1050).

DEFECTS OF ENTIRE ALA

For repair of defects of the entire ala, the following are available: free transplantation of a composite graft from the helix of the ear, flaps from the immediate neighborhood, and flaps from distant parts.

Composite grafts from the helix of the ear have been successfully used by Susloff and Fritz König. J. B. Brown revived the method and demonstrated its extraordinary success at Valley Forge General Hospital in many cases.

Technique (Fig. 182)

Healthy wound edges of the defect are imperative for success. They are the only source from which the graft receives its blood supply. The edges of the defect are excised until normal healthy tissue is encountered. Careful hemostasis, by pressure rather than by ligation, is next applied. A pattern of the defect is made, and a section of the helix of the ear corresponding in size and shape is removed (Fig. 182). The posterior skin of the graft is carefully sutured to the mucous-membrane edge of the defect with fine silk sutures on an atraumatic needle, the anterior skin to

A

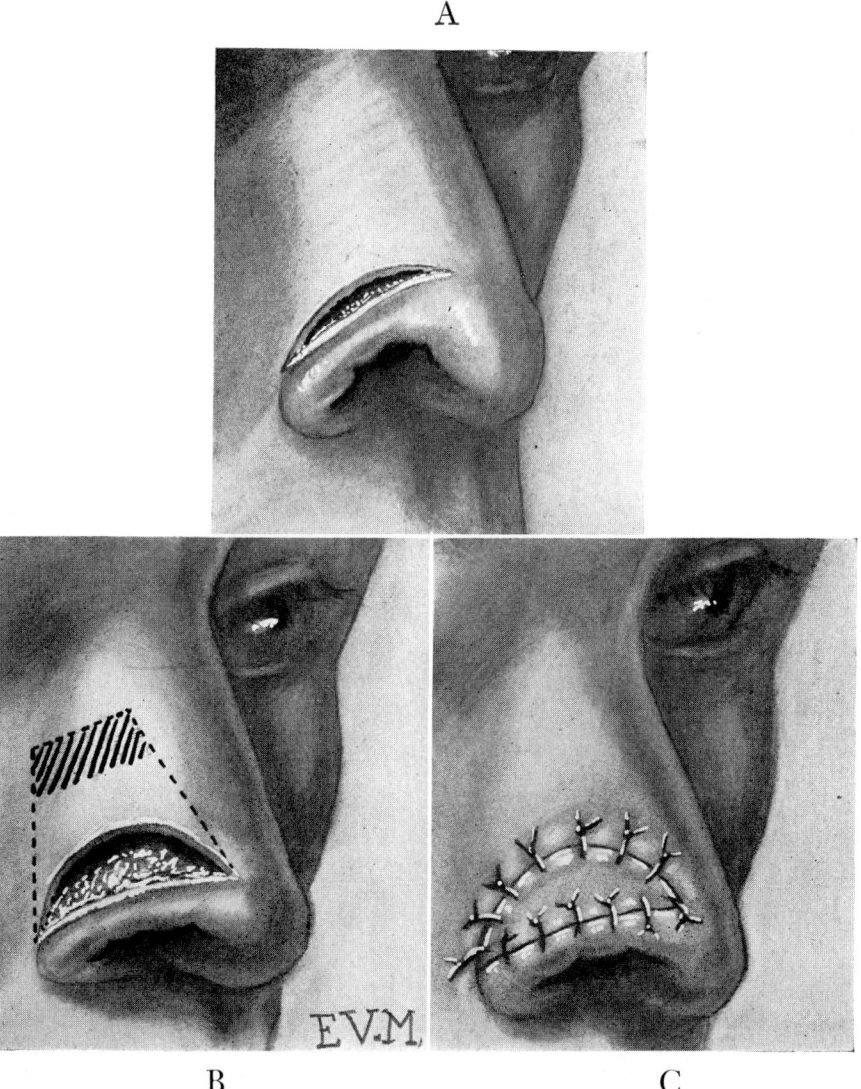

B   C

Fig. 181. *A:* Repair of defects of rim of ala (Kazanjian). A curved incision is made above margin of defect through skin and cartilage only. (V. H. Kazanjian: Trans. Amer. Acad. Ophth.) *B:* Mucous membrane is carefully separated from skin to extent outlined by dotted lines. Mucous membrane is severed along upper dotted line and moved downward. Defect from which mucous membrane has been shifted (shaded area) is left to granulate. *C:* Defect above alar rim is skin grafted.

389

the skin edge. The defect at the ear is closed either by making the ear slightly smaller (Fig. 251) or in larger defects by suturing the ear to a flap at the hairless mastoid region. (After three weeks, this flap is severed; its free end is hinged posteriorly [Case 75, p. 1089].) The graft at the nose must be carefully supported by packing the nostril and by the application of moderate pressure by tying the sutures, which have been left long over mechanic's waste.

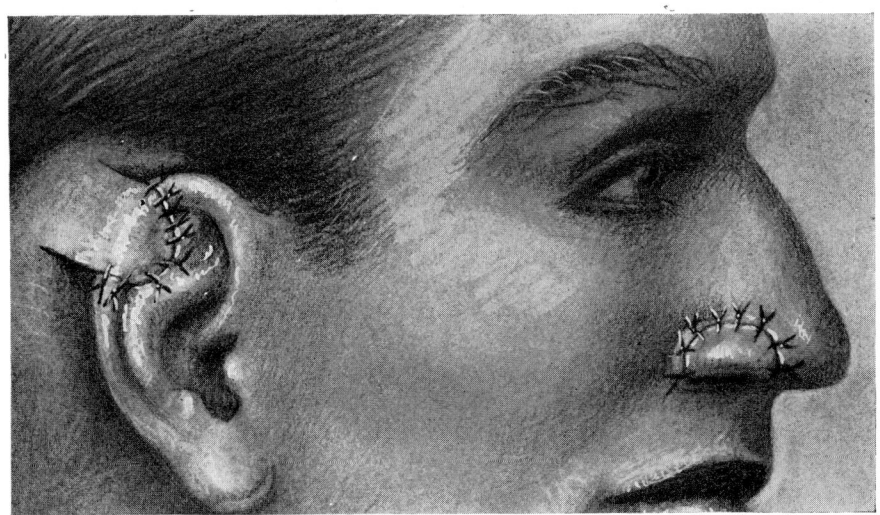

Fig. 182: Defect of entire ala repaired by free transplantation of composite graft from helix of ear (F. König). Defect at ear is immediately repaired with flap raised from hairless postauricular region. This flap is severed after three weeks and its posterior raw surface skin grafted or hinged posteriorly.

Rees, who confirmed McLaughlin's experience, warns against too much pressure, however, since composite grafts apparently receive their early blood supply from a direct vessel-to-vessel anastomosis. Too much pressure may result in occlusion of the vessels within the graft. Cooling may be of benefit by decreasing the metabolism within the graft (Converse, Conley and Vonfraenkel, and Schmid), although, as Symonds and Crikelair state, it may be difficult to maintain over a prolonged period of time.

Lexer's advice is recommended for the preparation of the host area. To increase the contact surface of graft and host area, the incision along the rim of the defect is curved so that a small skin flap can be turned downward and inward; this increases the wound surface. The skin surface of the graft which comes to lie inward must of course be made correspondingly small.

390

Technique (*Dieffenbach*) (Fig. 183)

If the skin of the cheek adjacent to the defect is healthy, rotation of a flap from the immediate neighborhood is possible. The flap is mobilized from the nasolabial region. The pedicle is placed so that after rotation of the flap it forms the base of the ala. Figure 183 is self-explanatory. The flap should be made wide enough to allow for shrinkage. It is elevated and lined with a split skin graft, returned to the donor area, and covered with a pressure dressing. After ten days the flap is transferred and the donor area is closed by skin sliding. This may cause a pull on the upper lip, but in the author's experience the tension is usually only temporary, although in one patient it took almost two years before the lip returned to its normal level.

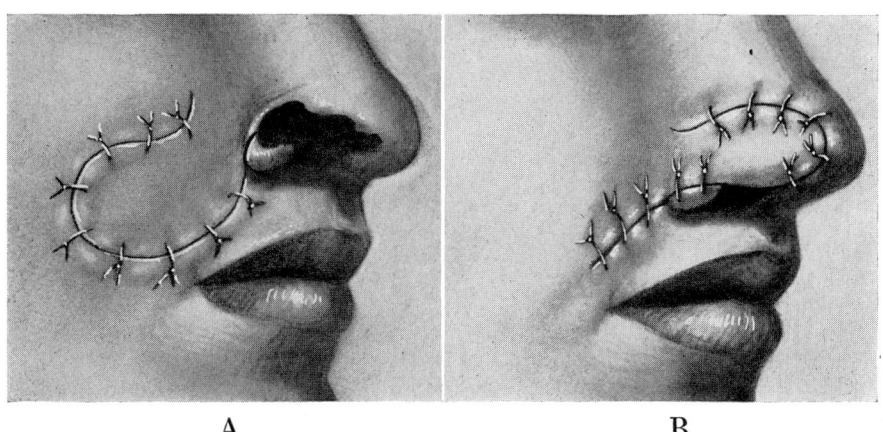

| A | B |

Fig. 183. *A:* Repair of defect of entire ala with flap which is rotated from adjacent cheek (Dieffenbach). Pedicle of flap is placed so that after rotation it forms base of ala. Unless an intranasal mucous membrane flap can be mobilized for lining, it is lined with a thick split graft and returned to its original site. *B:* Ten days after flap has been lined, it is rotated into the defect, and the secondary defect at cheek is closed by skin sliding.

In defects that are not too broad, a flap adjacent to the nose within the nasomaxillary area can be utilized. The pedicle is placed adjacent to the nostril.

Another very useful and simple method of transferring a nasolabial flap for reconstruction of large defects of the ala was originally described by Kilner and revised recently by McLarren.

Technique (Case 48, p. 1058)

A pattern is made of the defect, allowing for rolling the free end of the flap for the alar rim, and the flap is lined out. The pedicle of the flap is below the base of the lower eyelid. The flap, up to 1 inch broad and 3 inches long, comes to lie within the general direction of the nasolabial fold; part of its median edge is within the immediate neighborhood of the defect; the incision on the lateral side of the pedicle is curved outward to facilitate rotation of the flap (see p. 78). The flap should have only a very thin layer of subcutaneous tissue. After wide undermining, the donor area is closed. The edges of the nostril defect are pared and a triangular piece of skin above the defect is removed to provide a bed for the flap. The peripheral end of the flap is rolled inward and sutured to the lining of the defect edge; the remainder of the flap is sutured in place.

After all edema in the flap has subsided secondary refinements may become necessary, such as the removal of a "dog-ear" at the point of rotation of the flap; there may be a tenting of the nasolabial fold, which can be overcome by a Z-plasty. Insertion of a conchal cartilage graft seldom becomes necessary for support. Initial upward displacement of the upper lip has never been a problem since the lip returns to normal level after all swelling has subsided.

The method of Schmid, using a temporal flap attached to a supraorbital bridge flap, may also be used, although it comprises more stages than does the above method. Denecke and Meyer have described and illustrated various other possibilities useful in reconstruction of the ala (see also p. 384).

EXTENSIVE DEFECTS OF ALA

For extensive defects, particularly those which include portions of the tip and lateral wall of the nose, flaps from distant parts must be chosen. Suffice it to say that these flaps should be lined (by folding the peripheral end of the flap upon itself, for instance). A lateral (or, in women, a transverse) cervical tube flap from the upper anterior neck region or the acromiopectoral, arm, forehead, sickle flap, or an improved forehead flap (New) (Fig. 184) is available. Whenever possible, a forehead flap should be used.

Gillies' suggestion of lining the flap with a piece of skin plus cartilage taken from the concha of the ear seems to be excellent (Case 47, p. 1056; Fig. 184). Kazanjian advises the median forehead flap.

Technique (*Median Forehead Flap;* Case 44, p. 1052)

Two parallel incisions are made over the forehead from 1.2 to 2.5

cm. (½ to 1 inch) apart, extending from the hairline to just above the frontal eminence on both sides. The flap is raised; when it reaches the eyebrows, blunt dissection is carried downward almost to the root of the nose, thus saving the frontal vessels from injury. The donor area is closed by wide undermining and by making one or two incisions under the undermined skin parallel to the incised edges through the fascia but without penetrating all of the subcutaneous fat or any of the skin. This procedure of relaxation incisions through the fascia will allow approximation of the borders of the wound without undue tension. If a lining of the flap must be provided, the flap is raised in stages and lined as described below. Larger defects of the forehead are closed by advancing two forehead flaps from each side of the defect. The incisions for formation of these flaps are made just above the eyebrows for the lower borders and just within the hairline of the forehead for the upper borders.

Escoffier presented his personal experience with a large number and variety of forehead flaps. He states that edema due to twisting of the pedicle is likely to occur only if the pedicle has not been adequately freed to allow rotation of the flaps without tension. He advises that one of the lateral incisions of the pedicle should be prolonged on the side of the rotation into the nasopalpebral region.

With narrow foreheads where the hairline is low, the vertical forehead flap would be too short. One must then use the horizonal flap after Schmid (p. 384), which however is limited in size, or the so-called sickle flap after New. Gillies' way of lining the flap is readily applicable to this type of flap, and is demonstrated in Figure 184. The pedicle of the sickle flap is placed in the temple and scalp region. Only the peripheral part of the flap is in the forehead; hence, scarring in the forehead region is reduced to a minimum.

Technique (Fig. 184, Case 47, p. 1056)

The sickle flap of New is carefully measured, designed, and raised in stages. It contains the temporal artery. Converse believes that this flap, or any other forehead flap, should not be elevated from the undersurface in this first stage; he advises simply outlining it with an incision. This enhances its vascularization and, most important, induration of the flap and formation of scar tissue are avoided. The anatomical reason behind this is that blood supply of the scalp and forehead is derived from vessels which enter the circumference of the area, not from perforating vessels as in most other areas of the body. In the second stage, performed four weeks later, the peripheral end of the flap is lined.

The donor area, to provide the lining of the flap, is in front of the concha of the ear, where the skin is very closely adherent to the thin cartilage and where the curve of the cartilage is similar to that required in making the nostril. In making such a free graft, a piece of skin larger than the cartilage is cut. After its removal, it is buried beneath that part of the flap destined to make the new nostril. The part of the concha from which the graft has been taken, as well as the part of the forehead from which the flap has been raised, is skin grafted and a pressure dressing applied. Final transfer of the flap is performed after ten to fourteen days.

Another good method for replacement of large defects of the ala and adjacent regions is the scalping forehead flap after Converse (Fig. 187;

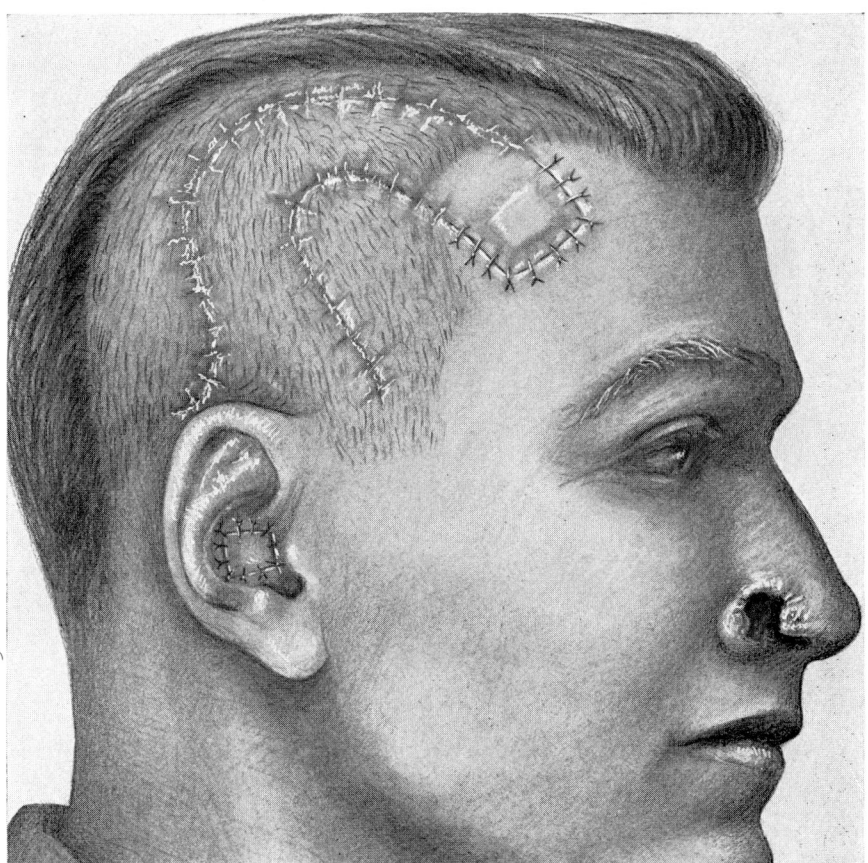

Fig. 184. Replacement of entire ala by so-called "sickle" flap (after New) and lining of flap with piece of skin plus cartilage taken from concha of ear (after Gillies). In the first stage the flap is circumscribed with an incision, but not undermined (see text). In the second stage, the peripheral part, or forehead part, of flap is raised and lined with piece of skin plus cartilage taken from concha of ear. This part is again returned to its original site, and defect in concha is skin grafted. Flap is ready for transfer one week after lining. (For more extensive defects, see Case 47, p. 1056.)

Case 49, p. 1059). It has the advantage of any temporal flap in that an angle, and therefore tension, is avoided. In addition, the flap does not extend over the eye (see also remark on p. 402).

Of other distal flaps, the author prefers the tube flap from the lateral or upper transverse cervical region or from the hairless median surface of the upper arm. The arm opposite to the defect is chosen. Denecke and Meyer have profusely illustrated a great many such possibilities. The peripheral end of the flap is lined with a hinge flap from the neighborhood of the flap bed or by the end of the flap folded upon itself. If a free graft is used for lining it tends to shrink, and thus may curl the flap (see also p. 98).

PERFORATIONS AND FULL-THICKNESS DEFECTS OF PARTS OF OSSEOUS OR CARTILAGINOUS VAULTS

For small holes, MacFee uses a composite graft from the auricular concha (see also pp. 388-390) after the wound edges have been broadened (for closure of the resultant hole in the ear, see pp. 506-507). Another method is to hinge a flap (in stages) from the immediate neighborhood into the defect to provide the lining and to use a split skin graft for coverage. A preoperative step similar to the one depicted in Figure 78 *A* should precede the actual turning over of the flap to ensure adequate circulation in the turnover flap.

Large full-thickness defects of parts of osseous or cartilaginous vaults require replacement of skin plus lining and, in some instances, of the supporting structures. Flaps, preferably a median forehead flap (pp. 388-390; Case 44, p. 1052) or a sickle flap (see above; Case 47, p. 1056) or the variety of other flaps described in the foregoing paragraph, are required to replace the outside skin. One may also use either a tube flap from the lateral or upper transverse cervical region or an open-pedicle flap (Fig. 189) from the upper arm (the side opposite the defect). The flap must be lined (see pp. 97-98) unless local flaps can be turned over. A preoperative step similar to that shown in Figure 78 *A* (2) should be performed before the flap is turned over as a means of enhancing its circulation. If support is needed, a cartilage or bone graft is inserted between skin and lining after the flap has healed in.

SUBTOTAL AND TOTAL DEFECTS OF NOSE

Subtotal defects of the nose comprise defects of either the cartilaginous or the bony part of the nose. In total defects, covering skin, lining, and entire framework are absent. The methods developed for replacing such large nasal defects are numerous. Although some of the older principles (Carpue) still govern modern technique, many details have been changed and improved. Comprehensive histories of this topic have been presented by Schmid of Stuttgart, Holdsworth and Pelly of London, and Millard of Miami. The latter has applied sound architectural principles as they are used in the construction of any building, and thus has put the various reconstructive steps in building a nose into correct sequence. In addition, he has introduced a new principle of support, the so-called cantilever principle. His beautiful results are convincing and speak for the soundness of his method.

For completeness, however, it is necessary to describe the various other methods of nasal reconstruction which are still used because they are still applicable, particularly in subtotal defects. The forehead flap is given preference for cover. It is fashioned and transported as a horizontal flap based on one of the supraorbital regions, or based as an "up-and-down flap" after Gillies-Penn, or as a "sickle flap" after New, or as a "scalping flap" after Converse. The next choice is the arm flap or an acromial-pectoral flap.

FOREHEAD FLAP

In constructing a new nose, the following requirements are necessary: replacement of the covering, lining, and supporting tissue; sufficient breathing space; and last, but not least, a pleasing cosmetic result. The formation of the columella, alae, nostrils, and their lining is achieved by folding the peripheral end of the flap over (Figs. 185 *B* and 186) as—according to Dubowitzky—first practiced by Labat (1830). (Somewhat later, however, in 1842, Calderini states that Petrali is the originator.) In addition to the advantages mentioned, this method almost guarantees maintenance of the prominence of the nasal tip without additional cartilaginous or bony support. The disadvantage is that the nostrils are more or less obstructed by bulky skin and subcutaneous tissue, requiring secondary correction. The lining of the upper half of the nose is provided by turning over local flaps or by lining the forehead with a full-thickness graft. Support of the ridge of the nose is provided by transplantation of a cartilaginous graft. Ivy advises inserting the cartilage as a finishing touch rather than placing it beneath the flap on the forehead before it is brought down, since it is much easier in the former case to judge the proper size, shape, and position to be given to the cartilage. Lexer and others advise insertion of bone grafts beneath the forehead flap before it is transferred. This method provides ample breathing space, but the shape of the nose may leave much to be desired. Millard considers both methods unsound and offers another solution to this problem (p. 405).

Technique (Fig. 185)

Step 1: The first requirement is a plaster cast of the face of the patient; upon this cast, the new nose is built up with clay. From this model, the shape of the new flap is outlined in the following way: A

A   B

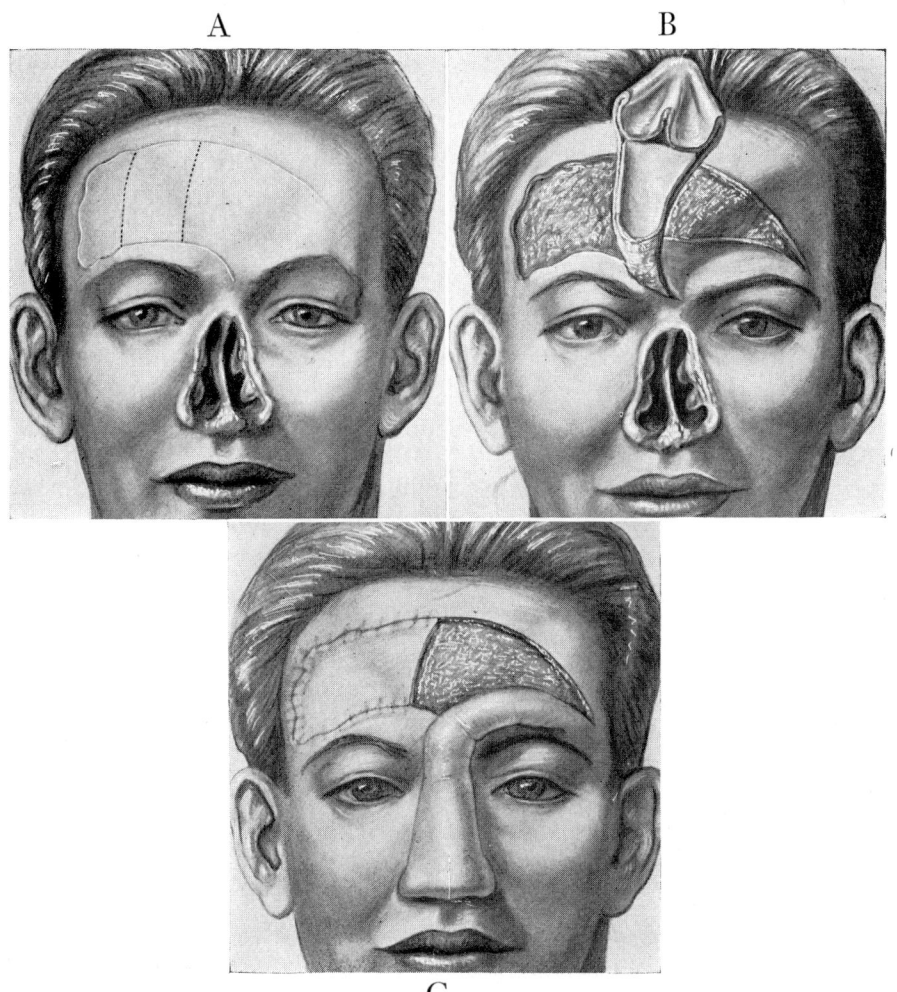

C

Fig. 185. *A:* Total loss of nose; forehead flap is outlined and prepared (for details, see text). Section between two dotted lines is to be lined, unless local flaps from nasal region can be turned inward. *B:* Flap is mobilized; lower end is folded in such fashion as to provide lining for lower portion of nose and columella. *C:* Flap is transplanted; secondary defect at forehead is covered with full-thickness skin graft.

piece of chamois is laid upon the model and held firmly against the glabella. The chamois is given the shape of the nasal pyramid; the lower part is folded in such a way as to provide the columella and the lining of the vestibule (see Fig. 185 B). The chamois pattern is unfolded and laid upon tinfoil and a second pattern is cut, similar in shape but one third larger, to compensate for immediate and later shrinkage. The tinfoil pattern is laid and outlined upon the forehead of the model, with the basic line in one temporal region. A pedicle connecting the nasal pattern with the opposite side of the forehead is drawn so that the pedicle contains the arteria frontalis, the arteria supraorbitalis, and the anterior branch of the arteria temporalis. Part of the pedicle, if necessary, may run within the hairy scalp. The whole figure is then traced upon another piece of chamois, cut out, and laid again upon the forehead; the peripheral end is again folded as described and the chamois flap rotated upon its pedicle to make sure that the pedicle is long enough to prevent tension or torsion. A tinfoil pattern is cut, according to the chamois pattern, and sterilized.

Step 2: A flap is outlined on the patient's forehead according to the tinfoil pattern. This flap should remain attached at two pedicles: at the central pedicle, which contains the arteries just mentioned, and at the peripheral pedicle in the opposite temporal region. The flap is now undermined between both pedicles, returned to its original site, and sutured in place. If the case is such that the lining of the upper half of the nose needs to be replaced and can be furnished by turning over local flaps, these flaps should be prepared in the same sitting by raising and returning them to their original site.

Step 3: Two weeks later, the peripheral pedicle is severed and, after hemostasis, sutured in place.

Step 4: Two weeks later, the entire flap is raised and returned to its original site for improving the circulation. According to Converse, Step 2 (preliminary raising of the flap) can be simplified, and Steps 3 and 4 may be eliminated (see p. 393).

Step 5: It is well to wait for at least two to three months before final transfer of the flap, that is, to delay transfer until all edema in the flap has disappeared and the flap is smooth and pliable. This will facilitate the folding of the flap. After two to three months the entire flap is raised and the peripheral end is folded to form the columella, alae, nostrils and their lining. The folded skin is held in place with mattress sutures (Fig. 186 B, C). The flap is rotated 90 degrees and sutured to the wound edges of the defect. The forehead defect, corresponding to the nose pattern, is covered with a full-thickness graft, which is cut according to the tinfoil pattern. A proper pressure dressing is applied to the forehead. The nose is loosely packed with plain gauze and covered with a dressing.

Step 6: After two weeks, the pedicle of the flap is partly severed; this is done in V-fashion, following the technique on Penn (Fig. 188 *B*). The separation is completed at the end of the third week. The pedicle is returned to its original site and the flap adjusted in place.

Step 7: If the ridge of the new nose needs support, a properly shaped and sized piece of cartilage is inserted after the wound healing is completed. An incision is made below the glabella, a pocket is made between skin and lining, and the cartilage graft is inserted into this pocket.

If nasal ridge and columella need support, a hinge graft is inserted according to the technique described on page 431. Other secondary corrective work may be needed to correct scars, to form the nostrils (see Fig. 186), and the like.

Variation

If the lining of the nose cannot be replaced by local turnover flaps, the forehead flap must be lined prior to its transfer (Figs. 185, 186). About two weeks before the final transfer, the peripheral end of the flap is raised

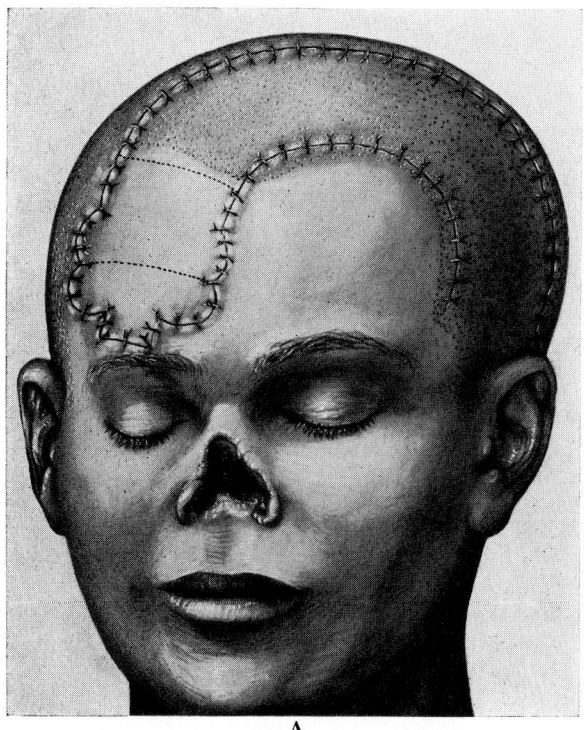

A

Fig. 186. *A:* Subtotal loss of nose; sickle flap with laterally placed peripheral end is outlined and raised in stages. Section between dotted lines is to be lined, unless local flaps from nasal region can be turned inward.

399

and a full-thickness graft is sutured to that part of the flap which needs to be lined.

The forehead flap described in the foregoing is the oblique type. For obvious reasons, it leaves scars across the forehead. To hide most of these scars, it may be possible to utilize the principle of the sickle flap (see p. 393). The peripheral end of the flap is placed either mediad (Case 50, p. 1060) or laterally (Fig. 186), depending upon the width of the fore-

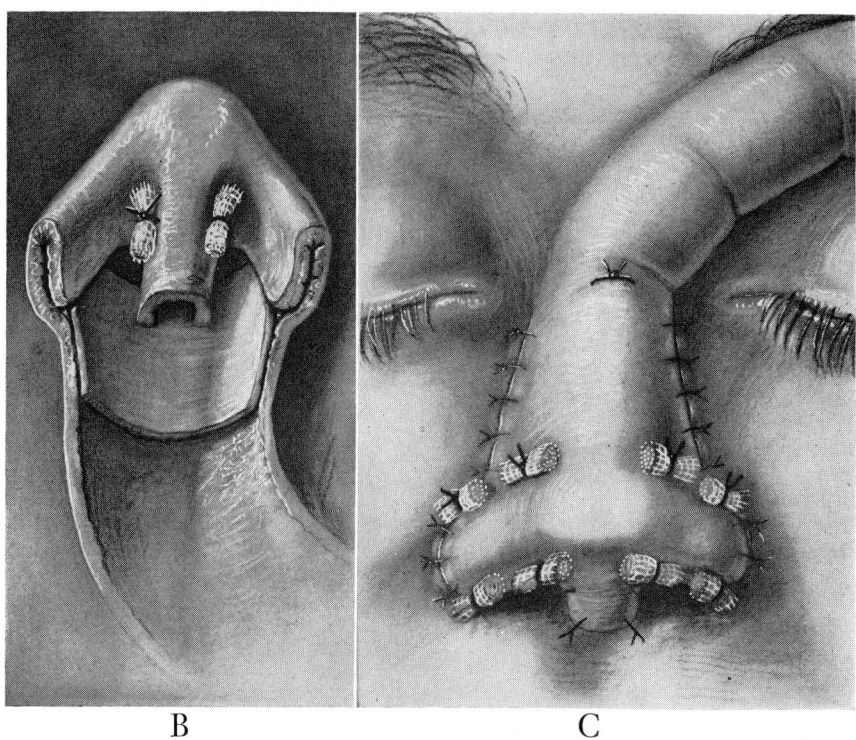

B   C

Fig. 186. *B:* The flap is raised and its lower end is folded to form columella, alae, nostrils and their lining. *C:* Folded skin is held in place with mattress sutures. Uppermost mattress suture above alae should go through both sides to form normal "pinch" above alae. Flap is sutured in place.

head. Such a flap must be raised in stages. Other flaps constructed on the same principle may be transplanted in one stage, i.e., the "scalping" forehead flap of Converse (Fig. 187) and the "horseshoe" flap, modified after Penn (Fig. 188). Since they are based on the supraorbital vessels, they have an excellent blood supply and need not be delayed unless lining of the flap is required. The peripheral end (forehead skin exclusive of scalp) of these three types of flaps, however, may not be of sufficient length and width to permit reconstruction of the whole nose. Converse reported

400

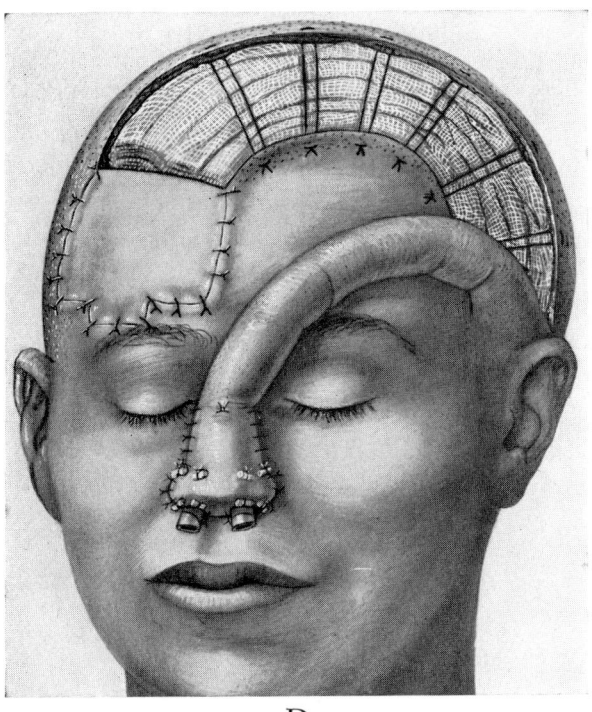

D

Fig. 186. *D:* Pedicle of flap is tubed; donor site at forehead skin grafted; periosteum of skull covered with ointment dressing; mattress sutures are laid to hold dressing in place and wound edges pulled together. For separation of the flap see Figure 188B.

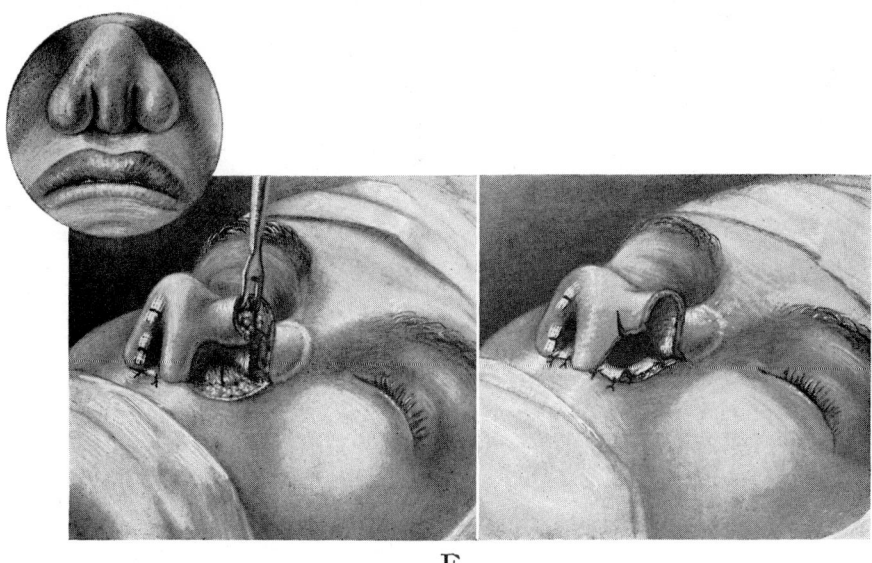

E

Fig. 186. *E:* Reduction of thickness of skin folds of columella and alae after all edema of flap has subsided.

401

recently his experience with the scalping flap demonstrating an amazing versatility in the use of this flap and new ways of providing lining and support.

Lexer and others insert bone grafts beneath the forehead flap before it is transplanted. The author has had personal experience with his former teacher's method: he agrees with others that his technique of total rhinoplasty results in an ample breathing space—if the bone grafts are made

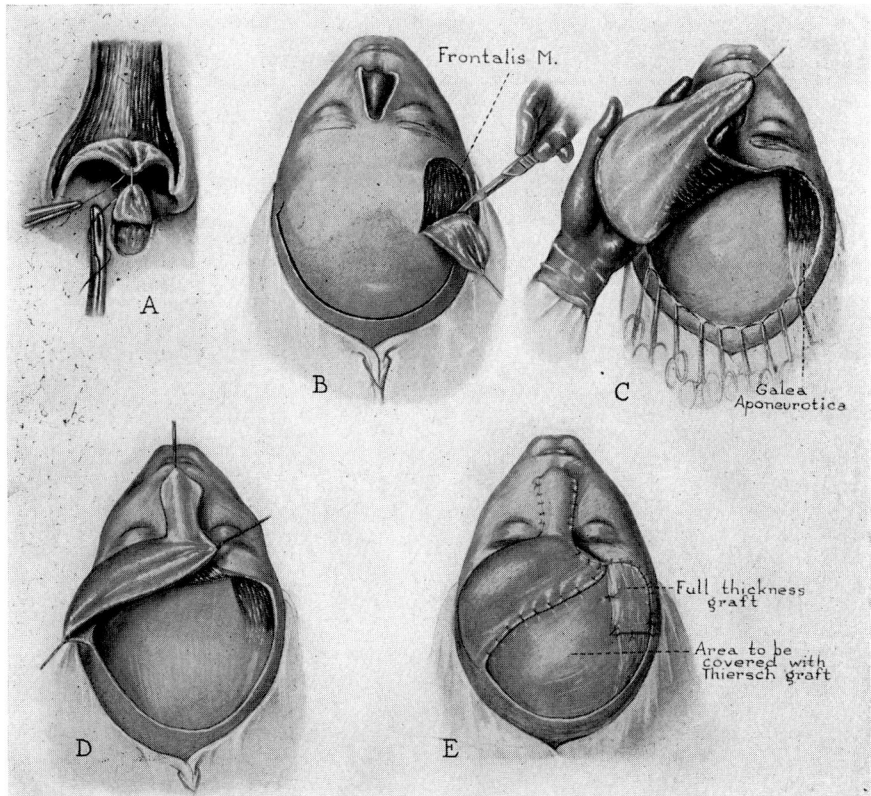

Fig. 187. Technique of the scalping forehead flap—after Converse. *A:* Nasal area prepared to receive the forehead flap. A small flap, raised from the upper lip, furnishes tissue for reconstruction of the columella. *B:* Outline of the flap. The portion of the flap serving for the nasal reconstruction is raised, care being taken to preserve the frontalis muscle. *C:* The scalping flap is raised. Note the splitting of the frontalis muscle; the frontalis is included in the base of the flap, a necessary precaution to preserve the blood supply. *D:* The flap is turned down into its position of transfer. The flap is folded, thus eliminating the raw area along its base. *E:* The area of the permanent defect on the side of the forehead is covered by a full-thickness retroauricular graft which insures good color and texture match. The temporary scalp defect is covered by a skin graft of intermediate thickness. (J. M. Converse: Proc. Roy. Soc. Med., 35:811, 1942; and V. H. Kazanjian and J. M. Converse: The Surgical Treatment of Facial Injuries. Williams & Wilkins.)

sufficiently broad—but the shape of the nose may leave much to be desired. Schmid limits this principle to the construction of the alae only.

Arm Flap

This flap has the advantage of avoiding facial scarring, but it offers two disadvantages: (1) color difference (paler than the face), and (2) cumbersome positions when being transferred. These disadvantages must be carefully weighed before the choice is made.

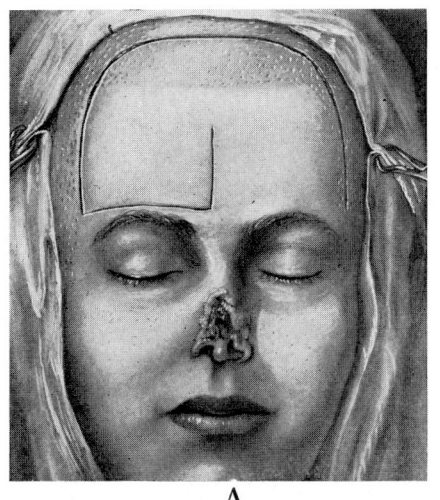 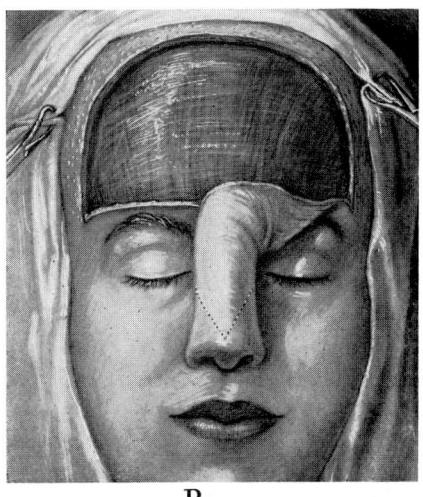

A   B

Fig. 188. *A:* "Horseshoe" flap for subtotal reconstruction of nose. Pedicle contains left supraorbital vessels. Pedicle plus peripheral end (the part of the flap above the eyebrow) should be at least 6 inches wide. If the entire columella is to be replaced by folding of the flap (see p. 396), it is good to curve the free end of the flap slightly. This provides more tissue for making the columella. The nasal part of the flap consists of skin only. The other part of the flap contains the supraorbital vessels. *B:* Flap transplanted; donor area to be skin grafted (compare with Fig. 187 *E*). V-shaped separation of flap outlined. Latter facilitates smoother adjustment of flap and remainder of nose. (J. Penn: S. Afr. Med. J.)

The outlining and preparation of the flap are as previously described (p. 397). The donor area is the median surface of the upper arm. The flap is prepared as an open double-pedicle flap, undermined between two longitudinal parallel incisions. It remains attached with a proximal and distal pedicle (see p. 83), and is returned to its original site. The proximal or distal pedicle—the choice is dictated by circumstances, and must be predetermined according to pattern—is severed after two weeks, and after hemostasis is sutured in place. Two weeks later, the entire flap is raised and returned to its original site. After all edema in the flap has subsided (from two to four weeks), the flap is ready for transfer. The flap is raised, the flap bed skin grafted, and the peripheral part of the flap sutured to the glabella and the lateral edges of the defect (Fig. 189). The

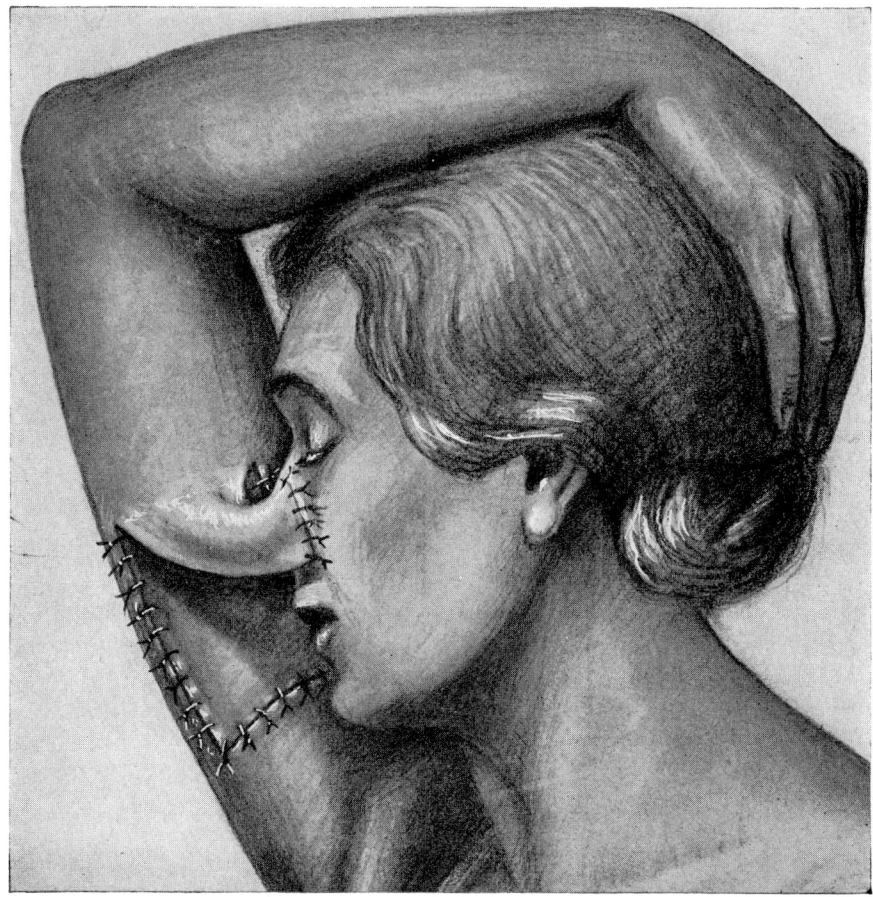

Fig. 189. Total loss of nose. Reconstruction with arm flap. Flap has been raised in stages from median surface of upper arm, donor area skin grafted. Arm is moved to face, and free end of flap is sutured to defect edges. Arm is held in position with plaster cast. Flap is to be gradually severed from its base after two weeks and its free end folded and sutured, as demonstrated in Figures 185, 186, after edema has receded.

arm is held in this position with a plaster cast. After two weeks, the flap is gradually severed from its base. Enough tissue should be left at the flap to allow folding of the lower end of the flap to provide lining of the lower portion of the nose and the columella (see Figs. 185, 186). The flap

404

should be folded, however, only after all edema in the flap has subsided. For insertion of cartilage grafts, for support and variation of lining, and for final formation of nostrils, see page 399.

TOTAL RECONSTRUCTION OF THE NOSE

Total loss of nose must be understood to mean a complete loss of all components of the nose, including all skin and bone of the nasal radix. Rebuilding a nose under those circumstances, giving it an esthetic appearance and adequate function, has intrigued every plastic surgeon for centuries, but none had really succeeded until Millard demonstrated his fascinating, well-thought-through method. His case reports demonstrate vividly the success of the technique.

The support phase is the most important feature of his method. In the absence of vertical support by the thin, strong septum, maintenance of a nasal pyramid calls for supportive struts embedded in the columella and sidewalls. These struts must be far thicker than normal alar cartilage, which condemns the nasal entrance to the unnatural bulkiness of one, two or three blobs. Thus it was thought that if the entire nose could be draped onto a rigid bridge beam, extending from the glabella to tip as one slender cantilever shaft, there would be no need for the extra props in the columella or sidewalls; the beam would lean at an angle like that of the gnomon on a sundial. After years of considering and testing, Millard finally decided that a slender, strong, autogenous bony cantilever—available and rigid from the moment of the initial repair—offered the best chance for reconstruction of a nose normal in appearance and function. For the details of the technique I refer the reader to Millard's article, which incidentally contains an exhaustive historical background of nasal reconstruction.

DEFORMITIES

The nose appears deformed if it differs in shape and in proportion from normal racial characteristics. However, a nose of normal size may be out of harmony with the rest of the face in a person with a retruding chin; and an enlarged nose may look normal if it is not grossly inharmonious with other facial features. Hence, the indication for a corrective operation and the operative plan itself must consider the relationship of the nose and the rest of the face in every instance. If a deformity is very noticeable and improvement by surgical reconstruction is possible, the advisability of an operation is clear cut. Far more difficult is the decision where the transition from abnormal to normal is slight. If such is the case, the surgeon must evaluate the patient's mental attitude carefully before making his decision, since even the finest surgical results may not please the patient. The assistance of a psychiatrist may be of great value. In some institutions such as Johns Hopkins Hospital in Baltimore, every patient seeking a rhinoplasty is routinely submitted to a psychiatric evaluation (Edgerton, Jacobson). Basing his reports on a painstaking study of one hundred and twenty patients, Jacobson (a psychiatrist) states that women are generally better risks than men for rhinoplasties because male motives are usually more complex than female motives and reflect a larger degree of psychiatric disorder. Men are less eager to change their own psychological outlook than to change that of others toward them. They are prone to "put all their eggs in one basket"—the operation—and may be disappointed in the result to such a degree that they are angered and even vindictive toward the physician.

Among women patients, Jacobson found a standard pattern: When children, they had rejected femininity as their mothers inadequately personified it, and embraced masculinity as their amiable fathers represented it. Sometime during adolescence, they decided they wanted to be women after all. The resultant conflict, said Jacobson, was expressed by a sense of nasal deformity (even if a serious deformity did not exist), because the women identified their noses with those of their fathers and felt that they were distastefully masculine. Women patients often told Jacobson that their noses "would look better on a man's face"; Jacobson got this remark even from married women. Jacobson also found that the success of the rhinoplasty depended a great deal on whether the patient's mother approved of the result. Hence, in many females seeking a rhinoplasty emotional rather than cosmetic motives are the reasons for the surgery.

A careful general and local examination should precede the operation. The patient must be in good health and free of any local infection. Photographs and in some cases casts of the face are of great aid in planning the operative procedures and in recording the case.

The object of the reconstructive operation is to bring the abnormal forms of a nose into harmony with the rest of the facial features. To achieve this, the surgeon must be able to imagine the final form of the nose. "Normal" and "abnormal" are terms which can be applied only in the light of the racial characteristics of the individual. The length of the normal average nose of an adolescent white person should equal the middle third of the distance between the hairline and the chin. The width of the nose (base of the ala) equals the space between the inner canthi.

The profile can be divided into three anatomical components: the bony component (*a* in Fig. 177), the upper cartilaginous component (*b* in Fig. 177), and the lower cartilaginous component (*c* in Fig. 177)

(Joseph). In a normal nose, all three components are of such proportions that they form a straight line from the root to the tip, and do not noticeably protrude or recede the nasal profile angle of about 20 to 38 degrees (30 degrees is ideal), and the nasolabial angle of 90 degrees. The nasal profile line is formed by the forehead, chin line, and the dorsum of the nose (Fig. 190). The normal profile line becomes disturbed if the three anatomical components protrude or recede the nasal profile angle singly or in combination. In Figure 190 *A*, the bony and upper cartilaginous components are protruding while the lower cartilaginous component (nasal tip) is receding. If one includes the length of the nose and its tilt in this scheme, the varieties of deformities become numerous.

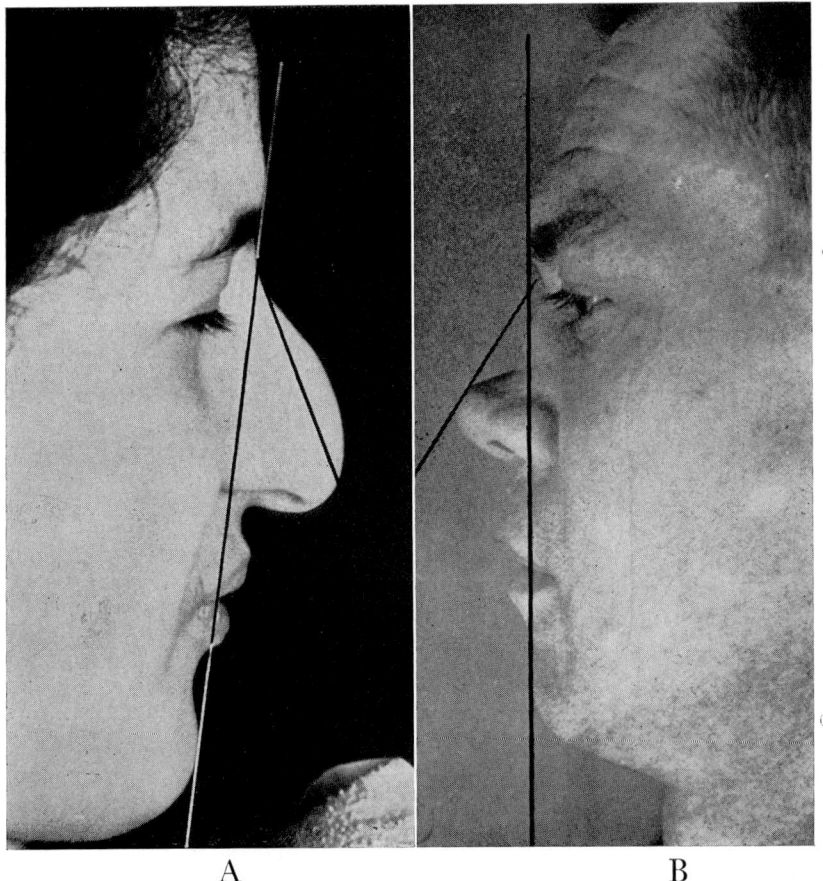

A   B

Fig. 190 Relation of nose to normal nasal profile angle. *A:* Upper and middle part of nose extending beyond normal nasal profile angle, while lower part of nose (nasal tip) is receding. *B:* Nasal ridge between nasal tip and glabella markedly receding from normal profile angle.

407

THE HEAD AND NECK

Classification

Berndorfer quotes Dufourmentel's division of the various nasal deformities:

1. Deformities due to insufficient skeletal support
    - (*a*) Depression of the bony structures (saddle nose)
    - (*b*) Depression of the cartilaginous framework (Negro nose)
    - (*c*) Depression of bony and cartilaginous framework (fat nose)
    - (*d*) Depression of the alae (nostril collapse)
    - (*e*) Stenosis of the nostrils
    - (*f*) Shortness of the alae
    - (*g*) Shortness of the nasal tip

2. Deformities of the bony and cartilaginous framework from hypertrophy
    - (*a*) Hypertrophy of the bony structure in the profile (hump nose)
    - (*b*) Hypertrophy in frontal direction (broad nose)
    - (*c*) Hypertrophy of the cartilaginous structures
        - (1) Elongation of the septum
        - (2) Prominence of the nasal tip
        - (3) Depression of the nasal tip (wide nostrils)

3. Deformities due to injury to the bony and cartilaginous framework
    - (*a*) Deviation of osseous structures
    - (*b*) Deviation of cartilaginous structures
    - (*c*) Deviation of nasal tip
    - (*d*) Subluxation of the septum
    - (*e*) Broadness of the nostrils

HUMP NOSE

A hump nose is a typical nasal deformity and, as a rule, can be satisfactorily repaired with rhinoplasty. Removal of the hump, however, is insufficient in the majority of cases without adjustment of the remainder of the external framework. Removal of the hump often causes broadness of the ridge, requiring narrowing, as well as reduction of the height of the ridge, which may make the nose appear too long, requiring shortening. The reduced height often causes prominence of the nasal tip, requiring reduction. All these operative steps, which should be planned preoperatively, require an adequate exposure of the nasal framework.

The procedure involves: (1) exposure of the nasal framework, (2) removal of the hump, (3) narrowing of the nasal ridge, (4) shortening of the nose, and (5) reconstruction of the nasal tip. The entire procedure is performed from intranasal incisions, and is based upon the ingenious work of Joseph of Berlin; the endonasal approach however had already been used previously by American surgeons Roe (1887), Weir (1892), and Goodale (1899). Improvements have been added, and much has been written about this subject (Aufricht and Safian having probably the largest experience in this field). The most extensive compilation of references has been made by McDowell, Valone, and Brown. Brown and McDowell of the United States and Denecke and Meyer of Germany and Switzerland have published monographs on rhinoplasty, each one a monumental piece of work.

Technique (Cases 52-55, pp. 1063-1066)

The operation can be performed under local as well as endotracheal anesthesia. Dingman has recently published an extensive article on local anesthesia for rhinoplasty. Both the outside and the inside of the nose are prepared. The hairs of the nostrils are cut with scissors, the face is gently washed with soap and water or pHisoderm, and the mucous membrane is painted with one of the nonirritating antiseptic solutions (Arnold's solution, see p. 4). The nose is then packed on both sides with plain gauze.

If general anesthesia is given, the endotracheal method under hypotension is used; this reduces bleeding to a minimum.

If local anesthesia is to be used, the patient is given 100 mg. of Nembutal the night before the operation. The same dosage is repeated two hours before the operation. One hour before the operation, 10 mg. of morphine are injected. The local anesthesia is preceded by packing each nasal fossa with a ½-inch strip of gauze, which is wrung dry after immersion in a solution of equal parts of 10 per cent cocaine and 1:1000 epinephrine. As a rule, 5 or 6 cc. of the solution will suffice. (If any solution is left, it should be discarded immediately to prevent confusion with the procaine solution used for local anesthesia. It is still better, and safer, to color the cocaine solution. Injected cocaine may cause instant death.) The packing is removed after thirty minutes. The local anesthetic (30 to 40 cc. of 2 per cent procaine solution to which 10 drops of 1:1000 solution of epinephrine is added) is injected first around and into the infraorbital foramina, then across the floor of the nostrils. The needle is now inserted intranasally between the upper and lower lateral cartilages and advanced subcutaneously to infiltrate the dorsum and glabella; it is then again inserted at the base of the ala, and the entire lateral wall of the nose is infiltrated. The same procedure is performed on the other side.

Exposure of Nasal Framework: The incisions necessary for this procedure are bilateral intercartilaginous incisions combined with an incision of the membranous septum. The intercartilaginous incisions are made first. The lower border of the upper cartilage is visualized by raising the tip of the nose with a small blunt retractor, which is held with the index finger and thumb of the left hand, while the middle finger presses the ala inside (Fig. 191 *A*). The mucous membrane is incised upon

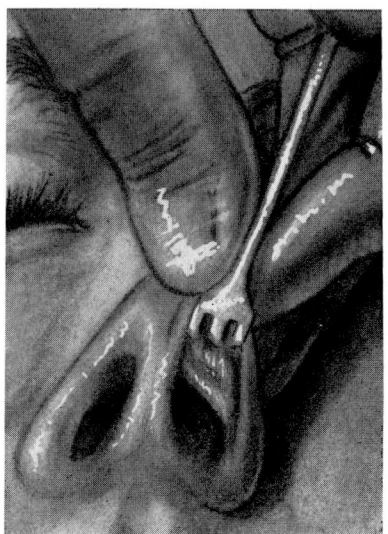

Fig. 191. *A:* Preparation for intranasal incisions in repair of hump nose. Lower border of upper lateral cartilage, along which intercartilaginous incision will be made, is visualized. (H. May: Plast. Reconstr. Surg.)

this ledge, starting posteriorly and reaching the tip cartilages anteriorly. The fibers between the upper and lower cartilages are severed. Thus, the lower border of the upper cartilage becomes exposed. A similar procedure is performed on the other side. With a curved pair of dissecting scissors, introduced through one of the incisions, the covering skin is freed from the nasal framework, anteriorly as well as laterally below the proposed line of reduction. The scissors are withdrawn. A two-pronged hook is inserted into the nostrils to elevate the nasal tip (Fig. 191 *B*). A pointed knife, Parker No. 11, is pushed through the interspace between the

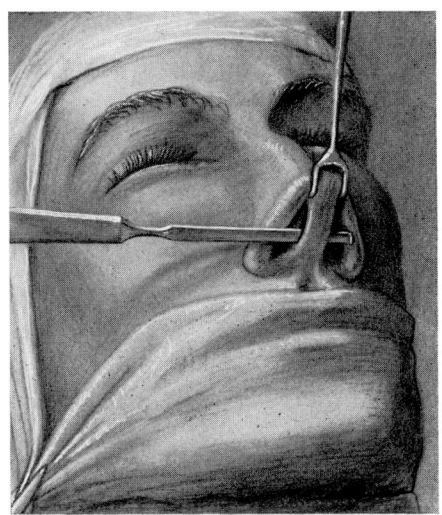

Fig. 191. *B:* Severance of columella cartilages from free edge of septal cartilage through membranous septum. (H. May: Plast. Reconstr. Surg.)

410

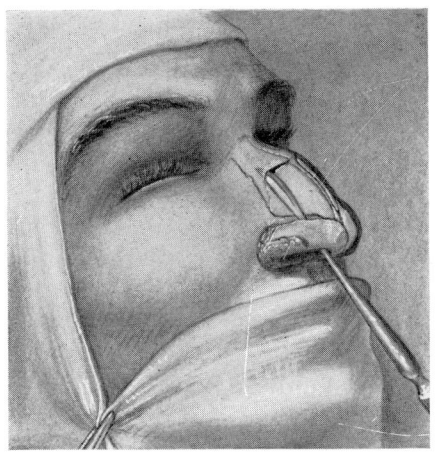

Fig. 192. *A:* Insertion of pointed knife through right intercartilaginous incision and incision of periosteum of nasal bones. (H. May: Plast. Reconstr. Surg.)

columella cartilages and the free edge of the septal cartilage; the pointed knife is then replaced with a dull-tipped knife, and the membranous septum is severed from the bottom to the tip (Fig. 191 *B*). At the tip, it is combined with the intercartilaginous incisions. The curved scissors are inserted through one, later through the other, intercartilaginous incision, and led from the root of the nose along the ridge, over the nasal tip and through the incision between columella and septum to make certain that no residual bands are left.

Removal of Hump: A pointed, slightly curved double-edged knife is inserted through the right intercartilaginous incision to incise the periosteum of the lateral wall of the anterior nasal bone (Fig. 192 *A*). The

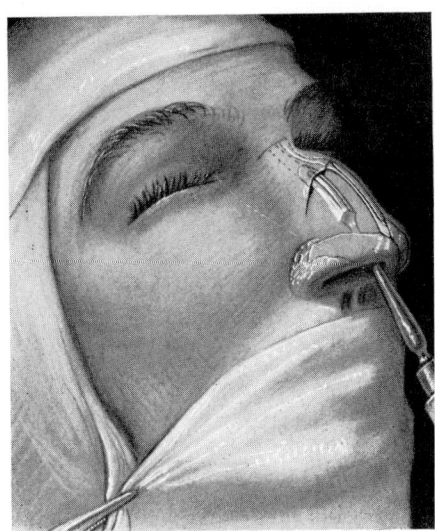

Fig. 192. *B:* Insertion of a small Joseph periosteal elevator to sever periosteum along the line of hump to be removed, closer toward face than the hump. (H. May: Plast. Reconstr. Surg.)

411

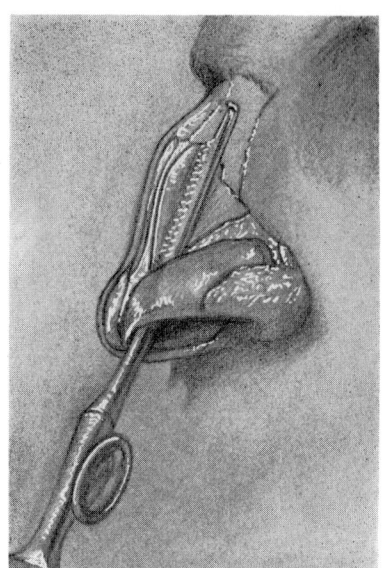

Fig. 192. *C:* Removal of hump with straight saw. (H. May: Plast. Reconstr. Surg.)

Joseph periosteal elevator is inserted into the periosteal incision, and the periosteum is elevated from the ridge and the lateral walls of the nasal bones along the line of the hump to be removed—closer, however, to the face than the hump (Fig. 192 *B*). The same procedure is performed on the

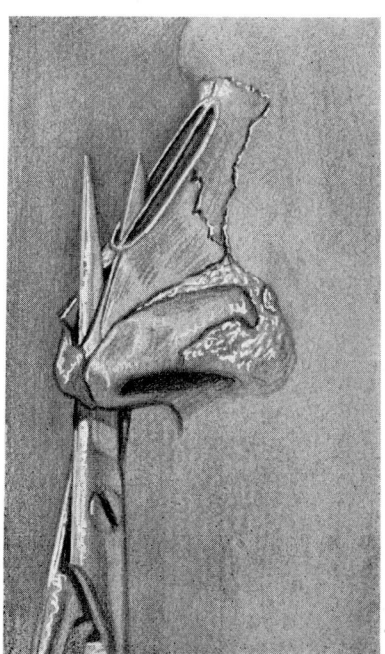

Fig. 192. *D:* Remaining attachments of upper lateral cartilages and septum are severed with pair of straight scissors. (H. May: Plast. Reconstr. Surg.)

412

other side. The hump is now removed, preferably with a straight nasal saw which is introduced through the left intercartilaginous incision (Fig. 192 C). The saw must be held horizontally to sever both nasal cartilages in the same plane. A guiding finger is placed upon the right side to prevent perforation of the skin. Any remaining attachments along the cartilaginous ridge can be severed with the angled drawing knife. The hump is now re-

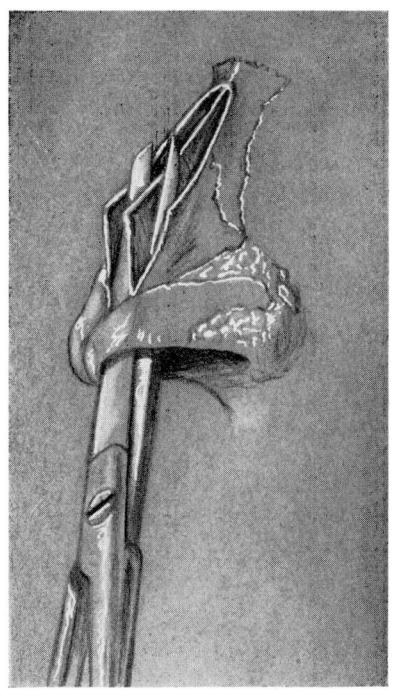

Fig. 192. *E:* Reduction of cartilaginous septal ridge which is followed by reduction of any protruding portions of the upper lateral cartilages. (H. May: Plast. Reconstr. Surg.)

moved with a grasping forceps. Although parts of the upper lateral cartilages which join the cartilaginous septum may have been removed with the hump, remaining parts may still be attached to the septal ridge; these are severed from the latter with a pair of straight scissors, which are held closely hugged to the septum (Fig. 192 D). With a nasal rasp, the sharp bony edges are smoothed; the debris is flushed out with water squirted from a bulb syringe. The skin over the dorsum is lifted with a long nasal retractor to permit inspection of the operative field; should the cartilaginous ridge of the septum or part of the upper lateral cartilages still be higher than desired, they can be reduced with a pair of straight scissors (Fig. 192 E). The anterior edges of the upper lateral cartilage, if too long and protruding, can be clipped at this stage.

413

Most noses do not require modification of the frontonasal angle, the dorsal hump being situated below the level of this angle. In some cases, however, further inspection and palpation may reveal a step-like bony protrusion remaining at the root of the nose above the area of the hump excision. This must be removed with a chisel to reduce fullness at the nasal root; further, infracture of the lateral nasal walls, which is to follow, would result in narrowing of the nose below the level of the undisturbed bony protrusion. To avoid this, Straatsma recommends the osteotome for removing the nasal hump because it provides an excellent glabellar notch and is accurate in removing small bony portions. The author fully agrees, but before using the osteotome he severs the upper lateral cartilages from the cartilagenous ridge and reduces the latter with straight scissors up the osseous ridge. He then inserts the osteotome and removes the hump in one piece (Figs. 193 *A* and *B*).

Narrowing: After removal of the lump, an elliptical defect is left, which usually broadens the nasal ridge (Fig. 194). To narrow it, the anterior processes of the maxilla, together with the nasal bone, must be mobilized to permit a median displacement of the nasal bones. This is done as follows:

The anterior processes of the maxilla, upon which the nasal bones rest, are severed; this can be done with a nasal saw or with an osteotome (Fig. 194). It is important to sever them flush with the face; if severed on a higher level, a bony ridge may become visible along the lateral nasal wall. Before the bones are severed, the skin and soft tissues are elevated along the base of the nose. A small intranasal incision is made at the right base of the anterior process of the maxilla at the piriform opening. The small Joseph periosteal elevator is pushed through the incision along the base of the lateral nasal wall, and the soft tissues are elevated. If an osteotome is used for severance, it is held in the right hand while thumb and index finger of the left hand protect the orbits; an assistant, with gentle blows on a mallet, drives the osteotome upward. If a saw is used (the bayonet type after Joseph), it is introduced with the help of Joseph's guiding elevator along the lateral wall of the frontal process of the maxilla, and the frontal process is sawed through in its entire length. The cutting should be done directly across the base of the lateral wall and not obliquely inward where it penetrates much thicker bone. The remaining anchorage of the nasal bone at the frontal process is now fractured. Before this is done, it may be necessary to sever or remove a segment of bone from the upper angle of the nasal bones with an osteotome (Fig. 195) to loosen the upper attachments and facilitate narrowing; if a segment of bone has been cut out, it is removed with a hemostat. The mobilization of the nasal bones is best done by inserting an osteotome between the septum and the

414

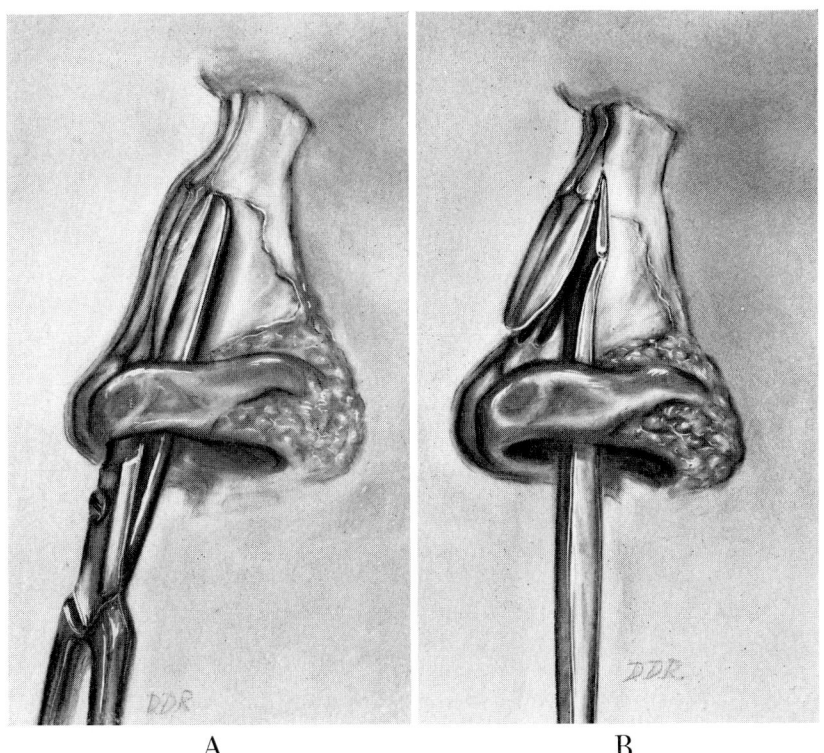

A   B

Fig. 193. *A:* Removal of cartilaginous hump with a pair of strong straight scissors inserted through an intercartilaginous incision. *B:* Completion of removal of bony hump with a chisel.

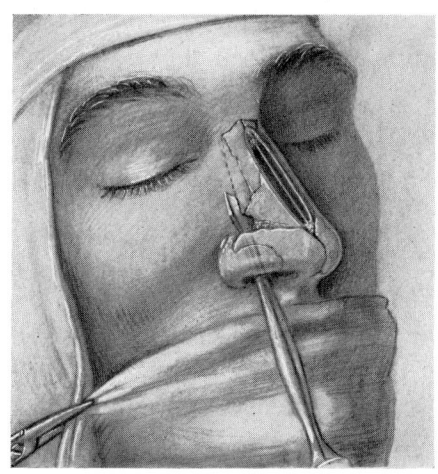

Fig. 194. To narrow elliptical defect of nasal ridge frontal processes of maxilla are severed. (H. May: Plast. Reconstr. Surg.)

415

nasal bone. When the osteotome enters the thick bone at the root of the nose, a dull sound is heard and the osteotome is then fixed in position without support. Using the septum as a fulcrum, the lateral nasal walls are pushed or broken outward, or the lateral walls are grasped with Walsham's nasal forceps and fractured outward. If the nasal bone is high at the root and thick, outward fracturing may occasionally become difficult. To facilitate this maneuver and to avoid fracturing the nasal wall too far below the root of the nose, a transverse osteotomy is performed with a

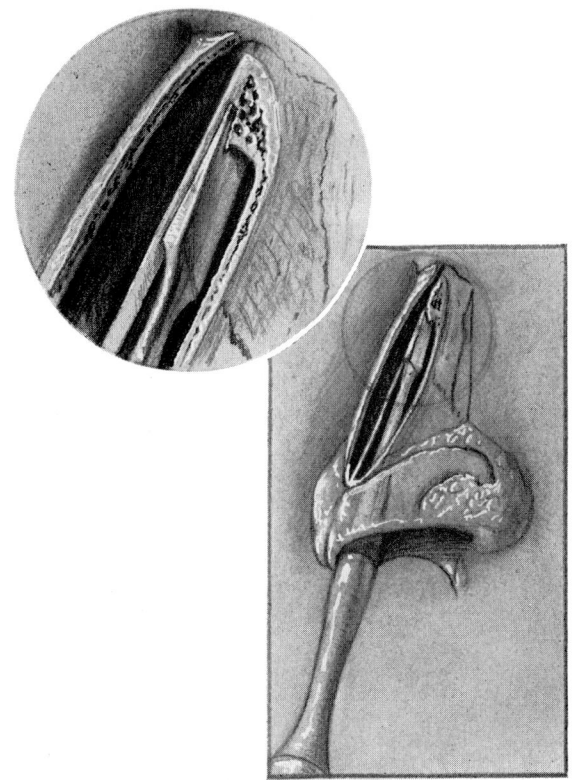

Fig. 195. Removal of triangular segment of bone of upper angle of nasal bones after Aufricht to loosen upper attachment of latter and facilitate narrowing. (H. May: Plast. Reconstr. Surg.)

straight osteotome inserted through a small horizontal incision which starts ½ cm. above and median to the inner canthus. A similar procedure is performed on the other side. The mobilized nasal bones are shifted into the midline by manual pressure (with the thumbs), thus narrowing the nasal ridge.

Shortening of Nose: This may or may not be necessary. The length of the nose is determined by the length of the septum and the thickness of the columella. Ideally, the length of the nose should equal the middle third of the distance between the hairline and the chin; the columella-lip

416

A

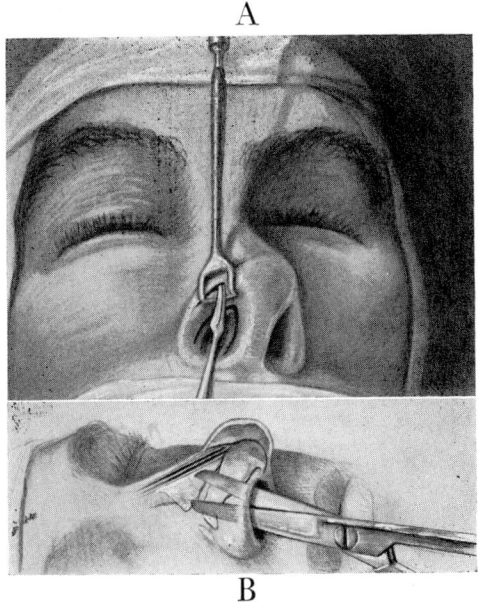

B

Fig. 196. *A:* Reconstruction of nasal tip. Intracartilaginous and transfixion incision is visible posteriorly. Alar cartilage to be exposed from rim incision. Nostril being steadied during the incision with ribbon retractor. *B:* With dissecting scissors skin is freed from alar cartilage. (H. May: Plast. Reconstr. Surg.)

angle should be about 90 degrees or slightly more, depending upon the length of the upper lip (in short upper lip, a tilt greater than 90 degrees will be more pleasing). If the nose appears too long, a quadrilateral strip of the free end of the septal cartilage is removed. Should, however, the anterior portion of the columella be "hanging," it is necessary to remove

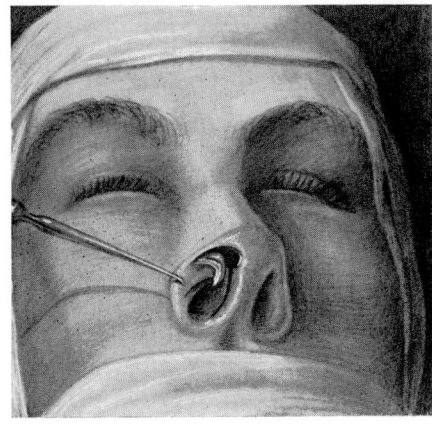

Fig. 197. Cartilage and mucous membrane incised near median crus below tip after Safian. (H. May: Plast. Reconstr. Surg.)

417

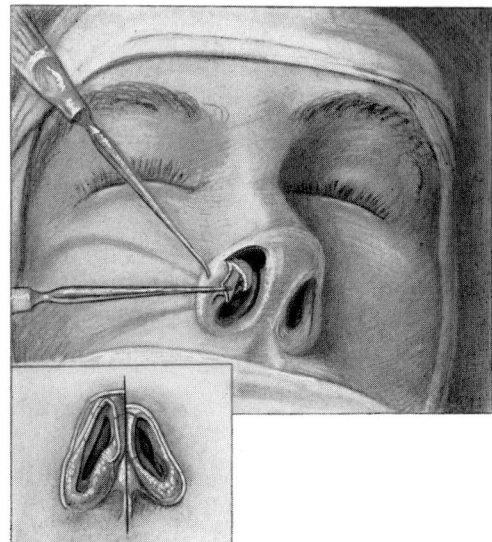

Fig. 198. Portion of cartilage to be excised freed from the underlying mucous membrane. Dotted lines of lower insert show incision along which dome is to be excised. (H. May: Plast. Reconstr. Surg.)

a triangular strip from the free end of the septum (base of the triangle anteriorly, tip toward the nasal spine) unless the hanging is due to excessive protrusion of the columellar cartilages, a situation that must be first corrected by proper trimming of the cartilages.

If the upper lip is too short due to protrusion of the anterior nasal spine of the vomer at the columella-lip junction, a quadrilateral strip of septum, including part of the anterior nasal spine, is removed. The columella is then suspended to the septum with a suture which passes through the base of the columella and through the skin, then back through the same suture opening and through the septum (Fig. 199).

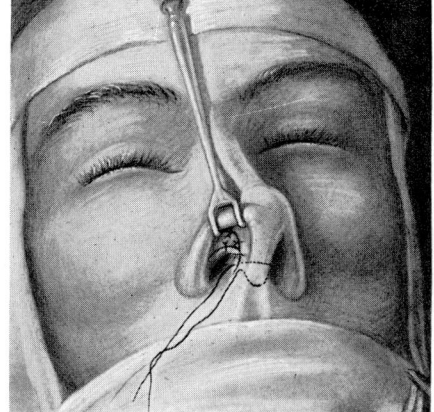

Fig. 199. Intranasal sutures and transfixion suture of columella and septum. (H. May: Plast. Reconstr. Surg.)

In all these excisions, one ought to be rather conservative; significant correction is often achieved after removal of small amounts of tissue. With a temporary stay suture, the columella is fastened to the free edge of the septum, thus shortening the midline of the nose. It now becomes noticeable that the lower rim of the upper lateral cartilages protrude into the nose through the intercartilaginous incision because the side walls are too long. These are shortened by excision of the protruding portions.

Reconstruction of Nasal Tip: After reduction of the height and the length of the septal-osseous framework of the nose, the tip as a rule is prominent and needs reduction. If the tip is not only prominent but wide and bulky, it must be reduced in height as well as in width and bulk. The lower lateral cartilages are exposed from an incision along the rim of the nostrils just within the nose. The insertion of a ribbon retractor, such as depicted in Figure 196, is of help to steady the nostril rim during the incision. The rim of the tip cartilage is exposed, and the covering skin is freed from the cartilage (Fig. 196) with a pair of dissecting scissors. The height of the tip cartilage is reduced by excision of a portion of the dome. This is done after Safian. Cartilage and mucous membrane are incised near the median crus just below the tip (Fig. 197). The portion of cartilage to be excised is freed from the underlying mucous membrane (Fig. 198); the exposed portion of cartilage is excised; the mucous-membrane flap is left behind, so that after proper shortening it can be reattached (Fig. 199). The same procedure is performed on the other side, care being taken to make the excisions of equal size.

If the lower lateral cartilages (the tip cartilages) require reduction not in height but in width, to make the tip more pointed, the excision does not include the median portion of the dome supplying the height, but only that part of the dome which gives breadth.

If reduction in bulk and height of the lower lateral cartilages is necessary, excision of the upper rim of the cartilage can be combined with the excision of the cross strip, after Brown and McDowell, so that the total excision consists of the removal of a single piece shaped like an inverted hockey stick, a procedure which the author favors. The cartilage is exposed by eversion and held everted on a pair of scissors (Fig. 200). The underlying mucous membrane should be left intact unless it is bulky and protruding. After the cartilages are repositioned, the rim incision is closed. The mucous membrane of the columella is sutured to that of the septum.

For correction of other tip and nostril deformities, see page 424.

Dressing and Immobilization: The packing is removed; the nasal vaults are cleansed with suction apparatus, and are packed again lightly with 1-inch strips of ointment gauze. One hundred and fifty units of hyaluronidase in 6 cc. of normal saline solution are injected into each side of the nose near the median canthi to prevent postoperative swelling (enzyme treatment is continued orally later). Final molding of the nasal walls and application of an immobilizing dressing follow. Of all the materials recommended for this purpose, the author finds the pressure dressing with halved corks efficient and simple: A medium-sized bottle cork is halved longitudinally. Each half is placed against the lateral wall of the nose, including the tip, and held in this position with adhesive strips (Fig. 201). The strip to hold the left cork in place starts on the right side

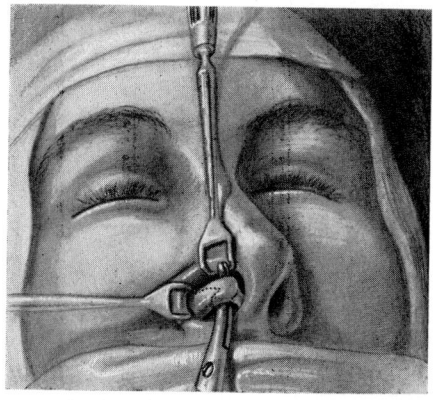

Fig. 200. Another method of reduction of heights and bulk (width) of alar cartilages—after J. B. Brown and F. McDowell. Cartilage is exposed from incision as in Fig. 190 and everted on a pair of scissors. Inverted hockey stick-like incision for removal of cross strip of the cartilage dome and upper rim of the tip cartilage is outlined. Underlying mucous membrane should not be excised.

of the forehead and proceeds over the left cork, then below the columella to the right side of the cheek. Readjustment of the strip may be necessary to place the flat side of the cork firmly and in its whole length against the nasal wall. A reverse procedure is performed with the right cork. One or two adhesive strips are placed transversely over the corks and attached to the cheek; to avoid depressing the nasal tip, they should not run over it. A piece of gauze is taped below the nostril for absorption of drainage.

After-Treatment

The dressings are changed on the third postoperative day. The packings are removed; the skin over the nose and the cheeks is gently cleansed with hydrogen peroxide solution and cold cream; the corks are firmly reapplied in the original manner. The dressings are removed on the fifth postoperative day. The nasal vaults are gently cleansed with swabsticks soaked in hydrogen peroxide solution, and the patient is discharged into ambulatory treatment.

Procedure for More Adequate Exposure of Nasal Framework

In the majority of cases, the classical intranasal incisions that derive from Joseph give adequate access to the nasal framework for the various steps of rhinoplasty. The Réthi incision, however, has been found extremely valuable when the cartilaginous framework, particularly of the nasal tip, is markedly and irregularly deformed and requires extensive

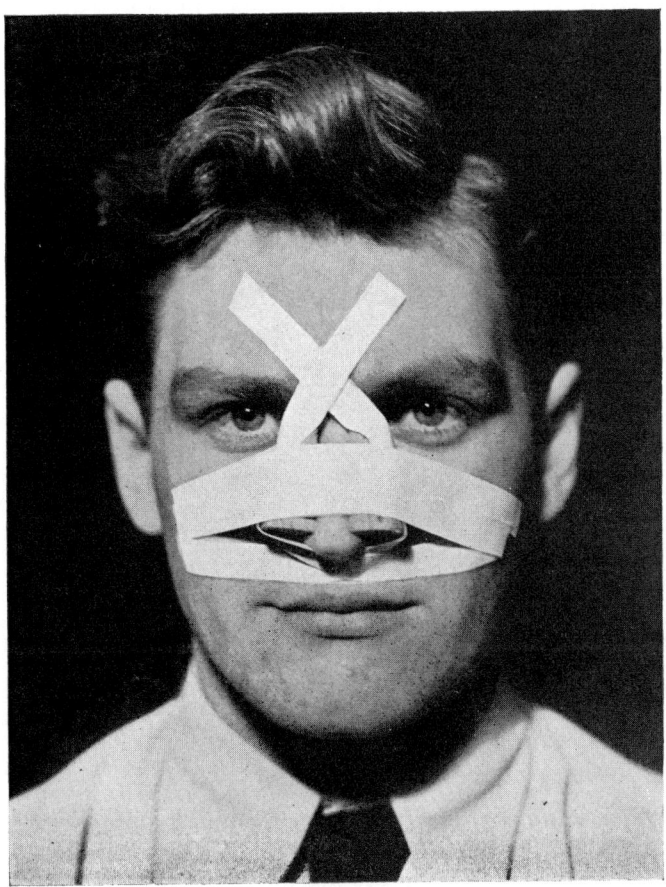

Fig. 201. Immobilization of nose with medium-sized cork, which has been halved. Each half is held firmly attached to nasal wall with adhesive strips which cross each other at forehead and below columella. One or two more adhesive strips are placed transversely over corks and attached to cheek.

421

reduction. The method is referred to in various textbooks, but its advantage of affording a much more adequate exposure of the lower half of the nose has not been widely appreciated.

Technique (Réthi) (Fig. 202; Case 51, p. 1062)

The Réthi procedure starts with a transverse incision through the columella. First, however, it is wise to make a longitudinal scratch with the scalpel through the middle of the columella. Later this will facilitate alignment of the wound edges. A transverse incision is made about 2 or 3 mm. (1/16 or 1/8 inch) posterior to the columella-alar angle; this penetrates the skin and to, but not through, the median crura. Two small arteries are encountered at each edge of the incision, and are ligated and severed. The direction of the incision is now changed abruptly toward the columella-alar angle, and from here runs parallel to and just inside the rim of the nostril, and circumscribes the anterior half of each rim. With the aid of traction sutures and under sharp and later blunt dissection, the skin overlying the median crura and the lower lateral cartilages is mobilized and retracted until the upper lateral cartilages are reached. This exposure offers an excellent access and view of the entire nasal framework. Whatever the nature of the deformity, the correction can be carried out under direct vision.

To separate the lower from the upper lateral cartilages, bilateral intercartilaginous incisions are made, unless they have already been made as the initial steps in exposure of the nasal framework in total rhinoplasty. After completion of the correction, the skin is reflected into its former position. The first suture of the wound edges is laid through the scratch-mark, followed by suturing of the remainder of the wound edges.

RHINOPLASTY AND CHIN AUGMENTATION

The nose and chin are conspicuous components of the profile line. The prominence of one will influence the other. It is well known that a receding chin will exaggerate the protrusion of the nose (see Case 54, p. 1065). If this is the case, reduction of the nose alone or additional build-up of the chin will greatly improve the appearance of the entire face. Aufricht routinely uses the resected osteocartilaginous hump and septal cartilage for augmentation of the receding chin, while Safian employs silastic implants inserting the implant from an outside incision. Millard uses an intraoral incision.

Technique (Case 55, p. 1066)

Before making the incision a vertical line is drawn from the center of the lower lip to the submental fold. To find the proper location for the protrusion of the chin, the soft tissues are manipulated and forced forward between the thumb and fingers and the proper location is marked out with a horizontal line. The incision is placed in the submental fold and should be not more than 1½ cm. long. The fat pad over the chin is dissected away down to the periosteum of the mandible. The periosteum is incised along the margin and elevated upward to create a pocket in the

A   B

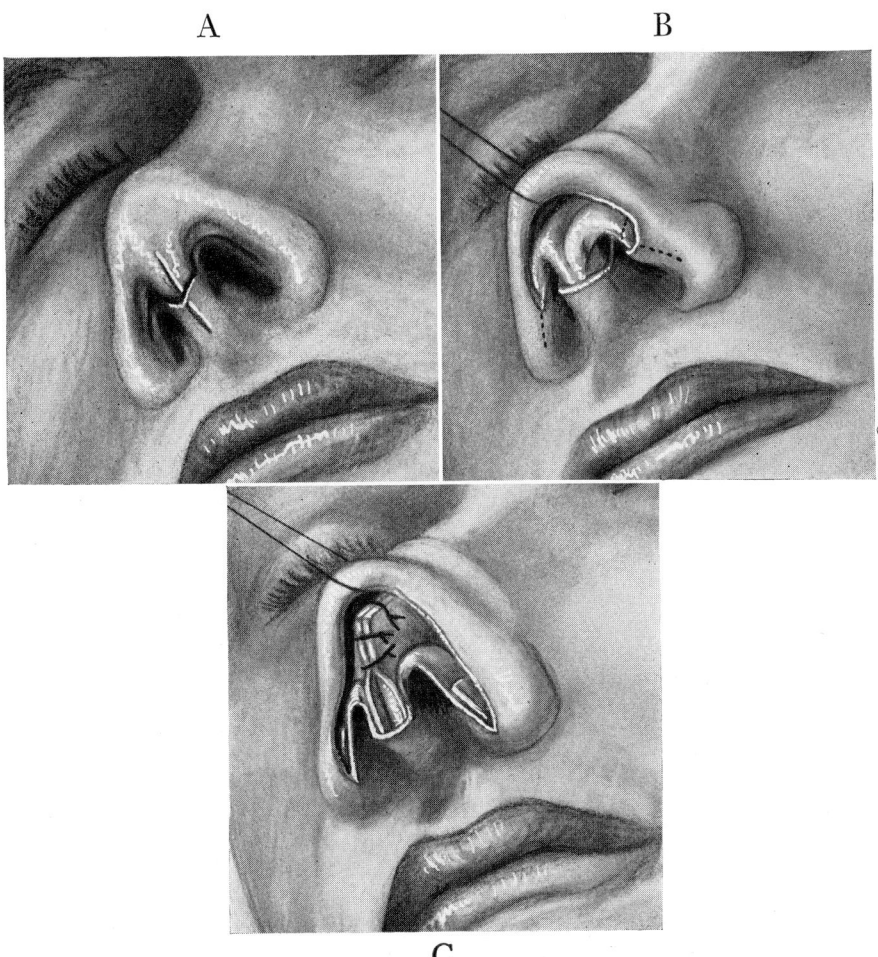

C

Fig. 202. *A:* Correction of retracted nasal tip (after Kazanjian and Straith). Exposure of lower and upper lateral cartilages (after Réthi). Intravestibular incision (internal incision) parallel to and just within nostril is combined with external incision across middle of columella. Small longitudinal line crossing columellar incision indicates landmark which should be scratched upon skin to facilitate accurate approximation later. *B:* Exposure of lower lateral cartilages by reflecting skin upward. *C:* After nasal mucous membrane has been dissected away, lateral crura are severed in proper level and everted and sutured back to back (Kazanjian, Straith).

423

exact location desired; it should be neither too large nor too small. The tissues below the margin of the mandible remain attached to form a shelf upon which the implant rests and to prevent it from slipping downward. The pocket is packed with gauze for several minutes prior to insertion of the implant to control whatever bleeding occurs. If a silastic implant is used—they come in various sizes—the implant is seized with a pair of sterile forceps and eased into the pocket. First one end is inserted toward the right side of the pocket and then, by traction on the left corner of the incision with the hooked retractor, the left end of the implant is guided into position. The implant rests subperiosteally on the mandible. The periosteum is now sutured as much as possible, thus holding the implant firmly in place. The small submental incision is closed with three or four silk sutures. A dressing similar to that described on page 581 is applied.

The trouble with the silastic implant is that it does not form an organic union and is thus apt to move around; this can be minimized by perforating the implant in several places with a perforator. Penn prefers the Kiel bone graft—denatured bovine bone after Maatz and Bauermeister (see also p. 75). He reports generally favorable results in a recent follow-up study.

It goes without saying that more radical procedures for building up a markedly retruding chin must be performed later, in a second stage (p. 579).

DEFORMITIES OF NASAL TIP

See also page 419.

Depressed (Wide) Tip

The tip cartilages are exposed from a Réthi incision. The lateral crura of the lower lateral cartilages are severed in the desired level (Fig. 202). Care must be taken to leave the underlying nasal mucous membrane intact. The mobilized lateral crura are then everted and sutured back to back (Kazanjian).

Depression (Shallow) above Tip

This depression is situated over the cartilaginous ridge, i.e., where the upper lateral cartilages join the cartilaginous septum. The upper lateral cartilages are exposed from a Réthi incision (Fig. 202), and are severed lateral to their insertion to the cartilaginous ridge. They are now everted and sutured back to back (Straith).

THE NOSE AND INTRANASAL REGIONS

Cleft Tip

In cleft tips, the soft tissues between the cartilages are removed by a Réthi incision; the width is reduced by excision of part of the dome from the lateral crura, and the cartilages are then firmly sutured together.

Retracting Tip

When the nasal tip is retracted, the columella is severed from the free edge of the septum and then pulled forward on the edge of the septal cartilage by an advancing mattress suture which reaches the columella at a more posterior level than the septal cartilage. This simple procedure, however, is usually not sufficient. It may take wide undermining of the ridge of the nose and shortening of the nose to accomplish a permanent result, i.e., a complete rhinoplasty.

DEFORMITIES OF NOSTRILS

See also page 419.

Bulging Nostrils

If the nostril is too bulging and outward curved at its base, a crescentic piece of ala is removed from its base with a pair of specially curved scissors which are inserted directly at the nasofacial groove. The latter can be better visualized by pressure upon the nostril. After suture of the wound, the suture line will come to lie along the groove of the base of the nostril.

Narrow Nostril Floor

If the floor of the nostril is too narrow, a triangular flap is made just lateral to the nostril (base toward the lip and tip toward nasofacial groove). The base of the nostril is severed as previously described, and the flap is switched from the outside to the inside (Fig. 203).

Wide Nostril Floor

When the floor is too wide, one may reverse the method just described. Another procedure is to excise a diamond-shaped piece of skin from the nasal floor, followed by wide undermining of the wound edges and suture of the skin.

Asymmetry of Nostrils

This is usually secondary to cleft-lip repair. (An excellent description of the pathological anatomy of the cleft-lip nose has been made by

Huffman and Lierle.) The lower lateral cartilage on the cleft side is below (posterior to) the level of the other side; the dome on the affected side is wide, causing a wide columella-alar angle, and the median crus is shorter than on the other side. Adjustment is made by repositioning the tip cartilage on the affected side as described on pages 316 to 317.

Atresia of Nostrils

This condition is due to destruction or absence of the mucous-membrane lining; it can be acquired or congenital. If congenital, it is usually associated with other deformities of the nose, requiring more or

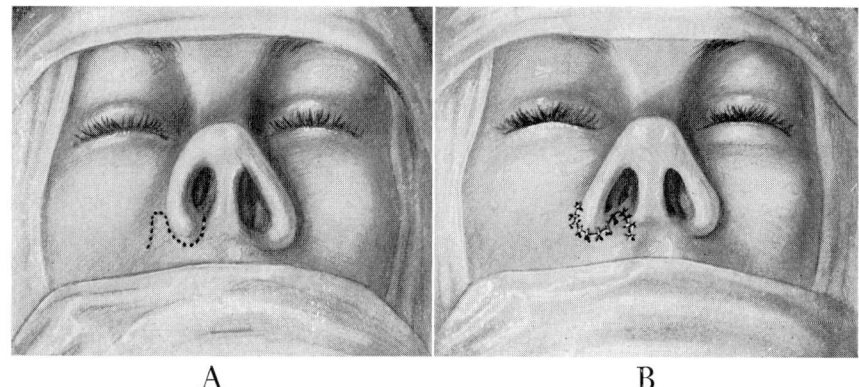

A   B

Fig. 203. *A:* Widening of floor of nostril; a triangular flap made just lateral to base of nostril. *B:* Base of nostril is severed and triangular flap switched from outside to inside.

less extensive reconstructive operations. If, however, the condition is due only to destruction of the mucous-membrane lining, the operation is simpler. It starts with excision of all scar tissue and formation of a normally shaped vestibule. A mold of dental compound is then formed of the latter with overcorrection, a thick split graft wrapped around it, raw surface outward, and inserted. The mold can be held in place by adhesive plaster or by a special dental prosthesis fastened to the upper teeth (see also pp. 433 to 434). The mold remains in place for ten days; it is then changed and replaced by another one, which is perforated to allow nasal respiration. The mold should be cleansed daily, and should be worn for at least two months to counteract shrinkage. In some cases of severely contracted nostril, better results are obtained by introduction into the floor of the nostril of a pedicled skin flap from the cheek alongside the nose.

426

DEFORMITIES OF COLUMELLA

Short Columella

The columella is freed from the lower edge of the septal cartilage by incising the entire membranous septum. The incision is continued toward the lip to form a V-shaped flap, which will lengthen the columella at the expense of the philtrum of the lip. The nasal tip is raised and the columella fastened to the septal cartilage; the wound edges of the lip are undermined and sutured together; suturing of the skin edges of the columella follows. For more extensive cases, a similar technique, as described on page 318, is applicable.

Oblique Columella

The columella may be displaced at its base or near its attachment at the nasal tip. The displacement is corrected according to the N-type of operation (compare with the method described on p. 360).

SADDLE NOSE

Saddle nose is due to destruction or displacement of the framework, particularly the ridge, of the nose.

In most cases, it is of traumatic or syphilitic origin, rarely congenital.

TRAUMATIC SADDLE NOSE

In saddle nose resulting from nasal injury, the bony framework is broad and flat; if the breadth is not too great, the depression of the nasal ridge is built up in one stage with a bone or cartilage graft. Otherwise, it may be necessary to elevate the displaced nasal bones and to narrow the abnormally wide base and ridge of the nose before introducing a graft. In this case, a two-stage operation is necessary.

Stage I (Reduction of Broad Nose)

From an intranasal incision (see p. 409), the nasal bones are exposed and separated anteriorly from their attachment at the septum by incising the bone on either side of the septum with the special straight broad dorsal saw (as devised by J. B. Brown and McDowell) from inward-outward. The upper lateral cartilages are then severed from their dorsal attachment to the septum and reduced in width. Then, from an incision along the lower border of the apertura piriformis, the anterior processes of the max-

427

illa are severed as described on page 414 and the nasal bones are brought into a more median position to approach each other in the midline above the nasal ridge, thus converting width into height; they are held in place with a cork dressing (Fig. 201) or with a mattress suture of stainless-steel wire, which is placed through either nasal bone and tied over lead plates.

Stage 2

Three weeks later, a properly shaped piece of cartilage or bone is inserted to fill out the depression. If only the nasal ridge is depressed, a simple graft is transplanted (Cases 59-60, pp. 1070-1071); if nasal tip and columella are also depressed, a columellar strut must be provided. The author prefers autogenous cartilage grafts, since they can be easily obtained and shaped, and also since they are not likely to become absorbed. The writer also prefers outside incisions at the nose for insertion of the graft, preferably the winged incision below the nasal tip. Curling of the cartilage graft has occurred occasionally and this indeed is a disadvantage. Gibson and Davis have counteracted this by a technique in which the cartilage is taken along a specified direction in the costal cartilage (see p. 64). The other popular graft material is bone which is taken from the iliac crest; it is shaped on the crest before its removal. Next in favor are cartilage homografts (Brown, McDowell) which however may gradually become absorbed. Least favored are foreign body implants, although silicone rubber has gained recently in popularity (see p. 76).

Technique (Fig. 205)

From a V-shaped incision below the nasal tip, the skin of the ridge of the nose is undermined, first with a small knife, then with a pair of curved scissors until the nasal bones are reached; from there the undermining is done subperiosteally. The undermining should be exactly in the midline and not too far laterally. At the glabella, the periosteum is raised to form a pocket. Hemostasis is now applied by pressure.

The cartilage graft is taken and prepared as described on page 63. The perichondrium is removed. The upper part of the graft is tapered so as not to obliterate the frontonasal angle. The lower part is also tapered to conform with the tip. The dorsum of the graft should be rounded and smooth. The graft is taken from the cartilaginous portion of the seventh, eighth, or ninth rib on the right side. For bulkier grafts as used in the majority of cases, a section of the whole thickness of the seventh rib is removed; this is the last to reach the sternum. The perichondrium is removed. One can now follow the advice of Gibson and Davis and cut the graft so that the transverse section is balanced (p. 64). The graft should

428

have the shape of the prow of a ship. The upper part of the graft is tapered so as not to obliterate the frontonasal angle. The lower part is also tapered to conform with the tip. The dorsum of the graft should be rounded and smooth. The graft is inserted, but may need removal for further shaping. To reduce trial insertions to a minimum, the author uses one of the commercially available silicone prostheses which come in various shapes and

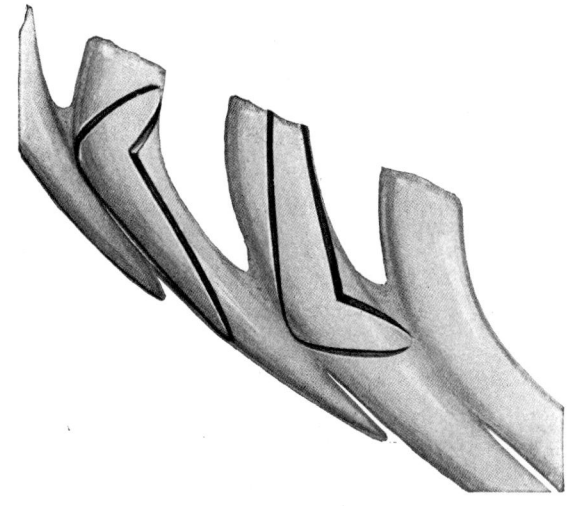

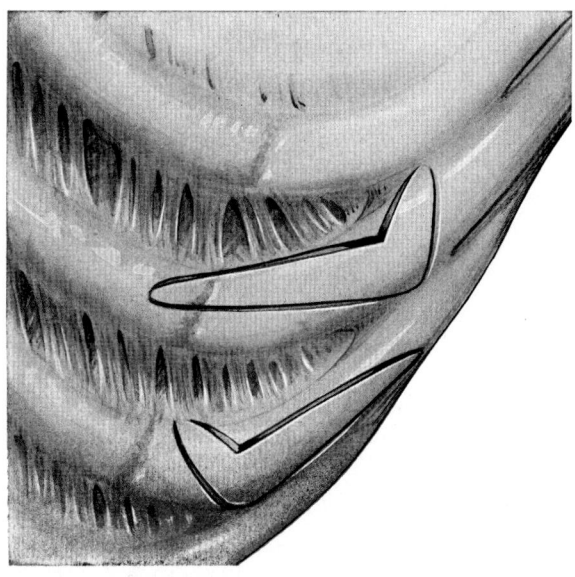

Fig. 204. Removal of angulated rib graft. For longer grafts bone must be included. (From H. J. Denecke and R. Meyer: Plastic Surgery of Head and Neck. Springer Verlag, New York, 1967.)

sizes; the one that fits best serves as a model according to which the cartilage graft is carved. After final insertion of the graft, the incision is closed (Cases 59-60; pp. 1070-1071). If there is a tendency for the graft to slip, a straight needle is pierced through skin, graft and underlying support. The needle is clipped short and removed after one week.

To prevent contamination of the chest wound, the author advises taking the cartilage graft before operating on the nose.

If the columella needs to be supported to maintain the prominence of the nasal tip, a Y-shaped incision is made, which is provided by a V-incision below the nasal tip and a longitudinal extension along the columella. From this incision, the entire columella is incised in the midline; in addition to the undermining of the nasal ridge, the cartilages of the columella are separated from each other, and posterior to them a pocket is prepared in the membranous septum reaching from the tip to the nasal spine of the maxilla (Fig. 205).

To provide a strut to the main graft, the use of an angulated piece of rib cartilage graft carved in one piece is satisfactory, although it takes patience and skill to provide it. E. Schmid advises either taking the graft from the eighth rib, with the short arm of the L at the angle of the rib and the long arm median to it, or from the eighth rib vice versa (Fig. 204); the long arm, if necessary, may be elongated into the bony part of the rib. The graft is outlined with the knife, which penetrates to about 2 mm. of the posterior layer of the rib. Along each edge of the long arm, a groove is cut away to permit insertion of a small Joseph periosteal elevator to undermine the graft posteriorly along the 2-mm. thin posterior layer of the rib. The short arm of the L is mobilized in a similar way. If the seventh rib is used as the donor area, removal of part of the eighth rib adjacent to the angle of the graft facilitates freeing of the short arm. The ribs are not fused in this area, as Denecke and Meyer point out correctly; they are only loosely connected. This syndesmosis should be carefully broken up with the elevator prior to removal of the adjacent part of the eighth rib. Routinely, another piece of cartilage graft should be removed in case the shorter arm needs to be built up, as will be pointed out later. If on the seventh rib bone must be removed for elongation of the long arm of the L, a chisel must be used for this purpose. The long arm of the L is now carved according to the previously inserted silicone prosthesis; the short arm should be broad, seen from the lateral view, so that it fills the entire membranous septum up to the anterior edge of the lamina quadrangularis. The angle between the short and long arms should be less than a right angle. The graft is now inserted. It is important that the short arm rests firmly upon the nasal spine and does not glide off it. Hence, it is good to reduce the spine to a shallow small groove with a narrow

430

rongeur. To facilitate this, the region of the spina nasalis and the lower rim of the apertura piriformis can be exposed from an incision along the upper gingivolabial sulcus. Link and Schmid use this approach for undermining the entire graft bed. The intraoral approach of the nasal spine is particularly useful when the short arm of the L-shaped graft cannot be cut long enough to provide sufficient support of the nasal tip. If this is the case, I cut a small square block from the additional cartilage graft removed previously, as long as necessary. A groove is made on the base of the addi-

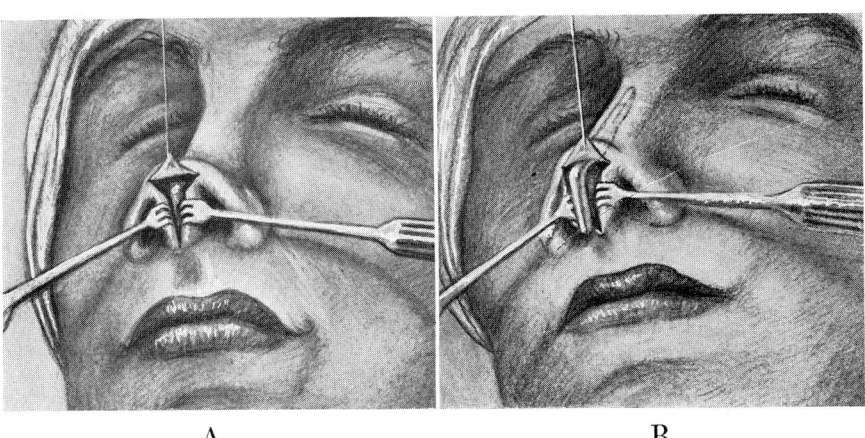

A.   B

Fig. 205. *A:* Reconstruction of traumatic saddle nose and depressed nasal tip by insertion of angulated cartilage graft. V-shaped incision is made below nasal tip with longitudinal elongation along columella. Columellar cartilages are retracted, exposing free end of septal cartilage. Triangular skin flap is lifted. Ridge of nose is undermined. *B:* From the cartilaginous part of the seventh or eighth rib, an angulated piece of cartilage is carved out. Its longer arm is inserted into dorsum of nose, the shorter arm posterior to columella resting upon nasal spine of maxilla.

tional strut to fit over the nasal spine, and another groove is made to receive the pointed part of the main strut. This square should be made broad enough to provide a solid basis for the main graft. All wounds are closed. Again it is stressed that rib cartilages be taken prior to the operation on the nose to prevent contamination of the chest wound.

Peer states that he prefers insertion of the columellar strut separately through a small incision in the buccal mucous membrane. The upper end of this cartilage strut is placed in front of the lower end of the dorsal graft, thus supporting the nasal tip at any height desired by the operator. This placement of the two cartilage grafts as separate segments enables the surgeon to obtain a soft, natural line for the nasal dorsum and tends to avoid a beaked appearance at the nasal tip.

431

The author has done this recently on two occasions (see Case 61, p. 1072) and recommends this method because he found it simpler and more satisfactory than the carving and insertion of an angulated cartilage graft. The strut graft, however, was inserted into a pocket of the membranous septum through a columella-splitting incision.

Some surgeons prefer bone grafts. The bone is taken from the crest of the ilium and removed with converging chisels (Seeley). The convergence is so arranged as to be entirely within the confines of the inner and outer table of the ilium. The graft is then carved L shaped or, if much of the cartilaginous septum is destroyed, a broader piece is left attached in shape of "a rudder of the common sailboat." One should make sure that the upper part of the graft comes to lie subperiosteally; hence, prior to the insertion, a chisel is inserted subperiosteally for the removal of a thin section of dorsal nasal bone for creation of such a pocket.

If there is a tendency of the graft to slip, a straight needle is pierced through skin, graft, and underlying support, thus anchoring the graft in a simple way. The needle is clipped short and removed after one week.

In some cases only the cartilaginous ridge is depressed as one sees it after an abscess of the septum. If this is associated with retraction of the nasal tip, the method of Kazanjian-Straith is suitable for correction (see Fig. 202). If unassociated with retraction of the tip, the depression is best corrected by a dermal graft which is inserted through the previously mentioned V-incision (Straatsma). For removal of dermal grafts, see page 46. Stark and Frilech use a conchal cartilage graft instead.

Syphilitic Saddle Nose

Before any operative work is done, one must be sure that the disease has been brought to a standstill; as a matter of fact, it is best to play on the safe side and submit the patient to thorough preoperative antiluetic treatment whether his Wasserman reaction is positive or negative.

Gillies divides the deformities of the syphilitic nose in three groups:

1. Syphilitic deformities from small losses of the cartilaginous septum, which are corrected by insertion of a cartilage graft as previously described.
2. Syphilitic deformities due to destruction of the framework and lining.
3. Syphilitic deformities due to destruction of skin, framework, and lining.

LOSS OF FRAMEWORK AND LINING

In these cases, it is necessary to replace first the lining of the nose and subsequently the framework.

Technique (*Gillies*)

To restore the nasal tip and alae to their normal position, it is necessary to sever them from the apertura piriformis and the underlying bone. The nasal skin can now be stretched forward to normal size and position. The resulting raw surface at the inside must be covered with a skin graft to prevent subsequent shrinkage.

Stage 1: A dental prosthesis to fit the upper teeth is designed by a dentist. To the center of this prosthesis, a removable flat splint is applied, which is broader at its end. The prosthesis is cemented to the teeth preoperatively.

An incision is made along the upper gingivobuccal sulcus from one fossa canina to the other. All soft tissues are severed until the nasal cavity is reached. While the nasal tip is pulled forward, the columella and the soft tissues of the nose—the septum is absent—are severed from the bone mediad and laterally until the root of the nose at the glabella is reached.

A mold of dental compound is made (see p. 39) to fit the new overdistended nasal cavity. After packing the piriform opening to prevent escape of the compound into the posterior nasal spaces, the softened compound is pressed through the buccal incision into the nasal cavity with one hand while the other one molds the compound from the outside. While the compound is still soft, the removable splint is warmed, pushed into it, and screwed to the dental prosthesis. After the mold has become hard, splint and mold are removed. It is recommended that one make a second stent at this time from which a permanent acrylic stent is later made. The stent is covered with a thin split graft, raw surface out (see p. 39), and reinserted after removal of the nasal packing; the splint is screwed to the prosthesis (Fig. 206). The usual after-treatment is carried out, as described on page 40. McLaren and Penny advise cutting the split graft thin and free of epidermal appendages to avoid sebaceous secretion and unpleasant odor later.

After two weeks the stent is removed and cleansed. The cavity is thoroughly irrigated with hydrogen peroxide and isotonic saline solution; any excess graft is removed and the stent, this time the acrylic stent, is reinserted. From then on, the same procedure is repeated every other day.

Stage 2: After two months, a cartilage graft is transplanted, as previously described; care must be taken not to perforate the new nasal lining while forming the canal for the graft. The opening between mouth and nose can be closed in the same sitting by simply denuding and suturing the wound edges.

Another way of lining the nasal cavity is by insertion of a median forehead flap. Cardoso (1945) and Kazanjian (1946) inserted such a flap from an incision over the dorsum of the nose. Loebe improved the method by pulling the flap through a tunnel beneath its own base at the root of the nose down into the nasal cavity. The flap is severed from its pedicle after four weeks and the pedicle is adjusted in place.

LOSS OF SKIN, FRAMEWORK, AND LINING

The reconstructive work in these cases is similar to that used for subtotal or total rhinoplasty.

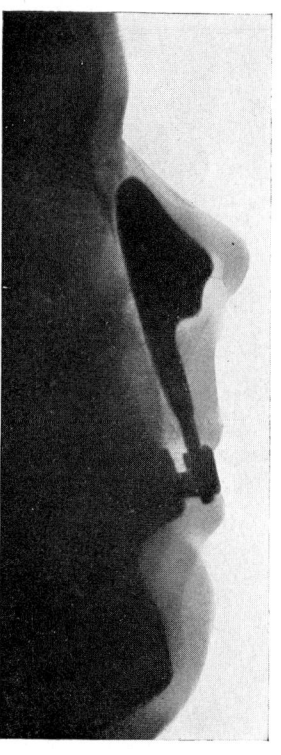

Fig. 206. Reconstruction of syphilitic saddle nose (after Gillies) (see text). (From H. D. Gillies: Deutsche Ztschr. f. Chir.)

In cases, however, in which columella, nasal tip, and parts of the skin of the dorsum of the nose are preserved—that is, the middle and upper portions of the nose destroyed—a transverse incision is made above the lower cartilaginous vault through the full thickness of the nasal wall. The lower portion is now pulled into normal position. The resulting defect is covered with a lined forehead flap, which is pedicled in the median third of one eyebrow (p. 392), or a sickle flap (p. 393). The lining may be provided by turning over a local flap (Nélaton and Ombrédonne, Lexer). A few weeks after the division of the pedicle of the flap, a cartilage graft is transplanted.

BIFID NOSE

Bifid nose, or cleft nose, is a rare congenital deformity (Case 56, p. 1067). Owing to its rarity and the complexity of its treatment, it will be considered only briefly. The reader is referred to the excellent articles on this subject by Webster and Demming, Peer, Gelbke, Marino and Davis, Denecke and Meyer, Wang and Macomber, and others.

As to the embryology of the midface, particularly of the upper central portion, the reader should refer to page 274 and Figure 86. It is evident that lack of fusion of the mesial nasal processes could cause not only the bifid nose but also, occasionally, a median cleft lip and palate and a median line dermoid cyst. A suggested hypertelorism may also be present, although seldom a real one. In most cases, marked improvement can be brought about by surgery. Delaying surgery until maturity avoids the possibility of disturbance of growth, but a delay is not suggested by most surgeons because the deformity may cause personality damage in early childhood. Later insertion of bone or cartilage grafts may then become necessary. All authors stress the necessity of an open surgical procedure. Webster and Demming have given a well-illustrated description of their various procedures in ten cases. After an alliptiform excision of skin and subcutaneous tissue, reaching from the hairline down to the base of the columella at the upper lip, the broad nasal structures are narrowed by excision of the broad top of the osseous and cartilaginous framework, followed by lateral osteotomies of the anterior processes of the maxilla, submucous narrowing of the wide septum, and suturing of the lateral walls together in the midline. When the tip is broad but not insufficient, a longitudinal strip of skin and subcutaneous tissue which lies between the cleft tip cartilages and median crura is excised, followed by approximation of the separated parts with 0000 chromic catgut. The wound edges are closed in layers after wide undermining. When the tip is insufficient and the nostrils are pointing upward, the oval excision should be delayed, and an inverted V-incision should be made instead. The tip of the V is on the forehead above the glabella; the arms of the V are on the lateral side, ending at the rim of the displaced nostrils lateral to the columella-alar angle. The enclosed skin is elevated as a flap, which is based inferiorly at the rim of the nostrils and the columella. The necessary reduction of width of the framework is then performed as described above. The flap is advanced downward, rolling on itself at the nasal tip. The wound edges are then closed resulting in an inverted Y-formation.

As mentioned above, in most cases any concomitant hypertelorism is only suggested and will improve after the nose is narrowed (Case 56,

p. 1067). Real hypertelorism is difficult to correct. I refer the reader to Converse and co-workers, Tessier and co-workers, and E. Schmid's ingenuity in this field.

DEFLECTION OF NOSE

Deflections of the nose are either congenital or due to malunited fractures. In the former case, the entire nose may be deflected toward one side; in deflections due to trauma, the osseous or the cartilaginous part may be involved singly or may be bent in different directions, resulting in a twist of the nose. There is, however, hardly any deflection where the cartilaginous septum is not involved. A correction must attack the external deformity as well as that of the septum. Unless the latter is straightened, the external deformity will recur. Trendelenburg, Goodale, and Joseph have done the pioneer work upon which the present reconstructive technique is developed. A good review of the subject has been provided by Elsbach.

Technique

Osseous Structures: The piriform openings are tightly packed with plain gauze. An intranasal incision is made along the lower border of the apertura piriformis, skin and periosteum are elevated from the lateral surface of the nasal bone, and the anterior process of the maxilla is severed as demonstrated in Figure 194. The same procedure is performed on the other side. A gauze pad is now laid upon the deviated or convex side; and, with the thumb, pressure is exerted upon the osseous structures of this side to sever the frontonasal attachment and fracture the perpendicular plate of the ethmoid. If the frontonasal attachment cannot be broken by manual pressure, a small incision is made over the root of the nose, just below the glabella, and the frontonasal attachment—together with the perpendicular plate of the ethmoid—is severed with a small chisel. The nose is now shifted into the midline.

In more severe cases of deflection, there is a discrepancy in the length of the nasal bones; the concave side is longer than the other. This can be rectified by shortening the elongated bone either at the base or along the ridge. The bone is shortened along the ridge if the deflection of the nose is accompanied by a hump. If this is the case, the hump is removed first (Case 46) in such a way that more of it is taken off the elongated side. The anterior process of the maxilla on the short side is now severed (Fig. 194) and shifted mediad. This alone, without severing the other side, may overcome the deflection; more often, however, the other side must also be severed and molded into correct position. If a hump is absent and

436

the elongated side must be shortened, a triangular piece of bone should be removed from the anterior process of the maxilla on the long side with its apex at the frontonasal suture and its base at the apertura piriformis. From an intranasal incision, described above, the anterior process of the maxilla is freed from its periosteum laterally and the nasal mucous membrane medially; the strip of bone is sawed out with the nasal saw, making the upper saw cut first. The bone is withdrawn with a grasping clamp. The anterior process of the maxilla on the short side is now severed; the frontonasal attachment may need severance (see above), and the nose is shifted into the midline, followed by repair of the deviated septum.

Cartilaginous Structures: In nasal deviations, the cartilaginous septum is also deviated, dislocated, or twisted, and, unless it is restored to its normal position, external deviation will recur. If the entire septal cartilage is dislocated from its midline insertion on the nasal floor, the entire cartilage must be freed anteriorly, posterior and above (Case 58, p. 1069). If in the first phase of the operation (see above) a hump was removed, the anterior attachments of the septum along the bony nasal ridge have already been freed; care must now be taken that the upper lateral cartilages are severed from their insertions at the ridge of the septum. In the absence of a hump, the necessary intranasal incisions must be made to sever the columella from the free edge of the septum and the upper lateral cartilages from the septal ridge. By retracting the columella to one side, the nasal spine and the base of the septum are visualized; the nasal mucous membrane is elevated with the Joseph elevator from the base of the septum all the way back; the same procedure is performed on the other side. With a small chisel, the septum is separated from its false position on the nasal floor; it is forcibly moved into the midline, and the perpendicular plate of the ethmoid bone may now be fractured. The insertion and spreading of a septal speculum is helpful in manipulating and freeing the septum. The septum may then remain in the midline without a return of the deviation.

Where the lower free border of the septum is laterally displaced and causes protrusion of it into one nostril, obstruction of the other nostril at the site of the angulation, and drooping of the nasal tip, the following procedure is added: From the previously mentioned incision through the membranous septum parallel to the free edge of the lower border of the dislocated septal cartilage, the mucous membrane is dissected away and reflected from the septal cartilage on each side until the site of the angulation of the septum is reached. At the angle of the deflection, the cartilage is incised vertically. Then the dislocated portion of the septum is separated from its false attachment at the maxilla with a small chisel. The thus mobilized septal cartilage, which is now as free as a graft, is reduced to normal position beneath the nasal tip, elevating the latter. It is sutured in this position with a mattress suture to the cartilages of the columella. The reflected mucous-membrane flaps are reduced to proper size and the wounds sutured.

Where the displacement of the lower end of the septum is associated with a long nose, Brown and McDowell advise cutting off the crooked lower end of the septum, chiseling off any deforming sector of the nasal spine, and shortening the nose (see p. 416).

After the deviation is corrected, a partial obstruction of the airways may still exist; this can be overcome later, after healing is complete, with a submucous resection.

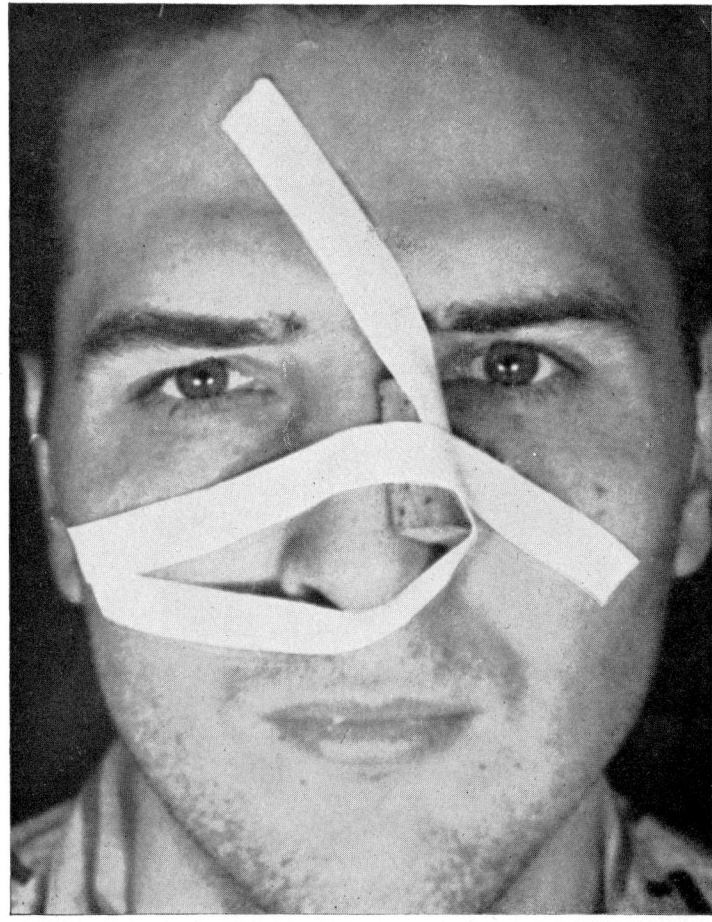

Fig. 207. Immobilization of nose after its severance for correction of deviation. Medium-sized cork is halved longitudinally. Its flat side is placed upon the formerly deflected side and held firmly with adhesive strips, pulling nose toward corrected side.

Immobilization: If after correction of the deviation, there is no tendency of the fragments to return to their former position, the nasal packings are replaced with packings of petrolatum gauze and the following simple immobilization applied (Fig. 207): A medium-sized cork is halved longitudinally. The flat side is placed upon the formerly deflected nasal side and held firmly in this position with adhesive strips, which also pull the nose toward the corrected side. Packings and immobilization device are removed after forty-eight hours, and the nasal vaults are cleansed with applicators dipped in hydrogen peroxide solution. The immobilization device is reapplied and worn for another week.

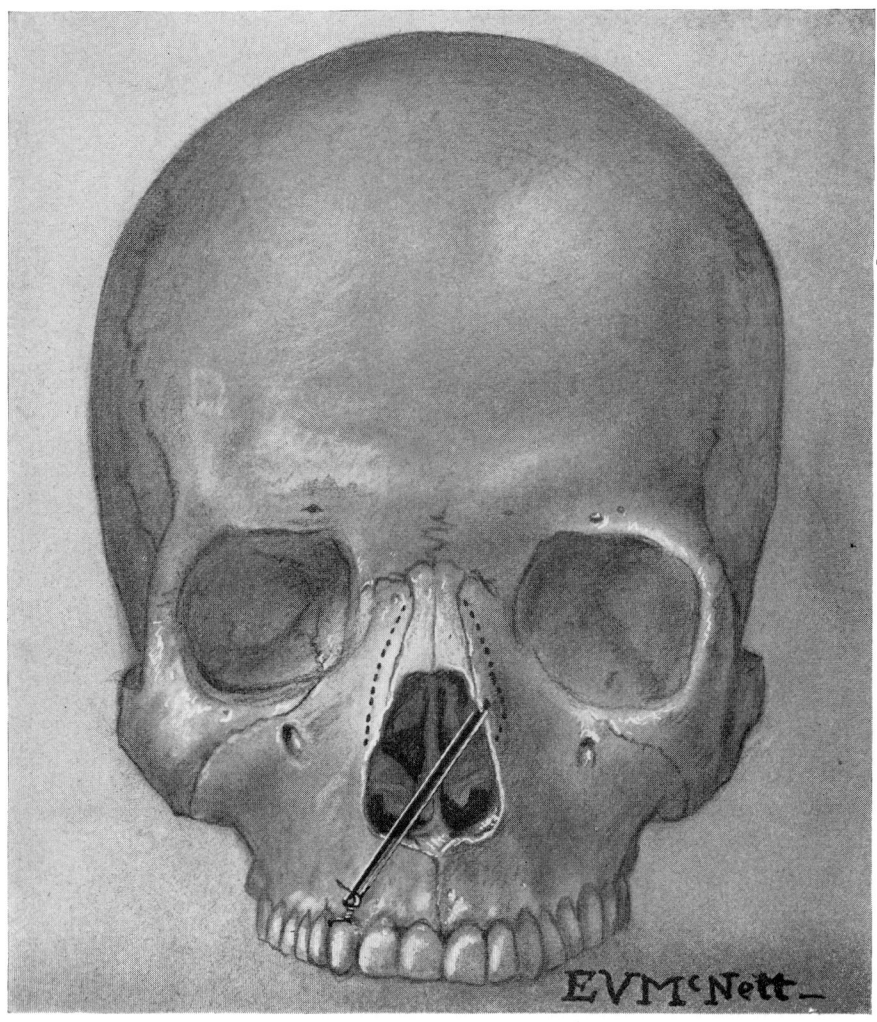

Fig. 208. Wire anchorage of severed nose (after Blair).

If after correction of the deviation there is a tendency for the deviation to recur, an adjustable nasal splint should be worn for several weeks. Blair's wire anchorage is also recommended (Fig. 208). From a small incision over the lateral aspect of the nasal bone of the deflected side, a small hole is drilled through the bone near its free border, and the ends of a loop of thin stainless-steel wire—slack end armed with a strong straight needle—are passed through the hole and around the free end of the bone, then obliquely through the septum and the mucogingival sulcus of the opposite side, where they are fastened to a wire loop applied to a molar or premolar tooth under tension. Obviously, the nasal packing must be removed before the wire is passed. The small skin incision does not require suturing. The wire should remain in place for four weeks.

RETRUSION OF MIDFACE (DISHFACE DEFORMITY)

Under this term are combined certain congenital or traumatic deformities in which a retroposition of nose and middle of the face is characteristic, but which, in the final analysis, vary a great deal. For this reason, the treatment or variety of treatments must be adapted to each case. In general, the deformities may be classified as follows:

Group 1

A typical situation is the retrusion of the upper lip in certain cases of secondary cleft lip and palate deformities, with a short, hanging columella, marked diminution of the columella-lip angle, and a drooping nasal tip. The retrusion of the upper lip is due either to faulty technique of primary lip repair or to lack of maxillary development after cleft-palate operation (see p. 280). The nasal deformities are usually due to lateral displacement of the septum, depriving the nasal tip and columella of support.

Group 2

To this group belong certain traumatic or more often congenital dishface deformities in which the entire midface is flattened, including the nose, and the columella is drooping over the recessed upper lip, producing a sunken-in impression. Often, the lower part of the cartilaginous septum and the nasal spine are found absent. The deformity may be accentuated by an associated protrusion of the mandible (Case 62, p. 1073).

Group 3

A third group of midface retrusion is due mainly to syphilitic destruction of the nasal bones and cartilages, as described on page 434. The treatment of this group is outlined on pages 432 to 434.

440

THE NOSE AND INTRANASAL REGIONS

Technique

The treatment, as already mentioned, must be adapted to each case. In a slightly retruding lip and drooping columella, an incision is made along the upper gingival sulcus, and the lip mucosa is advanced from each side toward the midline to make it protrude upon the nasal spine. The drooping of the columella is overcome by shifting a displaced lower septal cartilage into the midline (p. 437) or by advancing the columella (p. 427) or by transplantation of a strut (p. 431). In severe cases in which the retrusion of the upper lip is mainly due to shortness (tightness) (see Cleft-Lip Deformities) the lip is lengthened (loosened) with an Estlander flap from the lower lip (p. 251) or the Dieffenbach-Webster cheek-sliding operation (p. 259). The nose is "lifted" with a strut (pp. 431 and 432). In cases of retrusion of the maxilla in which the jaw is edentulous or the front teeth are missing (mainly after accidents), the lip can be advanced by deepening the gingivolabial sulcus with an inlay skin graft (p. 39). A prosthesis of acrylic resin or light metal, for instance, which pushes the lip forward, is inserted in this pocket. The prosthesis is fastened to a removable upper denture (Case 62, p. 1073). Any associated nasal deformity can be overcome in the same or a second stage. If teeth are present, the upper jaw itself is built up with the use of cartilage grafts, followed by reconstruction of the nose. The insertion of the grafts is best done after the method of Ragnell, who prefers bone-chip grafts to cartilage.

Technique (after Ragnell)

A columella split incision is made (p. 430) which, however, should be extended into the upper lip. From the incision, the nasal ridge is widely undermined, and this includes the lateral nasal walls; the space between columella and septum is opened. Dissection and undermining are continued at the base of the columella, over the nasal spine and over the anterior surface of the maxilla behind the ala. Care must be taken not to perforate the nasal or oral cavities; a Joseph periosteal elevator is of great help in this procedure. The entire cavity is now packed with bone chips (p. 74) while the soft tissues and the ala should be held elevated. By manipulation from the outside and also along the upper gingival sulcus, an even surface can be achieved. An L-shaped cartilage is then inserted to elevate columella and nasal ridge (p. 430). The two-stage procedure can also be used (p. 431) whereby only the ridge graft is inserted at this time while the columella strut is added later. Owing to the wide undermining over the nasal ridge, the ridge cartilage graft should be fastened either with a pin (p. 430) or by applying a cork splint (p. 420), to prevent slipping.

THE HEAD AND NECK

If the deformity is due to a pronounced retroposition of the maxilla with malocclusion of the teeth, a much more complicated procedure consisting of moving the maxilla forward must be resorted to (p. 571).

FRACTURES OF NOSE

For treatment of nasal fractures, the reader is referred to page 570.

RHINOPHYMA

Rhinophyma is, according to the present consensus, a hyperplasia on the basis of acne rosacea. (Adequate references have been compiled by Farina.) It consists of enlargement of the sebaceous glands, associated with an infiltration of hyperplastic fibrous tissue. The nasal tip and the lower nasal ridge are the usual sites of the nodular reddish-blue growth. Conservative treatment is unsuccessful.

Operative treatment consists of paring down the growth to proper nasal proportions without exposing the cartilages or rim of the nostrils, of thorough hemostasis, and of covering the raw surface with a full-thickness graft, from the posterior surface of the ear, or more often, because of the extent of the raw surface, with a thick split skin graft, preferably taken from the upper part of the chest, since this skin matches best the skin of the face (Case 57, p. 1068). In some cases, skin grafting may be omitted in the expectation that epithelium will regenerate from the remnants of the sebaceous glands; the raw surface is simply covered with bismuth tribromophenate (xeroform) gauze. Transplantation of a forehead flap is hardly ever indicated.

BIBLIOGRAPHY

ANDERSON, R., and DYKES, E. R.: *Surgical treatment of rhinophyma*. Plast. Reconstr. Surg., 30:397, 1962.

AUFRICHT, G.: *Combined nasal plastic and chin plastic*. J. Surg., 25:292, 1934. *A few hints and surgical details in rhinoplasty*. Laryngoscope, 53:317, 1943. *Combined plastic surgery of the nose and chin. Resume of twenty-seven years' experience*. Amer. J. Surg., 95:231, 1958. *Symposium on corrective rhinoplasty*. Plast. Reconstr. Surg., 28:241, 1961. *Rhinoplasty and the face*. Plast. Reconstr. Surg., 43:219, 1969.

BARRON, J. N., and EMMETT, A. J. J.: *Subcutaneous pedicle flaps*. Brit. J. Plast. Surg., 18:51, 1965.

BARSKY, A. J.: *Plastic Surgery*. W. B. Saunders, Philadelphia, 1938. *Principles and Practice of Plastic Surgery*. Williams & Wilkins, Baltimore, 1950.

BERNDORFER, A.: *Aesthetic of Nose*. Verlag Wilhelm Maudrich Wien 1949.

THE NOSE AND INTRANASAL REGIONS

BERSON, M. I.: *Rhinophyma.* Plast. Reconstr. Surg., 3:740, 1948.

BLAIR, V. P.: *Congenital atresia or obstruction of the nasal air passages.* Ann. Otol., Rhin., Laryng., 40:1021, 1931.

BLAIR, V. P., and BROWN, J. B.: *Nasal abnormalities, fancied and real.* Surg. Gynec. Obstet., 53:797, 1931.

BLAIR, V. P., and BYARS, L. T.: *"Hits, strikes, and outs" in the use of pedicle flaps for nasal restoration or correction.* Surg. Gynec. Obstet., 82:367, 1946.

BROADBENT, T. R., and MATHEWS, V. L.: *Artistic relationships in surface anatomy of the face: application to reconstructive surgery.* Plast. Reconstr. Surg., 20:1, 1957.

BROWN, J. B.: *Reconstructive Surgery of the Nose.* Nelson Loose-Leaf Surgery. Thomas Nelson & Sons, New York, 1940, Vol. 8, p. 237.

BROWN, J. B., and CANNON, B.: *Composite free grafts of skin and cartilage from the ear.* Surg. Gynec. Obstet., 82:253, 1946.

BROWN, J. B., and McDOWELL, F.: *Plastic Surgery of the Nose,* ed. 2. C. V. Mosby, St. Louis, 1965.

BYARS, L. T.: *Surgical correction of nasal deformities.* Surg. Gynec. Obstet., 84:65, 1947.

CALDERINI: Annali dell' Universita di Medicina, 104:520, 1842.

CARDOSO, A. D.: Rev. Med. Cir. S. Paulo, 5:271, 1945.

CARPUE, C.: *An account of two successful operations for restoring a lost nose.* London, 1816. Plast. Reconstr. Surg., 44:177, 1969.

CHAMPION, R.: *Reconstruction of the columella.* Brit. J. Plast. Surg., 12:353, 1960.

COHEN, S.: *Role of the septum in surgery of the nasal contour.* Arch. Otolaryng., 30:12, 1939.

CONVERSE, J. M.: *Corrective surgery of nasal deviations.* Arch. Otolaryng., 56:671, 1950.
A new forehead flap for nasal reconstruction. Proc. Roy. Soc. Med., 35:811, 1942.
The cartilaginous structures of the nose. Ann. Otol. Rhin. Laryng., 64:220, 1955.
Reconstruction of the nasolabial area by composite graft from the concha. Plast. Reconstr. Surg., 5:237, 1950.
Reconstruction of the nose by the scalping flap technique. Surg. Clin. N. Amer., 39:335, 1959.
Reconstructive Plastic Surgery. W. B. Saunders, Philadelphia, 1964.
Clinical application of the scalping flap in reconstruction of the nose. Plast. Reconstr. Surg., 43:247, 1969.

CONVERSE, J. M., and JEFFREYS, F. E.: *Nasomaxillary epithelial inlay for dish face deformity.* J. Oral Surg., 9:183, 1951.

CONVERSE, J. M., RANSOHOFF, J., MATTHEWS, E. S., SMITH, O., and MOLCUOAR, A.: *Ocular hypertelorism and pseudohypertelorism; advances in surgical treatment.* Plast. Reconstr. Surg., 145:11, 1970.

CONVERSE, J. M., and SMITH, B.: *An Operation for Congenital and Traumatic Hypertelorism.* In Troutman, R. C., *Plastic and Reconstructive Surgery of the Eye and Adnexa.* Butterworths, Washington, D. C., 1962.

THE HEAD AND NECK

CONVERSE, J. M., and WOOD-SMITH, D.: *Experiences with the forehead island flap with a subcutaneous pedicle*. Plast. Reconstr. Surg., 31:521, 1963.

DAVIS, W. B., THUSS, C. J., and NOBLE, J. H.: *Case report of unusual donor site of a composite graft*. Plast. Reconstr. Surg., 14:72, 1954.

DENECKE, H. J., and MEYER, R.: *Plastic Surgery of the Head and Neck: Corrective and Reconstructive Rhinoplasty*. Springer-Verlag, New York, 1967. *Plastische Operatinen an Kopf und Hals*, Vol. I. Korrigierende und reconstruktive Narenplastik. Springer-Verlag, Berlin, 1964.

DIEFFENBACH, J. E.: *Operative Chirurgie*. F. A. Brockhaus, Leipzig, 1845.

DINGMAN, R. O.: *Local anesthesia for rhinoplasty; and the nasal septum in rhinoplastic surgery*. Plast. Reconstr. Surg., 28:251, 1961.

DONLEY, J. J., and von FRAENKEL, P. H.: *The principle of cooling as applied to the composite graft in the nose*. Plast. Reconstr. Surg., 17:444, 1956.

DUBOWITSKY: Quoted by IVY, R. H.: *Repair of acquired defects of the face*. JAMA, 84:181, 1925.

DUPERTIUS, S. M.: *Free ear lobe grafts of skin and fat. Their value in reconstructions about the nostrils*. Plast. Reconstr. Surg., 1:135, 1946.

EDGERTON, M. T., and HANSEN, F. C.: *Matching facial color with split thickness skin grafts from adjacent areas*. Plast. Reconstr. Surg., 25:455, 1960.

EDGERTON, M. T., JACOBSON, W. E., and MEYER, E.: *Surgical-psychiatric study of patients seeking plastic (cosmetic) surgery: Ninety-eight consecutive patients with minimal deformity*. Brit. J. Plast. Surg., 13:136, 1960.

EITNER, E.: *Kosmetische Operationen*. J. Springer, Vienna, 1932.

ELLIOTT, R. A.: *Rotation flaps of the nose*. Plast. Reconstr. Surg., 44:147, 1969.

ELSBACH, E. J.: *Cartilaginous septum in the reconstruction of the nose*. Arch. Otolaryng., 44:207, 1946.

ESCOFFIER, J. B.: *The forehead flap in nasal repair*. Plast. Reconstr. Surg., 21:94, 1958.

FARINA, R.: *Rhinophyma: Plastic correction*. Plast. Reconstr. Surg., 6:461, 1950, and Arch. Otolaryng., 48:98, 1948.

FARINA, R., DIAS, J. V., and OSVALDO DE CASTRO, A.: *Development of bone graft integration, as established by x-ray follow-up in correction of deformity of nasal dorsum*. Plast. Reconstr. Surg., 20:297, 1957.

FOMON, S.: *The treatment of old unreduced nasal fractures*. Ann. Surg., 104:107, 1936. *The Surgery of Injury and Plastic Repair*. Williams & Wilkins, Baltimore, 1939.

FOMON, S., LUONGO, R., SCHATTNER, A., and TURCHIK, F.: *Cancellous bone transplants for correction of saddle nose*. Ann. Otol., Rhin., Laryng., 54:518, 1945.

GELBKE, H.: *Plastic operations for bifid nose*. Der Chirurg., 24:209-211, 1953. *The nostril problem in unilateral harelips and its surgical management*. Plast. Reconstr. Surg., 18:65, 1956. *Das Schüsselgesicht*. Langenbeck's Arch. u. Dtsch. Z. Chir., 286:1, 1957.

THE NOSE AND INTRANASAL REGIONS

GIBSON, T., and DAVIS, W. B.: *The distortion of autogenous cartilage grafts: Its cause and prevention.* Brit. J. Plast. Surg., 10:257, 1958.

GILLIES, H. D.: *Deformities of the syphilitic nose.* Brit. Med. J., 2:927, 1923.
Die Deformitäten der syphilitischen Sattelnase. Deutsche Ztschr. f. Chir., 250:379, 1938.
A new free graft applied to the reconstruction of the nostril. Brit. J. Surg., 30:305, 1943.

GOODALE, J. L.: *A new method for the operative correction of exaggerated roman nose.* Boston Med. Surg. J., 140:112, 1899.

GOUMAIN, A. J. M., and FEVRIER, J. C.: *Les transplants cutanes "en ilot" ou "island flaps" en chirurgie plastique de la face.* Ann. Chir. Plast., 10:174, 1965.

HAGE, J.: *Collapsed alae strengthened by conchal cartilage (the butterfly cartilage graft).* Brit. J. Plast. Surg., 18:92, 1965.
Surgical approach to the external and internal nose: with a supplementary report on two cases of nasal glioma. Brit. J. Plast. Surg., 12:327, 1960.

HEANLEY, C.: *The subcutaneous tissue pedicle in columella and other nasal reconstruction.* Brit. J. Plast. Surg., 8:60, 1955.

HOLDSWORTH, W. G., and PELLY, A. D.: *Forehead rhinoplasty.* Brit. J. Plast. Surg., 14:234, 1961.

HUFFMAN, W. C., and LIERLE, D. M.: *Studies on the pathologic anatomy of the unilateral harelip nose.* Plast. Reconstr. Surg., 4:225, 1949.

IVY, R. H.: *Plastic and reconstructive surgery.* Surg. Clin. N. Amer. 6:245, 1926.
Repair of acquired defects of the face. JAMA, 84:181, 1925.
Plastic and Reconstructive Surgery of the Face, Mouth, and Jaws. Nelson Loose-Leaf Surgery. Thomas Nelson & Sons, New York, 1940, Vol. 11, p. 679.

JACOBSON, W. E., EDGERTON, M. T., MEYER, E., CANTOR, A., and SLAUGHTER, R.: *Psychiatric evaluation of male patients seeking cosmetic surgery.* Plast. Reconstr. Surg., 26:356, 1960.
Screening of rhinoplasty patients from the psychologic point of view. Plast. Reconstr. Surg., 28:278, 1961.

JOSEPH, J.: *Nasenplastik und sonstige Gesichtsplastik.* Curt Kabitzsch, Leipzig. 1931.

KAZANJIAN, V. H.: *Nasal deformities and their repair.* Laryngoscope, 43:955, 1933.
Plastic repair of deformities about the lower part of the nose resulting from loss of tissue. Trans. Amer. Ophthal. Acad., 42:338, 1937.
The repair of nasal defects with a median forehead flap. Primary closure of the forehead wound. Surg. Gynec. Obstet., 83:37, 1946.
Nasal deformities of syphilitic origin. Plast. Reconstr. Surg., 3:517, 1948.

KAZANJIAN, V. H., and CONVERSE, J. M.: *The Surgical Treatment of Facial Injuries.* 2nd Ed. Williams & Wilkins, Baltimore, 1959.

KAZANJIAN, V. H., and HOLMES, E. M.: *Treatment of median cleft lip associated with bifid nose and hypertelorism.* Plast. Reconstr. Surg., 24:582, 1959.

KERNAHAN, D. A., and LITTLEWOOD, A. H. M.: *Experience in the use of arterial flaps about the face.* Plast. Reconstr. Surg., 28:207, 1961.

THE HEAD AND NECK

KILLNER, T. P.: *Plastic Surgery*. In MAINGOT, R.: *Postgraduate Surgery*. D. Appleton-Century Co., New York, 1937, Vol. 3.

KÖNIG, F.: *Zur Deckung von Defecten der Nasenflügel*. Berliner Klin. Wchnsch., 39:137, 1902.
Ueber Nasenplastik. Bruns' Beitr. z. klin. Chir., 94:515, 1914.

KUBACEK, F.: *Transposition of flaps in the face on a subcutaneous pedicle*. Acta Chir. Plast., 2:108, 1960.

LABAT, L.: *De la rhinoplastie et de la rhinoraphie soit dans les ças d'absence congénitale, on d'enlèvement accidental de la partie dorsale du nez*. Ann. Med. Phys., 24:619, 1833.

LAMONT, E.: *Reconstructive surgery of the nose in congenital deformity, injury, and disease*. Amer. J. Surg., 65:17, 1944.

LEXER, E.: *Die gesamte Wiederherstellungs-Chirurgie*. J. A. Barth, Leipzig, 1931.
Angeborene mediane Spaltung der Nase. Langenbeck's Arch. f. klin. Chir., 62:360, 1900.

LINK, R.: *Zur plastik des knorpeligen Nasengerüstes*. Z. Laryng. Rhinol., 30:84, 1951.

LOEB, R.: *Backward insertion of a median forehead flap in nasal deformities*. Brit. J. Plast. Surg., 12:349, 1960.

MacFEE, W. F.: *The surgical treatment of cancer of the nose, with emphasis on methods of repair*. Ann. Surg., 140:475, 1954.

MacGREGOR, F., ET AL.: *Facial Deformities and Plastic Surgery*. Charles C Thomas, Springfield, 1953.

MALBEC, E. F., and BEAUX, A. R.: *Reconstruction of the columella*. Brit. J. Plast. Surg., 11:142, 1958.

MARINO, H., and DAVIS, J.: *Hipertelorismo*. Tratmiento quirurgico. Rev. Lat. Amer. Chirig. Plast., 1:58, 1954.

MATTON, G., PICKRELL, K., HUGER, W., and POUND, E.: *The surgical treatment of rhinophyma*. Plast. Reconstr. Surg., 30:403, 1962.

McDOWELL, F., VALONE, J. A., and BROWN, J. B.: *Bibliography and historical note on plastic surgery of the nose*. Plast. Reconstr. Surg., 10:149, 1952.

McLAREN, L. R.: *Nasolabial flap repair for alar margin defects*. Brit. J. Plast. Surg., 16:234, 1963.

McLAREN, L. R., and PENNEY, D.: *The reconstruction of the syphilitic saddle nose: a review of seven cases*. Brit. J. Plast. Surg., 10:236, 1957.

McLAUGHLIN, C. R.: *Composite ear grafts and their blood supply*. Brit. J. Plast. Surg., 7:274, 1954.

METZENBAUM, M.: *Replacement of the lower end of the dislocated septal cartilage versus submucous resection of the dislocated end of the septal cartilage*. Arch. Otolaryng., 9:282, 1929.

MILLARD, D. R.: *Adjuncts in augmentation mentoplasty and corrective rhinoplasty*. Plast. Reconstr. Surg., 36:48, 1965.
Hemirhinoplasty. Plast. Reconstr. Surg., 40:440, 1967.
Total reconstructive rhinoplasty and a missing link. Plast. Reconstr. Surg., 37:167, 1966.

THE NOSE AND INTRANASAL REGIONS

NÉLATON, C., and OMBRÉDANNE, L.: *La Rhinoplastie*. G. Steinheil, Paris, 1904.

NEW, G. B.: *Total rhinoplastie*. JAMA, 91:380, 1928.

PALETTA, F. X., and VAN NORMAN, R. T.: *Total reconstruction of the columella*. Plast. Reconstr. Surg., 30:322, 1962.

PEER, L. A.: *An operation to repair lateral displacement of the lower border of the septal cartilage*. Arch. Otolaryng., 25:475, 1937.
A new method to correct saddle nose associated with retracted columella. Plast. Reconstr. Surg., 38:477, 1966.

PENN, J.: *Kiel-bone implants to the chin and nose*. Plast. Reconstr. Surg., 42:303, 1968.

PEGRAM, M.: *Repair of congenital short columella*. Plast. Reconstr. Surg., 14:305, 1954.

PETRALI: Quoted by CALDERINI: Ann. dell universal di Med., 104:520, 1842.

RAGNELL, A.: *A simple method of reconstruction in some cases of dish deformity*. Plast. Reconstr. Surg., 10:227, 1952.
Reconstruction of dishface deformity by bone grafts. Amer. J. Surg., 95:323, 1958.

REES, T. D.: *The transfer of free composite grafts of skin and fat: A clinical study*. Plast. Reconstr. Surg., 25:556, 1960.

REINHARDT, W.: Die Plastische Chirurgie, Stuttgart, F., Enke, 1953.

RÉTHI, A.: Quoted by KIRSCHNER, M.: *Operations-Lehre*. J. Springer, Berlin, 1935, Vol. III, pp. 505-509.
Ueber die Korrektiven Operationen der Nasenformitaten. Chirurg., 5:503, 1933.

ROE, F. O.: *The deformity termed "pug nose" and its correction by a simple operation*. The Medical Record, June 4, 1887. Republished in Plast. Reconstr. Surg., 45:18, 1970.

SAFIAN, J.: *Corrective Rhinoplastic Surgery*. Paul B. Hoeber, New York, 1935.
Fact and fallacy in rhinoplastic surgery. Brit. J. Plast. Surg., 11:45, 1958.
Progress in nasal and chin augmentation. Plast. Reconstr. Surg., 37:446, 1966.

SAVENERO-ROSSELLI, G.: Rev. Chir. Struct. (Belg.) 6:413, 1936.
La chirurgia plastica ne restauro di umbilazioni dopo exeresi di tumori maligni di tegumenti e del ma siccio faciale. Arch. Ital. Chir., 54:5, 491-501 (Donati-Festschr.) 1938.

SCHMID, E.: *Methods in Plastic Surgery of the Nose*. Beitr. Zur Klinischen Chirurg., 184:385, 1952.
Nasal Reconstruction. In Modern Trends in Plastic Surgery, T. Gibson, ed. Butterworths, Washington, D.C., 1964, p. 145.
Neue Gesichtspunkte und Ergebnisse bei partiellem und totalem Nasenersatz. Langenbeck's Arch. f. klin. Chir., 287:736, 1957.
Neue Wege in der plastischen Chirurgie der Nase. Brun's Beitr. Klin. Chir., 184:385, 1952.
Zur operativen Behandlung des angeborenen Hypertelorismus. Chir. Plast. et Reconstructiva, 3:130, 1967.
Die Verwendung von composite grafts bei Gesichtsverbrennungen. Fortschr. der Kiefer-und Gesichts-Chirurgie, 9:67, 1964.
Die Wiederherstellung des Nasengerüstes. Mschr. Obrenheilk., 89:27, 1955.

SCHUCHARDT, K.: in Bier-Braun-Kümmell's Chirurgische Operationslehre, 7th edition, Vol. 2, J. A. Barth, Leipzig, 1954.

THE HEAD AND NECK

SEELEY, R. C.: *Composite bone graft in saddle nose.* Plast. Reconstr. Surg., 4:252, 1949.

SELTZER, A. P.: *Fixity of facial expression following undermining of skin of nose, and a modified method by which it is avoided.* Amer. J. Surg., 48:326, 1945.
Plastic Surgery of the Nose. J. B. Lippincott, Philadelphia, 1949.

SERCERA, A., and MINDNICK, K.: *Plastische Operationen an der nase und Ohrmuschel.* Georg Thieme Verlag, Stuttgart, 1962.

SHEEHAN, J. E.: *Plastic repair of the syphilitic nose.* Laryngoscope, 35:22, 1925.
Plastic Surgery of the Nose. Paul B. Hoeber, New York, 1936.
General and Plastic Surgery. Paul B. Hoeber, New York, 1945.

SMITH, F.: *Total Rhinoplasty.* Warthin. Ann., 1927, p. 601.
Reconstructive Surgery of the Head and Mouth. Nelson Loose-Leaf Surgery, Thomas Nelson & Sons, New York, 1928.

STRAATSMA, C. R.: *Surgery of the bony nose: comparative evaluation of chisel and saw technique.* Plast. Reconstr. Surg., 28:246, 1961.
Use of the dermal graft in the repair of small saddle defects of the nose. Arch. Otolaryng., 16:506, 1932.

STRAATSMA, B. R., and STRAATSMA, C. R.: *The anatomical relationship of the lateral nasal cartilage to the nasal bone and the cartilaginous nasal septum.* Plast. Reconstr. Surg., 8:443, 1951.

STRAITH, C. L.: *Reconstructions about the nasal tip.* Surg. Gynec. Obstet., 62:73, 1936.

STRAITH, R. E., TEASLEY, J. L., von LINDE, M. G., and MOORE, L. T.: *The treatment of lateral deviations of the nose by pin fixation.* Plast. Reconstr. Surg., 15:346, 1955.

SYMONDS, F. C., and CRIKELAIR, G. F.: *Auricular composite grafts in nasal reconstruction.* Plast. Reconstr. Surg., 38:433, 1966.

TESSIER, P., GIRROT, G., ROUGERIE, F., DELBET, F. P., PASTORITZA, F.: *Ostéotomics cranio-naso-orbito-faciales.* Ann. Chir. Plast., 12:103, 1967.

TRENDELENBURG, F.: *Ueber die operative Behandlung schiefer Nasen.* Chir. Kongr. Verh., 1:82, 1889.

ULLIK, R.: *Die plast. Chirurgie des Gesichtes.* Wien 1948.

WANG, M. K. H., and MACOMBER, W. B.: *The Bifid Nose in Converse Reconstructive Plastic Surgery.* W. B. Saunders, Philadelphia, 1964, pp. 767-772.

WEBSTER, G. V.: *Randon reflections on rhinoplasty.* Plast. Reconstr. Surg., 39:147, 1967.

WEBSTER, J. P., and DEMING, E. G.: *The surgical treatment of the bifid nose.* Plast. Reconstr. Surg., 6:1, 1950.

WILSON, J. S. P.: *The application of the two centimetre pedicle flap in plastic surgery.* Brit. J. Plast. Surg., 20:278, 1967.

ZENO, L.: *Injerto libre de piel Acolchada en las pequenas rinoplastias.* An. de chir. 7:295, 1941.

ZIMANY, A.: *The bi-lobed flap.* Plast. Reconstr. Surg., 11:424, 1953.

THE EYELIDS,
EYEBROWS,   10
AND ORBITS

REPARATIVE surgery of the eyelids, eyebrows, and orbits is a part of ophthalmic plastic surgery, and thus belongs to this specialty. The general surgeon, however, confronted with traumatic wounds of the eyelids, must be informed about the proper ways of repair to avoid injurious consequences. The general plastic surgeon will find that repair in these regions encroaches upon his field, particularly if he is required to reconstruct regions around the eye as well as neighboring parts of the face.

ANATOMY OF THE EYELIDS

The eyelids are composed of two layers, which are combined at their peripheral end by the lid margin (Fig. 209). The outer layer consists of skin, musculus orbicularis, lashes and their glands, the inner layer of tarsus, meibomian glands, and conjunctiva. The septum orbitale reaches from the periosteum of the orbital rim to the upper border of the tarsus. The tarsus is a fibrocartilaginous plate which gives each lid stability. It is connected with the lateral wall of the orbit and, mediad, with the internal palpebral ligament. It is higher in the upper lid than in the lower lid.

The upper lid is lifted by the musculus levator palpebrae superioris, which is innervated by the nervus oculomotorius. The muscle originates in the vicinity of the canalis opticus, extends along the roof of the orbit,

THE HEAD AND NECK

and is inserted with a broad tendon to the upper rim of the tarsus. A few of its bundles penetrate the septum orbitale and musculus orbicularis to fuse with the skin. In addition to the levator, there is the smooth muscle of Müller, which is innervated by the sympathetic nerve. The musculus orbicularis, which is innervated by the nervus facialis, closes the lids.

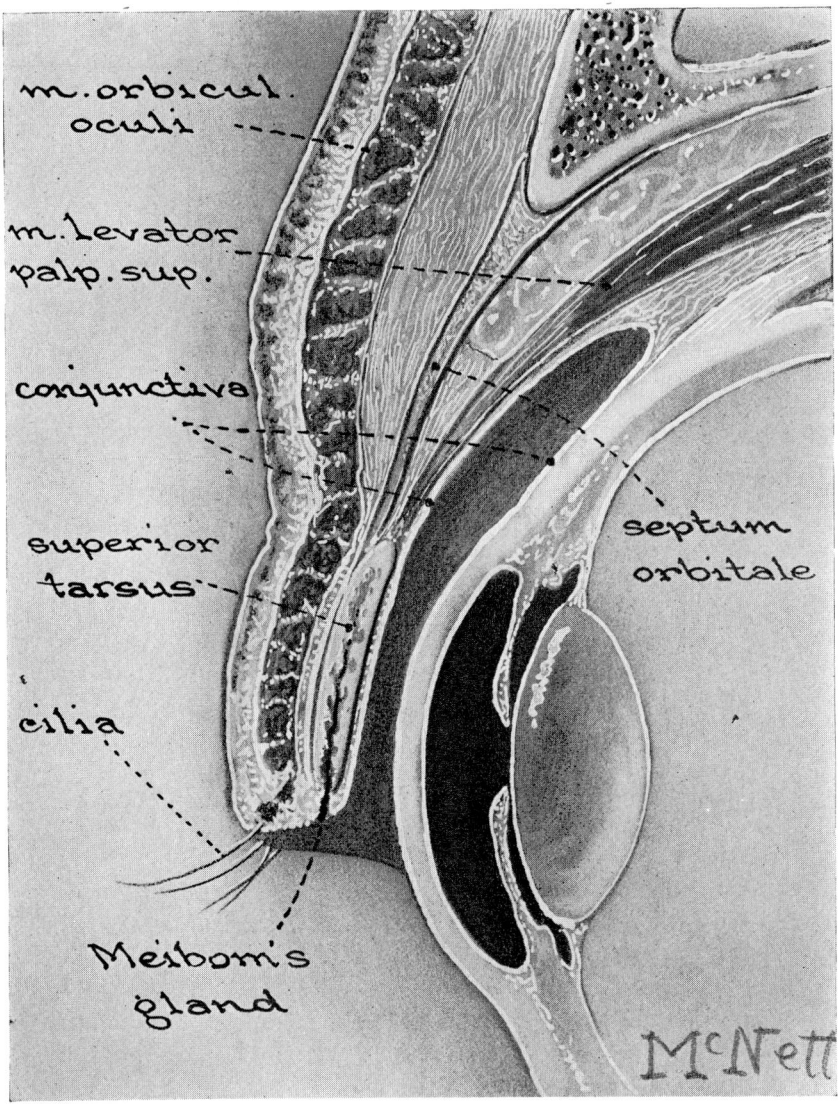

Fig. 209. Anatomy of eyelid (schematic).

450

DEFECTS

WOUNDS OF EYELIDS

The general principles of repair are the same as in wounds elsewhere on the body. It should be emphasized, however, that wounds of the eyelids should be closed as precisely as possible. While closure of horizontal wounds does not offer any difficulties, vertical wounds may involve problems, particularly if the full thickness of the lid is involved. If the wound edges are ragged, they should be excised, however, as sparingly as possible. If, in vertical wounds, parts of the lid are damaged and must be removed, the defect should if possible be made triangular, with the base of the triangle at the lid margin.

The wound edges are sutured in layers: The first suture, consisting of fine nylon on an atraumatic needle, is passed through the lid margins and approximates them as accurately as possible. The suture is not tied but used as a traction suture. If pull is now exerted upon this suture, the corresponding structures will fall in line with each other and are sutured. Conjunctiva and tarsus are approximated with buried sutures of 00000 chromic catgut in such a way that the sutures are passed through the tarsus only and tied upon it. Suture of the orbicularis muscle (with the same material) and of the skin (with fine nylon) follows. Finally, the marginal suture is tied. To avoid later notching of the lid margins, Wiener's suggestion is a good one: to give the skin defect an elliptical shape. Another good suggestion is to place the two rows of sutures in different planes, what is called in carpentry "halving" (Duverger, Wheeler) (Fig. 223; Case 63, p. 1074). After yellow mercuric oxide ointment is instilled into the conjunctival sac, the wound is dressed with sterile gauze and an eye pad is applied to both eyes to counteract overmotility. The skin sutures are removed on the fourth day, but the marginal sutures should remain in place for ten days.

DEFECTS OF SKIN OF EYELIDS

A defect of the covering skin of an eyelid must be replaced by skin to avoid contractures, unless the defect is small enough to permit simple closure by suturing. The skin defect can be closed either by skin grafting or by pedicle flaps. The skin of the eyelids, however, is so thin that whenever possible it should be replaced by a free graft rather than by a flap.

Wheeler has improved the grafting method to such a degree that results have been uniformly good. The two features which constitute the

451

improvement are the intermarginal suture with temporary closure of the eyelids—thus splinting and immobilizing the eyelids and protecting the cornea at the same time—and the use of a full-thickness graft from the sound eyelid.

Pedicle flaps are much less pliable than grafts and, therefore, less than ideal for replacing the skin of the lid. They are, however, of value in those cases of cicatricial ectropion of the lower lid in which the scar is thick and penetrates deep down to the orbital rim. A pedicle flap-particularly if anchored to the orbital rim—provides a suitable support and elevation of the lid. If possible, the flap should be taken from the immediate neighborhood (see p. 455) or, if the neighborhood is cicatricial, from distant parts (Case 68, p. 1080).

Technique (*Use of Skin Grafts, after Wheeler*) (Fig. 210; Cases 64-65, pp. 1075-1076)

The most suitable example is the correction of cicatricial ectropion. The first incision is led parallel to the rim of the distorted eyelid. Two traction sutures are placed through the lid margins, and while they are pulled every bit of scar tissue is removed to avoid future recontracture. If the inner canthus is drawn forward—a condition which occurs in eyelid burns associated with full-thickness loss of skin over the bridge of the nose and results in displacing the lacrimal puncta forward—all the contracting skin median to the median canthus must be removed until the lacrimal puncta rest upon the ocular globe. Care should be taken not to injure the orbicularis fibers. Bleeding is stopped by pressure rather than by ligatures. If the eyelid is relaxed, steps are taken to create intermarginal adhesions. With a small pair of scissors, the lid margins of upper and lower lids immediately posterior to the cilia are denuded exactly opposite each other. The small wounds are placed between middle and lateral and middle and median third of the lid margins. Mattress sutures are now passed through small plates of rubber (cut from sterile rubber tubing), overlying the skin of both upper and lower lids near their margins; alternatively, the mattress suture is tied over a second black silk suture, lying loose as a seton. These sutures are tied snugly, to assure firm apposition of the corresponding raw surfaces. Union of these raw surfaces causes adhesions, which hold the upper and lower lids together.

A pattern is now made of the defect. The grafts should preferably be taken from the opposite eyelid or from the eyelids of the opposite eye. As much as half of the skin can be removed without subsequent impairment of function. The pattern is laid upon the donor lid and circumscribed with an incision. Four traction sutures are passed through the graft edges opposite each other, and under constant traction and pull at

452

the lid the graft is removed. The same traction sutures are used to anchor the graft to the edges of the defect. If the defect is so large as to require additional grafts, these are taken from the posterior surface of the ears. If such is the case, the graft from the lid is used to replace the actual lid defect and the other grafts are used to cover the remaining raw surfaces. All grafts are sutured in place. If upper and lower lids are involved, a

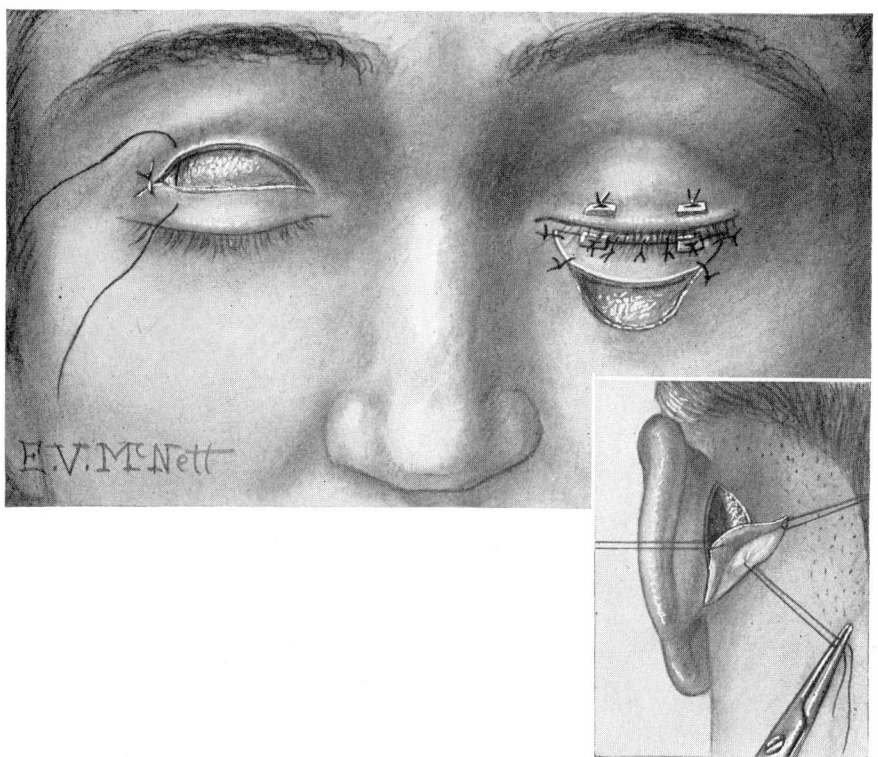

Fig. 210. Repair of cicatricial ectropion of left lower lid by use of skin grafts (Wheeler). After reduction of contracture by excision of all scar tissue, steps are taken to perform intermarginal adhesions (left eye). Lid margins of upper and lower lids immediately posterior to cilia are denuded exactly opposite each other, and held together with mattress sutures tied over small rubber plates. A full-thickness graft is removed from upper lid of right eye and sutured into defect below lid margin. An additional graft, taken from posterior surface of ear, is needed to close remainder of defect.

thick split graft, from the supraclavicular region or the hairless median side of arm or thigh (donor areas not to be shaved!), is used for each lid and sutured in place. Brown and Cannon consider full-thickness grafts from the neck and supraclavicular region superior because they are soft, provide good function, and have good color match (Case 3, p. 992). If these skin areas are too thick, split grafts rather than full-thickness grafts should be used.

The intermarginal adhesion technique is excellent in severe contractures. In less severe cases, however, it may not be needed. The graft is simply covered with mechanic's waste and pressure is applied by tying the skin sutures, which have been left long, over the mechanic's waste.

After-Treatment

A heavily padded pressure dressing is applied for ten days, care being taken to avoid undue pressure upon the eyeball. Upon the first change of the dressing the sutures are removed, with the exception of the mattress sutures, which should remain in place a few days longer to assure firm intermarginal union. The intermarginal adhesions are not severed for at least three months to counteract recontracture.

In severe ectropion of both eyelids, particularly of those in which the eyelid margins have been destroyed and the lower lid is short, Converse and Smith have employed successfully the tarsoconjunctival flap method of Dupuy-Dutemps in the reconstruction of the eyelids; the method is described on page 471. However, instead of using a flap for coverage they close the raw surface with a skin graft, as Macomber and co-workers had advised previously. The graft is covered with mechanic's waste and pressure applied by tying the skin sutures over it. Separation of the eyelids is carried out six to twelve weeks later.

DEFECTS OF FULL THICKNESS OF EYELIDS

The full-thickness defect may be partial or total. It may require replacement of cover and lining or of cover, lining, and support. The lining can be replaced by skin grafts or by mucous-membrane grafts. If the eyeball is still present and intact, the lower palpebral conjunctiva can be replaced by skin; however—as Spaeth emphasizes—to avoid approximation of the skin surface of the lid to the contiguous cornea, the bulbar conjunctiva of the lower, as well as the conjunctiva of the upper, lid should be replaced by mucous-membrane grafts from the buccal mucosa (see p. 46). The supporting tissue is provided by ear-cartilage grafts.

Although a distinct classification of full-thickness defects is impossible, owing to their great variety, the author groups them here as follows: (1) those involving the marginal parts of the lid; (2) vertical defects; (3) defects of the canthal angles; and (4) defects of the entire lid. The lower lid is involved more often than the upper.

DEFECTS OF MARGIN OF LOWER LID

Technique (*Kuhnt; Modification after Spaeth*) (Fig. 211)

The principle of this operation is the formation of a sliding bridge flap from the cheek.

Step 1: It is first necessary to form a pocket beneath the skin of the lid and to transplant a buccal mucous-membrane graft into this pocket at

A

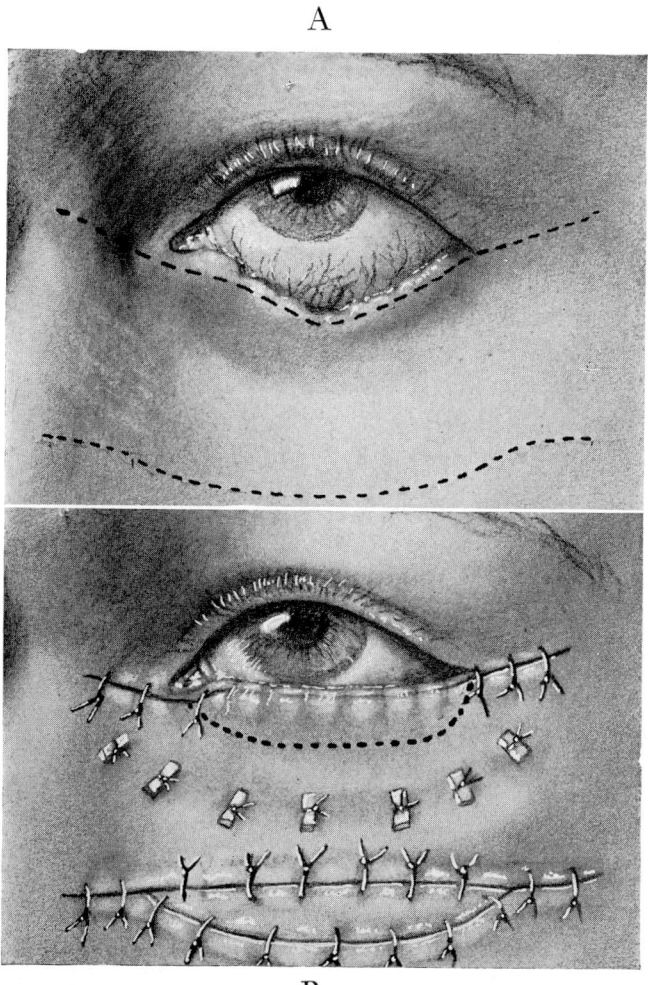

B

Fig. 211. Repair of defect of lower lid margin (Kuhnt, Spaeth). *A:* Outline of bridge flap to be shifted upward into defect. *B:* Bridge flap, its marginal end ten days previously lined with mucous-membrane graft, is anchored in place. Secondary defect below flap is covered with full-thickness skin graft; mattress sutures through flap anchor latter to orbital rim.

455

the site of the future new lid margin, with its epithelial side toward the conjunctiva. The graft is sutured not only to the raw surface of the flap but also to its superior margin.

Step 2: After ten days, the first incision is lengthened bilaterally, temporally, and medially for about 2 to 3 cm. ($1\frac{3}{16}$ to $1\frac{3}{16}$ inches) upward on a 45-degree angle. About 2 to 3 cm. below, another incision is made parallel to the first incision. The ends of this incision—unlike the upper incision—are made horizontal. Undermining of the bridge flap follows.

The flap is now moved upward. The inferior border of the mucous-membrane graft is sutured to the conjunctival margin of the

A

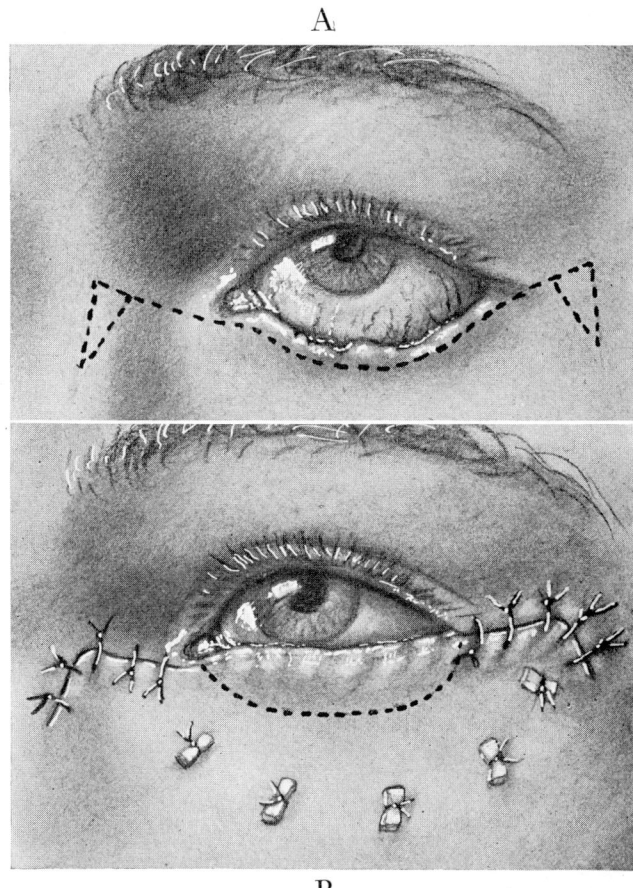

B

Fig. 212. Variation of technique of Fig. 211, without lower incision. Excision of lateral and median triangle of skin to facilitate skin shifting. Mattress sutures through flap anchor latter to orbital rim.

456

defect. Firm anchorage of the flap follows, with sutures to the periosteum of the inferior orbital rim. Mattress sutures are tied on small rolls of gauze, then to the internal canthal ligament, anteriorly and posteriorly, and to the periosteum of the lacrimal crest, then temporally at the outer rim of the orbit to the periosteum and into the upper lid. The secondary defect below the flap is covered with a flap from the immediate neighborhood or with a full-thickness graft from the posterior surface of the ear.

After the flap has healed in place well, a piece of ear cartilage 5 mm. ($\frac{3}{16}$ inch) wide is removed from a posterior incision along the concha,

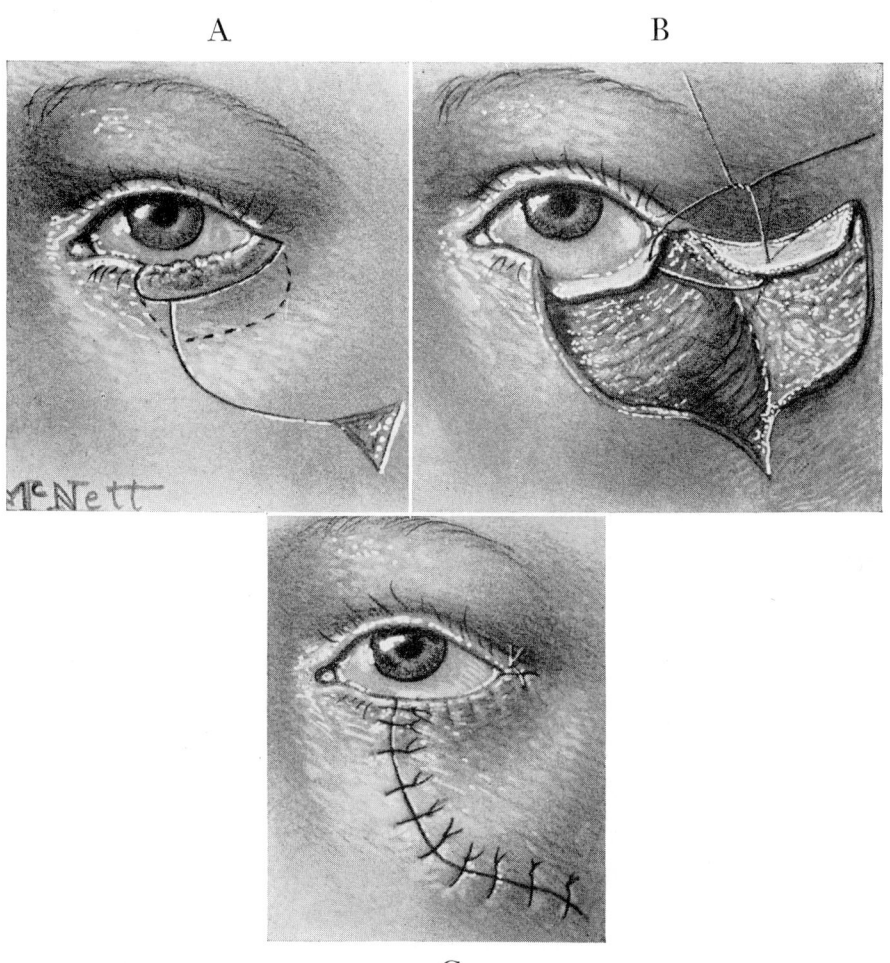

Fig. 213. Excision of carcinoma of lower lid and repair of defect (Imré). Principle of method is rotation of flap from immediate neighborhood. This is made possible by excision of triangle of skin at extremity of curved incision. Margin of flap has been previously lined with buccal-mucosa graft. (Compare with Figs. 225 and 226.)

457

thinned and shaped to replace the tarsus of the lower lid, and buried between mucous-membrane graft and flap.

Variation: In narrower defects, one may not need an actual flap but can cover the defect by skin sliding, as demonstrated in Figure 212. After the skin is moved upward, it is held in this position by suturing it to the inferior orbital rim and by resection of a triangle of skin from the median and lateral borders.

Technique (Imré) (Fig. 213; Case 67, p. 1078)

The principles of this ingenious method are based on the mobilizing of a flap from the immediate neighborhood of the defect and the sliding of the flap into the defect, which is made possible by the excision of a triangle of skin at the extremity of the incision. According to Katz, Imré has recently modified his method: Instead of an equilateral triangle, the apex is rounded and the side of the triangle nearest the defect curves gracefully over into the line of incision; this allows a greater displacement of the flap toward the defect and a smoother closure. The flap has previously been lined with a buccal-mucosa graft (see p. 454). The incision for the flap is bow shaped. The triangles of skin (after Burow; Fig. 13) are excised at the end of the incision. The narrower the defect, the greater should be the radius of the incision. The flap should be undermined well beyond the incision. After its rotation, it is sutured in place with obliquely placed sutures.

Manchester introduced a useful technique for closure of partial full-thickness defects of the lower lid. In his method, the conjunctiva is replaced by a conjunctival flap from the region of the lower fornix and lower part of the eyeball, and the skin covering is supplied by a double-pedicle flap from the upper lid, as advocated first by Landolt (1885).

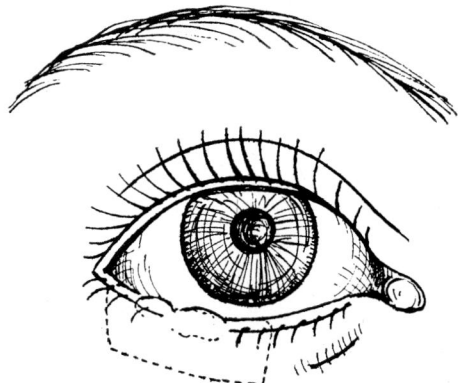

Fig. 214. Typical marginal neoplasm. The portion of lid indicated by the dotted line is excised through its whole thickness, giving the lesion a margin of ¼ inch (0.62 cm.) on all sides. (Manchester, W. M.: Brit. J. Plast. Surg.)

458

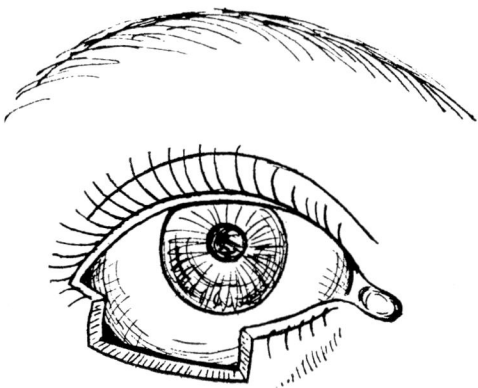

Fig. 215. Appearance of partial full-thickness defect requiring repair. (Manchester, W. M.: Brit. J. Plast. Surg.)

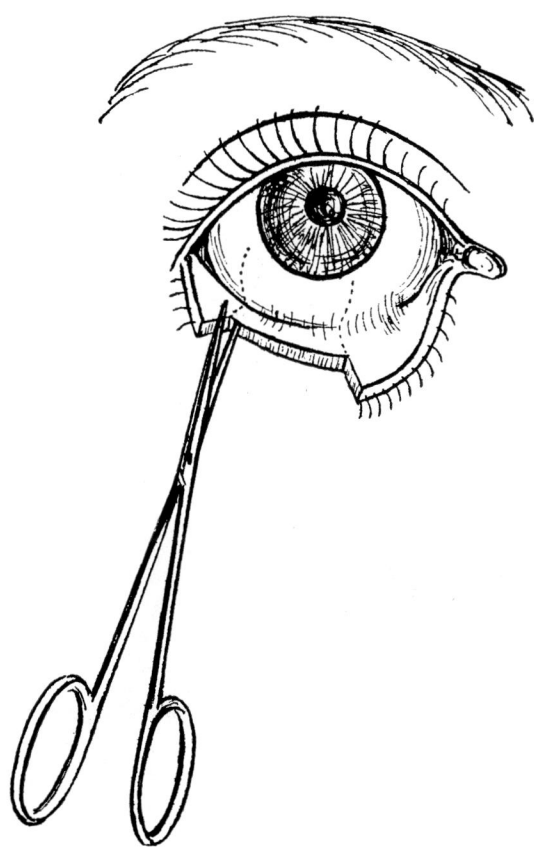

Fig. 216. A conjunctival flap corresponding in width to the defect is freed up from the lower fornix and lower bulbar conjunctiva. (Manchester, W. M.: Brit. J. Plast. Surg.)

459

Technique (*Manchester*)

The various operative steps are depicted in Figures 214-222, and are self-explanatory. This is the first stage of the operation. It is followed two weeks later by a second stage, which consists of division of the median and lateral pedicles of the flap and adjustment of flap and pedicles.

A similar procedure can be carried out for repair of partial full-thickness defects of the upper eyelid, as demonstrated. Hueston, McCoy and Crow, and Mustardé make use of the Estlander-Abbé principle and rotate a composite flap from the sound eyelid into the defect.

VERTICAL DEFECTS (COLOBOMAS)

Vertical notches or clefts of the lids, so-called "colobomas," are congenital or acquired. If acquired, they are due either to operations (removal of tumors) or to trauma.

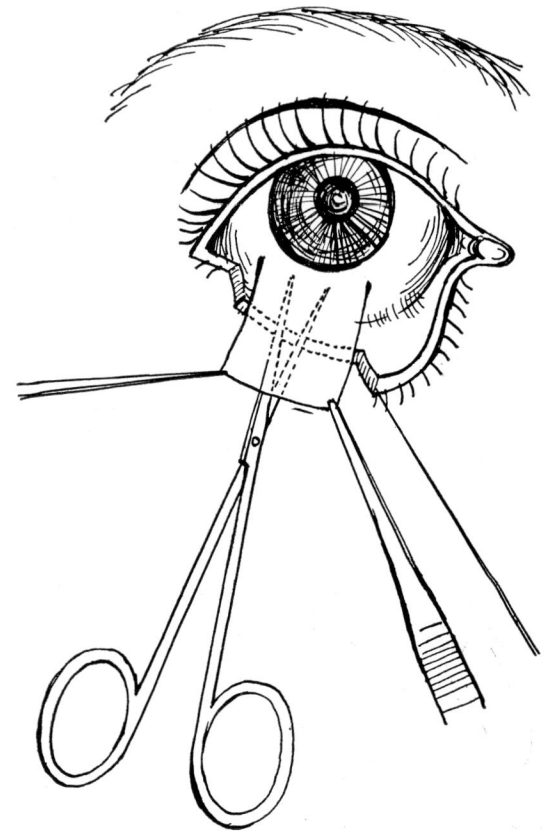

Fig. 217. The freeing may have to extend almost to the limbus. (Manchester, W. M.: Brit. J. Plast. Surg.)

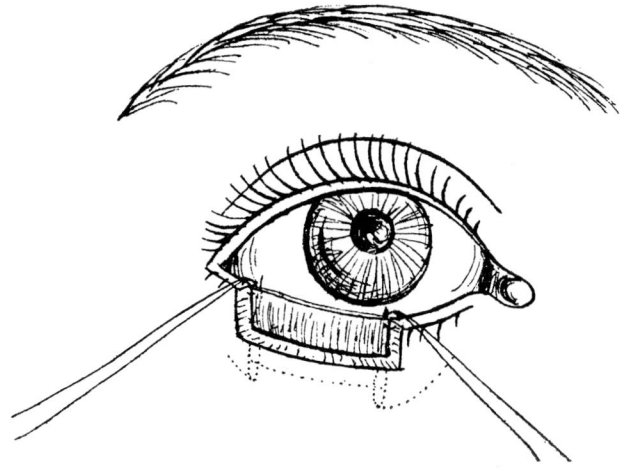

Fig. 218. The flap is folded on itself to recreate the fornix at a slightly higher level than that remaining untouched on either side. It is secured at each corner by a single black silk stitch. If the ends are left long they lie on the cheek and do not irritate the cornea. (Manchester, W. M.: Brit. J. Plast. Surg.)

CONGENITAL COLOBOMAS

V-shaped colobomas are best repaired by the so-called "halving" method (Duverger, Wheeler). The principle of this method is to overlap the skin and conjunctival wound flaps and to suture them at different planes, since simple approximation may be followed by recurrence of the notch.

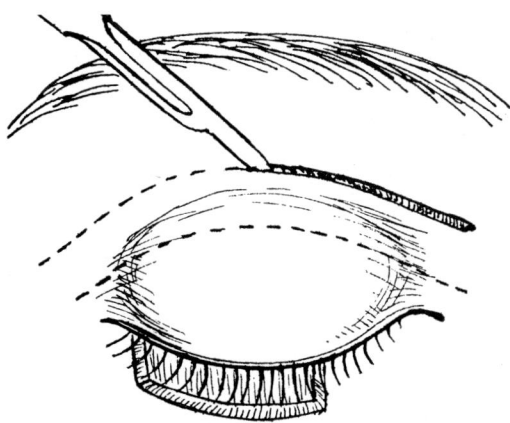

Fig. 219. Closure of the skin defect. A double pedicle flap of the Tripier type is outlined on the upper lid. (Manchester, W. M.: Brit. J. Plast. Surg.)

461

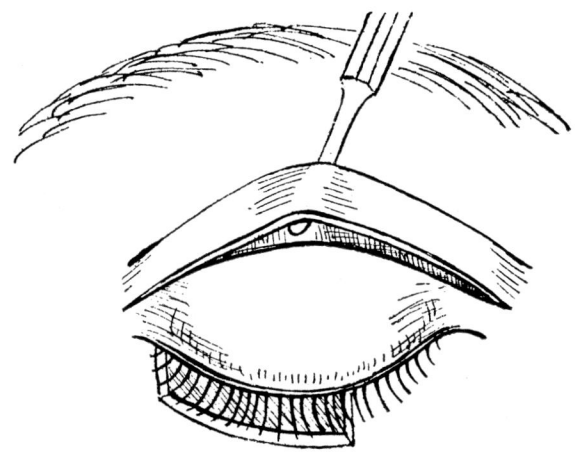

Fig. 220.   This double pedicle flap is freed. (Manchester, W. M.: Brit. J. Plast. Surg.)

Technique (Fig. 223; compare Case 63, p. 1074)

The edges of the colobomas are excised and the skin and orbicularis muscle separated from the tarsus and conjunctival layer. To avoid having the sutures for the conjunctiva and tarsus on the same plane as the skin sutures, the following procedure is carried out: A small, triangular piece of skin, including lid margin and orbicularis muscle, is excised from one wound edge (the base of the triangle is at the lid margin), and a similarly shaped piece of conjunctiva and tarsus is removed from the opposite wound edge. If the lesion is near the outer canthus, the skin-orbicularis excision should be made from the lateral wound edge; if the lesion is near the inner

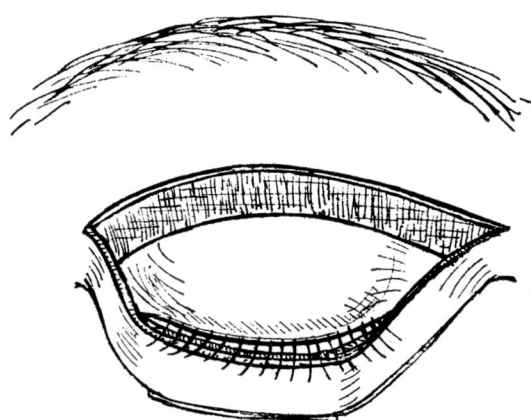

Fig. 221.   The double flap must lie easily in the defect without tension (Manchester, W. M.: Brit. J. Plast. Surg.)

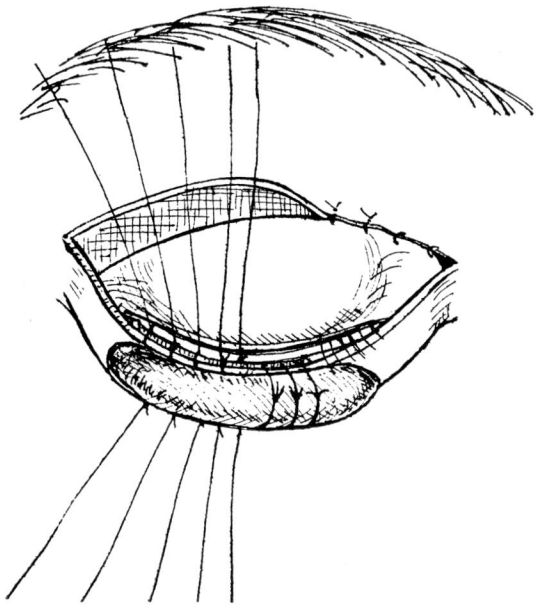

Fig. 222. Two series of stitches are left long to unite the upper border of the skin to the conjunctival flap and the lower border to the remaining eyelid skin, respectively. These are tied to each other over a tiny stent mold. The upper lid defect is closed with sutures. (Manchester, W. M.: Brit. J. Plast. Surg.)

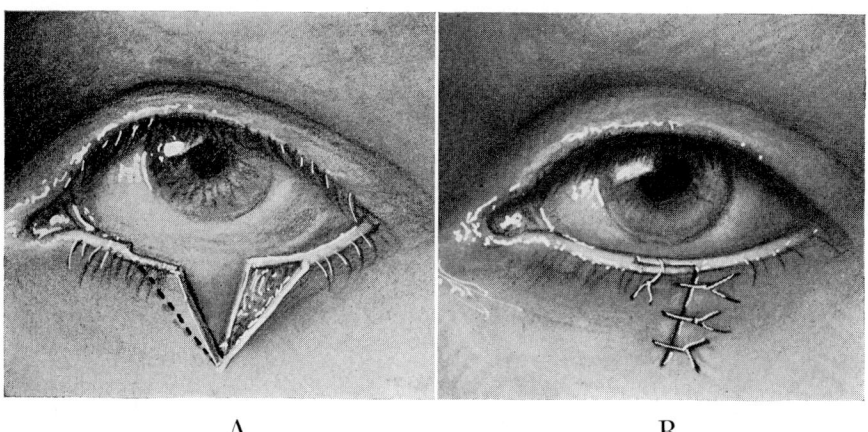

A   B

Fig. 223. *A:* V-shaped coloboma repaired by "halving" method (Duverger-Wheeler); that is, suturing skin and conjunctiva at different planes. Small triangular piece of skin (including lid margin) and orbicularis muscle is removed from lateral wound edge while similarly shaped piece of conjunctiva and tarsus is removed from median wound edge (dotted line). *B:* Closure of wound in layers.

463

canthus, it should be made from the median wound edge. The conjunctivotarsal layer is sutured first, with buried 00000 chromic catgut sutures (they should not pass through the posterior surface of the conjunctiva and be tied upon the tarsus). Accurate approximation of the wound edges is necessary. Suture of the orbicularis muscle follows. The skin sutures (fine nylon on an atraumatic needle) start at the margin with accurate marginal approximation; by leaving the suture long and using it as a traction suture, the wound edges fall in line. Thus, skin and orbicularis flap overlap the conjunctivotarsal flap. If the defect is wide, tension on the sutures can be lessened by performing a canthotomy of the external canthal ligament and subcutaneous myotomy of the orbicularis fibers. Dressing and after-treatment are as described on page 451.

ACQUIRED SURGICAL COLOBOMAS

These colobomas may have various forms. In many instances, they can be repaired according to Imré's principles (p. 458; see also Case 67, p. 1078, for comparison). The lining is replaced by a buccal mucous-membrane graft, which is transplanted ten days before the flap is rotated into place as described on page 454. If the tarsus needs to be replaced, a piece of ear cartilage, properly shaped and thinned, is later buried between the mucous membrane and skin (see p. 457).

Callahan describes the use of a free composite lid graft (taken from the sound lid), and recommends it particularly for colobomas of the upper lid. This is an ingenious but daring method. A less daring one is the rotation of a composite flap from the sound eyelid into the defect after the Estlander-Abbé principle (Hueston, McCoy and Crow, Mustardé; see also p. 251). Manchester's technique (p. 460) may also be applicable.

Technique (Kuhnt, after Dieffenbach-Szymanowski) (Fig. 224) (Case 66, p. 1077)

In triangular defects, this method is a good one. The principle is closure of a triangular defect with a square flap rotated from the immediate neighborhood (see Fig. 12). The flap consists of the lateral portion of the skin of the lid—leaving the orbicularis, tarsus, and conjunctival portions in situ—and of the bordering temporal region. The temporal incision, starting from the outer canthus, should be led obliquely upward. This not only elevates and supports the lid but also facilitates closure of the secondary defect (see Fig. 12). Preparatory to the formation of the flap, however (ten days previously), a buccal mucous-membrane graft of the size of the conjunctival defect is buried beneath the posterior surface of that part of the flap which is to cover the defect (see p. 454). A piece of ear cartilage to replace the tarsal defect is later buried between mucous membrane and flap (see pp. 457-458). If the flap is shifted into the defect, the graft of mucous membrane will form the posterior surface of the lid.

If neither Imré's nor Dieffenbach's method is suitable for closing partial full-thickness defects of the lids, temporal, cheek, or forehead flaps— similar to those used for replacement of entire lids (see below)—may be transplanted.

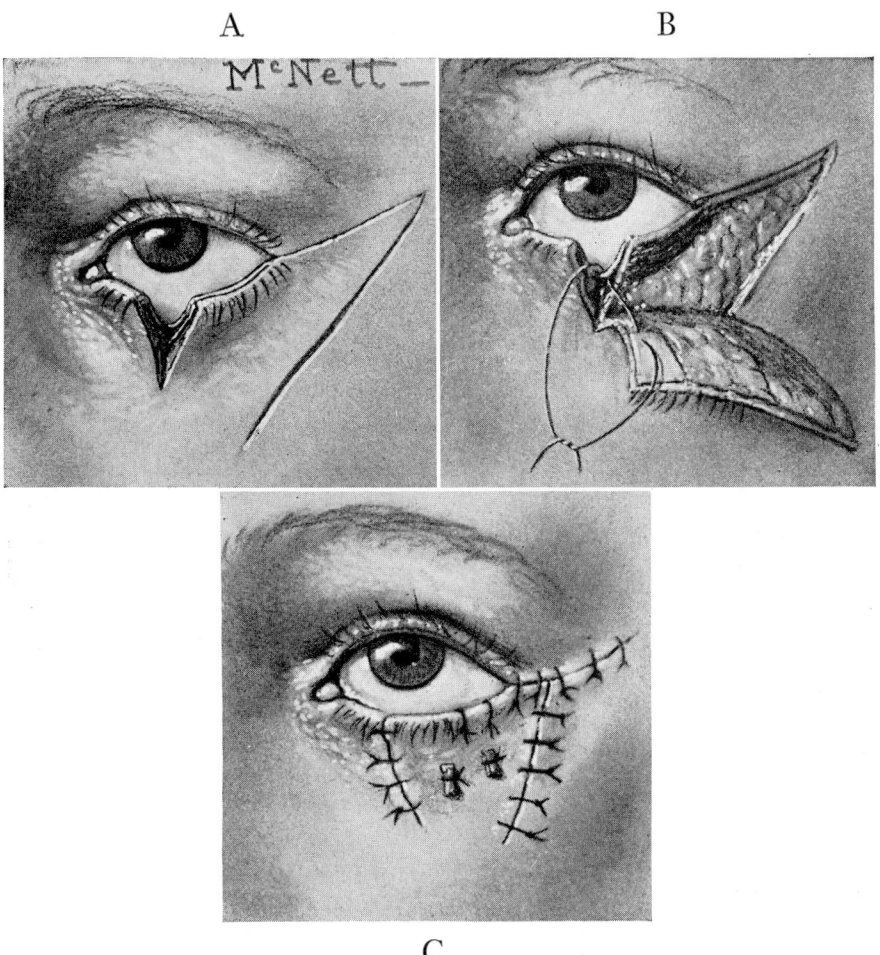

A   B

C

Fig. 224. *A:* Closure of triangular full-thickness defect of lower lid by rotating square skin flap from lateral portion of lid and temporal region (Dieffenbach, Szymanowski, Kuhnt). Preparatory to formation of flap (ten days before transfer), the part of flap which will cover defect is lined. *B:* Flap is mobilized, lining of flap being sutured to conjunctival defect edges. *C:* Flap sutured in place, secondary defect in temporal region closed by starting with closure of lateral corner; mattress sutures tied over small rolls of gauze anchor flap to orbital rim.

465

THE HEAD AND NECK

ACQUIRED TRAUMATIC COLOBOMAS

Traumatic colobomas have already been discussed (see above; see also Fig. 223; Case 63, p. 1074).

DEFECTS OF CANTHAL ANGLES

Some of these defects can be conveniently closed by Imré's method (see Figs. 225, 226). Other defects may be closed by single-pedicle flaps rotated from the neighborhood. Case 69, page 1082, demonstrates one example: Flaps for the lateral canthal angle may be taken from the temporal or malar region; for the inner canthal angle, from the glabella or nasal

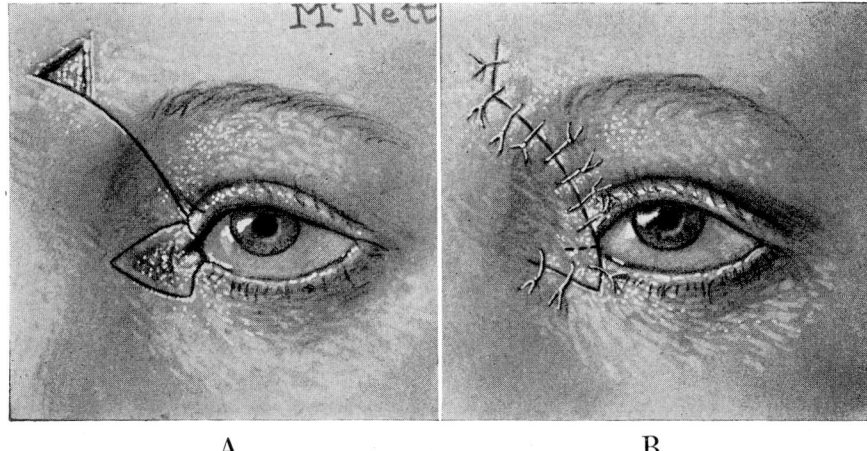

A   B

Fig. 225.   Closure of defect at median canthal angle by Imré's method. (See Fig. 213.)

region. Either the lining is supplied by local turnover flaps or, as in larger defects, the flap must be lined with a mucous-membrane graft. It is usually necessary to delay the transfer to improve the circulation in these flaps.

For more extensive defects, Byron Smith has devised several useful methods which, however, should be carried out by the ophthalmic plastic surgeon.

DEFECTS OF ENTIRE LID

For repair of defects of an entire lid, the pedicle-flap method offers the most versatile form of reconstruction (Fricke, 1829). In many instances, however, the defect is only subtotal, that is, a small stump of conjunctiva and skin is left. If this is the case, the lost eyelid structures can be replaced by eyelid structures from the opposite eyelid after an ingenious method which was originated by Landolt (1881) and further developed by Dupuy-Dutemps (1927), Hughes (1937), and others.

Technique (Pedicle Flap)

The flap, if possible, should be taken from the neighborhood. Only if the latter is cicatricial, a cervical (Case 68, p. 1080) or arm flap should be chosen. The basic forms and locations of flaps from the immediate neighborhood are illustrated in Figures 227 and 228. A temporal flap can be used for upper and lower lid, a malar flap for the lower lid, and a frontal flap for the upper lid.

The length and form of the flap are determined and outlined according to pattern; to counteract shrinkage, the flap should be made one third larger than required. The entire flap is raised. That part of the flap which is to replace the conjunctiva is lined with a buccal mucous-mem-

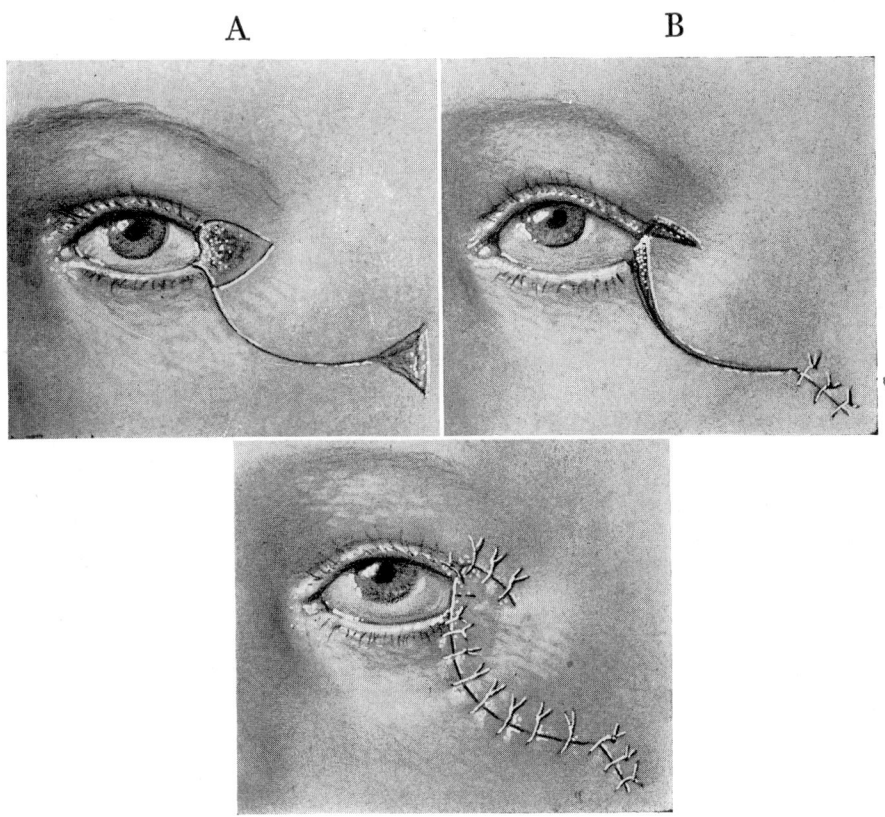

A   B

C

Fig. 226. Closure of defect at lateral canthal angle by Imré's method. (See Fig. 213.)

brane graft if the eyeball is intact, with a skin graft if the eyeball is absent (see p. 454). The flap is now returned to its original site, and is covered with a pressure dressing. Two weeks later, the flap is raised again and a piece of ear cartilage 5 mm. (³⁄₁₆ inch) wide, properly shaped and thinned to replace the tarsus, is buried beneath the subcutaneous tissue of the lining of the flap (see pp. 457-458). The flap is now rotated into the defect. The mucous-membrane lining is sutured to the conjunctival edge of the defect,

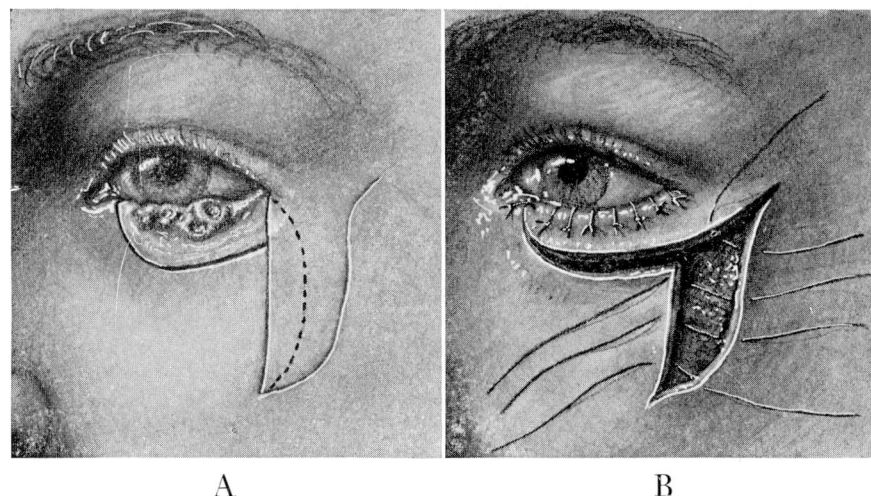

A   B

Fig. 227. *A:* Excision of entire lower lid. Malar flap to replace lower lid is outlined. Flap is made one third larger than required. Flap is raised and lined with buccal mucous-membrane graft to replace conjunctiva (dotted line) and returned to its original site. *B:* Two weeks later, flap is raised again and rotated into defect. Closure of secondary defect by undermining wound edges and skin sliding.

the skin to the skin edges. The wound edges of the secondary defect, left after elevation of the flap, are undermined and sutured together or the defect is covered with a thick split skin graft.

After eight weeks, the pedicle of the flap is severed and returned to its original site, and flap and pedicle are adjusted in place.

After the edema of the flap has subsided, the fold of the upper lid may be reconstructed by making an incision along the site of the fold and excising some of the subcutaneous tissue so that the resulting scar will become depressed.

Technique (Imré)

The basic features and principles of Imré's method have been discussed on page 458. This method is suitable only for subtotal defects of

468

the lower lid where a stump of conjunctiva and skin is still left. Lining and support are provided as outlined on pages 454 and 457.

In a case of subtotal defect of the lid where a stump of conjunctiva and skin is still left, the defect can be replaced by eyelid structures from the opposite eyelid after an ingenious method which was devised by Landolt (1881) and improved by Dupuy-Dutemps (1927) and by Hughes (1937).

Technique (Hughes) (Fig. 229)

The following procedure is for defects of the lower lid.

Stage 1: From an incision along the intermarginal white line of the upper lid (see p. 209), the upper lid is divided into two layers: the con-

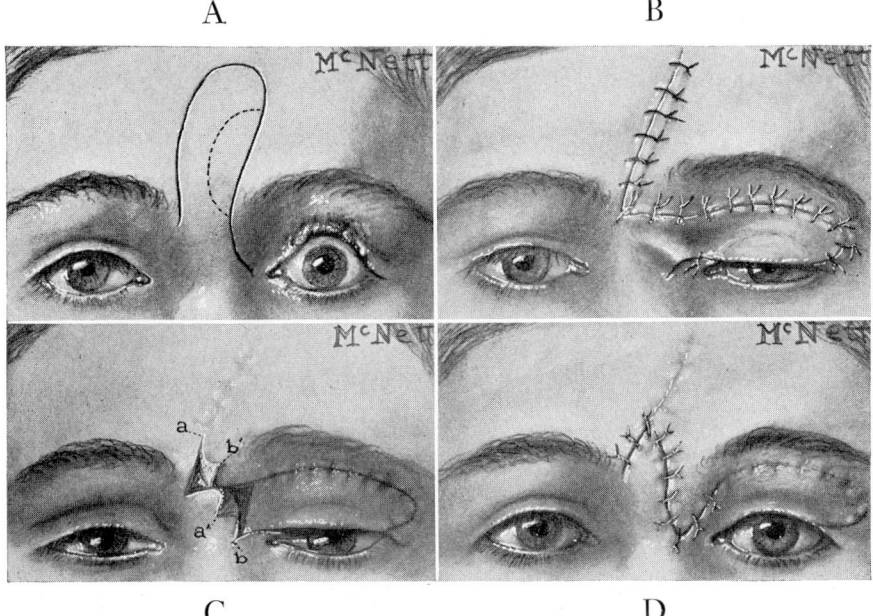

Fig. 228. *A:* Replacement of entire upper lid with frontal flap (Wiener). Flap is made one third larger than required. It is raised and lined with buccal mucous-membrane graft to replace conjunctiva (dotted line). *B:* After two weeks, flap is raised again and rotated into defect. Raw area of flap bed is closed by undermining wound edges and skin sliding. *C:* After two months, pedicle of flap is severed and adjusted as in Z-operation (see Fig. 52): formation of two triangular flaps, which are made so that their outlines form a Z. They are raised and exchanged so that *a* is approximated to *a'* and *b* to *b'*. *D:* After Z-operation.

junctivotarsal layer and the skin-orbicularis lamella. The separation is carried upward to about 3 mm. (⅛ inch) above the margin of the tarsus. The skin of the cheek bordering the defect of the lower lid is undermined sufficiently so that it can be pulled upward, without tension, to the level

469

A   B   C

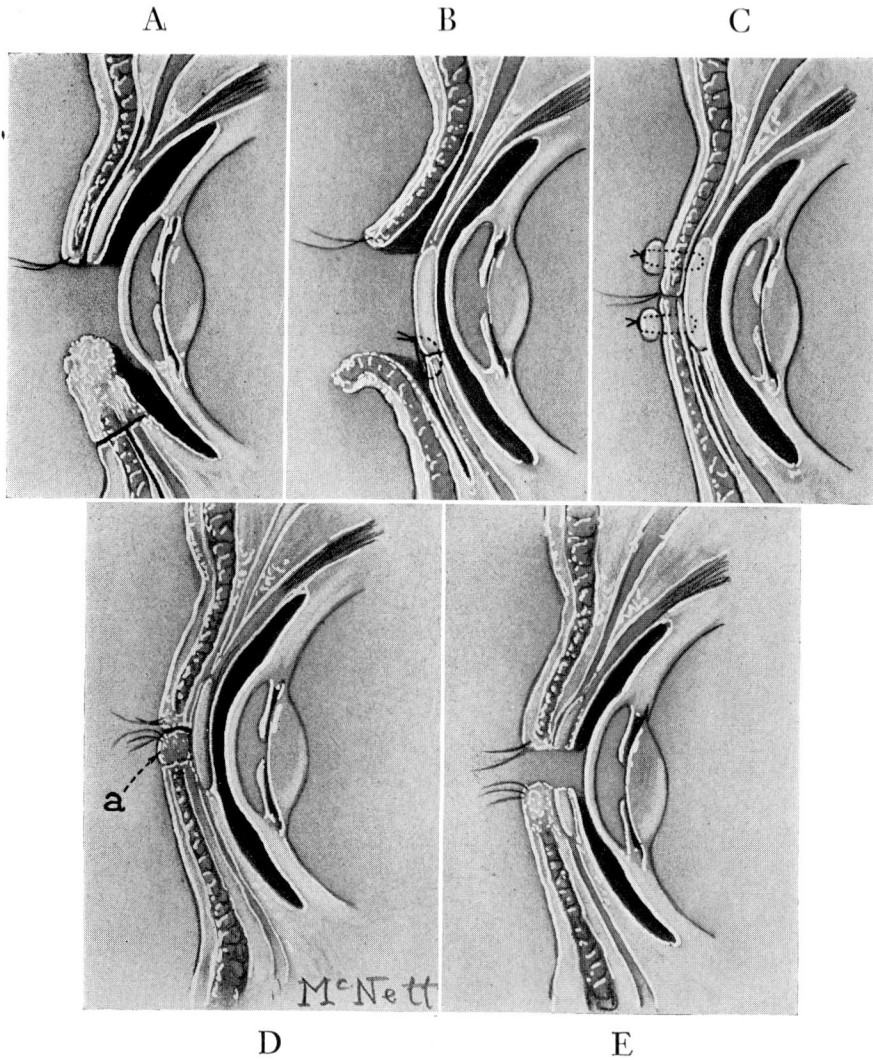

D   E

Fig. 229. *A:* Replacement of subtotal defect of lower lid (Hughes). Lower border of defect is marked by heavy horizontal line. Verticle lines indicate level of separation of lower lid and of upper lid. *B:* Conjunctivotarsal layer of upper lid is severed from orbicularis skin lamella and brought downward and sutured to conjunctival stump of lower lid. Skin of lower-lid stump is mobilized into cheek. *C:* Mobilized lower skin is drawn upward and attached to anterior surface of lower half of tarsus with mattress sutures tied upon rolls of gauze. Skin orbicularis layer of upper lid is attached to upper half of tarsus. *D:* Second Stage: Replacement of eyelashes of lower lid by hairbearing full-thickness graft (*a*) (see Fig. 231). *E:* Third Stage: Lids are severed between two rows of eyelashes with transverse incision through tarsus and conjunctiva.

470

normally occupied by the lower lid. The lower epithelial border of the upper tarsus is cut off, and the conjunctivotarsal layer is pulled downward. It is sutured to the conjunctival stump of the lower-lid defect with No. 36 stainless-steel wire in a continuous running suture, which can be pulled at either canthus. A second layer of reinforcing sutures (00000 chromic catgut) is laid over the first suture. The previously undermined skin is drawn upward and attached to the anterior surface of the lower half of the tarsus by means of three black silk sutures which are tied upon rolls of gauze. The superficial layer of the upper lid is then attached to the anterior surface of the upper half of the tarsus in the same manner. The two skin edges (lid margin and lower skin edge) are sutured together.

Stage 2: After an interval of four to six weeks, the eyelashes of the lower lid may be replaced if this seems desirable (for technique, see below). The hairbearing full-thickness graft is placed in a bed prepared just below and parallel to the margin of the upper lid.

Stage 3: Five to seven weeks later, an incision is made transversely, with a pair of blunt-nosed scissors, between the two rows of lashes through the full thickness of the lid. Whether the second stage is desirable or not, it is advisable to wait about three months before performing the third stage to allow the structures to stretch sufficiently.

A definite drawback of Hughes' method arises in cases where the lower skin (cheek) flap cannot be formed of sufficient width and mobility. It may later retract and shorten the new lower lid, and may even cause ectropion. The originator of this principle of eyelid reconstruction (Landolt) and his followers (Tripier, Dupuy-Dutemps) apparently were aware of this fact, and suggested replacement of the lower lid with flaps from the upper lid.

Technique (Dupuy-Dutemps) (Fig. 230)

Stage 1: Separation of the two upper-lid layers and suturing of the conjunctivotarsal layer to the conjunctival stump of the lower lid are performed as just described. The edge of the margin of the upper lid is now sutured to the raw edge of the skin bordering the lower-lid defect.

Stage 2: Three to six weeks later, the scar running between upper-lid margin and skin edge of lower lid is incised, and the skin of the upper lid is dissected free and pulled upward until its margin is at the normal level. A flap is now taken from above the upper lid, pedicled at the temporal side, rotated into the lower defect, and sutured into place; approximation of the upper-lid margin to the upper margin of the flap and closure of the donor site at the upper lid follow.

Stage 3: Three to six weeks later, the full thickness of the lid is severed along the margin of the upper lid, as described previously.

471

This method (Dupuy-Dutemps) can be facilitated by raising the upper-lid flap in stages before the first stage of the operation so that it can be transferred at the first stage, thus eliminating a second-stage operation. Even better, one may return to the originator's (Landolt's) advice

A   B

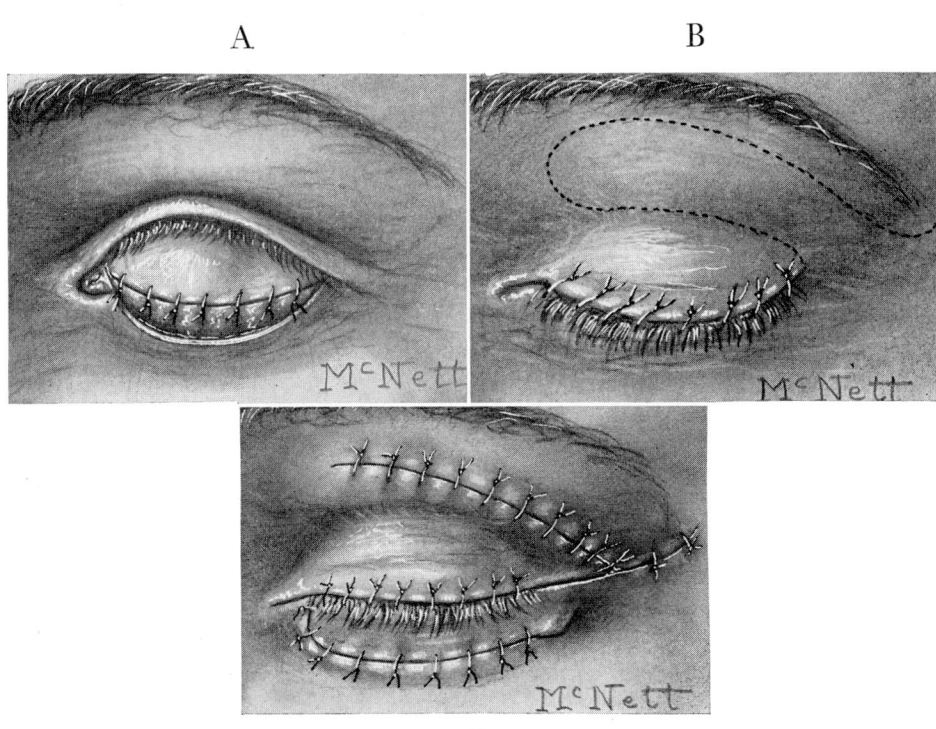

C

Fig. 230. *A:* Replacement of subtotal defect of lower lid (Dupuy-Dutemps) (compare also with Fig. 229). Conjunctivotarsal layer of upper lid is separated from orbicularis skin lamella and pulled downward and sutured to conjunctival stump of lower lid. *B:* Skin orbicularis layer of upper lid is sutured to skin bordering lower-lid defect. Flap above upper lid to replace skin of lower lid is outlined (see *C*). Raising it in stages is advisable to assure sufficient circulation. *C:* In second stage, skin orbicularis of upper lid is severed along former line of suture and moved upward. Flap previously prepared above upper lid is rotated into lower-lid defect, and sutured to wound edges of lower lid as well as to margin of upper lid. Raw surface of flap bed is closed by skin sliding. In third stage, full thickness of lids is severed between margin of upper lid and upper edge of flap (compare also with Fig. 229, *E*).

and shift a double-pedicle flap from the upper lid to provide skin cover for the lower lid (see Figs. 220-222). Such a flap is well vascularized, and does not need delaying. Before it is transplanted, the eyelash margin of the skin of the upper lid is sewn to the tarsus of the upper lid at such a

472

level that not more than the inferior one half of the tarsal plate is exposed. The flap is then shifted downward and sutured to the lower-lid margin as well as to the lid margin of the upper lid.

W. B. Macomber and co-workers provide skin coverage with a full-thickness (postauricular or clavicular) skin graft. In a second-stage operation, they provide eyelashes for the lower lid by means of a narrow single-pedicled flap (pedicled at the median canthus) that contains along its upper margin a single row of hair follicles from the eyebrow; it is raised in stages.

Manchester's method of developing a conjunctival flap (Figs. 216-218), appears to be another improvement in this principle of lid reconstruction. The conjunctiva is freed from the depths of the fornix and the lower part of the globe from canthus to canthus. The flap, corresponding to the entire width of the fissure, is folded upon itself and the fornix re-created. The remaining steps are the same as those described above.

Upper Eyelid

A technique similar to that described above can be used in reconstruction of the upper eyelid. D. B. Stark, Born and Hackleman shift an upper bipedicled flap, the lower edge of which is the upper defect edge, like a curtain over the united upper and lower conjunctiva flaps and suture it to the lower-lid margin. The defect above the flap is covered with a full-thickness skin graft from the upper eyelid of the sound eye. The lids are separated after four to six months. Cartilage grafts to replace the tarsus are not required.

DEFECTS OF EYELASHES AND EYEBROWS

Defects of eyelashes and eyebrows are replaced by free transplantation of hairbearing full-thickness grafts (Knapp, Lexer, Danternelle, Passot, Pirruccello, Mutou and Boo-Chai, and Longacre et al.) or hairbearing flaps.

Technique (Replacement of Eyelashes)

An incision is made slightly distal and parallel to the lid margin, and the wound edges are held separated by traction sutures. The graft bed is prepared by enlarging the incision. A hairbearing full-thickness graft 2 mm. ($3/32$ inch) wide is taken from the hairline posterior to the mastoid process, where the hairs are not so strong as elsewhere on the scalp. The donor area should be selected so that the hair will grow in the proper direction. Since the hair penetrates the scalp obliquely, the knife should be led in the same

473

direction so as not to destroy the hair follicles. The graft consists of the full thickness of the skin and some fat tissue. With a pair of scissors, the fat tissue is then trimmed away until all hair roots are exposed, recognizable as bulbous black protuberances; the roots must not be injured. The graft is inserted into the wound bed and anchored in place by sutures similar to those used in grafting eyebrows (Fig. 231). Mechanic's waste may be incorporated. The grafted area is covered with bismuth tribromophenate (xeroform) ointment; no other dressing is required. As a rule, the hair starts to grow after three weeks and has to be clipped regularly from then on. If the graft fails to take, the procedure should be repeated.

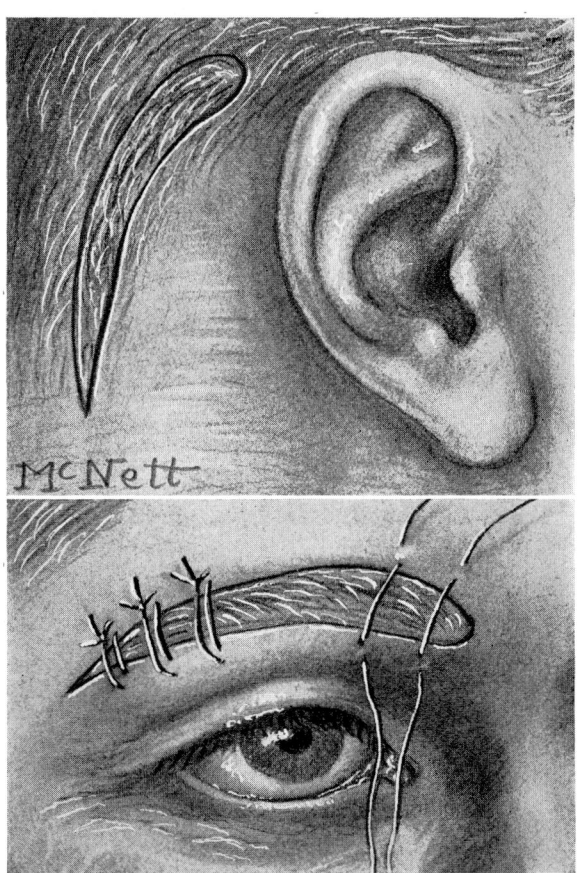

Fig. 231. Replacement of eyebrow with hairbearing full-thickness graft from neck hairline posterior to mastoid process. Graft is held in place with mattress sutures, which are inserted through wound edges of recipient area but not through graft. Mechanic's waste can be placed beneath the sutures and the latter tied over it to provide uniform pressure.

474

W. B. Macomber et al. replace the eyelashes by means of a narrow single-pedicle flap (pedicled at the median canthus) which contains along its upper margin a single row of hair from the eyebrows; the flap is raised in stages.

Technique (Replacement of Eyebrows) (Fig. 231)

The technique is similar to that used for replacement of eyelashes. The graft bed is prepared by excision of a wedge-shaped piece of skin of desired width. The graft is removed from the hairline posterior to the mastoid process, as described in the foregoing paragraph. The graft should be slightly larger than the defect and cut so that the hair will grow in the proper direction. After thorough hemostasis, the wound edges of the graft bed are held retracted. The graft is inserted and held in place by mattress sutures, which are inserted through the wound edges of the host area but not through the graft, or by simple single sutures laid through graft and skin edges and left long. Mechanic's waste is then laid over the graft and the sutures are tied over it, thus providing uniform pressure. The donor area is closed by simple suturing.

Variation: If the eyebrow of the other side is preserved and sufficiently wide, the lower half of it can be excised and used as a hairbearing full-thickness graft. The donor area is closed by simple suturing.

When eyebrow and eyelid must be reconstructed, Longacre, deStefano and Holmstrand used a postauricular-scalp graft in continuity and observed a better take of the scalp graft due to better circulation.

All methods in which hairbearing grafts are used may result in partial or complete necrosis of the graft, as the author can testify. This does not preclude the possibility of repeating the procedure. A more reliable method, if available, is the hairbearing arterial island flap.

Technique

The arterial island flap after Esser (p. 82) is the most satisfactory method of reconstructing an eyebrow if the pedicle can be made sufficiently long. The artery to be selected is the arteria temporalis of the same side. The hairs of the temporal region are clipped, not shaved. The vessel is followed up in front of the ear by digital palpation and exposed from a preauricular incision in all its length, starting almost level with the ear lobe. In the upper part, the hairbearing island of temporal skin is marked out in the shape of the eyebrow. It is incised all around; the incision becomes shallow at the lower end where the vessel approaches it. The wound edge anterior to the artery is dissected away from the artery, and this is followed by careful freeing of the temporal artery and vein up to

475

the outlined skin island after ligation and separation of the small branches. The skin island is carefully freed from deeper tissues and completely mobilized after ligation and severance of the vessels at the upper end. The flap bed at the site of the new eyebrow is incised. The island flap is drawn through a subcutaneous tunnel to the flap bed without torsion or twist of the vascular bundle, and the skinbearing part of the flap is sutured into place. Closure of the main incision follows. If necessary, a small drain is inserted.

DEFECTS OF ORBITS

Contracted Socket

The reconstruction of a socket for retention of an artificial eye becomes necessary after enucleation of the eyeball and subsequent obliteration of the socket through adhesions between lids and underlying structures. Many methods of reconstruction have been devised. The use of a free skin graft wrapped around a stent (Esser, Gillies, Killner, Wheeler, and others) has given most satisfactory results. Wheeler has contributed much towards the standardization of the method.

Technique (Fig. 232)

An incision is made between the margins of the eyelids; the margins are held apart by traction sutures. External canthotomy is performed by pushing one blade of a pair of straight scissors into the lateral cul-de-sac— the lids are held apart and pushed toward the nose with thumb and index finger of the right hand—and closing the other blade down on the skin; the tissues are severed with one snip. This facilitates introduction of the stent, since the sac is larger than the palpebral fissure. The lids are now dissected away from the underlying scar tissue. The dissection must be kept superficial on a plane along the tarsus of the lids so that only the lids proper are freed and no scar tissue is left on the posterior surface of the lids. Temporally and below, the dissection should be carried well to the orbital margin so that the graft will adhere to the periosteum of the anterior aspect of the orbital margin. Superiorly, the dissection is carried behind the orbital rim; the bony rim of the orbit, however, should not be touched so that the musculus orbicularis oculi and musculus levator palpebrae superioris can be saved. On the nasal side, the dissection is carried posterior to the plane of the normal caruncle and to the anterior crest of the lacrimal groove and the orbital rim above it. All scar tissue is removed from the cavity. The next step is thorough hemostasis, obtained by packing the cavity with moist gauze.

476

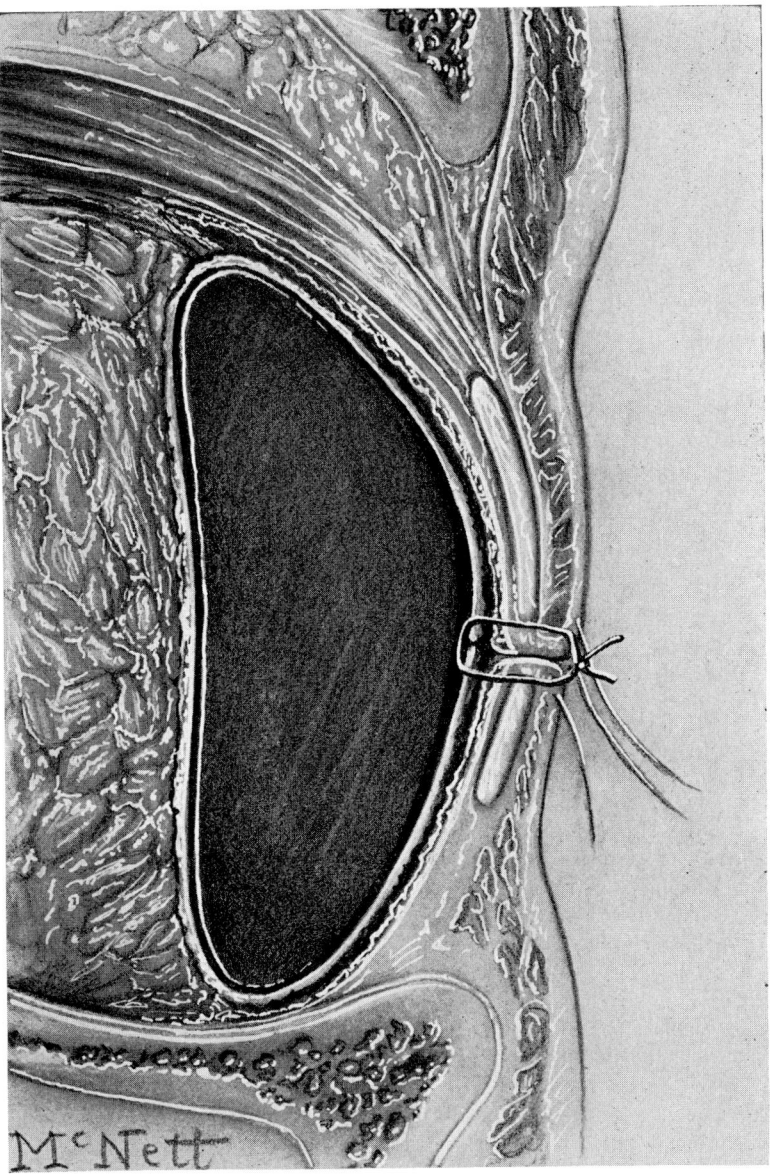

Fig. 232. Reconstruction of contracted socket. Lids are dissected away from underlying scar tissue. Plane of dissection is posterior surface of tarsus. Inferiorly, dissection is carried to periosteum of orbital margin. Superiorly, dissection is carried behind orbital rim. Bony rim of orbit should not be touched so that orbicularis and levator palpebrae muscles can be saved. Mold of dental compound is made of cavity. Split skin graft is wrapped around stent, raw surface outward (graft is indicated by white line around mold). Graft should be arranged in such a way that its overlap presents at palpebral fissure. Mold and graft are inserted and immobilized by suturing lids together so that each suture includes part of overlap of graft.

477

THE HEAD AND NECK

A mold of dental compound is now prepared. It is softened in hot water and introduced into the cavity. The dimensions of the mold are approximately: length, 3 to 4 cm. (1¾₁₆ to 1⁹₁₆ inches); width, 2.5 cm. (1 inch); thickness, 1 cm. (⅜ inch). While still soft, the mold is shaped to fit the cavity and left in place until it hardens; it is then removed. Upon the anterior surface of the mold, a point corresponding to the median or lateral canthal angle is marked out by scratching with a knife. This will facilitate correct reinsertion. Rough points are smoothed down with the knife. A split skin graft is removed from the hairless region of upper arm or thigh (donor area not to be shaved preoperatively!) and wrapped around the mold, raw surface outward, as described on page 39. The graft should be arranged in such a way that its overlap is at the palpebral fissure. Mold and graft are now inserted and immobilized by suturing the lids together so that each suture includes a part of the overlap of the graft. In cases of contracted socket in which there is sufficient conjunctiva to be worth conserving, the graft should consist of buccal mucous membrane and not of skin, since a combination of skin and mucous membrane has proved unsatisfactory. If insufficient conjunctiva is present, it should be removed and the entire graft be made of split skin.

After-Treatment

Bismuth tribromophenate (xeroform) gauze is placed upon the lids and a proper pressure dressing applied. Both eyes should be included. The dressing is changed after one week, but the mold is left in place for three weeks. Three weeks after the operation, the sutures are removed, the mold lifted out, and the canthotomy wound closed with sutures. An artificial eye may now be introduced. If a matched ocular prosthesis is not available at this time, the mold must be reinserted.

EXENTERATION OF ORBIT AND REPAIR

Exenteration of the orbital contents becomes necessary if malignant tumors infiltrate from the eyelids, the eyeball, the maxilla, or the sinuses into the orbit. In some cases, the eyelids must be removed at the time of the exenteration; in other cases, they, or at least their skin covering, can be spared.

Technique

Conservation of Full Thickness of Lids, Including Conjunctival Lining: If the full thickness of the eyelids, including their conjunctival lining, can be spared, the incision starts with separation of the fornices

478

of the upper and lower cul-de-sacs. The periosteum of the orbital rims is now incised and elevated, together with the orbital contents, and freed from the orbital wall until the apex is reached. Pressure against the bone should be avoided to prevent perforation of the bony wall, which in some places is quite thin. After mobilization of the orbital contents, the entire mass is removed from its pedicle at the apex; bleeding from the arteria ophthalmica can as a rule be arrested by pressure. To prevent necrosis of the bare bone, covering of the bone becomes necessary. For this purpose, the conjunctiva of the upper and lower fornices is dissected free and stretched until it can be pushed into the depth of the orbit and held in place by packing (Spaeth). Alternatively, it may be possible to suture the mobilized conjunctiva of upper and lower fornices transversely together, as is done after enucleation of the eyeball (Axenfeld).

Sacrifice of Conjunctiva of Lids: If the conjunctiva of the eyelids cannot be spared but must be removed together with the orbital contents, the incision starts at the lid margins; after the margins are penetrated, tarsus and conjunctiva are separated from the lids until the upper and lower cul-de-sacs are reached; the dissection from then on is the same as described in the foregoing. To cover the naked bony wall, the lids—after removal of their margins—are pushed with their denuded posterior surface into the depth of the orbit and held in place by packing. If not all the bone can be covered in this way, it is left to granulate. Reese and Jones cover the orbital walls with a flap of temporalis muscle which is pulled through a hole in the lateral wall of the orbit. The lid margins are then sutured together, and a pressure dressing is applied.

Sacrifice of Full Thickness of Lids: If the lids in their entire thickness must be sacrificed, the incision starts along the orbital rim and penetrates down to the bone. Lids and conjunctival sac are now removed, together with the orbital contents, as previously described. If the periosteum of the orbital bones can be left attached to them, an inlay skin graft can be used for coverage (Case 71, p. 1084). If the periosteum must be removed, the cavity is closed with a flap from the forehead (of proper size and shape, pedicled at the root of the nose, and containing the arteria supraorbitalis and arteria frontalis), or a flap from the temporal region (containing the anterior branch of the arteria temporalis) should be mobilized and rotated into the defect. The flap is sutured to the wound edges of the skin along the orbital rim. The secondary defect at the donor site is covered with a thick split skin graft. The pedicle of the flap is partly severed after three weeks. Final separation and adjustment of flap and pedicle are completed after four weeks.

Extension of Malignancy into Orbit: In cases where a malignant tumor of the maxilla or of frontal or other sinuses has broken into the orbit necessitating removal not only of the orbital contents but also of parts of the orbital wall, a large cavity is created which has a broad communication with the oral and nasal cavities. This cavity should not be closed primarily for two reasons: to prevent ascending infection of the sinuses and to prevent overlooking possible recurrences. Only if a sufficient interval, preferably five years, has elapsed, during which there is no evidence of recurrence and active infection is controlled, should closure be attempted. In the meantime, the patient is treated conservatively and infection controlled by cleansing the cavity with irrigation and application of local antiseptics. If possible, the cavity is temporarily closed with a latex or other type of prosthesis for cosmetic and functional purposes. The prosthesis may be simple or more elaborate, fixed to a pair of glasses, forming an upper and lower lid and holding an artificial eye. Final closure of the cavity is achieved by transplantation of a lined flap either from the forehead (Case 70, p. 1083) or from distant parts.

Bony Defects of Orbit

Bony defects of the orbit may need repair for functional or cosmetic reasons. Defects of the upper rim are not necessarily followed by functional disturbances, but may cause deformities for which the patient seeks plastic repair. Defects of the lower rim from old depressed fractures of the floor of the orbit or the malar bone, for instance, may cause a more or less marked ptosis of the eyeball with subsequent functional disturbance. This is usually absent in the so-called Treacher-Collins syndrome (p. 355; Case 17, p. 1016).

Technique

Bony defects of the entire upper rim are best repaired with cartilage grafts. The incision runs just within the eyebrow, which should not be shaved but covered throughout the operation. The incision penetrates through the soft tissue and the periosteum down to the bone. The periosteum is mobilized over the deformity to form a pocket into which an autogenous rib-cartilage graft is inserted (p. 62). The graft may be carved according to a pattern, which can readily be obtained with a mold of dental compound pressed into the defect. The graft is held in place with thin stainless-steel wires inserted through drill holes in graft and host bone. In partial defects of the upper rim, diced cartilage grafts (p. 64), dermal-fat grafts (p. 47; Case 12, p. 1006), or dermal grafts (p. 45) can be used to good advantage.

In defects of the lower rim of the orbit with ptosis of the eyeball, an incision is made through the eyelid within one of its wrinkles. The

480

fibers of the orbicularis oculi muscle are split and the anterior portion of the depressed orbital floor is exposed. The periosteum is elevated from the latter and from the floor of the orbit until the orbital contents can be raised sufficiently. A wedge-shaped graft of cartilage—with its base outward—is now driven into the subperiosteal pocket and held in place with sutures. Closure of the skin incision follows. (Compare also with Case 17, p. 1016.)

For treatment of so-called blow-out fractures of the floor of the orbit, see page 569.

DEFORMITIES

ECTROPION

Ectropion is a condition in which the eyelid is rolled outward so that the conjunctiva either partly or wholly is visible and exposed to the outside. It may affect one lid or both. It is either cicatricial or noncicatricial. Of the latter, the paralytic or senile form represents the majority of cases and constitutes a relaxation of the skin and muscles involving the lower lid only.

Cicatricial Ectropion

The repair of this condition has been described on page 451.

Paralytic or Senile Ectropion

Paralytic or senile ectropion may be either partial, involving only the lid margin, or complete. The type of repair depends upon the extent of the condition.

Technique (Partial Paralytic Ectropion) (Ziegler)

This is a simple and effective procedure, consisting in galvanopuncture of the conjunctiva and tarsus with the purposes of producing a scar which will cause contracture and thus elevation of the lid. The procedure can be done with the patient ambulant. The lid is everted; after an instillation of 1 per cent solution of tetracaine hydrochloride (Pontocaine), procaine is injected beneath the conjunctiva. A blunt-pointed galvanocaustic electrode heated to redness or an electrocoagulation needle is quickly pushed drawn at points 3 mm. (⅛ inch) apart along a line 5 mm. (³⁄₁₆ inch) away from and parallel to the lid margin. Yellow mercuric oxide ointment is then inserted into the lower cul-de-sac. This procedure may be repeated if necessary.

481

THE HEAD AND NECK

Technique (Complete Paralytic Ectropion)

Many operations have been devised for this condition. Some attempt to correct the condition by elevation of the lid, but neglect to correct the main factor, that is, shortening of the tarsus, which—particularly with a long-standing eversion—becomes stretched and elongated. Some devices are mainly concerned with shortening of the tarsus, leaving the elongated skin untouched. The following technique, a combination of various methods (Kuhnt-Dieffenbach-Szymanowski-Meller), takes care of the shortening of both the tarsus and the skin (Fig. 233).

The incision starts on the lid margin, somewhat mediad to its center. From here it runs along the lateral half of the margin on a line between the sharp posterior marginal edge, which is in contact with the eyeball, and the more rounded border, which contains the eyelashes. Care should be taken not to injure the meibomian glands (Fig. 209). The incision now penetrates deeper, separating the conjunctivotarsal layer from the orbicularis-skin lamella. The next step consists of excision of a proper-sized triangular piece from the middle section of the conjunctivotarsal layer with its base at the margin. From the outer canthus, the incision is now continued outward and obliquely upward for a distance equal to the length of the base of the excised conjunctivotarsal triangle. From here, an incision is carried downward which should be twice as long as the base of the triangle and led so that its terminal point comes to lie in a vertical plane with the outer canthus. Finally, both points, the terminal point of the former incision and the outer canthus, are connected with each other by another incision, thus outlining a triangular piece of skin which is excised. The skin mediad to this triangular defect is thoroughly mobilized until a triangular skin flap is formed.

Closure of the triangular tarsal defect with buried sutures of 00000 catgut or cotton now follows (see discussion on wounds, p. 451). The next step is suturing of the apex of the skin flap into the outer angle of the triangular defect, after the eyelashes and their roots have been removed between this point and the outer canthus. The remaining wound edges are sutured. The final suture should be a through-and-through suture at the center of the lid close to the lid margin, including skin and tarsoconjunctival wound edges. The suture is tied upon the skin over a small roll of gauze. A proper pressure dressing is applied over the side that has been operated upon. Since it is advisable to include the other eye in the dressing, it may be to the patient's advantage to correct the other side in the same sitting if it needs correction. The dressing is removed after four days, the sutures after five to seven days.

Edgerton and Wolfort recently developed a technique to create permanently a displaced external canthus and lower lid—not just the lid

482

A

B

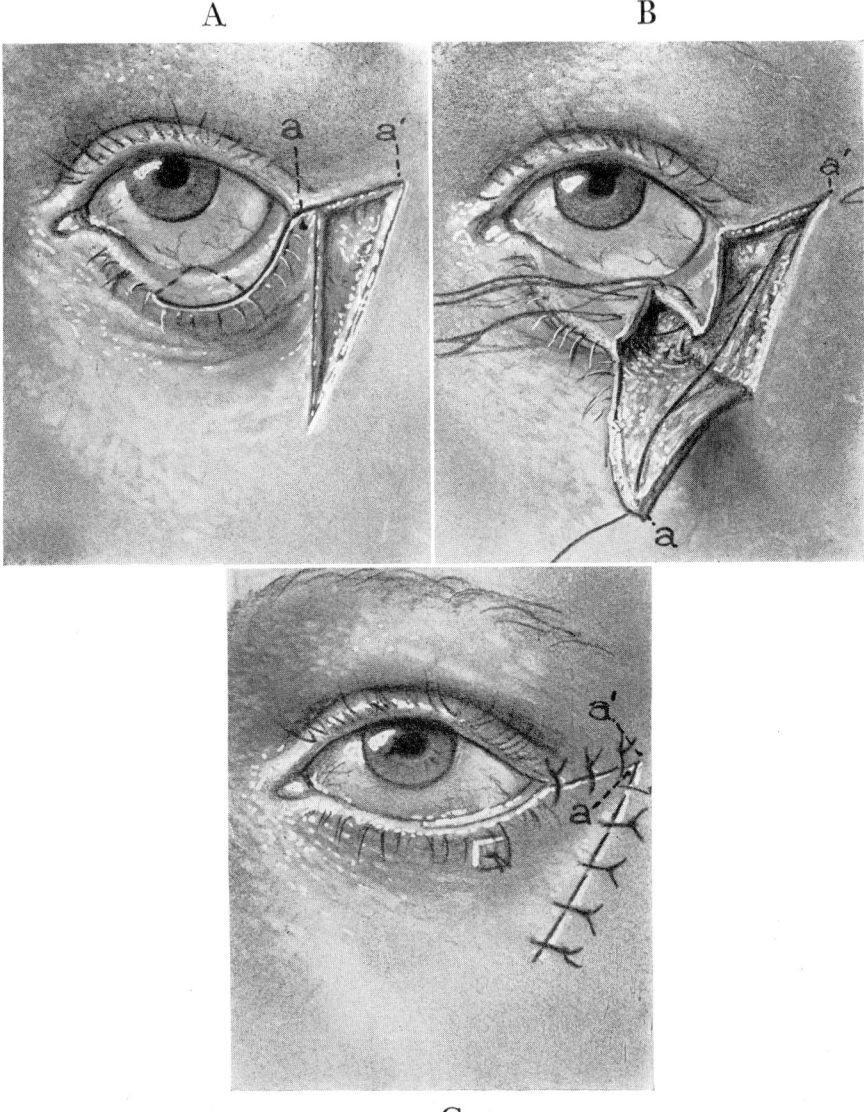

C

Fig. 233. *A:* Repair of complete paralytic ectropion (Kuhnt, Dieffenbach, Szy-manowski, Meller). From marginal incision along lateral half of lid, conjunctivotarsal layer is separated from orbicularis skin lamella. Triangular piece of middle section of conjunctivotarsal layer is removed (dotted line). From outer canthus, incision is continued obliquely outward and upward for distance equal to length of base of excised conjunctivotarsal triangle (*a-a'*). From here, incision is carried downward twice as long as *a-a'*. Terminal point comes to lie in vertical plane with outer canthus. This terminal point and outer canthus (*A*) are connected with another incision, thus outlining triangular piece of skin which is excised. *B:* Skin flap median to skin defect is mobilized. Conjunctivotarsal defect is closed by suturing wound edges together. *C:* Eyelashes are removed between point *a* and outer canthus. Point *a* is sutured to point *a'*. Mattress suture is placed at center of lid close to lid margin through skin and conjunctivotarsal wound edges.

alone. They use a ½ × 2½ cm. dermal flap which is taken from the region lateral to the lateral canthus and is based exactly at the lateral canthus. A bone groove is made at the lateral part of the bony rim of the orbit and a hole is drilled from the base of this concavity out into the infra temporal fossa. The flap is drawn through the bony canal and, after the paralyzed lid and sagging external canthus are lifted, it is flapped upon itself and returned. The author saw this method demonstrated by motion picture and was impressed by the good results.

The following technique is the simplest of all and reliable, but results in narrowing of the lid fissure. This disadvantage is, however, minor.

Technique (after Fuchs for Paralytic Ectropion after Facial-Nerve Palsy) (Fig. 234)

The extent to which it is desired to bring the lids together is marked out. The lower lid is split to the same extent in the marginal incision. This is the gray line that separates the orifices of the meibomian glands from the roots of the cilia (Fig. 209, p. 450). The lid is now split within the loose connective tissue that separates the tarsus and the muscular fibers of the orbicularis. The lid is split into two lamina—the anterior consisting of skin with the cilia, and the posterior the tarsus with the conjunctiva. From the median point of the incision, a short incision is carried downward through the skin so that a small triangular flap is formed (Fig. 234, A.) The ciliary follicles along the posterior border of the upper end

A   B

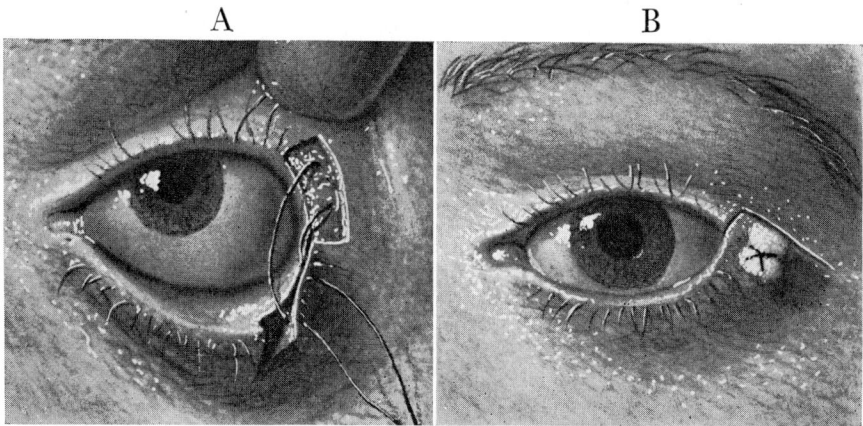

Fig. 234. *A:* Repair of paralytic ectropion after facial nerve palsy (Fuchs). Extent to which the lid to be brought together is marked out. Lower lid split to same extent and formation of a small triangular skin flap; removal of roots of cilia from follicles. Upper lid split to same extent as lower lid; a raw surface created by excision of hair follicles. Mattress suture to lift lower lid to upper lid. *B:* Mattress suture tied over small roll of gauze.

484

of the flap are removed by a pair of scissors so that the cilia may afterward fall out.

The upper lid is split by an intermarginal incision, in the same way and extent as was the lower lid. The bed of the hair follicles is excised, and in this way a raw surface is created to which the skin flap of the lower lid will fit. With a mattress suture the lower flap is firmly attached to the raw surface of the upper lid. With a few fine sutures, the remaining wound edges are sutured together.

ENTROPION

Entropion is a condition in which the lid margin is inverted. The entropion may be spastic or cicatricial.

SPASTIC ENTROPION

The inversion of the lid margin in spastic entropion is due to an overaction of the orbicularis muscle, and as a rule occurs in old age. Excision of a horizontal ellipse of skin and orbicularis muscle immediately below the lid margin may suffice. Ziegler's galvanopuncture, however, is said to be more effective. The method is similar to that described on page 481. The electrode, however, is inserted on the outside, and penetrates through skin and subcutaneous tissue.

Elliot believes that because the inferior tarsal plate is narrower than the superior one, it is apt to rotate on its long axis and to roll the lid margin inward when the orbicularis muscle advances upward on the tarsal plate upon closure of the lids. He counteracts this by inserting a fascial strip 3 mm. wide subcutaneously through the orbicularis fibers just below the tarsus. Laterally, the strip is fastened to the lateral rim of the orbit and medially to the median canthal ligament.

CICATRICIAL ENTROPION

The inversion of the lid margin in cicatricial entropion is due to destruction and replacement of the conjunctiva by scar tissue, resulting subsequently in deformity and shrinkage of the tarsus. It is nearly always due to trachoma. In the majority of cases, the condition can be repaired. Many operations have been devised but, in the more severe cases, only those procedures which attack the main factor of the deformity—the bent and deformed tarsus—can be regarded as effective. Hence, only tarsoplastic procedures may be considered and, of these, one is selected in which a wedge-shaped piece of tarsus is removed. This method, originally

485

devised by Streatfield (1858) and perfected later by Snellen (see Van Gils), has been modified in many ways.

Technique (for the Upper Lid) (Streatfield-Snellen) (Fig. 235)

The lid is steadied in a lid clamp which is long enough to include the entire tarsus. The skin is incised along the outer length of the lid margin and 3 mm. (⅛ inch) away from it. The upper wound edge is grasped and dissected free from the underlying orbicularis muscle to a point level with the upper border of the tarsus (Fig. 235, *A*). The fascia and orbicularis muscle covering the tarsus in the exposed section are grasped and excised from the tarsal plate. A wedge-shaped piece of tarsus is excised (with its base outward) from that region where it is most acutely bent (convex), that is, 3 mm. (⅛ inch) above the lid margin (Fig. 235, *A, B*). The width of the base of the wedge depends upon the severity of the deformity; as a rule, it is from 1 to 2 mm. wide. The incisions are outlined with a knife while the cartilaginous strip itself is removed with forceps and scissors; care should be taken not to perforate or excise the conjunctiva.

After completion of the excision, the lower part of the tarsus can be bent outward and held in this position by three mattress sutures, which are led in the following way: A silk thread is armed with two small, curved, cutting-edge needles. One needle engages the upper convex border of the tarsus vertically, and the other does the same thing a little away from the former stitch (Fig. 235, *A*). Both threads are now led downward upon the upper tarsal lamella (Fig. 235, *B, C*), and each thread is stitched through the skin of the lower wound edge, emerging above the cilia (Fig. 235, *A, B*). Two more such sutures are led in a similar way. The two ends of each suture are then passed through small plates of rubber (cut from sterile rubber tubing), the lid clamp is removed, and after hemostasis the sutures are tied (Fig. 235, *C*). Closure of the skin with a few fine silk sutures follows. The latter are removed after four days, the mattress sutures after three weeks.

BLEPHAROPTOSIS

The upper lid is lifted by the contraction of the musculus levator palpebrae superioris. In ptosis, the action of the muscle may be only weakened or it may be paralyzed completely. In the former case, ptosis is incomplete; in the latter, complete. Ptosis may or may not be associated with paralysis of the musculus rectus superior.

The medical profession is indebted to E. B. Spaeth for his efforts in clarifying the underlying physiological principles as related to proper

A

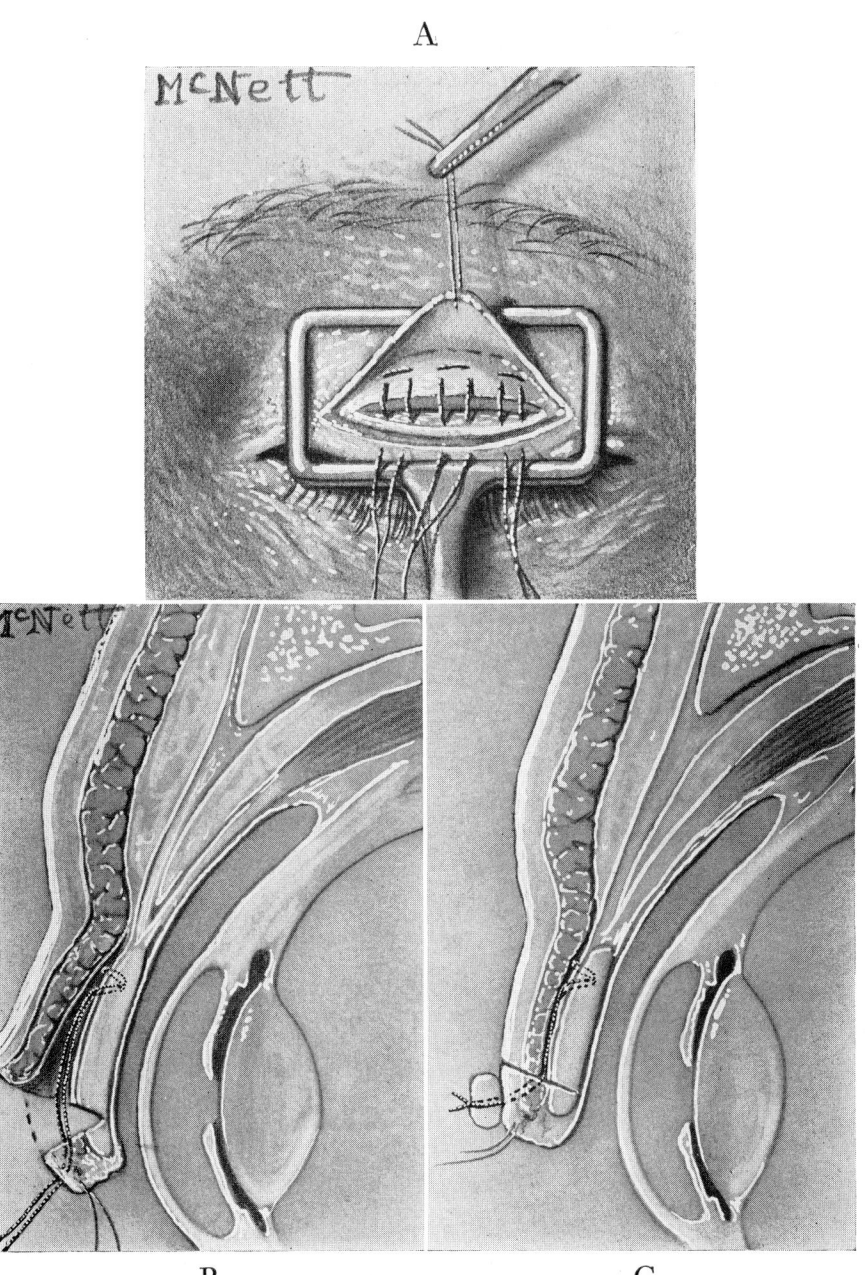

B   C

Fig. 235. Repair of cicatricial entropion by tarsoplasty after excision of wedge-shaped piece of tarsus (Streatfield, Snellen). (See text.)

therapy. This topic has been recently discussed in detail by Fox. Ptosis may be congenital or acquired, unilateral or bilateral.

Classification of Congenital Ptosis

Spaeth classifies the congenital cases into the following groups:
1. Unilateral ptosis without involvement of the superior rectus muscle.
2. Unilateral ptosis with involvement of the homolateral superior rectus muscle.
3. Bilateral ptosis without involvement of the superior rectus muscle.
4. Bilateral ptosis with involvement of the superior rectus muscle.
5. Unilateral ptosis with weakness of both superior rectus muscles.
6. Ptosis with more or less complete third-nerve and even sixth-nerve paralyses.
7. Ptosis with the classical jaw-winking reflex.
8. Ptosis with Duane's retraction syndrome.
9. Ptosis with neurofibromatosis.

Classification of Acquired Ptosis

Spaeth classifies the acquired cases into the following groups:
1. Traumatic (peripheral, cicatricial).
2. Traumatic (central and cerebrospinal), essentially sympathetic-nerve paralysis.
3. Third-nerve paralysis.
4. Third-nerve regenerating fibers (pseudo-Graefe syndrome).
5. Cervical sympathetic paralysis.
6. Atonic ptosis (senility, old enucleation).
7. Neuromuscular.
8. Degenerative. Blepharochalasis.
9. Neoplastic, as neurofibromatosis.
10. Hysterical.

Operative Procedures

It is beyond the scope of this book to mention all of the various operative procedures. None is entirely satisfactory, and no single procedure will meet all problems. Most of the operations belong strictly to the ophthalmic field, and should be performed only by those qualified in this field.

The main principles can be clarified by classifying the various operative procedures into three groups:

1. Advancement or shortening of the musculus levator palpebrae superioris, preferably in conjunction with resection of the upper part of the tarsus.
2. Utilization of the action of the musculus epicranius.
3. Utilization of the action of the musculus rectus superior.

Indications for the Various Procedures: The decisive factor is the degree of ptosis, whether incomplete or complete.

488

If the ptosis is incomplete—that is, the action of the musculus levator palpebrae superioris only weakened—advancement or shortening of the muscle with resection of the upper part of the tarsus is the operation of choice.

If the ptosis is complete and the paralysis of the musculus levator palpebrae superioris associated with the paralysis of the musculus rectus superior, utilization of the action of the musculus epicranius is the only choice. However, opinions of experts in this field are changing (see p. 491).

If the ptosis is complete and the musculus rectus superior functioning, utilization of the action of the latter is indicated, since it is followed by better functional results than are offered by utilization of the action of the musculus epicranius. This statement currently may not hold true entirely (see pp. 491, 495).

INCOMPLETE PTOSIS

ADVANCEMENT RESECTION OF MUSCULUS
LEVATOR PALPEBRAE SUPERIORIS

The precursor of this group of operations was the folding of the musculus levator palpebrae superioris, as devised by Everbusch (1883). This principle of shortening the muscle was quite unsatisfactory. Advancement of the muscle, with or without partial excision of the tarsoconjunctival lamella, was the next logical step.

Technique (Elschnig) (Fig. 236)

After application of a lid clamp, an incision is made 1.2 cm. (½ inch) above the lid margin and parallel to it, through skin and orbicularis muscle. The upper border of the tarsus and the septum orbitale are dissected free. The septum orbitale is severed 3 mm. (⅛ inch) above the tarsus along the entire length of the latter, exposing the levator lamella beneath. The levator lamella is secured with three silk mattress sutures, which are placed through the muscle 5 to 10 mm. (³⁄₁₆ to ⅜ inch) above the tarsus. Then follows subfascial dissection of the tarsus from the lower wound edge until the lid margin is reached. The musculus levator palpebrae superioris is severed below the sutures in its entire length.

The next step is the advancement of the levator; by retracting the lower wound lamella the tarsus is exposed; the three mattress sutures securing the upper levator lamella are placed as demonstrated in Figure 236. Each end of the mattress suture is passed through the anterior surface of the tarsus and conjunctiva about 4 mm. (⁵⁄₃₂ inch) above the lid margin; about 3 mm. (⅛ inch) below, the suture reenters the conjunctiva and tarsus, passes through the entire thickness of the lid, and emerges through the skin of the lid near the lid margin. The sutures are passed through a small piece of rubber (cut from rubber tubing) and tied. Closure of the fascia and skin follows. For after-treatment, see page 494.

The skin sutures are removed on the fifth day, the advancement sutures on the tenth day.

A   B

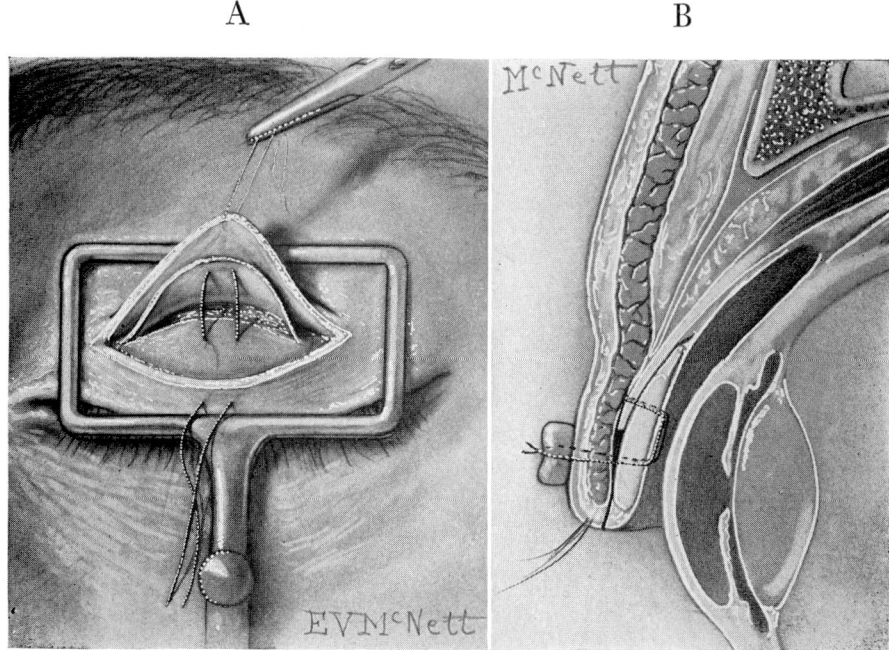

Fig. 236. *A:* Ptosis operation. Shortening and advancement of musculus levator palpebrae superioris (Elschnig). From horizontal incision, 12 mm. (½ inch) above lid margin, skin orbicularis and fascia are severed 3 mm. ($^3/_{32}$ inch) above tarsus and retracted (traction suture). Levator muscle is secured with three mattress sutures (only one depicted in drawing) 5 to 10 mm. ($^3/_{16}$ to ⅜ inch) above tarsus. Levator muscle is severed horizontally below sutures. After subfascial dissection of tarsus from lower wound edge, levator muscle is advanced as depicted in *B. B:* Each end of mattress suture is passed through anterior surface of tarsus and conjunctiva about 4 mm. ($^5/_{32}$ inch) above lid margin. About 3 mm. ($^3/_{32}$ inch) below, suture reenters conjunctiva and tarsus, passes through entire thickness of lid, and is tied over small piece of rubber.

A resection of a 2-mm. wide strip of the upper rim of the tarsus in addition to resection of the levator muscle can be more effective. The operation can also be carried out from the conjunctival side, as first recommended by Blaskovics and described in an improved way by Mustardé.

490

COMPLETE PTOSIS

UTILIZATION OF ACTION OF MUSCULUS EPICRANIUS

If the palsy is complete the levator palpebrae is totally paralyzed, as is the musculus rectus superior (see p. 450). Hitching up the lid to the frontalis muscle formerly was the operation of choice. However, shortening of the levator muscle is being used more and more—even if the muscle is completely paralyzed—and particularly in cases in which the superior rectus is functioning, thus taking advantage of the eye rolling upward beneath the lid in sleep. In transferring the action of an unparalyzed muscle to the paralyzed levator palpebrae, the musculus epicranius is used as a motor.

The results which Kirschner obtained in using fascia grafts to transfer the action of the musculus epicranius to the paralyzed musculus levator palpebrae superioris were so good that Pagenstecher's and similar sutures were abandoned. Lexer modified Kirschner's procedure and improved the cosmetic result. Wiener simplified Lexer's method.

Technique (Wiener) (Fig. 237)

An incision from 1 to 1.5 cm. (⅜ to ⅝ inch) long is made in the skin just above and parallel to the brow at about the middle of its outer half, and a similar incision at about the middle of its inner half, to expose the tendon of the musculus epicranius. An incision is now made in the lid, 4 mm. ($\frac{5}{32}$ inch) from and parallel to its border, through skin and musculus orbicularis oculi to the tarsus, the lid clamp having previously been applied to avoid bleeding (as in Fig. 236). The skin is freed from the underlying tissue, and that part of the musculus orbicularis oculi attached to the tarsal plate is removed with straight blunt-pointed scissors. The clamp is then removed and pressure exerted with a gauze sponge to control the bleeding.

A narrow strip of fascia is now removed from the thigh (see p. 48) and a mattress suture is placed through each end. A Reverdin needle or a small probe with an eye is passed from one of the openings over the brow subcutaneously under the skin of the lid, emerging at the opening over the tarsus. The threads attached to one end of the fascial strip are fastened to the needle, which is then withdrawn, pulling the end of the fascial strip out through the brow opening. This is then firmly sewed to the tendon of the musculus epicranius, the threads cut short, and the end of the strip tucked under the upper skin flap.

The instrument is then passed through the other brow incision under the lid skin, emerging at the opening over the tarsus, and the suture

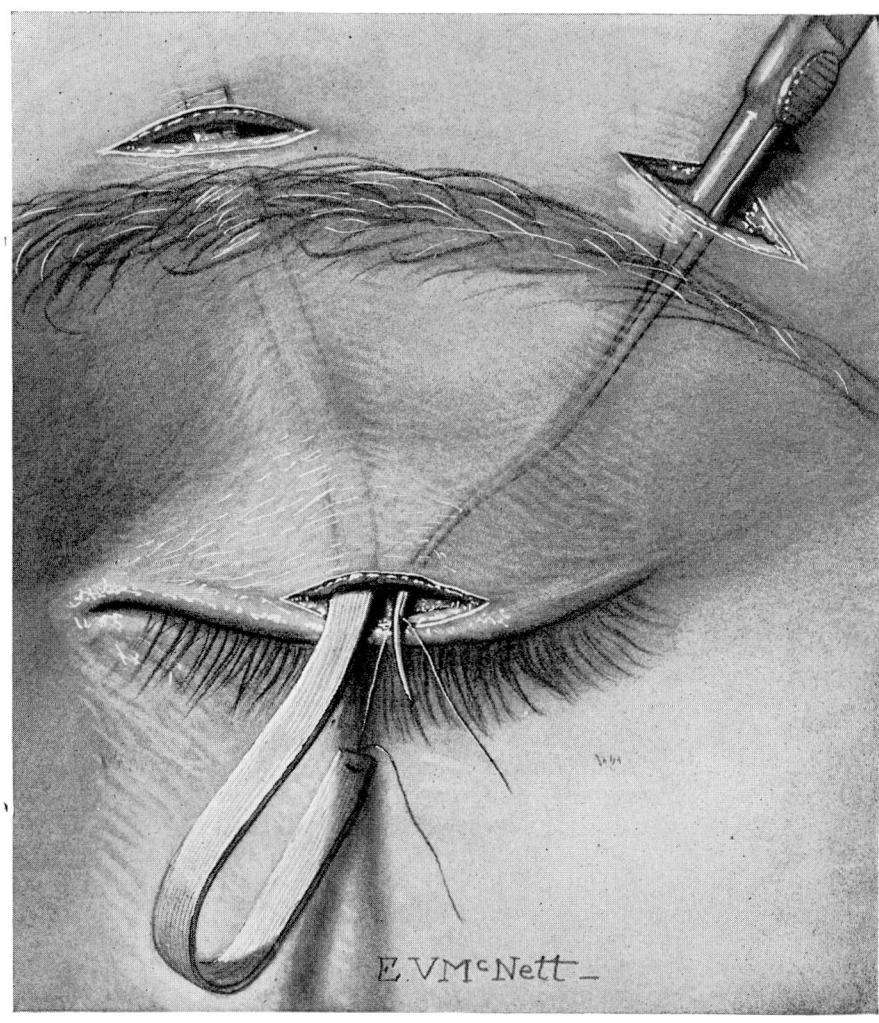

A

Fig. 237. *A:* Utilization of musculus epicranius in ptosis operation (Wiener). From two small incisions in skin just above brow, musculus epicranius is exposed. Another small incision is made 4 mm. (5/32 inch) from and posterior to lid border, exposing tarsus. Narrow strip of fascia is now inserted as follows: Mattress suture is placed through each end; Reverdin needle (or small probe with an eye) is passed from median opening over brow, subcutaneously under skin of lid and emerging at opening over tarsus. Thread is attached to one of fascial strips, fastened to needle which is then withdrawn, pulling fascial strip through brow opening. This free end is then firmly sewed to tendon of musculus epicranius. Same procedure is performed over lateral opening.

492

through the opposite end of the strip is attached to the instrument which is then withdrawn to the brow opening. Before it is pulled tight, a round toothpick or a section of a wooden applicator is passed through the loop of fascia. When traction is made on the fascial strip from the brow opening, the piece of wood passed under the loop prevents it from rising too far and disappearing under the skin fold.

Just enough traction on the strip is made to raise the lid to the degree judged by the surgeon to be adequate. The free end of fascia is then attached to the tendon of the musculus epicranius, as was the first. In this manner equal traction is exerted in raising the lid from each side of the brow. Two sutures are placed, fastening the loop of fascia securely to the tarsal plate, one on each side. Closure of the skin incisions follows.

The author (May) has slightly altered this technique (Fig. 237, *B*). After the fascial loop is placed, the toothpick inserted, and the loop placed under proper tension, one free end of the fascia is attached to the mus-

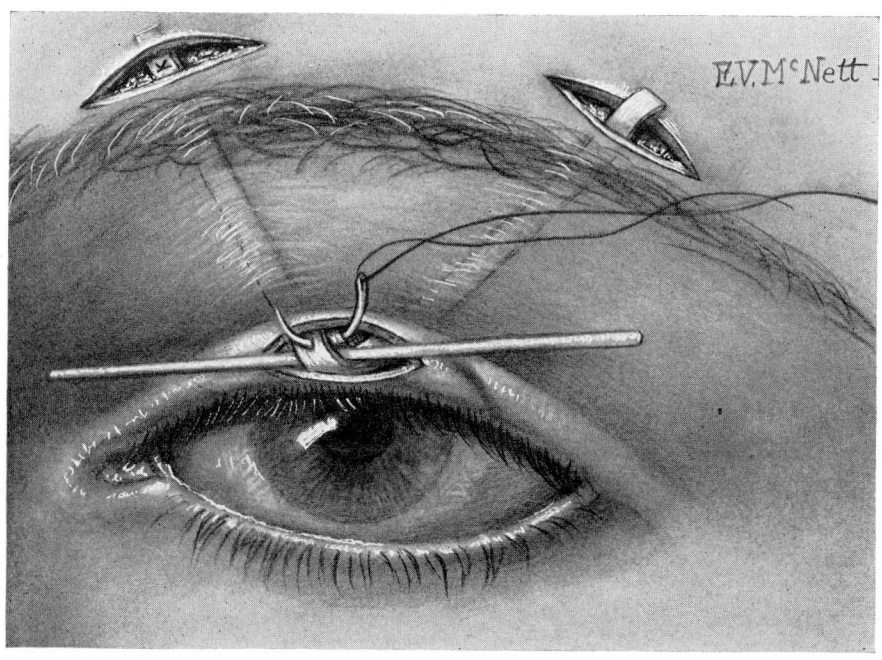

B

Fig. 237. *B:* Before pulling lateral strip tight, round toothpick is passed through angle of loop; traction is then made on fascial strip. Toothpick prevents loop from rising too far. One suture is now placed through median part of loop, fastening fascia graft to tarsus. After this suture is placed, toothpick is removed, equal pull is exerted on lateral part of fascial loop, and free end sutured to musculus epicranius. (Wiener and Alvis: Surgery of the Eye, W. B. Saunders.)

493

culus epicranius, the lower end to the tarsus. The toothpick is then removed, the other part of the loop pulled to assure equal tension, and its free end sutured to the musculus epicranius. A second suture may now be inserted to the other part of the angle of the loop. In this way puckering of the angle of the loop is avoided.

Wright (1922) inserted two separate fascial loops. This operation has been recently described with modifications by Crawford. I found this procedure also helpful.

Hendrix describes a simpler method which has been devised by Sawar, a British ophthalmologist. Instead of a strip of fascia, a transverse strip of the upper fibers of the orbicularis oculi is used as a sling and thus may act as a dynamic support.

Technique (Sawar)

Two parallel incisions are made: One is similar to the lower incision of Figure 237, A, only longer; the other one is immediately inferior to the supraorbital margin of the orbit. From this latter incision, the upper fibers of the orbicularis oculi muscle are exposed, and a strip 3 mm. (⅛ inch) in width and 3.2 to 4.4 cm. (1¼ to 1¾ inches) in length is raised. One side, median or lateral, is detached. A wide tunnel is made between orbicularis and levator muscles. The latter is severed from the upper rim of the tarsus, and the conjunctiva is detached from the posterior surface of the tarsal plate. A small incision is made through the tarsus near its superior border. A mosquito hemostat is now inserted through the slit in the tarsal plate and pushed upward through the previously made tunnel to grasp and pass the orbicularis strip downward through the tarsal plate and then upward upon the tarsal plate through the same tunnel toward the original insertion of the strip. The free end of the muscle strip is sutured back into the spot from which it had been attached, after the lid has been pulled up sufficiently.

Sawar believes that this kind of suspension is dynamic rather than static. Hendrix claims that the method is easily executed but depends much upon proper muscle training for good results; hence, it appears to be contraindicated in children.

After-Treatment

In applying a dressing, two thoughts must be held uppermost: (1) the cornea must be protected; and (2) there must be no traction or pull on the upper lid which will compromise the stitches placed to hold it in position. This is accomplished by covering the eyeball with the lower lid.

494

THE EYELIDS, EYEBROWS, AND ORBITS

After cheek and lower lid have been raised enough to cover the cornea, a broad piece of adhesive is attached to the cheek, a light gauze dressing placed over the upper lid and brow, and the other end of the adhesive strip fastened to the forehead. This protective dressing is required for only a few days, but it must be applied at night for protection as long as the lids will not close enough of themselves to cover the cornea during sleep. The patient must be observed during sleep to determine this.

UTILIZATION OF ACTION OF MUSCULUS RECTUS SUPERIOR

An entirely new principle in the treatment of complete blepharoptosis was introduced by Motais (1903) by transferring the musculus rectus superior, if it is functioning, to the paralyzed upper lid. Since that time, many modifications of the original operation have been devised. This operation is strictly an ophthalmic operation, to be performed by the ophthalmic surgeon. The principle, however, has been open to question. It is said that the failure of the cornea to roll up under the lid during sleep and an imbalance of the ocular muscles with production of diplopia are major disadvantages.

Technique (Motais) (Fig. 238)

The upper lid is everted. A fine retractor engages the sclera 3 or 4 mm. (⅛ or 5/32 inch) above the cornea and rotates the eyeball downward. A second retractor engages the free border of the tarsus, pulling the latter upward. Thus the upper fornix is exposed.

About 5 to 7 mm. (3/16 to 9/32 inch) above the margin of the cornea, a T-shaped incision is made through the conjunctiva. The wound edges are undermined until the tendon of the musculus rectus superior is exposed. The middle section of the tendon is now grasped with a forceps and a piece of it, 3 mm. (⅛ inch) wide, is severed from the sclera either with a fine scalpel or with fine, curved scissors. This section of the tendon is lengthened backward for about 1 cm. (⅜ inch). The peripheral end of this tendon flap, 3 mm. wide and 1 cm. long, is engaged in a double-armed fine-silk suture, the loop being made to lie posteriorly.

With a small scalpel an incision is made through the levator muscle in the upper extremity of the T-incision at the upper border of the tarsal plate and parallel to its upper border. The tarsal plate is pulled downward with a forceps, and the insertion of the levator, as well as the fascia, is severed with curved scissors from the tarsus for about 4 mm. (5/32 inch). From here, the anterior surface of the tarsus is dissected free to a point 3 to 4 mm. (⅛ to 5/32 inch) from the line of cilia.

495

The two needles of the double-armed suture are now passed through the levator incision between the anterior surface of the tarsus and the musculus orbicularis oculi to emerge through the skin 3 mm. (⅛ inch) from the lid margin. The conjunctival wound is closed, and the sutures are tied over a roll of gauze, tightly enough to overcorrect the ptosis slightly.

For after-treatment, see page 494.

EPICANTHUS

Epicanthus is a skin duplication due to vertical shortness of the tissue connecting the upper and lower lid at the inner canthus and bridging the latter. It may be congenital or acquired. It is a characteristic feature of some Mongolian races, although there is not the same degree of vertical shortage of skin across the canthus, and there is a fold extending into the

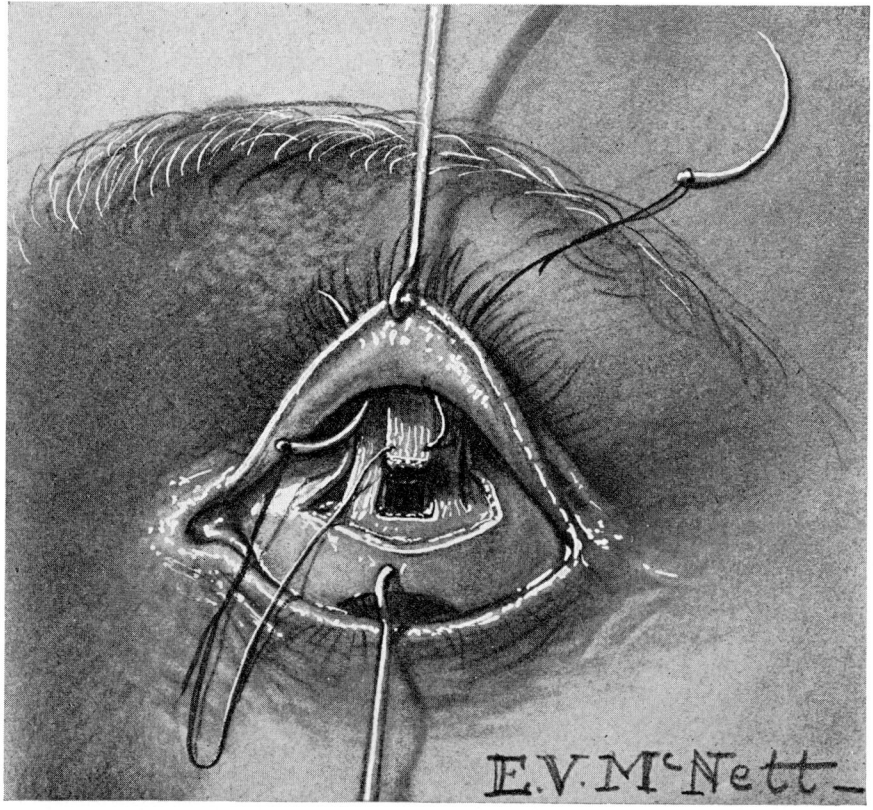

Fig. 238. Utilization of action of musculus rectus superior in ptosis operation (Motais). (See text.)

496

upper lid above the lashes (Fernandez). Correction of the congenital form of epicanthus can usually be obtained by flap switching, which adds vertical length at the expense of the transverse redundancy (Blair, Brown, and Hamm). In the traumatic type, a Z-operation (p. 185) may be sufficient, or excision of the scar and skin grafting or the use of local flaps may be required.

Technique (Blair-Brown-Hamm) (Fig. 239; Case 73, p. 1087)

The principle is the formation of two upper and two lower triangular flaps, which are interchanged as in a Z-operation. To form the two upper triangular flaps, a horizontal incision about 7 mm. (%32 inch) long is made through the skin nasally, starting from a point 5 mm. (%16 inch) away from the canthus. From the starting point a slightly curved incision is led upward and parallel to the fold of the epicanthus for about 7 mm. (%32 inch). From the termination of this incision another incision is led downward, ending at the margin of the upper lid 4 mm. (%32 inch)

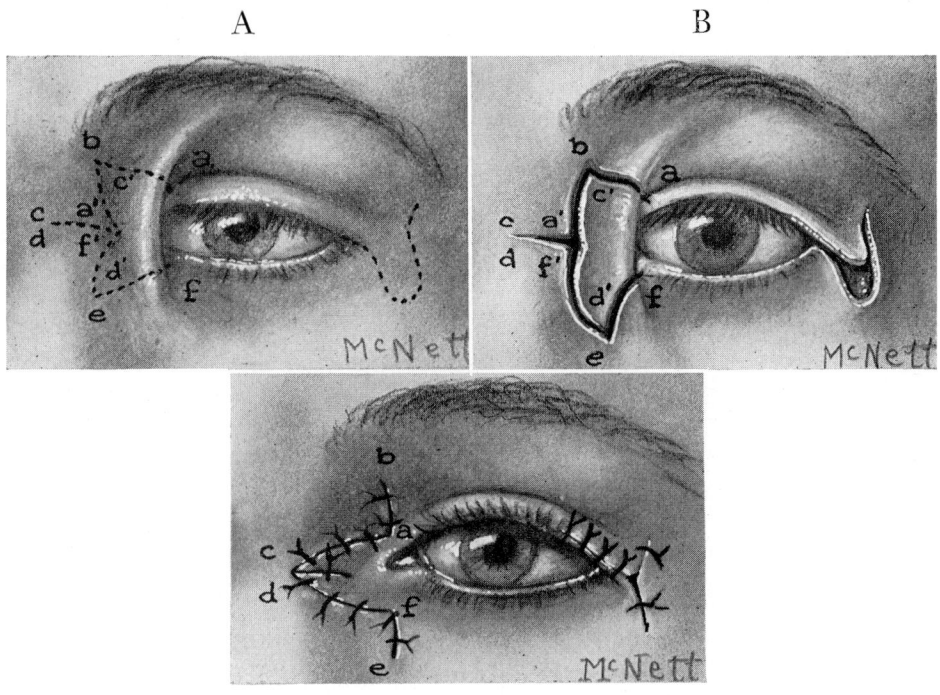

Fig. 239. *A:* Epicanthus operation (Blair, Brown, Hamm). Formation of two upper and two lower triangular flaps. Flap at outer canthus to widen lateral fissure. *B:* Flaps are being mobilized. *C:* Triangular flaps are exchanged. Lateral fissure is widened after elevation of upper lid and flap.

from the canthus. Two similar incisions are made in the lower half. Thus, four triangular flaps are outlined (the lateral two have one side in common), and are now thoroughly mobilized beyond their bases. They are then exchanged; first the two upper, second the two lower ones. They are held in position by sutures.

To widen the lateral fissure, a canthotomy about 3 to 4 mm. ($\frac{1}{8}$ to $\frac{5}{32}$ inch) long is made with scissors, separating skin, muscle, palpebral fascia, and conjunctiva; from here the incision curves downward and temporally for about 5 mm. ($\frac{3}{16}$ inch), then upward and medially, terminating about 7 mm. ($\frac{9}{32}$ inch) lateral to and 5 mm. ($\frac{3}{16}$ inch) above the canthus, separating skin, muscle, fascia, and external palpebral ligament. Thus, a rounded triangular flap is outlined, which is mobilized; the lateral (temporal) side of the wound edge is also mobilized by undermining, while the median wound edge (the continuation of the lower lid) is left intact. The conjunctiva is now undermined with scissors and sutured to the lower lid for about 3 to 4 mm. ($\frac{1}{8}$ to $\frac{5}{32}$ inch). At the upper lid, however, the conjunctiva is further sutured laterally to facilitate raising of the lid. The next step is approximation of the conjunctiva and skin of upper and lower lid to form the new canthus. The closure of the remainder of the wound follows.

Technique (Spaeth)

The anterior fold of the epicanthus is utilized for two horizontal Zs —one above and one below a horizontal line across the fold—with a common tip in the center of the fold and the bases of the triangular flaps of the Zs in the upper and lower parts of the fold. In other words, an X-shaped incision is made on the anterior surface of the fold. The upper of the two triangles is mobilized and moved into the upper lid, the lower of the two into the lower lid. To facilitate a smooth fitting of the flaps, additional incisions are made into the upper and lower lid across the edge of the epicanthal fold for a distance equal to the length of the triangular flaps, and the skin of upper and lower lid is undermined.

REDUNDANT SKIN AND POUCHES OF EYELID

Redundant skin may merely cause excessive lid wrinkles and be disturbing cosmetically, but the condition may be so marked that pouches are formed. These pouches are mainly due to herniation of intraorbital fat. Hence there are two conditions, and they are not synonymous. In the case of simple redundancy, only the skin of the lids is involved. With pouches, however, the intraorbital fat has herniated, causing the skin redundancy. This distinction has much bearing on therapy. In simple redundancy, excision of skin alone is enough; in herniation of fat, the fat pouches must be removed primarily. The subject has been extensively covered by Castanares, Reidy, Gonzalez-Ulloa, and others.

Technique

Upper Lid: The operation is carried out under local anesthesia, of which as little as possible is used, or, even better, under general anesthesia which does not distort the contours. The operation begins by marking the line which is to become the suture line. It should come to lie within

A   B

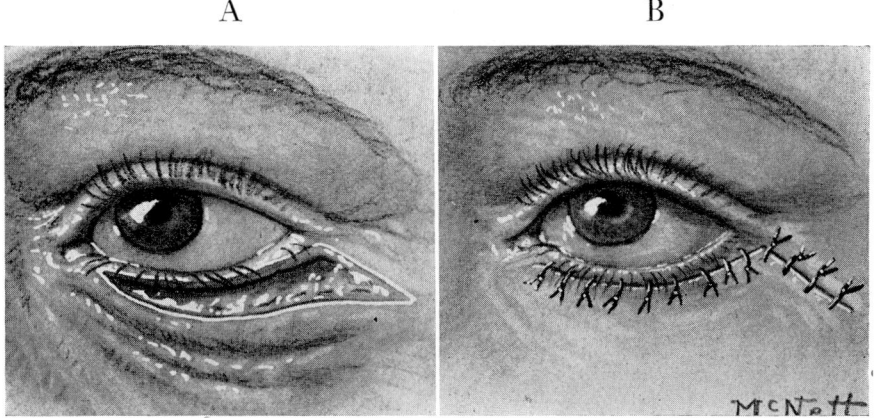

Fig. 240. *A:* Correction of redundant skin of lower lid. Removal of elliptical piece of skin. Upper incision runs close to lid margin. Lower incision diverges laterally, where triangular piece of skin is removed to avoid puckering. *B:* Wound edges sutured together.

an upper natural fold; a corresponding line should be drawn upon the upper lid of the other eye. With three or four Allis forceps which grasp the redundant skin fold superficially along the marked-out line, the redundant skin is lifted up as much as necessary to overcome the redundancy. The redundant skin is excised with a fine curved pair of eye scissors, and the wound edges are sutured with interrupted sutures of 000000 nylon sutures on an atraumatic eye needle.

Lower Lid: The upper incision is marked out with ink. It runs 2 to 3 mm. below and parallel with the rim of the eyelid. It continues laterally to the lateral canthus, diverging slightly downward within one of the crow-feet wrinkles. Three traction sutures are now laid through the eyelid margin and are clamped with hemostats; a moist 2 × 2 inch compress is laid upon the upper lid and the traction sutures, weighted by the hemostats, are laid upon it. An incision is then made along the marked-out line. The lower wound edge is grasped by mosquito hemostats and is dissected away from the underlying orbicularis muscle. If pouches are present from herniating fat tissue, they can be removed at the same sitting. The fat bags are, as a rule, divided in three parts. The median is removed from a nick in the median part of the orbicularis muscle; it bulges upon gentle digital pressure on the eyeball. The capsule is nicked with scissors, permitting the fat to protrude readily through the opening. The bulging fat is grasped with a hemostat, and under slight pull it is removed. The median and lateral fat bags are removed in a similar way from an incision in the middle part of the orbicularis muscles. Thorough hemostasis is imperative. It is not necessary to suture the ruptured fascia. The divided muscle fibers, however, should be closed with fine catgut sutures. The knots of the interrupted sutures should come to lie inside. The traction sutures are removed from the eyelid rim so that the rim is permitted to fall back into normal position. The redundant skin is now stretched, but only as much as the weight of the hemostats permit. The line of excision is marked out in projection of the lower eyelid rim. To prevent removal of too much skin, Rees advises having an assistant depress the eyeball slightly with his finger by pressing upon the upper lid in an open position. This maneuver elevates the tarsus and the lid margin of the lower eyelid to a safe position, from which one can safely assess the amount of skin to be excised. It is excised with a pair of straight-eye scissors. This still leaves a triangle of redundant skin lateral to the lateral canthus, which is then excised so that a triangular-shaped wound is created within the crow-feet wrinkles, as depicted in Figure 240. The first suture is laid through the angle lateral to the lateral canthus, followed by closure of the remainder of the wound edges with interrupted 000000 nylon sutures on an atraumatic eye needle.

If there is no redundancy of skin, and the pouches are near the base of the eyelids, they should be approached from small separate incisions which are laid so that the scars will come to lie along the lid wrinkles (Castanares). If there is much redundancy of skin, the latter is removed from an incision along a median lower lid wrinkle (Case 72, p. 1086).

After-Treatment

One hundred and fifty units of hyaluronidase are injected along the base of the eyelids to minimize postoperative swelling. A dressing is not necessary. Application of ice compresses to counteract ecchymosis may be necessary. The sutures are removed on the fourth postoperative day. If they are left too long in the eyelids they may cause thick suture marks. Converse points out that the epithelium tends to grow down the tracts around the sutures in the eyelids; when these tracts are epithelized, they collect sebaceous material and give the appearance of small cysts. Should this happen, Converse advises unroofing the suture tracts with a small pair of eye scissors.

500

OCULAR HYPERTELORISM

Hypertelorism may be defined as an abnormal spacing of the orbits with an increase in the interorbital distance. The size of the orbits is usually within the norm (Converse et al.). There are cases of apparent or pseudohypertelorism accompanying bifid nose deformities which will improve after the nose is narrowed. However, real hypertelorism is difficult to correct. The reader is referred to page 435.

BIBLIOGRAPHY

AXENFELD, K. T.: *Handbuch der aerztlichen Erfahrungen im Weltkriege*, 1914-1918. J. B. Barth, Leipzig, 1922.
Lehrbuch und Atlas der Augenheilkunde. Gustav Fischer, Jena, 1920.

BLAIR, V. P., BROWN, J. B., and HAMM, W. G.: *Correction of ptosis and of epicanthus.* Arch. Ophthal., 7:831, 1932.

BLASKOVICS, L.: Eingriffe am Auge. F. Enke, Stuttgart, 1938.

BOECK, J.: *Plastic replacement of the lower eyelid* (Uber den plastischen Ersatz des Unterlides) Wien. Med. Wschr., 99:375, 1949.

BROWN, J. B., and CANNON, B.: *Full thickness skin grafts from the neck for function and color in eyelid and face repair.* Ann. Surg., 121:639, 1945.

CALLAHAN, A.: *Free composite lid graft.* Arch. Ophthal., 45:539, 1951.
Surgery of the Eye: Injuries. Charles C Thomas, Springfield, 1950.
Reconstructive Surgery of the Eyelids and Ocular Adnexa. Aesculapius Publishing Co., Birmingham, 1966.

CASTANARES, S.: *Blepharoplasty for herniated intraorbital fat.* Plast. Reconstr. Surg., 8:46, 1951.

CASTROVIEJO, R.: *Total penetrating keratoplasty.* Amer. J. Ophthal. 34:1796, 1951.

CONVERSE, J. M.: *Clinical note: Treatment of epithelized suture tracts of the eyelid by marsupialization.* Plast. Reconstr. Surg., 38:576, 1966.

CONVERSE, J. M., and SMITH, B.: *Reconstruction of the floor of the orbit by bone grafts.* Arch. Ophthal., 44:1, 1950.
Repair of severe burn ectropion of the eyelids. Plast. Reconstr. Surg., 23:21, 1959.

CRAWFORD, J. S.: *Repair of ptosis using frontalis muscle and fascia lata.* Trans. Amer. Acad. Ophthal., 60:672, 1956.

DASILVA, G.: *Reconstruction after orbital exenteration.* Brit. J. Plast. Surg., 14:76, 1961.

DUPUY-DUTEMPS, L.: *Autoplastie palpébro-palpébrale intégrale.* Ann. d'ocul., 164:915, 1927.

DUVERGER: *Procédé permettant la refléction exacte du bord libre des paupières.* Arch. d'opht., 35:677, 1916.

THE HEAD AND NECK

ELLIOTT, R. A.: *Correction of senile entropion with fascialata graft.* Plast. Reconstr. Surg., 29:698, 1962.

ELSCHNIG, A.: *Die operative Behandlung der Ptosis.* Med. Klin., 1910, Vol. 20. *Augenärztliche Operationslehre.* J. Springer, Berlin, 1922. *Ptosis Operationen.* In AXENFELD, T., and ELSCHNIG, A.: *Handbuch der gesamten Augenheilkunde.* J. Springer, Berlin, 1922.

EVERBUSCH, O.: *Zur Operation der kongenitalen Blepharoptosis.* Klin. Monatsbl. f. Augenh., 21:100, 1883.

FERNANDEZ, L. R.: *Double eyelid operation in the oriental in Hawaii.* Plast. Reconstr. Surg., 25:257, 1960.

FOX, S. A.: *Ophthalmic Plastic Surgery.* Grune and Stratton, New York, 1958. *Surgery of Ptosis.* Grune and Stratton, New York, 1968.

FRICKE, J. C. G.: *Die Bildung neuer Augenlider (Blepharoplastic) nach Zerstörung und dadurch hervorgebrachten Auswärtswendung derselben.* Hamburg, 1829.

GAISFORD, J. C., and HANNA, D. C.: *Orbital exenteration.* Plast. Reconstr. Surg., 31:363, 1963.

GARCIA, F. A., and BLANDFORD, S. E.: *The use of the three-tailed fascial sling with pull-out wires to correct blepharoptosis.* Plast. Reconstr. Surg., 23:596, 1959.

GIFFORD, S. R.: *The Mashek operation for ptosis.* Arch. Ophthal., 8:495, 1932.

GILLIES, H. D., and KILNER, T. P.: *Symblepharon: Its treatment by Thiersch (contracted socket) and mucous membrane grafting.* Trans. Ophthal. Soc. UK, 49:470, 1929.

GONZALEZ-ULLOA, M.: *Correction of cicatricial ectropion.* Plast. Reconstr. Surg., 5:310, 1950.

GONZALEZ-ULLOA, M., and STEVENS, E.: *The treatment of palpebral bags.* Plast. Reconstr. Surg., 27:381, 1961.

GRUNERT, K.: *Ektropiumoperationen und Blepharoplastik.* In AXENFELD, T., and ELSCHNIG, A.: *Handbuch der gesamten Augenheilkunde.* J. Springer, Berlin, 1922.

HAGERTY, R. F., and SMOAK, R. D.: *Reconstruction of the lower eyelid.* Plast. Reconstr. Surg., 38:52, 1966.

HENDRIX, J. H.: *Orbicularis muscle strip for correction of ptosis of the eyelid.* Plast. Reconstr. Surg. 15:241, 1955.

HUESTON, G. T.: *Abbé flap technique in upper eyelid repair.* Brit. J. Plast. Surg., 13:347, 1961.

HUGHES, W. L.: *A new method for rebuilding a lower lid.* Arch. Ophthal., 17:1008, 1937.

IMRÉ, J.: *Lidplastik und plastische Operationen anderer Weichteile des Gesichts.* Studium Verlag, Budapest, 1928.

KATZ, D.: *Plastic surgery of the eyelids with special reference to the Hungarian school.* Arch. Ophthal., 12:220, 1934.

KAZANJIAN, V. H., and ROOPENIAN, A.: *The repair of full-thickness eyelid defects with special reference to malignant lesions.* Plast. Reconstr. Surg., 24:262, 1959.

KIRSCHNER, M.: *Die Praktischen Ergebnisse der freien Fascientransplantation.* Langenbeck's Arch., 92:888, 1910.

KUHNT, H.: *Plastische Operationen an Lidern und Bindehaut bei Kriegsverletzten.* In: Handbuch der aerztlichen Erfahrungen im Weltkriege, 1914-1918. J. B. Barth, Leipzig, 1922. *Beiträge zur operativen Augenheilkunde.* Jena, 1883.

LANDOLT, M.: *Nouveau Procédé de Blepharoplastic.* Arch. d'opht., 1881, p. 9.

LEXER, E.: *Wimpernersatz durch freie Transplantation behaarter Haut.* Klin. Monatsbl. f. Augenh., 62:486, 1919.
Ptosis operation, Herstellung der Oberlidfalte und Herstellung des Unterlides durch Faszienzügel. Klin. Monatsbl. f. Augenh., 70:464, 1923.

LONGACRE, J. J., DeSTEFANO, G. A., and HOLMSTRAND, K.: *Reconstruction of eyebrow: graft versus flap.* Plast. Reconstr. Surg., 30:638, 1962.

MACOMBER, W. B., WANT, M. K., and GOTTLIEB, E.: *Epithelial tumors of the eyelids.* Surg. Gynec. Obstet., 98:331, 1954.

MANCHESTER, W. M.: *A simple method for the repair of full thickness defects of the lower lid with special reference to the treatment of neoplasms.* Brit. J. Plast. Surg., 3:252, 1951.

MAY, H.: *Closure of defects after cancer surgery.* Clinics, 4:53, 1945.

McCOY, F. J., and CROW, M. L.: *Adaptation of the "switch flap" to eyelid reconstruction.* Plast. Reconstr. Surg., 35:633, 1965.

McLAUGHLIN, C. R.: *Surgical support in permanent facial paralysis.* Plast. Reconstr. Surg., 11:302, 1953.

MELLER, J.: *Augenaerztliche Eingriffe.* Vienna, 1919.
Ophthalmic Surgery. P. Blakiston's Son & Co., Philadelphia, 1923.

MINSKY, H.: *Surgical repair of recent lid lacerations.* Surg. Gynec. Obstet., 75:449, 1942.

MOTAIS, E.: *Etat actuel de la méthod opératoire du ptosis par la suppléance du muscle drost supérieur.* Bull. Acad. de Méd., 49:430, 1903.

MUSTARDÉ, J. C.: *Repair and Reconstruction in the Orbital Region, A Practical Guide.* Williams and Wilkins, Baltimore, 1966.
Reconstruction of the upper lid and the use of nasal mucosal grafts. Brit. J. Plast. Surg., 21:367, 1968.
The treatment of ptosis and epicanthal folds. Brit. J. Plast. Surg., 12:252, 1959.

MUTOU, Y., and BOO-CHAI, K.: *Transplantation of hair for eyelash replacement.* Plast. Reconstr. Surg., 29:573, 1962.

PAGENSTECHER, H.: *Eine neue Operation zur Heilung der Ptosis.* Internat. Kongr., London, 1881.

PIRRUCCELLO, F. W.: *Observations in the management of soft tissue injuries of the face: the reconstruction of eyebrows.* Plast. Reconstr. Surg., 25:584, 1960.

REES, T. D.: *Technical aid in blepharoplasty.* Plast. Reconstr. Surg., 41:497, 1968.

REESE, A. B., and JONES, I. S.: *Exenteration of the orbit and repair by transplantation of the temporalis muscle.* Amer. J. Ophthal., 51:217, 1961.

REIDY, J. P.: *Swellings of eyelids.* Brit. J. Plast. Surg., 13:1960 .

THE HEAD AND NECK

RYCROFT, B. W.: *Corneal Grafts.* C. V. Mosby Co., St. Louis, 1955.

SAWAR, M.: *A new operation for congenital and paralytic ptosis.* Brit. J. Plast. Surg., 4:293, 1952.

SCHOFIELD, A. L.: *A review of burns of the eyelids and their treatment.* Brit. J. Plast. Surg., 7:67, 1954.

SHEEHAN, J. E.: *Plastic Surgery of the Orbit.* The Macmillan Co., New York, 1927.

SHERMAN, A. E.: *Reconstruction of the upper eyelid.* Plast. Reconstr. Surg., 20:323, 1957.

SMITH, B.: *Eyelid Surgery.* Surg. Clin. N. Amer., 39:367, 1959.

SNELLEN (Quoted by VAN GILS): Klin. Monatsbl. f. Augenh., 10:33, 1872.

SNYDER, C. C.: *Eyelid ptosis.* Plast. Reconstr. Surg., 27:586, 1961.

SPAETH, E. B.: *The use of mucous membrane in ophthalmic surgery.* Amer. J. Ophthal., 20:897, 1937.
A review of some modern methods for ophthalmic plastic surgery. Amer. J. Surg., 42:89, 1938.
Principles and Practice of Ophthalmic Surgery. Lea & Febiger, Philadelphia, 1944, 1949.
Congenital blepharoptosis: A clarification. The principles of surgical correction. Trans. Amer. Acad. Ophthal., 1943.

STARK, D. B., BORN, G., and HACKLEMAN, G. L.: *Reconstruction of the complete upper eyelid defect.* Plast. Reconstr. Surg., 35:629, 1965.

STREATFIELD (Quoted by VAN GILS): Klin. Monatsbl. f. Augenh., 10:33, 1872.

TÖRÖK, E., and GROUT, G. H.: *Surgery of the Eye: a Handbook for Students and Practitioners.* Lea & Febiger, Philadelphia, 1913.

TUBIANA, R.: *Traitment chirurgical des cancers cutanés de la région oculaire.* Bull. Soc. Franc. Ophtal., 73:299, 1960.

VAN GILS: *Beiträge zur Behandlung gewisser Krankheiten der Augenlider.* Klin. Monatsbl. f. Augenh., 10:33, 1872.

WALSER, E.: *Plastische Chirurgie am Auge.* Lange und Springer, Berlin-Wilmersdorf, 1958.

WHEELER, J. M.: *Correction of cicatricial ectropion by use of true skin of the upper lid.* JAMA, 77:1628, 1921.
The use of the epidermic graft in plastic eye surgery. Int. Clin., 3:292, 1922.
Plastic operations about the eye. Proc. Int. Congr. Ophthal., 1922, pp. 443, 460.

WIENER, M.: *Surgical correction of defects due to paralysis of the muscles of the eyes and Lids.* Surg. Gynec. Obstet., 58:390, 1934.
Surgery of the Eye. Grune and Stratton, New York, 2nd ed., 1949.

WIENER, M., and ALVIS, B. Y.: *Surgery of the Eye.* W. B. Saunders, Philadelphia, 1939.

WIENER, M., and SCHEIE, H. G.: *Surgery of the Eye.* Grune and Stratton, 3rd rev. ed., New York, 1952.

ZIEGLER, S. L.: *Galvanocautery puncture in ectropion and entropion.* JAMA, 53:183, 1909.

THE EXTERNAL
AUDITORY 11
STRUCTURES

Lesions of the auricle may be congenital or acquired. For congenital lesions or lesions acquired in childhood, reconstruction should preferably be undertaken after the patient has matured. For psychological reasons, however, it may become necessary to operate earlier.

ANATOMY

The auricle, or pinna, is a skin duplication with a cartilaginous plate as a framework (Fig. 241). The skin is firmly adherent to the anterior surface of the cartilage but movable on the posterior side. The auricle is funnel shaped, and leads into the external auditory canal. The posterior and upper rim of the auricle, the helix, bends acutely forward. The anterior portion of the helix assumes a backward curve, called the crus helicis, which passes over into the concha. In front of the helix, almost parallel to it, is another rim, the anthelix. It commences in the upper part of the auricle with two converging limbs, the crura anthelicis, and in the lower part passes over into the antitragus. Between the latter and the tragus is the incisura intertragica. The tragus is a small cartilaginous plate which, like a valve, overhangs the external auditory canal. The deep fossa between tragus and anthelix is the concha.

505

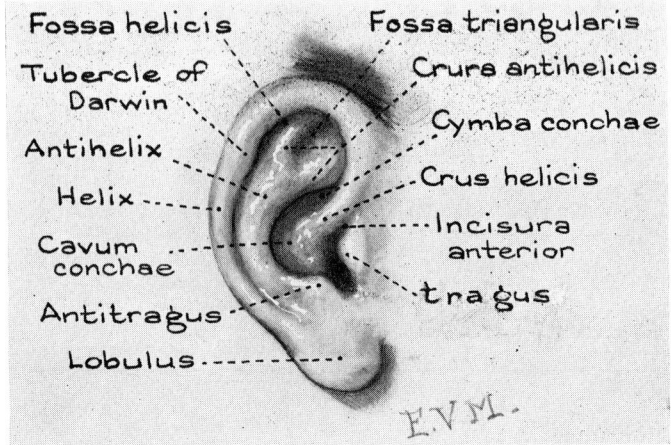

Fig. 241. Anatomy of auricle.

DEFECTS

Defects of the external ear may be partial or complete. Small defects can, as a rule, be closed by the use of local flaps. Large defects or absence of the entire auricle can also be corrected by local flaps in most cases but require more complicated procedures, making the reconstruction one of the most difficult tasks in reparative surgery.

HOLES IN CONCHA

Technique (*Small Hole*) (Case 74, p. 1088)

A double-pedicle flap is formed in the retroauricular region posterior to the hole in direct continuation of the defect. The site of the lateral pedicle is the skin of the posterior rim of the hole; that of the median pedicle is the mastoid region. The flap should be made one third wider than the defect. This bridge flap, remaining attached at the lateral and median pedicles, is undermined and returned to its original site. In the same sitting, a small rim of the skin surrounding the edge of the defect is mobilized from the underlying cartilage and returned to its original site. The reason for mobilization of this rim of skin is twofold: (1) to prepare hinge flaps of skin which later are turned inward and forward, forming the anterior covering of the hole; (2) to create, by exposing the cartilages, a firmer base on which the peripheral end of the bridge flap can rest more firmly than if sutured to the rim of the hole.

506

The lateral pedicle of the flap near the hole is severed after two weeks and sutured.

After two more weeks, the entire flap is mobilized; the rim of skin surrounding the defect is again mobilized and turned inward and forward; the flap is now sutured into the defect. Since the flap cannot be moved forward to reach the outer edge of the defect, the ear is tilted backward. After the flap is sutured in place, the ear is kept approximated to the skull with adhesive strips.

If after three weeks the ear is still tilted backward, the central pedicle of the flap in the mastoid region is severed. The median half of the flap is mobilized; the ear is moved to normal position; the flap is sutured to its new base; and the secondary defect resulting from moving the flap forward is skin grafted.

Technique (Large Holes) (Fig. 242)

Large holes are closed with a lined flap from the hairless mastoid region. A suitable flap, one third wider than the defect, is outlined as demonstrated in Figure 242, *A*. The posterior edge at the base is curved backward to facilitate later rotation. The peripheral half of the flap is mobilized, and returned and sutured to its original site.

After two weeks the entire flap is mobilized, and that part of the flap which is to cover the defect is lined with a skin graft. The flap is returned to its original site. After two more weeks the flap is again mobilized; a rim of skin surrounding the defect is removed from the underlying cartilage, and the flap is rotated into the defect and sutured in place. The peripheral part of the flap bed is covered with a full-thickness graft.

After three weeks, the pedicle of the flap is severed and returned to its original base; the flap itself is adjusted in place.

PARTIAL PERIPHERAL DEFECTS OF THE AURICLE

Except in burn cases where the mastoid skin is cicatricial, partial defects of the ear can be repaired by means of flaps from the mastoid area. In small defects, skin alone needs to be replaced; in large defects, cartilage grafts must be incorporated in the flap.

Technique (Small Defects of Helix and Anthelix not Requiring Cartilage Grafts) (Case 75, p. 1089)

The ear is pressed against the mastoid area and a flap somewhat larger and longer than the defect is outlined. The flap, pedicled posteriorly, is raised; the flap bed and undersurface of the flap are skin grafted, and the flap is sutured to the defect edges of the ear. A light pressure dressing is applied. There is a cutaneous tunnel behind the auricle which later must be cleaned with cotton-tipped applicators (Case 75, *B*). After three weeks, the pedicle of the flap lying some distance posterior to the rim of the ear is gradually severed; after separation is completed, the pedicle is turned backward and sutured posteriorly.

A   B

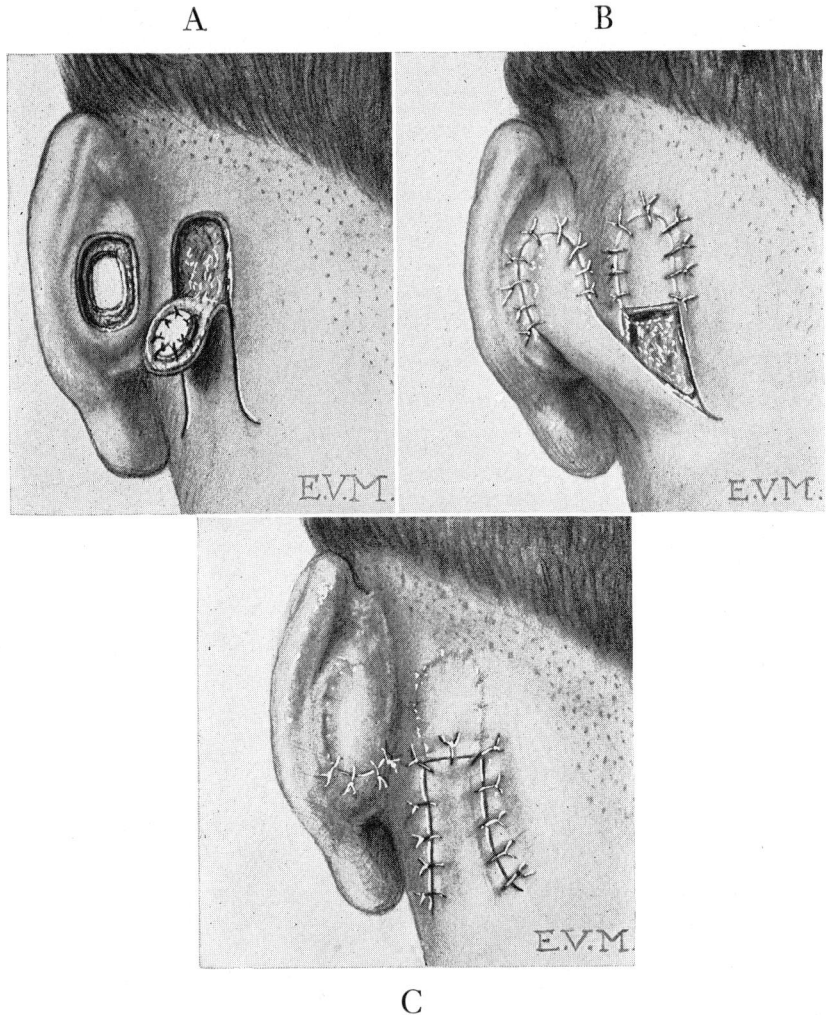

C

Fig. 242. *A:* Closure of hole in concha. Single-pedicle flap is raised in stages from hairless mastoid region. Its peripheral end is lined with skin graft and flap returned to its original site. *B:* Flap is raised again, rotated, and sutured into defect. Peripheral end of flap bed is skin grafted. *C:* After severance of pedicle and adjustment of pedicle and flap.

THE EXTERNAL AUDITORY STRUCTURES

Technique (*Absence of Entire Helix*) (Case 77, p. 1091)

If the entire helix is absent, usually owing to burns, it is replaced with a tube flap either from the cervical region or from the median side of the arm of the same side. The latter has the disadvantage of a slight color difference but can be made much thinner than the cervical-tube flap. The flap should be made $1\frac{1}{8}$ inch wide and constructed according to the technique described on page 87. If the cervical region is chosen, the base of the flap is in the mastoid area. It is made long enough to be carried over the ear. Its inferior pedicle is gradually severed after four weeks and transferred and sutured just above the tragus. Three weeks later the base of the flap over the mastoid process is gradually severed, the seam of the flap is opened, and the flap is draped around the auricle in such a way as to complete formation of the helix. In tube flaps from the arm, the upper pedicle is transferred and sutured just above the tragus. The arm is fastened to the head as described on page 80. After three weeks, the lower pedicle is gradually severed, and the flap is adjusted as described above.

Technique (*Ear Reconstruction After Burns*) (Case 77, p. 1091)

In addition to loss of the helix there may be adhesions between concha and mastoid region, causing a backward tilt of the auricle. This deformity must be overcome—by excision of the scar tissue, reduction of the contracture, and application of a skin graft as described on page 39—before a tube flap for replacement of the helix can be transferred as described above. In other cases there may be microtia from extensive loss of the auricle. Lueders describes some helpful ways of enlarging the ear by means of a composite helix cartilage flap which is pedicled on the postauricular skin; the anterior defect is covered with a full-thickness skin graft. A tube flap may be needed for replacement of the helix. In large defects (Case 22, p. 1021) the methods described on pages 510 or 521 must be employed.

LARGE DEFECTS OF EAR

The most satisfactory flap for replacement of the anterior skin is the mastoid flap, even if parts of the flap need depilation. In these large defects, the cartilaginous framework must also be replaced with autogenous rib cartilage grafts. As a rule, these grafts can be buried beneath the flap at the time the flap is raised and sutured to the defect edges. However, if depilation is needed, it is carried out first (p. 515) and the cartilage graft is buried three to four weeks later (Cases 76, 78, pp. 1090, 1092). I follow Converse's technique of reconstruction, which is simple and satisfactory.

*Technique (Large Defect of the Center and Upper Section
of the Auricle) (Case 76, 78, pp. 1090, 1092)*

The upper and lower defect edges are split by an incision (Fig.
243) into three layers: the posterior skin layer, the edge of the cartilage,
and the anterior skin layer. To start with the upper edge, the latter is
pressed against the mastoid area and an ink line is drawn on the mastoid
skin, the line being parallel and adjacent to the edge of the auricular defect.
An incision is now made through the skin along this line and both incisions
are connected with each other (Fig. 243, *D*). The same procedure is carried
out at the lower part of the defect. The mastoid skin is undermined between the two incisions (Fig. 243, *E*). In the upper part, the posterior auricular wound edge is sutured to the upper wound edge of the mastoid incision, and in the lower part, the posterior auricular wound edge is sutured to
the lower part of the mastoid incision (Fig. 243, *F*). A carved costal cartilage graft (Fig. 243, *A*, p. 62) is placed under the skin and anchored with
catgut sutures to the upper and lower auricular cartilage edges (Fig. 243,
G). Suture of the anterior wound edges follows (Fig. 243, *H*).

After two to three months, a curved incision is made at a distance
from the posterior edge of the cartilage graft. The entire composite flap is
raised. To avoid tearing the skin from the underlying cartilage graft while
raising the flap, it is well to place traction sutures through skin edges and
cartilage graft after the skin incisions are made. Further, in raising the flap
care must be taken not to expose the posterior surface of the graft but to
leave a sufficient amount of soft tissue upon it. A split skin graft with its
raw surface out is wrapped around a mold of dental compound and placed
upon the raw surfaces as described on page 39. The mold remains in place
for two weeks.

Variations of the technique may be necessary (Case 78, p. 1092). If
on the median (conchal) side of the defect there is an undesirable scar
needing excision and repair, this can be done at the same time the upper
and lower defect edges are anastomosed with the mastoid skin; however,
undermining the skin and transplanting the cartilage graft should be postponed for four weeks for obvious reasons. Transplantation of the cartilage graft should also be postponed if part of the mastoid skin must be
depilated (see Cases 76, 78, pp. 1090, 1092).

TOTAL AND SUBTOTAL RECONSTRUCTION
OF THE AURICLE

Total and subtotal reconstruction of an auricle remains one of the
most difficult tasks in reparative surgery. While formerly reconstruction

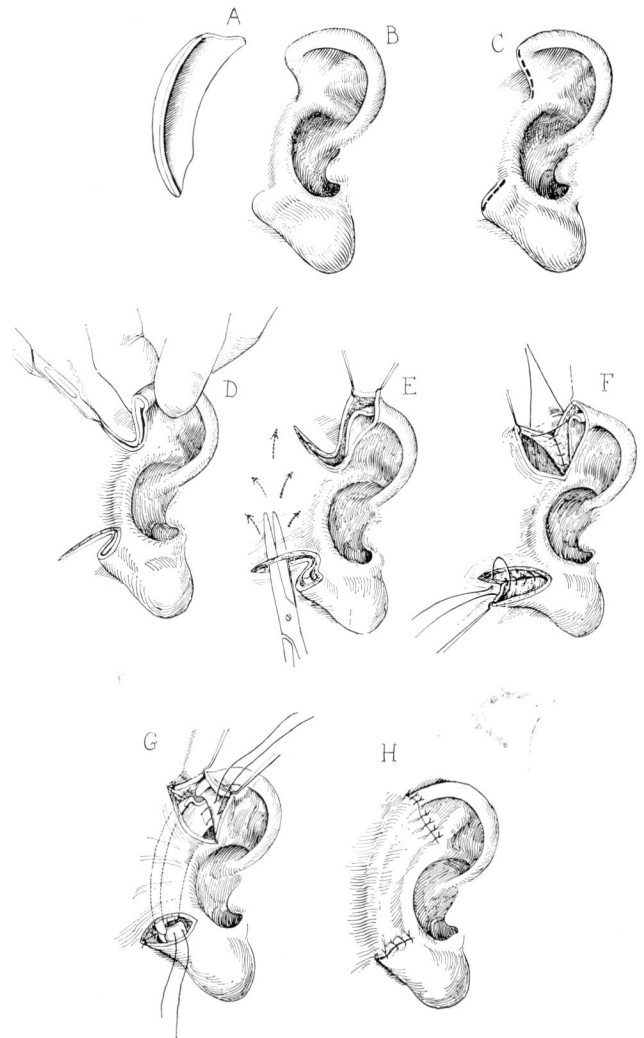

Fig. 243. Repair of a partial defect of the auricle. *A:* Diagram of carved costal cartilage graft. *B:* Diagram of the defect of the auricle. *C:* Outline of incisions through the margins of the defect. *D:* The incisions through the edge of the auricular defect are prolonged backward through the skin of the mastoid area. *E:* The skin of the mastoid area is undermined between the two incisions. *F:* The posterior edge of the incision at the border of the auricular defect is sutured to the upper edge of the postauricular incision. A similar type of suture is done at the lower edge of the defect. *G:* The cartilage graft is placed under the skin of the mastoid area anchored to the auricular cartilage by means of catgut sutures. *H:* Suture of the skin incisions. (J. M. Converse: Plast. Reconstr. Surg.)

resulted at best in a crude resemblance of a normal ear, recent refinements have improved greatly the overall appearance of the newly reconstructed ear. Among others (to name a few: Pierce, Gillies, Greeley, Padgett, Kirkham, Peer, Stephenson, Berson, Aufricht, Macomber and Cronin), we are indebted to the monumental work of Tanzer and Converse for perfecting the technique of ear reconstruction to such a degree that the difficult task is now crowned by much more gratifying results. As a rule, total reconstruction of the external ear is performed in congenital absence of the auricle, while subtotal reconstruction is usually required in traumatic cases or where ears have had to be resected for removal of pathological lesions. The principle of the method consists of raising a composite mastoid flap containing autogenous cartilage grafts. Cronin uses a silastic prosthesis instead of cartilage and reports good results.

In congenital absence of the ear, only the lobule or part of it and some rudimentary cartilages representing vaguely the anterior portion of the helix, the crus helicis or the tragus are present. As a rule, the external auditory canal is absent. Since the external and middle ear develop from the first and second branchial arch, absence of the auricle may be accompanied by other facial deformities and underdevelopments, such as of the mandible (see p. 276). The inner ear, however, is derived from the ectodermal plate near the hindbrain; hence it is almost never affected. The question therefore arises as to whether an attempt should be made to overcome the atresia of the external auditory canal to improve hearing. It is the consensus of opinion that this should not be done, since most children with a unilateral absence of the external auditory canal hear sufficiently well by bony conduction. Further, even under best conditions, the improvement in hearing after reconstruction of the canal is slight (Greeley, Bellucci, Converse, Tanzer), and inevitable scarring of the skin would hamper subsequent reconstruction of the auricle.

Another question arises as to when to start reconstruction in children. Since autogenous cartilage grafts are the only reliable material to be used for replacement of the missing framework, and cartilage grafts in the growing age grow slowly (Dupertuis, Peer), reconstruction should not be started too early. The author recommends starting no earlier than the age of seven, and also making the reconstructed ear somewhat larger than the normal one. The reconstruction consists of the following steps:

1. Making outline pattern of the unaffected ear.

2. Rearranging the cartilaginous rudiments into proper location and, if necessary, depilating the upper posterior part of the mastoid flap if it comes to lie within the hairy region of the scalp.

3. Transplanting autogenous rib cartilage grafts beneath a flap pedicled in front and in the mastoid region.

512

4. Raising composite mastoid flap and skin grafting the postauricular raw surfaces.

5. Reconstructing tragus, semblance of an external auditory canal, crus helicis; "retouching" procedures if necessary.

The author follows in general the principles of the technique of Converse and of Tanzer.

Technique (Figs. 244-247, Cases 79, 80, pp. 1093, 1094)

Step 1: A pattern is made over the normal ear either by tracing its outlines on transparent Pliofilm or by marking the contours of the ear with an aniline dye and pressing a piece of linen upon it before the dye has dried. The pattern is cut accordingly, reversed, and laid in the proper position upon the mastoid area of the other side. The auricle normally occupies a position below a horizontal line drawn from the upper border of the eyebrow and behind a vertical line extending upward from the angle of the mandible with the patient's teeth occluded. On the defective side this mandible, as already mentioned, may be underdeveloped, and hence the mandibular angle may be displaced. The upper line, however, can be drawn by comparison with the unaffected ear on full-face examination. Proper location of the vertical line may be facilitated if a rudimentary ear lobule is present and can be utilized. The line should then be drawn just in front of its lowest insertion point. Another guideline is the long axis of the ear, a line from the highest point of the helix to the anterior border of the lobule. This line normally runs parallel to the ridge of the nose. After the pattern has been properly positioned it is outlined on the skin, first with one of the dyes and then by scratching the skin with a scalpel.

Step 2: Before the repositioning of rudimentary ear cartilages is done, the sterilized pattern is reversed and laid in the proper position. The outline of the new ear is traced upon the skin. It is good to scratch the outlines deep enough to make the markings permanent. In most cases, enough rudimentary auricular tissue is present to provide an earlobe and anterior inferior portion of the helix; these rudiments usually are in a forward position and form an irregular vertical mass (Fig. 244, *A;* Case 79, p. 1093). They are divided into two thirds from the lower and one third from the upper portion (Fig. 244, *A*). The lower portion is to become the earlobe. To relocate it in the proper position, it has to be rotated backward and downward about 90 degrees on an inferior pedicle. It is detached and rotated into the proper position as demonstrated in Figure 244, *B.* The triangular mastoid flap is undermined. The posterior edge of the lobe flap is sutured to the inferior wound edge with 00000 chromic catgut sutures. The mobilized triangular mastoid flap is moved forward to close

513

Fig. 244. *A:* Congenital absence of ear (see Case 80, p. 1094). Lines for repositioning of ear rudimentary cartilages are lined out, corresponding roughly to a double Z. Lower two thirds consisting of ear lobule to be rotated backward and downward, upper third to be turned upward.

B: Ear lobule has been raised like a flap with an inferior pedicle and rotated downward and backward; inferior wound edges of incision are sutured to posterior wound edge of earlobe. The upper wound edge of the incision will be sutured to outer wound edge of earlobe. Incisions for rotation of upper segment are outlined. If both procedures are done in one stage a square mastoid flap may be formed which after mobilization can be easily advanced forward for closure of the entire anterior vertical wound.

C: After completion of rotation of rudimentary ear cartilages.

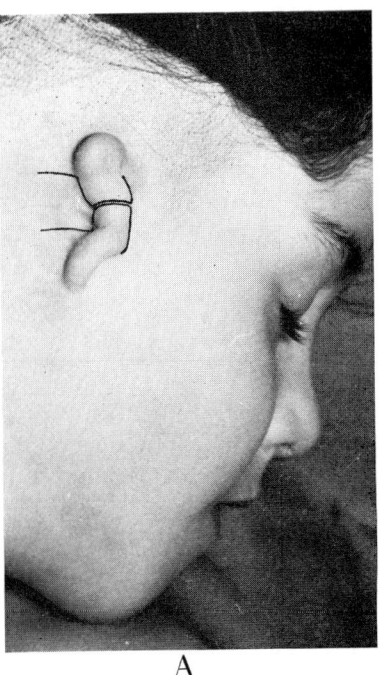

A

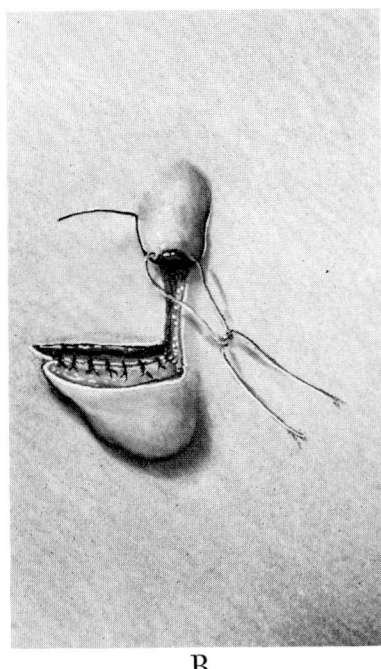

B

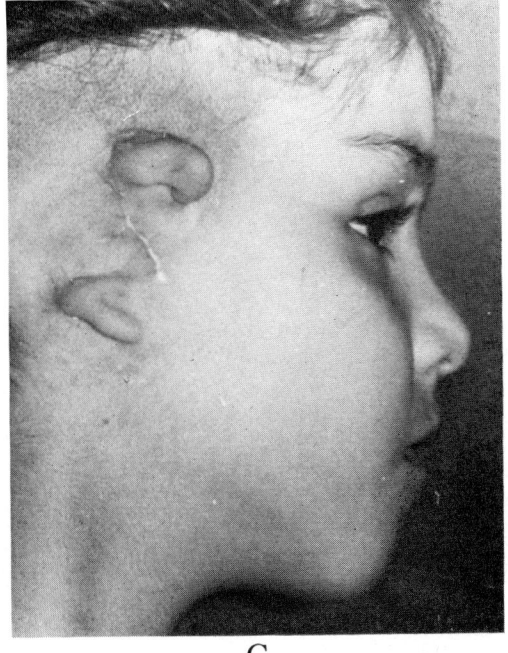

C

514

the anterior wound edge. Finally, the anterior edge of the lobe is sutured to the mastoid flap. This leaves the upper third of the rudiment behind; this is used to form the anterior inferior insertion of the helix including the crus of the helix. It may be in the proper position; otherwise, it must be repositioned upward and forward in a similar way as described above for the earlobe (Fig. 244, C). If both procedures are done a square mastoid flap may be formed which after mobilization can be easily advanced forward for closure of the anterior vertical wound.

Depilation may or may not be necessary, depending upon the position of the hairline. It can be carried out either in the same stage of repositioning the cartilages or somewhat later. If the hairline is low and part of the mastoid flap to be used for reconstruction of the upper part of the helix comes to lie within the scalp, this area must be depilated. This is done in one of two ways. Either the hairbearing part of the skin is removed like a full-thickness skin graft and the raw surface is covered with a full-thickness skin graft from the supraclavicular area (see p. 204), or the involved scalp area is raised as a flap not thicker than full thickness of the skin, but bearing the hair follicles and folded upon itself (similar to, but not as extensive as White et al. recommend). The raw subcutaneous tissue surface is covered with a skin graft as described above. After reconstruction of the ear, the folded scalp flap is unfolded to restore the former hairline.

Step 3: After the graft has healed and all induration has subsided (this may take many weeks), the cartilaginous auricular framework is inserted in two parts: anthelix-concha and helix-fossa. The grafts are taken from the junction of the eighth, ninth, and tenth costal cartilages of the same side of the chest as the ear deformity. In this way, they can be turned inside out to reproduce the outward curvature and inclination of the auricle. The perichondrium of the outer surface then becomes the inner surface and serves as a splint, binding adjacent cartilages together. The costal area is exposed as described on page 63. The pattern, which should have been preserved or is newly made prior to this step, is placed upon the surface of the fused portion of the costal cartilages. It is turned inside out, so that, as already mentioned, the outer surface becomes the inner surface to serve as a binding splint, and a generous amount of full-thickness rib graft is removed. Another full-thickness costal cartilage graft consisting of a single rib is removed, which will be made into an anthelix, and a third generous amount of rib (if still available) is removed to be stored beneath the skin incision for later use. The anthelix is carved first. The second rib cartilage which had been removed is laid upon its base and sliced repeatedly through two thirds of its thickness along its external

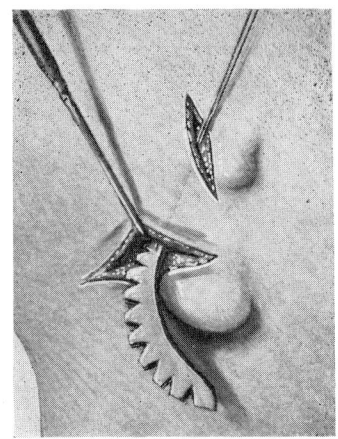

Fig. 245. *A:* Outline of skin incisions for insertion of rib cartilage grafts. Before the latter are inserted the skin is undermined along a superficial level. The anthelix graft is inserted first. It has been sliced through two thirds of its thickness along the external border to permit bending for conforming to the curved shape of the anthelix which outlines the concha.

A

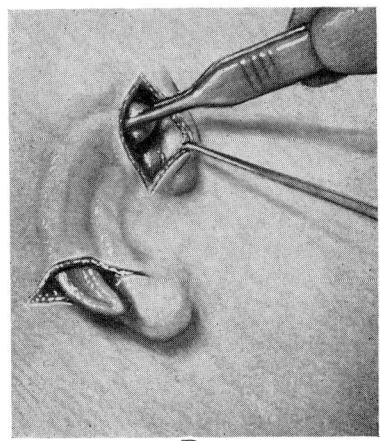

Fig. 245. *B:* Insertion of the helix fossa unit from above to below. The thin (median) part of the section comes to lie beneath the anthelix graft.

B

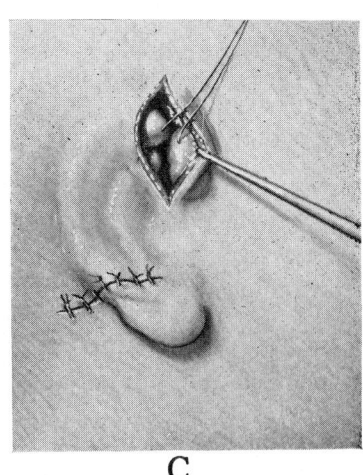

Fig. 245. *C:* Both sections, i.e., helix fossa unit and anthelix graft, are sutured above to the rudimentary cartilage. The lower tip of the helix fossa unit is inserted into the earlobe; the lower end of the anthelix graft is held in forward position with a fine catgut suture.

C

516

border. This procedure permits bending the cartilage to conform to the curved shape of the anthelix which outlines the concha (Fig. 245, A).

The graft which is to become the helix-fossa part is turned inside out. The pattern is laid upon it and it is cut according to pattern. The graft is now carved by gouging out certain parts and leaving others as thick as possible. The part to be left thick is the rim of the graft which is to form the helix. Because the thin, close-fitting skin coverage of the normal auricular cartilage cannot be duplicated, the indentation of the new auricular framework should be as deep, and the portions in relief as sharp, as possible. Hence, the portion of the auricle between helix and anthelix should be carved as thin as possible. The auricular framework may be fenestrated (Stephenson) to insure adhesion of skin on lateral and median surface for sufficient anchorage. If the cartilage piece to form the helix-concha part is of insufficient size, another piece should be added.

The two cartilage units are now inserted from incisions as outlined in Figure 245, *A*. Undermining the skin is done along a superficial level, but a thin layer of subcutaneous tissue must be included to safeguard the circulation of the skin. The first unit to be inserted is the anthelix graft, which is bent and anchored above and below to the rudimentary cartilages with fine chromic catgut sutures. Insertion of the helix-fossa unit follows, from above to below (Fig. 245, *B*). Two precautions must be taken. First, since all of the structures of the auricle are situated posteriorly to a vertical tangential to the lobe—the tragus and anterior portion of the helix and the contour of the auricle may be compared with a question mark (Gillies)—it is important to position the auricular framework correctly (see Step 1). Second, it is important to make sure that the thin median part of the helix-fossa unit comes to lie beneath and not above the anthelix unit. The helix-fossa unit is sutured above to the upper rudimentary cartilage, and its tip is inserted below into the earlobe (Fig. 245, *C*). The wounds are then sutured. Pieces of wet mechanic's waste are placed behind and in front of the helix and in front of the anthelix, a piece of gauze is placed upon the top, and a moderate pressure dressing is applied. After all induration has subsided, one must judge whether or not the rim of the helix is sufficiently prominent. In most cases it is not, since insertion of a too-prominent rim in the preceding stage might endanger the circulation of the mastoid flap. Hence, one should not hesitate to remove a suitable part of the rib graft which had been previously stored beneath the incision at the chest (the remainder to be left behind for later use for reconstruction of the tragus and crus helicis) and to carve a narrow-based, well-rounded malleable piece of cartilage graft at the site of the prominence. From a small incision in front of the helix and at the earlobe, the skin is elevated with a small periosteal elevator (the Joseph type, as used in rhinoplasties) along the rim

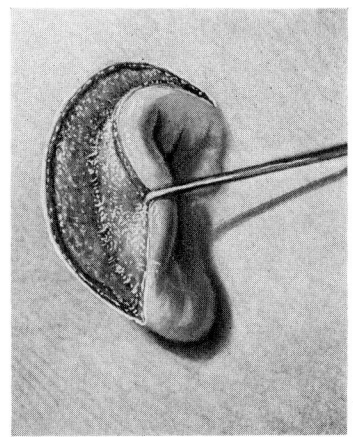

Fig. 246. *A:* Raising of the composite mastoid flap after an incision around and several millimeters away from the auricular framework.

of the helix; the additional helix graft is now inserted. If it is too thick, the overlying skin will blanch; hence, it must be reduced in thickness. The ends of the graft are bevelled and inserted beneath the anterior wound edge and the earlobe.

Step 4: Three months after insertion of the main cartilaginous framework, the composite mastoid flap is raised (Fig. 246, *A*). An incision is made around and several millimeters away from the auricular framework. In raising the flap, care must be taken not to expose the graft but to leave a sufficient amount of soft tissue upon it. The groove between the flap and the flap bed is made as deep as possible, since there is a tendency for the groove to become more shallow during the healing process. A mold of dental compound (see p. 39) is now made of the posterior raw surface with the new ear in protrusion; a thick split skin graft is taken from the gluteal region and wrapped with its raw side outward around those parts

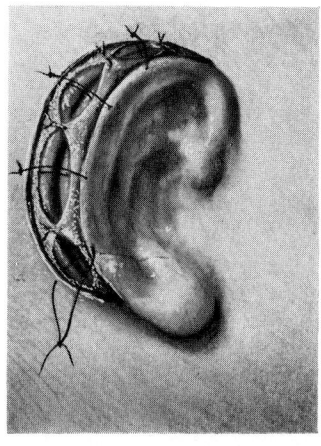

Fig. 246. *B:* A mold of dental compound is made of the posterior raw surfaces with the ear in protrusion and covered with a skin graft—raw surface out—and inserted and held buried with sutures.

of the mold which come to lie upon the posterior raw surfaces (Fig. 246, *B*). Mold and graft are now inserted and held in place, with sutures through the rim of the flap and skin graft and through the posterior edge of skin graft and flap bed. A protective dressing is applied. Unless there is evidence of discharge from beneath the mold, the mold is left in place from two to three weeks. It is then removed and replaced with a well-padded dressing which is held in place with adhesive strips which keep the newly formed auricle protruding Since there is a tendency toward posterior contraction, this forward pull should be maintained as long as possible.

Step 5: In this stage, the tragus and a semblance of the external auditory canal and crus helicis are formed; additional "retouching" is done if necessary, and re-skin grafting of the posterior surface, if it is contracted, is performed. These additional operations are carried out in one stage about three months after Step 4. First the tragus and a semblance of the external auditory canal are formed. At times, there is enough rudimentary cartilage present for formation of the tragus; more often, however, a cartilage graft must be used from the stored source beneath the original chest incision. A flap of skin with an anterior pedicle is raised from the conchal area and folded upon itself after insertion of a piece of cartilage. The edges of the folded flap are sutured together while the folded terminal end of the flap is sutured to the base; the sutures are left long. Subcutaneous tissue is removed from the conchal area until the periosteum of the mastoid is reached (Fig. 247, *A*). A split skin graft is removed and laid into the cul-de-sac of the new canal and fastened with sutures; these sutures are left long (Fig. 247, *B*). The cavity is tightly stuffed with mechanic's waste, which is held in place by tying the sutures over it (Fig. 247, *C*). If necessary, the crus helicis is now formed (compare with Fig. 241). This must be

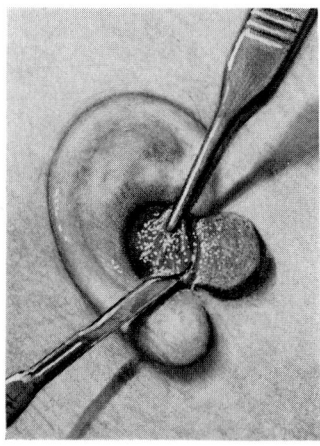

Fig. 247. *A:* Reconstruction of tragus and semblance of external auditory canal. A U-shaped flap with an anterior pedicle is raised from the conchal area. The auditory canal-conchal area is being deepened.

519

improvised according to the situation. The crus helicis may have already been formed after switching the cartilaginous rudiment in Step 1, or it can be done now by inserting a cartilage graft from the stored source subcutaneously, thus defining the anterior-inferior position of the helix.

If "retouching" becomes necessary to accentuate the helix and anthelix, the fossa helicis can be reconstructed in the same stage (Cronin; Fig. 247, C). The incision is made median and parallel to the helix. The skin is undermined laterally. A sufficient amount of subcutaneous tissue is removed between the helix and anthelix; a thin layer of connective tissue should be left on the underlying cartilage. The lateral skin edge is now sutured to the base of the helix; the sutures tied anteriorly are left long. A full-thickness skin graft is removed from the posterior side of the sound ear and laid upon the raw surface; it is sutured to the base of the helix and to the rim of the anthelix. The latter sutures are left long and, together

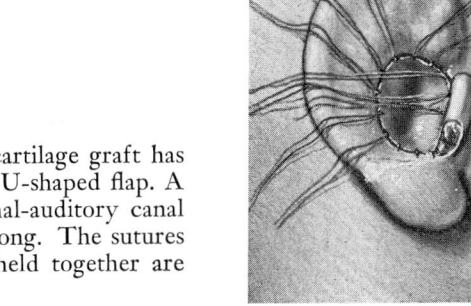

Fig. 247. *B:* A small piece of cartilage graft has been inserted within the folded U-shaped flap. A skin graft is laid into the conchal-auditory canal area and held with sutures left long. The sutures with which the folded flap is held together are also left long.

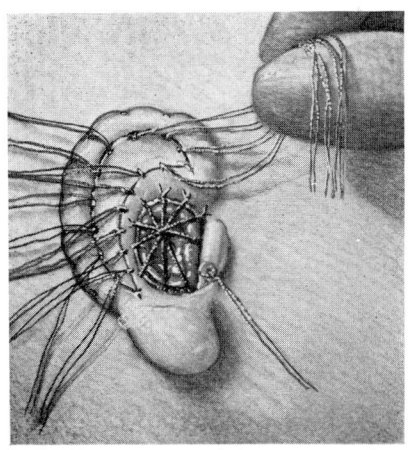

Fig. 247. *C:* Mechanic's waste is stuffed into the conchal-auditory canal cavity and held firmly in place by tying the sutures which have been left long. A groove (fossa helicis) has been made to accentuate helix and anthelix. The lateral skin edge is sutured to the base of the helix; the sutures are left long. A skin graft is laid upon the raw surfaces and sutured in place. The sutures on the median side are left long so that all sutures which have been left long can be tied over the mechanic's waste.

520

with the first sutures along the helix, are used to tie a pressure dressing in place.

Further "retouching" may be necessary to overcome a notch between the earlobe and the helix with "stepping" the area of junction (Z-plasty-like) and inserting the pointed portion of the lobule into the helix border by the tongue-groove method.

As a rule, one more step becomes necessary: to give the new ear the suitable degree of protrusion. The original step to achieve this consisted of skin grafting the posterior raw surface of the ear and mastoid region; in most cases, however, the new ear is pulled against the head by the progressive retraction of the skin graft. If this happens, another skin graft should be performed after contracture is released. This serves one of two purposes: (1) the ear may now remain protruding; (2) if the auricle retrudes again—this time as a rule not from shrinkage of the graft but from lack of support—there is now a sufficient amount of skin present beneath which a cartilage graft for support can be buried. The graft is taken from the concha of the sound ear, removed from a posterior incision. The edges of the remaining concha are sutured together. This causes a certain degree of retrusion of the sound ear, which aids in equalizing the protrusion of both ears. An incision is now made along the posterior fold of the reconstructed auricle. Under sharp dissection the ear is retracted laterally, care being taken not to perforate the anterior surface. The conchal graft is inserted cupping anteriorly. It is held with two mattress sutures which are laid through the ends of the axis of the elliptiform-shaped graft. The anterior and posterior skin edges are mobilized and sutured over the graft.

If there is tension on the suture lines, or if skin coverage over the cartilage graft is not sufficient, a narrow flap can be transferred from an area just in front of the ear to the posterior side. The pedicle is based just below the earlobe. The donor area is closed after undermining the skin anteriorly. This step, however, is rarely necessary.

As already mentioned, the external auditory canal is usually absent and does not need to be reconstructed for reasons explained on page 512. In one of the author's cases, the other ear had a marked narrowing and virtual closure of the external auditory canal. To enlarge this opening, I used the inlay skin grafting method over a strut with only little improvement. Macomber, Wang, and Lueders, and Gingrass and Pickrell seem to have much more success with the use of neighboring skin flaps for reconstruction of a stenosed external auditory canal.

Variation: If the skin of the mastoid region is destroyed, it must be replaced by an arm, neck, or chest flap before reconstruction of the ear can be started (see Case 11, p. 1004). It is also possible to transplant the cartilage graft beneath the flap before the flap is transferred, but the author

521

advises against this, since, in his experience, permanent impairment of circulation may occur in this part of the flap and graft. It is safer to transplant the flap first and then to reconstruct the ear, as suggested previously.

ABSENCE OF LOBE

Technique (Gavallo) (Fig. 248)

A flap is used from the mastoid region with an anterior pedicle at the cheek. The flap, which is one third larger than the defect, is outlined as shown in Figure 248. The posterior half, *A*, is raised and returned to its original site. After two weeks, the entire flap is raised and returned to its original site. After two more weeks, the entire flap is raised and folded upon itself so that the posterior half of the flap forms the median surface of the flap. The upper wound edge of the posterior half of the flap is sutured to the posterior wound edge of the defect, the upper wound edge of the anterior flap to the anterior wound edge of the defect. The raw surface of the flap bed is closed either by undermining and skin sliding or by skin grafting.

DEFORMITIES

PROTRUDING EARS

Protrusion of the external ear is the most common deformity of the auricle. It is usually congenital. The base of the concha of a normal ear projects from the head in less than a 30-degree angle. The body of the concha then rounds forward until it reaches the anthelix. Here the auricle bends sharply backward, forming the ridge of the anthelix (Fig. 241). In the majority of protruding ears, the deformity is due to absence of this ridge (Case 81, p. 1095). The cartilage, instead of folding backward to form the ridge, is flat. The object in correcting the deformity in these cases must be the restoration of the ridge of the anthelix. In some cases, the deformity is accentuated by overdevelopment of the concha, together with an increase of the angle between concha and head (Case 82, p. 1096). This deformity must also be overcome in the same operation.

Numerous procedures have been devised for repair of protrusion of the ears. The author follows the Davis-Kitlowski technique if the cupping of the ears from absence of the anthelix is not too pronounced; in all other cases, however, the author prefers the Converse technique. With this method, the ridge of the anthelix becomes well rounded and more normal looking than with the Davis-Kitlowski procedure, which is apt to produce a sharp-edged anthelix edge.

A   B

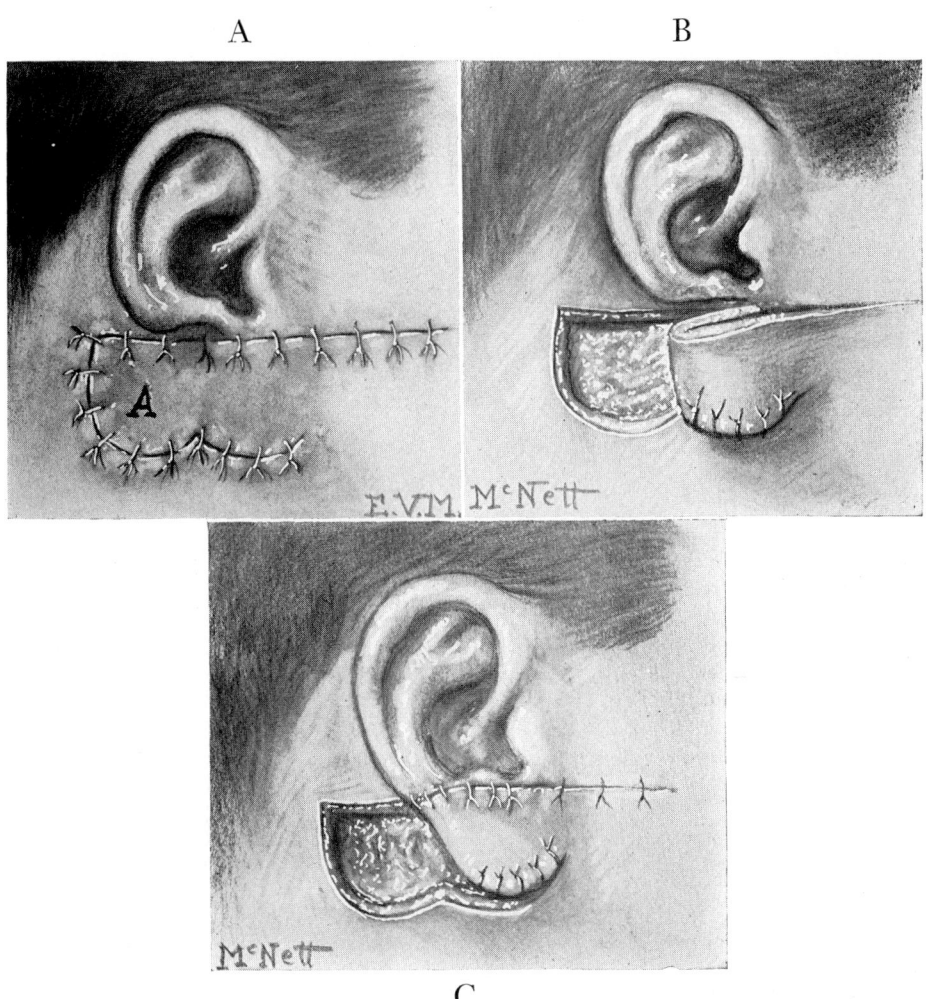

C

Fig. 248. *A:* Reconstruction of lobule (Gavallo). Flap is used from mastoid region with anterior pedicle. In first stage, posterior half, *A*, is raised and returned. In second stage, entire flap is raised and returned, as depicted in drawing. *B:* In third stage, flap is raised and folded upon itself. *C:* Upper edges of flaps are sutured to defect's edges. Raw surface of flap bed is closed by undermining and skin sliding or skin grafting.

THE HEAD AND NECK

Technique (after Davis-Kitlowski) (Fig. 249)

With the patient under general anesthesia, the operative field is prepared in the usual way; only one ear is prepared and draped initially. The ear is brought closer to the head by folding the unfolded portion of the anthelix upon itself, thus forming the ridge of the anthelix. When the ear is

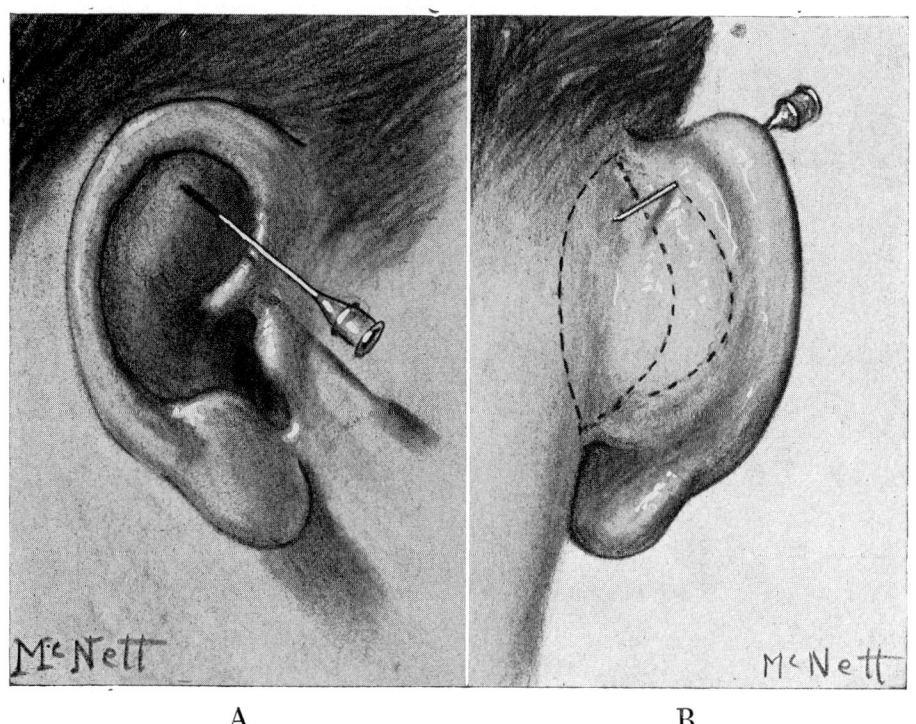

A   B

Fig. 249. *A:* Protruding ears. Restoration of ridge of anthelix (Davis-Kitlowski). Ridge of anthelix is marked out by series of punctures made with hypodermic needle dipped in aniline dye. *B:* Needle is pushed through ear. Before withdrawal, it is touched with aniline dye to stain posterior surface of cartilage. Lateral dotted line is line of punctures or posterior projection of ridge of anthelix. The elliptical piece of skin to be excised is outlined by other dotted lines.

in this position, the ridge of the anthelix is marked out on the anterior surface of the ear with one of the aniline dyes. Then along the full length of this line a series of punctures is made in the following manner: A hypodermic needle is placed at right angles to the anterior skin surface and thrust completely through the ear from front to back, coming out at a corresponding skin point on the posterior surface. When the needle emerges through the skin of the back of the ear, its point is touched with a toothpick swab dipped in an aniline dye before it is drawn back again.

524

In this way, sufficient dye is carried through the tissues to make the required marks on the cartilage.

An elliptical piece of skin is now excised from the posterior surface of the auricle. The vertical axis of this piece lies in the sulcus of the cephaloauricular angle, and should extend along the entire sulcus. At its greatest width its lateral border should not be too far away from the puncture marks of the skin; if necessary, more skin can be removed at the end of the operation.

The posterior surface of the cartilage is now exposed by undermining and reflecting the lateral wound edge. When the cartilage is exposed, a line of puncture points stained with the aniline dye can be seen in the cartilage itself. This is the line along which the spring of the cartilage must be divided. Sometimes, it is merely necessary to incise the cartilage along this line; at other times, excision of a small elliptical piece of cartilage is necessary, care being taken by the guiding finger on the anterior surface not to perforate the skin.

It is important to see that all cartilage spring is divided so that there will be no resistance or tension when the margins are turned in to form a supporting ridge. The cartilages are folded over upon themselves to form the ridge of the anthelix. They are held together in this position by a Lembert type of suture: A cotton suture is passed through the perichondrium on one side, beginning about 0.5 cm. (³⁄₁₆ inch) from the cartilage margin, and coming out close to the margin. The needle is then carried across the defect and thrust into the perichondrium a similar distance from the margin and then out about 0.5 cm. (³⁄₁₆ inch) from the defect. Four or five of these sutures are placed but not tied. A Babcock clamp is placed on the anterior surface of the new ridge in front of the first suture, thus holding the folded cartilages rigidly together. The suture is now tied. Just before the knot is drawn tight, the clamp is removed temporarily. The other sutures are tied in a similar way. The skin is then closed with sutures. If, however, the skin is redundant, more skin is removed from the anterior wound edge. The skin sutures are on-end mattress sutures of 000 chromic catgut, and the suturing should include the periosteum of the mastoid region. After they are tied, the skin edges are drawn into the sulcus of the ear. (If the periosteum is not included, the skin would drape like a tent over it.) The ends are cut short; the sutures usually bury themselves and do not need to be removed.

Should there also be an enlarged concha, it is possible to overcome its protrusion simply by taking a wider "bite" of skin edges with the mattress sutures. Hence, it is possible to control the degree of retrusion with this type of suture. Seldom is it necessary to excise a strip of cartilage from the base of the concha. This may result in breaking of the skin at

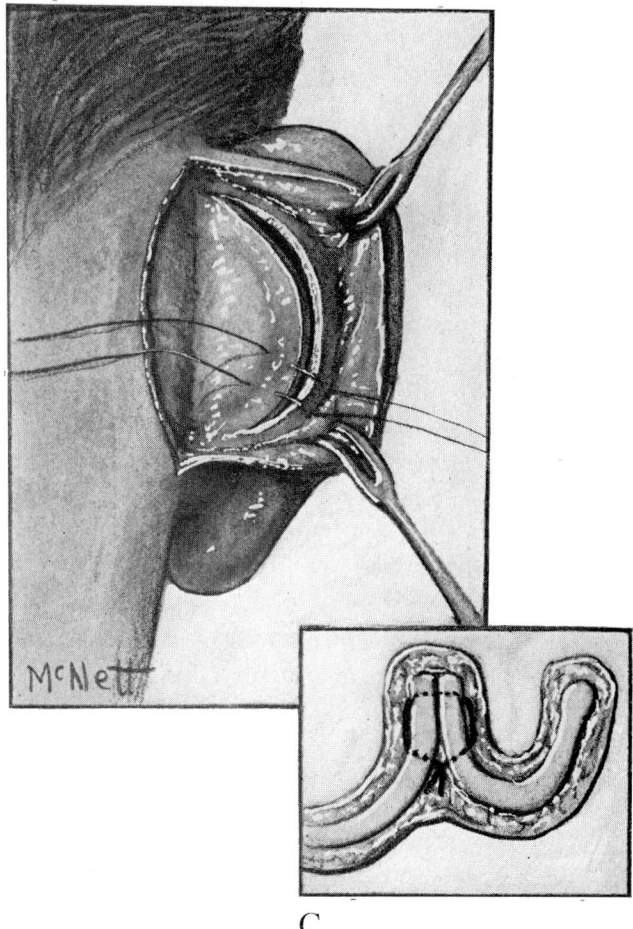

C

Fig. 249. *C:* Lateral wound edge is undermined and reflected. Cartilage is divided along line of punctures. Cartilages are folded upon each other (insert) and held
together with Lembert-type sutures.

the anterior surface from shortening of the concha. This roll of skin
should be excised immediately, as the resulting scar will become inconspicuous.

If at the end of the operation there should be a difference in the
degree of protrusion of the two ears, the skin sutures of the more protruding side should be removed. Then either more skin is excised before
resuturing is done or—more often—it is possible by simply taking a wider
"bite" of the skin edges with the now end-on mattress sutures to match the
degree of protrusion with the other ear just by controlling the tension of
the sutures.

After-Treatment

The dressing is important. A piece of ointment gauze and a narrow strip of sterile dressing gauze are laid upon the wound. In front, all convolutions of the ear are packed with pieces of wet cotton or mechanic's waste. A piece of gauze is then placed on top, held with adhesive plaster, and over this a firm head bandage. If possible, the dressing is allowed to remain in place for ten days. Another dressing is applied just over the posterior wound edges for one more week. The patient is then instructed to hold the ears close to the head at night for three weeks with an elastic skullcap.

As already mentioned, the Davis-Kitlowski procedure is apt to produce a sharpness of the ridge of the anthelix if the protrusion is pronounced. Efforts have been made to overcome this by tubing the anthelial fold (Barsky, Becker, Converse and associates, followed by Tanzer, who has refined the method and achieved excellent results; the author recommends it highly).

Technique (After Converse) (Fig. 250, Cases 81, 82)

After the patient is anesthetized (the author prefers general anesthesia) and the operative field prepared and draped (only one ear is initially prepared), the ear is folded back until a normal appearance of the anthelix curvature is achieved. The outline should be carried well up into the superior scapha, but not so far laterally that the helix buckles. It is also important that the future anthelix form a graceful curve and not a straight line. The anterior and posterior limits of the anthelix are outlined with ink on the anterior side of the auricle. They form a pear-shaped area, the anterior-superior aspect reaching a point immediately above the fossa triangularis and extending downward into the concha medial to the anthelix. On the lateral side, a rim of at least 3 mm. of scaphal cartilage should be preserved. The height of the future anthelix or the axis of the pear-shaped outline is transferred to the posterior side with punctures made with a hypodermic needle dipped in aniline dye (compare with Fig. 249, *A* and *B*). An elliptiform incision is now made on the posterior side of the ear similar to the one demonstrated in Figure 249, *A*. The elliptical piece of skin is excised, and the cartilaginous framework is exposed by wide dissection and undermining of the lateral wound edge (Fig. 250, *F*). Now that the cartilage is exposed and the row of punctures representing the axis of the pear-shaped outline becomes visible, the pear-shaped outline is also transposed from the anterior to the posterior surface of the cartilage (Fig. 250, *G, H*) with multiple puncture dots; incisions are made through the cartilage along the anterior and posterior limits of the pear-

527

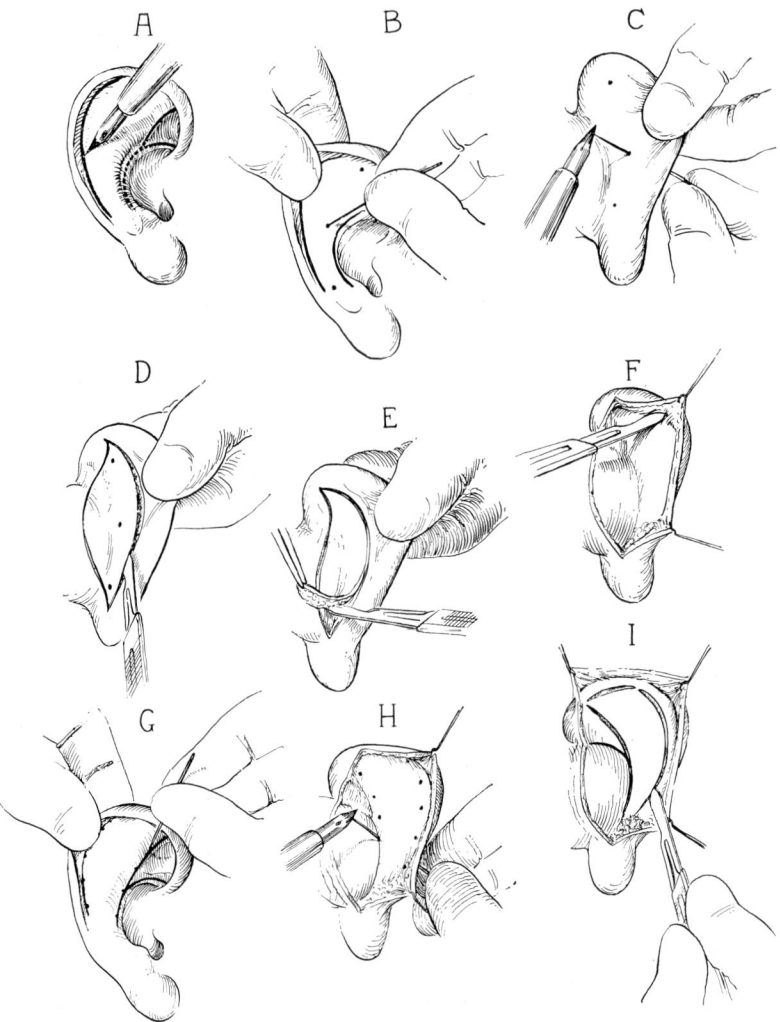

Fig. 250. *A:* The deformed ear has been folded back. The anterior and posterior limits of the antihelix are outlined with ink. An additional ink line outlines the crus helicis. The dotted line represents the portion that extends into the concha behind the antihelix fold. *B:* The needle is placed through the center of the outlined pear-shaped area at the upper, middle and lower portions. *C:* The needle transpierces the ear and is tipped with ink in order to leave a mark upon the skin. *D:* The three ink dots indicate the center of the elliptical area of skin to be removed. *E:* The ellipse of skin and subcutaneous tissue is resected. *F:* The skin edges are undermined in order to obtain adequate exposure of the auricular cartilage. *G:* The limits of the pear-shaped segment are outlined by another series of perforations with a straight cutting needle. *H:* The needle is tipped with ink in order to leave a mark upon the cartilage, indicating the outline of the pear-shaped segment. *I:* Incisions are made through the cartilage along the anterior and posterior limits of the pear-shaped area. Additional incisions are made, one superiorly following the curve of the helix and another through the crus anthelicis. Note that the incision which follows the curve of the helix superiorly does not join with the

528

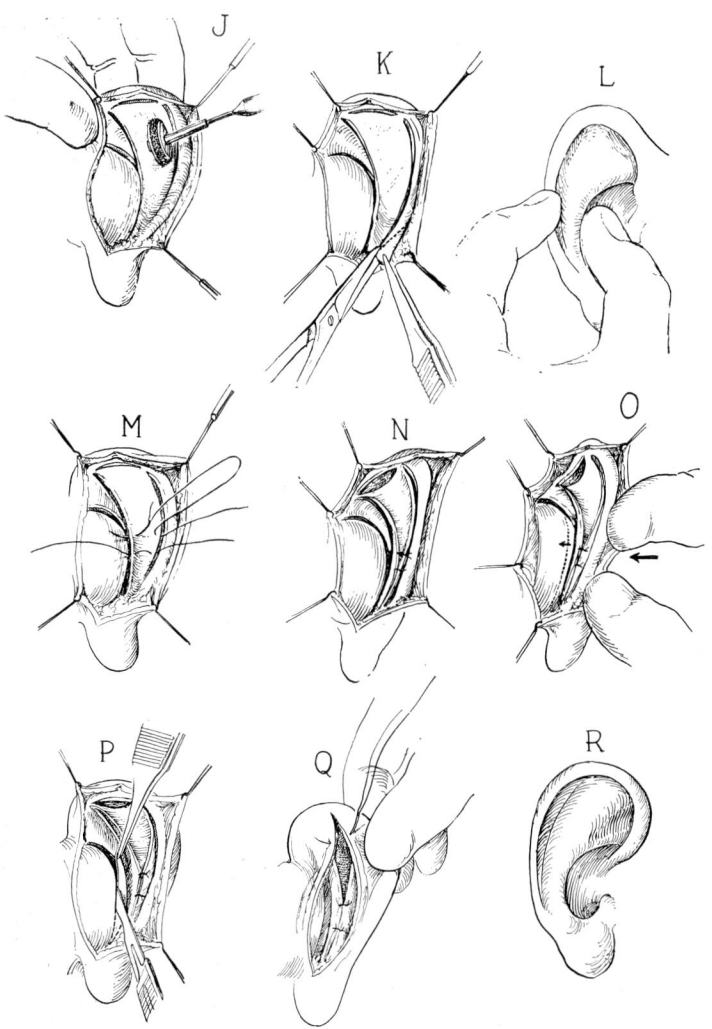

vertical incisions. *J:* In certain cases the auricular cartilage is thick and cannot be readily folded back. In such cases thinning of the cartilage is accomplished by means of a wire brush, electrically driven, similar to that used for abrasion of the skin. *K:* In many cases resection of a portion of or of the entire cauda helicis is necessary to correct the protrusion of the lower part of the ear. *L:* The auricular cartilage may now be folded back, simulating an adequate antihelix. *M:* The sutures are placed in order to tube the cartilaginous pear-shaped segment. *N:* A sufficient number of sutures are placed in order to produce the adequate amount of curvature. *O:* In most cases there remains a protrusion of the lower half of the ear due to an excessively cupped concha. By pressing the antihelix inward it is possible to evaluate the amount of conchal cartilage to be resected to correct the protrusion. *P:* An adequate segment of conchal cartilage is resected. *Q:* The operation is completed by suturing the margins of the postauricular skin defect. *R:* An adequately curved antihelix has been formed and excessive cupping of the concha has been corrected. (J. M. Converse et al.: Plast. Reconstr. Surg., 1955.)

shaped area up to but not through the anterior skin. Additional incisions are made, one superiorly following the curve of the helix above (Fig. 250, *I*) (note that this does not join with the vertical incisions), the other through the lower crus of the anthelix (compare with Fig. 241) unless this is present. In older individuals, in whom the cartilage is thick, folding of the cartilage may be facilitated by thinning it with an electrically driven wire brush, similar to that used for dermabrasion (Fig. 250, *J*). The cartilage is now folded and tubed to itself in the lower portion of the pear-shaped area, cotton sutures being used to maintain the tubing (Fig. 250, *M*). Sometimes it is necessary to resect protruding portions of the cartilage of the cauda helicis (Fig. 250, *K*). The auricle is examined from the anterior surface, and additional sutures are laid until the tube of cartilage presents the appearance of a well-formed anthelix. At this stage, the upper portion of the auricle is in its corrected position; the concha, however, remains prominent. To overcome this, the auricle is pressed against the side of the head until the protrusion is corrected. The amount of excess of conchal cartilage is visualized from the degree to which the anthelix overlaps the conchal cut edge (Fig. 250, *O*), and the excess is excised. If the inferior part still protrudes, the original incisions should be elongated into the inferior part of the concha and the antitragal base and a segment of cartilage excised. This completely breaks the spring of the cartilage inferiorly, allowing the lower portion of the ear to sink inward. This, however, has one disadvantage: it leaves in almost every case an unsightly fold of skin rolled up on the anterior side. This should be excised immediately, as the resulting scar will become inconspicuous. In most of the author's cases, it was not necessary to reduce the width of the concha; its protrusion was simply overcome by proper trimming and suturing of the skin edges. The skin sutures are on-end mattress sutures of 000 chromic catgut, and the suturing should include the periosteum of the mastoid region. After they are tied, the skin edges are drawn into the sulcus of the ear. (If the periosteum were not included, the skin would drape like a tent over it.) The ends are cut short; the sutures usually bury themselves and do not need to be removed. Thus, the degree of retrusion can be controlled simply by the amount of "bite" and tension which is taken at the skin edges with the on-end mattress sutures. (See remarks on page 526 on correction of difference in protrusion of the ears at the end of the operation.)

After-Treatment

See page 527.

CORRECTION OF THE CONGENITAL LOP EAR

The lop ear is not a protruding ear. "Lop" means to hang limply, and the protruding ear does not hang. The term "lop" ear should be applied only to the rather rare downward folding of the top of the ear caused by acute folding of the helix with absence of the anthelix. Hence, a lop ear is often combined with a certain degree of protrusion of the ear. K. L. Stephenson devised a good method to overcome this deformity, to which Musgrave added a valuable improvement.

Technique

This consists first of overcoming the "lopping" and the protruding. From a posterior incision, the posterior surface of the auricle is exposed. The undermining of the skin is carried over the folded helix to its anterior aspect. After reflecting the skin well forward, three to four radiating incisions approximately 1 cm. in length are made through the crumpled helix. The helix can now be unfolded, and the cartilage strips fan out like spokes from an axle. However, without further support they tend to fall back into the former crumpled position; even with proper dressings they may not unfold completely again, as the author has experienced. Musgrave overcomes this difficulty in the following way: He removes a strip of cartilage from the area of the absent anthelix (see previous section on protruding ears) and fashions the graft into a curved strut. The strut is carefully sutured with fine silk to the anterior side of the periphery of each fanned-out cartilage strip, just as the rim of a wheel is attached to its spokes. To form the anthelix the cartilages are folded upon each other along the line of the excised cartilage strip. Instead of holding them together with the type of suture depicted in Figure 249, C, the author simply lays mattress sutures through the cartilages on the anterior side and ties them over small rolls of vaseline gauze. The skin is now draped over the newly positioned framework. Some excess skin will need to be removed. The posterior wound edges are sutured as described on page 525. The after-treatment is the same as that described on page 527.

LARGE EARS

The external ear may only appear large or may actually be large. In the first type, the appearance is caused by a protrusion of the auricle. Correction of the protrusion, as previously described, will correct the apparent enlargement. Genuinely large ears, however, need actual reduction.

Technique (Lexer) (Fig. 251)

An anterior incision is made along the sulcus of the helix. A skin flap is dissected downward until the anthelix is reached. This exposes the anterior surface of the fossa between helix and anthelix, leaving the posterior skin covering and that of the helix intact. The next step consists of excision of a wedge-shaped piece of the full thickness of the helix and skin, with the base of the wedge at the helix; to prevent later notching of the rim, the excision at the rim should be made staircase-like. The wound edges of the helix and the remainder of the cartilaginous wound edges are

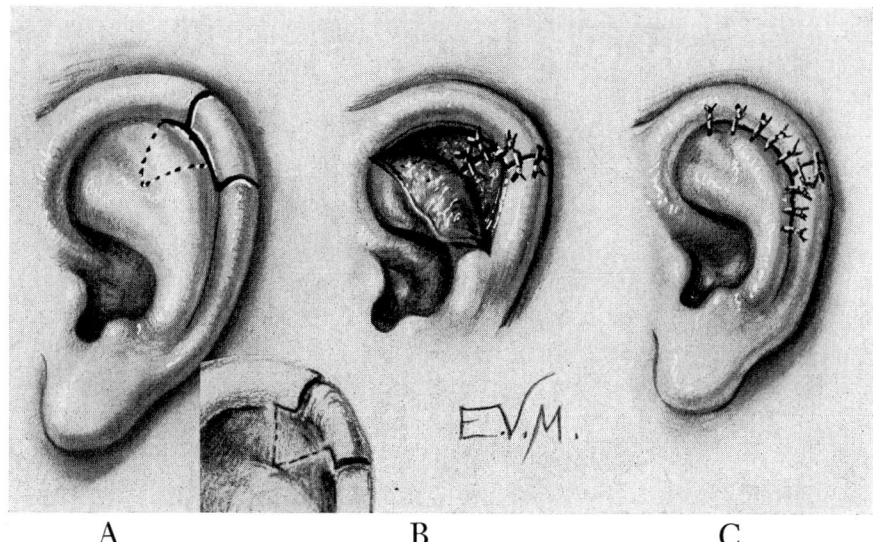

A.   B   C

Fig. 251. *A:* Reduction of large ears (Lexer). Excision of wedge-shaped piece of helix and anthelix in staircase-like manner outlined. *B:* Skin flap below helix is mobilized, wedge-shaped piece of helix, anthelix and posterior skin excised in staircase manner and wound edges sutured together. *C:* Flap trimmed and sutured in place.

now sutured together. The anterior skin flap is trimmed to proper proportions and sutured to the skin edges of the helix. Thus, the two excisions shorten the ear longitudinally and vertically. The last step consists of trimming the wrinkles of the posterior skin to fit the new shape of the ear. If the ears are not only large but also protruding, protrusion can be overcome at the same time the ears are made smaller. After reduction in size an incision is made along the proposed anthelix of the anterior surface of the ear cartilage; the cartilages are folded upon each other (compare with Fig. 249 insert) and held in this position with a few mattress sutures. The anterior skin flap is then draped over and sutured in place. (Compare with Case 43, p. 1050.)

THE EXTERNAL AUDITORY STRUCTURES

CAULIFLOWER EARS

This deformity, as commonly seen in wrestlers, is due to the invasion of fibrous tissue by subcutaneous hematomas; the cartilage itself may increase in size and change the ear into a cauliflower-like shape. Operative correction consists of elevation of an anterior or posterior skin flap, excision of cicatricial tissue, shaping of the cartilage, and replacing of the skin flap. The ear is well padded and a pressure dressing applied.

BIBLIOGRAPHY

ALEXANDER, G.: *Zur plastischen Korrektur abstehender Ohrmuscheln.* Wien. Klin. Wchnschr., 41:1217, 1928.

AUFRICHT, G.: *Total ear reconstruction.* Plast. Reconstr. Surg., 2:297, 1947.

BARSKY, A. J.: *Plastic Surgery.* W. B. Saunders, Philadelphia, 1938.

BECKER, O. J.: *Correction of the protruding ear.* Brit. J. Plast. Surg., 5:187, 1952.
Surgery of the protruding ear. Arch. Otolaryng., 72:758, 1960.

BELLUCCI, R. J.: *The problem of congenital auricular malformation. I. Construction of the external auditory canal.* Trans. Amer. Acad. Ophthal. 64:840, 1960.

BERSON, M. I.: *Complete reconstruction of auricle.* Amer. J. Surg., 60:101, 1943.

BROADBENT, T. R., and MATHEWS, V. L.: *Artistic relationships in surface anatomy of the face: Application to reconstructive surgery.* Plast. Reconstr. Surg., 20:1, 1957.

CONVERSE, J. M.: *Construction of the auricle in congenital microtia.* Plast. Reconstr. Surg., 32:425, 1962.
The problem of congenital auricular malformation. II. Construction of the auricle in congenital microtia. Trans. Amer. Acad. Ophthal. Otolaryng., 64:853, 1960.
Reconstruction of the auricle (Part I). Plast. Reconstr. Surg., 22:150, 1958.
Reconstruction of the auricle (Part II). Plast. Reconstr. Surg., 22:230, 1958.

CONVERSE, J. M., and WOOD-SMITH, D.: *Technical details in the surgical correction of the lop ear deformity.* Plast. Reconstr. Surg., 31:118, 1963.

CONWAY, H., ET AL.: *Reconstruction of the external ear.* Ann. Surg., 128:266, 1948.

CRONIN, T. D.: *One stage reconstruction of the helix: Two improved methods.* Plast. Reconstr. Surg., 9:547, 1952.
Use of a silastic frame for total and subtotal reconstruction of the external ear. Plast. Reconstr. Surg., 37:399, 1966.

CRONIN, T. D., GREENBERG, R. L., BRAUER, R. O.: *Follow-up study of silastic frame for reconstruction of external ear.* Plast. Reconstr. Surg., 42:522, 1968.

533

THE HEAD AND NECK

DAVIS, J. E.: *Congenital atresia of the external auditory meatus.* Plast. Reconstr. Surg., 8:173, 1951.

DAVIS, J. S., and KITLOWSKI, E. A.: *Abnormal prominence of the ears: A method of readjustment.* Surgery, 2:835, 1937.

DUNTON, E. F., BLOCKER, T. G., LEWIS, S. R., and PADEREWSKI, J.: *A compromise approach to total ear reconstruction.* Plast. Reconstr. Surg., 34:247, 1964.

DUPERTUIS, S. M.: *Actual growth of young cartilage transplants in rabbits.* Ann. Surg., 43:32, 1941.

FROMM, B. E., KNUTSON, P., and STENSTROM, S. J.: *Prosthetic ears: Two methods of fixing to a reconstructed auditory meatus.* Plast. Reconstr. Surg., 34:252, 1964.

GAVALLO: In NÉLATON and OMBRÉDANNE: *Les Autoplasties.* J. Steinheil, Paris, 1907.

GELBKE, H.: *Ohrplastiken.* Lehrbuch der Chirurgie und Orthopadie des Kindesalters, A. Oberniedermayr, Springer-Verlag, Berlin, 1959.

GILLIES, H.: Referred to by GREELEY, P. W.: *Reconstructive otoplasty.* Surgery, 10:457, 1941.

GINGRASS, R. P., and PICKRELL, K. L.: *Techniques for closure of conchal and external auditory canal defects.* Plast. Reconstr. Surg., 41:568, 1968.

GONZALEZ-ULLOA, M.: *An easy method to correct prominent ears.* Plast. Reconstr. Surg., 9:386, 1952 (Abstract). Article in Brit. J. Plast. Surg., 4:207, 1951.

GREELEY, P. W.: *Reconstructive otoplasty.* Surgery, 10:457, 1941.

GROTTING, J. K.: *Otoplasty for congenital cupped protruding ears using a postauricular flap.* Plast. Reconstr. Surg., 22:164, 1958.

KIRKHAM, H. L. D.: *The use of preserved cartilage in ear reconstruction.* Ann. Surg., 111:896, 1940.

LEXER, *Die gesamte Wiederherstellungs-Chirurgie.* J. A. Barth, Leipzig, 1931.

LUEDERS, H. W.: *One stage enlargement of the burned ear.* Plast. Reconstr. Surg., 37:512, 1966.

MACOMBER, D. W.: *Plastic mesh as a supporting medium in ear construction.* Plast. Reconstr. Surg., 25:248, 1960.

MACOMBER, W. B., WANG, M. K. H., and LUEDERS, H. W.: *Reconstruction of the traumatically stenosed external auditory canal.* Plast. Reconstr. Surg., 22:168, 1958.

McNICHOL, J. W.: *Total helix reconstruction with tubed pedicles following loss by burns.* Plast. Reconstr. Surg., 6:373, 1950.

MILLARD, D. R.: *The chondrocutaneous flap in partial auricular repair.* Plast. Reconstr. Surg., 37:523, 1966.

MUSGRAVE, R. H.: *A variation on the correction of the congenital lop ear.* Plast. Reconstr. Surg., 37:394, 1966.

NÉLATON, C., and OMBRÉDANNE, L.: *Les Autoplasties: lèvres, joues, oreilles, tronc, membres.* G. Steinheil, Paris, 1907.

PADGETT, E. C.: *Total reconstruction of the auricle.* Surg. Gynec. Obstet., 67: 761, 1938.

PATTON, H. S.: *The use of a mastoid gouge as a tool to simplify bilateral otoplasty.* Plast. Reconstr. Surg., 29:702, 1962.

PEER, L.: *Cartilage grafting.* Surg. Clin. N. Amer., 24:404, 1944.
Experimental observation of growth of young human cartilage graft. Plast. Reconstr. Surg., 1:108, 1946.
Reconstruction of the auricle with diced cartilage grafts in a vitallium ear mold. Ibid., 3:653, 1948.

PENNISI, V. R., KLABUNDE, H., and PIERCE, G. W.: *The preauricular flap.* Plast. Reconstr. Surg., 35:552, 1965.

PIERCE, G. W.: *Reconstruction of the external ear.* Surg. Gynec. Obstet., 50:601, 1930.

PIERCE, G. W., KLABUNDE, E. H., and BROBST, H. T.: *Further observations on reconstruction of the external ear.* Plast. Reconstr. Surg., 10:395, 1952.

ROUND, H.: *Prosthetic appliances: A new method of fixation.* Proc. Roy. Soc. Med., 36:486, 1943.

SMITH, F.: *Manual of Standard Practice of Plastic and Maxillofacial Surgery: Military Surgical Manuals National Research Council.* W. B. Saunders, Philadelphia, 1942.
Plastic and Reconstructive Surgery. W. B. Saunders, Philadelphia, 1950.

STEPHENSON, K. L.: *Correction of a lop ear deformity.* Plast. Reconstr. Surg., 26:540, 1960.

STRAITH, R. E.: *Correction of the protruding ear.* Plast. Reconstr. Surg., 24:277, 1959.

TANZER, R. C.: *The reconstruction of acquired defects of the ear.* Plast. Reconstr. Surg., 35:355, 1965.
An analysis of ear reconstruction. Plast. Reconstr. Surg., 31:16, 1963.
The correction of prominent ears. Plast. Reconstr. Surg., 30:236, 1962.
Total reconstruction of the external ear. Plast. Reconstr. Surg., 23:1, 1959.

YOUNG, F.: *Correction of abnormally prominent ears.* Surg. Gynec. Obstet., 78:541, 1944.

THE OSSEOUS FRAMEWORK OF THE FACE

12

OF the defects of the facial bones, only the traumatic defects, comprising fractures and nonunions, will be considered here. There are numerous excellent monographs available on this subject. One of the older ones is a classic treatise by two pioneers in this field, Ivy and Curtis. The latest one, a monumental piece of work, is published by Dingman and Natvig.

FRACTURES OF MANDIBLE

Fractures of the mandible constitute the majority of fractures of the facial bones, for the mandible is exposed and poorly protected. The injury as a rule is due to direct, less often to indirect, trauma.

ANATOMY

The mandible, or lower jaw, consists of the body, which is convex anteriorly, and the two rami ascending from the two ends of the body (Fig. 252).

Embryologically, the body consists of two halves which unite in the midline, forming the symphysis. It is the carrier of the teeth, which are supported by the alveolar process. After loss of the teeth, this process disappears. The protuberantia mentalis forms the lower border of the symphysis, and is the most prominent part of the chin. The foramen

537

mentale, a frequent site of fractures, is situated at the outside below the alveola of the second premolar. It forms the exit of the canalis mandibulae, from which the nervus alveolaris inferior and vessels escape.

Each ramus forms an angle with the body of about 130 degrees. Its lateral surface is roughened for the attachment of the masseter muscle.

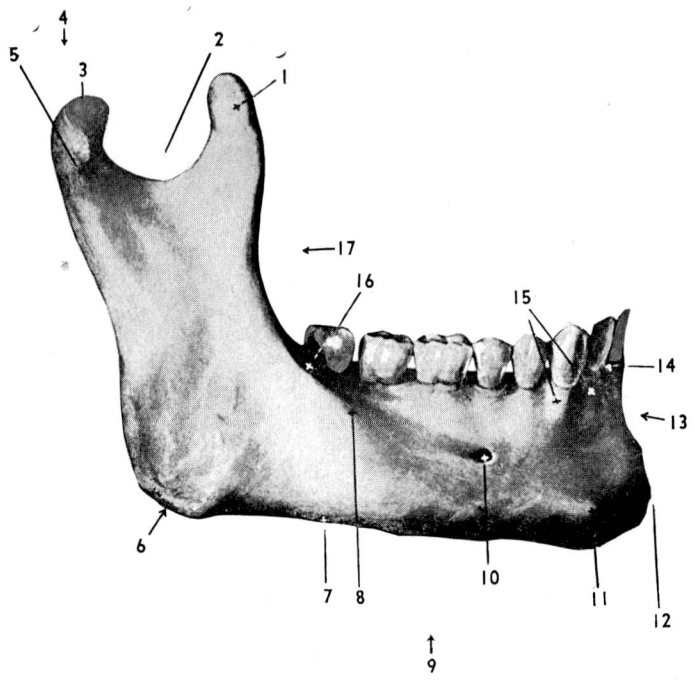

Fig. 252. *A:* Anatomy of mandible.

1: Processus coronoideus	10: Foramen mentale
2: Incisura mandibulae	11: Tuberculum mentale
3: Capitulum	12: Protuberantia mentalis
4: Processus condyloideus	13: Pars alveolaris
5: Collum	14: Limbus alveolaris
6: Angulus mandibulae	15: Juga alveolaria
7: Basis mandibuli	16: Crista buccinatoria
8: Linea obliqua	17: Ramus mandibuli
9: Corpus mandibulae	

(W. Spalteholz: Handatlas der Anatomie der Menschen. S. Hirzel, Leipzig.)

The center of the median surface contains the foramen mandibulare. This is the entrance of the canalis mandibulae, through which the nervus alveolaris inferior and vessels pass. The upper end of the ramus carries two processes which are separated by an incisure. The anterior process is called the "processus coronoideus," which is the inserting point for the musculus temporalis; the posterior process, the processus condyloideus, carries the capitulum mandibulae, which forms the lower half of the mandibular joint. Below the capitulum is a constriction called the "collum mandibulae," a frequent site of fractures.

The muscles inserting at the mandible can be divided roughly into elevators and depressors. The *elevator* group consists of the musculus masseter, the musculus temporalis, and the musculi pterygoideus internus and externus. This group inserts at the angle and the ramus of the mandible; the musculus masseter, at the lateral surface; the musculus temporalis, at the processus condyloideus; the musculus pterygoideus internus, at the median surface of the angle and ramus; and the musculus

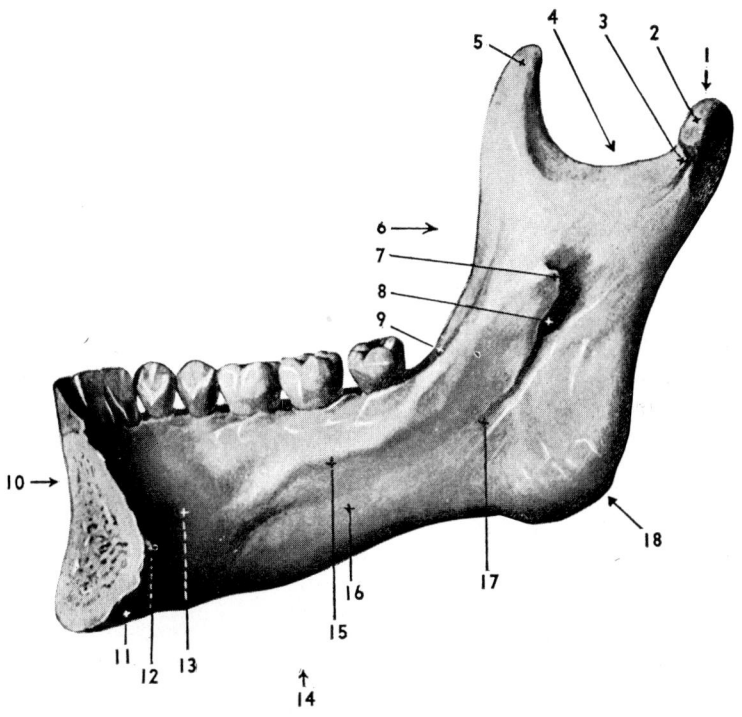

Fig. 252. *B:* Anatomy of mandible.

1: Processus condyloideus	10: Pars alveolaris
2: Capitulum	11: Fossa digastrica
3: Fovea pterygoidea	12: Spina mentalis
4: Incisura mandibulae	13: Fovea sublingualis
5: Processus coronoideus	14: Corpus mandibulae
6: Ramus mandibuli	15: Linea mylohyoidea
7: Lingula mandibulae	16: Fovea submaxillaris
8: Foramen mandibulare	17: Sulcus mylohyoideus
9: Crista buccinatoria	18: Angulus mandibulae

(W. Spalteholz: Handatlas der Anatomie der Menschen. S. Hirzel, Leipzig.)

pterygoideus externus, at the neck of the processus condyloideus. The *depressor* muscles are the musculus digastricus, the musculus geniohyoideus, the musculus genioglossus, and the musculus mylohyoideus. They all arise from the lingual or inner surface of the body, and form the floor of the mouth.

SYMPTOMS, SIGNS, AND DIAGNOSIS

The patient with a fracture of the mandible is as a rule unable to open and close his mouth to a normal extent, owing to the interruption of the continuity of the bone and to pain. Bleeding from a tear of the mucous membrane, swelling, and tenderness over the injured place are seldom missing. Abnormal motility, malocclusion, and deformity, if present, confirm the diagnosis.

Fractures of Symphysis
If the fracture line runs through the midline, a deformity may be absent. If there is marked comminution, however, and a loss of bone, a considerable narrowing of the mandibular arch may be the consequence.

Fractures of Mandibular Body
The most common fracture runs through the region of the foramen mentale. The anterior fragment is displaced downward, owing to pull of the depressor muscles; the posterior fragment is pulled upward and out-ward, owing to action of the elevator group. There may be a deviation of the chin toward the fractured side.

Fractures of Ascending Ramus, Processus Condyloideus, and Processus Coronoideus
The displacement of the fragments of the ramus is slight; the de-formity may consist only of a deviation of the chin toward the fractured side. In the majority of fractures of the processus condyloideus, a deform-ity is not noticeable. Fractures of the processus coronoideus are rare and without visible displacement.

Double Fractures
The most common fracture runs through the foramen mentale on one side and through the angle on the other side. The anterior fragment (chin fragment) is displaced downward and backward, owing to the pull of the lingual muscles; the posterior fragments are pulled upward by the elevators.

THE OSSEOUS FRAMEWORK OF THE FACE

While in most cases the clinical diagnosis of fracture of the mandible is obvious, the exact location and form of the fragments can be defined only by x-ray examination. X-ray pictures should be taken from two planes, should possibly be three dimensional, and must include the entire jaw together with the condyles.

TREATMENT

Therapy may be primarily an emergency treatment followed by a final treatment. In a simple fracture of the mandible, the *emergency* treatment consists merely of the application of a head bandage, such as that shown in Figure 253. No turn should go around the anterior surface of the

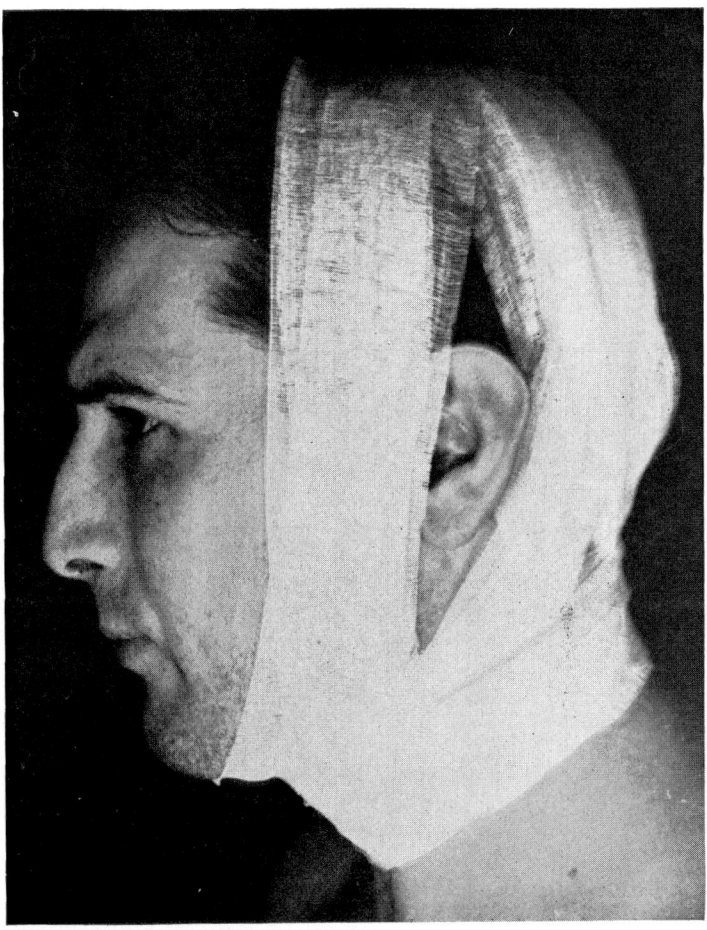

Fig. 253. Emergency dressing for fractured mandible, similar to Barton bandage. Anterior part of chin should not be included in dressing to avoid posterior displacement.

541

chin, since this would inevitably increase the displacement. Such a bandage achieves sufficient temporary immobilization to keep the patient comfortable until final treatment can be undertaken. The emergency treatment of compound fractures of the jaw has been discussed on page 132.

The *final* treatment consists of reduction of the fragments and of retention. Certain preliminary steps, however, are necessary. The mouth should be thoroughly cleansed with hydrogen peroxide. If the fracture line runs through the socket of a tooth, the latter should be removed unless loss of the tooth would increase the displacement of the fragments and make reduction difficult. The best example is a fracture in front of the last molar tooth. Loss of this tooth would favor upward displacement of the posterior fragment. In such a case, the tooth should be left in place for ten to fourteen days or even longer; the fixation is then temporarily removed and the tooth carefully lifted out of its socket.

Reduction of Fragments

Reduction of the fragments may require anesthesia. General anesthesia should be avoided if possible. Local anesthesia, either as block anesthesia of the nervus alveolaris inferior or as infiltration anesthesia, is the method of choice. If general anesthesia must be used, the intravenous

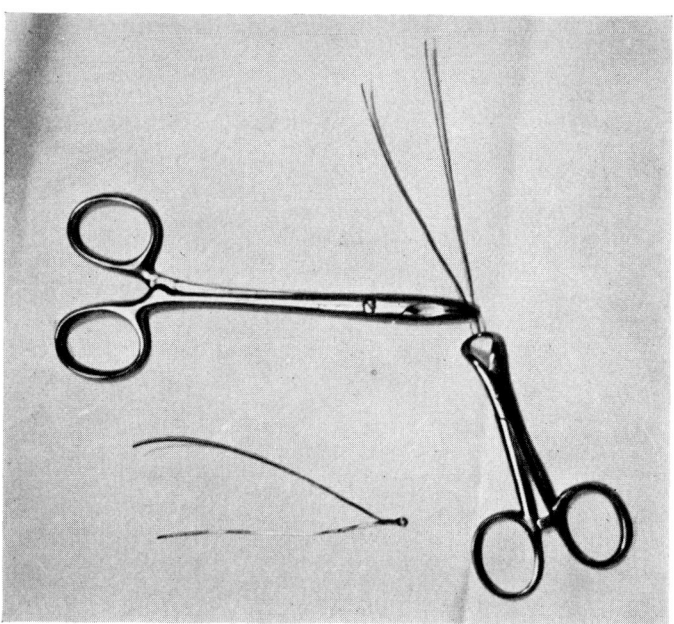

Fig. 254. Making eyelet in No. 24 gauge soft brass wire. The wire, 15.2 cm. (6 inches) long, is folded at its middle around towel clamp. Two twists are made with hemostat.

injection of sodium pentothal is preferable. The object of reduction is to achieve a normal occlusion of lower and upper teeth if they are present. In edentulous jaws, however, a proper alignment of the fragments is difficult to obtain.

Immobilization

The object of immobilization is to retain the reduced fragments in position until healing has occurred. This is best achieved by using the upper jaw as a splint and fastening the teeth of the lower jaw to those of

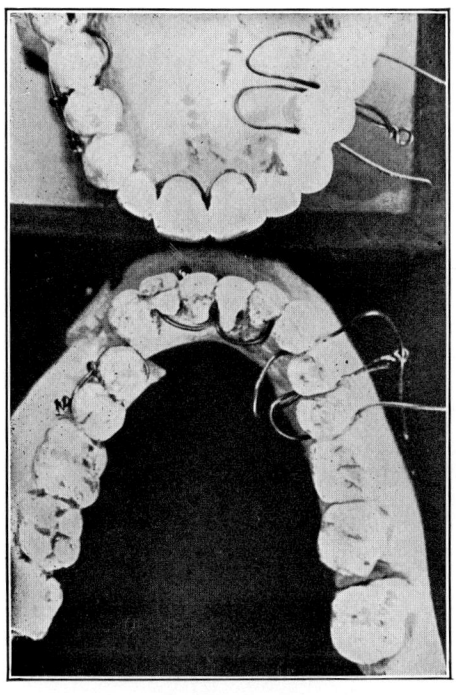

Fig. 255. *A:* (R. H. Ivy and L. Curtis: Fractures of the Jaws. Lea & Febiger.)

the upper jaw with wires. If teeth are missing, the problem of immobilization becomes more difficult.

Interdental Wiring: Many methods have been described. The author prefers the eyelet-wire method that has been described by Ivy and Curtis. This is a simple way of fixation in uncomplicated cases where a sufficient number of teeth are present and where the fragments can easily be reduced and maintained in position.

The wire used for the procedure is No. 24 gauge, of soft brass. A wire 15.2 cm. (6 inches) long is folded at its middle around a towel clamp, and two twists are made with a hemostat to form a small eyelet (Fig. 254).

The teeth usually selected for attaching the wires are the premolars above and below on each side and the incisors in front, or other opposing teeth if the aforementioned are absent. Both ends of the eyelet wire are inserted from the vestibular aspect through the interproximal space of a pair of these teeth until only the eyelet is visible buccally, the ends lying lingually. Each end of the wire is now passed around the neck of the adjacent tooth so that both ends emerge on the vestibular aspect (Fig. 255, *A, above*). One end of the wire is threaded through the eyelet lying between the teeth (Fig. 255, *A, below*). Each free end is now grasped with a hemostat and pulled snugly around the necks of the teeth. Then the wires are twisted as tightly as possible. All twists should be made in one direction, so that one will know how to tighten the wires should it become necessary later. The ends are cut short and bent against the teeth.

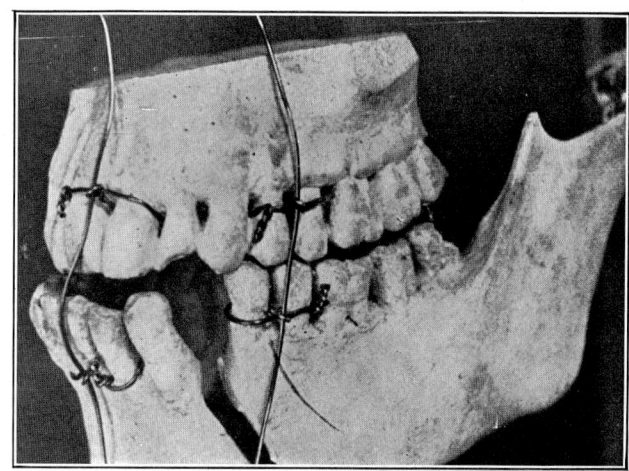

Fig. 255. *B:* (R. H. Ivy and L. Curtis: Fractures of the Jaws. Lea & Febiger.)

The same procedure is undertaken at the other selected pairs of teeth. Thus, three points of attachment are prepared. Through each of the three pairs of eyelets is passed a single strand, 30.5 cm. (12 inches) long, of the same No. 24 gauge brass wire (Fig. 255, *B*). The patient is instructed to bring the teeth together while an assistant, with the palms of both hands beneath and around the mandible, aids in reducing the fragments. The corresponding ends of the wires are twisted, and the ends are cut short and turned away from cheeks and lips. Some tightening of the wires may be necessary after twenty-four hours.

Alternative Method: When good reduction of the fragments is difficult to achieve and maintain, or when teeth are not sufficient in number, application of upper and lower arch bars and intermaxillary rubber band

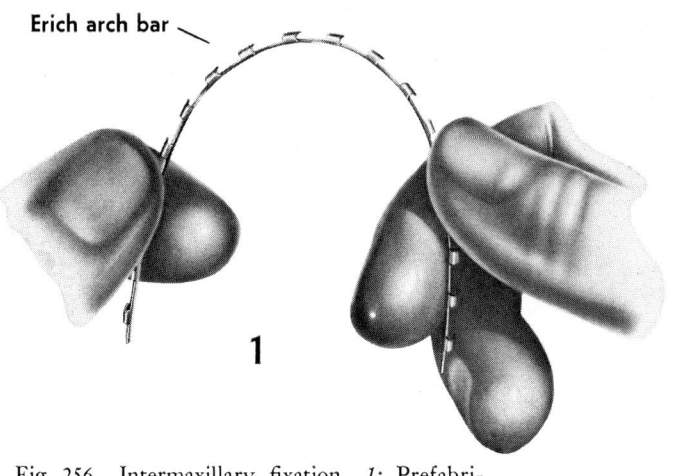

Erich arch bar

1

Fig. 256. Intermaxillary fixation. *1:* Prefabricated arch bars of malleable metal are available commercially in pre cut lengths. These can be contoured easily by hand to fit the outer surfaces of the maxillary and mandibular arches. The bars are designed with small hooked attachments for the reception of rubber bands. Care should be taken to place the arch bar with the hooks in a direction favorable for reception of the rubber bands between the upper and lower arches. The hooks are directed toward the gums on each arch.

2: By grasping the horseshoe-shaped bent arch bar with forceps, it can be laid over the surfaces of the teeth to determine the exact length desired. The bar should extend completely around the dental arch from the left molars to the right molars and should be of sufficient length to permit ligating to all available teeth.

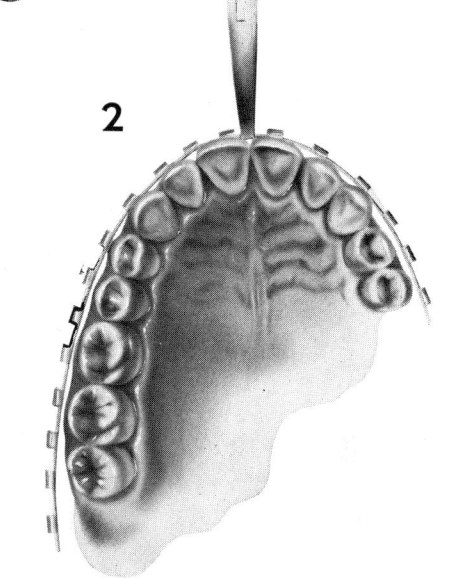

2

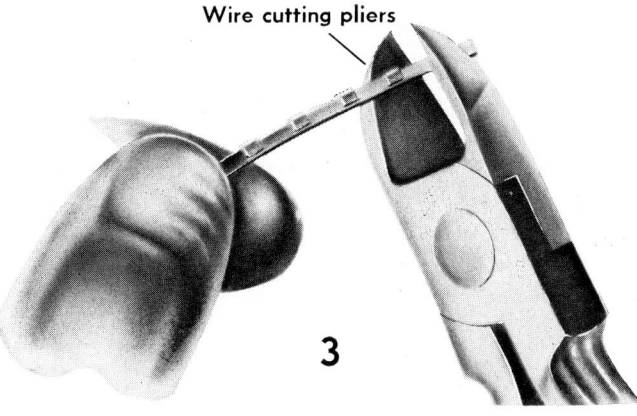

Wire cutting pliers

3

3: The arch bar is soft enough to cut with a pair of heavy cutting pliers. The arch bar should be kept long enough so that the very end of it can be bent toward the posterior surface of the last available tooth.

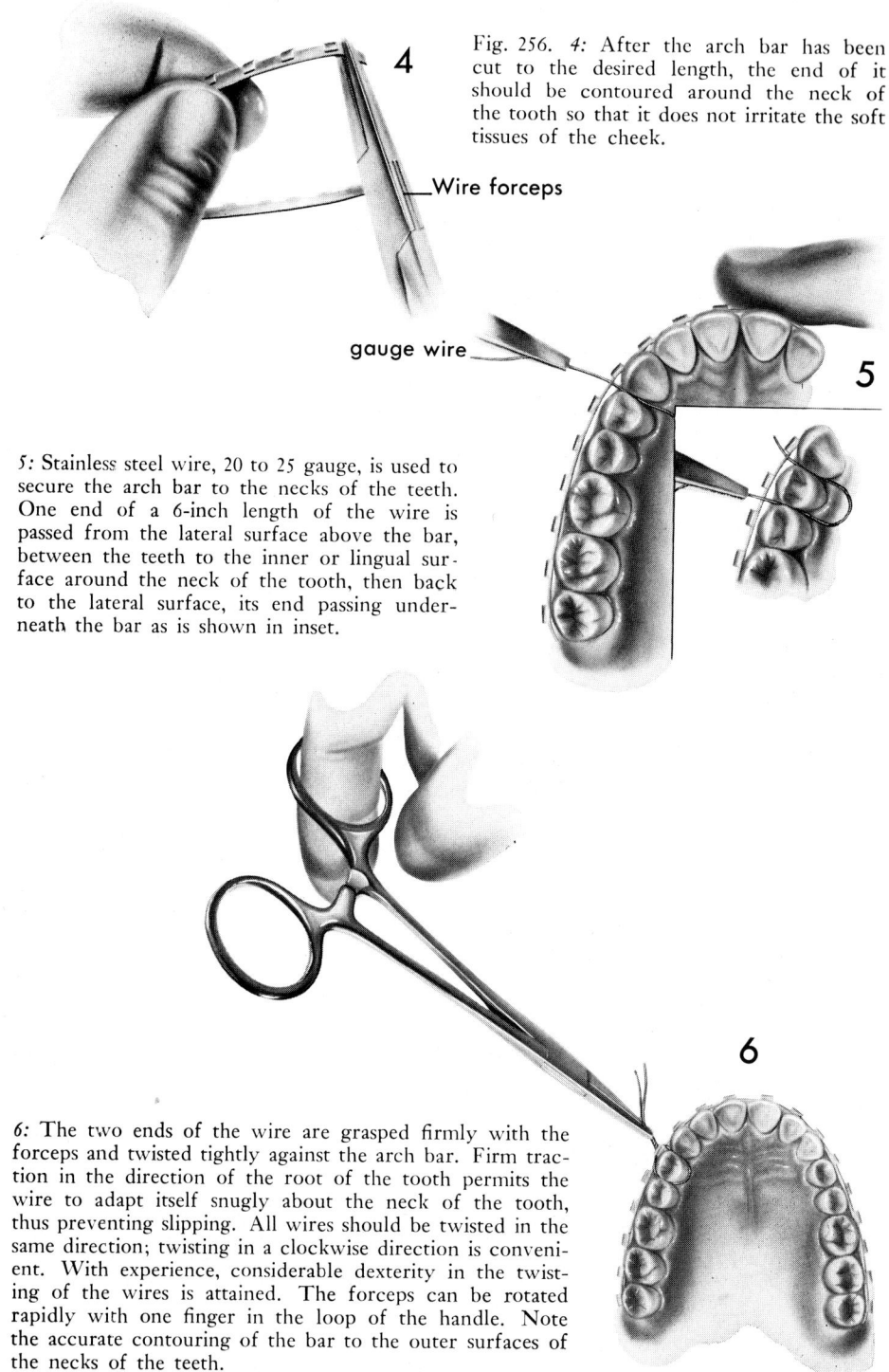

Fig. 256. *4:* After the arch bar has been cut to the desired length, the end of it should be contoured around the neck of the tooth so that it does not irritate the soft tissues of the cheek.

Wire forceps

gauge wire

5: Stainless steel wire, 20 to 25 gauge, is used to secure the arch bar to the necks of the teeth. One end of a 6-inch length of the wire is passed from the lateral surface above the bar, between the teeth to the inner or lingual surface around the neck of the tooth, then back to the lateral surface, its end passing underneath the bar as is shown in inset.

6: The two ends of the wire are grasped firmly with the forceps and twisted tightly against the arch bar. Firm traction in the direction of the root of the tooth permits the wire to adapt itself snugly about the neck of the tooth, thus preventing slipping. All wires should be twisted in the same direction; twisting in a clockwise direction is convenient. With experience, considerable dexterity in the twisting of the wires is attained. The forceps can be rotated rapidly with one finger in the loop of the handle. Note the accurate contouring of the bar to the outer surfaces of the necks of the teeth.

546

Fig. 256. 7: The bell-shaped crowns of the posterior teeth permit use of the simple loop in wiring the arch bar to the teeth. The bell-shaped crown favors the seating of the wire loop under the gingiva and prevents downward slipping when traction is applied. This figure shows the wire passing over the top of the bar on one side, around the neck of the tooth, and upward under the bar on the opposite side. Pulling in an upward direction also favors seating of the wire at the smallest circumference of the crown of the tooth. This permits strong force to be applied with the rubber bands without dislodgement or slipping of the arch bar.

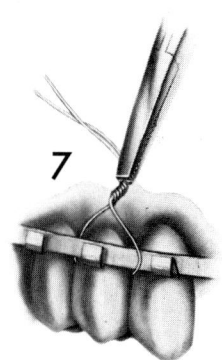

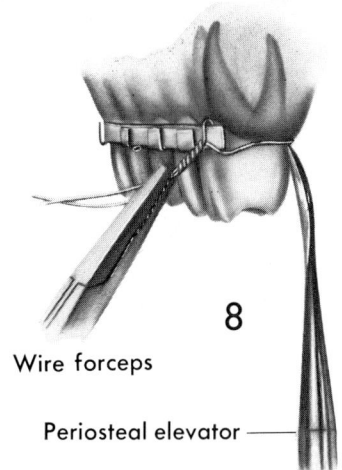

Wire forceps

Periosteal elevator

8: This cutaway section illustrates the placement of the wire around the neck of the tooth. If the wire has a tendency to slip downward while it is being twisted, it can be held firmly against the neck of the tooth or pushed under the gingival margin by the use of a sharp-pointed periosteal elevator. This places the wire in the position of least diameter about the neck of the tooth so that it will not slip. When applying the arch bar, it will usually be most convenient to start the wiring in the premolar region. The bar can be secured with one wire on each side to start the wiring procedure. This stabilizes the bar so that the wiring of subsequent teeth becomes less difficult. At this stage the bar can be rechecked for length and can be contoured to fit accurately against the necks of all the teeth in the dental arch.

9: The canine is a key tooth in retaining the arch bar, since its root is long and the surrounding bone is dense. Thus this tooth can withstand great stress. The shape of the tooth, however, is somewhat unfavorable for the retention of the ligature wire, because the crown is narrow at the gingival line and the wire has a tendency to slip, loosen, and permit movement of the arch bar. A special wire loop is effective in maintaining stability of the bar. Both ends of the wire are passed above the bar, one on each side of the tooth, and one of the ends is twisted around the bar in the form of a loop. When this wire is tightened, it has a tendency to adapt itself, beneath the gingival margin, to the root of the tooth, where usually it remains secure without slipping. The simple wire loop as shown in 7 is ineffective in ligating the arch bar to the canine teeth.

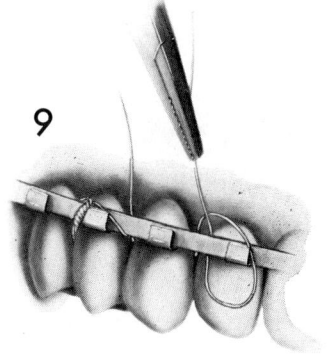

547

10

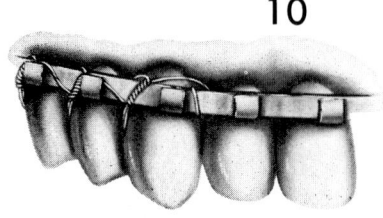

Fig. 256. *10:* As the individual wires are tightened securely about the necks of the teeth, they are cut at a convenient length with the wire cutter but are left long enough so that the ends can be tucked down between the teeth away from the soft tissues to prevent irritation. All the available teeth in the dental arch should be ligated to maintain accurate and adequate stability. However, the conical shape of the roots of the eight incisor teeth do not lend themselves well to the placement of ligatures. Strong intermaxillary forces with rubber bands may cause them to loosen from their sockets.

11

Latex rubber band

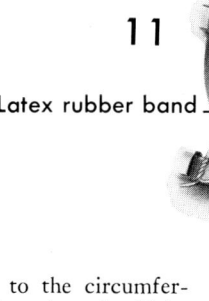

11: After fixing the arch bars securely to the circumferences of the upper and lower dental arches, they should be grasped with a forceps to test their stability. If either is loose, the wires should be tightened further and additional wires applied if necessary. Loosening of the arch bars, or movement of them during the postoperative period of fixation, is distressing and many times is difficult to correct by adjustment. Good quality, small rubber bands with high resiliency should be used. A few rubber bands on each side will exert strong traction. The direction of the rubber bands may vary with the individual case to produce the desired direction of movement of the segments.

Mosquito hemostat

12

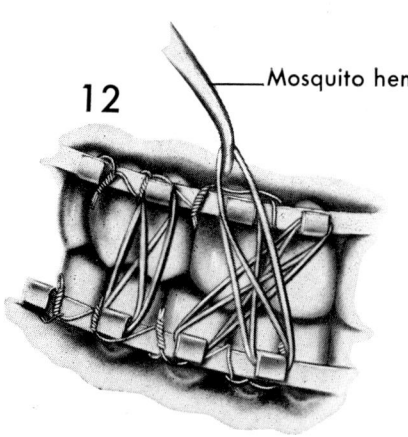

12: If the application of rubber bands in single loops does not seem to give adequate traction, the bands can be stretched and passed from the upper to the lower arch bar and again to the upper bar; in some instances bands can be stretched far enough so that they pass again to the lower arch bar. A small, curved hemostat is helpful in manipulating the rubber bands.

fixation constitute the method of choice. The prefabricated arch bar after Erich, made of malleable metal and supplied with hooks, can be shaped to the outer surface of the upper and lower dental arches. It provides an effective way to attach the rubber bands. The method of application is well described by Dingman and illustrated in Figure 256. In case of instability of the lower arch bar, one or two additional circumferential wires may be passed around the arch bar and the mandibular bones. The method of passing the circumferential wire is described on page 552. In cases of instability of the upper arch bar, Dingman recommends passing a wire through a small burr hole in the bony margin of the pyriform aperture of the maxilla on the left and right sides and, if necessary, through the anterior nasal spine; the regions are exposed from vertical incisions over the canine areas and at one side of the frenulum. The wires are firmly attached to the upper arch bar.

In cases of fracture with considerable displacement, it is advisable to place a separate arch bar on the teeth of each segment with elastic rubber-

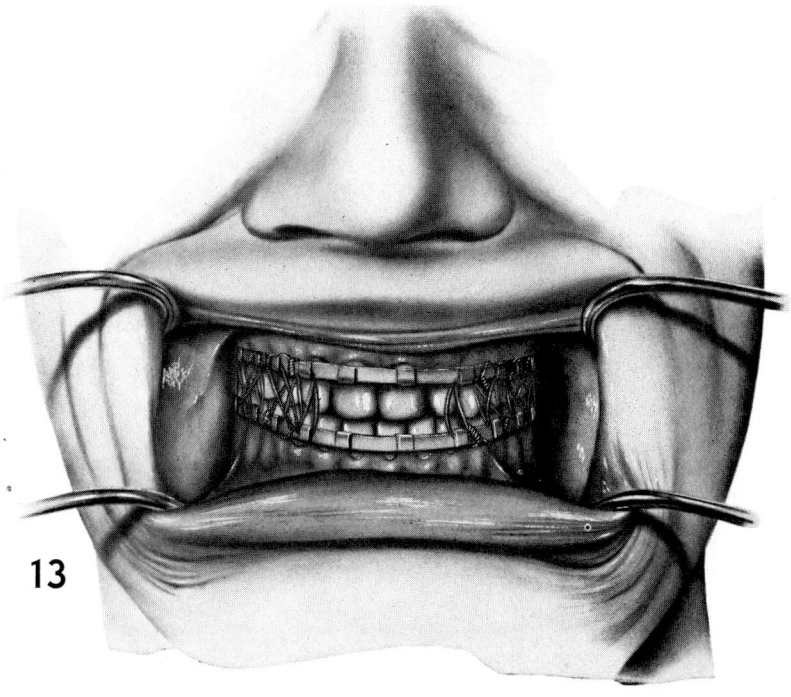

13

Fig. 256. *13:* Arch bars placed carefully on the dental arches, and ligated securely with all sharp ends of wire turned in against the teeth, provide excellent anchorage for intermaxillary fixation and are quite comfortable. The neat, thin bars and fine wire take up little room in the mouth and the patient adjusts to them quickly. (R. O. Dingman and P. Natvig: Surgery of Facial Fractures, W. B. Saunders.)

549

band pull until complete reduction has been obtained, and then to replace the separate arch bars by a single arch (Fig. 257).

If reduction of the fragments cannot be accomplished by the closed method, one should not hesitate to resort to open reduction and fixation of the fragments with bone sutures of thin stainless-steel wires. This is followed by immobilization of the fragments with interdental wiring or with the arch-bar method.

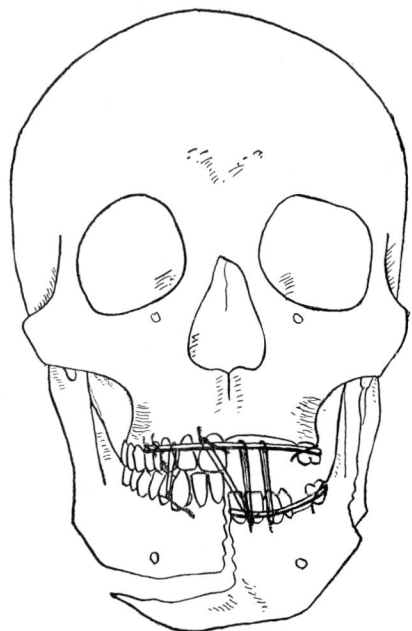

Fig. 257. (R. H. Ivy and L. Curtis: Fractures of the Jaws. Lea & Febiger.)

In simple transverse fractures, particularly those without much displacement of the fragments, internal fixation by means of a Kirschner-type wire, drilled from a small skin incision through the longitudinal axis of the fragments, as recommended by Ipsen (1933) and J. B. Brown and F. McDowell (1942), is a simple and effective method (Figs. 258 and 264). The end of the wire is buried beneath the skin. Additional fixation is unnecessary. The wire is removed after healing has taken place.

Interdental wiring is also effective in fractures through the neck of the condyle. Open reduction is hardly ever necessary. It has frequently been stated that this fracture, if the condyle becomes displaced, is followed by ankylosis or deformity unless open reduction is performed. Ivy, Curtis, MacLennan, and Wilde, however, who base their recommendations on great experience, treat the fractures at the neck of the condyle, with or without displacement of the head fragment, by the usual

550

THE OSSEOUS FRAMEWORK OF THE FACE

methods of wiring the teeth in occlusion and have invariably had good results. The author also agrees with J. B. Brown that in a number of cases the fracture is oblique with the posterior obliquity at the head fragment, thus preventing a forward displacement of the latter.

Cleansing, Feeding, Duration of Immobilization

A simple and effective way of cleansing the teeth and mouth is by application of hydrogen peroxide in any of the ordinary antiseptic mouthwashes. The vestibular surface of the teeth is cleaned with an applicator, while the lingual surface is taken care of by the patient himself by the use of his tongue and the same solution.

Feeding, as a rule, is possible by drinking tube; a liquid or semisoft, high-caloric, vitamin-rich diet is essential. Rarely, and then only during

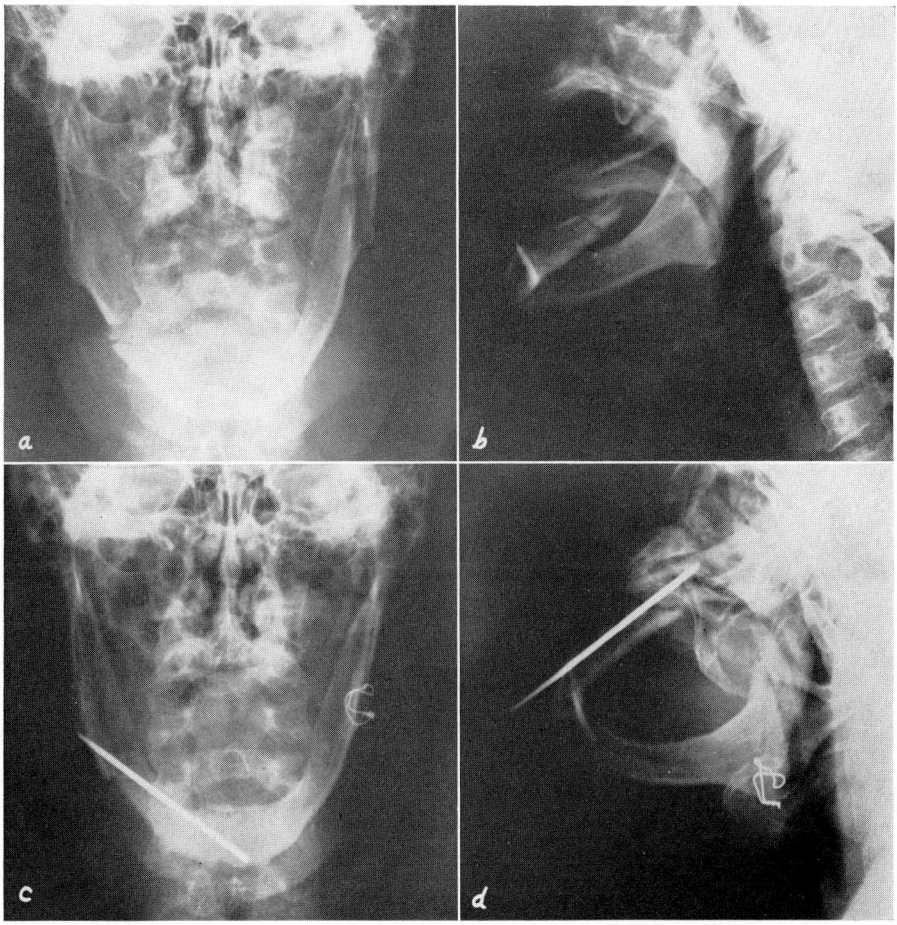

Fig. 258. *a-d:* Bilateral fracture of mandible; left side stabilized with intramedullary wire; fracture through angle of right side fastened with wire suture.

551

the first few days after the trauma, feeding through a nasal catheter may be utilized. An excellent small booklet that outlines the details of dietary management and contains suggestions for variations in the diet is published by Dingman. The manual is also useful to the ambulatory patient.

The fragments must remain immobilized until sufficient callus has formed, which in a simple fracture usually occurs between three and six weeks.

TREATMENT IN SPECIAL CASES

Fractures with Long Edentulous Posterior Fragments

In this case, the posterior fragment, owing to lack of opposition, is displaced upward by the pull of the elevator muscles.

For the majority of these cases, open reduction and fixation of the fragments with bone sutures of thin stainless-steel wire is a simple and effective procedure. This is followed by immobilization of the fragments by means of interdental wiring. Intramedullary wire fixation (see p. 550) will not be applicable, as a rule, owing to the obliquity of the fragments. Extraoral skeletal pin fixation (see p. 553) may rarely be considered.

Fractures through Angle of Mandible

These fractures are often impacted, requiring no special treatment. Otherwise, open reduction and fixation of the fragments with a bone suture of thin stainless-steel wire or insertion of an intramedullary wire (Fig. 258, *a* to *d*) may be indicated. If the former method is used, additional immobilization of the fragments by means of interdental wiring is usually required.

Fractures of Edentulous or Almost Edentulous Mandible

If the fragments are displaced, circumferential wiring of the mandibular bone (G. V. Black) over a vulcanite splint (Ivy and Curtis) provides sufficient stability. A vulcanite splint is first made like a saddle, to cover the alveolar ridge on each side of the fracture. In some cases, the patient's denture may serve as the splint.

From the lingual (posterior) side of the mandible, a curved suture-carrier (Fig. 268) is led along the posterior surface of the bone in close contact with the latter until the tip is felt beneath the skin of the chin. A small incision is made at this point, the instrument pushed through the opening, and then armed with No. 24 gauge brass wire. Instrument and wire are withdrawn, and the wire is disengaged. The instrument is reinserted, this time along the anterior surface of the bone until the tip can be pushed through the same small incision. The other end of the wire loop is engaged into the instrument and the latter withdrawn. Using the same entrance allows the wire loop to rest on the bone with no skin between; conducting the wire in the direction described makes its twist lie inside the mouth, facilitating later removal. The same procedure is performed around the other fragment. The fracture is now reduced, the vulcanite splint is placed upon the alveolar ridge bridging the line of fracture, and the wires are twisted tightly upon the splint.

In some cases, intramedullary fixation (see p. 550) may be a simpler and more effective method of stabilization of the fragments (Fig. 258, *a* to *d*). On the other hand, insertion of the wires may be more difficult than had been anticipated. If this is the case, the following method should be applied.

Extraoral Skeletal Pin Fixation: The indications for extraoral skeletal fixation are—according to Thoma—as follows: if a patient, as in wartime, has to be transported; if there is an insufficient number of teeth for interdental fixation; if many teeth are broken or loose, unsuitable for wiring or splinting; if jaws are edentulous; if there is displacement of an edentulous posterior fragment; if there are multiple fractures; if the jaw is to be stabilized when large parts of bone have been lost; if compound fractures are associated with extensive wounds; if bone grafting is indicated; if bone infection or dental infection is present; or if there are wounds which require irrigation and other local treatment.

The underlying principle is that of the dual transfixation of each fragment (after Roger Anderson, Converse and Waknitz, Stroub and others). Under anesthesia with intravenous sodium pentothal, endotracheal nitrous oxide and oxygen, or ether, and under aseptic precautions, two pins of medium-sized wire are inserted with a hand drill at an angle of about 75 degrees to each other at an elected position of one of the fragments. The pins must penetrate the outer cortex and also, slightly, the inner cortex. An assistant, not belonging to the aseptic operating team, steadies the fragment from the oral side. A pin clamp with a universal joint is slipped over each pin; a rod of proper size and length is slipped through the pin clamps and fastened by tightening the screw of the joint. The rod should project 1.2 cm. (½ inch) toward the fracture side. The same procedure is performed at the other fragment. Double universal-movement clamps are slipped over the contiguous ends of the rods. The fracture is reduced; a fixation rod is slipped through the double universal-movement clamp and locked by tightening the screws of the latter. In double fractures, one unit on each side is necessary for proper stability and fixation with an additional crossbar, which unites the two units (Fig. 259).

This method has the advantage of satisfactory immobilization, and it permits the use of the mandible. It also allows subsequent improvement of the position of the fragments, if necessary, since the universal-movement clamps may be unlocked and the fixation rod adjusted.

Nonunions and Bone Defects

Nonunions of the mandible, as with nonunions in general, are due to absence or lack of stimulation of the local osteogenetic forces. Actual bone defects are due to infection, destruction, or tumors of the mandible.

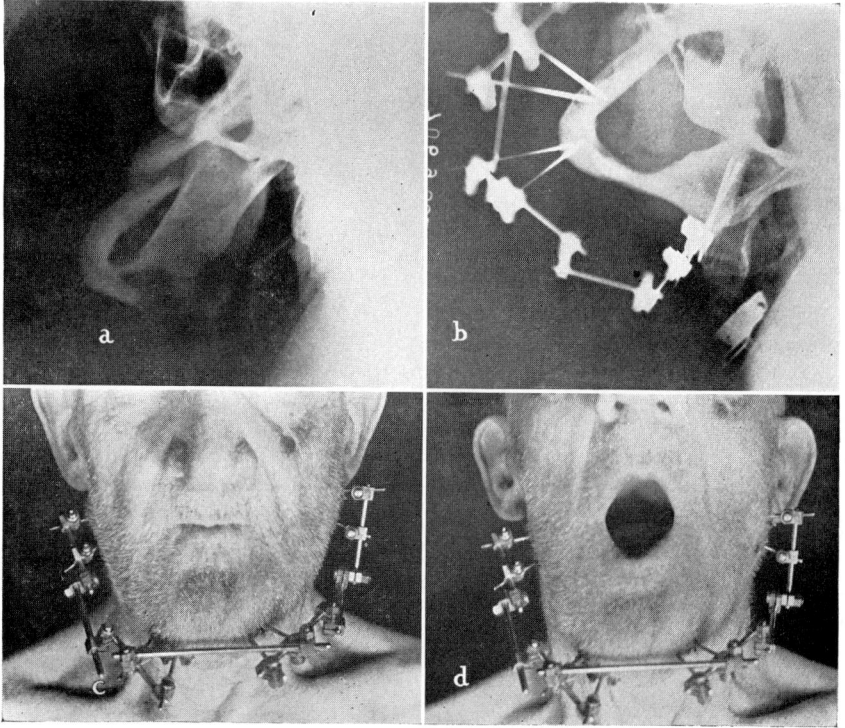

Fig. 259. Double fracture of an endentulous mandible. After reduction of the fragments, extraoral skeletal pin fixation was applied.

In these cases, the treatment consists in bone grafting, as first recommended by Sykoff (1900), whose technique was improved and standardized by Lexer, Garrè, Payer, Lindemann, Gillies, Risdon, Ivy and Epes, Blocker and Weiss, Stout, Macomber, and others. Ivy has presented a collective review of the literature on this subject up to 1951 and McDowell and Ohlwiler up to 1962. The principles do not differ from those for bone grafting in other regions: absence of infection for at least six months (preoperative and postoperative administration of antibiotics), presence of sufficient skin covering, removal of all scar tissue—particularly of all atrophic and sclerotic bone tissue—and prolonged immobilization. Immobilization, when enough upper and lower teeth are present, is not difficult to obtain, but may become a problem in edentulous or almost edentulous jaws. Hence, the problem of immobilization should be of primary concern; it should be solved preoperatively.

Preoperative Preparation for Immobilization: If interdental wiring is possible, the arch-bar method (see p. 545) should be used, since it guarantees better stabilization than the eyelet method.

The arch bars should be applied preoperatively, but upper and lower teeth should not be connected with each other until the patient is well out of anesthesia. In edentulous or almost edentulous jaws, special splints should be made of acrylic resin or other substance, fitting the upper and lower jaws and providing a feeding space; the splints are kept in place by supporting the lower jaw with a head bandage. Alternately, an acrylic splint is made like a saddle to cover the alveolar ridge on each side of the defect and held in place with circumferential wires as described on page 552. Extraoral skeletal pin fixation (see p. 550) may be the method of choice in certain cases. In any case, the ingenuity and collaboration of a skillful dental colleague are paramount.

Choice of Graft (Including Consideration of Foreign-Body Prostheses): The selection of the proper type of graft depends upon the location and size of the defect. Available are grafts from the anterior surface of the tibia, crest of the ilium, and occasionally a section of a rib and a metatarsal bone.

Iliac cancellous bone chip grafts have been introduced by Mowlem. Since then, cancellous bone from the crest of the ilium, either in blocks or combined with bone chips, have been found widely successful. The author prefers a massive graft from the crest of the ilium from which much of the cortical substance is removed. Such a graft is useful for filling the majority of mandibular defects. In cases where the ascending ramus must be replaced together with the condylar head, the fifth metatarsal bone with its articular surface is used (Fig. 260). Dingman reports a brilliant case of bilateral replacement of the mandibular condyles with metatarsal bone grafts (the fifth) from Risdon incisions. If the fifth metatarsal is too short to fill the defect, a piece of the eighth or ninth rib with a thin cartilaginous attachment is used; the latter replaces the condyle, and the curved part of the rib replaces the angle of the mandible. The graft should be transplanted with its periosteum. In still larger defects, bone grafts may not be available. If this is the case, one may use vitallium prostheses (recommended by Conley) or a stainless-steel mesh prosthesis (by Abbie et al.)

555

or an acrylic implant (after Healy et al.). Lovett, Brintnall and Grandon use an appliance consisting of a Steinman pin with a fabricated acrylic condyle head processed on one end and a separate thimble-type receptacle for insertion into the mandibular fragment. The thimble receptacle prevents forward migration of the Steinman pin. (The thimble may be re-replaced with nuts and washers as described by Warren and by Hamilton and Hardy.)

Technique (Fig. 261): From a curved incision (curved posteriorly) below the mandible, the bone fragments are exposed. All scar tissue is

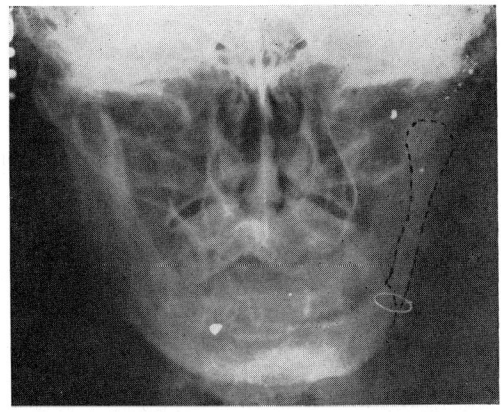

Fig. 260. Loss of left ascending ramus of mandible replaced with fifth metatarsal bone (including articular head). Immobilization of edentulous jaws with a splint of acrylic resin, fitting to upper and lower jaws and providing feeding space. Bony union after three months with full function.

removed, and—no matter how large the resulting defect—all atrophic and sclerotic bone ought to be resected until bleeding bone is encountered. Care is taken not to perforate the buccal mucous membrane.

The fragments to receive the bone graft are prepared in one of two ways: either by the staircase-like method (Fig. 261) or by effecting a broad transverse section. In small defects only the former method is suitable, while the fragments of large defects can be prepared in either way.

In the *staircase-like method*, the periosteum is elevated from the outer lower borders of the bone stump to form a pocket; with a bone rongeur, the lower cortex of the bone is removed for a distance of 1 to 2 cm. (⅜ to 1¾6 inch) until the medullary cavity is exposed. A bone graft is removed from the crest of the ilium, as demonstrated in Figure 32. It is advisable to remove all cortical bone to obtain a cancellous-bone graft, since cancellous bone regenerates more quickly than cortical bone. The cancellous graft is now prepared to fit into the prepared graft bed. All cancellous fragments should be saved so that they can later be packed into the dead spaces of the graft bed. Although the periosteal pockets of the host bone may hold the graft in place, the author prefers additional wiring by drilling transverse burr holes through the end of each fragment, feeding a thin stainless-steel wire through each hole, and twisting the wires upon the graft. The wires are cut short and bent backward.

In *large defects* the ends of the host bone are shaped so as to present a broad transverse section of bleeding healthy bone. A bone graft is re-

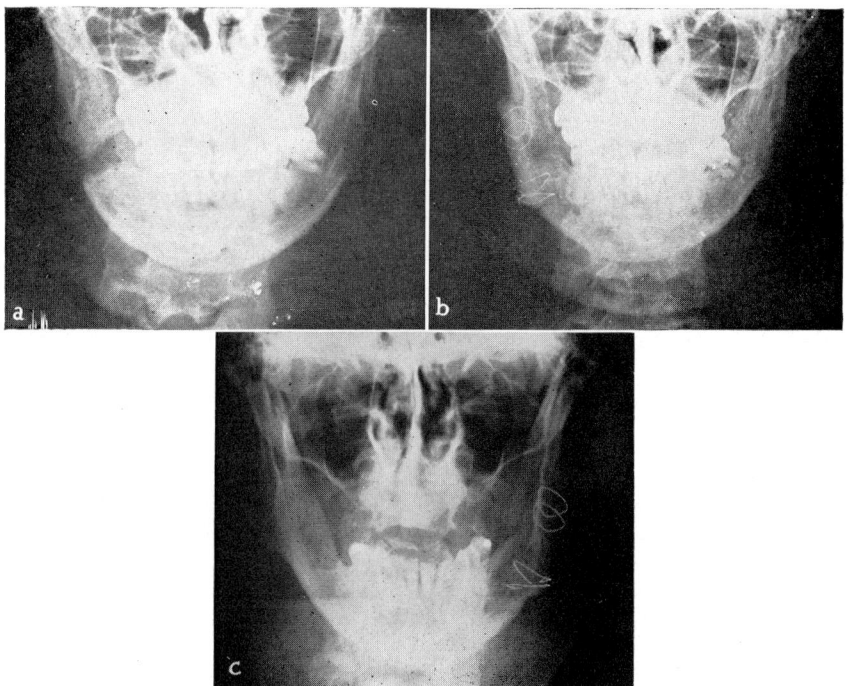

Fig. 261. *a:* Bone defect after sequestrotomy (osteomyelitis). *b, c:* Eight months and ten years after insertion of periosteum covered bone graft. Immobilization of jaws by interdental wiring for three months. (*c* is inadvertently reversed.)

moved from the crest of the ilium (Fig. 32), and shaped to fit snugly into the defect. To afford better stability in these large defects, it is advisable not to remove the cortical part of the ilium graft. A transverse burr hole is drilled through the end of each fragment and each end of the graft. A thin stainless-steel wire is threaded through the corresponding canals, twisted, and cut short. Closure of the soft tissues in layers follows.

In cases where the oral cavity has had to be opened temporarily—for instance, after resection of large mandibular tumors—Marino et al., Edger-

557

ton et al., Castio et al. (mentioned by Ivy), Conley, Millard, Obwegeser and others have reported success after immediate correction of the defect with a bone graft. It may be safer, however, to bridge the gap with a temporary prosthesis until healing has taken place, thus preventing shortening of the mandible from contracture. Freeman uses vitallium plates. Byar's method of insertion of a bar of stainless steel is simpler and just as effective (Fig. 262). Drill holes are made in the most dense part of the bone ends, and a thick Kirschner wire is snugly inserted into them. If pos-

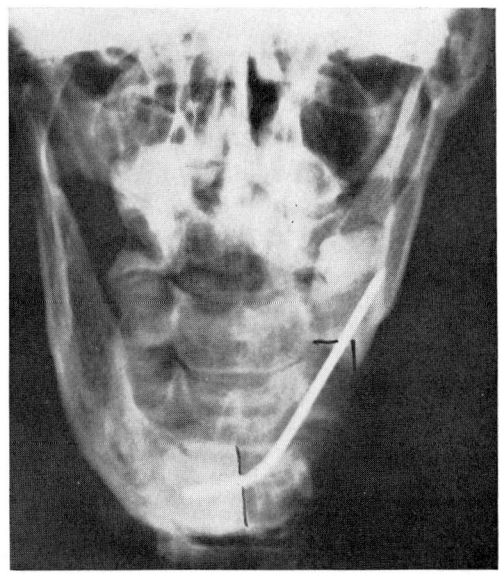

Fig. 262. Defect of horizontal ramus of left side of mandible after radical resection of cancer of floor of mouth. Temporary stabilization of fragments by insertion of stainless-steel bar inserted into drill hole of end of each fragment, eight years after insertion.

sible, the bar should be inserted so that the ends, contained in the bone, are slightly bent. Thus, the stress is distributed so that the metal ends stop boring through the rather soft bone. Yet perforation of the wire through the bone may occur. Hamilton and Hardy recommended the use of the webb bolt and Masson nuts and washers on a threaded Kirschner wire to prevent perforation. In one case the author used a single pin clamp as used in extraoral skeletal pin fixation (p. 553) as washer. The bar should be left in place as long as it is tolerated.

Time of Immobilization: The grafted mandible should be immobilized until an organic union has formed between host bone and graft, which—as a rule—occurs after the third month.

THE OSSEOUS FRAMEWORK OF THE FACE

FRACTURES OF MAXILLA

These fractures may involve the body of the maxilla or may be complicated, involving in addition the facial bones, such as the zygoma, orbit, nasal bones, and septum. They may be unilateral or bilateral. They are, as a rule, due to direct trauma and, in most instances, are compound fractures.

Fractures of Alveolar Process

The fractures either are due to direct hits or occur in the extraction of teeth. As a rule, they can be easily reduced by manipulation and held in alignment with arch bars fastened to the teeth of the fragment and those of the sound part of the upper jaw; interdental wiring with occlusion of the teeth may occasionally also be needed.

Unilateral Fractures of Body of Maxilla

In this type, a longitudinal fracture occurs through the midline of the maxilla, separating the fragment through the apertura piriformis, laterally somewhere above the level of the teeth and mediad through the midline of the hard palate. The fragment is usually pushed backward and either overrides and overlaps the sound side or is displaced laterally.

Treatment

Treatment of the fracture should be instituted only after shock or other complications, such as lacerated tissues, have been taken care of. The mechanical treatment consists of reduction of the fragments under general anesthesia (intravenous sodium pentothal) and retention of the fragments by wiring the teeth of the sound side of the maxilla to the corresponding ones of the mandible by arch bars.

Badly impacted mediad displaced fragments may need separation with chisel and mallet before manipulation is possible. In laterally displaced fragments which resist manipulation, Ivy and Curtis narrow the dental arch by elastic bands running transversely or diagonally across the palate, the bands being attached on each side to an arch bar on the teeth. The ends of the brass-wire ligatures attaching each arch to the teeth are twisted on the palatine side of the teeth to form hooks, which afford attachments for the elastic bands. Interdental wire fixation is needed after reduction is completed.

The internal-wire fixation method (p. 564) may also be possible.

559

THE HEAD AND NECK

Bilateral Fractures of Body of Maxilla

These fractures are either horizontal (low transverse, LeFort I) or pyramidal (LeFort II) or there is a complete separation of the facial bones from their cranial attachment (high transverse, LeFort III) (Fig. 263). The horizontal or low transverse type (LeFort I) runs either level with the apertura piriformis or higher and more or less parallel to the hard palate but below the orbital floor. The fragment (or fragments) is displaced backward and sags down posteriorly. In the pyramidal maxillary fracture (LeFort II), in addition to the above-described fragment which forms the base of the pyramid, the fracture line runs through the frontal process of the maxilla and the nasal bones through the lacrimal bone and the median part of the orbit; it then continues downward and outward through the wall of the frontal sinus and the zygomaticomaxillary suture to reach the pterygomaxillary suture and the pterygoid process. In the LeFort III case, the fracture is a high transverse one which separates the bones of the middle face from the cranium at the level of the floor of the orbital cavity through the zygomaticofrontal, maxillofrontal and naso-frontal sutures and through the ethmoid and the sphenoid.

The diagnosis is made according to the history (e.g., a heavy frontal blow), the clinical examination, which may however be handicapped by the massive swelling of the entire face, and roentgenographic evaluation. The clinical examination is the most important. Swelling of the face from subcutaneous hematoma, bleeding from the nose, conjunctival and scleral ecchymosis are always present; there may be malocclusion of the teeth and a marked downward displacement of the fragments, resulting in elongation of the face. If the fracture runs above the floor of the orbit, the eyeballs are displaced downward also; the face looks elongated. If a fragment is loose, as is usually the case, the fragment and the eyeballs move upward and downward when the patient opens and closes his mouth. If the fragments are impacted there may be a "dishface" deformity. A combination of maxillary fractures and fractures of the base of the skull may cause drainage of clear fluid from the nose. Palpation for abnormal motility and difference of contours is important.

Maxillary fractures, particularly the extensive ones, are often accompanied by such severe complications as concussion, shock, intracranial hemorrhage, severe lacerations, and emphysema of the cellular tissue of the face. Naturally, these complications deserve primary attention before the fractures are treated. Obstruction of the upper airways, if present, needs immediate attention by forward traction of the tongue and removal of obstructing material (fractured prosthesis, bone fragments, etc.). Trache-

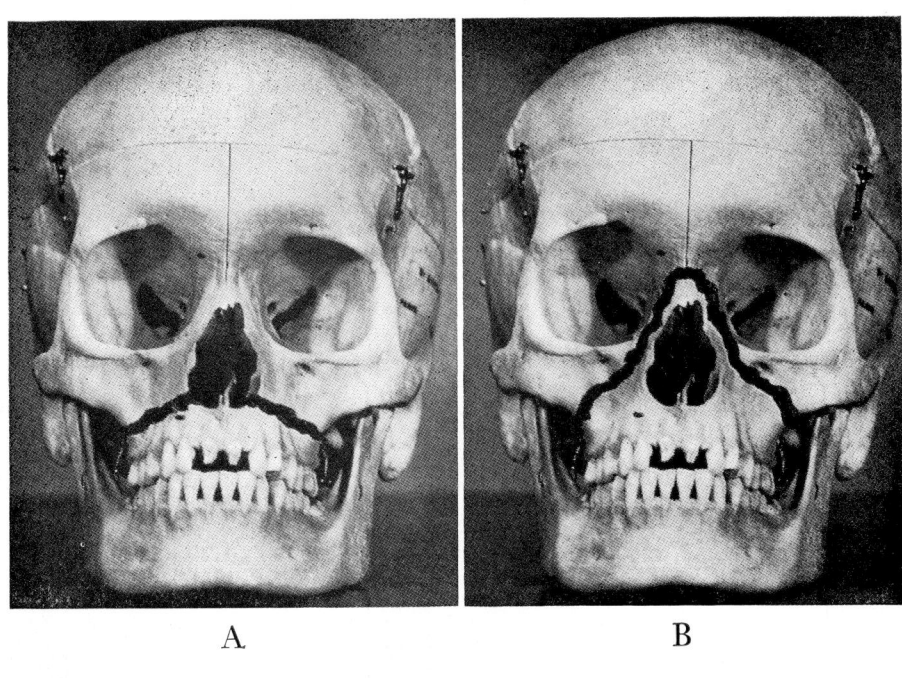

A.   B

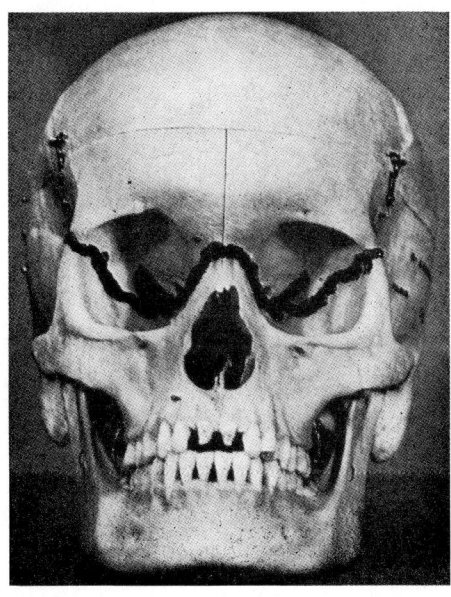

C

Fig. 263. *A:* Low transverse fracture (LeFort I). *B:* Pyramidal fracture (LeFort II). *C:* High transverse fracture (LeFort III). (Hogeman, K. E., and Illmar, K.: Acta Chirurg. Scand.)

ostomy may be necessary; it will also facilitate administration of inhalation anesthesia when the local treatment is carried out.

Treatment

The mechanical treatment starts with reduction of the fragments, which in posterior impaction should be done forcibly. No matter what direction the fragments are displaced, the teeth must be brought in apposition such that normal occlusion can be established with the teeth of the lower jaw. This occlusion is maintained by application of anteromaxillary

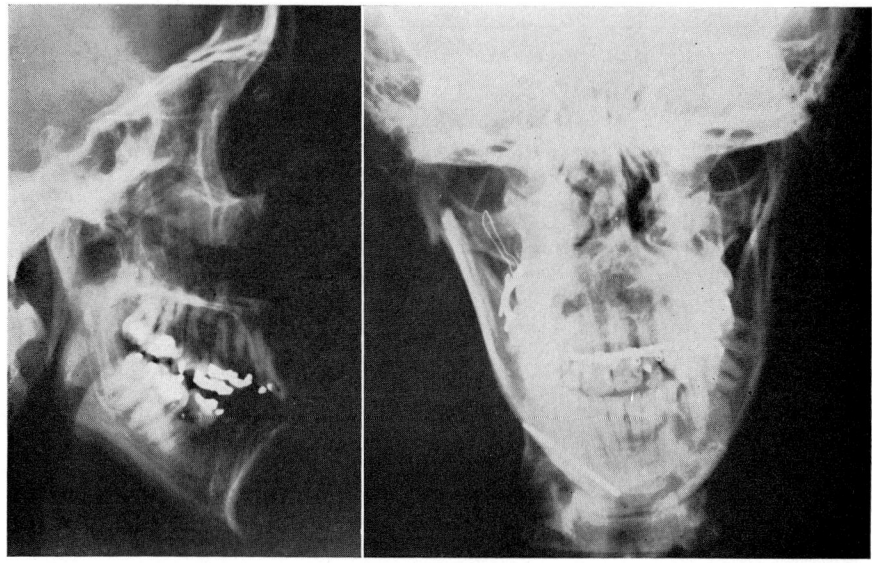

Fig. 264. *A:* Multiple fractures (four fragments, no loss of teeth!) of maxilla; separation of fragments from orbital floor (Le Fort I type). Fracture of mandible. *B:* Insertion of intramedullary wire for stabilization of fracture of mandible. Fragments of maxilla gathered and held together with arch bar. Interdental wiring. Maxilla suspended with a wire loop through hole in right orbital rim. (Compare with Case 50, p. 1060.)

arch-bar fixation (p. 545); thus the maxillary fragments are guided in the sagittal plane. Therefore, an intact mandible is of the utmost importance; if the mandible is fractured also the mandibular fragments must be reduced and stabilized before the maxillary fractures are treated (p. 545). The next step consists of suspension and fixation of the maxillary-mandibular compound to the neurocranium. This can be done in one of two ways: either by extraoral fixation to a skullcap of plaster of Paris or by internal wire fixation. The latter method, originally devised by Adams (1942) and enthusiastically endorsed by Dingman and Alling, Hogeman and others, is superior. The skullcap is cumbersome to apply and to wear.

562

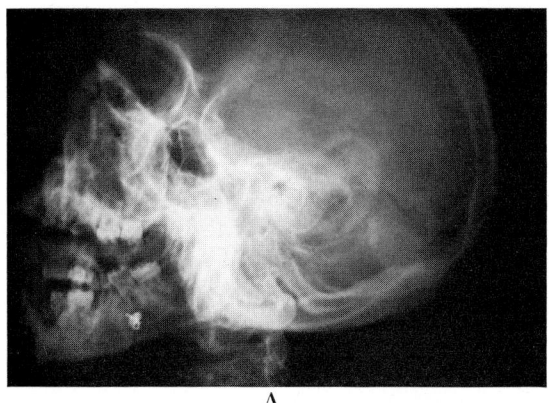

A

Fig. 265. *A:* Fractures of the upper jaw and facial bones of the LeFort III type (Fig. 263, C) and the angle of the left side of the mandible. Note tilting forward and downward of entire middle face fragment.

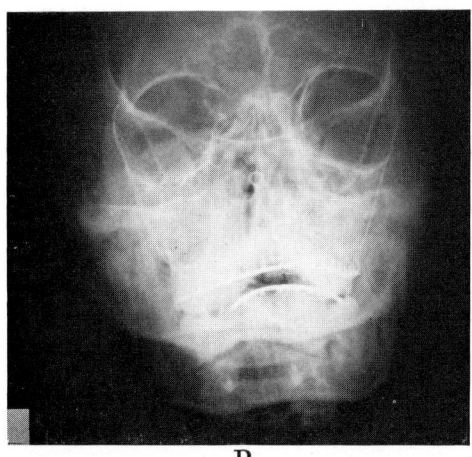

B

Fig. 265. *B:* After open reduction and wiring of mandibular fracture (see C) the upper jaw fragments were reduced and held together with an arch bar and interdental wiring. Then followed suspension of the upper jaw complex bilaterally with a wire through the upper lateral orbital rim above the zygomaticofrontal fracture line.

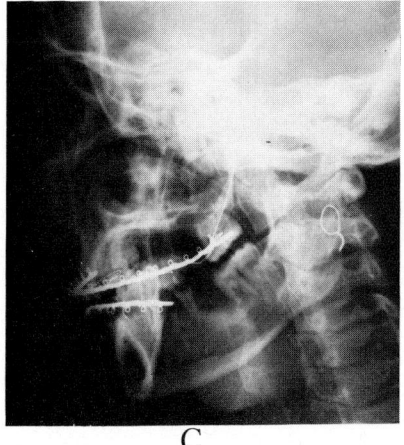

C

Fig. 265. *C:* Lateral view after reduction and suspension.

THE HEAD AND NECK

Internal-Wiring Fixation (Figs. 264, 265): By this method, fixation is achieved by suspending the maxilla with thin wires to the first solid structure above the fracture site. In transverse fractures below the floor of the orbit the lower rim of the latter (Fig. 264) or the zygoma is used for support. In higher fractures, the lateral wall of the orbit above the zygomaticofrontal suture is chosen for support. In low transverse fractures (Fig. 264), an incision is made along one of the wrinkles of the base of the lower eyelid; the intraorbital rim is exposed and the periosteum elevated. A drill hole of sufficient size to accommodate a No. 25 stainless-steel wire is made through the infraorbital ridge lateral to the infraorbital foramen. The wire is then threaded through the opening, looped over the ridge, and both ends armed on a long, straight needle are passed together along the anterior wall of the antrum into the upper sulcus opposite the second molar tooth. The same procedure is performed on the other side.

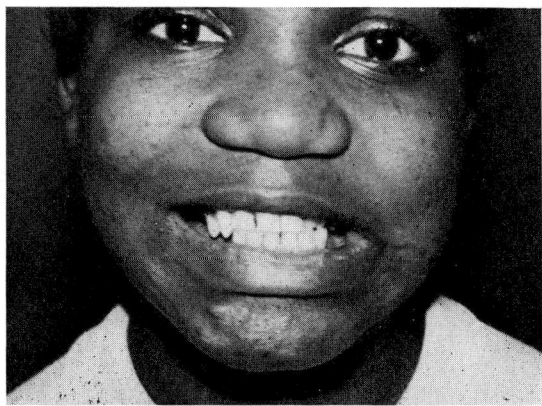

Fig. 266. Patient whose roentgenograms are shown in Fig. 265, two years after injury. Good occlusion of teeth.

An assistant pushes the chin upward—the teeth have been fastened in the meantime in occlusion by intermaxillary rubber-band traction—and the wires are looped around the upper arch bar drawn taut and twisted tightly. In edentulous patients the wires are tightened through drill holes in the prosthesis, which is sutured to the alveolar ridges.

In higher fractures (Fig. 265) with involvement of the lower orbital rim, the first solid structure above the fracture site which is the lateral wall of the orbit above the zygomaticofrontal suture must be chosen. The orbital rim is exposed through a small incision in the upper lateral part of the eyelid, just within the lateral extension of the eyebrow, and a drill hole is made. The suspension wire is passed through this hole and both ends armed on a long darning-like needle are passed down through the soft tissues median to the zygoma into the upper sulcus, where they are secured to the upper arch bar as described above. Wire suspension and intermaxillary suspension should be maintained for at least six weeks (Fig. 266).

564

FRACTURES OF MALAR BONE AND
ZYGOMATIC ARCH

These fractures are due to direct trauma. While the body of the malar bone seldom breaks, since it is strong, its processes are frequently fractured. The body may become separated from all its attachments (frontal, orbital, maxillary, and zygomatic processes) and depressed. Knight and North classify these fractures as follows: Group I, fractures with no significant displacement; Group II, arch fractures; Group III, unrotated fractures; Group IV, medially rotated body fractures; Group V, laterally rotated body fractures; Group VI, complex fractures. Freeman also points out that fractures of the orbital floor are more often associated with these fractures than formerly recognized. Even excellent stereo-roentgenograms do not reveal the true status of the orbital floor. Often only direct exposure and exploration of the orbital floor will show the need for correction (see blowout fractures, p. 569).

There is as a rule much swelling of the malar region so that it is impossible to evaluate the extent and details of the injury. After the initial swelling has disappeared the cheek is found depressed just below the lateral canthus of the eye, while lower down it may appear swollen. Involvement of the orbital floor results in dysfunction of the eyeball. Loss of sensation in the distribution of the infraorbital nerve is often found.

Treatment consists of reduction and retention of the fragments. The Gillies-Killner method is applicable only for depressed fractures of the zygomatic arch. Those isolated fractures, however, are encountered infrequently. Antral packing by gauze or balloons to elevate and stabilize the malar body becomes more and more obsolete because of inaccuracy and instability of reduction of the fragments, but it may still be useful in certain types of fractures. In most cases, however, open reduction is the method of choice. The author follows the technique of Dingman and Natvig.

Technique

Under endotracheal anesthesia the fracture sites are exposed from two incisions. The upper one, to expose the zygomaticofrontal suture line, is made through the lateral end of the eyebrow—brow not to be shaved—directly down to the bone of the orbital rim; with a periosteal elevator the periosteum is stripped away and the entire lateral orbital rim and thus the fracture site can be identified. Before attempting to elevate the zygoma the lower incision is made following the lower wrinkle line of the lower eyelid level with the crest of the infraorbital ridge. The fibers of the

565

musculus orbicularis oculi are split and the periosteum is incised along the rim of the orbit, care being taken not to injure the orbital septum. The periosteum is elevated from the upper surface of the infraorbital ridge, followed by elevation of the periosteum and preorbit from the floor of the orbit. This permits wide exposure of the orbital floor, to demonstrate any fracture in that region and to detect herniation of orbital contents into the maxillary sinus. (For treatment of fractures of orbital floor see page 569). A heavy periosteal elevator is passed through the brow incision into the temporal fossa on the median side of the zygoma (compare with Fig. 267). With the palpating hand placed over the prominence of the zygoma and with one of the fingers in the inferior wound, the zygoma is manipulated upward anteriorly and laterally into position. Depressed fractures of the zygomatic arch can be elevated through the same incision (or through an incision as illustrated in Fig. 267). After the fracture has been reduced, drill holes are made on each side of the fracture; the small burr is directed from the anterolateral surface of the orbital rim backward into the temporal fossa. A No. 25 gauge stainless-steel wire is passed through these holes so that the ends will come through on the posterior side, i.e., the temporal side of the zygoma. In the lower orbital rim the wire is passed so that the ends will escape on the anterior side. The wires are twisted tightly and cut; the cut ends are pressed against the bone. The periosteum is then sutured, followed by accurate approximation of the deep structures and suture of the skin edges.

As mentioned above, it may happen that the zygomatic arch alone has been fractured and becomes depressed without involvement of the malar body. If this is the case, restoration of the zygomatic arch can be accomplished by the Gillies-Killner technique.

Technique (Fig. 267)

The hair is shaved in the corresponding temporal region. From a small incision 2.5 cm. (1 inch) above and anterior to the upper attachment of the ear within the hairline of the temporal region, the temporal fascia is exposed and incised. A bone elevator is now inserted beneath the fascia; the instrument comes to lie upon the musculus temporalis, which inserts at the processus coronoideus. If the instrument is pushed downward, between fascia and muscle, it inevitably finds its place mediad to the depressed fragments of the zygomatic arch. A gauze pad is laid upon the scalp, posterior to the instrument, to act as a fulcrum and protector for the temporal bone. Downward pressure is now exercised upon the instrument, thus elevating the fragments. The reduced fragments usually remain in position without support, for there are no strong muscles attached to them. The wound is closed in layers.

In multiple fractures of the zygomatic arch, the fragments tend to fall back into the former depressed portion. They should again be elevated and while held in this position a No. 25 Kirschner wire should be introduced about 1 cm. anterior to the line of fracture. The wire is guided tangentially and superficially to the multiple fragments in the deep muscle layer adjacent to the bone until the stable posterior third is met (Adamson,

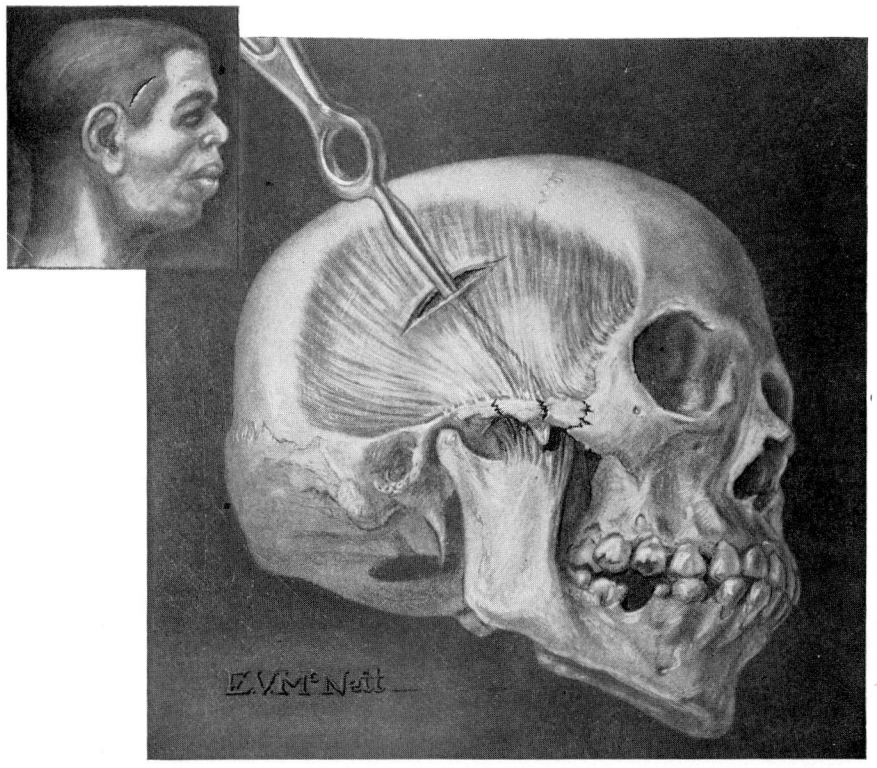

Fig. 267. Depressed fracture of zygomatic arch (reduction after Gillies). From incision within hairline of temporal region, temporal fascia is exposed and incised. Above elevator is passed between fascia and musculus temporalis until it finds its place median to depressed fragments. Pressure upon handle of instrument elevates tip of instrument and thus the fragments.

Horton, Crawford "external" pinning of the zygomatic arch). The wire is cut 1 cm. outside the skin and the end is protected with a cork; it is removed two weeks later.

In badly comminuted fractures of the malar body and fractures of the antrum and orbital floor, stabilization of the fragments with bone sutures may not suffice. Supporting stabilization can then be achieved by packing the antrum or by the internal wire-pin fixation. For packing the

567

antrum, iodoform gauze with balsam of Peru on it has been recommended. The author, however, favors a water-inflated balloon (rubber-glove finger on a No. 14 catheter after Johnson or a Foley catheter after Oakey). This is a more versatile method and permits adequate drainage; hence, elevation of the fragments can be carried out over a period of weeks instead of days.

Technique (Use of Foley Catheter after Oakey)

From an incision in the gingivobuccal fold above the second molar, a hole in the antrum is made with a chisel in the same manner as in the Caldwell-Luck procedure. If the fragments are badly impacted and cannot be elevated from the outside (by a pull or hook which is inserted beneath the zygoma or the orbital rim if the latter is depressed), reduction is aided by direct push with elevators from the antrum. A No. 20 to 24 Foley catheter is now selected and its tip is cut off; part of the main tubing is also removed, but the small tube which leads into the balloon part is retained. The catheter is inserted through the hole in the antrum and gradually inflated. When this is done, the position of the fragments must be controlled by outside molding; this includes the canthal region when the orbital borders are displaced. One word of caution: When the fragments are loose, there is more danger from over- than undercorrection.

Technique (Internal Wire-Pin Fixation after
Brown, Fryer, McDowell)

This method consists of stabilization of the fragments with a regular Kirschner wire, which is drilled from a solid area into the loose fragment. In comminuted fractures, it may be drilled through loose fragments without such a support, since there is the advantage of holding the fragments together. Before the wire or wires are inserted, the fragments must be reduced as outlined in the foregoing technique. The exposed end or ends of the wire are covered with adhesive or corks.

After-Treatment

Through postoperative x-ray films, the position of the fragments is checked. If a Foley catheter has been used and reduction of the fragments is found over- or undercorrected, further correction can be easily accomplished by inflating or deflating the balloon; this cannot be done after internal-wire fixation without removing the wire. Elevation is maintained for three weeks, and the balloon is then deflated. If the fragments remain in place, the catheter is removed; the hole in the maxilla closes quickly. With internal-wire fixation, it is well to leave the wire in place for at least four weeks.

THE OSSEOUS FRAMEWORK OF THE FACE

BLOWOUT FRACTURES OF THE ORBIT

Although sporadic publications of cases of depressed fractures of the orbit can be found in the literature prior to 1957, credit goes to Converse and Smith who have alerted the profession to the significant clinical entity which they call the blowout fracture of the orbit. Originally they considered the blowout through the thin areas of the orbit without fracture of the orbital rim a specific syndrome, not to be confused with other types of fractures of the orbital floor which are associated with fractures of the adjacent facial bones; later, however, they conceded that the blowout fracture can accompany multiple facial fractures. Cramer, Tooze and Lerman termed the isolated blowout fracture as pure and the other impure. Converse, Smith, Obear and Wood-Smith have recently reported about their ten-year experience.

Early diagnosis is extremely important but may be difficult because of orbital and preorbital edema and hematoma within the orbit and antrum. Initial diplopia may be misleading because of the edema of the orbital contents. The patient's inability to rotate the affected eye upward is a strong sign of blowout fracture. Exophthalmos is a significant diagnostic sign but may not be initially apparent due to swelling. Special roentgenological techniques to obtain a radiologic diagnosis of blowout fractures have been developed to show which of the various types of fracture the patient has incurred: a lowering of the thin areas of the orbital floor of the medial wall; the "hanging drop" seen in the small blowout fracture; the trapdoor fracture, which is a bone fragment hanging into the sinus on a periosteal hinge or the massive extension of the orbital contents within the maxillary sinus. In addition there may be fractures of the zygomatico-maxillary bodies. If roentgenograms are inconclusive but the clinical signs suggest a blowout fracture, treatment should be undertaken as early as possible to counteract imbalance and shortcoming of the extraocular muscles.

Technique

Under endotracheal anesthesia the orbital floor is approached transorbitally from an incision within one of the lower lid wrinkles in level with the crest of the orbital rim. The fibers of the musculus orbicularis oculi are split and the periosteum along the rim of the orbit is incised, care being taken not to injure the orbital septum above. Following elevation of the periosteum from the upper surface of the infraorbital ridge, the preorbita is elevated from the orbital floor until the blowout fracture is exposed. The inferior rectus muscle and other orbital structures are freed

569

from the area of the blowout. The bone may be delivered by means of a small hook and the continuity of the floor is restored with autogenous bone grafts or alloplastic material. The latter seems to be preferred by most authors. Freeman uses Teflon sheets 0.015 inch thick, Cramer employs silicone rubber (silastic (R)) less than ⅛ inch thick placed subperiosteally without suturing. The author uses silicone discs also (the latter should be cut large enough to bridge the defect and restore the stable adjacent portion of the floor). In impure blowout fractures (those associated with other fractures of the orbital floor and the middle face) multiple approaches are required (see p. 565) including possibly an intraoral antrostomy. These fractures should be treated as described on pages 565-568; restoration of the orbital floor will follow.

FRACTURES OF NASAL BONES

Fractures of the nasal bones are due to direct trauma. The resulting displacement of the fragments is in the line of force.

A force striking laterally separates the nasal bones from the frontal process of the maxilla or breaks the latter off, and severs the frontonasal sutures. The nasal pyramid is displaced in the line of force. The septum becomes deviated; in extreme displacements, it may even become dislocated from its insertion in the vomerine groove.

If the striking force is directed anteriorly, the nasal bones become displaced posteriorly and between the frontal process of the maxilla; they may also become displaced laterally, causing the flat, broad nose. In either case, the nasal bones become separated from their anterior and frontal attachments; the septum may break or become dislocated and deviated, causing marked obstructions and additional deformities.

Most nasal fractures are compound and comminuted, causing hemorrhage and marked swelling of the surrounding soft tissues. The swelling may be so marked that a correct clinical diagnosis is impossible. Intranasal examination for disclosure of any deviation of the septum may be of value. X-ray pictures may reveal the line of fracture, but—as a rule—are of little value concerning the relationship of the fragments.

Treatment

Fractured nasal bones without displacement do not need any treatment except that applied in injuries of soft tissues. Fractures with resulting displacement, however, should be reduced as soon as possible. The reduction is performed under local (cocainization) (see p. 409) or general anesthesia (intravenous injection of sodium pentothal).

Lateral Displacement: Reduction is accomplished either manually by pressure of gauze-padded thumbs on the deviated side or with a well-padded Kelly forceps. The forceps grasps the side which is nearest the midline (concave side). Since the fragments are not only displaced laterally but resting posteriorly and beneath the maxilla, the direction of the reduction must be anteriorly and outward (Fomon). After reduction of the fragments, the nasal septum should be inspected. If it is still dislocated, it should be forced into proper position with a forceps; if this fails, the dislocated edge should be lifted with an elevator and forced into the vomerine groove (p. 437). Immobilization is achieved by packing the nose with iodoform gauze, which should be removed after forty-eight hours. A medium-sized cork is halved longitudinally and placed with its flat side upon the deflected side and held with adhesive strips (see p. 438). Another method of immobilization is that of Blair, described on page 439.

Horizontal Displacement: In fractures due to forces striking from an anterior direction, the flattened nasal pyramid must be elevated. A bone elevator or any other suitable instrument, inserted beneath the fractured nasal bones, lifts the latter while thumb pressure molds the pyramid from the outside. A bilateral cork application (p. 421) may hold the fragments in alignment. In comminuted fractures with a tendency to spread, the fragments are kept in alignment with a mattress suture of thin wire, which is passed through skin, nasal bones, and mucosal septum on one side, then passed through the other side and back. The suture should be passed through lead plates on both sides.

Correction of septal deformities should follow the reduction of the bony fragments.

For treatment of old, unreduced nasal fractures, see page 436.

DEFORMITIES AND IMPROPER FUNCTION

MANDIBULAR PROGNATHISM

Mandibular prognathism is a protrusion of the mandible. Sometimes the external deformity is caused not by a protrusion of the mandible but by retrusion of the under- or malformed maxilla—secondary or pseudomandibular prognathism as classified by Hogeman. Such deformities are results of operations for clefts of lip and palate and are post-traumatic. They may require relatively simple procedures for revision as previously described for correction of the dishface deformity (p. 440), extensive rearrangement of the maxilla in form of the Le Fort I or Le Fort III fracture (p. 560), or even a combination of the two. It is beyond the scope of this book to go into details of these highly specialized procedures. The reader is referred to the works of such experts in this field as Wassmund, Axhausen, Gillies, Schuchardt, Converse, Wunderer, Hogeman, Murray and Swanson, Jabley and Edgerton, to the ingenious methods of Tessier, and Obwegeser's recent summary of his experience with this type of surgery. The following is concerned mainly with correction of mandibular prognatism by surgical procedures on the mandible.

If extensive, the protrusion of the mandible not only produces a deformity but also causes malocclusion of the teeth. The incisor teeth of the mandible are from 1 to 2 cm. ($\frac{3}{8}$ to $1\frac{3}{16}$ inch) in advance of the upper teeth. This, in turn, causes functional disturbances, such as disturbances of mastication and phonation. The condition may be congenital or due to developmental errors, such as faulty eruption of the teeth, or to endocrine disturbances (acromegaly). It is seldom the cause of trauma or infection. Before the ages of twelve to fourteen years, moderate degrees of prognathism can be corrected by orthodontic treatment. Later, and in severe cases, only surgery can correct the problem.

Many methods have been devised to overcome the deformity and to obtain occlusion of the teeth. The various operations can be divided into two groups, ostectomy and osteotomy. Although no single method is applicable in all cases, the preference of the surgeon for one technique may outweigh any slight advantage of alternate methods if satisfactory occlusal relationship can be achieved. A large list of references concerning this subject is published by Sarnat and Robinson. *Ostectomy* is performed from the body or angle or condyles of the mandible (Blair, Pickerill, Harsha, Dufourmentel, Schultz, Kazanjian, Henschen and Schwartz, New and Erich, Kitlowski, Dingman, Converse, Gonzalez-Ulloa, Smith, and others). *Osteotomy* is performed through the ascending ramus between the foramen and incisura mandibulae (Babcock, Pichler, Lindemann-Bruhn, Kostecka, Ivy, Scher, Schuchardt, Newman, Henry, Hogeman, and others).

The correction of various jaw deformities including prognathism has been well covered by Waldron, Kazanjian, Dingman, Converse and Shapiro. The author prefers bilateral ostectomy through the ascending ramus in cases of moderate protrusion and malocclusion; if accompanied by severe malocclusion, osteotomy of the body of the mandible is performed. This latter procedure is also apt to narrow the mandibular arch, which in more severe cases is usually larger than the alveolar arch of the maxilla.

Babcock was the first to devise osteotomy through the ascending ramus; he used an osteotome. Kostecka modified the method by using the

Gigli saw. The section is performed through the inferior alveolar foramen, thus preserving joint function and the integrity of the nervus alveolaris inferior. The thinness of the bone at this level may cause loss of contact of the fragments and nonunion, particularly after use of a Gigli saw. The author has not encountered this, but became aware of the possibility after a postoperative displacement of the fragment due to vomiting. To counteract this, the operation should be performed under local or sodium pentothal anesthesia. Others (Kazanjian, Pomroy and Cabrol, Converse) have advised an oblique osteotomy of the ascending ramus, establishing an outward and upward level in the lower fragment, and thus counteracting the pull of the external pterygoid muscle and preventing median rotation of the condyle and loss of bony contact. Other possible complications following osteotomy are serious hemorrhage from the internal maxillary artery and injury to branches of the facial nerve (frontal, mandibular); there is also the possibility of auriculotemporal syndrome (perspiration and reddish discoloration of the skin of temple and cheek area upon mastication) which Hogeman overcomes by resection of the damaged nervus auriculotemporalis. However, the advantages—namely, extraoral approach, avoidance of possibility of injury to the alveolar nerve, avoidance of extraction of teeth, and sacrifice of bone—outweigh the disadvantages.

The surgical treatment of prognathism can be divided into three stages, preoperative measures, the operation, and after-treatment. For the preoperative preparation and after-treatment, the congenial collaboration of a competent dental colleague is indispensable.

Preoperative Measures

These procedures consist of making casts of the denture, providing x-ray pictures, and splinting. With the casts on hand, the degree of protrusion is determined. The x-ray pictures are of value to define the position of the foramen mandibulare. Preoperative splinting in preparation of adequate postoperative immobilization can be performed in various ways. The most satisfactory retention splint is the half-round arch-bar splint to upper and lower teeth, as described on page 545.

Technique (*Transverse Section of Ascending Ramus after Kostecka*) (Case 84, p. 1098)

Before the operation, the previously attached arch bars of the jaws are connected to each other by elastic bands, thus counteracting sudden gross displacement of the mandible after the second side of the mandible is severed. A stab wound is made through the skin at the posterior border of the mandible, about 2 cm. ($1\frac{3}{16}$ inch) below an imaginary horizontal line passing through the center of the meatus acusticus externus. Blair's

573

full-curved special needle (Fig. 268) is introduced into the wound and passed around the posterior border of the mandible. It is then pushed forward between the median surface of the ramus and the musculus pterygoideus internus, in close contact with the bone, and emerges through a stab wound through the skin of the cheek at the anterior border of the ramus. In this way, neither the nervus facialis, the nervus alveolaris inferior, nor

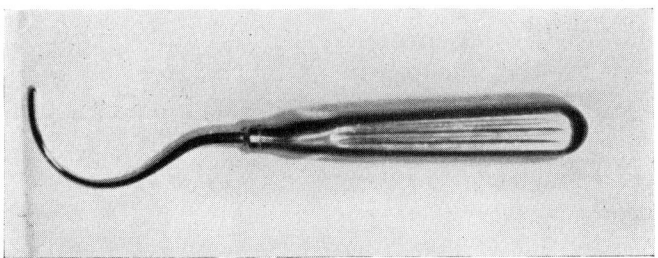

Fig. 268.   Blair's full-curved suture-carrier needle.

larger vessels are in danger of being injured; the oral cavity is not penetrated. The eye of the needle is armed with a strong silk thread, which is attached to a Gigli saw. Needle, thread, and Gigli saw are withdrawn through the first incision. With the Gigli saw in place, the ramus is severed between foramen mandibulare and incisura mandibulae (compare with Fig. 252). The same procedure is carried out on the other side. Bleeding is arrested by pressure.

The body of the mandible is then pushed back until satisfactory occlusion of the teeth is obtained. The previously attached arch bars of upper and lower teeth are connected with brass tie wires (compare with Fig. 255).

After-Treatment

Postoperative care does not differ from that of mandibular fractures (see p. 551). Position of fragments should be checked by x-ray examination. The connecting wires should be tightened weekly. Immobilization is required for eight to ten weeks.

Technique (Oblique Section of Ramus after Pomroy-Cabrol, Kazanjian-Converse) (Fig. 269)

A vertical incision about 1.5 cm. (⅝ inch) in length is made through the skin along the posterior border of the ramus, just above the angle where the ramus is felt immediately beneath the skin, thus avoiding the parotid gland and facial nerve. Following the incision, the subcutaneous tissues

574

are separated by blunt dissection and the periosteum is exposed and incised widely; the insertions of the masseter muscle are then elevated subperiosteally. The soft tissues are raised and the lateral surface of the ramus exposed by means of an elongated retractor. With a narrow osteotome

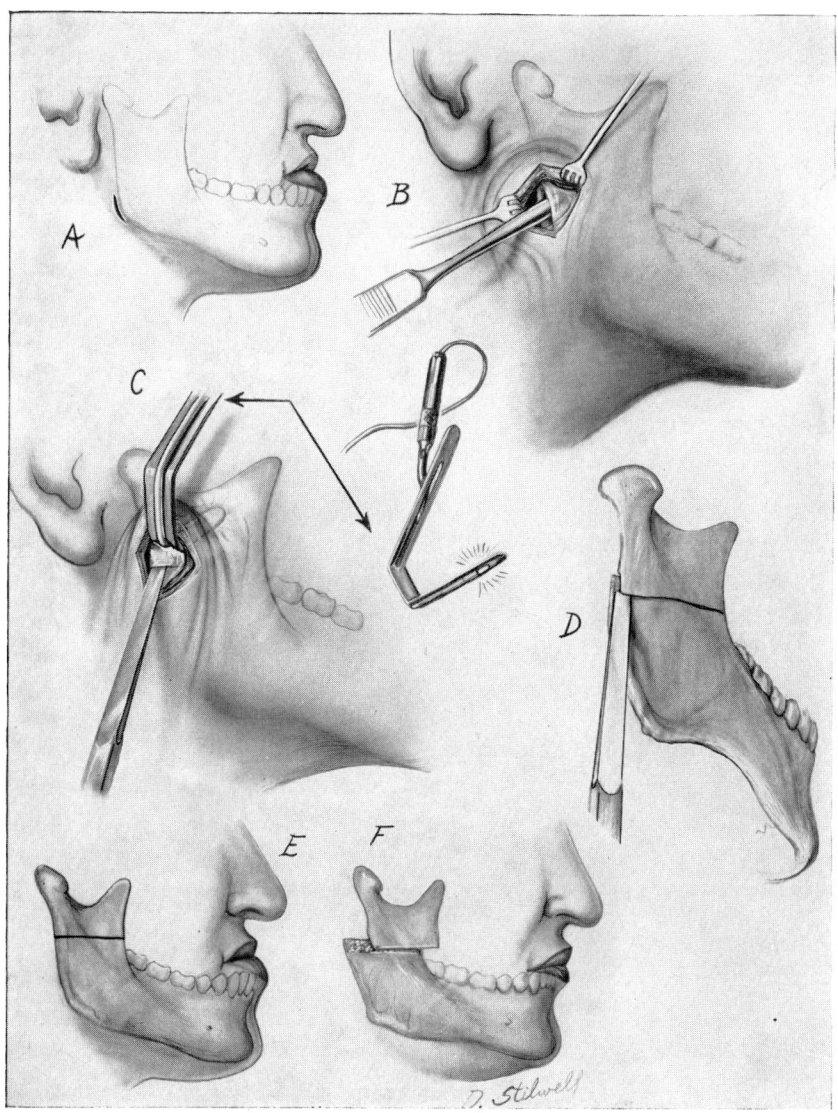

Fig. 269. Technique of osteotomy of the ramus for correction of mandibular prognathism. *A:* Small external incision made above the angle of the jaw. *B:* The periosteum and masseter muscle are raised from the outer aspect of the ramus. *C:* Subperiosteal retraction, with an illuminated retractor, gives exposure for osteotomy. *D:* The osteotome, introduced from below, cuts through the ramus obliquely. *D,* *F:* Backward displacement of the mandible after osteotomy. (Converse, J. M.: Plast. Reconstr. Surg.)

under direct vision, the ramus is cut on the bevel obliquely from below upward; the line of section is established above the inferior alveolar foramen. It lies about 2 cm. (¾ inch) below an imaginary horizontal line passing through the center of the meatus acusticus externus. The level of the inferior alveolar foramen may be located on the outside of the face previous to the osteotomy (the lateral x-ray film of the skull should be noted). For the steps following repositioning and the after-treatment, see previous technique.

Technique (Intraoral Step Osteotomy of Body of Mandible after Kazanjian-Converse) (Figs. 270-272) (Case 85, p. 1099)

The indication for this operation has been discussed on page 572. Antibiotics are routinely employed pre- and postoperatively. It is usually necessary to extract a bicuspid tooth on each side. A large horseshoe-shaped incision is made through the mucosa of the cheek, just lateral to the gingival sulcus from the mental to the retromolar region. The mucosa is dissected away from the underlying muscle until the lower border of the mandible is exposed. The periosteum is incised along the lower border and a mucoperiosteal flap is raised to expose the lateral surface of the mandible, the foramen mentale being located and exposed. This indicates the level of the inferior alveolar canal, which can be exposed by removing the outer table of bone with a large, round dental burr. Thus, the inferior alveolar bundle comes into view and can remain under direct vision and be safeguarded during the following procedure (should the nerve be accidentally severed, as happened in one of the author's cases unilaterally and in another bilaterally, regeneration does occur after varying periods of time). A step osteotomy is now performed through the mandible, with removal of an upper and a lower segment of bone (Fig. 271). The upper one is posterior to the alveolar foramen and above the alveolar canal; the lower one is anterior and inferior to the foramen. The tooth above the bone to be resected, if it is present, is extracted. The segments are marked out on the cortex of the mandible by a groove made with the electrically driven burr. With the same burr, the mandible is perforated along the step-like line of osteotomy (Fig. 270, *E*), at first vertically from the posterior border of the socket of the extracted tooth to a point some distance below the mental foramen (to avoid damaging the roots of the teeth), then forward in the horizontal plane to the anterior border of the lower bone segment, which is to be removed later. From here, a vertical line of perforation is extended downward to the lower border of the mandible. The upper and the lower bone segments are now outlined with perforations (Fig. 271, *A*). The bone between the holes is cut through with a fissure burr, and the fracture and excision of the two bone segments are completed with a

576

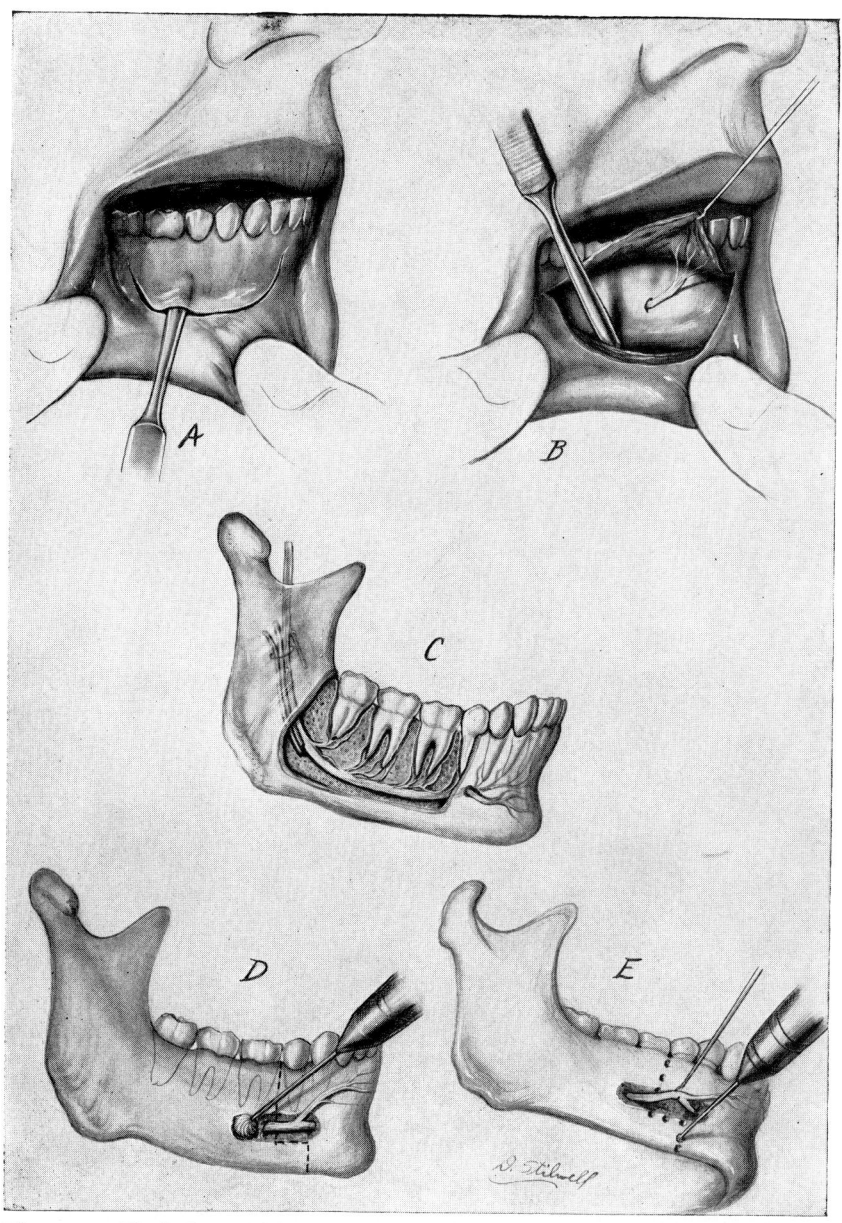

Fig. 270. Technique of intraoral step osteotomy of the body of the mandible for correction of mandibular prognathism. *A:* Wide flap to expose the lateral aspect of the body of the mandible. The periosteum is being raised. *B:* The outer aspect of the body of the mandible is exposed; the branches of the mental nerve are preserved. *C:* Drawing, representing the inferior alveolar nerve trunk, showing the mental nerve and the anterior inferior alveolar branch (shaded). *D:* The inferior alveolar canal is uncovered by removing the outer plate, thus exposing the neurovascular bundle. *E:* Step osteotomy is performed without sectioning the inferior alveolar neurovascular bundle. (Converse, J. M.: Plast. Reconstr. Surg.)

narrow osteotome. However, before the section of the bone it is helpful to make drill holes for wiring the bones together. The separated rami are approximated and fixed by wiring the bone ends together and by interdental wiring appliances made and secured to the teeth before the operation (compare with Fig. 272). These consist of a mandibular splint of arch bar constructed in three parts (see also p. 545) and an arch bar to the upper teeth.

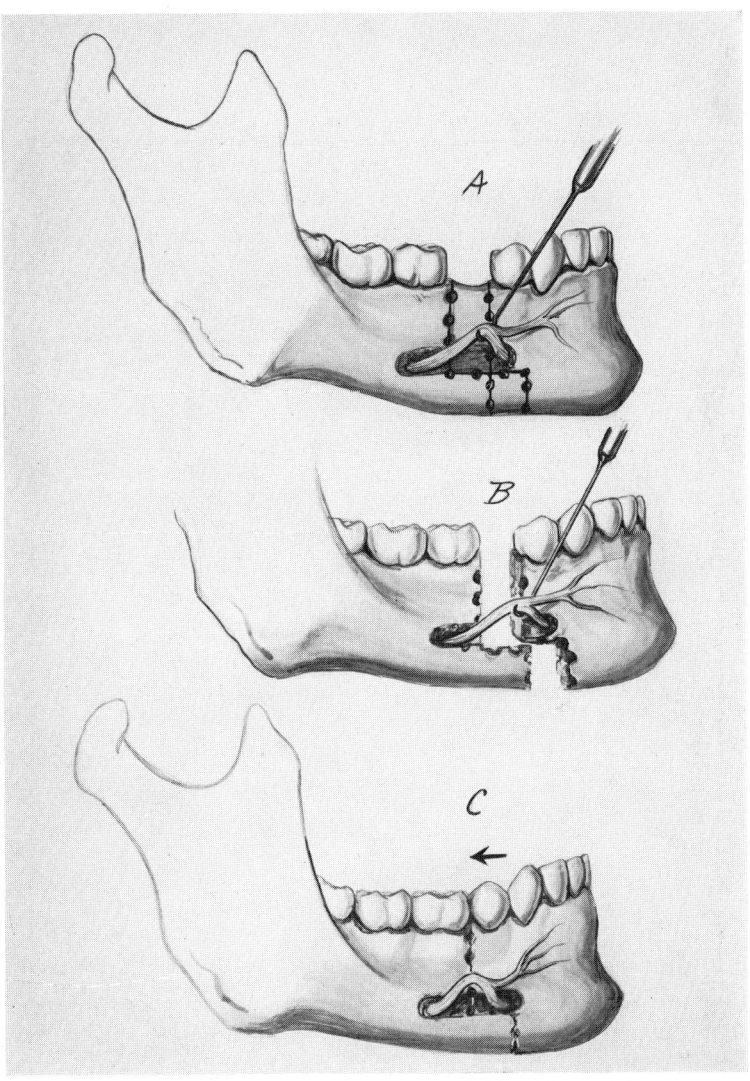

Fig. 271. Step osteotomy with resection of a bone segment to shorten the body of the mandible. *A:* The inferior alveolar canal and neurovascular bundle are exposed. *B:* A segment of bone, determined preoperatively, is removed. *C:* The anterior segment is moved posteriorly, achieving contact of the fragments. Pinching of the inferior alveolar nerve is avoided. (Converse, J. M.: Plast. Reconstr. Surg.)

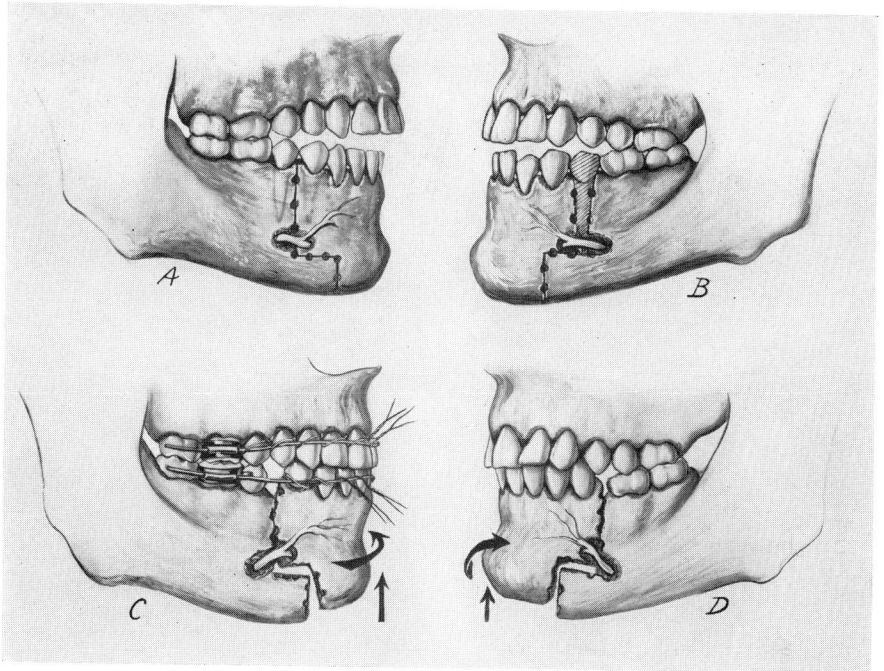

Fig. 272. Technique for surgical correction of open-bite. *A:* Step osteotomy follow-ing exposure of the inferior alveolar nerve on the right side. *B:* On the left side, removal of a tooth permits the resection of a V-shaped segment of bone. Step osteotomy follows. *C, D:* The anterior segment of the body is displaced upward and rotated forward and toward the left side. (Converse, J. M.: Plast. Reconstr. Surg.)

Crushing or pinching of the nervus alveolaris is avoided by wide decom-pression of the canal. The two mucoperiosteal flaps are reflected back and sutured. A figure-of-8 Barton bandage (Fig. 253) is applied for pressure to prevent hematoma and to aid in fixation.

Dingman uses the staircase type of section only in cases where the posterior fragment is edentulous; in other cases he uses a straight section through the mandible. He also operates from an inside incision for sever-ance of the upper half and from an outside incision (well below the man-dibular branch of the facial nerve) for section of the lower half of the bone. The fragments are held together with a wire suture.

RETRUSION OF MANDIBLE

Shortening of the mandible may occur on one or both sides. It is rarely congenital; in the majority of cases, it is due to trauma or disease or to faulty eruption of the teeth. In some cases, especially in ankylosis

579

of the jaw from accidents during childhood, it is due to failure of development because of lack of muscle function (Thoma). The retrusion may or may not be associated with malocclusion of the teeth. In the former case, it causes a deformity plus functional disturbances, such as disturbance of mastication and phonation. In the absence of malocclusion, retrusion constitutes a deformity only. In retrusion unassociated with malocclusion, the deformity is corrected by building up the chin contours with grafts, such as fat (Lexer, Newman), bone or cartilage (New, Erich), or alloplastic material such as silicone implants, or by a horizontal osteotomy of the mandible through the mandibular body below the inferior alveolar canal with forward sliding of the fragment (Hafer, Obwegeser, Converse).

The various methods for correction of retrusion associated with malocclusion can be divided into: osteotomies through the ramus (Blair and Ivy, Padgett, Scher, and others), through the body (Bruhn, Kazanjian, and others), through the body associated with transplantation of bone grafts (Limberg), insertion of cartilage implants behind the head of the condyles (Babcock), and intraoral insertion of prosthetic appliances into an epithelium-lined pocket between lip and mandible (Gillies).

Technique (Retrusion Unassociated with Malocclusion)

In slight to moderate retrusions, particularly those associated with hump noses, the techniques described on page 422 are applicable. In more advanced cases either Converse's intraoral technique of inserting an iliac bone graft is used, thus obviating an external scar—the method has its limitations—or the external approach is chosen.

Intraoral Approach (Fig. 273; Case 86, p. 1100): In using this approach, certain precautions must be taken. A bone graft is used to build up the chin. The bone graft is taken before the intraoral exposure of the mandible; it is placed subperiosteally, which causes an advancement of the lower lip and the musculature. This places tension upon the mucosa of the lower lip, and may result in gaping of the mucosal wound edges. Hence, the incision must be placed high above the cul-de-sac of the sulcus to permit easy closure. A thick mucosal flap is dissected to the periosteum; the latter is incised and raised with a sharp periosteal elevator, exposing the mandible. Elevation of the periosteum is extended downward to the lower border of the symphysis, and may be extended laterally to the mental foramen or even beyond. An incision about 2 cm. (¾ inch) in length, usually placed to the side of the frenulum, gives adequate exposure for small implants. For wider exposure when larger grafts are used, an incision about 5 cm. (2 inches) in length is required, extending across the inner surface of the lower lip. Even in the wider exposures, the mental nerve and vessels remain attached to the soft tissue, thus permitting bone grafting either anterior or posterior to the foramen. An iliac bone graft (from median plate of ilium) (for removal of graft, see p. 70), comprised of cortical and cancellous portions, is removed and suitably shaped by trimming the cancellous part and placing the cortical portion against the mandible. The cortical part may be bent to yield to the contours of the mandible. Numerous chips of cancellous bone are used to supplement the main bone graft. These chips are placed between the bone graft and the mandible to support the graft and to provide projection to the implant. Such chips are also packed in the interstices between the bone graft and the host bone to eliminate dead space. Flat pieces of bone are used to shape the contour of the lateral areas of the body of the mandible. Traction-guide sutures are useful when placing chin implants (Fig. 273). These are removed at the end of the operation. The implants are further maintained in correct position by strips of elastoplast on the skin over the grafts. The first strip is placed in the labiomental groove to maintain the graft over the symphysis. Successive strips of elastoplast are then placed over the chin. These are anchored by strips of adhesive to maintain firm immobilization for five to seven days. Instead of bone graft, diced cartilage graft (see p. 64) can also be used. The grafts can be molded to conform to the contours. Safian, Millard and others use silicone implants which, however, do not become an organic unit with the host bone and are apt to slide (see also p. 422, Case 55).

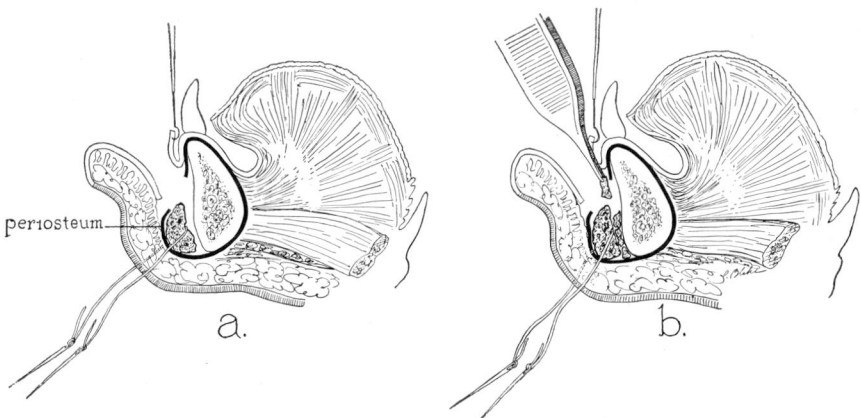

Fig. 273. Intraoral approach for bone grafting in correction of mandibular retrusion. Use of traction sutures for the placing of bone grafts in the region of the symphysis via the intraoral approach. *a:* The bone graft is held in correct position by guide-traction sutures placed through the soft tissues of the chin. *b:* Bone chips are packed between the host bone and the bone graft in order to provide sufficient projection of the graft. (Converse, J. M.: Plast. Reconstr. Surg.)

THE HEAD AND NECK

Extraoral Approach (Cases 87, 88, pp. 1101, 1102): An incision is made below the chin through skin, subcutaneous tissue, and muscles. Either two superimposed cartilage grafts (for removal, see p. 63) or an iliac bone graft (from crest of ilium) is used (for removal, see p. 70); the latter consists of cortical and cancellous portions. It is suitably shaped by trimming the cancellous part. The cortical part comes to lie against the body of the mandible. A pocket is prepared in front of the mandible by stripping of soft tissues and periosteum from the bone. The graft is fastened to the bone by drilling holes through graft and bone in such a way as to allow the passage of two mattress sutures of stainless steel (Fig. 274). Or two Kirschner wires may be drilled obliquely (about 75 degrees to each other) through the graft or grafts into the mandible which they should penetrate. The wires are cut short and bent upon the graft. For use of silicone implants see page 422.

HORIZONTAL OSTEOTOMY OF THE MANDIBLE

Hofer in 1942 described a technique for horizontal osteotomy through the mandibular body below the level of the inferior alveolar canal with forward sliding of the lower mandibular segment. He used the extraoral approach and left platysma, digastric and geniohyoideus muscle attached to the horseshoe-shaped section of the bone. Obwegeser improved the method by using the intraoral approach and severed the muscles to avoid an effacement of the chin-neck line. Converse endorses this method and has used it also for correction of chin deviation and reduction of excess vertical height of the mandible, whereby the sectioned bone is used as a graft and placed upon the mandible. The bone is exposed as shown in Figure 273. Since, however, a wider exposure is required, great care must be taken not to sever the mental nerve also. The horizontal osteotomy is made with the Stryker sagittal plane saw along a level immediately below the inferior alveolar canal terminating at a point immediately anterior to the mental foramen; from there a right angle extension to the inferior border of the mandible is made. When an oblique section is planned, the line of section continues backward beyond the level of the mental foramen. The platysma and the digastric muscle are severed from the sectioned bone and the geniohyoideus muscle is incised. If the lateral portions of the segment are broad and overlapping, the mandibular body when slid forward should be adjusted with a rongeur. The detached segment of the mandible is then advanced anteriorly. Bone grafts may be employed to fill the lateral gaps. Fixation is achieved by the use of circumferential wires. The mucosal flap is sutured into position with catgut sutures. An elasto-

582

plast dressing is applied to the mental region as described on page 581. The circumferential wires are removed between four to six weeks.

Technique (Retrusion Associated with Malocclusion)

If the retrusion of the mandible is associated with ankylosis of the temporomandibular joints, arthoplasty should be performed first (Kazanjian) (see p. 586). In bilateral ankylosis, a two-stage procedure is preferable. It is also important to make provision for immobilization of the mandible following operation (see p. 545). For correction of the retrusion, the author prefers the osteotomy through the ramus and sliding the mandible forward (pp. 573-574) (Lindemann, Axhausen, Wassmund, Schuchardt). The step osteotomy through the body of the mandible, as described on page 576, is also available (compare with Fig. 271). To permit good coaptation of the bone, the horizontal fracture line must be made sufficiently long. The step of the osteotomy line also needs reversal, namely, posteriorly instead of anteriorly to assure a longer horizontal fracture line and fragments. The alveolar nerve should be safeguarded. The line of the osteotomy then runs as follows: With a dental burr, the mandible is cut from the alveolar ridge downward in front of the mental foramen, backward below the alveolar canal, and then downward again across the posterior border of the mandible. The extended fragments are held together by a bone suture of wire and by interdental wiring. If teeth are absent, a circumferential wire is passed around the symphysis, brought out through the skin of the chin, and twisted to form a loop. The loop is then attached to a special headgear under traction, as described by Kazanjian. In unilateral retrusion, only the short side is elongated unless occlusion of the teeth remains unsatisfactory, whereupon the other side must also be severed.

Technique (for Severe Retrusion) (Case 88, p. 1102)

In severe retrusion, particularly where the lip is pulled back by its attachment to the gums, osteotomy is either insufficient or not possible at all owing to thinness of the mandibular bone. The method of choice in these cases is the intraoral insertion of a prosthetic appliance into an epithelium-lined pocket between lips and mandible (after Gillies). If the mandible is sufficiently thick, a step osteotomy is performed first; otherwise (as in Case 88, p. 1102), a platform must be built first in front of the mandible with an iliac bone graft on which the intraoral prosthesis will later rest (Fig. 274). After the bone graft has healed in place, the intraoral epithelium-lined pocket is made. Between lip and mandible, a cavity is prepared and lined by insertion of a skin graft wrapped around a stent, as described on page 39. The pocket should extend down to the lower border of the mandible, and should be made large enough to improve or possibly correct the deformity. After six days, the stent of dental compound is removed and replaced by a prosthetic appliance which carries artificial teeth. The latter are attached to the prosthesis in such a way that

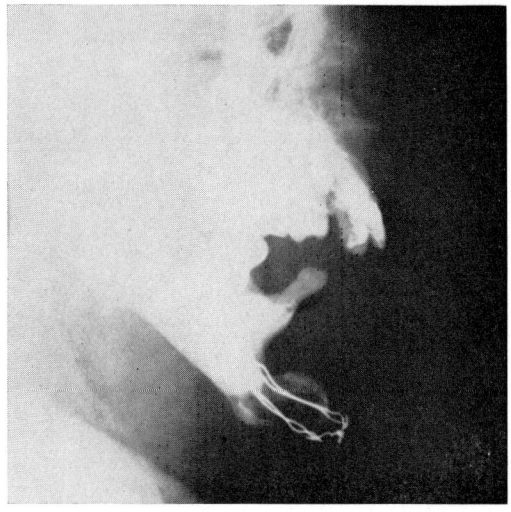

Fig. 274. Marked underdevelopment and retrusion of mandible. Onlay bone graft from crest of ilium fastened to anterior part of mandible (compare with Case 88, p. 1102).

they are in occlusion with the teeth of the maxilla and hide the teeth of the retruded mandible. For a few days after the appliance is inserted, the lower lip, which is stretched and tense, has a tendency to contract downward. To counteract this retraction, New and Erich advise the use of adhesive tape to hold the lower lip in the desired position until the contracture is overcome.

OPEN BITE

Open bite is a condition in which after closure of the jaws the frontal teeth cannot be brought into occlusion. In rare instances, the condition is due to a malunited fracture. The most common cause is a developmental fault whereby the anterior part of the mandible is bent downward in front of the second molar. In some cases, the maxilla is the seat of the deformity. Before the age of twelve, the condition may be corrected by orthodontic treatment; in older patients, however, surgery may become necessary if the functional disturbance demands correction.

THE OSSEOUS FRAMEWORK OF THE FACE

Technique (Blair)

The principle is bilateral excision of a V-shaped section of the mandible just in front of the first occluding tooth. The apex of the V-shaped section is at the lower border of the jaw, and usually a tooth must be extracted from the site of the section on each side; the tooth extraction should be performed several months prior to the operation. Plaster reproduction of the denture will reveal the size of the piece of bone to be resected. An incision is made below the mandible at the selected site; the mandible is exposed, and the V-shaped piece of bone—together with its

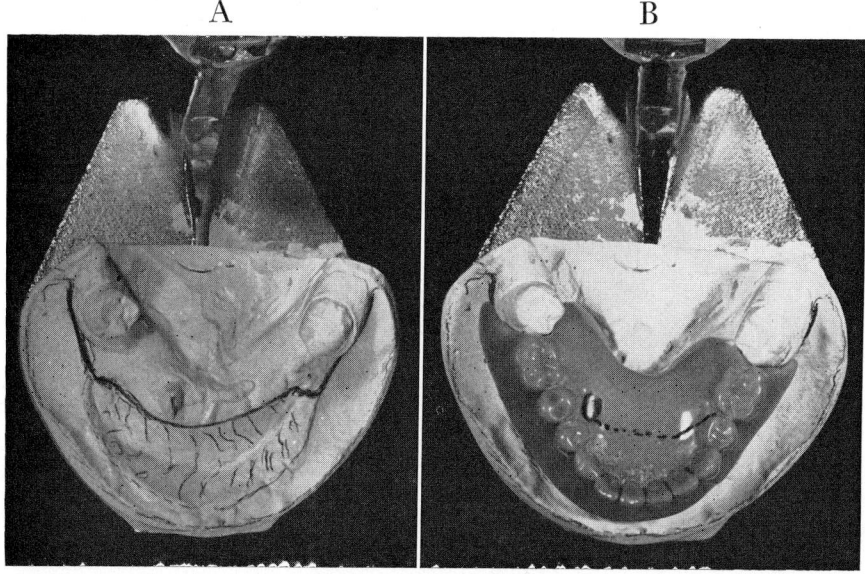

Fig. 275. Moulages before and after skin inlay grafting of case of Fig. 274 (compare with Case 88, p. 1102). *A:* Heavy line indicates original sulcus; broken line and shaded area marks out skin-lined pocket in front of mandible. *B:* Prosthesis inserted into pocket; broken line indicates original alveolar ridge.

periosteum—is resected with a straight or electrically driven saw from below upward into the mouth. The same procedure is undertaken on the other side. A drain is inserted externally and the wounds are closed. The anterior fragment is brought into occlusion with the upper teeth and immobilized by intermaxillary splinting.

If the open bite is associated with retrusion or protrusion of the mandible, the techniques described in the former paragraphs (p. 576) (compare with Figs. 270-272) should be considered. If the maxilla is the seat of the deformity, osteotomy of the maxilla must be performed (see p. 571).

585

THE HEAD AND NECK

BONY ANKYLOSIS OF TEMPOROMANDIBULAR JOINT

This condition may be unilateral or, seldom, bilateral. It may be congenital—rarely however—or acquired. If acquired, it is due either to trauma or to infection. The ankylosis is more often intra-articular than extra-articular. To overcome the ankylosis, arthroplasty is necessary, and requires the removal of a section of bone followed by interposition of local tissue or tissue grafts or alloplastic material to prevent reunion. The bone is removed either from the condyle (Helferich, Murphy, Blair) or from the ramus (Risdon). Whenever possible the author prefers removal of the bone from the condyle. A great variety of tissue and material has been recommended for interposition to prevent reunion. Trauner followed up the large number of arthroplasties of the temporomandibular joint at the Pickler Clinic and found that reankylosis could be prevented by interposition of cartilage (Dufourmentel) or alloplastic material. Trauner employs an acrylic plastic which is placed on the lower jaw like a cap or into the joint cavity in the shape of a cup; since it is a self-hardening material it can be shaped during the operation. The author uses polyurethan for the same purpose. This material is easy to handle, shapes itself well during and after the operation, has not caused any irritation or infection in eleven consecutive cases, and has prevented reankylosis.

Technique (Resection of Condyle)

An incision is made in front of the ear just anterior to the tragus downward level with the ear lobule and upward level with the top of the helix. The superficial temporal vessels are identified and ligated and severed. The next step is to identify the zygomatic process of the temporal bone. For better exposure of the joint the periosteum with the posterior insertion of the masseter muscle is elevated from the lower border of the zygomatic process. The temporomandibular joint is located just below and deep to the zygomatic arch and directly in front of the external auditory canal. The joint is opened from a horizontal incision. The joint, however, may be obscured by adhesions or replaced by a mass of bone between the ramus and the zygomatic arch. The upper part of the ramus must then be approached posteriorly and freed. This is best done with the Joseph periosteal elevator. Unless there is a mass of bone present in front, the anterior part of the condyle can now be freed. With a Joseph periosteal elevator in front and another one posteriorly, inserted so that both meet behind the condyle, a piece of bone 1 cm. wide is removed with burrs and chisels. The periosteal elevators protect the internal maxillary artery during this maneuver. If this artery should be injured, ligation of the vessel in this area is impossible; hence, one should not hesitate to ligate the external carotid artery. If there is a mass of bone present in front between the zygomatic arch and the condyle, the mass of bone must be resected with gauge chisels and bone-cutting instruments before resection of the condyle is performed. Rarely the entire ramus in level of the sigmoid notch will need resection. A suitable piece of polyurethan is pressed into the resected space; since it molds itself easily, it can be adapted readily to the configuration of the adjoining bony structures. Since it remains soft for a long time, postoperative movements will mold it even further. The wound is closed and a pressure dressing applied. The patient receives a full liquid diet for one week and is permitted to move the jaw cautiously and more vigorously later. Those patients in whom the mouth could be opened to its full extent during the operation regain full function without the use of passive exercises; otherwise the use of such applicances (after Ivy, Kazanjian, Schuchardt, Trauner) are recommended.

In extreme cases of ankylosis of the temporomandibular joint, in which it would be most difficult to resect the upper part of the ramus from an incision anterior to the ear without risking injury to the facial nerve and large vessels, Risdon has advised a lower approach resecting a piece of the ramus.

Technique (Resection of Ramus) (Risdon)

An incision is made starting behind the angle of the mandible and running forward about 4 cm. (1⅝ inches). It can be lengthened upward, but must remain superficial to the parotid gland to safeguard the facial nerve. It can be lengthened anteriorly, but must remain below the border of the mandible to safeguard the mandibular branch of the facial nerve. Enough skin and subcutaneous tissue are reflected upward to obtain access to the inferior attachment of the musculus masseter. The latter is stripped from the mandible almost to the bony deformity that caused the ankylosis. Then under direct vision, the ascending ramus is divided transversely with a Gigli saw (see p. 573) or with dental burrs of various sizes beneath the sigmoid notch. The cut is enlarged by using a large fissure burr. When the inner plate of the bone is reached, great care must be taken in dividing it since the arteria maxillaris interna may lie close to the ramus. It may be necessary to cut the inner plate with a chisel. After the division of the ramus, a piece of bone, about 1 cm. (2 inch) wide, is removed from the lower fragment with a rongeur.

A piece of plastic material—polyurethan—is inserted into the space between the fragments as described above and the wound is closed. After-treatment is the same as that described above.

587

BIBLIOGRAPHY

ADAMS, W. M.: *Internal wiring fixation of facial fractures.* Surgery, 12:523, 1942.

ADAMS, W. M., and ADAMS, L. H.: *Internal wire fixation of facial fractures. A fifteen year follow up report.* Amer. J. Surg., 92:12, 1956.

ADAMSON, J. E., HORTON, C. E., and CRAWFORD, H. H.: *External pinning of the unstable zygomatic arch fracture.* Plast. Reconstr. Surg., 36:343, 1965.

v. ALSTINE, R. S., and DINGMAN, R. O.: *Correction of mandibular protrusion in the edentulous patient.* J. Oral Surg., 11:273, 1953.

ATTIE, J. N., CATANIA, A., and RIPSTEIN, M. B.: *A stainless steel mesh prosthesis for immediate replacement of the hemimandible.* Surgery, 33:712, 1951.

AXHAUSEN, W.: *Leitfaden der zahnarztlichen Chirurgie.* Munchen, 1950.
Zur Behandlung veralteter disloziert geheilter Oberkieferbrüche. Dt. Zahn-Mund-Kieferhk., 1:334, 1934.

BABCOCK, W. W.: *Surgical treatment of certain jaw deformities.* JAMA, 53:833, 1909.
Advancement of the receding lower jaw. Ann. Surg., 106:1105, 1939.

BARROW, G. V., and DINGMAN, R. O.: *Orthodontic considerations in the surgical management of developmental deformities of the mandible.* Amer. J. Orthodont., 36:121, 1950.

BETHMANN, W.: *Bilateral resection of the mandible with replacement of it by alloplastic material (Doppelseitige Unterkieferresktion mit alloplatsichem Ersatz des Unterkiefers).* Zbl. Chir., 84:889, 1959.

BLAIR, V. P.: *Surgery and Disease of the Mouth and Jaws.* C. V. Mosby Co., St. Louis, 1917.

BLAIR, V. P., and IVY, R. H.: *Essentials of Oral Surgery.* C. V. Mosby Co., St. Louis, 1944.

BLOCKER, T. H., Jr., and STOUT, R. A.: *Mandibular reconstruction World War II.* Plast. Reconstr. Surg., 4:153, 1949.

BLOCKER, T. H., Jr., and WEISS, L. R.: *Use of cancellous bone in the repair of defects about the jaws.* Ann. Surg., 123:622, 1946.

BRAITHWAITE, F., and HOPPER, F.: *Ankylosis of the temporo-mandibular joint.* Brit. J. Plast. Surg., 5:105, 1952.

BROMBERG, B. E., WALDEN, R. H., and RUBIN, L. R.: *Mandibular bone grafts.* Plast. Reconstr. Surg., 32:589, 1963.

BROWN, J. B.: *Fractures of the bones of the face.* Surg. Gynec. Obstet., 68:564, 1939.
Fractures of the Jaws and Related Bones of the Face. In KEY, J. A., and CONWELL, H. E.: C. V. Mosby Co., St. Louis, 1942.
Internal wire fixation of jaw fractures with note on external bar fixation. Surg. Gynec. Obstet., 75:361, 1942.

588

THE OSSEOUS FRAMEWORK OF THE FACE

BROWN, J. B., FRYER, M. P., and McDOWELL, F.: *Internal wire-pin fixation for middle third facial fractures.* Plast. Reconstr. Surg., 9:276, 1952.

BROWN, J. B., and McDOWELL, F.: *Internal wire fixation for fractures of jaws, preliminary report.* Surg. Gynec. Obstet., 74:227, 1942.

BRUHN, CHR.: *Ueber die Beseitgung der Progenie durch chirurgische und zahnaerztlich orthopaedische Massnahmen.* Deutsche Monatschr. f. Zahnh., 38:50, 1920.
Ueber chirurgische und zahnaerztlich orthopädische Mass-Nahmen zum Ausgleich der Makrognathie (Progenie) und Mikrognathie des Unterkiefers. Deutsche Monatschr. f. Zahnh., 39:385. 1921.

BÜRKLE DE LA CAMP, H.: *Operationen au den Kiefern.* Chir. Op. lehre, Bier-Braun-Kümmel Vol. I. Barth, Leipzig, 1933.

BYARS, L. T.: *Preservation and reconstruction of mandibular function and contour.* Ann. Surg., 127:863, 1948.
Surgical management of mandible invaded by oral cancer. Surg. Gynec. Obstet., 98:564, 1954.

CONLEY, J. J.: *The use of vitallium prostheses and implants in the reconstruction of the mandibular arch.* Plast. Reconstr. Surg., 8:150, 1951.
A technique of immediate bone grafting in the treatment of benign and malignant tumors of the mandible and a review of 17 consecutive cases. Cancer, 6:558, 1953.

CONVERSE, J. M.: *Technique of bone grafting for contour restoration of the face.* Plast. Reconstr. Surg., 14:332, 1954.
Micrognathia. Brit. J. Plast. Surg., 16:197, 1963.

CONVERSE, J. M., HOROWITZ, S. L., GUY, C. L., and WOOD-SMITH, D.: *Surgical orthodontic correction in the bilateral cleft lip.* Cleft Palate J., 1:153, 1964.

CONVERSE, J. M., and SHAPIRO, H. H.: *Treatment of developmental malformations of the jaws.* Plast. Reconstr. Surg., 10:473, 1952.

CONVERSE, J. M., SMITH, B., OBEAR, M. F., and WOOD-SMITH, D.: *Orbital blowout fractures: A ten year survey.* Plast. Reconstr. Surg., 39:20, 1967.

CONVERSE, J. M., and WOOD-SMITH, D.: *Horizontal osteotomy of the mandible.* Plast. Reconstr. Surg., 34:464, 1964.

CRAMER, L. M., TOOZE, F. M., and LERMAN, S.: *Blowout fractures of the orbit.* Brit. J. Plast. Surg., 18:171, 1965.

DAWSON, R. L. G., and FORDYCE, G. L.: *Complex fractures of the middle third of the face and their early treatment.* Brit. J. Surg., 41:254, 1953.

DINGMAN, R. O.: *Surgical correction of developmental deformities of the mandible.* Plast. Reconstr. Surg., 3:124, 1948.
Osteectomy of the mandible in cleft lip and palate habilitation. Plast. Reconstr. Surg., 25:213, 1960.

DINGMAN, R. O., and GRABB, W.: *Reconstruction of both mandibular condyles with metatarsal bone grafts.* Plast. Reconstr. Surg., 34:441, 1964.

DINGMAN, R. O., and NATVIG, P.: *Surgery of Facial Fractures.* W. B. Saunders, Philadelphia, 1964.

DITCHFIELD, A.: *Interosseous wiring of mandibular fractures: A follow-up of fifty cases.* Brit. J. Plast. Surg., 13:146, 1960.

THE HEAD AND NECK

DUFOURMENTEL, L.: *Le Traitement chirurgical du prognathisme.* Presse Méd., 29:235, 1921.
Chirurgie de l'Articulation Tempero Maxillaire. Paris, 1929.

ERICH, J. B., and AUSTIN, L. T.: *Traumatic Injuries of Facial Bones: An Atlas of Treatment.* W. B. Saunders, Philadelphia, 1944.

FEDERSPIEL, M. N.: *Maxillo-facial injuries.* Wisconsin Med. J., 33:563, 1934. *Extreme open-bite malocclusion resulting from improper care of a complete horizontal fracture of the maxilla and a bilateral of the mandible.* Wisconsin Med. J., April, 1949.

FREEMAN, B. S.: *The use of vitallium plates to maintain function following resection of the mandible.* Plast. Reconstr. Surg., 3:73, 1948.
The direct approach to acute fractures of the zygomatic-maxillary complex and immediate prosthetic replacement of the orbital floor. Plast. Reconstr. Surg., 29:587, 1962.

FRY, W. K.: *The Dental Treatment of Maxillo-facial Injuries.* J. B. Lippincott, Philadelphia, 1934.

GARRÉ: *Kieferersatz.* Niederrh. Ges. f. Natur. -u. Heilkunde Bonn., 22:7, 1907.

GEORGIADE, N. G., and QUINN, G. W.: *Newer concepts in surgical correction of mandibular prognathism.* Plast. Reconstr. Surg., 27:185, 1961.

GILLIES, H. D.: *Plastic Surgery of the Face.* H. Frowde, London, 1920.

GILLIES, H. D., KILNER, T. P., and STONE, D.: *Fractures of the malar-zygomatic compound.* Brit. J. Surg., 14:651, 1927.

GONZALEZ-ULLOA, M.: *Temporomandibular arthroplasty in the treatment of prognathism.* Plast. Reconstr. Surg., 8:136, 1951.
Some important details in the correction of prognathism. Ibid., 9:391, 1952.

GONZALEZ-ULLOA, M., and STEVENS, E.: *The role of chin correction in profileplasty.* Plast. Reconstr. Surg., 41:477, 1968.

GORN, S. B., STRAUSS, R. B., and OSBORN, O. B.: *Blowout fractures of the orbital floor.* Amer. J. Ophthal., 61:893, 1966.

HAMILTON, J. M., and HARDY, S. B.: *The use of the webb bolt as a space maintaining appliance in defects of the mandible.* Plast. Reconstr. Surg., 22:296, 1958.

HARRIS, A. H., BROMBERG, B. E., and SONG, I. C.: *Fractures of the malar compound.* Surg. Gynec. Obstet., 122:541, 1966.

HARSHA: *Bilateral resection of the jaw for prognathism.* Surg. Gynec. Obstet., 15:51, 1912.

HEALY, M. H., JR., ET AL.: *The use of acrylic implants in one-stage reconstructions of the mandible.* Surg. Gynec. Obstet., 98:395, 1954.

HELFERICH, H.: *Ein neues Operationsverfahren zur Heilung der Kiefergelenksankylose.* Verhandl. d. deutsch. Gesellsch. f. Chir., 1894, pp. 504-510. Arch. f. klin. Chir., 48:864, 1894.

HENRY, T. C.: *The surgical correction of mandibular protrusion and retrusion.* J. Bone Joint Surg., 36B:62, 1954.

590

THE OSSEOUS FRAMEWORK OF THE FACE

HENSCHEN, C., and SCHWARZ, R.: *Die operative Behandlung der Progenie nach cephalometrischem Princip.* Chirurg., 1:56, 1928.

HINDS, E. C., SPIRA, M., SILLS, A. H., and GALBREATH, J. C.: *Use of tantalum trays in mandibular surgery.* Plast. Reconstr. Surg., 32:439, 1963.

HOFER, O.: Dtsch. Ztschr. f. Zahn-Mund-Kieferheilkunde 9:121, 1942.

HOGEMAN, K. E.: *Surgical-orthopedic correction of mandibular protrusions.* Acta Chir. Scand., Suppl. 159, Stockholm, 1951.
Indikation und Technik der operativen Progeniebanhandlung. Fortschritte der Kiefer- und Gesichts-Chirurgie, Vol. 1, 178, 1955.
Die Behandlung von Oberkieferfrakturen ohne extraorale Stützvërbande. Forschritte der Kiefer- und Gesichts-Chirurgie, Vol. 2:49, 1956.

HOGEMAN, K. E., and ILLMAR, K. (Malmö, Sweden): *Internal wire fixation of maxillary fractures.* Acta Chir. Scand., 129 (Plastic Surgery Issue IV) 300, 1965.

HOGEMAN, K. E., RYDEN, B., and SARNAS, K. V.: *Surgical orthodontic correction of maxillary protrusion.* Forschritte der Kiefer- und Gesichts-Chirurgie, Vol. 1, 1955.

HOGEMAN, K. E., and SARNAS, K. V.: *Surgical and dental protrusion of Angle class II division I malocclusion.* Scand. J. Plast. Reconstr. Surg., 1:101, 1967.

HOGEMAN, K. E., and VILMAR, K.: In Schuchardt, K.: *Fortschritte der Kiefer-Gesichtschirurgie.* Bd. XII. Georg Thieme, Stuttgart, 1967.

IPSEN, J.:*Eine Behandlung von Kieferbrüchen, Zentralbl.* J. Chir., 60:2840, 1933.

IVY, R. H.: *Observations on fractures of the mandible.* JAMA, 79:295, 1922.
Surgery of the Mouth and Jaws: In Nelson Loose-Leaf Surgery. Thomas Nelson & Sons, New York, 1927, Vol. 2, Chap. XI.
Practical method of fixation in fractures of the mandible. Surg. Gynec. Obstet., 34:670, 1922.
Surgery of the Mouth and Jaws: In Nelson Loose-Leaf Surgery. Thomas Nelson & Sons, New York, 1932, Vol. 2.
Collective review—Bone grafting for restoration of defects of the mandible. Plast. Reconstr. Surg., 7:333, 1951.

IVY, R. H., and CURTIS, L.: *Fractures of the Jaws.* Lea & Febiger, Philadelphia, 1945.

IVY, R. H., and EPES, B. M.: Bone grafting for defects of the mandible. Mil. Surgeon, 60:286, 1927.

JOHNSON, M. R.: *Depressed fracture of the orbital rim.* Surg. Clin. N. Amer., 24:340, 1944.

KAZANJIAN, V. H.: *Surgical treatment of mandibular prognathism.* Int. J. Orthodont., 18:1224, 1932.
The interrelation of dentistry and surgery in the treatment of deformities of the face and jaws. Amer. J. Orthodont., 27:10, 1941.
Ankylosis of the temporo-mandibular joint. Surg. Gynec. Obstet., 67:333, 1938.
Mandibular retrusion with ankylosis of the temporomandibular joint. Plast. Reconstr. Surg., 17:91, 1956.
Temporomandibular joint ankylosis with mandibular retrusion. Ann. Surg., 90:905, 1956.

591

THE HEAD AND NECK

KAZANJIAN, V. H., CONVERSE, J. M.: *Surgical Treatment of Facial Injuries.* Williams & Wilkins, Baltimore, 1949, 2nd ed. 1959.

KELIKIAN, H.: *A method of mobilizing the temporomandibular joint.* J. Bone Joint Surg., 32A:113, 1950.

KITLOWSKI, E. A.: *The surgical correction of mandibular prognathism.* Ann. Surg., 115:647, 1942.

KNIGHT, J. S., and NORTH, J. F.: *The classification of malar fractures: An analysis of displacement as a guide to treatment.* Brit. J. Plast. Surg., 13:325, 1961.

KOHLER, J. A.: *Diagnostik und Therapie der Kieferfrakturen.* Heidelberg Dr. Alfred Huttig, 1951.

KOSTECKA, F.: *Zahnärztl.* Rundschau., 40:670, 1931.

LeFORT, R.: *Étude expérimentale sur les fractures de la machoire supérieur.* Rev. Chir., Paris, 23:208, 1901.

LENORMANT, C., and DARCISSAC, M.: *Le procédé des "anses métalliques trans-osseuses" pour la contention der branches montantes, dans les fractures du maxillaire inferieur; son application dans un cas de fracture double. Rétrodentaire de la mâchoire inferieure.* Bull. et mém. Soc. nat. de chir., 53:503, 1927.

LEWIS, G. K.: *The fractured mandible.* J. Oral Surg., 8:95, 1950.

LEXER, E.: *Die Verwendung der freien Knochenplastik.* Chir. Kongr. Verh., 1908, p. 188.
Gesichtsplastik, Kieferverletzungen. Beitr. z. klin. Chir., 101:233, 1916.
Die gesamte Wiederherstellungschirurgie. J. A. Barth, Leipzig, 1931.

LIMBERG, Λ. Λ.: *A new method of plastic lengthening of the mandible in unilateral microgenia and asymmetry of the face.* J. Amer. Dent. Assoc., 15:851, 1928.

LINDEMANN, A.: *Die gegenwärtigen Behandlungswege der Kieferschussverletzungen.* Bruhn Ergebnisse aus dem Düsseldorfer Lazarett, Wiesbaden, 1916, p. 243.

LONGACRE, J. J., and GILBY, R. F.: *Further observations on the use of autogenous cartilage graft in arthroplasty of the temporomandibular joint.* Plast. Reconstr. Surg., 10:238, 1952.

LOVETT, D. W., BRINTNALL, E. S., and GRANDON, E. L.: *Mandibular reconstruction in cases of partial mandibulectomy with disarticulation.* Plast. Reconstr. Surg., 30:74, 1962.

MACLENNAN, W. D.: *Consideration of 180 cases of typical fractures of the mandibular condylar process.* Brit. J. Plast. Surg., 5:122, 1952.

MACOMBER, W. B., SHEPHARD, R. A., CROFUT, V. E.: *Mandibular bone grafts.* Plast. Reconstr. Surg., 3:570, 1948.

MAJOR, GLENN: *Fractures of the Jaws and Other Facial Bones.* C. V. Mosby Co., St. Louis, 1943.

MASSON, J. K.: *A variation of kirschner wire prosthesis for reconstruction of mandible after partial mandibular resection for intraoral malignancy.* Plast. Reconstr. Surg., 35:457, 1965.

MAY, H.: Kinnaufbau bei Mikrognie Zentralbl. f. Chir., 86:2097, 1961.

McDOWELL, F., BROWN, J. B., and FRYER, M. P.: *Surgery of Face, Mouth and Jaws.* C. V. Mosby Co., St. Louis, 1954.

McDOWELL, F., and OHLWILER, D.: *Collective review: Mandibular resection and replacement*. Int. Abstr. Surg., Surg. Gynec. Obstet., 115:103, 1962.

McKEE, D. M.: *Immediate reconstruction of the mandible in tumor surgery*. Southern Med. J., 54:620, 1961 (Int. Abstr. Surg., Surg. Gynec. Obstet., Oct. 1961, p. 338).

MILLARD, D. R.: *A new approach to immediate mandibular repair*. Ann. Surg., 160:306, 1964.

MILLARD, D. R., MAISELS, D. O., and BATSTONE, J. H.: *Immediate repair of radical resection of the anterior arch of the lower jaw*. Plast. Reconstr. Surg., 39: 153, 1967.

MOWLEM, R.: *Cancellous chip bone graft*. Report on 75 cases. Lancet, 2:746, 1944.

MURPHY, J. B.: *Arthroplasty for intra-articular bony and fibrous ankylosis of Temporomandibular articulation: Report of nine cases*. JAMA, 62:1783, 1914.

MURRAY, J. E., and SWANSON, L. T.: *Midface osteotomy and advancement for craniosynostosis*. Plast. Reconstr. Surg., 41:299, 1968.

NEW, G. B., and ERICH, J. B.: *Retruded chins, correction by plastic operations*. JAMA, 115:186, 1940.
The surgical correction of mandibular prognathism. Amer. J. Surg., 53:2, 1941.

NEWMAN, J.: *Repair of prognathic and retruded Jaws*. Amer. J. Surg., 58:35, 1942.

OBWEGESER, H. L.: *Primary repair of the mandible by the intraoral route after partial resection with and without pre-operative infection*. Brit. J. Plast. Surg., 21: 282, 1968.
Operation on the maxilla for the correction of progenia. Zahnheilkunde, 75:365, 1965.
Vorteile und Möglichkeiten des intraoralen Vorgehens bei der Korrektur von Unterkieferanomalien. In Fortschritte der Kiefer- und Gesichts-Chirurgie edited by Karl Schuchardt, M.D., Vol. 7, Georg Thieme Verlag, Stuttgart, 1961.
Surgical correction of small or retrodisplaced maxillae. The "dish-face" deformity. Plast. Reconstr. Surg., 43:351, 1969.
Zur Behandlung der veralteten Oberkieferfrakturen. In Schuchardt, K.: *Fortschritte der Kiefer-Gesichtschirurgie*. Bd. XII. Georg Thieme, Stuttgart, 1967.

PADGETT, E. C.: *Surgical Diseases of the Mouth and Jaw*. W. B. Saunders, Philadelphia, 1938.

PARKER, D. B.: *Synopsis of Traumatic Injuries of the Face and Jaws*. C. V. Mosby Co., St. Louis, 1942.

PAYR, E.: *Ueber osteoplastischen Ersatz nach Kieferresektion*. Zentralbl. f. Chir., 1908, No. 16.

PICHLER, H.: *Die operative Behandlung der Progenie*. Ztschr. f. Stomatol., 1927, p. 1166.

PICKRELL, K. L.: *Double Resection of the Mandible*. Dental Cosmos, 1912, p. 1114, Vol. 54.

PICKRELL, K. L., ET AL.: *The correction of ankylosis of the jaw and associated deformities of the face*. Ann. Surg., 134:55, 1951.

RISDON, F.: *Treatment of non-union fractures of mandible by free autogenous bone grafts*. JAMA, 79:297, 1922.
Ankylosis of the temporo-maxillary joint. J. Amer. Dent. Assoc., 21:1933, 1934.

593

THE HEAD AND NECK

ROWE, N. L., and KILLEY, H. C.: *Fractures of the Facial Skeleton*, 2nd ed., Williams & Wilkins, Baltimore, 1968.

SARNAT, B. G.: *The Temporomandibular Joint.* Charles C Thomas, Springfield, 1951.

SARNAT, B. G., and ROBINSON, I. B.: *Surgery of the mandible.* Plast. Reconstr. Surg., 17:27, 1956.

SARNAT, B. G., and LASKIN, D. M.: *Diagnosis and Surgical Management of Diseases of the Temporomandibular Joint.* Charles C Thomas, Springfield, 1962.

SCHER, S. R.: *The deformed chin and lower jaw.* Ann. Surg., 115:869, 1942.

SCHUCHARDT, K.: *Ein Beitrag zur chirurgischen Kieferorthopädie usw.* Dtsch. Zahn, Mund u. Kieferhk. 9, Vol. 2, 1942. In Bier-Braun-Kümmell's Chirurgische Operationslehre, 7th Edition. Vol. 2. J. A. Barth, Leipzig, 1954.
Die Behandlung der Kiefergelenksankylose. Zahnärztliche Wschr., 11:121, 1946.
Formen des offenen Bisses und ihre operativen Behandlungsmöglichkeiten. Fortschritte der Kiefer-und Gesichts-Chirurgie, Vol. 1, 22:1955.

SCHUCHARDT, K., KAPOVITS, M., and SPIESSL, B.: *Technik und Anwendung des Drahtbogenkunststoffverbandes.* Deutsche Zahnarztliche Zeitschrift, 16:1241, 1961.

SCHUCHARDT, K., and WASSMUND, M.: *Fortschritte der Kiefer- und Gesichts-Chirurgie*, A. Yearbook, Vol. I. Georg Thieme, Verlag, Stuttgart, 1956.

SCHULTZ, L.: *Bilateral resection of mandible for prognathism.* Surg. Gynec. Obstet., 45:379, 1927.

SCHWARTZ, L., D. D. S.: *Disorders of the Temporomandibular Joint.* W. B. Saunders, Philadelphia, 1960.

SMITH, A. E., and ROBINSON, M.: *A new procedure in bilateral reconstruction of condlyes.* Plast. Reconstr. Surg., 9:393, 1952.

SPADAFORA, A.: *Mandibular prognathism; personal technique (Prognatismo mandibular; tecnica personal).* Prensa Med. Argent., 47:2235, 1960.

STEIN, M., TEUBES, M. N., SHER, S.: *Results of treatment of fractured mandibles by the Anderson splint.* Surg. Gynec. Obstet., 95:289, 1952.

SYKOFF: *Zur Frage der Knochen-plastik am Unterkiefer.* Zentralbl. f. Chir., 1900, p. 881.

TESSIER, P.: *Osteotomies Totales de la Face Syndrome de Crouzon, Syndrome D'Apert Oxycephalies. Saphocephalies. Turricephalies.* Ann. chir. plast., 12:273, 1967.
Transactions of the Fourth International Congress of Plastic Surgery in Rome, 1967. Excerpta Medica Co., Amsterdam, 1968.

TRAUNER, R.: *Trans. Inter. Cong. Plast. Surg.*, 546. Excerpta Medica Foundation, Amsterdam, 1964.

TRAUNER, R., and WIRTH, F.: *Therapie der Kiefergelenksankylose.* Fortschritte der Kiefer- und Gesichts-Chirurgie. Band VI Georg Thieme Verlag, Stuttgart, 1960.

TRAUNER, R., and OBWEGESER, H.: *The surgical correction of mandibular prognathism and retrognathia with consideration of genioplasty.* J. Oral Surg., 10:889, 1957.

THE OSSEOUS FRAMEWORK OF THE FACE

THOMA, K. H.: *Principal factors controlling the development of the maxilla and mandible.* Amer. J. Orthodont., 24:171, 1938.
Traumatic Surgery of the Jaws. C. V. Mosby Co., St. Louis, 1942.
Oral Surg. Vol. I and II, 2nd Edition. C. V. Mosby Co., St. Louis, 1952.

WALDRON, C. W., KAZANJIAN, V. H., and PARKER, D. B.: *Skeletal fixation in the treatment of fractures of the mandible.* J. Oral Surg., 1:59, 1943.

WALDRON, C. W., KARLEEN, C. I., and WALDRON, C. A.: *Fundamentals in the surgical treatment of mandibular prognathism.* Plast. Reconstr. Surg., 4:163, 1949.

WASSMUND, M.: *Lehrbuch der Prakt. Chirurgie des Mundes und der Kiefer.* Leipzig, 1935.

WINTER, L.: *Operative Oral Surgery.* C. V. Mosby Co., St. Louis, 1943.

WUNDERER, S.: *Die Prognathieoperation mittels frontal gestieltem Maxillafragment.* Oesterr. Ztschr. Stomat., 59:98, 1962.

THE NECK
AND LARYNX   13
AND TRACHEA

DEFECTS

WOUNDS, burns, tracheal fistulas, and defects of pharynx and upper esophagus are the principal defects of the neck that require reparative and reconstructive procedures.

WOUNDS

Treatment does not differ from that already outlined in Chapter 3. A few special points, however, should be emphasized. The normal creases of the skin of the neck run horizontally. Hence, vertical wounds crossing the normal creases heal with less cosmetic and functional satisfaction than horizontal wounds. They are apt to contract and to form a web, which may require later repair by a Z-operation. For the same reason, wounds which need lengthening should be extended horizontally and not vertically. The same principle holds good for all operative incisions around the neck. Deep wounds at the anterior surface of the neck, often the results of suicidal attempts, are complicated by injuries to the larynx, trachea, muscles, and—surprisingly less often—to major vessels and nerves. Each structure requires special attention. If larynx or trachea is injured, tracheotomy must be performed below the injury before the perforation is closed.

597

THE HEAD AND NECK

BURNS

Here again the therapeutic principles are the same as those for burns in other regions (Chap. 4). In third-degree burns, skin grafting should be performed as soon as possible to prevent contractures, which inevitably lead to poor functional and cosmetic results. Difficult to deal with are those deep burns in which the platysma is destroyed. Even if early skin grafting has been performed, a contracture and an obliteration of the chin-neck line may result. The degree of contracture, however, is definitely less after skin grafting. It should be pointed out that the graft on the anterior surface of the neck must be laid horizontally and not vertically so that, for the reasons mentioned in the preceding paragraph, the scars between the grafts come to lie within the creases of the neck.

TRACHEAL FISTULAS

Tracheal fistulas are of several kinds, and the technique of their closure varies accordingly. The fistula that remains after simple tracheotomy for acute laryngeal obstruction, necessitating the wearing of a cannula for only a few days or weeks, presents no problem for it closes spontaneously and almost immediately. On the other hand, if the cannula has been worn for a number of months or years, it will not, as a rule, close tightly without a plastic procedure. In such cases, after at least a week or two has been allowed for partial spontaneous closure, the epithelized fistulous tract is dissected down to the tracheal wall, ligated, and amputated, after which the subcutaneous tissues and the skin are closed without drainage. Larger openings, such as those used for the insertion of laryngotracheostomic apparatus in the treatment of severe chronic laryngeal stenosis, must be closed with special precautions to avoid narrowing the airway; of course, closure must not be attempted at all until suitable tests have been carried out to prove that sufficient permanent dilatation has been accomplished. Such openings must be closed by simply covering them, as with a lid, care being exercised to avoid sutures that tend to pull the lateral margins of the opening together. This can be accomplished, in most cases, by making an elliptical incision about the opening and then inverting the inner skin edges in such a way as to roof over the opening with skin. The outer skin edges are then undermined and united in the midline.

In the case of some larger openings, it is wise to make the closure in stages, closing the part of the opening over the narrowest point in the airway first, so that if there should be temporary narrowing from post-operative inflammatory reaction the patient can still breathe through the

598

part remaining open. In a second stage, this remaining opening can be closed with no fear of obstruction in the postoperative period. Occasionally, a more elaborate type of plastic procedure may be deemed preferable, using a pedicle flap (Erdelyi, Champion), with or without a cartilage implant and lining (Serrano, Ortiz-Monasterio, and Andrado-Pradillo).

RECONSTRUCTION OF DEFECTS AFTER LARYNGOPHARYNGOESOPHAGECTOMY

These large cervical defects result as a rule from removal of malignant tumors. Depending upon the extent of the defect, reconstruction can be carried out in one of four ways: by means of a free skin graft wrapped over a stent, the stent to be removed after a few weeks through the mouth (Negus, Edgerton as quoted by Krogh and Devine); by reconstruction of skin flaps from the neck, the Wookey type procedure (Wookey, Krogh and Devine, Till and Cameron and others); by reconstruction with skin flaps from neck and chest (Cowan and MacDougall, Silver and Capozzi et al. and others); by an autograft of a section of the lower intestinal tract which is revascularized by immediate anastomosis to appropriate vessels in the recipient site, as recommended by Nakayama, who was preceded by others (Jurkiewicz etc.). Since many methods are available, and the method of choice must be selected according to a given situation, they will not be described in detail here. I refer the reader to the above references.

DEFORMITIES

CONGENITAL BANDS (PTERYGIUM COLLI)

Designated "pterygium colli" by Finkle in 1902, these bands stretch from the mastoid region to the acromion. They may be unilateral or bilateral, and may or may not be associated with other congenital conditions, such as concomitant axillary webs or malformations of the cervical spine (Klippel-Feil syndrome). Bettman described these bands picturesquely, "as though a rope had been spanned across . . . and the skin then draped over it and allowed to hang in a graceful festoon." Between the leaves of pterygium colli one finds connective tissue and even muscle tissue. The latter, however, has no connection with the skeletal muscles outside the pterygium.

To correct such a web, one may be tempted to give Z-plasty a chance; but unless multiple Zs are used the operation will not be successful,

599

since the hairline becomes displaced to the anterior surface of the neck, and relaxation may not be sufficient. The author has followed Bettman's advice with gratifying results.

Technique

The crest of the web is brought into prominence by pushing the head toward the other shoulder. An incision is made along and through the entire crest down to the skeletal muscles. Two incisions, about 3.8 to 5 cm. (1½ to 2 inches) long, are made at right angles to the first (longitudinal) incision at different levels—the upper one on the posterior side, about one-third the length of the primary incision, the lower one on the anterior side, about two-thirds the length of the primary incision. All incisions go through the subcutaneous layer and connective-tissue bands to the muscular layers. The flaps are widely undermined. Care must be taken not to injure the nervus accessorius, which lies on the splenius muscle. The point of one flap of skin will automatically fall into the angle of the opposite incision, and vice versa. Additionally, one or more similar but shorter right-angle incisions are made above or below or both, followed by interchanging flaps and closure of the wounds. If both sides are affected, they are operated upon in the same stage. A voluminous pressure dressing is then applied. If the Klippel-Feil syndrome is associated with deformities of the shoulder girdle, additional bone operations may become necessary (Bonola).

CICATRICIAL CONTRACTURES

Cicatricial contractures of the neck constitute the majority of deformities. The scars causing the contractures are, as a rule, due to burns, and run longitudinally on the anterior and lateral surfaces of the neck. They obliterate the chin-neck line, causing an awkward, straight profile. In extensive cases involving the deeper tissues, chin and lip are pulled on the chest, causing ectropion of the lip and marked limitation of motion.

Technique

The patient is operated upon in the dorsal position, with the shoulder elevated on a pillow to cause a backward tilt of the head and stretching of the neck. The correction depends entirely upon the depth and extent of the cicatricial changes. In mild cases—that is, the scar being soft and weblike—the deformity can be corrected by one or several Z-operations (p. 185). The triangular flaps for the formation of the Z should include skin only, while the underlying platysma should be excised

600

and removed. In cases with numerous webs, the Z-operation is not likely to be successful. In one of the author's cases, the immediate cosmetic effect was good but the webs recurred. In such cases there appears to be too much skin, while the actual seat of the contracture is the platysma. In the aforementioned case, the author improved the condition by making a T-incision (the horizontal part in the chin-neck line, the vertical part over the trachea) and dissecting two triangular skin flaps. They were reflected laterally. This opened the entire anterior surface of the neck. The platysma was excised, and the skin flaps were reflected back in place and trimmed to conform to the new contours.

In very extensive cases with ectropion of the lower lip, relaxation incisions to overcome the contracture are not sufficient. The entire scar must be excised until normal tissue is reached. Only then is one able to release the contracture. The raw surface is covered with a thick split graft. A full-thickness graft is contraindicated for reasons mentioned on page 27 (Case 89, p. 1103). For the reasons given on page 598, the grafts on the anterior side of the neck must be laid horizontally and not vertically; thus, the adjoining scars come to lie within the creases of the neck. To avoid lateral contracting webs, it is also important to break up the lateral vertical borders of the wound edges spirally and Z-like.

Only rarely will it be found necessary to use a flap which, owing to length, must be "delayed." The flap, tubed or untubed, is prepared from the back, chest, or thoracoepigastric region, a method which the author has chosen to replace x-ray-damaged skin of the anterior side of the neck. The long tube was constructed in two stages and transferred via one "jump." The only disadvantage was that in this female patient her abdominal striae were also transplanted and became quite noticeable at the neck.

After-Treatment

A heavily padded pressure dressing is applied, and the patient is placed in bed with the head tilted backward. The dressing is changed on the eighth day; the sutures are removed.

Proper splinting holds the clue to the success of the skin grafting, and here Cronin has provided a most helpful suggestion. As is frequently the case, recurrence of some of the contracture, with wrinkling of the graft, is almost certain unless the neck is splinted properly and continuously for about six months. Cronin advises construction of a well-fitting brace one week after the operation. He demonstrates several types, from a simple collar to an elaborate adjustable splint as depicted in Figure 276. The brace is formed from a plaster-cast mold which is made at the time the first dressing is changed. While the mold is being made, the grafts are covered with ointment gauze. The patient is then allowed to sit up with the neck in slightly extended position. A strip of malleable metal is laid along each side of the neck and shoulders. This is used to cut against when removing the cast. A complete circular cast is applied closely to the neck and shoulders and clavicular areas and over the chin and inferior border of the mandible. As the plaster begins to warm it is cut through on one side and removed. If the plaster has already set, both sides are cut and the cast can be removed. The brace to be made from this mold consists of silastic which is lined with a thin layer of foam rubber

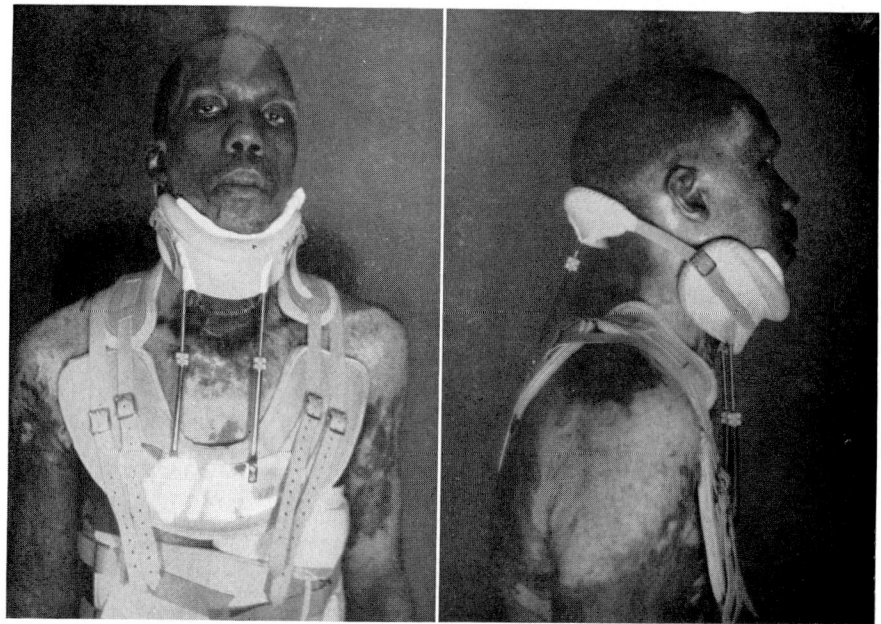

Fig. 276. Adjustable brace (after Cronin) individually made to splint the neck after repair of cicatricial contractures of the neck with skin grafts.

and covered by soft calfskin. As the lining is applied to the splint, great care must be taken to avoid loss of the desired contour. The brace should be worn for approximately six months.

Ousterkout and co-workers constructed an inflatable splint to be used with a standard myocervical collar. They claim that this is superior to all other splints.

BIBLIOGRAPHY

ASHLEY, F. L., BRIGGS, J. D., and AFFLEY, H. J.: *Reconstruction of pharynx.* Plast. Reconstr. Surg., 16:362, 1955.

THE NECK AND LARYNX AND TRACHEA

BETTMAN, A. G.: *Congenital bands about the shoulder girdle.* Plast. Reconstr. Surg., 1:205, 1946.

BONOLA, A.: *Surgical treatment of the Klippel-Feil syndrome.* J. Bone Joint Surg., 38B:440, 1956.

CAPOZZI, A., FEIERABEND, T. C., DAVENPORT, G., BERNARD, F. D.: *Cervical esophageal reconstruction.* Plast. Reconstr. Surg., 38:347, 1966.

CHAMPION, R.: *Reconstruction of cervical trachea: Case report.* Brit. J. Plast. Surg., 12:259, 1959.

COWAN, R. J., and MACDOUGALL, J. A.: *Reconstruction of the pharynx following laryngo-pharyngo-oesophagectomy.* Plast. Reconstr. Surg., 21:362, 1958.

CRONIN, T. D.: *Successful correction of extensive scar contractures of the neck using split-skin grafts.* Trans. Proc. First Int. Congr. Plast. Reconstr. Surg., p. 123. Baltimore, Williams & Wilkins Co., 1955.
The use of a molded splint to prevent contracture after split skin grafting on the neck. Plast. Reconstr. Surg., 27:7, 1961.

DAVIS, A. D.: *Congenital webbing of the neck.* (Pterygium colli). Amer. J. Surg., 92:115, 1956.

ERDELYI, R.: *Tubular flap procedure for the closure of a large pharyngeal fistula.* Brit. J. Plast. Surg., 9:72, 1956.

GONZALEZ-ULLOA, M., and GONDA, T. F.: *Klippel-Feil syndrome.* Plast. Reconstr. Surg., 4:109, 1949.

KRAGH, L. V., DEVINE, K. D.: *Reconstruction of the pharynx and upper esophagus.* Surgery, 46:319, 1959.

NAKAYAMA, K., ET AL.: *Experience with free autografts of the bowel with a new venous anastomosis apparatus.* Surgery, 55:796, 1964.

OUSTERKOUT, DOUGLAS K., ET AL.: *Inflatable splint: An adjunct to prevention and treatment of cervical scar contractures.* Brit. J. Plast. Surg., 22:185, 1968.

SCHMIDT-TINTEMANN, U.: *Sekundarplastische Massnahmen nach Verbrennung im Bereich der unteren Gesichtshälft und des Halses.* Chirurgia Plastica et Reconstructiva, 1:149, 1966.

SERRANO, A., ORTIZ-MONASTERIO, F., and ANDRADO-PRADILLO, J.: *Reconstruction of the cervical trachea.* Plast. Reconstr. Surg., 24:333, 1959.

SILVER, C. E., SOM, M. I..: *Reconstruction of the cervical esophagus after total pharyngolaryngectomy.* Ann. Surg., 165:239, 1967.

SPINA, V.: *Tratamento Cichurgica das Cicatrizes do Pescoco Pos-Qucimadura.* Sao-Paulo 1955.

TILL, H. J., and CAMERON, J. M.: *A method of reconstruction of the neck after* esophagectomy and laryngectomy. *Surg. Gynec. Obstet.,* 114:120, 1962.

WOOKEY, H.: *Surgical treatment of carcinoma of the hypopharynx and oesophagus.* Brit. J. Surg., 35:249, 1948.

DIVISION
THREE
THE
TRUNK

INTRODUCTORY
ASPECTS OF   14
THE TRUNK

THE general principles of repair and reconstruction are those which have been discussed in detail in the first part of the book, and will not be stressed.

The problems selected are of special nature and of interest to the general surgeon as well as the general plastic surgeon. The subject is divided into anatomical regions and discussed in the following five chapters.

ANESTHESIA

Ether is used in operations on the trunk, alone or in combination with gases such as nitrous oxide and halothane. Local anesthesia is provided with Xylocaine or Carbocaine, either alone or in combination with sodium pentothal. Spinal anesthesia may be used in operations below the diaphragm. For long operations, continuous spinal anesthesia is infrequently used; continuous epidural anesthesia is preferred since Xylocaine, Carbocaine, etc. have been introduced. For short anesthesia, sodium pentothal, alone or in combination with nitrous oxide, is used. Endotracheal methods of anesthesia are not necessary for surgery on this section of the body unless absolutely indicated.

For details concerning the various agents and methods mentioned here, the reader should refer to standard textbooks on anesthesiology.

607

BIBLIOGRAPHY

CLEMENT, F. W.: *Nitrous-Oxide-Oxygen Anesthesia*. Lea & Febiger, Philadelphia, 1951.

DAGLIOTTI, A. M.: *Anesthesia; Narcosis, Local, Regional, Spinal*. S. B. Debour, Chicago, 1937.

DRIPPS, R. D., ECKENHOFF, J. E., and VANDAM, L. D.: *Introduction to Anesthesia: The Principles of Safe Practice*. W. B. Saunders, Philadelphia, 1957.

FLAGG, P. F.: *The Art of Anesthesia*. J. B. Lippincott, Philadelphia, 1944.

GILLESPIE, N. A.: *Endotracheal Anesthesia*. The University of Wisconsin Press, Madison, 1948.

GUEDEL, A. E.: *Inhalation Anesthesia: a Fundamental Guide*. The Macmillan Company, New York, 1937, and 2nd Edition, 1951.

HALE, D. E., and Forty American Authors: *Anesthesiology*. F. A. Davis Company, Philadelphia, 1954.

LABAT, G.: *Regional Anesthesia, Its Technic and Clinical Application*. W. B. Saunders, Philadelphia, 1928.

LEIGH, M., DIGBY, M., and BELTON, M. K.: *Pediatric Anesthesia*. The Macmillan Company, New York, 1949.

LUNDY, J. S.: *Clinical Anesthesia: a Manual of Clinical Anesthesia*. W. B. Saunders, Philadelphia, 1943.

MINNITT, R. J., and GILLIES, J.: *Textbook of Anesthetics*. Williams & Wilkins, Baltimore, 1948.

MOORE, D. C.: *Regional Block: A Handbook for Use in the Clinical Practice of Medicine and Surgery*. Charles C Thomas, Springfield, 1953.

PITKIN, G. P.: *Conduction Anesthesia*. J. B. Lippincott, Philadelphia, 1950.

WYLIE, W. D., and CHURCHILL-DAVIDSON, H. C.: *A Practice of Anesthesia*. Year Book Medical Publishers Inc. 1966.

608

THE ABDOMINAL WALL AND THE BACK

15

OF THE defects of the abdominal wall, the incisional hernia requiring tissue grafts for closure has been selected as a typical example. The same technique is applicable for other large defects, such as inguinal hernias with defective structures or defects resulting from removal of tumors.

INCISIONAL HERNIA REQUIRING TISSUE GRAFTS FOR CLOSURE

Indication for the use of a strong tissue graft in repairing an incisional hernia arises in cases where the hernial defect is so large that over-lapping the aponeurosis of the defect's edges is impossible. The graft most suitable for this purpose is the derma, that is, the epithelial denuded skin (see p. 45). It is stronger than fascia or any other connective tissue, and owing to metaplasia assumes the characteristics of the tissue surrounding it (Rehn); a further advantage is that it is readily available. G. B. Mair employed whole-thickness skin grafts, that is, he included the epidermis. He states that the epidermis atrophies and that inclusion cysts do not form. Others (Massden, Zavaleta et al., M. and A. Behrend, and Vasquez) have confirmed his findings. The reasons for the author's preference for the dermal graft have been given on page 45. Foreign-body material, such as tantalum mesh (Koontz), Teflon (Luding-

609

ton and Woodward) and pliable plastics (Moore and Siderys), have also been suggested. The foreign-body meshes are known to have broken and caused considerable distress to the patient when bending forward.

Technique (Case 105, p. 1130)

An incision is made over the hernia; if possible, the former scar is excised. The hernial sac is dissected free from the surrounding structures until the fascial ring is well defined. The sac is then opened, care being taken not to injure abdominal contents which may be adherent to the sac.

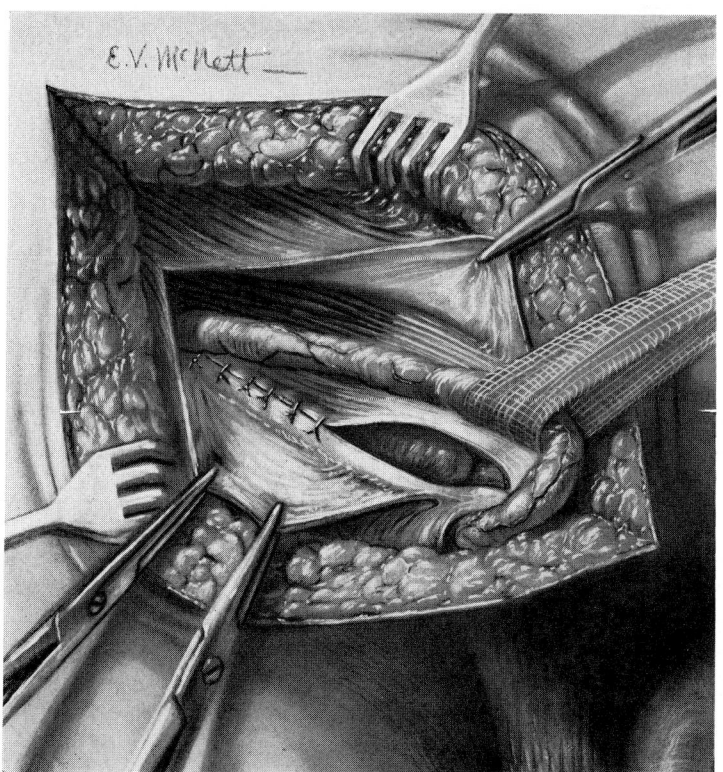

Fig. 277. Recurrent inguinal hernia. Incomplete closure; tension on sutures of conjoined tendon and Poupart's ligament.

The sac may or may not need removal. In the latter case, its edges can later be utilized for closure. All adhesions on the peritoneal side are severed for a distance of 12.5 to 14 cm. (about 5 to 6 inches) from the hernial ring. The hernial opening is now reduced as much as possible by Mayo's overlapping method. To facilitate the overlapping of the aponeurosis, a transverse or longitudinal incision is made on each side of the ring, thus

610

forming two flaps of aponeurosis. If the transverse incision is used, the upper flap is pulled over the lower flap ("vest over pants"). The edge of the lower (under) flap is held well drawn up to the overlap (upper) flap by mattress sutures (for insertion of mattress sutures, compare with Figs. 280, 281). The edges of the overlap flap are then sutured to the fascia,

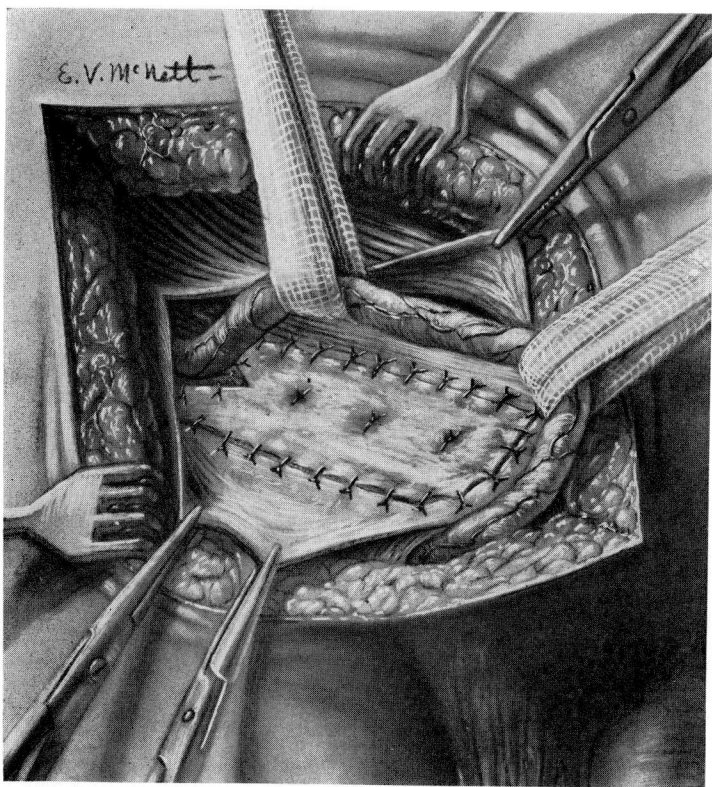

Fig. 278. Reinforcement of suture line and closure of remaining inguinal gap with dermal graft. Fascia of musculus obliquus externus to be sutured over the graft beneath the spermatic plexus.

upon which they lie. In longitudinal incisions, the side-to-side overlap is similar. In this way, the hernial opening is made as small as possible.

A pattern is now made of the remaining defect, and a dermal graft 2.5 cm. (1 inch) wider than the pattern is removed from the abdomen or one of the thighs (for technique of removal of dermal graft, see p. 45). The graft is placed upon the fascia surrounding the edges of the defect. Since the graft has been cut larger than the defect, it overlaps the edges. Interrupted sutures of silk are placed through the graft and the edges of the hernial defect beneath it. The graft is held under as much tension as possible. Suture of the overlapping graft edges to the aponeurosis follows. The overlying subcutaneous tissue and skin are coapted. To facilitate an intimate contact between graft and overlying subcutaneous tissues and to avoid dead spaces, the subcutaneous-tissue sutures should include the graft surface. Suture of the skin edges follows.

The technique for repair of an inguinal hernia with a dermal graft is shown in Figures 277 and 278.

Even massive full-thickness abdominal wall defects can be successfully closed with split-thickness skin grafts as demonstrated by Meadick, Pickrell, Royer, McCraw and Brown and by Millard, Pigott and Zies. The grafts are placed directly upon the exposed viscera from which they receive their blood supply.

After-Treatment

A firm dressing is applied, and is changed after seven days; the skin sutures are removed at that time. The patient is allowed out of bed ten days after the operation.

DECUBITAL ULCERS

Decubital ulcers, developing as common bedsores or from spinal injuries followed by paraplegia, may heal under conservative treatment. More often, however, particularly in the paraplegic group, they may resist medical management. Skin grafting has been successful in closing these ulcers (Barker, Elkins, and Poer) including the reversed or "upside down" dermis grafts (Wesser and Kahn). A more reliable closure, with better padding of the ulcerated area, is established by the use of pedicle flaps (Croce, Schullinger, and Shearer, White and Hamm, Gibbon and Freeman, Kostrubala and Greeley, Conway et al., Gelb, Guttman and others). Before such a closure is attempted in the debilitated patient, his general condition should be improved by local and systemic measures. These include relieving pressure on the site of the lesion (placing the patient on a Stryker frame, on which he can be turned every two hours, is valuable), combating infection and inflammation, establishing a positive nitrogen balance, and providing an adequate intake of vitamins (Rossak and Krahn). The patient should be given a diet high in calories and proteins, supplemented by vitamins, together with infusions of plasma, whole blood, and amino acids (Berger). It has been pointed out that a true metabolic imbalance occurs in paraplegic patients. Cooper, Ryerson, et al., and Langston have counteracted this with testosterone propionate, varying from 25 mg. three times weekly to 100 mg. once a day. The whole topic has been recently covered by Bailey in a monograph.

The ulcer should be cleansed with hydrogen peroxide and covered with wet dressings of Dakin's or saline solution. Only after the patient's general condition has been improved and the ulcerated area is covered with healthy granulations, free from sloughing, should the operation be per- formed. It consists of excision of the ulcer and all scar tissue, removal of underlying bony prominences—a valuable innovation made by Blocksma, Kostrubala, Greeley and Cannon—and closure of the defect with sliding flaps. The various flaps have been outlined in detail by Croce et al. and Gelb.

Large sacral defects must be covered with four sliding flaps, as Case 97, page 1111, demonstrates. Smaller defects should be closed with two flaps, as demonstrated by Case 98, page 1112. The two-flap method has the advantage that the suture lines do not meet in a center point over the ulcer site, and thus a locus minoris resistentiae is avoided. Constant vacuum drain- age for two days with a plastic tube brought through a stab wound well away from the suture line is of value (Rossak and Krahn), In trochanteric ulcers, the flap is outlined on the anterior lateral aspect of the upper thigh, with its base at the femoral triangle. It is shifted laterally over the resected trochanter region and the flap bed is covered with a split graft. In ischial ulcers, one performs a wide resection of the tuberositas ischii and portions of the superior and inferior rami ischii and inferior rami pubi. The musculus obturator internus is sutured to the cut end of the biceps, and the wound is closed by simple approximation (Arregui, Cannon, Murray, O'Leary). Shifting of a flap from the posterior aspect of the thigh may occasionally be necessary.

DEFORMITIES

ADIPOSE ABDOMEN

In the majority of cases, the deformity of the adipose abdomen is a combination of hyperadiposity and other aggravating factors, such as re- laxation of the abdominal fasciae and muscles, diastasis recti abdominis, or abdominal hernia. Hence, reduction of skin and fat tissue would not suffice unless the other underlying conditions were corrected. Schepel- mann divides the adipose abdomen into two varieties, the globular and the pendulous. The globular abdomen is mostly due to rectus diastasis or large umbilical hernia. Approximation of the recti and longitudinal overlap of the anterior rectus sheaths, followed by reduction and adaptation of the overlying subcutaneous fat tissue and skin, is the operative procedure for correction of the globular abdomen due to rectus diastasis. The transverse overlap of the aponeurosis ("vest over pants") and reduction and adaptation of subcutaneous tissue and skin is the method of choice in umbilical hernia (see foregoing remarks on technique in incisional hernia, p. 610).

The pendulous abdomen, or fat apron, however, has a different cause. It is mostly due to hyperadiposity associated with relaxation of the fasciae and muscles. Hence, the operation of correction is divided into two phases: (1) transverse shortening of the fasciae and muscles, (2) excision of fat tissue and skin.

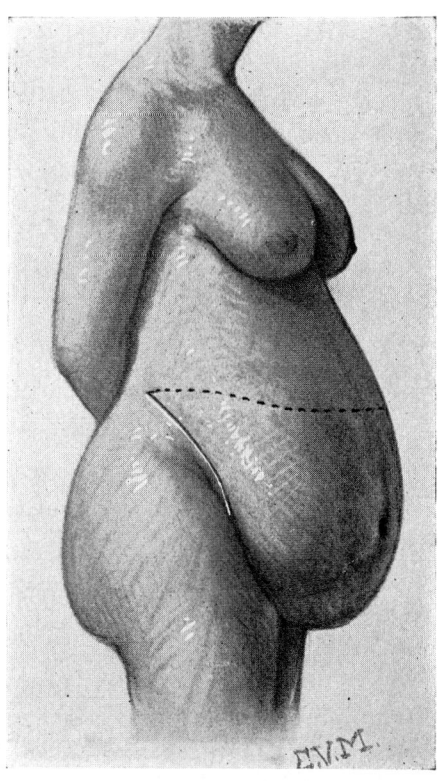

Fig. 279. Plastic correction of adipose abdomen associated with relaxation of fasciae and muscles. A curved incision, passing from one loin through inguinal region, mons pubis, other inguinal region to other loin, is made, penetrating skin and subcutaneous tissue. Dotted line indicates base of flap of skin and fat tissue to be lifted up. (E. Schepelmann.)

614

Technique (*Schepelmann*) (Figs. 279-282) (Case 104, p. 1128; Case 106, p. 1130)

A curved incision—passing from one loin through inguinal region of same side, mons pubis, and inguinal region of other side to the other loin —is made, penetrating skin and subcutaneous tissue. Skin and subcutaneous fat tissue are dissected free from the aponeurosis, and a large apron of tissue is lifted to a line above the umbilicus. A transverse, downward-curved incision is now made through the aponeurosis covering the abdominal muscles. The aponeurosis on each side of the incision is dissected away from the muscles, forming an upper and a lower flap. A midline incision may be added above the umbilicus. Any diastasis of the recti muscles is corrected at this stage by tucking the so-called "middle field" (posterior aponeurosis, fascia transversalis, peritoneum) inward and suturing the median borders of the recti muscles together, thus shortening the abdominal wall transversely. The longitudinally stretched recti are short-

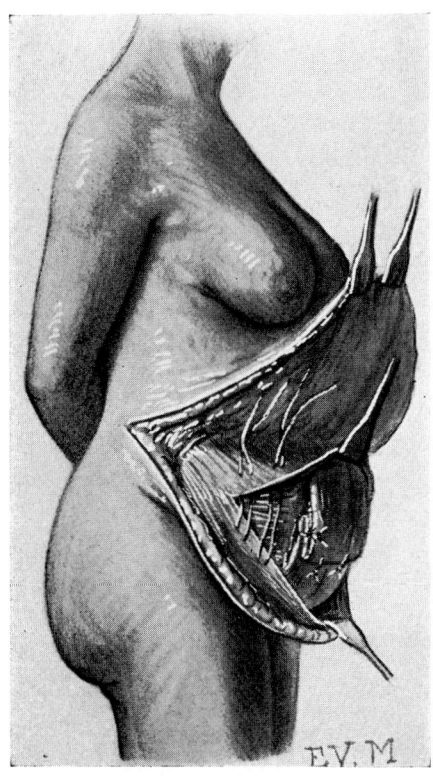

Fig. 280. Flap of skin and fat tissue is lifted up. An upper and lower flap of aponeurosis covering abdominal muscles are formed. Longitudinally stretched recti are "pleated." Edge of lower aponeurosal flap is to be lifted upward beneath upper flap. Mattress sutures are laid as in Mayo's overlap technique of hernial repair.

ened by "pleating" the muscles. The edge of the lower aponeurosal flap is then lifted upward beneath the upper flap. (Above the umbilicus the aponeurosal flaps are overlapped longitudinally.) The edge of the lower (under) flap is held well drawn up to the upper (overlap) flap by mattress sutures, according to Mayo's overlap technique. The edges of the overlap flap are then sutured to the aponeurosis upon which they lie.

The skin and fat-tissue flap is reflected downward and shortened to proper size. Castanares and Goethel and also Pitanguy shorten it by removal of a wedged-shaped portion of the middle section of the flap, which was found helpful in a recent case. Suction drainage is inserted at either lower lateral angle of the wound, and the wound is closed in layers.

If the umbilicus is to be preserved, it is circumscribed by a transverse elliptical incision as the first step of the operation. The incision penetrates to the posterior sheath of the rectus muscle. Thus, the umbilicus is left in place when the skin and upper aponeurosal flaps are lifted up. The latter have corresponding elliptical holes. When the aponeurosal

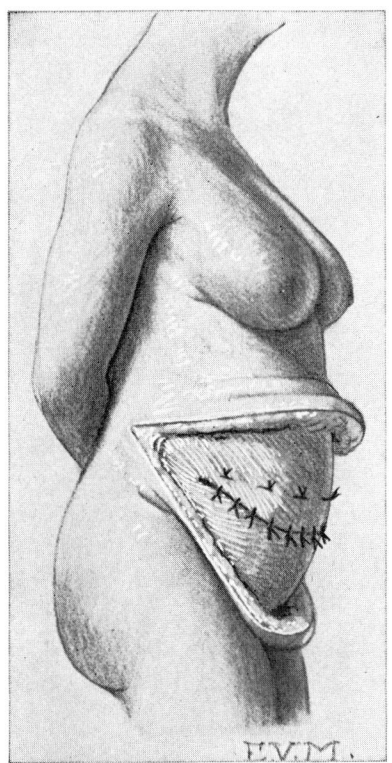

Fig. 281. Mattress sutures are tied. Edges of overlap flap are sutured to aponeurosis upon which they lie.

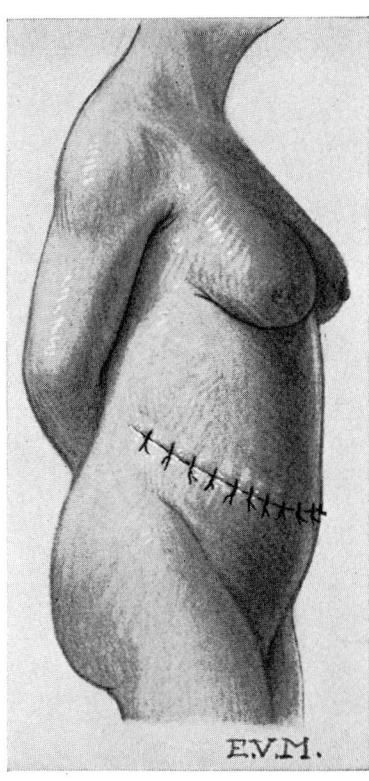

Fig. 282. Skin and fat-tissue flap is reflected downward and trimmed; wound is closed in layers.

616

flaps are overlapped, elliptical holes must be cut for the reception of the umbilicus. The same holds true when the skin flap is adjusted.

BIBLIOGRAPHY

THE ABDOMINAL WALL

BEHREND, M. A.: *Full thickness skin graft in the repair of voluminous hernias.* J. Int. Coll. Surg. 13:41, 1950.

CASTANARES, S., and GOETHEL, J. A.: *Abdominal lipectomy: A modification in technique.* Plast. Reconstr. Surg., 40:378, 1967.

GRAY, D. B., MANSBERGER, A. R., and YEAGER, G. H.: *The fate of buried full thickness skin: An experimental study.* Ann. Surg., 134:205, 1951.

GUY, C. C., and WERELIUS, C. K.: *The use of tantalum mesh in hernia repair.* Arch. Surg., 62:867, 1951.

KOONTZ, A. R.: *Tantalum mesh in the repair of large ventral hernias.* Surg. Gynec. Obstet., 93:112, 1951.
An operation for large incisional epigastric hernias. Surg. Gynec. Obstet., 114:117, 1961.

LESNICK, G. J., and DAVIDS, A. M.: *Repair of surgical abdominal wall defect with a pedicled musculo fascial flap.* Ann. Surg., 137:569, 1953.

LUDINGTON, L. G., WOODWARD, E. R.: *Use of teflon in the repair of musculofascial defects.* Surgery, 46:364, 1959.

MAIR, G. B.: *The Surgery of Abdominal Hernia.* Williams & Wilkins, Baltimore, 1948.

MAY, H., SPANN, R. G.: *Cutis grafts for repair of incisional and recurrent hernias.* Surg. Clin. N. Amer., 517, April 1948.

MILLARD, D. R., PIGOTT, A., ZIES, P.: *Free skin grafting of full-thickness defects of abdominal wall.* Plast. Reconstr. Surg., 43:569, 1969.

MEADICK, R. A., PICKRELL, N. L., ROYER, F. R., McCRAW, F., BROWN, I.: *Skin graft reconstruction of massive full-thickness abdominal wall defect.* Plast. Reconstr. Surg., 43:587, 1969.

MOORE, T. C., and SIDERYS, H.: *The use of pliable plastics in the repair of abdominal wall defects.* Ann. Surg., 142:973, 1955.

MORAES, C. C., and RIBEIRO, F. M.: *Skin grafts in treatment of hernia and eventration of abdominal wall.* Rev. Brasil, cir. 26:273, Sept., 1953. (In Portuguese.)

PITANGUY, IVO: *Abdominal lipectomy: An approach to it through an analysis of 300 consecutive cases.* Plast. Reconstr. Surg., 40:384, 1967.

SCHEPELMANN, E.: *Ueber Bauchdenkenplastik mit besonderer Berücksichtigung des Hängebauches.* Beitr. z. klin. Chir., 111:372, 1918. Zentralbl. f. Gynäk., 1924, p. 2289.

VASQUEZ, M. J.: Prensa Med. Argent., 36:1283, 1326, 1396, 1458, 1949.

617

THE TRUNK

ZAVALETA, D. E., and URIBURU, J. V.: *Whole thickness skin grafts in treatment of hernias, analysis of 211 cases.* Surg. Gynec. Obstet., 91:157, 1950.

ZIMMERMAN, L. M.: *Anatomy and Surgery of Hernia.* Williams & Wilkins, Baltimore, 1953.

THE BACK

ARREGUI, J., CANNON, B., MURRAY, J. E., and O'LEARY, J. J., Jr.: *Long term evaluation of ischiectomy in the treatment of pressure ulcers.* Plast. Reconstr. Surg., 36:583, 1965.

BAILEY, B. N.: *Bedsores.* London, Edward Arnold, 1967.

BARKER, D. E., ELKINS, C. W., and POER, D. H.: *Methods of closure of decubitus ulcers in the paralyzed patient.* Ann. Surg., 123:523, 1946.

BERGER, J. C.: *Surgical treatment of decubitus ulcers.* Plast. Reconstr. Surg., 20:206, 1957.

BLOCKSMA, R., KOSTRUBALA, J. G., and GREELEY, P. W.: *The surgical repair of decubitus ulcer in paraplegics; further observations.* Plast. Reconstr. Surg., 4:123, 1949.

CONWAY, H., et al.: *The plastic surgical closure of decubitus ulcers in patients with paraplegia.* Surg. Gynec. Obstet., 85:321, 1947.
Complications of decubitus ulcers in patients with paraplegia. Plast. Reconstr. Surg., 7:117, 1951.

CONWAY, H., and GRIFFITH, B. H.: *Plastic surgery for closure of decubitus ulcers in patients with paraplegia: Based on experience with 1000 cases.* Amer. J. Surg., 91:946, 1956.

CROCE, E. J., SCHULLINGER, R. H., and SHEARER, T. P.: *Operative treatment of decubitus ulcers.* Ann. Surg., 123:53, 1946.

GELB, J.: *Plastic surgical closure of decubitus ulcers in paraplegics as result of civilian injuries.* Plast. Reconstr. Surg., 9:525, 1952.

GIBBON, F. H., and FREEMAN, L. U.: *The primary closure of decubitus ulcers.* Ann. Surg., 124:1148, 1946.

GRIFFITH, B. H., and SCHULTZ, R. C.: *The prevention and surgical treatment of recurrent decubitus ulcers in patients with paraplegia.* Plast. Reconstr. Surg., 27:248, 1961.

GUTTMAN, L.: *The problem of treatment of pressure sores in spinal paraplegics.* Brit. J. Plast. Surg., 7:196, 1955.

LANGSTON, R. G.: *Testosterone in the treatment of decubitus ulcers.* Plast. Reconstr. Surg., 9:543, 1952.

ROSSAK, K., and KRAHN, J.: *Surgical treatment of decubitus ulcers in paraplegics (Ueber die chirurgische Behandlung von Decubitalgeschwueren bei Paraplegikern).* Langenbeck's Arch. Klin. Chir., 1965, 312:125.

WESSER, D. R., and KAHN, S.: *The reversed dermis graft in the repair of decubitus ulcers.* Plast. Reconstr. Surg., 40:252, 1967.

WHITE, F. C., and HAMM, W. G.: *Primary closure of bedsores by plastic surgery.* Ann. Surg., 124:1136, 1946.

MAMMAPLASTIC PROCEDURES 16

MAMMAPLASTY IN THE FEMALE

BREASTS are deformed, according to the female patient, because they are either hypertrophic or too small. The causation in either type is not well understood, but the condition is probably the result of endocrine dysfunction. In the hypertrophic type, additional factors such as pregnancy or obesity may lead to deformity.

HYPERTROPHIC PENDULOUS BREASTS

For about fifty years numerous methods for correction of hypertrophy of the female breast have been recommended. The initial techniques, consisting of partial amputations, suspensions or simple resections of the skin, were inadequate. Only those methods in which the resection and reconstruction of the breast are combined with displacement of the areola can be considered effectual. Before Thorek devised his method of transplantation of the areola as a free graft, Lexer's dictum was generally accepted, namely, a breast plasty must aim at reconstruction of the deformity while preserving the function of the gland.

The numerous methods, starting with Lexer's (1920, described by Kraske in 1923), can be divided into two groups:

619

THE TRUNK

a. The areola is circumscribed by an incision, i.e., severed from its circulation from the surrounding skin, and resection of the redundant part of the breast is carried out in such a way that the glandular blood supply to the areola is not impaired (Lexer, Biesenberger, Gillies and McIndoe, Bürkle de la Camp, Ragnell, Aufricht, Maliniac, Penn, to mention only a few; for a more detailed list of references the reader is referred to the monographs of Biesenberger, Thorek, Ragnell and Maliniac).

b. Only part of the circumference of the areola is severed from the surrounding skin; the other part forms a pedicle which is freed from its epidermis and transplanted subcutaneously (1930, Schwarzmann). Hence, the circulation of the areola is safeguarded by glandular as well as cutaneous sources. Strömbeck (1960) in taking advantage of this principle constructed two broad dermoglandular bridges for the areola. The author modified Lexer's method in 1945 after similar (Schwarzmann) principles but gave it up in favor of a method described later in this text.

An entirely different procedure from those described above, in which the glandular function is preserved, is Thorek's, in which the areola is removed and transplanted as a free graft. Hence, the function of the gland becomes interrupted. Since introduction of this new principle the various procedures of breast plasty must be divided into two main groups: those in which the function of the gland is preserved and those in which it is interrupted. Among the latter are Thorek's original method and one more recently (1963) devised by Skoog. While in Thorek's procedure the areola is excised in the beginning of the operation and preserved to be transplanted after completion of the reconstruction, Skoog leaves it attached at one or two cutaneous pedicles from which—as in Schwarzmann's method—the epithelium is removed. To give the areola more motility it is severed from the underlying glandular tissue, and after resection of the breast it is sutured into the place selected at the beginning of the operation; the pedicles are buried subcutaneously.

According to ample personal experience with Thorek's procedure I have no doubt that in big breasts a free transplantation of the areola permits a much more effective reconstruction of the breast than do methods in which the areola remains in contact with the glandular circulation. Fear that interruption of the function of the gland may lead to cystic degeneration or such other pathological changes as malignancy of the breast is unfounded (Davis, Snyderman and Lizardo, Crikelair, Richey and Symonds), particularly since most of these large breasts have little if any glandular tissue. If after the operation the woman becomes pregnant, as did three of the author's patients, the function of the gland can be promptly stopped by the administration of diethylstilbestrol. I have no experience with Skoog's method by which—as already mentioned—the areola is severed from the

620

underlying gland but remains attached to dermal pedicles. However, I feel that the modified Thorek method in which the areolae are transplanted as free grafts is simpler and more effective. Even the largest breasts can be reduced to normal size since the resection of the breast can be carried out without considering the circulation to the areolae; secondly, there is freedom to choose the most favorable site for the areolae at the end of the operation. I do not recommend a permanent interruption of the function of the gland in the reconstruction of medium-sized hypertrophy of the breasts. In these cases sufficient amount of breast tissue can be resected without endangering the glandular blood supply to the areola.

The blood supply of the breast is derived from three sources: branches of the arteria axillaris, of the arteria mammaria interna, and the arteriae intercostales. According to Cruveilliers, Kaufman, Maliniac, Edholm and Strömbeck, and others, the third and fourth branches of the arteria mammaria interna carry the main blood supply, not only to the gland but also to the areola. While the branches of the arteria axillaris supply only the lateral superficial parts of the breast, the intercostal arteries are insignificant (Anson, Wright, and Wolfer). Thus, the areola receives its blood supply from beneath—from the branches of the arteria mammaria interna and also from the surrounding skin. If the areola is separated from the surrounding skin but left attached to its base, a sufficient blood supply is guaranteed from beneath. If, however, in addition to the skin incisions, much breast tissue needs to be removed, the deep blood supply of the areola may become insufficient unless proper precautions are taken, such as resecting

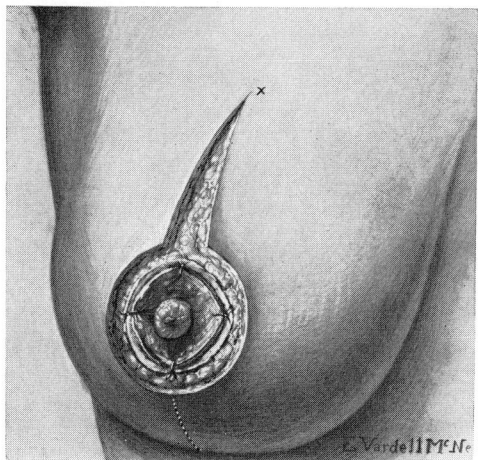

Fig. 283. Breast plasty with preservation of function of the gland. New site of the areola is marked out (x). Areola circumscribed with an incision through partial thickness of skin; a wider rim of entire thickness of skin circumscribed; areola fastened to rim of latter with holding sutures. Incision from upper pole of areola incision to x and from lower pole downward.

621

only the lateral parts of the breast tissue, leaving the median half intact to form a median pedicle (Biesenberger, Gillies, and McIndoe), and leaving the areola attached to a pedicle flap which is freed from epidermis and transplanted subcutaneously after the two-pedicle procedure of Strömbeck. For correction of medium-sized and fairly large breasts, the author

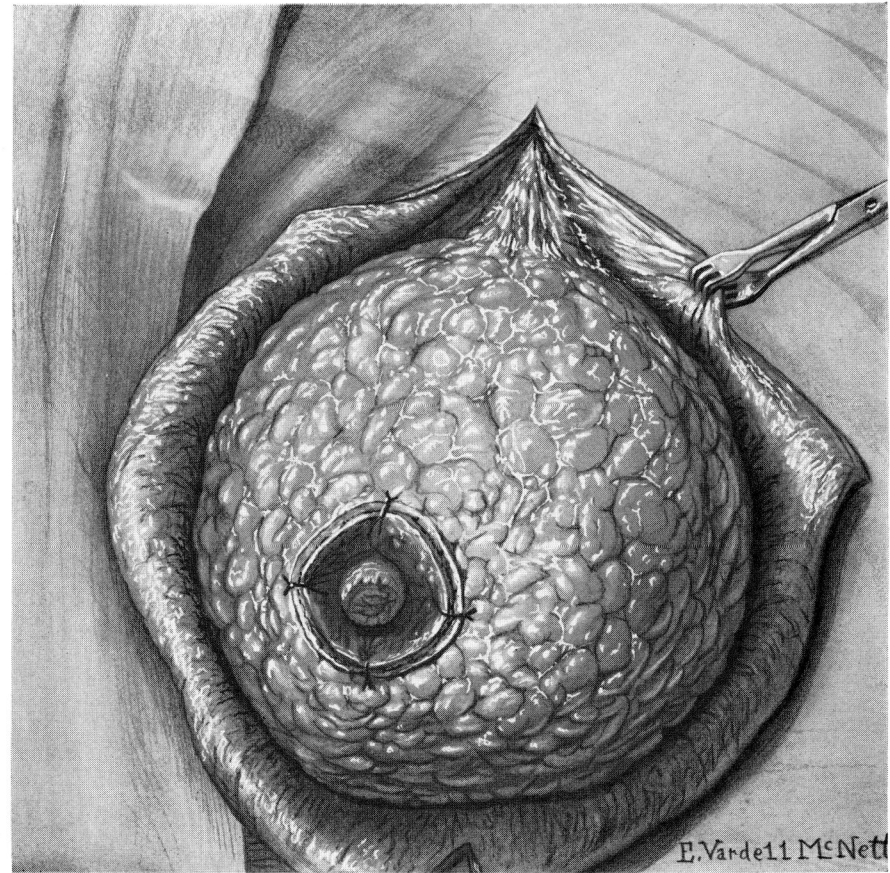

Fig. 284. Skin and thin layer subcutaneous fat tissue dissected away from breast.

recommends an operation which is based upon Biesenberger's principle in combination with certain favorable features taken from other techniques (Lexer's, Aufricht's, for example).

Technique (Correction of Medium-Sized and Fairly Large Pendulous Breasts) (Figs. 283-289; Cases 90, 91, pp. 1104, 1105)

The patient is operated upon in a half-sitting position under endotracheal anesthesia; a blood transfusion is running through a vein of the foot. The new site of both nipples is selected and marked with a drop of methylene blue injected intracutaneously (Fig. 283). An assistant now stretches the areola lightly. An ordinary medicine glass, the rim of which is painted with methylene blue, is placed over the areola, thus outlining its new size. An incision is made around the inscribed circle, but is not

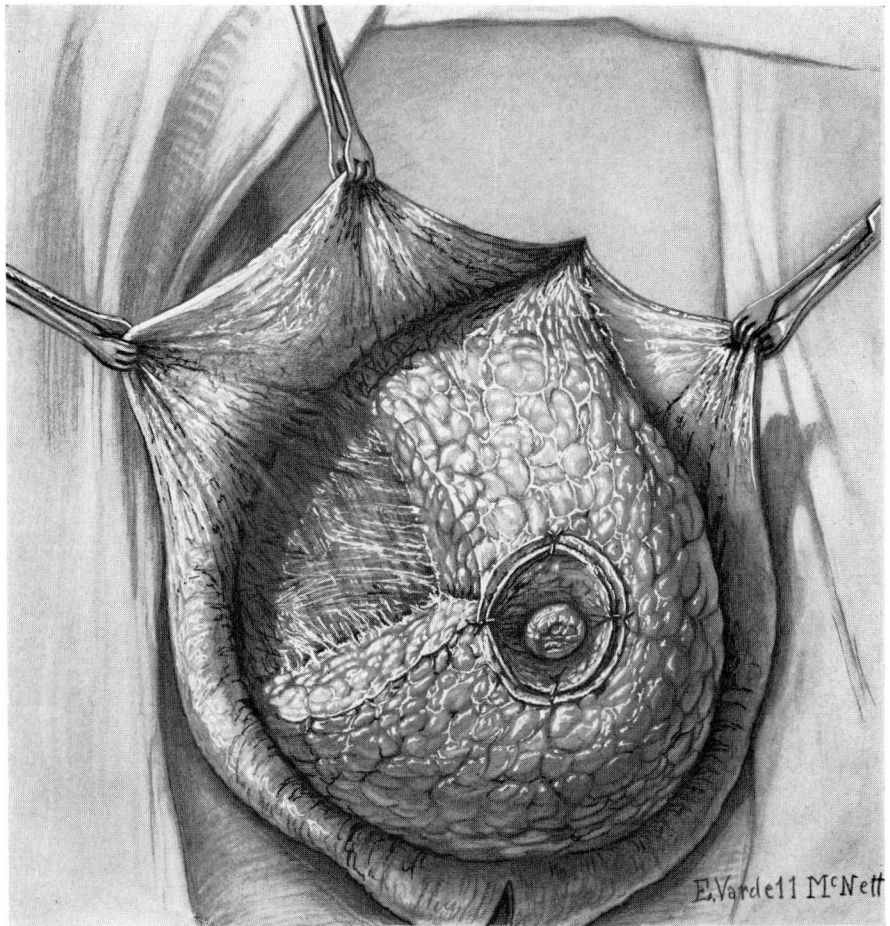

Fig. 285. Excision of wedged piece of breast tissue from lateral parts of upper and lower quadrants.

carried through the entire thickness of the skin. The skin around the areola is stretched tightly so that the subcutaneous tissue becomes exposed; this is incised about 1.2 to 2.5 cm. (½ to 1 inch) away from the original areolar incision (Aufricht); thus, when the skin is subsequently placed around the areola, the subcutaneous ring anchors it and prevents bulging and herniation. A few catgut stitches through the rim and the underlying

623

breast tissue will prevent tearing of the areola during the subsequent dissection (Fig. 283). An incision is made from the newly selected site of the nipple to the upper pole of the areolar incision and from the lower pole, two-thirds of the distance between nipple and mammary fold (Fig. 283). The skin and a thin layer of subcutaneous fat tissue are now dissected away

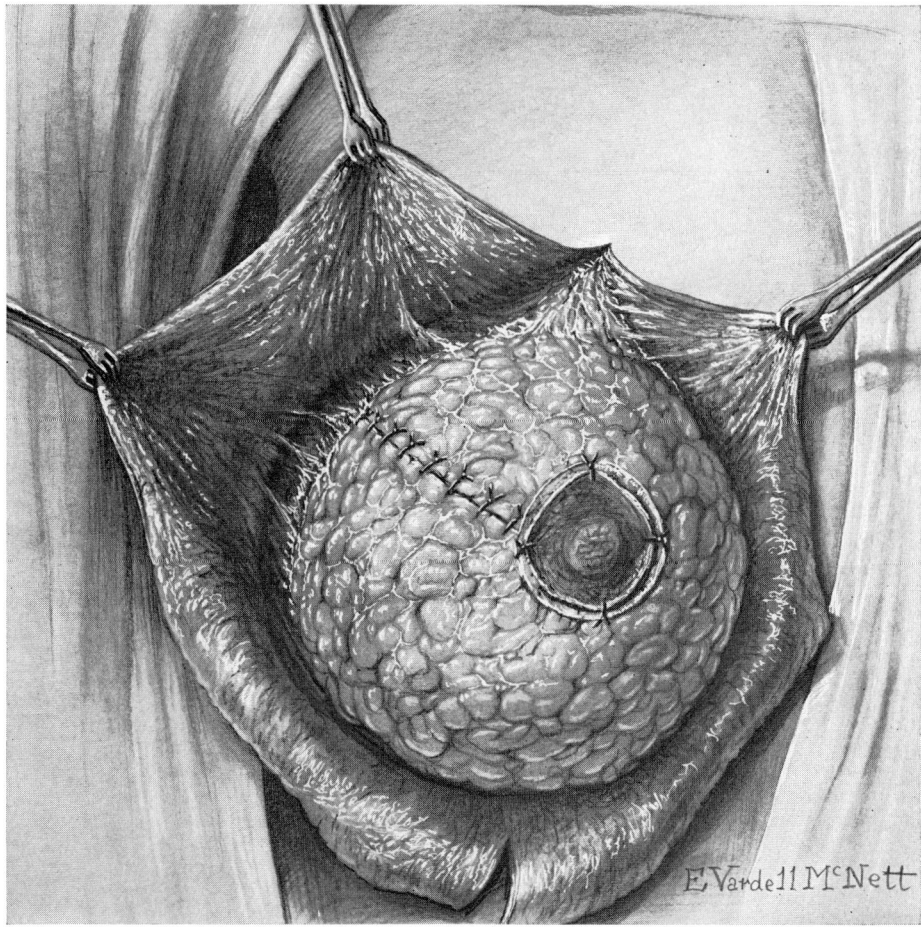

Fig. 286. Adaptation of wound edges of breast.

from the breast, mostly by blunt stripping, until the whole body of the breast is developed (Fig. 284). A wedge-shaped piece of tissue is removed from the upper and lower lateral quadrants. The wound edges of the breast tissue are approximated with a few sutures (Figs. 285-286). The patient can now be changed from a half-sitting to a more horizontal position to facilitate the following steps. The skin is draped around the breast like a brassiere (Fig. 287). Thus, the nipple becomes temporarily buried beneath the skin. The skin is held snugly together with towel clips or special clamps as demonstrated in Figure 287. The lowest clamp should be placed not at the base of the breast but about 2.5 cm. (1 inch) above the mammary fold. A running wire mattress suture is temporarily laid just beneath the clips, and the latter are then removed. The redundant skin

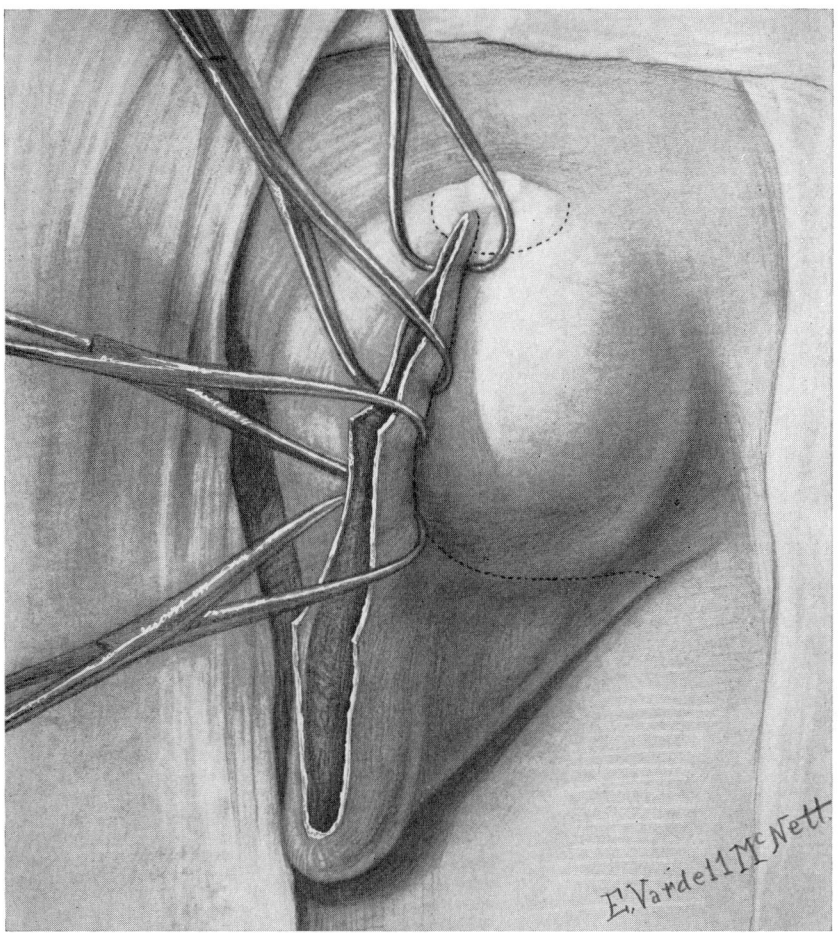

Fig. 287. Skin draped around breast, areola temporarily buried; lines of excision of redundant parts outlined.

is excised in front of the wire suture, and the skin edges are sutured together with interrupted nylon sutures. The lowest suture is about 2.5 cm. (1 inch) away from the base of the breast. The wire suture is then removed. From the points of the lowest suture, a curved incision is made laterally and medially. A triangular flap is made, as outlined in Figure 288, *insert*, with its base along the mammary fold. It is trimmed to fit into the

625

THE TRUNK

remaining triangular defect at the base of the breast. This triangular flap affords a good support. Even if the triangular flap is not made, the excision of the lower part of the redundant skin should be carried out one fingerbreadth above the original mammary fold because the new mammary fold will shift upward after reduction of the breast. The patient is placed

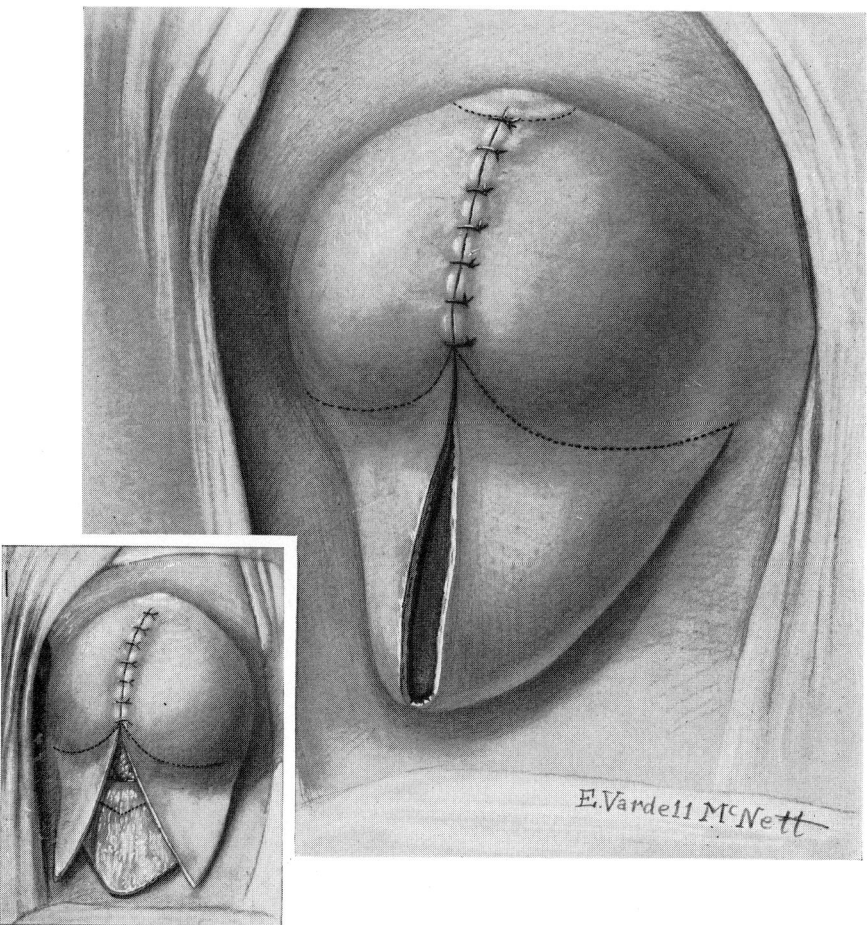

Fig. 288. Curved incisions outlined for formation of narrow triangular flap beneath breast.

again in a half-sitting position, and the same procedure is performed on the other side. The final step is the excision of skin over the buried areola and the adjustment of the areola to the wound edges. The possibility of rechecking and adjusting the new site of the areola at the end of the operation is a definite advantage of this procedure over methods in which the areola is sutured into the new position at the beginning. The proper

626

position of the skin to be excised is visually rechecked, and the incision is marked out with one of the dyes. Since it should have the same width as the buried areola, it is advisable to use the medicine glass for the pattern again. The new position of the nipple should not be at the top of the

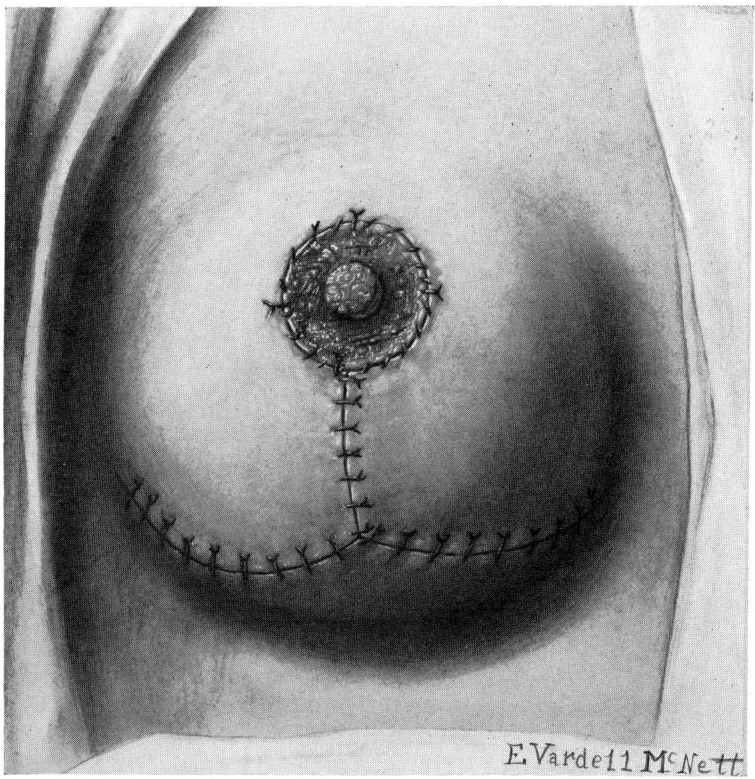

Fig. 289. Triangular flap beneath breast sutured in place. Skin over buried areola excised. Areola sutured in place.

conic breast but slightly below. The marked-out skin is excised and the areola drawn out and sutured to the wound edges (Fig. 289). The cutis ring surrounding the areolar incision (see Fig. 283) remains subcutaneously buried for firmer anchorage and prevention of bulging and herniation of the areola. A drain is inserted into each lateral wound corner.

After-Treatment

A firm, uplifting pressure dressing is applied to both breasts. The drains are removed on the third day, preferably without disturbing the remainder of the dressing. The sutures are removed on the eighth postoperative day. As soon as possible the patient should wear an uplifting brassiere in which the dressings can be incorporated.

THE TRUNK

Technique (Mammaplasty for Large Pendulous Breasts with Free Transplantation of the Areolae)
(Figs. 290-294; Cases 92-94, pp. 1106-1108)

Thorek excises the areola and transplants it at the beginning of the operation. Adams, however, points out correctly that one should select the new site for the areola at the end of the operation, since only after the partial amputation and reshaping of the breast is an accurate estimate possible. The author agrees also with Adams that both sides should be operated upon at one sitting.

The patient is operated upon in a half-sitting position under general anesthesia. The areola is stretched by an assistant, who squeezes the

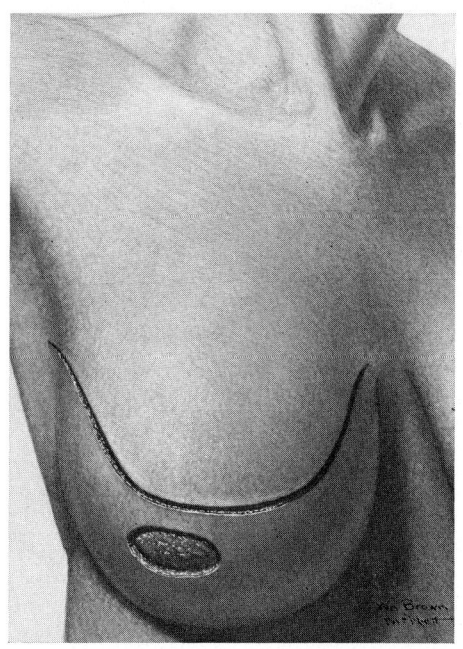

Fig. 290. Breast plasty with free transplantation of the areola. The latter has been excised as a free full-thickness skin graft and is temporarily preserved between cool saline-soaked compresses. The upper downward curved horizontal incision for resection of the redundant parts of the breast is indicated.

breast between his two hands. An ordinary medicine glass, the rim of which is painted with methylene blue, is placed over the areola, thus outlining the new size. The areola is now excised like a full-thickness graft, the operator carefully avoiding any subcutaneous or fat tissue. Near the nipples, the dissection is gradually made deeper in order to obtain some of the smooth-muscle tissue. The areola is carefully wrapped in gauze wet with isotonic saline solution, care being taken that the solution is not hot or even warm. The graft, wrapped in the gauze, is laid on a separate instrument table as a precaution against its being discarded. An anterior horizontal semicircular incision is made, from

628

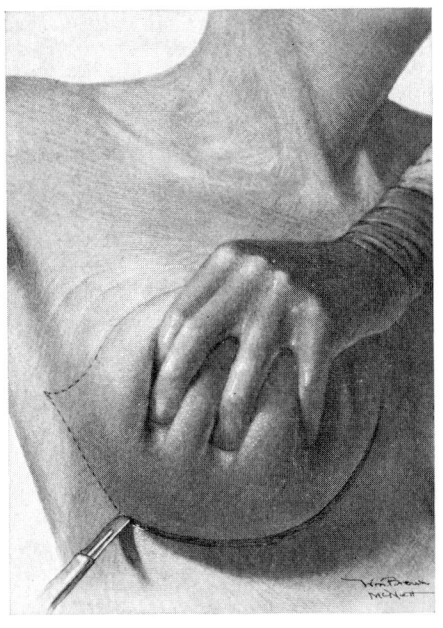

Fig. 291. The lower incision is made one inch above the mammary fold since the latter will inevitably become displaced upward after resection.

which the redundant parts of the breasts are to be removed. The incision is downward and convex, with its extremities rounded. A line connecting the two extremities of the incision should be on a level with the mam-

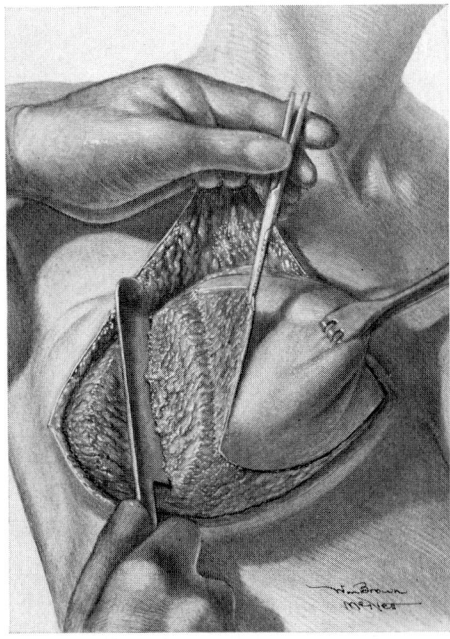

Fig. 292. From the upper incision a skin flap is dissected upward. The redundant skin and breast tissue are removed from a wedge-shaped excision.

629

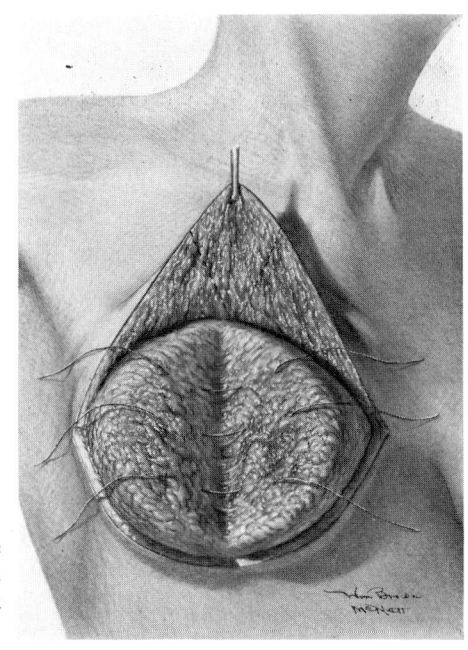

Fig. 293. The large wound edges of the breast tissue are loosely sutured together. Note outline of wedge-shaped excision of upper skin flap.

mary fold on the posterior side of the breast. The breast is elevated and an incision is made on the posterior side parallel to and about 2.5 cm. (1 inch) above the mammary fold. The skin edges are undermined along

Fig. 294. After adaptation of the wound edges of the breast with catgut sutures. The upper wound flap is draped over the reduced breast. A wedge-shaped excision is necessary to adapt the wound edge of the upper flap to the shorter lower wound edges. After both breasts have been operated upon, the new site of the areolae is selected. The skin for reception of the areola graft is excised so that a thin layer of derma is left behind (a free skin graft heals better on derma than on fat tissue). The interrupted sutures are left long and used to tie a pressure dressing over the areola in place.

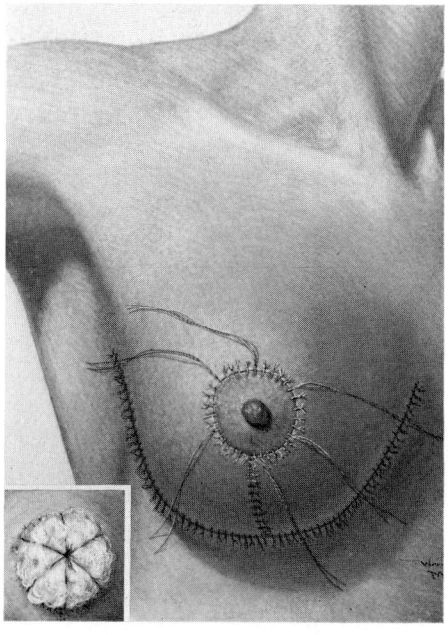

the anterior and posterior incision. The redundant mammary tissue together with the skin between the two incisions is now excised in wedge-shaped fashion; the broad wound surfaces are sutured together with heavy catgut sutures to rebuild the remaining breast tissue to a conic shape. The upper skin flap, which invariably is broader and longer than the lower one, is reduced in size by a vertical wedge-shaped incision (Fig. 293) to shorten it horizontally and to shape it brassiere-like. The wound edges are sutured together and a drain is inserted into the lateral wound corner. The other breast is operated on in the same way.

The site to which the areola is to be transplanted is selected and marked out with one of the aniline dyes. Since it should have the same width as the areola graft it is advisable to use the medicine glass again. The new position of the nipple should not be at the top of conic breast but slightly below. The host area should be made slightly smaller than the areola graft, since some immediate shrinkage of the graft always occurs. The skin of this circular host area is dissected away as with a thick split graft, leaving a thin basal layer of derma behind. The subcutaneous fat tissue should not be exposed, since adipose tissue is not as well vascularized as the derma of the skin. The previously excised areola is placed upon the host area, and carefully sutured in place with interrupted sutures of 000 nylon which are left long and continuous sutures of 00000 Dermalon on an atraumatic needle. One piece of bismuth tribromophenate (xeroform) gauze is now laid over the areola followed by a thick layer of mechanic's waste, which is held in place by tying the nylon sutures over it.

Same procedure is performed on the other side.

After-Treatment

A firm pressure dressing is applied. The pressure dressing over the grafts should not be changed for at least ten days, unless there is evidence of infection, while the other part of the dressing is changed and the drains are removed on the third day. As soon as possible the patient should wear an uplifting brassiere, in which the dressing can be incorporated.

SMALL BREASTS

Indications for reconstructive operation in small breasts are: smallness of breasts due to removal of breast tissue (cystic mastopathia, tumor) and genuine small breasts (hypomastia). Czerny, as far as can be ascertained, was the first to perform a reconstructive operation for correction of a small breast. For an actress from whom cystic tissue of the left breast had been removed, he replaced the tissue by a lipoma from the patient's lumbar region. The breast remained well formed, and the lipoma did not grow.

THE TRUNK

Until polymerized plastics were introduced as filling material and proved relatively harmless to the body tissues, dermal fat-tissue grafts, preferably taken from the gluteal fold (Winkler and others), were transplanted. The great disadvantages of these grafts are shrinkage and the creation of another wound. Hence, insertion of Ivalon or silicon sponges is preferred for build-up of small breasts (Edgerton and McClery, Conway and Dietz, Schmidt-Tintemann, Cronin, Peras, Clarkson, Gurdin and Carlin). The objection of course is the large amount of foreign-body material inserted. Further, Ivalon tends to shrink and to become hard and heavy. The polyurethan-silicon rubber prosthesis however seems to remain pliable and soft. It comes in five standard sizes in sealed containers and needs only to be autoclaved. None of the materials has caused malignancies, according to long-term follow-up examinations (Hoopes, Edgerton and Shelley), but do occasionally cause complications (Gurdin and Carlin) of which inflammation and infection are the most frequent. If infection becomes uncontrollable the prosthesis must be removed.

Technique

A 2½-inch long incision is made one inch below the mammary fold through the skin only; the dissection is carried caudalward above the subcutaneous fat for one inch in order to create a pendant fat pedicle attached to the superior border of the incision. This fat flap is of considerable value in giving a cross-lapped closure after the sponge has elevated the breast tissue away from the chest wall. With the superior margin of the wound edge retracted upward and forward an incision is made in the superficial fascia, and with blunt dissection a space is created between the breast capsule and the pectoral fascia. Bleeding is controlled with electrocoagulation. The prosthesis is inserted after folding it on the longitudinal axis. After insertion it is smoothed into place and the incision is closed; only the wound itself is dressed.

To counteract infection Edgerton injects 600,000 units of penicillin solution into the center of each sponge. Perras routinely aspirates the breast implants twice weekly until the breast regains a normal appearance. If infection does occur it should be controlled with a vigorous regimen of aspiration and instillation of the appropriate antibiotics.

TRAUMATIC ASYMMETRY

After mastectomies or destruction of the breasts from burns, the patient may be unduly self-conscious of the asymmetry in spite of shielding with a foam-rubber prosthesis. Gillies, also Holdsworth, devised a rather simple technique for replacing the mammary prominence. The method consists of transferring the circumumbilical skin and fat pad by means of a tube pedicle to form the new prominence. The umbilicus is turned out to form the new nipple.

Technique (Gillies)

Three stages and one substage are required. In the first stage, a tube flap is constructed on the affected side similar to the thoracoepigastric tube flap described on page 98. It starts in the midaxillary line at the level of the sixth rib. Its direction is toward the abdominal prominence which surrounds the umbilicus. In a substage two weeks later, the circumumbilical fat pad is elevated except for 5 cm. (2 inches) on its far side. The umbilicus is freed and everted, and the hollow beneath it is filled out by gathering small fat pads from the neighborhood and suturing them together. (As an alternative method, Gillies recommends burying a firm substance such as cartilage beneath the everted nipple.) The edges of the elevated flap are sutured together, thus continuing the tubed pedicle. Two weeks later, the abdominal end of the flap is severed gradually. A few days later, the flap is partly opened out and sutured into the place prepared for it. In the third and last stage, three weeks after the transfer of the flap, the pedicle is severed and discarded. Insertion of polymerized plastic sponges beneath the flap may be considered to increase the breast prominence.

In a suitable case Edgerton transplanted the flap from the normal breast and used it to enclose a mammary prosthesis.

LOSS OF AREOLA

Loss of the areola is more often due to impairment of circulation after mammaplasties than to trauma such as burns. If replacement is warranted, the Adams method appears feasible. He used the skin of the labium minus, which is picked up with a thumb forceps and clipped off with a pair of scissors, as a free graft. This skin is brownish and has a rough surface, and is thus most suitable to replace an areola.

INVERTED NIPPLES

Pfaundler distinguishes two varieties of inverted nipples: the genuine and the spurious. The former is considered to be a developmental hypoplasia in that the nipple failed to grow forward above the plane of the areola. The spurious form is due to hypertrophy of the muscles of the areola which hold the nipple back. Hence, in the first form, the nipple is not developed or at least not sufficiently developed; in the second form, the nipple is well built, but hidden behind the areolar muscles. Inverted nipples not only are a deformity but may also lead to inflammation of nipples and breasts and may make nursing difficult or impossible. Hence, operative correction may become necessary. Sellheim, improving Kehrer's and Barth's procedures, devised a good method, which is carried out as follows:

Technique (*Sellheim*) (Fig. 295)

The incisions are outlined with one of the aniline dyes, as illustrated in Figure 295, 2. The long horizontal incisions are made first, and should penetrate the entire thickness of the skin. The smaller radial incisions and the circular incisions are then added (Fig. 295, 3). The nipple is grasped with a traction suture and pulled forward. The entire areola is circumscribed with an incision which should reach the smooth muscle layers. While the nipple is held under constant pull, the skin of the areola is severed with circular incisions from the muscles (Fig. 295, 4). Some of

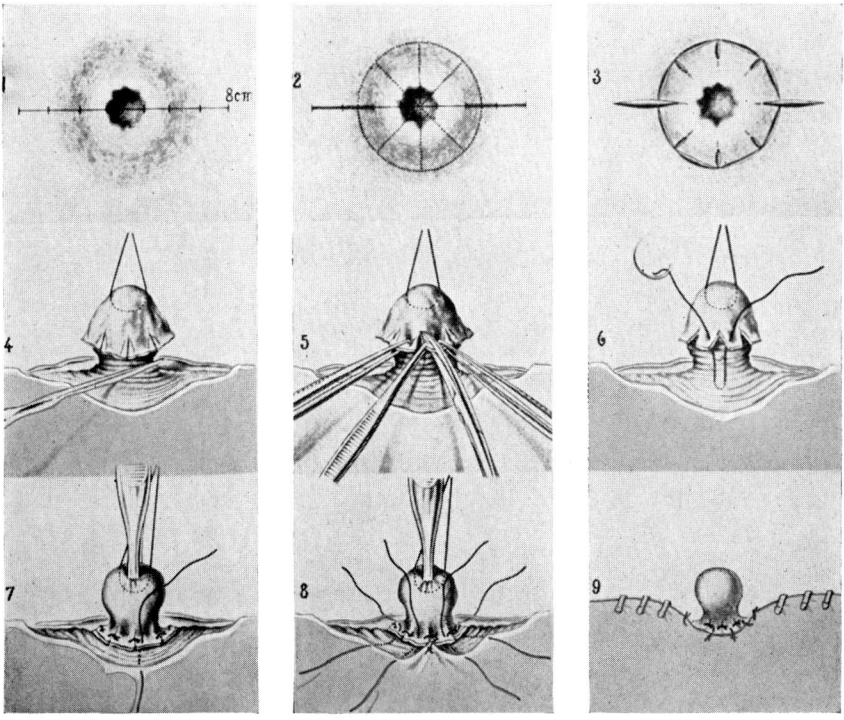

Fig. 295. Correction of inverted nipples (after Sellheim). (H. Sellheim: Zentralbl. f. Gyn.)

the muscle bundles, whenever restricting, should be divided. Galacto-phorous ducts and major vessels, however, should not be injured. Dissection is best carried out with the knife blade directed vertically to and not paral-lel to the base, and proceeds until the everted nipple and adjacent skin look like a folded umbrella.

Excision of small triangles of skin from the edges of the areola and subsequent suturing of those defects shorten the circumference of the areola and prevent retraction of the nipple (Fig. 295, *5, 6*). Figure 295, *6*, shows the tightening of the collar around the neck of the nipple.

With silk sutures, the wound margins of the everted areola are now united with those of the surrounding skin. The first suture is placed through the middle of the upper half, the second through that of the lower half (Fig. 295, *7*). From there the sutures are placed fanwise, mediad and laterally (Fig. 295, *8*). Whatever the size of the remaining defects, they can be closed by pulling the long horizontal incisions together with sutures (Fig. 295, *9*).

Spina covers the denuded area around the nipple, i.e., the denuded areolar region, with a skin graft from the labium minus (see p. 633), thus avoiding deformities from suturing of the horizontal incisions.

MAMMAPLASTY IN THE MALE

Mammaplasty in the male is performed in cases of benign gyneco-mastia. Conservative treatment, such as irradiation and endocrine therapy, fails as a rule to reduce the enlarged breast. Surgical treatment offers the greatest promise, and eliminates the threat of subsequent malignant changes and the development of psychic trauma. The author is familiar with the operation devised by J. Webster, and has found it very satisfactory. A slight modification facilitates the removal of the breast tissue.

Technique (*J. Webster*) (Fig. 296; Case 95, p. 1109)

The operation is performed under general anesthesia. If both sides are involved, they are operated upon in the same stage. The areola is dis-tended by pressure, and a semicircular incision is made just within the margin of the pigmented area of the areola. The areola is dissected away from the underlying ducts and glandular tissue. Traction is now applied on the divided ductal stumps, and a cone-shaped piece of breast tissue is dissected away from the subcutaneous fat tissue partly under blunt and partly under sharp dissection. Enough adipose tissue must be left behind to be drawn eventually beneath the areola. Bleeders should be clamped and ligated. To facilitate separation of the conic breast tissue from the pectoral fascia, the author makes a small incision at the lower base of the breast, and inserts an amputation knife between the base of the breast and the pectoral fascia, upon which a layer of fat tissue should be left attached (see dotted line in Fig. 296, B). With the left hand held against the breast as a

A   B

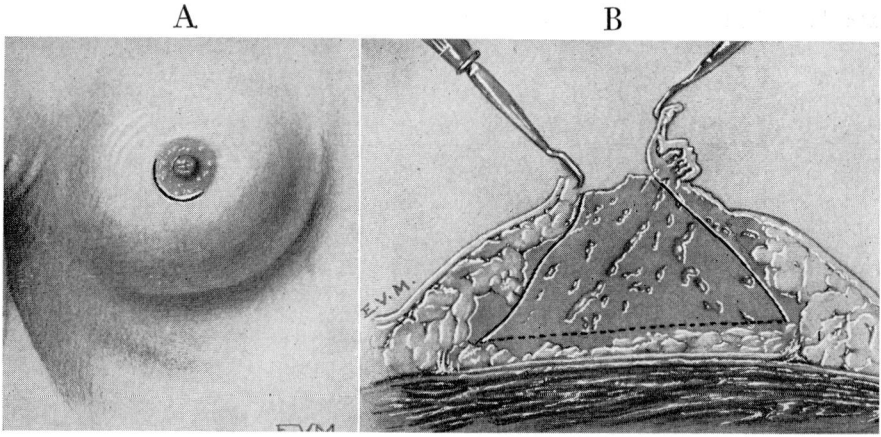

Fig. 296. Breast plasty for gynecomastia after Webster. *A:* Semicircular incision just within pigmented area of areola. *B:* Areola dissected away from ducts and glandular tissue. Lines of conic excision of breast tissue marked with heavy lines; broken line indicates separation of base of breast with amputation knife inserted through separate incision below breast.

protecting measure, and with pull exerted on the breast tissue, the breast tissue is severed from its base with long sweeps of the amputation knife. Pull should be relaxed before severing the central part to avoid removal of too much tissue where the areola will come to lie. The cone-shaped tissue is pulled through the opening at the areola; it may need halving or quartering if the tissue is too large to be drawn in toto through the opening at the areola. After thorough hemostasis, the wound is closed in layers. This is one of the most difficult phases of the operation. To prevent the nipple from becoming adherent to the underlying fascia, sufficient fat tissue must be sutured together, often by a trial-and-error method. After this is accomplished, the areola wound is closed. If the edges of the areolar flap look devitalized through pressure of the retractors, débridement of the devitalized rim should be performed first. A drain is placed into the small wound through which the amputation knife was inserted, or suction drainage, if necessary, through a small stab wound, and a heavily padded pressure dressing is applied. It is changed after five days, and drain and sutures are removed.

636

BIBLIOGRAPHY

ADAMS, W. M.: *Free transplantation of nipples and areolae.* Surgery, 15:186, 1944. *Labial transplantation for correction of loss of the nipple.* Plast. Reconstr. Surg., 4:295, 1949.

ANSON, B. J., WRIGHT, R. R., and WOLFER, J. A.: *Blood supply of the mammary gland.* Surg. Gynec. Obstet., 69:468, 1939.

AUFRICHT, G.: *Mammaplasty for pendulous breasts.* Plast. Reconstr. Surg., 4:13, 1949.

BIESENBERGER, H.: *Deformation und Kosmetische Operationen der weiblichen Brust.* Wilhelm Maudrich, Wien, 1931.

BLUMBERG, J. B., GRIFFITH, P. C., and MERENDINO, K. A.: *The effect of specific compression on soft-tissue response to formalinized polyvinyl alcohol (Ivalon) sponge.* Ann. Surg., 151:409, 1960.

BÜRKLE DE LA CAMP, H.: *Mammaplastik.* Chirurgiche Operationslehre, Vol. II, Urban and Schwarzenberg, Germany, 1955.

CLARKSON, P., and JEFFS, J.: *Modern mammaplasty.* Brit. J. Plast. Surg., 20:297, 1967.

CONWAY, H., and DIETZ, G. H.: *Augmentation mammaplasty.* Surg. Gynec. Obstet., 114:573, 1962.

CONWAY, H., and SMITH, J.: *Breast plastic surgery: Reduction mammaplasty, mastopexy, augmentation mammaplasty, and mammary construction.* Plast. Reconstr. Surg., 21:8, 1958.

CRIKELAIR, G. F., RICHEY, D., SYMONDS, F. C.: *Histologic studies of the female breast before and after free nipple transplant.* Plast. Reconstr. Surg., 34:590, 1969.

CRONIN, T., GEROW, T. J.: Augmentation mammoplasty: A new "natural feel" prosthesis. Third Internat. Congr. Plast. Surg., Washington, 1963.

DAVIS, H. H.: *Effects on the breast of removal of the nipple or severing of the ducts.* Arch. Surg., 58:790, 1949.

EDGERTON, M. T.: *Breast reconstruction after radical mastectomy for cancer.* South. Med. J., 60:719, 1967.

EDGERTON, M. T., and McCLARY, A. R.: *Augmentation mammaplasty.* Plast. Reconstr. Surg., 21:279, 1958.

EDGERTON, M. T., MEYER, E., JACOBSON, W. E.: *Augmentation mammaplasty. II. Further surgical and psychiatric evaluation.* Plast. Reconstr. Surg., 27:279, 1961.

EDHOLM, P., and STRÖMBECK, J. O.: *Influence of mammaplasty on the arterial supply to the hypertrophic breast. Angiographic studies before and after operation.* Acta Chir. Scand., 124:521, 1962.

GALTIER, M.: *Chirurgie Esthetique Mammaire.* G. Doin & Co., De L'Odeon, Paris, 1955.

THE TRUNK

GILLIES, H.: *Operative replacement of the mammary prominence.* Brit. J. Surg., 32:377, 1944.

GILLIES, H., and McINDOE, A. H.: *Technique of mammaplasty in conditions of hypertrophy of Breast.* Surg. Gynec. Obstet., 68:658, 1939.

GILLIES, H., and MILLARD, D. R.: *The Principles and Art of Plastic Surgery,* 2 *vols.* Little, Brown & Co., Boston, 1957.

GOHRBANDT, E.: *Mammaplastik, Langenbeck's Archiv für Klinische Chirurgie.* Deutsche Zeitschrift für Chirurgie, 282:607, 1955.
Mamma-Plastik. Zentralblatt für Gynäkologie, 69:1147, 1947.

GURDIN, M., and CARLIN, G. A.: *Complications of breast implantations.* Plastic Reconstr. Surg., 40:530, 1967.

HOLDSWORTH, W. G.: *A method of reconstructing the breast.* Brit. J. Plast. Surg., 9:161, 1956.

HOOPES, J. E., EDGERTON, M. T., and SHELLEY, W.: *Organic synthetics for augmentation mammaplasty: Their relation to breast cancer.* Plast. Reconstr. Surg., 39:263, 1967.

KAUFMAN, M. R.: *A propos de la chirurgie esthetique mammaire.* Bull. et Mem. Soc. méd. d. hóp. de Paris. 1935, p. 484.

LAMONT, E. S.: *Plastic surgery in reconstructing enlarged breasts.* Surgery, 17:374, 1945.

LESSING, M.: *Zur Mammaplastik.* Langenbeck's Archiv für Klinische Chirurgie. Deutsche Zeitschrift für Chirurgie, 282:613, 1955.

LETTERMAN, G., and SCHURTER, M.: *The surgical correction of inverted nipples.* South. Med. J. 60:724, 1967.

LEXER, E.: *Die gesamte Wiederherstellungschirurgie.* J. A. Barth, Leipzig, 1931.

LONGACRE, J. J.: *Correction of the hypoplastic breast with special reference to reconstruction of the "nipple type breast" with local dermo-fat pedicle flaps.* Plast. Reconstr. Surg., 14:431, 1954.
Surgical reconstruction of the flat discoid breast. Ibid., 17:358, 1956.

MacBRYDE, C. M.: *The production of breast growth in the human female.* JAMA, 112:1045, 1939.

MALINIAC, J. W.: *Arterial blood supply of the breast: Revised anatomical data relating to reconstructive surgery.* Arch. Surg., 47:329, 1943.
Breast Deformities and Their Repair. Grune and Stratton, New York, 1950.

MASSAPUST, L. C., and GARDNER, W. D.: *Infrared photographic studies of the superficial thoracic veins in the female: Anatomical considerations.* Surg. Gynec. Obstet., 91:717, 1950.

MAY, H.: *A plastic operation on the breast.* Arch. Surg., 38:113, 1939.
Reconstruction of breast deformities. Surg. Gynec. Obstet., 77:523, 1945.
Breast plasty in the female. Plast. Reconstr. Surg., 17:351, 1956.

McINDOE, A. H.: *Review of eighty cases of mammaplasty.* Rev. de chir. structive, 8:39, 1938.

638

MAMMAPLASTIC PROCEDURES

O'CONNOR, G. B., McGREGOR, M. W., and LONG, A. H.: *Mastoplasty in the last decade; a review.* Plast. Reconstr. Surg., 17:484, 1956.

PENN, J.: *Breast reduction.* Brit. J. Plast. Surg., 7:357, 1955.

PERRAS, C.: *The prevention and treatment of infections following breast implants.* Plast. Reconstr. Surg., 35:649, 1965.

PITANGUY, I.: *Mammaplasties (study of a sequence of 245 cases and presentation of a personal technique). Mammaplastias (estudo de 245 casos consecutivos e apresentacao de tacnica pessoal).* Rev. Brasil. Cir., 42:201, 1961.

RAGNELL, A.: *Breast reduction and lactation.* Brit. J. Plast. Surg., 1:99, 1948. *Transactions of the First Congress of the International Society of Plastic Surgeons.* Williams and Wilkins, Baltimore, 1957.

REINHARDT, W.: Die Plastische Chirurgie., Stuttgart, F. Enke, 1953.

SCHÖRCHER, F.: *Mammaplastik.* Verlag der Rieger'schen Universitätsbuchhandlung, München, 1951.

SCHMIDT-TINTEMANN, U.: *Erfahrungen mit Silikon-Kautschuk.* Langenbeck's Archiv für Klinische Chirurgie, 304:951, 1963.

SCHWARZMANN, E.: *Technik der Mammaplastik.* Chirurg., 2:932, 1930.

SELLHEIM, H.: *Brustwarzenplastik bei Hohlwarzen.* Zentralbl. f. Gynäk., 41:305, 1917.

SKOOG, T.: *A technique of breast reduction.* Acta Chir. Scand., 126: 1963.

SNYDERMAN, R. K., and LIZARDO, J. G.: *Statistical study of malignancies found before, during, or after routine breast plastic operations.* Plast. Reconstr. Surg., 25:253, 1960.

SPINA, V.: *Inverted nipple–contribution to the surgical treatment.* Plast. Reconstr. Surg., 19:63, 1957.

STRÖMBECK, J. O.: *Mammaplasty: Report of a new technique based on the two-pedicle procedure.* Brit. J. Plast. Surg., 13:79, 1960.

THOREK, M.: *Plastic Surgery of the Breast and Abdominal Wall.* Charles C Thomas, Springfield, 1942.

WATSON, J.: *Some observations on free fat grafts: With reference to their use in mammaplasty.* Brit. J. Plast. Surg., 12:263, 1959.

WEBSTER, J. P.: *Mastectomy for gynecomastia through a semicircular intra-areolar incision.* Ann. Surg., 124:557, 1946.

WINKLER, E.: *Mammaplastic.* Langenbeck's Archiv für Klinische Chirurgie. Deutsche Zeitschrift für Chirurgie, 282:609, 1955.
Subtotale Mammektomie mit freier Mamillentransplantation bei chronischer Mastopathie und Mammahypertrophie. Langenbeck's Arch. u. Dtsch. Z. Chir., 286:14, 1957.

CONSTRUCTION
OF ESOPHAGUS 17

An esophagus is constructed for reestablishing deglutition in patients with cicatricial atresia of the esophagus following chemical burns, with neo-plasms, and with congenital tracheoesophageal fistulas. This can be achieved in various ways either via the extrathoracic or intrathoracic route. The direct replacement of the esophagus with a plastic tube (after Berman) is the latest innovation but carries a high mortality from leakage. The extrathoracic route, popular as it has been, is seldom used nowadays. With the great advances that have been made in the field of anesthesiology and chest surgery, the intrathoracic esophagoplasty is given preference, and is an operation which belongs strictly to the field of general or thoracic surgery. However, for historic reasons and for the occasional cases where extrathoracic methods must be used, those methods are described in detail. The various techniques of replacement of the cervical esophagus have been described on page 599.

CONSTRUCTION OF
EXTRATHORACIC ESOPHAGUS

SURVEY OF PROCEDURES

Various procedures have been recommended to connect the cervical part of the esophagus in an extrathoracic manner with the stomach

(Fig. 297). Bircher (1894) was the first who attempted to circumvent a malignant stricture of the esophagus with an antethoracic skin tube, which was to connect the stomach with the cervical part of the esophagus.

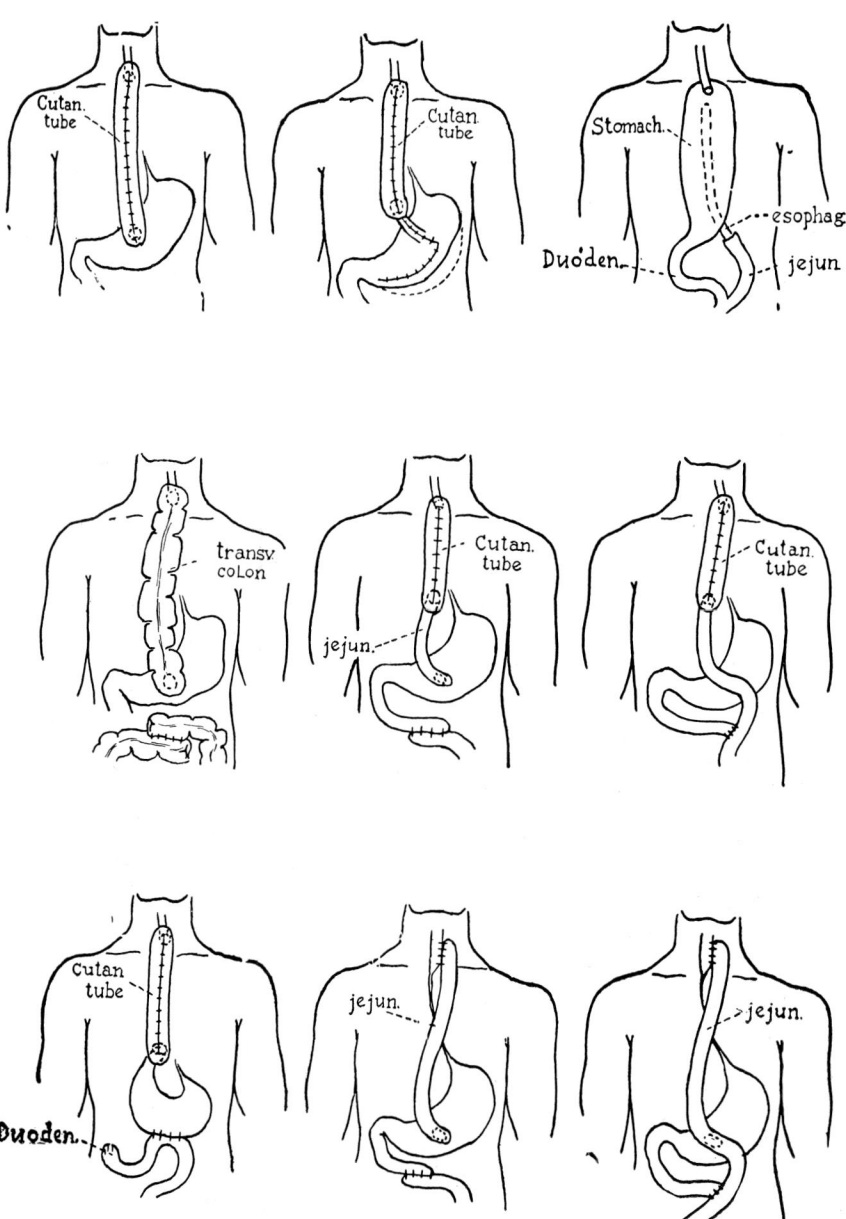

Fig. 297. *A:* Various procedures of extrathoracic esophagoplasty. (S. S. Yudin: Surg. Gynec. Obstet.)

He could not complete the operation, since the patient died from a pulmonary embolism. Wullstein (1904), from cadaveric studies, suggested the first jejunodermatoesophagoplasty. He severed the jejunum a short distance below the ligament of Treitz; the proximal loop of the jejunum was anastomosed to the distal part about 30 cm. (11¾ inches) below the division with an end-to-side anastomosis. The distal part of the jejunum above the anastomosis was pulled through the mesocolon, lesser sac, and gastrocolic omentum, led in front of the stomach and through a subcutaneous tunnel anterior to the thoracic muscles, and made to escape through a small skin incision at the level of the cartilage of the sixth rib. In a second operation, he suggested formation of a skin tube which was to connect with the jejunal opening and to reach the sternoclavicular joint. In a third operation, he suggested severing the cervical part of the esophagus and connecting its proximal part with the skin tube. In this way, the food would pass through the jejunum, but not through the stomach.

Roux, in 1907, was the first to demonstrate a successful case of jejunoesophagoplasty. He mobilized a loop of jejunum, displaced it antecolicly, anastomosed one end to side with the anterior surface of the stomach, and led the other end through a subcutaneous tunnel in front of the

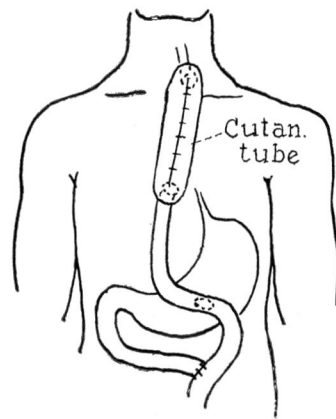

Fig. 297. *B.*

thorax to the suprasternal notch, where he left it subcutaneously. The afferent and efferent ends of the abdominal jejunal loops were anastomosed side to side with each other. In a second operation, the proximal end of the displaced jejunal loop was anastomosed with the mobilized esophagus.

Herzen (1907), following Roux's suggestion, improved the method first by leading the mobilized proximal end of the efferent loop through a slit of mesocolon and gastrocolic omentum in front of the stomach, thus shortening the distance and preventing torsion of the pedicle, second by excluding the jejunal loop unilaterally—suggestions previously made by Wullstein. While the latter did not join the jejunum with the stomach, Herzen anastomosed the mobilized jejunal loop with the stomach by an anterior side-to-side anastomosis.

F. Torek (1913) utilized the greater curvature of the stomach to form an esophagus and Kelling (1911) and von Hacker (1914) a loop of colon and a skin tube. Orsoni and Toupet (1950) reported the first successful case of an antethoracic cervical esophagocolostomy.

Lexer, in 1911, published his first successful case of jejunodermato-esophagoplasty. He excluded the upper jejunal loop, displaced it antecolicly, anastomosed it end to side with the anterior surface of the stomach, and led it subcutaneously anterior to the thoracic muscles upward. In a second stage, he formed the skin tube and joined it with the jejunal opening; in a third stage, the esophagus was opened laterally and the opening sutured into the cervical skin wound. In a fourth stage, the upper end of the skin tube and the cervical opening of the esophagus were joined. Lexer's reason for making a lateral opening in the esophagus instead of transversely sectioning it was twofold: (1) to lessen the danger of mediastinitis from the retracting distal end of the severed esophagus; and (2) to prevent stagnation of esophageal secretion in the blind section (Fig. 297, A [center], and Fig. 298).

Since that time, various other suggestions have been made. Ochsner and Owens published an exhaustive and critical review of the literature up to 1934 and presented their own case, the first successfully completed jejunodermatoesophagoplasty recorded in America. Davis and Stafford in 1942 added valuable information. Since then, additional articles have been published and modifications recommended (Longmire and Ravitz, Stevenson, Watson and Converse, Ivy and Hawthorne, Hardin, Ashley et al.). Axhausen reported a long-term follow-up examination of three patients with total esophagoplasty.

In 1944, Yudin of Moscow published his enormous experience of eighty-eight completed antethoracic esophagoplasties. Of these eighty-eight cases, twenty-one were total intestinal esophagoplasties, the remainder jejunodermatoesophagoplasties. The total intestinal esophagoplasty is, of course, the ideal method. The whole operation can be accomplished in two stages. However, as Yudin states, the procedure can be very difficult, very risky, or absolutely impossible owing to excessive fat in the mesentery, shortness of the mesentery, or particularly unlucky disposition of the radial vessels and of the mesenteric arcades.

JEJUNODERMATOESOPHAGOPLASTY

Technique (after Lexer) (Fig. 298)

Stage 1: The abdomen is opened from an upper paramedian incision through the left rectus muscle. Unless a gastrostomy has been already made, it is performed now on the left side and the gastrostomy tube led out of the abdomen pararectally on the left side. Then the proximal loop of the jejunum is located and severed 10 to 12 cm. (4 to 4¾ inches) from the ligament of Treitz. Both ends are closed in the usual way. The purse-string suture of the efferent end is left long for later use. The next step consists of mobilizing and lengthening the efferent loop of the jejunum by ligation and separation of some of the vascular trunks in the root of the mesentery while the peripheral arcades are carefully preserved. The vessels should be severed only after they have been compressed with an elastic clamp and no changes in color peripheral to the compression have been observed. After the jejunal loop has been lengthened sufficiently, but not unduly, its distal end is divided; thus the mobilization and isolation of the

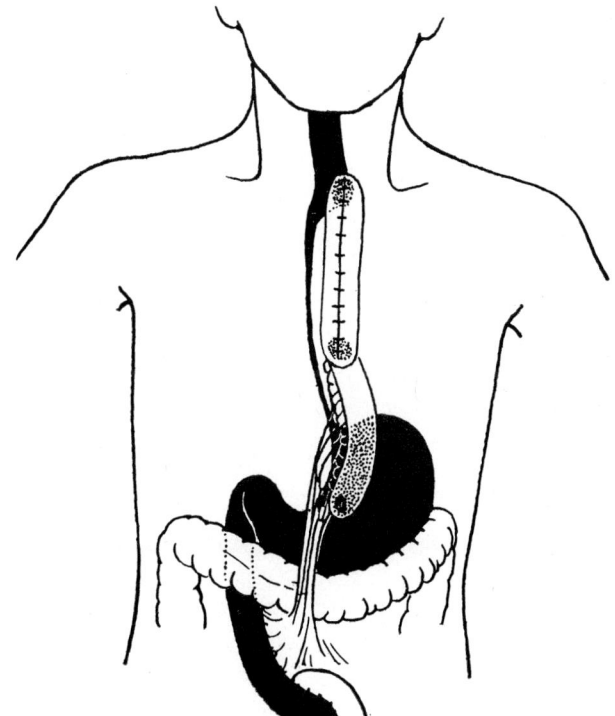

Fig. 298. Diagram of jejunodermatoesophagoplasty (Lexer).

645

intestinal loop are completed. The immobilized afferent and efferent jejunal loops are joined by a side-to-side anastomosis (Fig. 298).

The isolated loop is now displaced upward either antecolicly (Fig. 298) or, if the omentum is heavy, retrocolicly through a slit in an avascular field of the mesocolon and gastrocolic omentum; the open, distal end of the loop is anastomosed end to side to the anterior surface of the stomach near the middle of the lesser curvature (Fig. 298). From the upper edge of the abdominal incision, the skin is tunneled, anteriorly to the thoracic muscles and somewhat to the left of the midline, for a distance equal to the length of the isolated jejunal loop. The tunneling is best done by pushing a Graser or Payer type of gastric clamp upward beneath the skin and then opening the branches. The jejunal loop is laid upon the undermined skin and a small transverse incision is made through the skin on a level with its upper end. From this perforation, a Kelly clamp is passed through the tunnel, the purse-string suture of the closed jejunal end is grasped, and the jejunal loop is passed through the tunnel and through the upper small incision, where it is sutured to the skin without opening it.

Stage 2: About four weeks following the first operation, after all wounds have healed, the skin tube is formed and connected with the jejunum (Fig. 299).

Two parallel incisions, 8 cm. (3 inches) apart, are made on each side of the proximal end of the jejunum, leading upward, somewhat toward the left from the midline, and ending from 3 to 5 cm. ($1\frac{3}{16}$ to 2 inches) above the left sternoclavicular junction. Below the level of the closed jejunal end, the incisions approach each other gradually (Fig. 299). Between these two parallel incisions, skin, subcutaneous tissue, and deep fascia of the median margins are undermined one third until a lateral and a median skin flap are made for the formation of the skin tube. A broad base must be left attached to insure sufficient circulation in the flaps. The flaps are sutured together with silk sutures, which are tied on the inside (Fig. 299). A second row of 00 chromic catgut sutures approximates the subcutaneous fat tissue and fascia at the outside over the first row. (A good suggestion is to form the flaps eccentrically, one broader than the other, which will avoid placing the suture line directly beneath the future skin suture line.) Before the distal part is completed, the jejunum is opened at its exit from the skin. The skin tube is now connected with the jejunal opening, as depicted in Figure 299.

To cover the raw areas on and around the skin tube, one of three procedures is available: (1) mobilization of skin and subcutaneous tissue on each side of the raw areas until the wound edges can be shifted over the skin tube; (2) skin grafting; or (3) transplanting a tube flap which must be constructed in a previous stage (a valuable suggestion of Ivy). The first method is given preference, but only if the undermined skin portions are freely movable so that there will be no tension on the suture lines. To facilitate mobilization, relaxation incisions along the anterior axillary lines may be necessary (Fig. 299). If this is the case, the resulting secondary defects along the anterior axillary lines may be narrowed by skin sliding or closed by skin grafting (Fig. 300) after healing. If, however, there is

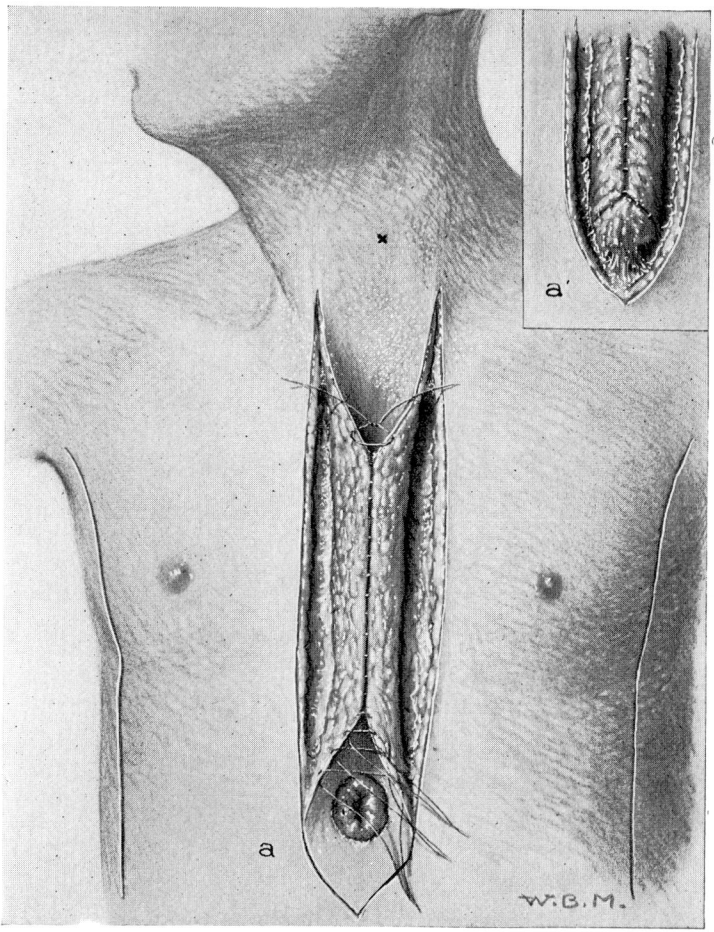

Fig. 299.   Drawing depicts second stage of procedure four weeks after upward displacement and gastroanastomosis of jejunal loop. Upper end of jejunal loop where it escapes through chest wall is opened (*a*). Skin tube is made by inverting skin edges of lateral and median skin flaps. Lower end of tube is connected with jejunal opening by forming a small pointed lower flap and hinging it upward like an envelope flap (*insert*). Raw surfaces are covered by skin sliding. Longitudinal incision in preparation for skin sliding is depicted on left and right sides of patient. Lateral secondary defects resulting from skin sliding are covered with skin grafts (see Fig. 300).

the slightest tension, skin sliding is abandoned, and skin grafts are used to cover the raw areas on and around the skin tube. With the plasma-contact method of Sano available (see p. 36), thick split grafts are glued to the raw areas. This method does not require dressings. Hence, the usual pressure dressing to hold the grafts firmly in place becomes unnecessary, a definite advantage, of course, in this particular case. The distal end of the tube, however, where it joins the jejunum, should preferably be

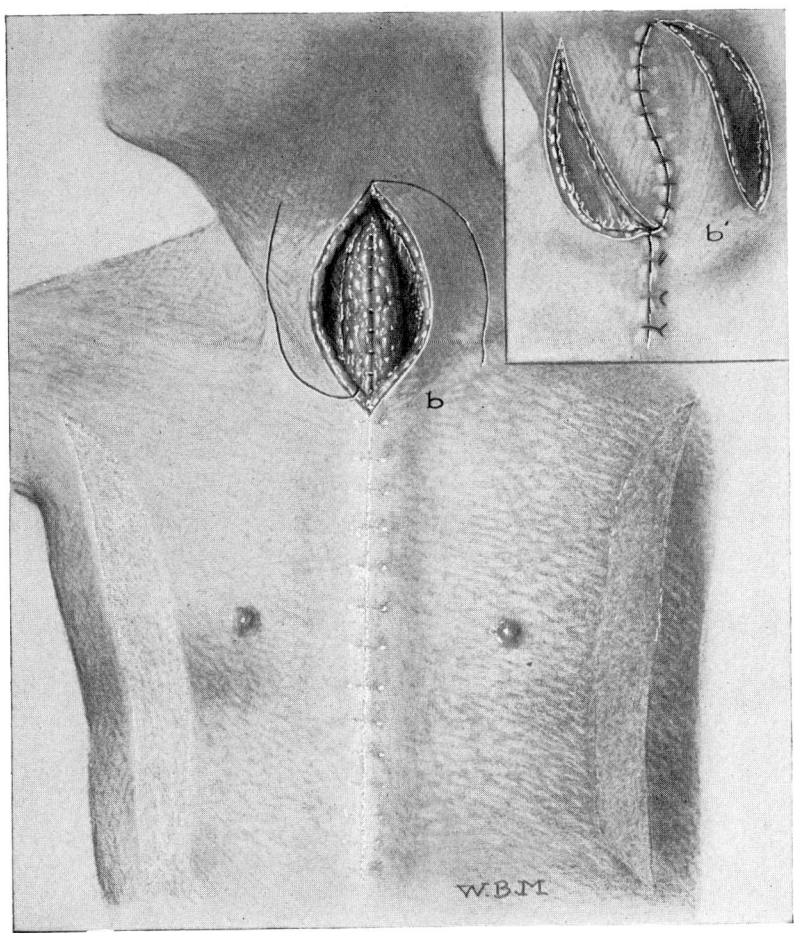

Fig. 300. In third stage of procedure, cervical part of esophagus has been mobilized and sutured to skin wound at left side of neck. In fourth stage, as depicted in this drawing, esophageal opening has been connected with skin tube, either by simple lengthening and closing of skin tube over it or by swinging an envelope flap downward (compare with *insert*, Fig. 299). (See also former figure, upper part of skin tube; *x* at lateral part of neck indicates point where esophageal opening is to escape.) To close raw surface at neck, two flaps are made, as outlined. They are shifted over raw surfaces (see *insert*). The secondary raw surfaces resulting from shifting the flaps are skin grafted.

648

covered with pedunculated flaps unless the skin sliding method is possible. The flaps to be used are those outlined for closure of the junction at the neck (Fig. 300). At this stage, the gastrostomy is kept open on bottle drainage to prevent any regurgitation of gastric juice while the wounds are healing.

Stage 3: About two months following the last stage, after all wounds have healed, the esophagus is mobilized. A longitudinal incision is made on the left side of the neck, starting at the level of the upper border of the left thyroid cartilage and leading downward toward the opening of the skin tube. From this incision, the anterior border of the musculus sterno-cleidomastoideus is exposed and retracted laterally. After incision of the deep cervical fascia, the carotid sheath is exposed—but not incised—and retracted laterally. The musculus sternothyreoideus and musculus sterno-hyoideus are incised, thus exposing the lateral border of the thyroid gland. The superior thyroid artery is ligated and severed, and the thyroid gland retracted medially. With blunt dissection, the esophagus is now located behind the trachea, anterior and somewhat to the left of the cervical spine, and mobilized.

The question now arises whether (1) to divide the mobilized esophagus transversely, closing the distal end blindly with a two-row suture and suturing the proximal lumen into the skin wound, or (2) to make an opening into the lateral wall and suture the opening into the skin wound. Each method has advantages and disadvantages. The disadvantages of the former method are possible accumulation and retention of secretion in the lower blind segment, with possibility of rupture and the higher chance of mediastinitis. The disadvantage of the latter is the diverticulum-like formation of the lower pouch. Lexer originally advocated the lateral opening, but also has used transverse sectioning in later cases (unpublished). The choice of the method depends mainly upon the motility of the cervical esophagus. In either case, the esophageal opening is sutured into the skin wound and the wound closed in layers.

Stage 4: The connection between the upper end of the skin tube and the esophageal opening should be made only after the latter has well healed without evidence of stenosis. The skin tube is lengthened by continuing the two original parallel incisions upward on each side of the esophageal fistula. Above the level of the fistula, the incisions approach each other gradually. Two flaps are raised, inverted, and sutured together as previously described, ending proximally in a small blind pouch above the fistula; or the upper end is closed by swinging an "envelope" flap downward (compare with Fig. 299, *insert*), thus avoiding the blind pouch. To cover the raw areas and to provide sufficient protection of the anastomosis, two lateral flaps are made which, if pulled together, will

649

cross the tube obliquely (Yudin) (Fig. 300). The secondary defects are either covered with skin grafts (Fig. 300, *insert*) or closed or at least narrowed by undermining the lateral wound edges, shifting the wound edges mediad, and suturing them to the cervical fascia (not to the free edges of the flaps!).

Stage 5: Closure of the gastrostomy opening should be performed only after deglutition through the newly formed esophagus is well established.

TOTAL JEJUNAL EXTRATHORACIC ESOPHAGOPLASTY

Technique (Fig. 301)

Yudin modified the Roux-Herzen type of replacement of the esophagus by a loop of the jejunum. The principle of this method is the mobilization of a long loop of jejunum (not anastomosed with the stomach), which is drawn through a subcutaneous antethoracic tunnel and anastomosed with the cervical part of the esophagus. The main advantages of

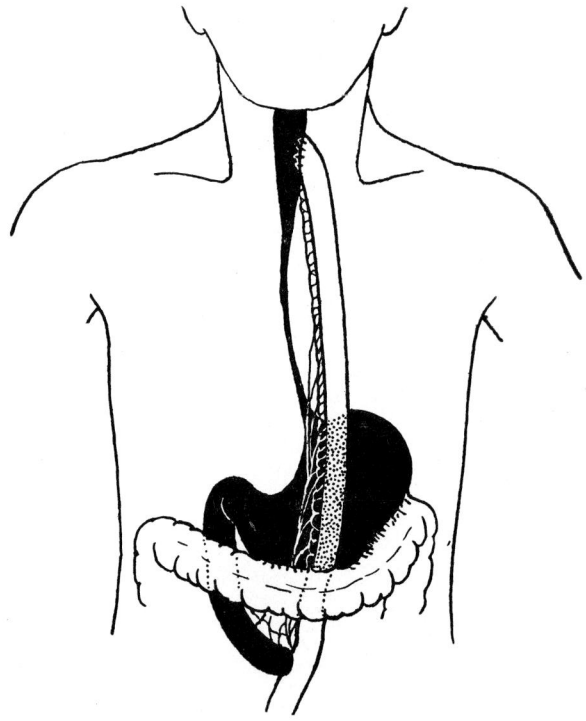

Fig. 301. Diagram of Yudin's modification of the Roux-Herzen type of extrathoracic total intestinal esophagoplasty.

omitting the anastomosis between stomach and jejunum are the simplification of the first step of the operation and the better motility of the jejunal loop. According to Yudin's experience, exclusion of the stomach had no ill effects on the patients. The method is possible only if a sufficiently long, viable loop of jejunum can be obtained.

If, owing to shortness or retraction of the jejunal loop or to the high level of the esophageal obstruction, the intestine cannot be joined with the esophagus directly, the opening of the esophagus and that of the jejunum are sutured into the skin wound. In a third stage, both are joined by a skin tube, which is constructed similarly to, but much shorter than, the one described. The raw surfaces are covered with two flaps, as outlined in Figure 300.

CONSTRUCTION OF
INTRATHORACIC ESOPHAGUS

The intrathoracic route of esophagoplasty, at first approached hesitantly, is becoming more and more popular because of the great advances that have been made in the fields of anesthesiology and chest surgery. Of the three sections of the intestinal tract which have been used for replacement, i.e., stomach (Adams and Phemister, Garlock, Sweet), jejunum (Rienhoff, Harrison, Robertson and Sarjeant, Johnson, Schwegman and Kirby, and others), colon (Kergin, Mahoney and Sherman, Dale and Sherman, Neville, Smith, and Storer, Patterson and Robbins, Hatson, Linder and Hecker, Gregorie and Othersen and others), a loop of the transverse colon appears to be preferred for replacement of part or the entire esophagus. The anastomosed stomach has caused peptic esophagitis and regurgitation of gastric contents into the pharynx. The jejunum has a variable blood supply, which may become insufficient in jejunal loops used for high esophageal anastomoses. The transverse colon has an excellent blood supply and is of sufficient length to reach the neck. (Flavel's and Postlethwait's monograph provide considerable coverage of the surgical management of esophageal replacement. See also page 599 for reconstruction of the cervical esophagus.) Neville, Smith, and Storer emphasize that careful dissection of the middle colic artery and vein down to their origin from the superior mesenteric vessels and division of the mesentery so as to preserve the marginal vessels will assure viability of the bowel. They outline the general technique as follows:

THE TRUNK

Technique (Use of Transverse Colon for High Esophageal Anastomosis)

Under endotracheal anesthesia the abdomen is opened and the lesser peritoneal cavity is entered through the gastrocolic omentum. The proximal transverse colon is dissected free from liver and duodenum, and the distal end is mobilized to the splenic flexure. The avascular lateral peritoneal attachments of the ascending colon and cecum are divided. The colon is divided at the splenic flexure and 10 cm. (4 inches) above the ileocolic junction; the mesentery is transected from either end of the segment to the middle colic vessels. The ascending colon and that of the splenic flexure are anastomosed. The cervical esophagostomy is dissected free. A tunnel is made in the anterior mediastinum behind the periosteum of the sternum from below and above. A long clamp is passed from the neck down to the mediastinal tunnel. Stay sutures which have been applied to the proximal end of the isolated colonic segment are grasped and the colon is pulled through this tunnel into the neck. The anastomosis of the colon to the upper esophageal segment is then performed. If two teams are available the other team can anastomose the distal end of the colon to the stomach just proximal to the pylorus. Just before completing the anterior suture line of the upper anastomosis, a Levin tube should be passed through the nose down through the transplanted segment of the bowel into the stomach. The neck muscles are then reapproximated over the anastomosis after a small drain has been inserted. The Levin tube should stay in place for about five days, at which time oral feedings can be begun. The gastrostomy tube should stay in place until the patient is eating normally.

BIBLIOGRAPHY

ADAMS, W. E., and PHEMISTER, D. B.: *Carcinoma of lower thoracic esophagus: Report of a successful resection and esophagogastrostomy.* J. Thorac. Surg., 7:621, 1938.

AXHAUSEN, G.: *Late reports of total esophagoplasty.* Der Chirurg., 23:4, 1952.

BERMAN, E. F.: *The plastic esophagus.* J. Int. Coll. Surg., 18:695, 1952.

BIRCHER, E.: *Ein Beitrag zur plastischen Bildung eines neuen Oesophagus.* Zentralbl. f. Chir., 34:1479, 1907.

DALE, W. A., and SHERMAN, C. D., JR.: *Late reconstruction of congenital esophageal atresia by intrathoracic colon transplantation.* J. Thorac. Surg., 29:344, 1955.

DAVIS, J. S., and STAFFORD, E. S.: *Successful construction of an antethoracic oesophagus.* Tr. Eleventh Annual Meet. Amer. Soc. Plast. Reconstr. Surg.

CONSTRUCTION OF ESOPHAGUS

FLAVELL, G.: *The Oesophagus*. Butterworth, London, 1963.

FRANKLIN, R. N.: *Surgery of the Esophagus*. Williams & Wilkins, Baltimore, 1952.

GARLOCK, J. H.: *Resection of thoracic esophagus for cancer located above arch of aorta. Cervical esophagogastrostomy.* Surgery 24:1, 1948.

GIBBON, J. H., JR., ET AL.: *Carcinoma of esophagus and gastric cardia.* JAMA, 145:1035, 1951.

GREGORIE, H. B., and OTHERSEN, H. B.: *Total esophagectomy and esophago-coloplasty.* Surg. Gynec. Obstet., 115:153, 1962.

HACKER, F. VON: *Ueber Oesophagoplastik im allgemeinen und über den Ersatz der Speiseröhre durch antethorakale Haut-Dickdarmschlauchbildung im besonderen.* Arch. f. Klin. Chir., 105:973, 1914.

HARDIN, C. A.: *Reconstruction of the cervical esophagus by means of an arm flap.* Ann. Surg., 142:121, 1955.

HARRISON, A. W.: *Transthoracic small bowel substitution in high stricture of the esophagus.* J. Thorac. Surg., 18:316, 1949.

HERZEN, P.: *Eine Modifikation der Roux schen Oesophago-jejuno-gastrostomie.* Zentralbl. f. Chir., 35:219, 1908.

HIEBERT, C. A., and CUMMINGS, G. O.: *Successful replacement of the cervical esophagus by transplantation and revascularization of a free graft of gastric antrum.* Ann. Surg., 154:103, 1961.

HONG, P. W., SEEL, D. J., and DIETRICK, R. B.: *The use of colon in the surgical treatment of benign stricture of the esophagus.* Ann. Surg., 160:202, 1964.

IVY, R. H., HAWTHORNE, H. R., and RITTER, J. A.: *Construction of skin-tube esophagus, following surgical treatment of tracheoesophageal fistula.* Plast. Reconstr. Surg., 3:173, 1948.

JOHNSON, J., SCHWEGMAN, C. W., and KIRBY, C. K.: *Esophageal exclusion for persistent fistula following spontaneous rupture of the esophagus.* J. Thorac. Surg., 32:827, 1956.

KELLING, G.: *Oesophagoplastik Mit Hilfe des Querkolon.* Zentralbl. f. Chir., 38:1209, 1911.

KERGIN, F. G.: *Esophageal obstruction due to paraffinoma of mediastinum.* Ann. Surg., 137:91, 1953.

LEXER, E.: *Oesophagoplastik.* Deutsche med. Wchnschr., 34:574, 1908.
Vollständiger Ersatz der Speiseröhre. München. med. Wchnschr., 58:1548, 1911.
Verhandl. d. deutsch. Gesellsch. f. Chir., 40:119, 1911.

LINDER, F., and HECKER, W.: *Oesophagusersatz durch Colon.* Arch. f. klin. Chir., 301:316, 1962.

LONGMIRE, W. P., JR.: *A modification of the Roux technique for antethoracic esophageal reconstruction.* Surgery, 22:94, 1947.

MAHONEY, E. B., and SHERMAN, C. D., JR.: *Total esophagoplasty using intrathoracic right colon.* Surg., 35:937, 1954.

MONTENEGRO, E. B., CUTAIT, D. E.: *Construction of a new esophagus by means of the transverse colon and its application for caustic atresia, carcinoma and varices of the esophagus.* Surgery, 44:785, 1958.

THE TRUNK

NEVILLE, W. E., SMITH, A. E., and STORER, J.: *The use of the transverse colon for reconstruction of the esophagus in tracheo-esophageal fistula.* Ann. Surg., 144:1045, 1956.

OCHSNER, A., and OWENS, N.: *Antethoracic oesophagoplasty for impermeable stricture of the oesophagus.* Ann. Surg., 100:1055, 1934.

ORSONI, P., and TOUPET, A.: *Utilisation du colon déscendant et de la partie gambe du colon transverse pour l'Oesophagoplastie prethoracique.* Presse med., 58:804, 1950.

PALMER, E. D.: *The Esophagus and its Diseases.* P. B. Hoeber, Inc., New York, 1952.

PATTERSON, R. H., and ROBBINS, S. G.: *Substitution of right colon for the esophagus.* Ann. Surg., 147:854, 1958.

PORIES, W. J., GERLE, R. D., SHERMAN, C. D., and HINSHAW, J. R.: *The danger of esophageal replacement with antiperistaltic loops of small bowel.* Ann. Surg., 156:68, 1962.

RIENHOFF, W. F., JR.: *Intrathoracic esophagojejunostomy for lesions of the upper third of the esophagus.* South Med. J., 39:928, 1946.

ROBERTSON, R., and SARJEANT, T. R.: *Reconstruction of the esophagus.* J. Thorac. Surg., 20:689, 1950.

ROUX: *L'oesophago-jéjuno-gastrostomose, nouvélle opération pour rétrécissement infranchissable de l'oesophage.* Semaine méd., 27:37, 1907.

SCANLON, E. F., and STALEY, C. J.: *The use of the ascending and right half of the transverse colon in esophagoplasty.* Surg. Gynec. Obstet., 107:99, 1958.

STEVENSON, T. W.: *Reconstruction of the esophagus by a skin-lined tube.* Surg. Gynec. Obstet., 84:197, 1947.

SWEET, R. H.: *A new method of restoring continuity of the alimentary canal in cases of congenital atresia of the esophagus with tracheo-esophageal fistula not treated by immediate primary anastomosis.* Ann. Surg., 127:757, 1948.

THOREK, P. H.: *Diseases of the Esophagus.* J. B. Lippincott, Philadelphia, 1952.

TOREK, F.: *First successful case of resection of the thoracic esophagus.* Surg. Gynec. Obstet., 16:614, 1913.

WATSON, W. L.: *Substitution for the esophagus.* J. Int. Coll. Surg., 27:761, 1957.

WATSON, W. L., and CONVERSE, J. M.: *Reconstruction of the cervical esophagus.* J. Plast. Reconstr. Surg., 11:183, 1953.

WULLSTEIN, L.: *Uber antethorakale Oesophago-jejunostomie und Operationen nach gleichem Prinzip.* Deutsche med. Wchnschr., 31:734, 1904.

YUDIN, S. S.: *The surgical construction of eighty cases of artificial esophagus.* Surg. Gynec. Obstet., 78:561, 1944.

THE GENITALIA
IN MALE   18
AND FEMALE

LOSS OF SKIN OF PENIS AND SCROTUM

Loss of skin of the male genitalia is due either to trauma or to infection. Such a defect may involve the penis, the scrotum, or both. In traumatic cases in which the wound can be treated within the stage of contamination, surgical restoration can be started almost immediately. Before reconstruction can be undertaken in defects due to infection (necrosis of skin from infection following circumcision, gangrene from erysipelas, lymphogranuloma inguinale, etc.), the infection must be combated by local and general means and the granulations thoroughly prepared until they are healthy, pinkish, and flat. The literature on this subject has been thoroughly discussed up to 1942 by Neal Owens, up to 1950 by the author, and more recently by Beverly Douglas.

The missing skin of the penis can be replaced with skin flaps or skin grafts. According to early reports on the restoration of penile skin, surgeons have apparently preferred pedicle flaps rather than free grafts. Lexer, Brown, Owens, Byars, Hamm, and others, however, have demonstrated clearly that a thick split skin graft has an excellent chance of regeneration. It remains pliable, develops normal sensation, and does not hinder erection. The operation can be performed in one stage. In traumatic defects where the torn penile skin is still available, it may, unless it is dirty and ragged, have a chance to heal in place and regenerate. However, the prospect of success in replacement seems better if the skin

655

remains attached even by a small bridge (Case 99, p. 1114). Flaps require multiple operations, and when taken from thigh or abdomen are thick and may grow hair. Scrotal skin flaps are pliable, but the source is limited, and they can be used only for partial defects. If the surface is cicatricial, all scar tissue, and in the case of a granulating surface the entire granulating area, together with the cicatricial base, must be excised until the penis can be developed to full length. A Foley catheter is then inserted and the penis covered with a thick split skin graft, unless the defect is deep and involves the corpora cavernosa. If such is the case, flaps must be employed.

In total reconstruction of the penis, flaps must always be used. The literature of this subject was reviewed by Gelb, who also reported a case.

In scrotal defects the use of free skin grafts to cover the testicles has been recently revised (Balakrishnan, Watson, Campbell). It may be worthwhile for either an initial or permanent coverage of the testicles although the coverage seems to be rather thin to provide adequate comfort. The simplest way to provide initial coverage for the plexus and the testicles is to form a subcutaneous pocket on the median surface of the thighs (rarely on the abdomen) and bury the two structures beneath the skin (Seeman, Thierry, Krug, Owens, and others). This is usually done from a longitudinal incision or by undermining the skin from the former base of the scrotum near the groin. It has been often and reliably stated (Moore, Harrenstein and others) that sterility ensues in a testicle that maintains a temperature equal to body heat instead of one degree less. This, however, appears not to be the case as demonstrated by Brown and Fryer and others. However, the patients, particularly the younger ones, may object to the deformity and develop a psychological handicap. Hence, the testicles should not remain buried permanently and a new scrotum should be constructed unless the patient accepts the deformity.

The author has reconstructed a scrotum by means of two oblique pedicle flaps of the thighs beneath which the testicles were buried. The flaps were raised in stages and combined, thus deviating from the technique of König, who enveloped each testicle with the adherent flap and formed two separate units. The author's method requires three or four stages over a period of four weeks. The functional and cosmetic result is very satisfactory. A different principle was employed by Douglas. He formed two large oblique, fan-shaped flaps with fairly broad pedicles left attached below in the upper median thigh regions, adjacent to the perineum, their axes paralleling the inguinal canals and their free ends being on the upper anterior thighs near the level of a horizontal line through the base of the penis. They were rotated toward the midline and around their axes to receive the testicles and the cords, and they were sutured together. Since the pedicles remain attached, the method is cosmetically inferior to the method outlined above. It has, however, the distinct advantage of being a one-stage procedure.

Technique (Traumatic Avulsion of Skin of Penis and Scrotum)
(Case 99, p. 1114)

Stage 1: After the entire area has been prepared in the usual way (soap and water), a thorough excision of ragged wound edges and débridement are performed.

The next step consists of supplying a protective covering for the exposed testicles, hanging free on their spermatic cord, and the preparation of oblique thigh flaps for the reconstruction of the scrotum. A double-pedicle oblique bridge flap is formed on the anteromedian surface of the thigh. The upper incision is made just below (about 2.5 cm. distally—1 inch) and parallel to the crease of the groin. Each flap is 15 by 8 cm. (6 by 3⅛ inches). Both flaps are elevated from the fascia lata. The testicle and the spermatic cord are now buried beneath the flap. The proximal and posterior part of the plexus rests upon the narrow strip of skin of the crease of the groin. The remainder of the posterior part of the plexus and the testicle lie upon the raw surface of the thigh. To prevent the testicle from growing to the donor area and also to prevent the flap from becoming reattached to its donor area, the donor area should be skin grafted at this stage by using a nylon-backed thick split graft, cut with the dermatome from the median surface of the same thigh (p. 34). The flap is now sutured to the wound edges of the flap bed. In the region of the spermatic cord, it is sutured to the raw pubic area.

The denuded penis is now covered with a thick split skin graft (Case 100, p. 1118). First, an indwelling catheter is inserted and a traction suture placed through the glans. A thick split skin graft is removed from a hairless region of the abdomen (the donor area should not be shaved preoperatively) and wrapped around the penis. Where the free edges of the long sides of the graft meet, a new raphe is formed. The raphe, however, should not be straight but zigzag; this shape is provided by making incisions on one side of the graft and leaving projections on the other side. Thus, a Z-like plasty is performed to counteract contractions. It is simpler, however, to make the suture line unbroken. If this is preferred, the scars should be placed on the dorsum of the penis in case light contracture should occur. The graft is sutured to the base of the penis. The sutures are left long. The penis is held stretched by means of a holding suture through the glans and the graft is sutured longitudinally. The distal part of the graft is then trimmed and sutured to the corona glandis.

657

THE TRUNK

These sutures are left long. A heavily padded pressure dressing is applied which is held in place by tying the sutures over it, reinforced by strips of Elastoplast. A pressure dressing is applied upon the thighs by means of figures-of-8 around thighs and abdomen. Aside from postoperative administration of antibiotics, bromides and other sedatives are given to prevent erections.

Stage 2: Nine days after the operation, the dressings are changed, sutures and catheter are removed, and the median pedicle of each bridge flap is severed under local anesthesia, one third from each side, and a laboratory clamp is applied to the median third (Case 99, c, p. 1115). The penis is redressed with moist normal saline solution dressings. Within the following few days, the median third is crushed with the clamp.

Stage 3: Five days after the second operation, the same procedure as in Stage 2 is carried out at the lateral pedicles.

Stage 4: One week after Stage 3, the flaps with the testicles closely attached are elevated; the nylon backing of the skin grafts is removed. Should the flaps become cyanotic, they are returned to their former site for another week. Otherwise, the operation can be completed by anastomosing the flaps in the following manner: The lateral pedicles become the posterior raphe, and the median pedicles the anterior raphe; the lower oval openings of the flaps are sutured together, thus forming the bottom of the new scrotum. The posterior rim of the upper oval opening is sutured posteriorly to the perineal region; the anterior rim is sutured to the pubic region.

It is quite conceivable that an extensive traumatic avulsion of the skin of the male genitalia must, in some patients, result in profound psychological and endocrine disturbances, regardless of the surgical reconstruction. Baxter and co-workers have recently stressed these consequences and described in detail the proper treatment.

ABSENCE OF VAGINA

Absence of the vagina is a congenital abnormality usually associated with a rudimentary development of uterus and adnexa, yet the external genitalia, as well as sex instinct and secondary sex characteristics, may be well developed. Hence, construction of a vagina may be indicated to offer the patient the possibilities of a normal sexual relationship and to prevent development of an inferiority complex.

Another group of patients occasionally requiring construction of an artificial vagina are the so-called "pseudohermaphrodites." For the historical background and the details of the subject, I refer to the classic treatise of H. H. Young and more recent publications by Jones and Scott and by Overzier. The author has presented the highlights, together with the latest research developments and his own experience, in a symposium (see also Case 102, p. 1122; Case 103, p. 1124).

Various methods of construction of a vagina have been developed, such as transplantation of a section of the intestine (Baldwin, Schubert), pedicle flaps (Heppner, Graves, Frank, and Geist), free skin grafting Abbé, Esser), and gradual stretching of the rudimentary organ (Frank). The subject has been critically reviewed by Owens, by Counsellor, by Fletcher, by McIndoe, and more recently by Blocker and associates and by Cali and Pratt and Evans who followed up a large series of cases treated by inlay skin grafting. The most recent review of this subject is by Goldsmith, who includes a comprehensive list of references. The most popular method is the use of an inlay skin graft; that is, the use of a thick split graft wrapped around a stent.

Technique (Fig. 302; Case 101, p. 1120)

The patient's bowels should be prepared two days prior to operation by saline enemas twice daily. The patient is placed on a liquid diet. She also receives 1 gr. of neomycin every six hours for six doses, and paregoric (5 cc.) at 8 P.M. that evening and the same amount at 7 A.M. of the day of the operation. A retention (Foley) catheter is inserted in the urethra and the patient is placed in lithotomy position. From a transverse incision midway between urethral meatus and anus, the space between

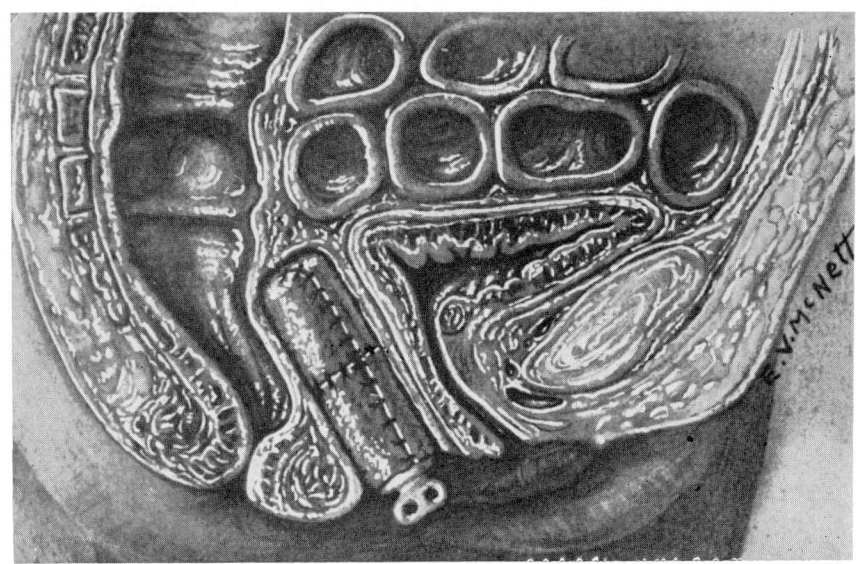

Fig. 302. Reconstruction of vagina with inlay skin graft over a stent. Stent of plexiglas (10 × 4 cm.) and skin graft inserted. For details of shape of stent see page 660.

659

the urethra and the juncture of the labia majora is opened. An assistant should now reach beneath the drapes and insert a finger into the rectum. Along this guiding finger, under blunt dissection, a cavity is created between bladder and urethra on one side and the rectum on the other side, care being taken not to perforate either organ, not to enter the peritoneal cavity, and not to make the cavity too roomy. It is good to start the cavity by inserting rectal dilators. A few spurting bleeders are usually encountered at the level of the broad ligaments; they should be ligated. Oozing from the cavity is controlled by insertion of hot moist sponges. The size of the cavity is finally made to fit snugly over a previously prepared solid cylindrical mold of plexiglas or other material. The average mold measures about 10 by 4 cm. (4 by 1⅝ inches) (Case 101, *b*, p. 1121). The upper end lies toward the peritoneum. The lower end, which lies against the urethra, has a trough-like depression 1 cm. (⅜ inch) in width and 3 cm. (1³⁄₁₆ inch) in length. This lower end also has a projecting disk attached with two openings for the reception of two rubber tubes to keep it firmly in place later, as described in the following paragraph. A thick split skin graft is removed from a hairless region of thigh or abdomen (donor area not to be shaved) and—with its raw side out—is wrapped around the mold and fastened to itself with catgut sutures through its edges. The moist sponges are removed from the newly formed cavity. Should oozing persist, hot moist sponges are again inserted for a few minutes; they are then removed, the cavity is flushed with thrombol (see p. 37), and mold and graft are correctly inserted into the cavity. The freshened edges of the labia are sutured over the mold to hold it firmly in place.

After-Treatment

The patient is kept postoperatively on a liquid diet. She receives 5 cc. of paregoric every two hours for six doses. On the fifth postoperative day, the diet is changed to soft foods, and 30 cc. of mineral oil are administered. If there has been no bowel movement on the sixth postoperative day, an enema is administered. Sutures and mold are removed on the tenth postoperative day, and the newly lined cavity is cleansed by irrigation. The mold is then reinserted and held in place with two rubber tubes, which are threaded through the openings in the mold and fastened anteriorly and posteriorly to an abdominal belt. The belt should be fitted preoperatively (see Case 101, *c*, p. 1121). The mold is removed every day for irrigation of the cavity. Later, this can be easily done by the patient herself. The mold should be worn continuously for three months to avoid contracture. For the following three months, it is worn at night. If the patient does not plan early marriage, dilatation should be carried out at regular intervals to avoid subsequent shrinkage.

DEFORMITIES

By David M. Davis, M.D.

HYPOSPADIAS

Hypospadias cases are classified as follows, according to the location of the external urethral meatus:

1. Glandular
2. Frenal
3. Penile
4. Penoscrotal
5. Scrotal (sometimes subdivided into anterior scrotal, midscrotal, and posterior scrotal)
6. Perineal

The glandular type requires no treatment, the frenal type only for the sake of appearance, since the urinary and sexual functions can be satisfactorily carried on in both. All other types require plastic correction.

Hypospadias may occur in the female, the meatus being posterior to its usual location in the vulva, or on the anterior wall of the vagina. Since incontinence is a rare complication, no treatment is necessary unless it is present (von Bouwdijk).

The surgical procedures for the cure of hypospadias vary with the type and degree of malformation. Before describing the different operations, it would be well to emphasize that adherence to a few principles is necessary for success. They are as follows:

1. The penis must be thoroughly straightened, with the urethal orifice set back away from the tip if necessary.
2. The urine must be clear and sterile.
3. The urine (according to most surgeons) should be diverted so that it does not come in contact with the tissues concerned in the plastic operation.
4. The skin from which the new urethra is made must be hairless.
5. The new urethra must be of sufficient caliber at all points.
6. The new urethra must be covered as deeply as possible and the sutures arranged so that one row does not lie directly over another.
7. Erections should be avoided during convalescence.

THE TRUNK

Before beginning plastic operations, the operator must assure himself beyond all possible doubt that the patient is really a male. If the testes are undescended, laparotomy is necessary for complete assurance. Chromosome patterns are helpful. Hormonal tests are not conclusive, but when quantitative may be interesting and suggestive.

The first question is usually that of the proper age for operation. Practically all surgeons agree that the penis should be straightened or at least the straightening commenced as early as possible. The plastic reconstruction of the urethra is delayed until the organs are larger. Some believe it may be commenced at the age of four or five, some prefer a year or two before the onset of puberty, and a few wait until after puberty so that the penis may attain its full growth. This last is particularly necessary if free grafts are used, since they do not grow with the penis as do plastic reconstructions and pedicle flaps. The writer believes that the years from five to eight, depending on the size of the child, are the most favorable.

The literature on the surgical treatment of hypospadias records a remarkable series of original ideas, patient and meticulous craftsmanship, amazing success, and, sad to say, many pompous and immodest ex cathedra statements and ill-natured disparagements of other persons' methods. While the surgical correction of hypospadias has always been regarded as very difficult, a study of the latest reports shows that excellent and practically identical results can be obtained with any of the presently recognized methods (Barcat, Browne, Byars, Carrai, Culp, Davis, Dodson, Douglas, Fogh-Anderson, Havens, Kiefer, Pariente, Schaefer, Smith, and Young). A great deal of the improvement in results must be ascribed to the antibiotic drugs and their conquest of postoperative infection.

Preliminary Search for Complications

Rectal Examination. The purposes of this examination are to make sure that a prostate is present and to exclude the possibility of a postprostatic utricular or Müllerian duct cyst. The latter is not an infrequent complication. The cyst may be removed suprapubically or perineally, with danger of impotence in either case, or it may, if not too large, be opened transurethrally into the urethra.

Cystourethroscopic Examination: If urinary tract infection is present, one must search for any obstructive cause. Sterile urine is absolutely necessary if plastic procedures are to succeed. However, there are other important reasons why this examination should never be omitted. In the bladder, tumor, stone, diverticulum etc. may be present. Contracture of the vesical orifice or posterior urethral valves can be detected, as well as vaginas of various sizes or enlarged utricles. In any event the utricle

662

can be probed to detect cystic enlargement. Stricture of the urethra can be found and treated. All of these lesions must be corrected before attempting the urethral reconstruction, except perhaps a small vagina opening freely into the urethra, which may be left undisturbed.

Methods

The following table will help to put the various methods in their proper relations:

1. Straightening of penis with displacement of preputial skin to ventrum
   (*a*) Transverse incision closed longitudinally (Heinecke-Miculicz) (Fig. 303, *1, 2*)
   (*b*) Freeing and longitudinal splitting of prepuce (Edmonds) (Fig. 303, *3, 4, 5*)
   (*c*) Freeing and buttonholing of prepuce (Nesbit, Ombrédanne) (Fig. 303, *14, 15, 16*)
   (*d*) Freeing and oblique displacement of prepuce (Davis) (Fig. 303, *11, 12, 13*)
2. Plastic construction of new urethral tube
   (*a*) Production of tube from ventral skin, without tunneling
       (1) Sutured tube (Thiersch-Duplay-Marion) (Fig. 304, *1, 2, 3, 4*)
       (2) Flat flap (Browne) (Fig. 305, *1, 2, 3, 4, 5, 6*)
       (3) Circular flap with purse-string suture (Ombrédanne)
   (*b*) Production of tube from ventral and scrotal skin (Bucknall)
   (*c*) Production of tube from dorsal preputial skin with tunneling (Mayo, Young, Davis) (Fig. 306)
   (*d*) Production of tube by free graft with tunneling (Nové-Josserand, McIndoe, Havens) (Fig. 307)
3. Covering of tube when not buried in tunnel
   (*a*) By flaps of penile skin
       (1) Straight edge flaps (Thiersch, Duplay, Marion, Blair) (Fig. 304, *1, 2, 3, 4*)
       (2) Staggered edges (Cecil) (Fig. 304, *5, 6, 7*)
       (3) Mattress sutures plus dorsal counterincision (Browne) (Fig. 305)

Straightening of Penis

The surgeons who earliest attempted surgical correction discovered at once that the down-curved penis must, in order to give a good result, be straightened before being supplied with the new urethra. The straightening, to be effective, demands the absolute removal of all adhesions, fibrous bands, or other structures, whatever their embryological origin may be, which hold the corpora cavernosa in the curved position. This sometimes involves the removal of the ventral portion of the septum between the corpora cavernosa, but must nevertheless be prosecuted most radically until perfect straightening is achieved. When this is accomplished, the lengthening of the ventral surface requires more skin to cover it; there are various ways of doing this.

Transverse Incision with Longitudinal Closure: The most primitive method is associated with the names Heinecke and Miculicz. One or more transverse skin incisions are closed longitudinally (Fig. 303, *1, 2*). This

663

method has fallen into disuse because its lengthening is accomplished at the expense of the circumference, and is apt to lead to constriction and distortion.

Freeing and Longitudinal Splitting of Prepuce: In most cases, there is abundant thin, hairless, mobile skin in the hooded prepuce. This is highly suitable for constructing the new urethral tube, since hairs in the urethra are to be avoided, but many surgeons prefer to transplant it first to the ventrum of the penis before actually constructing the tube. In one method of doing this, a ventral median longitudinal incision is made; the cut then passes around both sides of the coronary sulcus to separate the glans entirely from the penile skin, and finally the median longitudinal incision is continued dorsally (Fig. 303, 3, 4, 5). The preputial skin is then freed and elevated and pulled around to the ventrum, the glans fitting into the proximal angle of the median dorsal incision. This method is associated with the name of Edmonds, but it is now used by

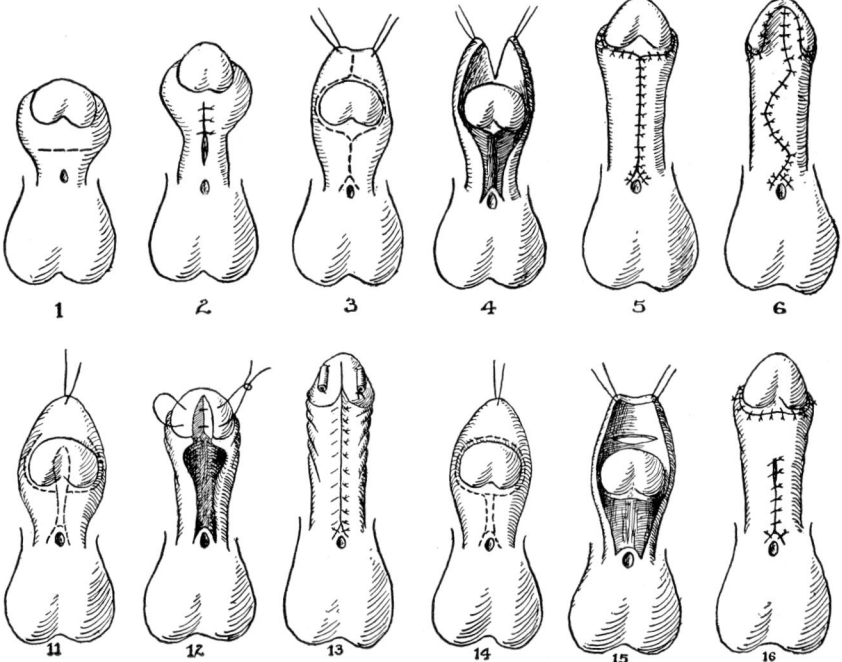

Fig. 303. Methods of straightening penis. (1, 2) Heinecke-Miculicz method. (3, 4, 5) Edmonds' methods. Adhesions shown in 4 must be thoroughly removed. (6) Byars' modification. The glans is deeply incised, and the cleft so made is lined with preputial skin. (11, 12, 13) Davis' method. Cleft in glans is denuded, the two halves of the glans brought together by mattress suture. (14, 15, 16) Nesbit's method. The preputial skin is completely freed from the penis, a dorsal incision made as in 5, the glans thrust through this opening, bringing much of the prepuce onto the ventral surface. The original incision is closed.

664

very many surgeons. Byars has modified this procedure by (1) cutting the edges of the incision so that it can be closed in a zigzag line, which he thinks lengthens the ventral scar; and (2) splitting the glans ventrally and lining the split with an excess of preputial skin, so that this skin-lined groove can be used to construct the urethra all the way to the tip of the penis (Fig. 303, *6*).

Freeing and Buttonholing of Prepuce: A similar effect is achieved by Nesbit who, instead of using a dorsal median longitudinal incision, makes a buttonhole in the prepuce dorsally and thrusts the glans through this buttonhole, the edges of which are sutured to the narrow collar of the skin remaining in the coronary sulcus (Fig. 303, *14, 15, 16*). Ombrédanne also buttonholes the prepuce, but merely uses it to cover the funnel-shaped urethra produced by placing a purse-string suture around the edges of a circular ventral skin flap.

Freeing and Oblique Displacement of Prepuce: Davis extends his coronary-sulcus incision only part way around the glans, then pulls the preputial skin obliquely downward and ventrally on each side of the glans. In this manner, he aims to utilize the lateral parts of the preputial skin to cover the ventrum and at the same time preserve the full length of the median portion of the preputial skin, from which the pedicle tube flap will subsequently be made. If there is a ventral groove in the glans he removes the skin lining it, and draws the two halves of the glans together with a mattress suture. The purpose of this is to give the glans a nearly circular outline and so make it more suitable for the tunneling procedure to be carried out later. Young and Benjamin recommend the same procedure as a preliminary to their free-graft method of reconstructing the urethra (Fig. 303, *11, 12, 13*).

The results of straightening operations must be appraised carefully; if the straightening is not perfect, the procedure must be repeated as many times as necessary to make it so. The straightening is not entirely satisfactory, in a certain number of cases, at the first attempt. This is a weighty argument against one-stage procedures. If a new urethra is constructed in an inadequately straightened penis, a very difficult situation is created.

Since the preputial skin is so important in the plastic correction of hypospadias, all physicians should be aware that a hypospadias patient must *never* be circumcised, and rabbis should be urged to make their ritual circumcisions in such cases as vestigial as possible.

Plastic Construction of Urethral Tube

Sutured Tube: The oldest and simplest method of constructing a urethral tube is to raise the edges of a rectangular skin flap on the ventrum of the penis and suture it into a skin-lined tube as shown in Figure 304,

THE TRUNK

1, 2, 3, 4. This method is usually known by the coupled names of Thiersch and Duplay, but it has been used and modified by many others, and in the United States the name of Blair is particularly associated with it. Marion modified it by using one set of sutures to produce the tube and to mattress the skin edges. The sketches in Figure 304 show the simplest closure. Subcutaneous tissues are brought together over the tube by interrupted sutures of very fine catgut, and the skin edges are closed by fine nonabsorbable

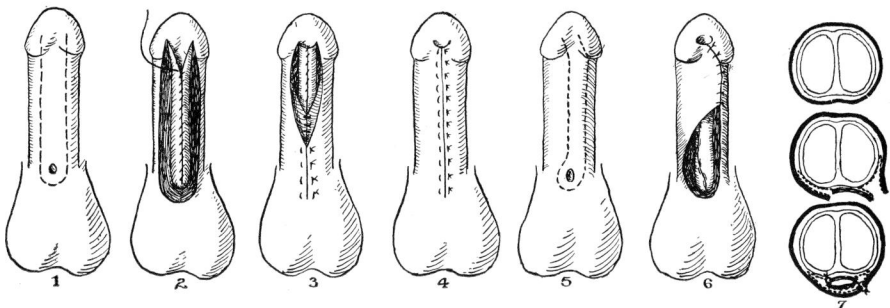

Fig. 304. Thiersch-Duplay method of constructing new urethra: (1) incision; (2) strip of skin formed into a tube; (3) subcutaneous tissue closed over new tube; (4) skin closed. (5, 6, 7) Cecil modification. (5) The strip is cut to one side of the midline; (6) in closing, the skin incision does not lie over the suture line in the tube; (7) cross sections. Note that only one side of the rectangular strip is freed up from the underlying tissue.

sutures, which may be plain or mattress, and may or may not be tied over small rubber tubes, beads, or other devices to prevent them from cutting into the skin (Fig. 305, 7). Tubes have the advantage of holding the penis straight, of keeping the sutures in proper relationship with one another, and of facilitating their removal. This method is therefore recommended. It will be noted, however, in Figure 304, *3,* that no matter how carefully they are placed the sutures all lie in the same plane, each line superimposed on the previous one, so that any failure of primary union will surely produce a fistula. The successful covering of the tube by skin without fistula formation has, for these reasons, its difficulties, and we shall presently consider the various procedures which have been suggested to make it more certain. It is also difficult to bring the external meatus of the new urethra to its proper position at the tip of the glans. Byars' method of splitting the glans (see above) is designed to overcome this objection.

Flat Flap: Denis Browne omits the suturing of the ventral rectangular flap into a tube, and does not even free the lateral edges of the flap from the underlying tissues. He does free the lateral flaps of the penile skin very extensively, and in addition makes a median longitudinal counter-

666

incision on the dorsum so that the skin edges can be drawn easily over the flat flap and deeply mattressed with nonabsorbable sutures passing through beads held in place by metal clips on the sutures (Fig. 305, *1, 2, 3, 4, 5, 6*). The object is to produce a wide approximation of denuded subcutaneous tissues over the flat flap which, in the experience of Browne, tends to produce primary healing without fistulas. The buried flat flap, by proliferation of its edges, forms itself into a tube. According to the

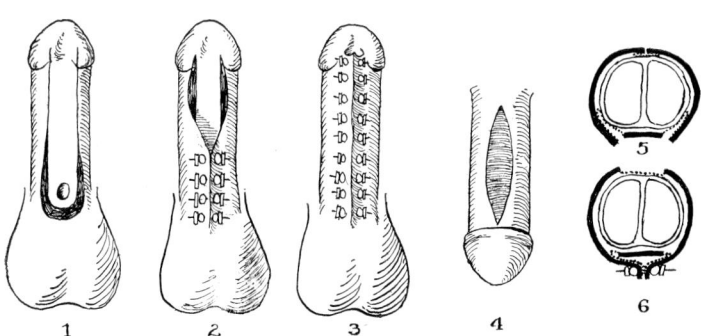

Fig. 305. Denis Browne method of constructing new urethra. (1) The rectangular strip outlined. (2) It is not freed, but the lateral skin edges are deeply undermined and drawn over the strip by mattress sutures. (3) Operation finished. (4) Dorsal counterincision to mobilize lateral skin edges. (5, 6) Cross sections. Note that the rectangular strip is not freed up from the underlying tissue at all.

experiments of Nesbit, the flat flap should be cut of a width equivalent or almost equivalent to the circumference desired for the completed urethra; Browne feels that it need not be quite so wide.

Formation of Tube from Ventral and Scrotal Skin: Bucknall described a method in which the new urethra is formed from two narrow strips of skin, one from the ventrum of the penis and the other from the scrotum. The lateral penile flaps and the lateral scrotal flaps are then sutured together, temporarily burying the new urethra between penis and scrotum. This means that the new urethra has two longitudinal suture lines, instead of one, and that its floor, being of scrotal skin, will give forth an abundant growth of hair. For these reasons, the Cecil modification shown in Figure 308, *1, 2, 3, 4, 5, 6, 7, 8,* is now usually preferred. Variations of this method for penile hypospadias have been described by Mathieu and Leveuf.

Tube Made from Dorsal Preputial Skin with Tunneling: Mayo and Young described operations in which a tube made from preputial skin and remaining attached by a pedicle at one of its ends was drawn through a subcutaneous tunnel in the glans. The object of this was to do away with the possibility of fistula formation. However, thinking to have the pedicle as near the tip of the penis as possible, they left the tube flap attached by its distal end, and it proved that the blood supply so provided was inadequate. For this reason, the tube flap often sloughed, and the method was not satisfactory. Davis modified the method by leaving the tube flap attached at its proximal end, which preserved the dorsal artery of the penis and prevented sloughing. The tunnelized penis was then bent over backward to receive the tube flap. The tunnel must be large enough to admit the tube flap perfectly freely and at its distal end an oval piece of glandular skin must be removed to prevent contracture of the new meatus. Experience showed that this method was practical and that erections did not interfere with its success. It further demonstrated that tube flaps made in this manner could be cut the entire length of the dorsum of the penis back as far as the point where pubic hair follicles began to appear. The long tubes are perfectly viable and permit the penile tunnel to be made as long as the tube flap, often reaching all the way to a meatus at the penoscrotal junction. Anastomosis with the preexisting urethra can be made at the time of the original operation or later. The pedicle of the tube flap is divided about three weeks after its formation, by which time the tube itself will be receiving an adequate blood supply through anastomosis with vessels within the penis (Fig. 306). The advantages claimed for this method are (1) that the meatus is always at the tip of the glans in a perfectly normal position; (2) that there is no chance of fistula formation except at one point only—namely, the site of anastomosis with the preexisting urethra; and (3) that the urethra, being made of full-thickness penile skin, will grow with the penis.

Production of Tube by Free Graft with Tunneling: The method of producing a tube by lining a penile tunnel with a free graft of split-thickness skin is associated with the name of Nové-Josserand, and its chief present-day exponents are McIndoe and Havens. The graft is wrapped about a catheter with a diameter about one third of that of the penis, and sutured thereto with fine absorbable sutures. The catheter so wrapped is passed into the penile tunnel, fastened in place by nonabsorbable sutures at each end of the tunnel, and left for a considerable time, usually about two weeks (Fig. 301, *1, 2, 3, 4, 5*). The tunnel is subcutaneous in the shaft but passes directly through the erectile tissue. Havens then keeps a large lucite obturator in the urethra for six months, to insure against stricture formation, before anastomosing the new urethra with the old. He further feels that, since the split-thickness free graft does not grow with the penis, operation should be deferred until the age of sixteen or seventeen, when it may be assumed that the penis has reached its full size. One great advantage of this operation is that it does not depend upon the presence

668

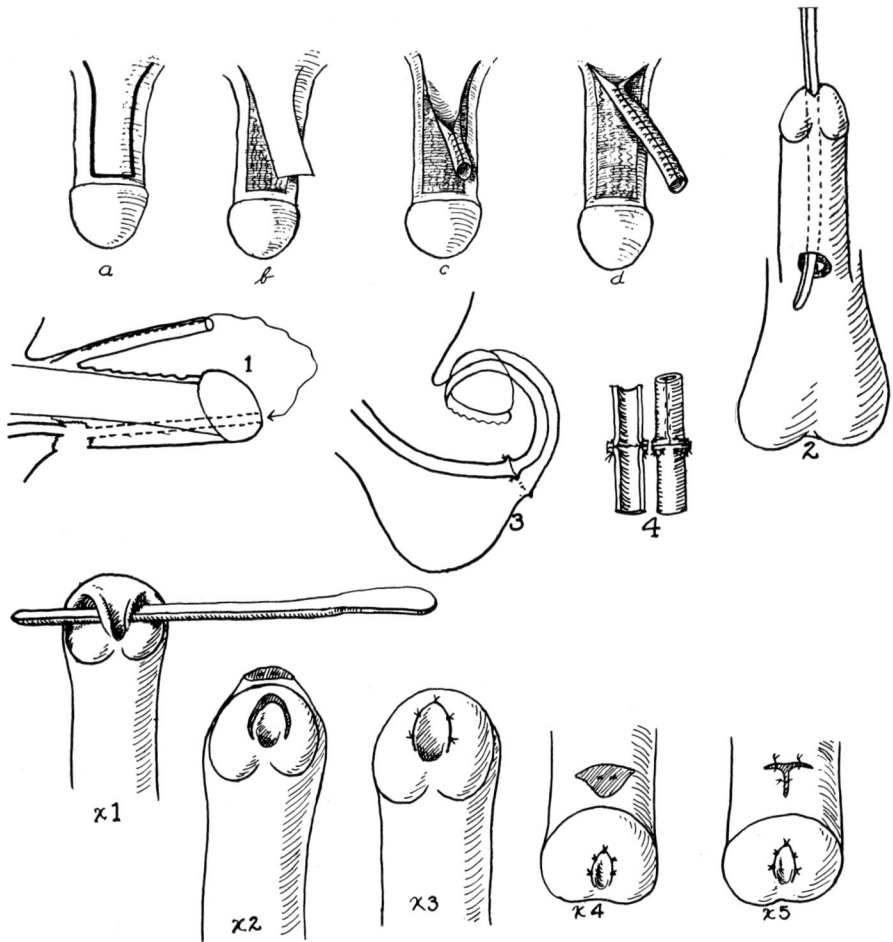

Fig. 306. Davis method of constructing new urethra. *a:* Rectangular flap cut on dorsum of penis. *b:* Flap raised including dorsalis penis artery. *c* and *d:* Flap sutured into skinlined tube. (1) Diagrammatic sagittal section showing tunnel prepared for tube flap. (2) Tunnel being dilated. (3) Diagrammatic sagittal section showing tube flap drawn into tunnel and anastomosed to preexisting urethra. The muco-cutaneous junction has been trimmed off slightly obliquely. The glans is pushed down to the pedicle of the tube flap and held there by a few cutaneous sutures. (4) Mucosa-to-mucosa suture of new to old urethra. Edges of incision around meatus are undermined. The anastomosis is buried as deeply as possible. The skin is closed with mattress sutures. (x1) Grooved director placed beneath pedicle of tube flap after healing is complete. (x2) Pedicle severed. A small rosette of skin should be left above level of surface of glans to prevent later contracture. (x3) Lining of tube flap sutured to skin of glans. (x4) and (x5) Ligature of vessels in stump of pedicle, suture of skin.

669

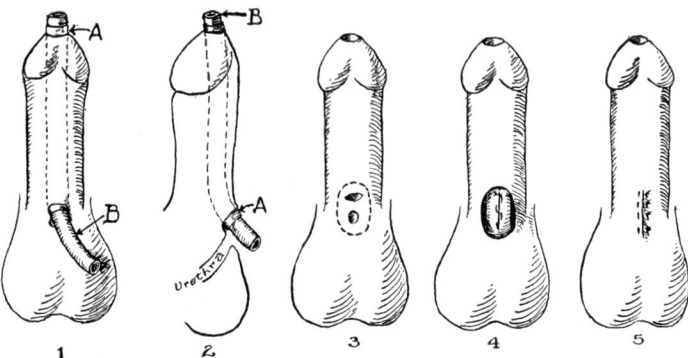

Fig. 307. Nové-Josserand method of constructing new urethra. (1, 2) After tunnel is made in penis, catheter about which split-thickness skin has been sutured is drawn into tunnel and sutured in place; *a*, tubular graft of split-thickness skin, *b*, catheter. (3) After urethra is well established, oval incision is made about it and meatus. (4) Skin edges are freed and sutured into a tube. (5) Lateral edges are undermined and sutured over anastomosis.

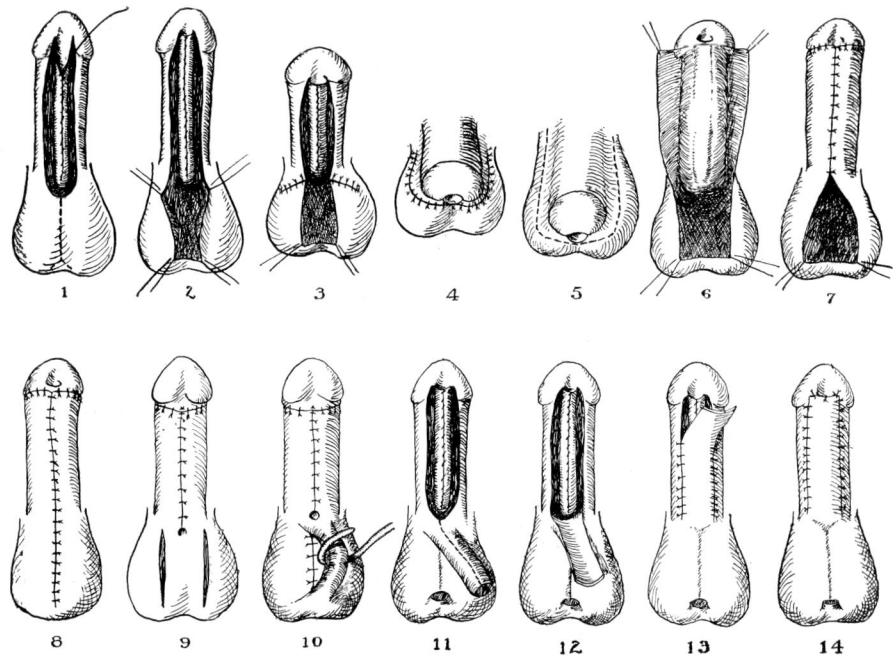

Fig. 308. Methods of covering new urethra. (1 to 8, inclusive) Cecil-Cabot method. (1) Incision extended on scrotum. (2) Edges undermined. (3, 4) Penis sutured to scrotum. (5) After healing, incision made providing flaps of scrotal skin sufficient to cover ventrum of penis as shown in 6. (7 and 8) Closure of penis and scrotum. (9 to 14 inclusive) Wehrbein method. (9, 10) Double pedicle tube flap raised on scrotum. (11, 12) After healing; lower pedicle is divided, tube incised on ventral surface, unrolled into a flat flap and used to cover Thiersch-Duplay plastic as shown in 13 and 14.

670

of a large amount of preputial skin, and may therefore be used where the prepuce is deficient or has been previously removed. Others have used, in place of split-thickness skin, full-thickness skin, strips of bladder mucosa (Marshall and Memmelaar), of vaginal mucosa (Legueu), and of intestinal mucosa, the vermiform appendix (Lexer, Weitz), portions of the patient's own ureter (necessitating unilateral nephrectomy) (Biebl), preserved human urethra from fresh cadavers (Bourque), and large veins (Tuffier). None of these methods has proved satisfactory.

Covering of Tube

Flaps of Penile Skin: The simplest method of covering the newly made urethra when it is not buried in a tunnel is to suture over it the straight-edged lateral flaps of penile skin (Fig. 304, *3, 4*). Plain or mattress sutures may be used, as shown in Fig. 304, *4, 6*, and Fig. 305, *6* and the flaps may be freed by a counterincision on the dorsum of the penis, as shown in Figures 305, *4, 5, 6*.

Separation of Suture Lines: Cecil proposed that the rectangular flap be cut mostly to one side of the midline, and that only the edge farther from the midline be freed up. This edge is then drawn over across the midline and sutured to the opposite, unfreed edge. Thus, when the lateral penile flaps are drawn over the new urethral tube and sutured together, the skin suture line will not lie directly over the urethral suture line but will be separated from it by a considerable distance (Fig. 304, *5, 6, 7*).

Covering Tube by Burying in Scrotum: Other surgeons have gone to even greater lengths to provide abundant cover for the new urethral tube. A method ascribed to Cecil, and also used by Cabot, is to make a midline incision in the anterior surface of the scrotum continuous with the incisions outlining the rectangular flap of skin from which the new urethra is to be constructed (Fig. 308, *1, 2*). The edges of this incision are deeply undermined and, at the time of closure, they are sutured to the corresponding lateral penile skin flaps (Fig. 308, *3, 4*) so that the urethral tube is deeply buried between penis and scrotum (Fig. 308, *4, 5*). Some weeks later, after healing is complete and the urethra intact, penis and scrotum are cut apart, leaving some scrotal skin, sufficient to cover its ventrum, attached to the penis on each side (Fig. 308, *5, 6*). These flaps are then sutured together over the urethra, and the scrotal incision is closed longitudinally (Fig. 308, *7, 8*).

Covering of Tube by Pedicle Tube Flap of Scrotum: Another ingenious method was described by Wehrbein. At least several weeks before the construction of the new urethra, two parallel longitudinal incisions are made in the anterior surface of the scrotum and extended up to the level of the base of the penis (Fig. 308, 9). The skin between these incisions is undermined and sutured into a tubular structure, attached at both ends and with the skin outside. The scrotal halves are sutured together beneath it (Fig. 308, 10). After healing is complete, the new urethral tube is constructed. Before closure of the penile incision, the tubular structure is cut away from its lower pedicle, incised along its anterior aspect, and unrolled into a rectangular skin flap (Fig. 308, 11, 12). This flap is then turned up, applied over the new urethra, and sutured to the lateral penile skin edges (Fig. 308, 13, 14). This flap, being of scrotal skin, will bear hairs, but this is of little importance, since it involves only the outer surface of the penis and not the urethra.

Special Considerations

The above-described methods may be applied whenever the urethral meatus is at any point on the penis, including the penoscrotal junction. If the orifice lies farther back, in the midscrotal, posterior scrotal, or perineal positions, the Thiersch-Duplay principle may be used with no fear of fistula formation, since in this region it is easy to bury the new urethra very deeply.

If, as often happens, a midline strip of hairless skin is present (Fig. 309), this procedure is comparatively simple; if hair follicles are present, careful and thorough depilation must be carried out before fashioning the new urethra. Individual destruction of hair follicles by electrocoagulation is more satisfactory than x-ray. Havens pulls on the hair to tent the skin, and then snips off with fine scissors a bit of skin containing the follicle.

In perineal hypospadias, a vagina, shorter or longer, is often present. If short, it is easily removed (Fig. 310). If longer, its removal may be more complicated, since it may run very close to the anterior wall of the rectum. A number of authors attest that such a vagina may be left in place without ill effects (Cecil). In all such cases, it is essential to be absolutely certain before proceeding with urethral construction that the real sex of the patient is male.

Almost all authors recommend diversion of the urine during the healing stage of the plastic urethral construction. In cases of perineal hypospadias, it may be necessary to perform cystostomy. If so, the drain should be kept in place until the plastic procedures are completed. In all other cases, perineal urethrostomy will suffice. A Foley catheter should be used as a drain, and may be removed as soon as the operative incision is healed, even if further operation is to be carried out, since the reestablishment of a perineal urethrostomy is very easy. In posterior scrotal hypospadias, the drainage tube may be brought out from the operative incision through a stab wound in the perineum (Fig. 309). Douglas trains his patients to void slowly to avoid excessive pressure in the new urethra, and finds that this often makes urinary diversion unnecessary.

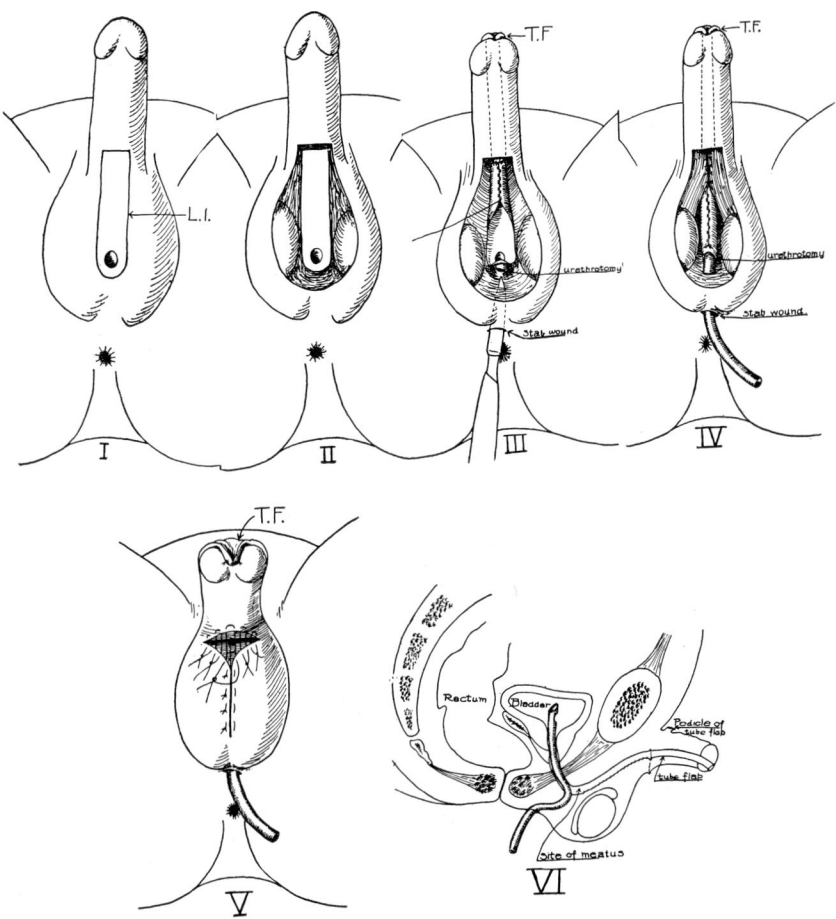

Fig. 309. Method of operating on midscrotal hypospadias (Davis). (I) Median rectangular flap cut as usual for Thiersch-Duplay type of tube formation, ending distally at a point which can be reached by a Davis-type pedicle tube flap brought through a penile tunnel. (II) Edges of flap raised, edges of incision deeply undermined. (III) Davis-type pedicle tube flap formed, brought through penile tunnel and anastomosed to Thiersch-Duplay type of tube formation in scrotal area. Stab wound made from perineum through scrotal tissues, urethrostomy opening made proximal to preexisting meatus. (IV) Urethral tube completed, drainage catheter (Foley) inserted to bladder through urethrostomy, scrotal tissues drawn together over new urethra to bury it as deeply as possible. (V) Scrotal incision closed. In distal part scrotum and penis are sutured together according to the Cecil-Cabot principle (Fig. 308), the resulting web to be divided later. (VI) Diagrammatic sagittal section of conditions after division of the pedicle of the tube flap three weeks after its formation.

673

If urethral fistula does occur, its closure may be somewhat difficult. The usual procedure is to cut around the fistula, free it down to the urethra, and amputate it. The tissues are then closed over the opening in the urethra by a purse-string suture of fine catgut, reinforced by a number of individual subcutaneous sutures. The edges of the skin incision are then closed by mattress sutures of nonabsorbable material.

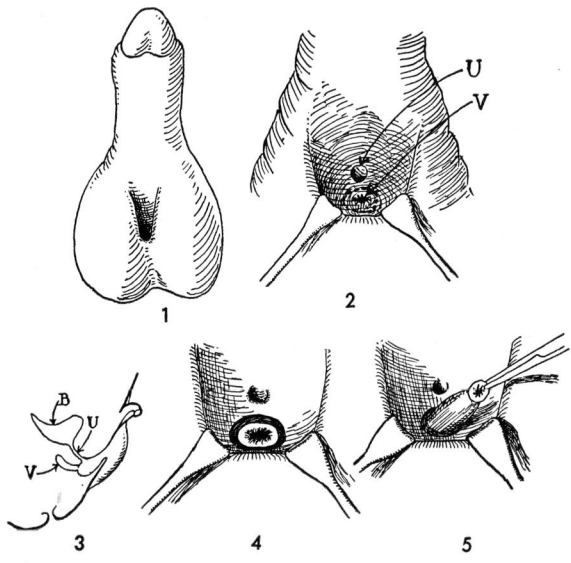

Fig. 310. Case of perineal hypospadias. (1) External appearance after straightening of penis. (2) Edges of skin lappet covering urogenital sinus retracted showing vagina, V, and urethra U. Dotted line is incision circumscribing vagina. (3) Diagrammatic sagittal section. (4, 5) Dissection and complete removal of vagina.

Byars modifies this procedure by using fine nonabsorbable material tied over a bit of rubber tissue or tubing. Davis does not amputate the fistula after carefully freeing it, but takes a mattress suture in the outer edges of the fistula, brings the ends of the suture out through the urethra, and by traction on these ends turns the fistula inside out into the lumen of the urethra. This inversion of the fistula is maintained by fastening the ends of the inverting suture to the abdominal wall by means of another suture and a light elastic band so that slight elastic traction is exerted continuously (Fig. 311). The subcutaneous tissues and the skin incision are then closed over the site of the fistula described above. Diversion of the urine, usually by perineal urethrostomy, is most important and is advised by practically all surgeons.

674

The author believes that in hypospadias surgery the administration of antibiotic drugs immediately before operation and during the post-operative period is of the utmost value, since a slight infection can impair an otherwise perfect result. Since coccal infections are the most damaging, one should give not only a wide-spectrum antibiotic but also one particularly active against staphylococci and streptococci. If the patient

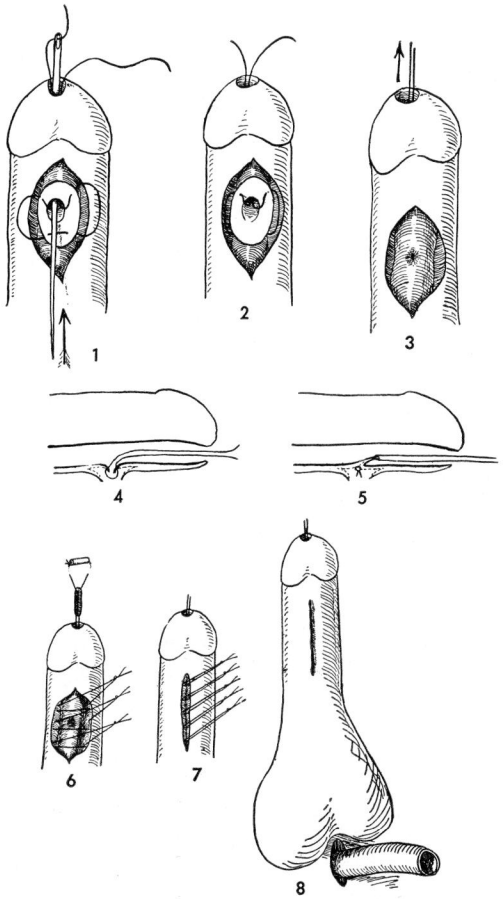

Fig. 311. Davis operation for closing small fistulas. (1) Double mattress silk suture taken in edge of small flange around outer end of fistula, needle passed butt first and out through urethra and meatus; (2) suture ready to be pulled out; (3) suture pulled and fistula turned inside out; (4) diagrammatic sagittal section, suture in place; (5) same, suture pulled and fistula inside out; (6) silk suture holding fistula inside out fastened to abdomen by rubber band, purse-string about site of fistula, subcutaneous sutures placed; (7) subcuticular sutures placed. Mattress sutures may be used, with protection from cutting (rubber tubes or beads), or, if covering tissue is inadequate, penis may be sutured down to scrotum according to Cecil-Cabot principle (see Fig. 308, 1-8). (8) Incision closed by subcuticular sutures, catheter in perineal urethrostomy.

675

is sensitive to penicillin, erythromycin or novobiocin with ampicillin is satisfactory.

In the surgery of hypospadias, one is dealing with very delicate and highly elastic integument. It is therefore very easy to distort the flaps in the process of cutting them, and the greatest care must be exercised to avoid this. Exactly equal tension must be exerted upon the skin in all directions during the entire process of cutting the flap; otherwise its edges

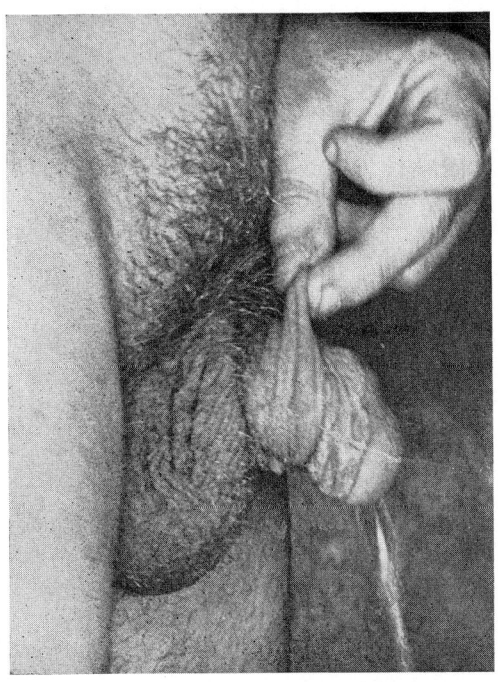

Fig. 312. End result of surgical treatment in penoscrotal hypospadias.

will not be parallel. The author has found curved sharp-pointed scalpel blades of great value in this connection. For handling the delicate tissues, particularly in children, the small forceps and scissors used in ophthalmic surgery are ideal.

Seventy-four articles on the treatment of hypospadias published between 1962 and 1967 have been reviewed. Of these, thirty authors prefer the Denis-Browne, twenty-two the Thiersch-Duplay, ten the Nové-Josserand-McIndoe and seven the Cecil-Cabot-Bucknall procedure. Other surgeons describe experiences in which they have obviously tried many methods in search of a satisfactory one. This I think is a mistake. After a careful reading of the literature, one should select the method which seems to oneself the most reasonable and then proceed to perform it, exactly according to directions, until one is able to procure results at least as good as anyone else has had with that method. Then and only then is the surgeon qualified to begin making changes in the technique. Too many have begun to introduce hoped-for improvements at much too early a stage of their surgical development. Further, it is quite evident that excellent results can now be obtained by any one of a number of methods provided the execution is skillful and the technique faultless—which can come only as the result of experience.

Three authors try to avoid diversion of the urine. Crawford uses the Denis-Browne method closing with a continuous suture made water tight. Persky and Broadbent and their collaborators use the latter's method, a spiral Thiersch-Duplay with its terminal portion laid into a split glans. The case experience for all of these papers is small.

Farkas describes an interesting instrument for making a penile tunnel, and, if desired, introducing a tubular free graft. Mustardé mentions a Thackeray clamp favorably. Gross uses a spring clamp to close Denis-Browne incisions. Barcat and Godard find a delicate retractor useful in placing sutures or skin clamps accurately. Lenko has devised two identical acrylic perforated strips which protect a continuous suture for closing after a Thiersch-Duplay and at the same time hold the penis straight. Incidentally, Lich and Pers find a continuous suture desirable for Denis-Browne closures, Lich using three layers. Schober and Panzner prefer the Davis method of straightening the penis, and hold it extended with a wire bridge attached to a pelvic plaster cast.

Suction drainage is mentioned in three papers. Michalowski and Modelski drain their straightening operations through a stab wound; Bartrino and Gyarmathy use suction drainage after Denis-Browne operations, the latter placing his tube in the new urethra.

The original Bucknall operation using scrotal skin appears to be almost entirely abandoned. Lombardi describes a case in which a profuse growth of hair caused complete urinary retention.

Six authors like the Wehrbein procedure for covering Denis-Browne or Thiersch-Duplay reconstruction. Marshall and his collaborators, Lewis and Kenneth, and Farina, Campos-Freire and their collaborators present reasonably convincing statistical data. Barcat and Stephan, Szkodny and Serafino and collaborators, Marino, Gupta, Mustardé, Mariani and Salata, Dalessio and Coffola present methods for constructing a glandular urethra from the internal layer of the prepuce.

Five authors report methods for one-stage procedures. Singer, Aronoff, and Mustardé use different attacks. Persky and his collaborators use the Broadbent method, reporting thirteen cases with three fistulas and three strictures. Devine and Horton use a free preputial graft laid in a split glans, reporting twenty-eight cases with seven fistulas and sixteen

677

primary healings; the fate of the other five cases is not given. The arguments against one-stage procedures are given above.

The Davis pedicle tube flap method of reconstruction has been used by comparatively few surgeons, but they continue to use it and obtain excellent results.

Montagnani and Frittelli report a case of Thiersch-Duplay reconstruction in which the totally denuded penile shaft was buried in a tunnel under the skin of the prepubic area. The penis was freed later along with enough pubic skin to cover it. We have used this method successfuly, but it produces a penis covered by a growth of pubic hair.

The value of a good many papers is destroyed or reduced by the failure of authors to give exact data as to some or all of the following: (1) the number of cases operated on, (2) the number of each type of hypospadias, (3) the number of operations necessary in each case, and (4) the end results in detail. Photographs of patients while voiding give the most convincing evidence of good results, and are seldom given. They should be required in all serious reports.

EPISPADIAS

In epispadias, the defect in the urethra may involve only the glandular part or it may extend back any distance. The entire penile urethra may be open dorsally without any incontinence, but if the anomaly involves the deep urethra there may be great widening of the channel and complete incontinence. In some cases, it may even be possible to insert a finger into the bladder. Naturally, if such conditions are present, the plastic operation on the penis must be supplemented by further procedures on the deep urethra and vesical orifice to provide urinary control.

The penile part of the operation is the same in principle regardless of the extent of the deformity. It is the writer's opinion that only one method needs to be described: namely, Young's modification of Cantwell's procedure. It is superior to other methods in that it preserves the blood supply of all parts, it brings the urethra to its proper ventral position, and it reconstructs the broad, spadelike penis to an essentially normal form. The use of grafts and flaps to cover the new urethra only serves to preserve or increase the deformity of the penis.

Technique (Young's Modification of Cantwell's Procedure)
(Fig. 313)

The urethra is constructed according to the same principles as those used in the Thiersch-Duplay procedure for hypospadias. When the incision

678

is made outlining the strip from which the new urethra is to be built, one limb of this incision is extended deeply down between the corpora cavernosa to the ventral part of the penis, as shown in the small cross sections in Figure 313. This leaves the new urethra firmly attached to one corpus for its blood supply, and mobilizes the corpora so that they can be rotated. The urethra is formed by suture in the usual manner, using continuous or interrupted sutures of the finest plain catgut. The corpus

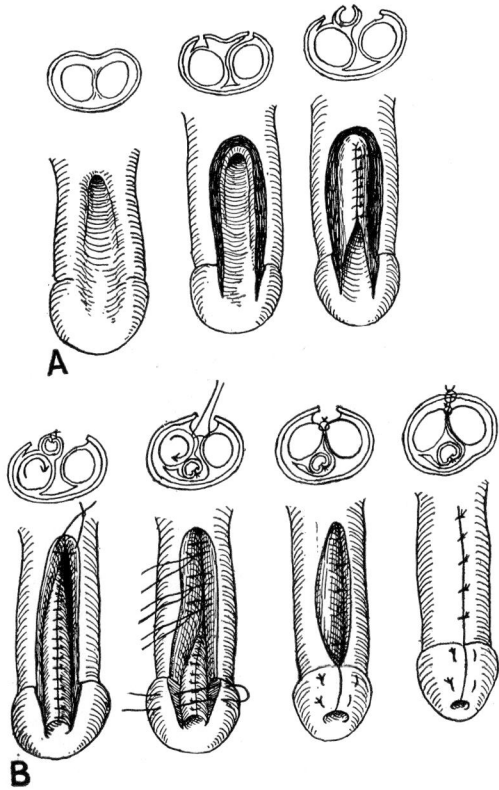

Fig. 313. *A:* Young-Cantwell operation for epispadias. U-shaped incision, formation of new urethra by suture. Cross sections show how incision is extended down between corpora cavernosa almost to ventral surface. *B:* Urethra completed, corpora cavernosa drawn together over it. Arrows in cross sections show how one corpus cavernosum is rotated to bring new urethra to ventral surface of penis.

to which the urethra remains attached is then rotated until the urethra lies under the ventral skin of the penis in its normal position, and is held in this position by numerous sutures of fine chromicized catgut penetrating the tunica albuginea and holding the two corpora closely together. This apposition may be further insured by through-and-through stay sutures of nonabsorbable material if desired. The two halves of the glans are then sutured together over the urethra, and here one or two nonabsorbable mattress stay sutures are desirable. They should be tied over small, soft rubber tubing, not as shown in Figure 313.

If the epispadias is complicated by dilatation of the deep urethra and incontinence, a corrective operation, such as that seen in Figure 314, should be performed. When the bladder is opened suprapubically, the greatly widened vesical orifice is seen, and a segment, *a-b*, marked for removal.

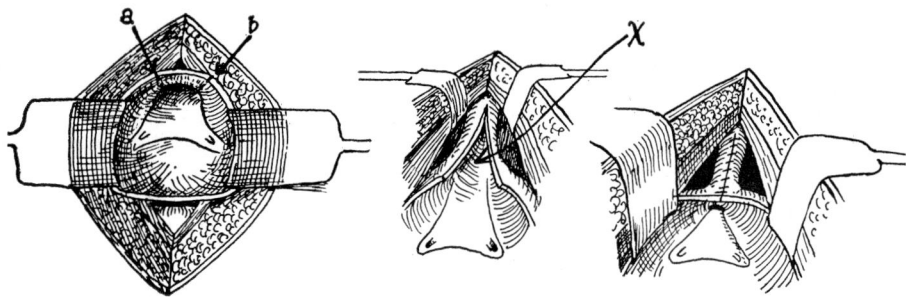

Fig. 314. Young operation for epispadias with incontinence. From left to right: (1) Bladder opened. (2) Triangular area excised at X to reduce vesicle orifice to normal size. (3) Urethra reconstructed by sutures. Other mattress sutures are used to draw rudiments of internal sphincter over new vesicle orifice. *a, b:* Tissue to be removed. X. Site of new vesicle orifice.

One should aim to leave enough behind to make an orifice a little smaller than normal. The cutting of this wedge-shaped segment should be continued down the urethra until well away from the bladder, as shown in the middle panel of Figure 314 at X. One should try to make the reconstructed urethra, in an adult, about the size of a No. 12 French catheter. The closure of the urethra is accomplished by interrupted suture of fine chromic catgut. At the site of the vesical orifice, every effort must be made to bring up as much muscle tissue as possible from the muscular wall of the bladder and suture it over the new vesical orifice. If the urethra is too large, incontinence will continue; if it is too small, it can easily be dilated.

The results of operations for epispadias are usually good, even to restoration of urinary control. Diversion of the urine is necessary here, as in surgery for hypospadias. Perineal urethrotomy can be used only in the mild forms of glandular epispadias; in all other cases, suprapubic cystostomy is necessary. The methods described here are useful for restoration of the penis in cases of extrophy of the bladder. The urethra should be carefully reconstructed back as far as the verumontanum, even when the ureters are to be transplanted into the rectum and the bladder excised, in order to make sexual relations possible and provide egress for the semen.

PHIMOSIS

The most common congenital malformation of the penis is phimosis. This name is properly applied only to those cases in which the preputial orifice is so small that retraction of the prepuce is difficult or impossible. Phimosis is treated by circumcision or posthectomy, which consists of the removal of a part of the prepuce, including the narrow preputial orifice. It must be remembered that this same operation is often performed for redundant or elongated prepuce, even when no real phimosis is present.

Circumcision is a simple, innocuous procedure but it can be, and too often is, done incorrectly. The necessities for a proper circumcision are as follows:

1. The lines of incision must be traced beforehand, so that they will be even and symmetrical, and that neither too much nor too little will be cut away (Fig. 315).

2. Phimosis is often complicated by an adherent prepuce. All adhesions between prepuce and glans must be completely separated.

3. Phimosis is often complicated by congenital stenosis of the meatus (Fig. 316). This must be detected and, if present, treated by meatotomy.

4. The skin must be left longer in the frenal region to avoid tension on the frenum during erection and intercourse, and yet not too long.

5. Hemostasis must be good.

6. The skin edges must be accurately approximated.

Technique

Circumcision is performed as indicated in Figure 315. In newborn babies, no anesthesia is used. With older children, general anesthesia is usually necessary. With adults (or children with unusual composure), local anesthesia is the choice. Procaine, 0.5 per cent, is the agent most often used. The injections are usually made near the base of the penis, and through four wheals, one dorsal, one ventral, and two lateral. Special attention is paid to the dorsal cord of lymphatics and nerves. The tunica albuginea of the penile corpora should not be penetrated. After the anesthetic is injected, a tourniquet may be applied if desired. For this a No. 10 or No. 12 rubber catheter is satisfactory. It is important to note that the foregoing injections will not anesthetize the inner leaf of the prepuce. Further subcutaneous injections must therefore be made around the coronary sulcus after the prepuce is retracted (Fig. 315). At this time, any adhesions to the glans should be completely separated. Firm wiping with gauze is usually sufficient; if it is not, a fine-pointed hemostat may be thrust in along the coronary sulcus, and the blades spread. If retraction of the prepuce is difficult or impossible, a dorsal

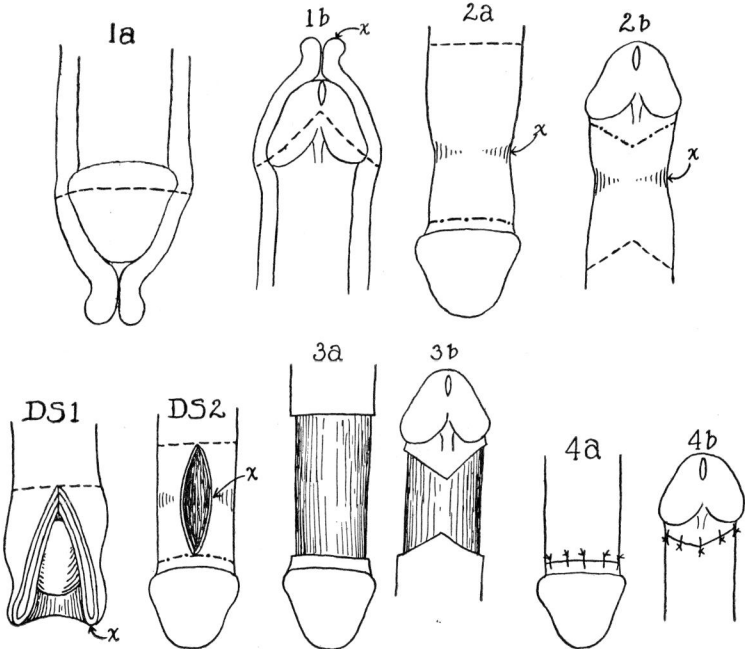

Fig. 315. Circumcision (posthectomy). 1a: Line of incision on dorsum of penis. 1b: Line of incision on ventrum of penis. x: Edge of contracted preputial orifice. 2a: Prepuce drawn back. Preputial orifice x, now surrounds and constricts shaft. Second incision now made close to glans dorsally. 2b: Ventrally, this incision is made V-shaped to avoid frenum. DS1: If preputial orifice is too small to permit retraction both layers of prepuce are incised in midline dorsally to level of coronary sulcus (dorsal slit). DS2: Prepuce is then retracted and second incision around penis made as in 2a and 2b. 3a, 3b: All of skin between two incisions around penis is removed, bleeding points ligated or coagulated. 4a, 4b: Skin edges drawn together and closed by interrupted sutures, leaving glans uncovered.

slit is made with scissors. The slit should extend all the way from the circular line of incision about the shaft to the line of incision in the coronary sulcus. The skin included within these lines of incision is then dissected away from the underlying tissues. There will usually be several bleeding arteries, especially in the midline dorsally and in the frenum ventrally. They are seized with fine-pointed clamps, and may be tied with fine plain catgut or the clamps may be touched with a coagulating electrode. The skin edges are then drawn together with interrupted sutures. Silk may be used, but must be removed later. The usual practice is to use 00 or 000 plain catgut, which does not require removal. Eight sutures usually suffice, but more may be put in if the line of suture gapes. At this time, the meatus should be carefully examined; if any stenosis is present, meatotomy should be carried out as described in Meatal Stenosis below.

Innumerable modifications of the operation of circumcision have been proposed, and it would be impossible here to describe them all. If the principles outlined in the foregoing are adhered to, good results are assured. An ingenious device called the "Gomco clamp" has proved useful. It clamps the outer and inner layers of skin so tightly together that, after the excision is completed, they do not separate, and the sutures can be placed without any bleeding.

After-Treatment

Since it is difficult to keep a dressing in place over a circumcision, it is wise to leave the ends of the skin sutures long, and tie them over a strip or bundle of petrolatum gauze about 1 cm. (⅜ inch) in diameter. This holds the gauze in place. Dry gauze can be placed over the petrolatum gauze and held in place with strips of adhesive plaster running spirally about the penis and then along the groins. This is not necessary in infants. The end of the glans is left uncovered to permit voiding. The long ends of the sutures and the petrolatum gauze are usually removed on the fourth day. Little or no further attention is required. Ordinarily the patient is not kept from his usual occupation.

MEATAL STENOSIS

This condition is not quite so common as phimosis, but is all too frequently neglected. A pinpoint meatus can cause serious trouble, particularly by keeping up infection in the urethra and higher in the urinary tract. The usual types are shown in Figure 316. The type shown in Figure 316, *3,* is particularly deceptive, since the blind pouch is often taken for a normal urethral meatus.

Technique

The types shown in Figure 316, *1, 2,* are the most common. The diagram shows how the membrane partly covering the meatus is slit ventrally. In the type shown in Figure 316, *3,* the septum separating the

683

urethra from the blind pouch is divided. If two small orifices are present, they are joined (Fig. 316, 4). If the stenosis is at the termination of a glandular hypospadic urethra, so that it is desirable not to extend it farther in the proximal direction, it can be widened without displacing it farther backward by making a small incision laterally on each side of the meatus (lateral meatotomy). Sometimes the stenosis extends some distance down the urethra, as shown in Figure 316, 2b. If so, the stricture must be divided throughout its entire length. A blunt or probe-pointed

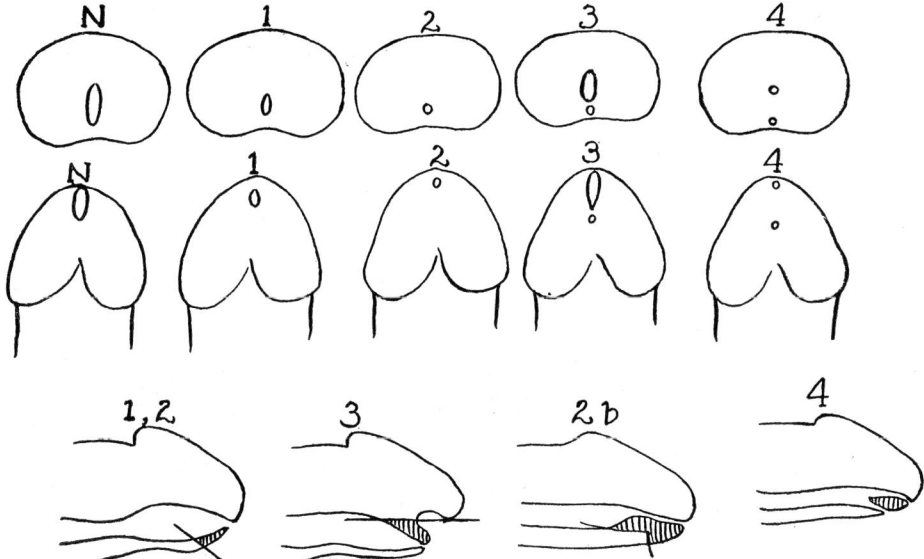

Fig. 316. Meatotomy. N: Normal. *1:* Small meatus. *2:* Pinpoint meatus. *3:* Pinpoint meatus with blind meatal gutter. *4:* Double pinpoint meatus. In sagittal sections, shaded areas represent tissues to be incised. *2b:* Procedure when meatal stricture extends some distance down urethra.

bistoury is desirable for this. After meatotomy, a single, plain catgut suture may be placed in the angle of the incision to prevent reclosure. If the narrowing extends far down the urethra (Fig. 316, 2b) it may be necessary to assure that the edges of the cut do not heal together. This can be done by inserting in the urethra a short piece of tubing, preferably silastic, and fastening it in place by a mattress suture through the glans, tied over a small piece of tubing or sponge rubber. The patient voids through this, and it may be left in place as long as two or three weeks until the urethra is completely healed.

Bleeding from the cut edges may be arrested by pressure, a silver nitrate stick, or electrocoagulation. The incision itself may be made with the electric cutting current, which obviates bleeding. For meatotomy, sufficient anesthesia is usually obtained by placing in the meatus for a few minutes a cotton swab soaked in cocaine, 10 per cent; tetracaine (Pontocaine), 2 per cent; or any other good local anesthetic. If more is required, a few drops of procaine, 1 per cent, can be injected about the meatus with a fine hypodermic needle.

ACCESSORY URETHRA

The variety of forms of accessory urethra is almost endless. The treatment, if treatment is necessary, can only be complete excision. If the accessory urethra reaches the bladder, the procedure is more complicated, and must be planned according to the conditions present.

OCCLUSION OF MEATUS

This condition is rare. Often the occlusion is membranous, and needs merely to be slit open. In other cases, the whole distal part of the urethra is obliterated, so that cystotomy is necessary to find its extremity. With these more advanced forms, umbilical fistula may be present and give exit to the urine.

BIBLIOGRAPHY

ABBÉ, R.: *New method of creating a vagina in a case of congenital absence.* Med. Rec., New York, 54:836, 1898.

ADAMS, W. M.: *Construction of an artificial vagina.* Surg. Gynec. Obstet., 76: 746-751, 1943.

ATAKAM, ASIL MUKBIL: *A case of hermaphrodismus masculinus internus.* Ann. Surg., 140:216, 1954.

BALAKRISHMAN, C.: *Scrotal avulsion: A new technique of reconstruction by split-skin graft.* Brit. J. Plast. Surg., 9:38, 1956.

BALDWIN, F.: *The formation of an artificial vagina by intestinal transplantation.* Ann. Surg., 40:398, 1904.

BANHAM, A. R.: *Total denudation of the penis.* Brit. J. Surg., 36:268, 1949.

BANKOFF, G.: *Plastic Repair of Genito-Urinary Defects.* Philosophical Library Inc., New York, 1956.

BARCAT, and PETROPOULOS. *Résultats du traitement des hypospadias antérieurs par la.* Tranchée Balanique. Mém. Acad. Chir., 78:896, 1952.

THE TRUNK

BARCAT, J., and GODARD, F.: *Ecartepinces autostatique pour la chirurgie de l'hypospadias.* Ann. Chir. Infantile, 3:71, 1962.

BARCAT, J., and STEPHAN, J. C.: *Clinical and therapeutic study of 140 cases of hypospadias,* J. Chir., 81:551, 1961.

BARTRINA, JOSÉ: *Modification de la technique de traitment de l'hypospadias.* Acta Urol. Belg., 31:569, 1963.

BENZADON, J.: *Hipospadia Peneana. Procedimiento de Leveuf Y Godard Modificado.* Bol. Soc. Cir. de Rosario, 13:339, 1946.

BERGONZELLI, V., RUFFA, P., and MARTEN-PEROLINO, R.: *Surgical treatment of hypospadias.* Minerva Chir., 17:869, 1962.

BIEBL, M.: *Gestielte Ureterplastik bei Hypospadie.* Ztschr. f. Urol., 44:657, 1951.

BLAIR, V. P., and BYARS, L. T.: *Hypospadias and epispadias.* J. Urol., 40:814, 1938.

BLOCKER, T. G., LEWIS, S. R., and SNYDER, C. C.: *Plastic construction of the artificial vagina.* Plast. Reconstr. Surg., 11:177, 1953.

BOURQUE, J. P.: *New surgical procedure for cure of scrotal hypospadias: Grafting of a male human urethra taken from a fresh cadaver.* J. Urol., 67:698, 1952.

v. BOUWDIJK BASTIAANSE, M. A.: *Hypospadie met Uitmonding van eén Ureter in de Vagina met Congenitale Totale Incontinentia Urinae.* Ned. Tijdschr Verlok en Gynaec., 47:144, 1946-47.

BRADY, L.: *Methods of constructing vagina.* Ann. Surg., 121:518, 1945.

BROADBENT, T. R., and WOOLF, R. M.: *Hypospadias one-stage repair.* Brit. J. Plast. Surg., 18:406, 1965.

BROWN, J. B.: *Restoration of the entire skin of the penis.* Surg. Gynec. Obstet., 65:362, 1937.

BROWN, J. B., and FRYER, M. P.: *Peno-scrotal skin losses, repaired by implantation and free skin grafting.* Ann. Surg., 145:656, 1957.

BROWNE, D.: *Hypospadias.* Postgrad. Med. J., 25:367, 1949.
A comparison of the Duplay and Denis Browne techniques for hypospadias operations. Surgery, 34:787, 1953.
Campbell Urology. W. B. Saunders, Philadelphia, 1954.

BRYAN, A. L., NIGRO, J. H., and COUNSELLOR, V. S.: *One hundred cases of congenital absence of the vagina.* Surg. Gynec. Obstet., 88:79, 1949.

BYARS, L. T.: *Functional restoration of hypospadias deformities: With a report of 60 completed cases.* Surg. Gynec. Obstet., 92:149, 1951.
A technique for consistently satisfactory repair of hypospadias. Surg. Gynec. Obstet., 100:184, 1955.

CABOT, H.: *The treatment of hypospadias in theory and practice.* New Eng. J. Med., 214:871, 1936.

CALI, R. W., and PRATT, J. H.: *Congenital absence of vaginal reconstruction in 175 cases.* Amer. J. Obstet. Gynec., 1968, 100:752.

CAMPBELL, R. M.: *Dermatome grafting on the totally denuded testes.* Plast. Reconstr. Surg., 19:509, 1957.

THE GENITALIA IN MALE AND FEMALE

CARRAI, P. E., and PALCHETTI, G.: *Su 60 Casi di Ipospadia Operati col Metodo dell 'Ombrédanne.* Arch. Ital. Chir., 74:157, 1951.

CECIL, B.: *Surgical management of the vagina in male construction in hermaphrodites.* J. Urol., 62:709, 1949.
Modern treatment of hypospadias. Ibid., 67:1006, 1952.

COUNSELLOR, V. S.: *Congenital absence of the vagina.* JAMA, 136:861, 1947.

COUNSELLOR, V. S., and FLETCHER, S. S.: *Treatment for congenital absence of the vagina.* Surg. Clin. N. Amer., 24:938, 1944.

CRAWFORD, B. S.: *The treatment of hypospadias.* Proc. Roy. Soc. Med., 54:1013, 1961.

CRONIN, T. D., GUTHRIE T., and HERR, D.: *Experiences in the surgical correction of hypospadias.* Amer. J. Surg., 110:818, 1965.

CULP, O.: *The treatment of hypospadias.* Henry Ford Hosp. Med Bull., 14:17, 1966.

CULP, S.: *Early correction of congenital chordee in hypospadias.* J. Urol., 65:264, 1951.

D'ALESSIO, E., and COPPOLA, M.: *Treatment of distal hypospadias.* Minerva Chir., 17:856, 1962.

DAVIS, D. M.: *The pedicle tube-graft in the surgical treatment of hypospadias in the male.* Surg. Gynec. Obstet., 71:790, 1940.
A new operation for mid-scrotal hypospadias. J. Urol., 52:340, 1944.
The surgical treatment of hypospadias, especially scrotal and perineal. Plast. Reconstr. Surg., 5:373, 1950.
Results of pedicle tube-flap method in hypospadias. J. Urol., 73:343, 1955.

DEVINE, C. J., JR., and HORTON, C. E.: *One stage hypospadias repair.* J. Urol., 85:166, 1961.

DICKIE, W. R.: *A simple modification in technique of urethral reconstruction by the buried skin strip method.* Brit. J. Plast. Surg., 14:185, 1961.

DODSON, A. I.: *The treatment of hypospadias.* J. Urol., 61:116, 1949.

DODSON, A. I., and FROHBOSE, W. J.: *Hypospadias.* J. Mich. Med. Soc., 51:852, 1952.

DOUGLAS, B.: *One-stage reconstruction for traumatic denudation of the male external genitalia.* Ann. Surg., 133:889, 1951.
Recent experiences in the operative and post-operative management of hypospadias. Plast. Reconstr. Surg., 11:107, 1953.

EVANS, T. N.: *The artificial vagina.* Amer. J. Obstet. Gynec., 99:944, 1967.

FARINA, R.: *Total reconstruction of the penis.* Plast. Reconstr. Surg., 14:351, 1954.

FARINA, R., DE CAMPOS FREIRE, G., KEPPKE, E. M., PEGGEON, A., and BARONDI, R.: *Surgical handling of hypospadias.* Chirurg, 32:125, 1961.

FARKAS, L. G.: *Circumstances affecting the method and the results of the surgical treatment of hypospadias.* Plast. Reconstr. Surg., 36:191, 1965.
Hypospadias. Academia, Prague, 1967.

FISCHER, H. W., LISCHER, C. E., and BYARS, L. T.: *True hermaphroditism.* Ann. Surg., 136:864, 1952.

687

THE TRUNK

FOGH-ANDERSON, P.: *Hypospadias: 34 completed cases operated on according to Denis Browne.* Acta Chir. Scand., Stockholm, 105:414, 1953.
Transvestism and trans-sexualism, surgical treatment in a case of auto-castration. Acta Medicinae Legalis et Socialis, 9:33, 1956.

FRANK, R. T.: *The formation of an artificial vagina without operation.* Amer. J. Obstet. Gynec., 35:1053, 1938.

FRANK, R. T., and GEIST, S. H.: *The formation of an artificial vagina by a new plastic technic.* Amer. J. Obstet. Gynec., 14:712, 1927.

FRASER, K.: *A Queensland review of 31 major hypospadias repairs using a uniform technique.* Brit. J. Surg., 51:167, 1964.

GELB, F., MALAMENT, M., and LOVERME, S.: *Total reconstruction of the penis. A review of the literature and report of a case.* Plast. Reconstr. Surg., 24:62, 1959.

GIBSON, T.: *Traumatic avulsion of the skin of the scrotum and penis: Use of the avulsed skin as a free graft.* Brit. J. Plast. Surg., 6:283, 1954.

GONZALEZ-ULLOA, M.: *Severe avulsion of the scrotum in a bullfighter: reconstruction procedure.* Brit. J. Plast. Surg., 16:154, 1963.

GOLDSMITH, I. M.: *Vaginal aplasia.* Surg. Gynec. Obstet., 123:361, 1969.

GRAVES, W. P.: *Gynecology.* W. B. Saunders, Philadelphia, 1917, p. 385.

GROSS, R.: *Treatment of hypospadias with an apparatus of my own construction.* Chirurg, 34:225.

GUPTA, S. J.: *A preliminary report of a method for treatment of subglandular hypospadias.* Brit. J. Plast. Surg., 18:193, 1965.

GYARMATHY, F.: *Our experiences with the hypospadias operation of Denis Browne.* Ztschr. f. Urol., 56:223, 1963.

HAMBLEN, E. C., ET AL.: *Male pseudohermaphroditism: Some endocrinological and psychosexual aspects.* Amer. J. Obstet. Gynec., 61:1, 1951.

HARRENSTEIN, R. J.: *Uber die Funktion des Scrotums und die Behandlung der Retentio Testis beim Menschen.* Zentrlbl. f. Chir., 55:1734, 1928.

HASLINGER, K.: *Doppelbildungen der Männlichen Harnöhre.* Ztschr. f. Urol., 33:24, 1939.

HAVENS, F. Z., and BLACK, A. S.: *The treatment of hypospadias.* J. Urol., 61:1053, 1949.

HEIM, W.: *Erkenntnisse aus der Hypospadiebehandlung.* Zentbl. f. Chir., 74:757, 1949.

HINMAN: *Practice of Urology.* 1935, pp. 129-139, pp. 398-476.

HOWARD, F. S.: *Hypospadias with enlargement of prostatic utricle.* Surg. Gynec. Obstet., 86:307, 1948.
The surgery of intersexuals. J. Urol., 65:636, 1951.

HUFFSTADT, A. J. C.: *Surgical correction of female pseudohermaphroditism due to adrenal hyperplasia.* Brit. J. of Plast. Surg., 20:359, 1967.

THE GENITALIA IN MALE AND FEMALE

JOHANSON, B.: *Reconstruction of the male urethra in strictures. Application of the buried intact epithelium technic.* Acta. Chir. Scand. Supplementum 176, Stockholm, 1953.

JONES, H. W., and SCOTT, W. W.: *Hermaphroditism—Genital Anomalies and Related Endocrine Disorders.* Williams and Wilkins, Baltimore, 1958.

JUDD, E. S., and HAVENS, F. Z.: *Traumatic avulsion of the skin of penis and scrotum.* Amer. J. Surg., 112:246-252, 1943.

KIEFER, J. H.: *Construction of the terminal urethra in correction of hypospadias.* J. Urol., 59:1164, 1948.

LADD, W. E., and LANMAN, T. H.: *Exstrophy of the bladder and epispadias.* New Eng. J. Med., 222:130, 1940.

LEGUEU, F.: *Repair of urethral defects by tubal grafts of vaginal mucosa.* J. Urol., 2:369, 1918.

LENKO, J.: *Personal modification of Duplay operation for hypospadias.* J. Urol. Med. et Chir., 66:278, 1960.

LEVEUF, J.: *Le Traitement de l'Hypospadias.* Jour. de Chir., 62:90, 1946.

LEVEUF, J., and GODARD, H.: *La Greff Temporaire de a Verge sur le Serotum dans la Cure de l'Hypospadias.* Jour. de Chir., 48:328, 1936.

LICH, R., JR., and HOWERTON, L. W.: *Hypospadias or urethral fistula.* South. Med. J., 57:1136, 1964.

LOMBARDI, R.: *Concerning a complication in a plastic operation for hypospadias.* Minerva Med., 55:2477, 1964.

LOUGHRAN, A. M.: *Observations on hypospadias, including the late results of Ombrédanne's urethroplastic operation.* Brit. J. Plast. Surg., 1:147, 1948.

LOWSLEY, O. S.: *Accessory urethra. Report of two cases with a review of the literature.* New York State J. Med., 39:1022, 1939.

LOWSLEY, O. S., and KIRWIN: *Clinical Urology.* 1940, Vol. 1, pp. 298, 591.

MARSHALL, M., JR., JOHNSON, S. H., III, and PRICE, S. E., JR.: *Problems of hypospadias repair.* Penn. Med. J., 68:45, 1965.

MARSHALL, V. F., and SPELLMAN, R. M.: *Construction of urethra in hypospadias using vesical mucosal grafts.* J. Urol., 73:335, 1955.

MAY, H.: *Reconstruction of scrotum and skin of penis.* Plast. Reconstr. Surg., 6:134, 1950.
The metamorphosis of a male pseudohermaphrodite. Ibid., 15:143, 1955.
Reconstruction and rehabilitation of pseudo- and true hermaphrodites including a case of testicular feminization. Ibid., 16:201, 1955.
A follow-up study of hermaphrodites after their reconstruction and rehabilitation. J. Germantown Hosp., Feb., 1963.
Reconstruction and rehabilitation of hermaphrodites. Pacif. Med. Surg., Vol. 73, Jan./Feb., 1965, No. 1.

MAYS, H. B.: *Hypospadias: Complete correction.* J. Urol., 85:55, 1961.

McCORMACK, R. M.: *Simultaneous chordee repair and urethral reconstruction for hypospadias.* Plast. Reconstr. Surg., 13:257, 1954.

THE TRUNK

McGOWAN, A. J., and WATERHOUSE, K.: *Mobilization of the anterior urethra.* Bull. N. Y. Acad. Med., 40:776, 1964.

McINDOE, A. H.: *The treatment of congenital absence or obliterative conditions of the vagina.* Brit. J. Plast. Surg., 2:254, 1950.
The treatment of hypospadias. Amer. J. Surg., 38:176, 1937.

McKENNA, C. M.: *Hypospadias. Observations on its surgical correction.* JAMA, 113:3128, 2143, 1939.

MEMMELAAR, J.: *Use of bladder mucosa in a one-stage repair of hypospadias.* J. Urol., 58:68, 1947.

v. D. MEULEN, J. C. H. M.: *Hypospadias.* Charles C Thomas, Springfield, 1964.

MICHALOWSKI, E., and MODELSKI, W.: *Operative treatment of hypospadias.* J. Urol., 89:698, 1963.

MILLARD, D. R.: *Scrotal construction and reconstruction.* Plast. Reconstr. Surg., 38:10, 1966.

MONTAGNANI, C. A., and FRITTELLI, G.: *Method for surgical correction of posterior hypospadias.* Ospedali d'Italia Chir., 12:83, 1965.

MOORE, C. R., and QUICK, W. J.: *The scrotum as a temperature regulator for the testis.* Amer. J. Physiol., 68:70, 1924.

MOORE, F. T.: *A review of 165 cases of hypospadias.* Plast. Reconstr. Surg., Transplantation Bull., 22:525, 1958.

MUSIANI, and SALATI: *Personal method of reconstructing distal urethra.* J. d'Urol. et Nephrol., 72:109, 1966.

MUSTARDÉ, J. C.: *One stage correction of distal hypospadias and other people's fistulas.* Brit. J. Plast. Surg., 18:413, 1965.

NESBIT, R. M., BUTLER, W. J., and WHITAKER, W. L.: *Production of epithelial lined tubes from buried strips of intact skin.* J. Urol., 64:387, 1950.

NOVÉ-JOSSERAND, and GAYET: *Encyclopaedie Française d'Urologie.* 1914, Vol. 5, pp. 827-931.

OVERZIER, C.: *Intersexuality.* Translated from the German: *Die Intersexualität.* Academic Press Inc., New York, 1963.

OWENS, NEAL: *Reconstruction for traumatic denudation of the penis and scrotum.* Surgery, 12:88-96, 1942.
Simplified method for formation of an artificial vagina by split skin graft. Surgery, 12:139-150, 1942.
A suggested pyrex form for support of skin grafts in the construction of an artificial vagina. Plast. Reconstr. Surg., 1:350, 1946.

PARIENTE, R.: *La Tecnica di McIndoe per la Cura Chirurgica dell'Ipospadia.* Policlinico, Sez. Chir., 60:196, 1953.

PERROT, A., and TAILLARD, W.: *Traitement Chirurgical de l'Hypospadias.* Rev. Med. Suisse Rom., 7:589, 1950.

PERS, M.: *Skin shaving in the treatment of hypospadias, etc.* Acta Clin. Scand., Suppl., 313:209, 1965.

PERSKY, L., KIEHN, C. L., and DES PREZ, J. D.: *One stage hypospadias repair.* J. Urol., 88:259, 1962.

PFEIFFER, D. B., and MILLER, D. B.: *Traumatic avulsion of skin of penis and scrotum.* Plast. Reconstr. Surg., 5:520, 1950.

PIGNALOSA, D. M.: *Le Obliterazioni Congenite de Meato e dell'Uretra Anteriore.* Arch. Ital. di Chir., 53:847, 1938.

PRPIC, I., and PASINI, M.: *Beitrag der Operation der Hypospadie.* Chirug, 33:370, 1962.

RITCHIE, H. P.: *Hypospadias. A discussion of the subject from the viewpoint of reconstructive surgery and a report of the use of a depilated scrotal flap.* Surgery, 5:911-931, 1939.

ROBERTSON, J. F.: *Avulsion and reconstruction of the scrotum.* South. Med. Surg., 93:527, 1931.

ROBINSON, D. W., STEPHENSON, K. L., and PADGETT, E. C.: *Loss of coverage of the penis, scrotum and urethra.* Plast. Reconstr. Surg., 1:58, 1946.

RUKSTINAT, G. J., and HASTERLIK, R. J.: *Congenital absence of the penis.* Arch. Path., 27:984-993, 1939.

SCHAEFFER, A. A., and ERBES, J.: *Hypospadias.* Amer. J. Surg., 80:183, 1950.

SCHOBER, K. L., and PANZNER, R.: *Experiences with the Denis Browne operation.* Ztschr. F. Urol., 55:83, 1962.

SCHOFIELD, A. L.: *The Denis Browne repair of hypospadias.* Brit. J. Plast. Surg., 18:188, 1965.

SCHUBERT, G.: *Concerning the formation of a new vagina in the case of congenital malformation.* Surg. Gynec. Obstet., 193:376, 1914.
Anatomic and topographic considerations for my operative method in vaginal defect. Zentralbl. f. Gynäk., 47:347, 1923.

SCHUMANN, E.: *Röntgenuntersuchung zur Abgrenzung der Einfachen Hypospadie von der Hypospadie bei Hermaphroditismus.* Fortschr. Geb. Roentgenstrahlen, 78:576, 1953.

SERAFINO, G., CIARPELLA, E., SCATAFASSI, S., and CARACCIOLO LA GROTTERIA, F.: *Use of preputial skin in the surgical treatment of balanic hypospadias.* Policlinico (Chir.), 72:102, 1965.

SERFLING, H. J.: *Die Hypospadie und ihre Behandlung.* Georg Thieme, Leipzig, 1956.

SMITH, J. R.: *Hypospadias repair with preputial free inlay graft urethroplasty.* J. Urol., 96:73, 1966.

SMITH, R. D., and BLACKFIELD, H. M.: *A critique on the repair of hypospadias.* Surgery, 31:885, 1952.
Surgical treatment of hypospadias. J. Urol., 73:329, 1955.

THOMPSON, H. T., GEORGE W. REPER, T., and SEGERSON, J. E.: *Hypospadias: The principle of the third degree.* J. Urol., 94:582, 1965.

TUFFIER: *Traitement de l'Hypospadias; Par la Tunnellisation du Penis et l'Application des Greffes Ollier-Thiersch.* Ann. des Org. G. U., 17:370, 1899.

THE TRUNK

WATSON, J.: *Loss of the skin of the scrotum: Treatment by free skin graft.* Brit. J. Plast. Surg., 8:333, 1956.

WEITZ, H.: *Zur Hypospadiebehandlung.* Deut. Med. Woch., 41:1064, 1915.

WEHRBEIN, H. L.: *Hypospadias.* J. Urol., 50:335, 1943.

WHARTON, L. R.: *Spontaneous perforation of the recto-vaginal septum, five weeks after construction of the vagina.* Ann. Surg., 121:530, 1945.

WOUDSTRA, S. T.: *Hypospadie—Behandelung en Vooruitzichten.* Geneesk Gids, 31:439, 1953.

YOUNG, F., and BENJAMIN, J. A.: *Pre-school age repair of hypospadias with free inlay skin graft.* Surgery, 26:384, 1949.

YOUNG, H. H.: *Genital Abnormalities, Hermaphroditism and Related Adrenal Diseases.* Williams & Wilkins, Baltimore, 1937.
Note on treatment of hypospadias. J. Urol., 42:470, 1939.
Operative treatment of true hermaphroditism. A new technic for changing hypospadias. Arch. Surg., 41:557, 1940.

YOUNG, H. H., and DAVIS, D. M.: *Young's Practice of Urology.* Vol. II, pp. 70-136, 596-647. W. B. Saunders, Philadelphia, 1926.

ZVYAGINTSEV, A. E., ZHELEZNYAKOVA, F. I., and GADZHIMIRZAEV, G. A.: *Operative treatment of hypospadias in children.* Urologia 29:3, 1964.

DEFECTS OF
SPHINCTER   19
ANI MUSCLE

ANAL incontinence is due to injury or absence of the musculus sphincter ani. Various procedures have been offered for repair or replacement of the sphincter. The choice depends on whether the muscle is totally absent or destroyed or whether larger parts of the muscle are intact. The number of patients in whom the muscle is absent or totally destroyed is small. In such cases, restoration of control of the anal outlet can be achieved only by transfer of voluntary-muscle action. Far more numerous are the patients in whom the sphincter muscle is only partly destroyed. Direct suture of the divided muscle may be attempted if the rent is small; in larger defects, however, where up to half of the sphincter muscle is missing, a two-stage plastic procedure—as devised by Blaisdell—has been found successful.

In determining the extent of the defect, the anatomical appearance is of greater value than the clinical picture. Wherever the muscle is destroyed, the overlying skin tends to be smooth and depressed, while the skin over intact muscle is folded.

TOTAL DEFECT OF SPHINCTER MUSCLE

Function of the anal outlet is controlled by the voluntary external and the involuntary internal sphincter muscles. If the internal sphincter is paralyzed—sometimes after a "pull-through" operation for instance in cases of imperforated anus or cancer of the rectum—the external sphincter is strong enough to control continence, but can act only as an emergency brake since it cannot be kept contracted voluntarily for any length of time. For more details of the motor action of the sphincter mechanism I refer the reader to the work of Bacon, Courtney, Gaston, Smith and Gross. If the external sphincter is paralyzed or destroyed also and a sphincter plasty is contemplated, one must remember that only the action of the external sphincter can be restored, i.e., only the emergency action. In such a case the patient must rely also on regulating his bowel habits and irrigations every other day. Hence, control of the anal outlet by a sphincter plasty is much more reliable if only the external sphincter action is absent while the internal sphincter function is intact.

In total defects of the sphincter, various procedures, consisting of transfer of voluntary-muscle action, have been offered. Shoemaker's transfer of gluteal-muscle flaps has been modified in various ways. Stone, having tried many procedures without much success, developed a method which was based upon an original idea of the Russian orthopedic surgeon, R. R. Wreden. Stone and others who have had considerable experience with this operation report gratifying results in the majority of cases. The author has used it in the absence of both sphincters. The result was a complete failure after the first operation, with marked improvement after a second attempt. In the first operation foreign material (ox fascia) was used, which became completely absorbed. This may be the reason for the failure. No trace of the fascial strips could be found at the second operation, two years after their insertion. In the second operation autogenous fascia-lata strips were used, which seem to hold well; the parents report marked improvement of the child's condition, with only occasional soiling.

Technique (Wreden-Stone)

Preoperative preparation: The patient is admitted to the hospital a few days before the operation. The bowels are prepared two days prior to the operation by saline enemas twice daily; the patient is placed on a liquid diet and receives 1 gr. of neomycin every six hours for six doses and paragoric (5 cc.) at 8 P.M. that evening and the same amount at 7 A.M. the day of the operation.

Procedure (Figs. 317–319): Two fascia-lata strips are removed from the patient's thigh with the fascia stripper (see p. 48). They should be 15 cm. (5⅞ inches) long and 0.5 cm. (³⁄₁₆ inch) wide. They are wrapped in moist gauze. The small incisions are closed with silk sutures and the patient placed in the lithotomy position.

694

DEFECTS OF SPHINCTER ANI MUSCLE

Small incisions are made on the left and right sides, along a line joining the tip of the coccyx to the tuberosity of the ischium, and about
2 cm. (¾ inch) posterior to the anal margin. These wounds are deepened
bluntly into the subcutaneous fat. By blunt dissection, a curved Kelly
clamp is pushed from one incision to the other, in front of the rectum, in
the subcutaneous fat, care being taken to avoid injury to the rectum, anal
canal, or vagina. The clamp is then opened and made to grasp and
lock on the ends of the two fascial strips, the other ends being secured

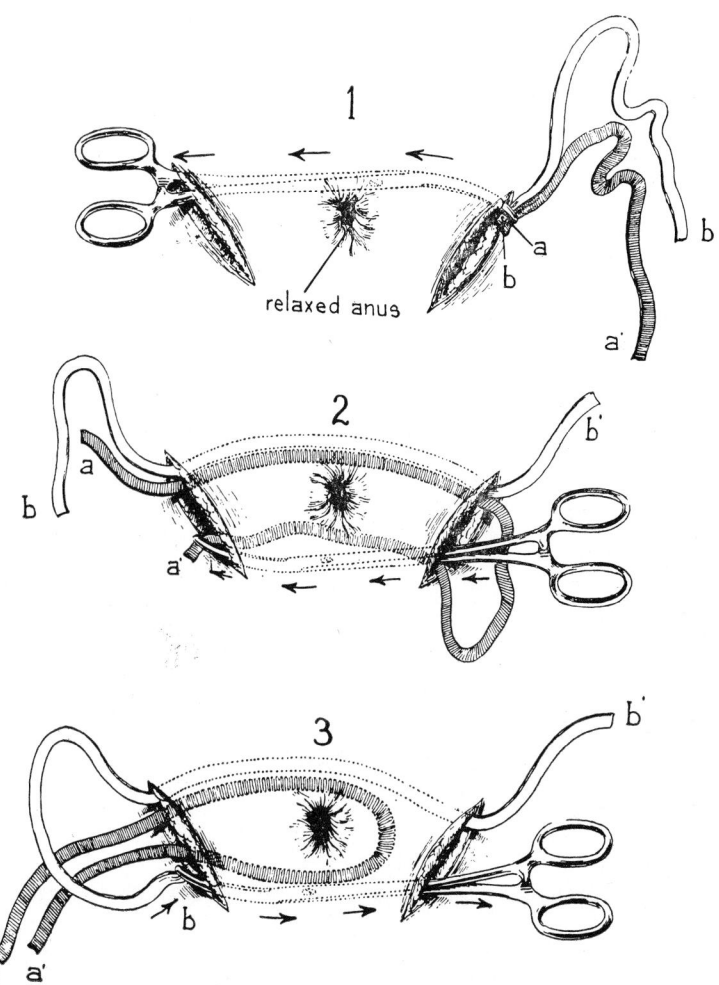

Fig. 317. Anal-sphincter plastic procedure (Stone). *1:* Two fascial strips are to be
passed subcutaneously in front of anus. Clamp holding free ends of fascia is shown
in position. *2:* One fascial strip, *b*, is in front of anus. Other one is being passed
posteriorly around anus. *3:* Fascial strip is being passed around anus in opposite
direction. (H. B. Stone: Arch. Surg.)

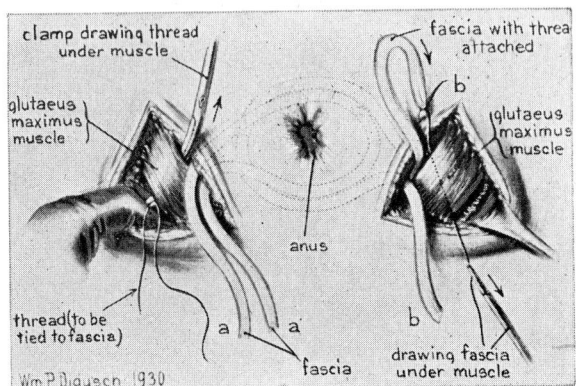

Fig. 318. One free end of each fascial strip is passed around a substantial bundle of gluteus muscle. (H. B. Stone: Arch. Surg.)

with a hemostat. This clamp, holding the strips of fascia, is pulled back through the tunnel that it has made, which thus places two fascial strips in front of the anal canal in the subcutaneous tissues. The free end of one of the fascial strips is grasped with a Kelly clamp, which is pushed, in similar fashion, from one incision to the other in the subcutaneous tissue behind the anus. The clamp is released, and the fascial end is drawn out of the second incision so that this strip enters one incision, encircles the anus under the skin, and emerges from the same incision. Before the clamp is drawn back, it grasps the end of the other strip. It is then withdrawn, pulling this second strip with it. Thus, the second strip also encircles the anus, but from the opposite side, and its two ends emerge from the opposite incision. The finger is then inserted into one of the incisions and feels outward and backward until the mesial margin of the musculus gluteaus maximus is defined. An aneurysm needle or clamp carrying a strong guide thread is then pushed around a substantial bundle of the gluteus muscle. This thread is tied to one of the ends of fascia lying in the incision, and the strip is pulled around

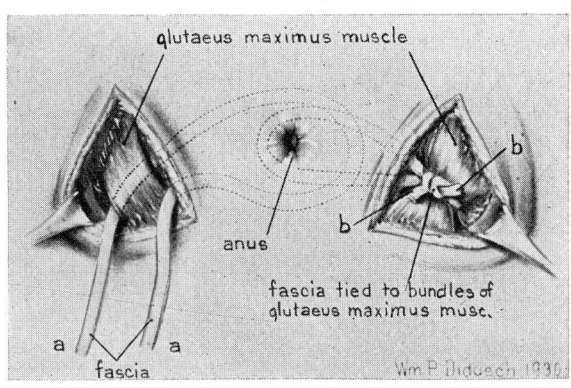

Fig. 319. Fascial ends are tied on right side, ready to be tied on left side. (H. B. Stone: Arch. Surg.)

696

the bundle of gluteus fibers. This end of the strip is then tied to the other end of the same fascial strip, in a firm square knot, with enough tension to close the anal opening snugly but not with strangulating tightness. A similar maneuver is carried out on the other side. Thus, the two fascial strips form closed rings which encircle the anal canal on their inner or mesial curves and provide a bundle of gluteus fibers on their outer curves, but pull against each other and firmly close the anal canal. The wounds are closed.

After-Treatment

The patient is given a liquid diet. He receives 5 cc. of paregoric every two hours for six doses and antibiotics. On the fourth postoperative day, the diet is changed to soft foods, and he receives 30 cc. of mineral oil every night. If there has been no bowel movement on the sixth postoperative day, an enema is administered. After the second week, the patient is told to exercise the gluteal muscles at regular intervals daily. (See also p. 701 of following chapter.)

Pickrell and co-workers reported an ingenious method of sphincter reconstruction by means of a gracilis muscle transplant. They found this new principle effective even in cases of anal incontinence resulting from absence or interruption of the nerve supply to the perineal muscles (spina bifida, etc.); however, according to the author's experience, it is not successful in cases of dense scarring around anus and rectum.

Technique (Pickrell, et al.) (Figs. 320–322)

After consultation with the urologist and neurologist and preoperative studies and preparation (see p. 694), the lower extremity that has the stronger gracilis muscle is chosen. With the legs widely abducted the muscle is palpated as the most superficial muscle along the median aspect of the thigh. Three incisions are made at the thigh as outlined in Figure 320. From the middle incision while the thigh is held adducted and the knee slightly flexed, the gracilis tendon is identified just posterior to the sartorius tendon. It is freed distally by blunt dissection as it passes behind the median condylus femoris and curves around the median condylus tibiae. By pulling the muscle the insertion of its tendon can be visualized through the lowermost incision. The entire fishtail-like part is preserved and severed from its insertion at the tibia and withdrawn through the middle incision. From the uppermost incision the muscle is freed bluntly and withdrawn. Care must be taken to avoid injury to the neurovascular bundle that enters the muscle at its highest part from the deep lateral aspect (Fig. 320 insert). The patient is now placed in lithotomy position

697

and the perineal incisions are made as shown in Figure 321. At 12 and 6 o'clock the incisions are deepened on each side of the raphae without injuring or perforating the latter. The incisions are now connected with each other with a subcutaneous tunnel. A tunnel is also made to connect the incision at 12 o'clock with the highest incision at the thigh. The tunnels should be wide enough to allow free insertion of two fingers.

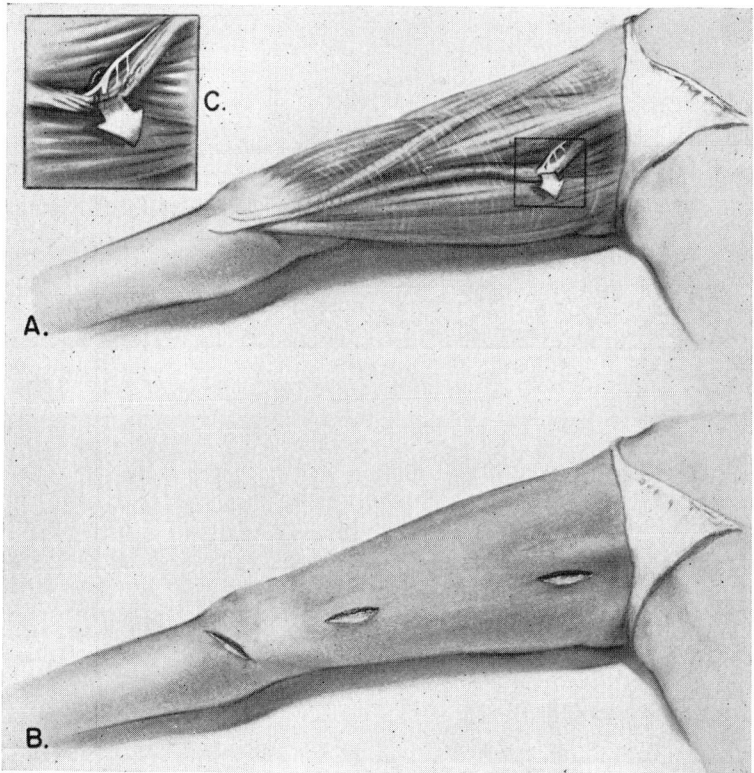

Fig. 320. Anal sphincter plasty with gracilis tendon transfer (K. Pickrell). *A:* The gracilis is the most superficial muscle along the inner aspect of the thigh, being located at its origin just medial to the tendon of the adductor longus. It arises from the lower half of the symphysis and pubic arch and extends below the knee to insert into the tibia in dovetail fashion. *B:* The highest incision in the thigh is made just medial to the tendon of adductor longus in he adductor-gracilis groove or trough. The proximal part of the tendon is mobilized with finger dissection to avoid injury to the neurovascular bundle which enters from the lateral side. A second incision is made parallel to the muscle over its lower third. Traction placed on the muscle through the highest incision will disclose the path of the muscle. A third incision is made in an oblique direction along the upper and medial aspect of the tibia to preserve the dovetail insertion of the gracilis into the periosteum of the tibia. All incisions are connected by subcutaneous tunnels through which the muscle is mobilized. *C:* The innervation (L2, 3, 4) and blood supply (profunda femoris) enter the gracilis high on its lateral side as a neurovascular bundle. Care should be exercised to avoid injury to it. (K. Pickrell, et al., Surgery.)

698

The gracilis muscle is then threaded through the thigh to the perineal tunnel and beneath the anterior raphae (Fig. 321, *C*). As the muscle is placed under tension the neurovascular bundle will be seen to enter from the deep lateral aspect of the origin of the gracilis (Fig. 321, *A*). If it is not seen the muscle has not been mobilized high enough. The tendon and muscle are threaded around the anus in a clockwise direction to make a complete circle. The tendon is passed beneath the anterior raphae

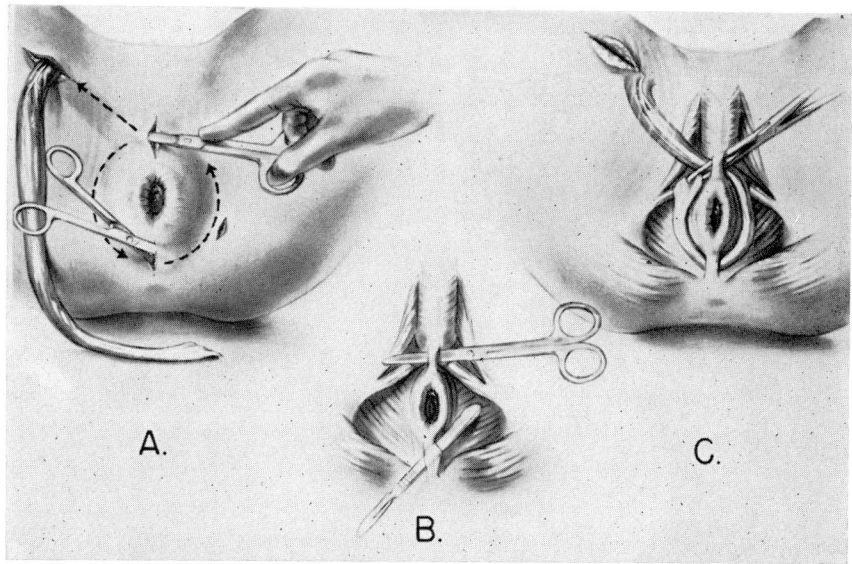

Fig. 321. *A:* With absence of muscle tone and structural support, the perineal floor will bulge when the patient is placed in exaggerated lithotomy position. Incisions are made in the anterior (12 o'clock) and posterior (6 o'clock) commissures, care being taken to avoid injury to the raphae. A subcutaneous tunnel is made around the anus. A tunnel is also made to connect the highest incision in the thigh with the incision at 12 o'clock. *B:* When possible, pulleys are constructed from the anterior and posterior raphae. They are not essential, however. *C:* The gracilis tendon and muscle are threaded through the tunnels and beneath the pulleys, if they have been constructed. (K. Pickrell, et al., Surgery.)

at 6 o'clock. If possible the tendon is threaded beneath the anterior pulley a second time. When the muscle is large and bulky there is not sufficient space beneath the raphae at 12 o'clock to admit the tendon a second time; then the tendon is passed externally to the raphae. The meticulous closing of the subcutaneous tissue and skin is of utmost importance.

An incision is made over the tuberosity of the left ischium, in other words, opposite to the donor leg (the right leg being the donor leg in this case). An opening is made at 3 o'clock to expose the tuberosity as well as the lateral aspect of the levator ani (Fig. 321, *A*). A periosteal

699

flap or pulley is elevated from the tuberosity of the ischium (Fig. 322, *A*). A pulley is also made from the levator ani. The dovetail tendonoperiosteal insertion of the gracilis is then split for one centimeter or more. Half of the dovetail is anchored with sutures of silk either beneath or into the periosteal flap over the prominence of the ischium, while the remaining half is anchored securely to a pulley of levator ani (Fig. 322, *A*).

In patients who are heavy or obese, it is somewhat easier to anchor the tendon end to the medial end of the inguinal ligament, the lacunar liga-

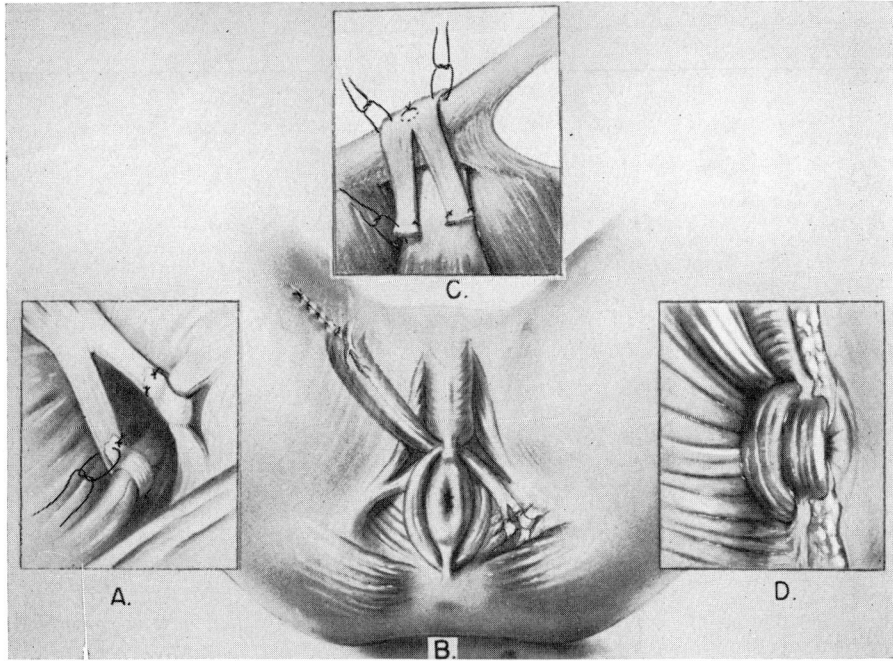

Fig. 322. *A* and *B:* The dovetail tendinoperiosteal insertion of the gracilis is split to form a Y. If the gracilis is to be anchored into the tuberosity of the ischium on the opposite side, an incision is made directly over the tuberosity at approximately 3 to 4 o'clock. One end is anchored around a pulley or a periosteal flap elevated from the tuberosity of the ischium. The remaining limb of the dovetail is anchored around a pulley or bundle of levator ani muscle, using sutures of silk. *C:* In heavy or obese patients, it is easier and better to anchor the gracilis to the adductor tendon or to the lacunar ligament. An incision is made in the groin on the side opposite the transplant. A subcutaneous tunnel is formed to connect it with the incision at 12 o'clock. The tendon is threaded through the tunnel and beneath the lacunar ligament or tendon of the adductor on the opposite side. The gracilis tendon is then anchored to itself and to the ligament on each side, using sutures of silk. *D:* The anal orifice is constricted and closed by a collar of contractile muscle. Sufficient tension should be placed on the gracilis to insure that the orifice is very tight—like a cervix. Remember that the orifice must be air- and watertight and must be able to withstand considerable pressure upon it. (K. Pickrell, et al., Surgery.)

ment or the fixed heavy portion of the adductor longus tendon of origin, on the side opposite the muscle transplant (Fig. 322, C). The tendon is anchored in the following manner. An incision approximately two inches in length is made just below the fold of the groin, over the medial end of the inguinal (Poupart) or lacunar (Gimbernat) ligament. The incision is deepened to expose the ligament just lateral to the pubic tubercle, as the spermatic cord in the male is retracted superiorly. By retracting the inferior skin edge downward, the adductor longus tendon is exposed. A subcutaneous tunnel is then formed by finger or blunt scissors or clamp dissection to connect this incision in the groin with the incision at 12 o'clock in the perineum. A pulley or tunnel is made beneath the lacunar ligament or the adductor tendon. The tendon end of the gracilis is then pulled through the subcutaneous tunnel into the groin, then beneath and over the pulley of the lacunar ligament or the tendon of the adductor longus. The tendon end of the gracilis is anchored securely both to itself and to the lacunar ligament on each side (Fig. 322, C), using sutures of silk. The incision in the groin is then closed in layers using interrupted sutures of silk.

The final insertion of the muscle is not decided upon or fixed until the legs have been brought down into line with the body, then adducted and abducted to make absolutely sure that the anus is tight and very snug. When attempting to insert the finger, over which a second glove has been placed, a cervix-like channel should be encountered. All operative incisions are closed without drains in layers with sutures of silk. The perineal incisions are sealed with collodion. No perineal dressing is required. A snug compression dressing is applied to the thigh.

After-Treatment

The urological consultant will advise regarding the removal or insertion of a catheter. Antibiotics are administered. Patient is given only liquids for the first several days, then is placed on a low-residual diet. On the seventh day well-balanced meals are begun and are supplemented with mineral oil at bedtime. Within several days the patient will become conscious of a feeling of abdominal fullness. He is then placed on a commode and with the thighs adducted and the trunk flexed he is taught to relax the perineum and apply manual kneading pressure to the lower abdomen. If cramps are felt it is possible that the gracilis cuff is too tight; gentle dilation will cause it to relax. Subsequently, daily training periods should be scheduled each morning; an oil retention enema may be necessary if a fecal mass develops in the rectum.

PARTIAL DEFECT OF SPHINCTER MUSCLE

Partial defects of the sphincter can be successfully bridged by Blais-dell's procedure, which consists of a gradual transplantation of sphincter-bearing flaps. The method has been found simple, versatile, and effective.

Technique (Figs. 323-324)

For preoperative preparation of the patient, see page 694.

Stage 1: (Fig. 323, *A-B*): A "goblet" incision is made on each side of the defect, with the cavity of the goblet surrounding the respective edge of the preserved part of the sphincter. The incision is made deep enough to include functioning muscle. After separation of the wound edges, a tongue-shaped flap, *A* (Fig. 323, *A*), of muscle-bearing tissue is formed, mobilized, and moved downward to point *A'*. It is held in this position with a buried suture of stainless-steel wire. The skin wound is closed

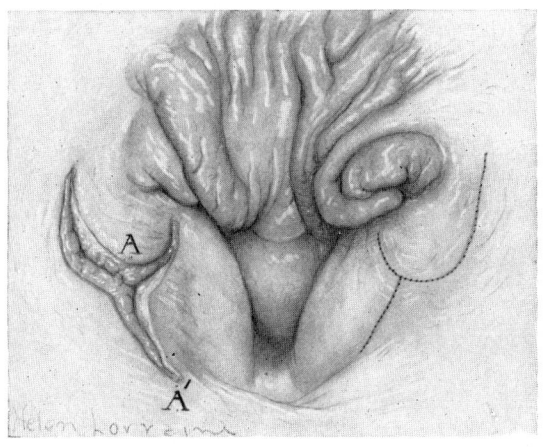

Fig. 323*A*. Anal-sphincter plastic procedure (Blaisdell). Stage 1: "Goblet" incision is made on each side of defect. Cavity of goblet surrounds respective edge of pre-served part of sphincter, thus forming tongue-shaped flap, *A*, of muscle-bearing tissue. *A* is to be transplanted to *A'*. (P. C. Blaisdell: Surg. Gynec. Obstet.)

with silk sutures. The same procedure is performed on the other side. To counteract tension, a purse-string suture is inserted around the anus, as depicted in Figure 323, *B*, and is pulled and tied tightly.

Stage 2 (Fig. 324): After a few weeks, a curved incision is made over the remaining gap. Again the incision is carried the greatest depth of the sphincter muscle. After separation of the wound edges, the extreme ends

702

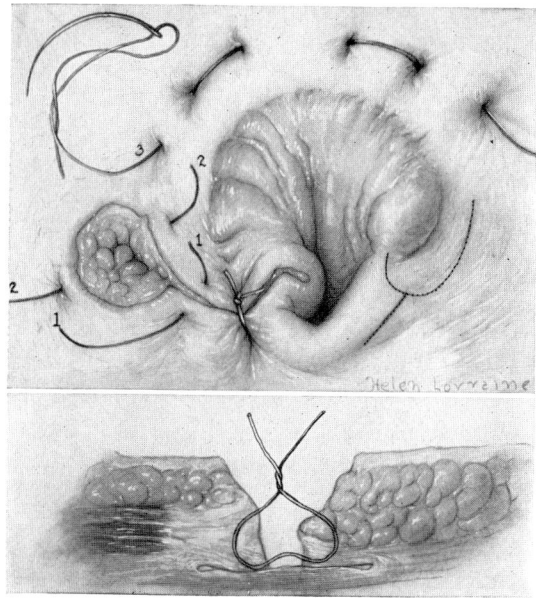

Fig. 323B. Deep-buried wire sutures of fine stainless steel hold *A* approximated to *A'* (*lower*) (see also Fig. 323A). Wound is closed with silk sutures. Purse-string suture is inserted around anus to counteract tension.

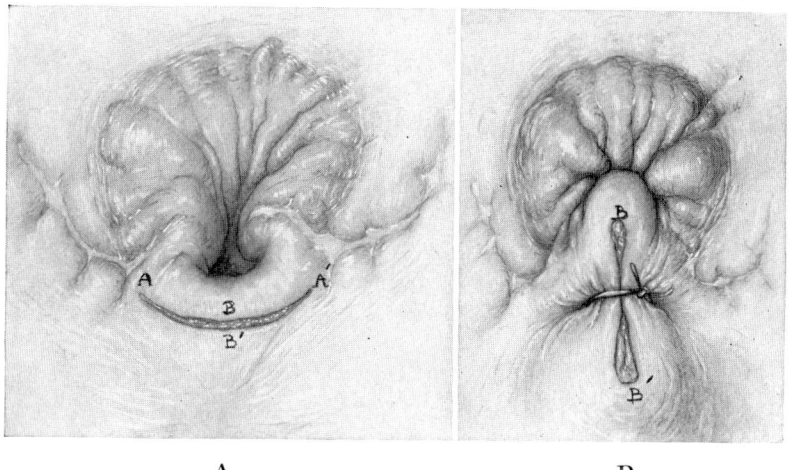

A

B

Fig. 324. *A:* Anal-sphincter plastic procedure (Blaisdell). Stage 2: A curved incision is made over remaining gap. It is carried to the greatest depth of sphincter muscle. *B: A* has been approximated to *A'* with deep-buried wire suture. Wound is closed with silk sutures. (P. C. Blaisdell: Surg. Gynec. Obstet.)

of the incision, with the free edges of the functioning sphincter beneath, are united with buried wire sutures, thus changing the transverse direction of the wound into a longitudinal one. The skin edges are united with silk sutures. A purse-string suture is inserted around the anus.

Variation

For larger defects, more than two stages are recommended; in small defects, only one stage—the second stage, as just described—may be needed.

BIBLIOGRAPHY

BACON, H. E.: *Cancer of the Colon, Rectum and Anal Canal.* J. B. Lippincott, Philadelphia, 1964.

BLAISDELL, P. C.: *Repair of the incontinent sphincter ani.* Surg. Gynec. Obstet., 75:634, 1942.

COURTNEY, H.: *Anatomy of the pelvic diaphragm and anorectal musculature as related to sphincter preservation in anorectal surgery.* Amer. J. Surg., 79:155, 1950.

GASTON, E. A.: *The physiology of fecal continence.* Surg. Gynec. Obstet., 87:669, 1948.

KIESEWETTER, W. B., and TURNER, C. R.: *Continence after surgery for imperforate anus: A critical analysis and preliminary experience with the sacro-perineal pull-through.* Ann. Surg., 158:498, 1963.

PICKRELL, K. L., ET AL.: *Construction of a rectal sphincter and restoration of anal continence by transplanting the gracilis muscle; A report of four cases in children.* Ann. Surg., 135:853, 1952.
Rectal sphincter reconstruction using gracilis muscle transplant. Plast. Reconstr. Surg., 13:46, 1954.
Gracilis muscle transplant for rectal incontinence. Surgery, 40:349, 1956.

SMITH, E. I., and GROSS, R. E.: *The external sphincter in cases of imperforate anus: A pathologic study.* Surgery, 49:807, 1961.

STONE, H. B.: *Plastic operation for anal incontinence.* Arch. Surg., 18:845, 1929; Arch. Surg., 24:120, 1932.

STONE, H. B., and McLANAHAN, S.: *Results with the fascia plastic operation for anal incontinence.* Ann. Surg., 114:73, 1941.

WREDEN, R. R.: *Method of reconstructing voluntary sphincter ani.* Arch. Surg., 18:841, 1929.

DIVISION FOUR
THE EXTREMITIES

INTRODUCTORY
ASPECTS
OF THE   20
EXTREMITIES

THE principles of reparative and reconstructive surgery as applied to the extremities are applicable to all parts of the extremities. From the functional standpoint, however, the hand must be considered as a distinct unit, necessitating a certain variation and specification in some of the reconstructive principles. Hence, reparative and reconstructive surgery of the extremities are discussed under the following section headings: (1) the Extremities Other than Hand, and (2) the Hand. The problems discussed are those in which the general surgeon, as well as the general plastic surgeon, is interested. Those matters belonging strictly to other specialized fields, such as orthopedics, have been omitted.

To furnish a proper division of this rather broad field, the material is divided into anatomical units; certain reparative problems applicable to those units have been selected, and are discussed under the following headings: Skin, Subcutaneous Tissue, and the Fasciae; the Muscles and Tendons; the Nerves; the Blood Vessels; the Bones; the Articulations.

ANESTHESIA IN SURGERY OF EXTREMITIES

The agents and methods for operation on the upper extremities are *ether*, either alone or in combination with the gases, and the *gases*, such as nitrous oxide and halothane, either alone or in combination with solution of sodium pentothal. Local anesthesia is obtained less often with *pro-*

caine, more frequently with newer agents, such as Xylocaine and Carbocaine, either by infiltration or by nerve block or by a combination of both. The various nerve blocks which are possible are the brachial plexus block, a block distal to the elbow or distal to the wrist, a block distal to the metacarpophalangeal joints of the fingers.

For anesthesia of the lower extremities, the agents and methods used are the same as the aforementioned. However, field blocks and nerve blocks are rarely used, since spinal anesthesia dispenses with them. For long operations continuous, spinal anesthesia is infrequently used; continuous epidural anesthesia is preferred instead since Xylocaine, Carbocaine, etc., have been introduced.

For details concerning the various anesthetic agents and methods, the reader should refer to standard textbooks on the subject.

BIBLIOGRAPHY

CLEMENT, F. W.: *Nitrous-Oxide-Oxygen Anesthesia.* Lea & Febiger, Philadelphia, 1951.

DAGLIOTTI, A. M.: *Anesthesia: Narcosis, Local, Regional, Spinal.* S. B. Debour, Chicago, 1937.

DRIPPS, R. D., ECKENHOFF, J. E., and VANDAM, L. D.: *Introduction to Anesthesia: The Principles of Safe Practice.* W. B. Saunders, Philadelphia, 1957.

GILLESPIE, N. A.: *Endotracheal Anesthesia.* The University of Wisconsin Press, Madison, 1948.

GUEDEL, A. E.: *Inhalation Anesthesia, a Fundamental Guide.* The Macmillan Company, New York, 1937.
Inhalation Anesthesia, 2nd Ed. The Macmillan Company, New York, 1951.

HALE, D. E., *Editor and Forty American Authors: Anesthesiology.* F. A. Davis, Philadelphia, 1954.

LABAT, G.: *Regional Anesthesia, Its Technic and Clinical Application.* W. B. Saunders, Philadelphia, 1928.

LEIGH, M., DIGBY, M., and BELTON, M. E.: *Pediatric Anesthesia.* The Macmillan Company, New York, 1949.

LUNDY, J. S.: *Clinical Anesthesia: a Manual of Clinical Anesthesia.* W. B. Saunders, Philadelphia, 1943.

MINNITT, R. J., and GILLIES, J.: *Textbook of Anesthetics.* Williams and Wilkins, Baltimore, 1948.

MOORE, D. C.: *Regional Block: A Handbook for Use in the Clinical Practice of Medicine and Surgery.* Charles C Thomas, Springfield, 1953.

PITKIN, G. P.: *Conduction Anesthesia.* J. B. Lippincott, Philadelphia, 1950.

WYLIE, W. D., and CHURCHILL-DAVIDSON, H. C.: *A Practice of Anesthesia.* Year Book Medical Publishers Inc., 1966.

Section One
The Extremities
Other Than
The Hand

SKIN, SUBCUTANEOUS TISSUE, AND THE FASCIAE

21

DEFECTS

ACCIDENTAL DEFECTS

IN THE majority of cases, acute defects of skin and subcutaneous tissue are due to trauma. The treatment of wounds and burns has been discussed (pp. 121-149) (see also Cases 107, 108, pp. 1132-1135). Open for discussion then are those wounds which have resulted in actual loss of tissue. The type of closure depends entirely upon the width and depth of the defect.

Superficial Defects

Superficial losses involving only the skin are best closed by skin grafting. The type of graft ordinarily used is a *thick split graft*. The full-thickness graft is applicable only under strictly aseptic conditions—after removal of tumors, for instance. Full-thickness grafts are contra-indicated in all traumatic wounds, since the latter are potentially infected (see p. 26). In traumatic loss of skin, the raw area, unless grossly infected, is properly cleansed and débrided, and then covered immediately with a split skin graft, regardless of the lapse of time. Antimicrobic therapy is instituted postoperatively. Such a skin graft has a good chance to take.

If the graft takes, the healing process of the wound is shortened and the cosmetic and functional results are much better than they would be

711

if the wound were left to granulate. It is unfortunate that the popular conception that one should wait for granulations to develop still prevails. The results are comparable to those of wound healing by primary intention. If the graft does not take, no further damage occurs except that the superficial raw area of the donor site is added. The principle of immediate skin grafting in acute surface defects is applicable not only to losses involving the skin alone but also to deeper defects of the subcutaneous tissue which cannot be closed by skin sliding and which do not require a flap. The grafts may then be considered as biological dressings promoting quick and better healing.

Deep Defects

These defects, exposing important structures such as tendons and bones, require *flaps* for their closure. If a flap cannot be applied immediately the defect may be closed temporarily with a skin graft, which provides protection against infection and necrosis. In some instances, the flap can be taken from the immediate neighborhood. A typical example is the closure of a longitudinal defect of the covering tissue in front of the tibia after compound fracture or osteomyelitis. Such a defect is closed with two longitudinal bridge flaps, which are mobilized from the immediate neighborhood and, after being shifted into the defect, are held together with sutures. The secondary defects lateral to the flaps are covered with skin grafts (Case 121, p. 1156). In the majority of cases, however, flaps must be transplanted from distant parts. Wherever a direct transfer is possible— as, for instance, an abdominal flap to the arm (Case 120, p. 1154) or a flap from the thigh or leg of one side to the leg of the other side (Cases 122-124, pp. 1158-1162)—the open-pedicle flap method is used (p. 82). (For details see p. 720 and p. 808.) If the flap is to be transferred by an intermediate carrier, such as the wrist (Cases 116, 119, pp. 1146, 1150), the tube-flap method is chosen (p. 95). However, Cannon et al. and Edwards have demonstrated that even in those cases the open-jump flap method, using the forearm as a carrier, may be applicable. In selected cases of surface defects of the leg, in which sliding flaps are not applicable and distant flaps seem to be the only choice, Deming was able to close them with tube flaps from the calf of the same side.

CHRONIC LEG ULCERS

Chronic ulcers—in most cases involving the lower extremity—are of various origins: disturbance of circulation (varicose veins, arteriosclerosis), metabolic disorders (diabetes), trauma (pressure, compound fractures), infection (osteomyelitis, tuberculosis, syphilis, conditions caused by anaerobic organisms), and neuropathic disorders (Raynaud's disease, malum perforans).

Concerning treatment, two general principles are outlined: (1) The local treatment should be preceded by or at least accompanied by a treatment of the underlying cause. No permanent local cure can be expected unless the causative factors are eliminated. (2) An ulcer, after elimination of the underlying cause, should be resurfaced with transplanted skin, unless it shows a tendency to spontaneous healing. The type of transplant depends upon the depth of the ulcer. Ulcers in soft tissues can be closed successfully with free skin grafts. Ulcers in which tendons or bare bone (without periosteum) are exposed require the transfer of a pedunculated flap.

CHRONIC ULCERS FROM DISTURBANCE OF CIRCULATION

The most common ulcer resulting from disturbance of circulation is the so-called varicose ulcer. As the name implies it is due to circulatory disturbances from varicose veins. Too often, however, the varicosities are taken as the obvious cause while other underlying factors are overlooked, as has been extensively discussed by Linton, Rutter, and others as well as by Barrow and by Sigg in their short but comprehensive monographs. It is generally conceded that the vast majority of these ulcers are due to faulty venous circulation and less often by obliterative arterial diseases. The veins of the lower extremity consist of three systems: the superficial, the deep, and the communicating veins. The superficial system consists of the saphena magna on the median side and the saphena parva on the lateral side. The deep venous system consists of the vena femoralis communis, superficialis, and venae popliteae in the thigh; of the venae tibiali, anterior and posteria, and venae peronealis in the leg. The communicating veins connecting the superficial and the deep venous system are few in the thigh and numerous in the leg. It has been the common belief that the skin and subcutaneous tissues of the leg are normally drained of blood chiefly by the veins of the superficial system. Stasis in this system, resulting from incompetence of the valves, causes atrophy of the skin over the anterior surface of the tibia and in the malleolar region. The atrophic skin, if damaged by trauma or infection, breaks down and—owing to impairment of regenerative ability of the surrounding skin—the defect does not become resurfaced. This is the origin of a varicose ulcer. Its chronicity or recurrence, however, is caused by other factors. Local infection is one of them. The disturbed circulation and the local necrosis provide excellent soil for the growth of organisms. The ulcer becomes enlarged and deeper, and cicatricial changes take place and may become so extensive as to involve the entire surrounding skin (Case 118, p. 1149). The skin becomes brownish, hard, and fixed to the underlying tissue. These changes lead to an aggravation of the circulatory disturbance, to edema, and finally to elephantiasic chronic edema.

This classic form of varicose ulcer is most often seen in elderly people and, as already pointed out, has been blamed on incompetence in the saphenous or superficial system. Recently, it has become clear that not all of these ulcers can be blamed on varicosities of the superficial veins, particularly in younger people; attention has been turned to the deep venous circulation. Bauer, Linton, and others developed the thesis that thrombosis and obliteration of the main deep venous channels of the leg are followed by canalization of these veins, with resultant incompetence of the valves in the deep communicating and superficial veins, and thus become the cause of the leg ulcer.

Treatment

It is essential to submit each patient with a leg ulcer to a careful history and clinical examination, including various tests to provide corrolatory evidence of superficial or deep venous incompetence. It is beyond the scope of this book to go into these details. The fundamental principle in treating a leg ulcer based on venous incompetence is elimination of venous stasis and edema. The patient may either be ambulatory or require hospitalization. The local applications recommended for treatment of the ulcer are numerous. The nature of the local application is immaterial. If the ulcer is grossly infected the patient should be hospitalized—strict rest in bed with the leg elevated is essential. The ulcer is dressed with gauze soaked in Dakin's solution and alternated with normal saline solution; the dressing should be kept moist constantly (see also pp. 28-30). In addition, the infecting organisms should be identified, their sensitivity to the various antibiotics estimated, and proper antibiotic treatment initiated. After the infection has subsided the ulcer is covered with xeroform gauze (p. 36), and a supportive leg dressing such as an elastic bandage, rubber stocking, or Unna's paste boot is applied. If the ulcer is not infected the patient can be ambulatory with pressure dressings such as the "closed" Elastoplast technique, which has become popular in Great Britain, Unna's paste boot, and Linton's dressing, which aims to obliterate the superficial veins of the lower leg by means of a large spongy dressing held in place with a very firm dressing.

These measures alone, however, cannot be permanently successful unless the underlying cause of the ulcer, namely, the venous incompetence,

714

is corrected by an operation. If possible, the operation should be delayed until the ulcer is healed. If the superficial venous system is at fault, the long saphenous vein and its uppermost branches are ligated at the sapheno-femoral junction, the remaining larger veins are "stripped" and excised, and an incompetent perforation is ligated. Single incompetent veins communicating between deep and superficial venous systems below the knee are usually associated with varicose ulcers (the so-called "feeder" vein); these should be taken care of at the time of the ulcer repair. Multiple incompetent communicating veins are usually the sequelae of deep thrombophlebitis and should be treated as outlined later.

If the deep venous system is at fault, in other words, thrombosis and obliteration of the deep veins are present, it has been thought dangerous to ligate the superficial system. The large experience of Rutter, Linton, Barrow, and others contradicts this opinion. Linton not only ligates and strips the superficial veins of the lower leg but also ligates the communicating veins between the posterior tibial and the superficial veins, interrupts the vena femoralis superficialis at its junction with the profunda, and ligates and strips the long saphenous veins. Rutter, however, advocates only ligation of the superficial system, in most cases, while ligation of the deep system (popliteal vein) is carried out only when the following four requirements are fulfilled: *a.* chronic or recurring ulceration not responding to other less radical treatment, including the obliteration of all superficial varicose veins; *b.* severe and crippling pain, especially if it is of the "bursting" type; *c.* absence of severe edema; *d.* positive venographic evidence of dilatation and irregularity of outline of the popliteal vein.

Under such treatment the ulcer, which as a rule is situated in the malleolar region or over the anterior surface of the tibia, may remain healed. However, the resulting scar, which is often surrounded by atrophic skin, may be unstable and break down after trauma or infection and—owing to impairment of regenerative ability of the surrounding skin—the defect does not become resurfaced. The ulcer then becomes chronic; cicatricial changes take place beneath and around the ulcer, and may become so extensive as to involve the entire surrounding skin. The skin becomes brownish, hard, and fixed to the underlying tissues. These changes lead to an aggravation of the circulatory disturbance, to edema, and finally to the elephantiasic chronic edema.

Preparation of Local Area: As mentioned in the foregoing, elimination of the venous stasis and edema must be the preliminary treatment. The patient is kept in bed, with the leg elevated. As a rule, in chronic cases, the veins have been ligated and injected previously. If not, this should be performed unless contraindications, such as cellulitis and phlebitis, exist. The next step is the control of any infection, as outlined above.

Then follows the preparation of the granulations for skin grafting. A daily bath of the leg in warm saline solution, with washing of the area surrounding the ulcer with pHisoderm G-11, followed by pressure dressings and elevation of the extremity, is of the utmost importance. The granulations themselves are treated as has already been described on pages 28-30.

The question now arises as to whether or not the ulcer should be excised prior to the application of the graft. The following rules have proved valuable: If the granulations are flat and pinkish red and the skin surrounding the ulcer is atrophic but movable and not indurated, the graft is applied directly on the granulations. The most suitable type of graft to cover such an ulcer is the small deep graft (p. 44). If the granulations are of the sluggish or hypertrophic type, they should be sliced down to a yellow vascularized layer, which constitutes the base of the granulations prior to the application of the grafts. If the surrounding skin is indurated by cicatricial changes, the entire involved area—no matter how large—must be excised, together with the base of the ulcer, down to the deep fascia, care being taken not to expose tendons or bone. The raw area is covered with a large split graft (Case 118, p. 1149). Removal of the damaged surrounding skin eliminates the tendency to recurrence and leads to improvement of the local circulation by relieving constriction. The grafted area is covered with a pressure dressing, and the leg is elevated.

After-Treatment

The dressing is changed after seven days. The leg should remain elevated, with a pressure dressing applied for at least two weeks. If parts of the graft do not take, wet dressings (Dakin's and isotonic saline solution alternately) are applied, and the extremity is kept elevated until the entire area has healed. When the patient is up and around, he is advised to wear a supportive dressing until the graft has assumed normal color.

If the graft does not take or takes only partially the healing process will result eventually in a shiny, adherent, atrophic scar which is apt to break down upon the slightest trauma. In such cases, Webster, Peterson and Stein have developed the so-called overgrafting technique. The scarred area is dermabraded until an actively bleeding surface is encountered, upon which a skin graft 0.015 inch thick is laid and held with a pressure dressing.

Chronic Undermining, Burrowing Ulcers from Infection

In 1935, Meleney described a type of ulcer which he called the "chronic undermining, burrowing ulcer." He found its cause to be the

716

microaerophilic hemolytic streptococcus, which may enter the tissues either through an accidental wound or an operative wound or through a lymph gland from a distant source. He reported successful treatment of the lesion with zinc peroxide. His findings and success with the zinc peroxide treatment have been confirmed—often dramatically.

This ulcer can occur on any part of the body surface. The lesion is characterized by prolonged suppuration, with the gradual development of an ulcer with undermined rolled-in skin margins and sinuses which tend to burrow beneath the skin or into the deeper tissues, along lymphatic channels, veins, or fascial planes. The base of the ulcer is covered with grayish, gelatinous, anemic, and shaggy granulations. Gangrenous processes are entirely absent. The author has also found the anaerobic hemolytic streptococcus in chronic ulcers without undermined rolled-in skin margins and for which no other cause could be established (Case 117, p. 1148). They have invariably responded to the zinc peroxide treatment.

By careful anaerobic as well as aerobic studies Meleney found the microaerophilic hemolytic streptococcus to be invariably present. Laboratory studies showed them existing between the aerobic hemolytic streptococci and the strictly anaerobic hemolytic streptococci. The diagnosis depends upon thorough aerobic and anaerobic cultivation.

Treatment

The antibiotics, in spite of acting dramatically in the early stages of an acute infection caused by the hemolytic streptococcus, are of little value in the chronic stage, when the hemolytic streptococcus becomes adapted to an anaerobic environment. It is in this stage of the disease where application of *zinc peroxide* has proved to be of enormous value, since it provides a high oxygen tension in the tissues for a considerable period of time.

The secret of the success of zinc peroxide, however, depends upon three fundamental requirements, as Meleney emphasizes. The first is the material itself. The du Pont Company, which manufactured the zinc peroxide originally used and found to be effective, has been the only chemical company consistently able to manufacture effective material. The importance of certain physical properties of this material are fundamental because, while the chemical content of zinc peroxide in the powder may be high, the oxygen may not be mobilized or made available. Preliminary heating in a dry oven at 140° C. for four hours not only sterilizes the powder but mobilizes the oxygen. When added to sterile distilled water after the sterilization and activation process, effective material always flocculates quickly as a soft, curdy mass, leaving a clear supernatant fluid, and it is soon lifted up by the formation of oxygen bubbles. This test should always be made before using any preparation.

717

THE EXTREMITIES

The second most important feature of the treatment is to obtain close contact between the zinc peroxide and the infection. With many of these ulcers, there are deep, undermined skin flaps and deep sinuses which prevent close contact of the medication unless the advancing margins of the infections are excised.

The third essential feature of the treatment is the prevention of evaporation. The oxygen is conveyed from the zinc peroxide to the tissue by means of water. When zinc peroxide is suspended in water, oxygen is given off into the water, hydrogen peroxide is formed, and the oxygen is then transferred to the surroundings. This leaves H_2O, which then takes up more oxygen from the zinc peroxide. If the zinc peroxide dressing is allowed to dry, this action stops or is greatly diminished, and the dry material may mechanically irritate the wound whenever the patient shifts his position. The tissue fluids and the body exudates may act as catalytic agents, but the activity of the zinc peroxide suspension is at its best only when extraneous moisture is present. For that reason, not only must the zinc peroxide be applied to every part of the wound surface but the wound surface must be covered with a double layer of fine-meshed gauze soaked in the suspension. This helps to maintain contact, but must, in turn, be covered by gauze compresses or sheet cotton wet with water. The whole dressing is sealed with petrolatum gauze or, better still, gauze impregnated with zinc oxide ointment, which is more impermeable to the air and does not irritate the surrounding skin. The impermeable covering should have a wide margin around the wet compresses, so that any slight movement of the part will not displace them. In leg or forearm ulcerations, it is possible at times to use rubber sheeting to seal the dressing, but this is not practical on other parts of the body.

This dressing is changed daily. Antibiotic treatment is imperative. In those ulcers with overhanging skin edges and undermined areas and sinuses, proper excision should be carried out to provide adequate contact of the material with the tissues. As soon as the area is clean and covered with pinkish, flat granulations and, thus, the ulcer changed into a clean granulating wound, a thick split skin graft should be applied to the raw area. The graft is applied directly upon the granulations and as a rule takes extremely well.

Chronic Ulcers of Foot

The preferred seat of deep chronic ulcers of the foot is over the heel and the metatarsal pads. They are due to excessive pressure (decubital sores, pressure from plaster cast), vascular disturbances (arteriosclerosis, diabetes), infection (osteomyelitis), or to unsuccessfully treated plantar

718

wart. The cause of the latter is still obscure. It originates as a papilloma beneath the derma. If growing, it gradually perforates the horny plate of the skin and appears at the outside. Various treatments are recommended such as cauterization, electrocoagulation, freezing, application of caustics, excision, and irradiation; the latter appears to be the most successful. The use of vitamin A has also been recommended, and seems to be worth trying, particularly in cases of multiple warts (see Bibliography under May). Occasionally, the defect from destruction of the growth fails to heal, forming a deep, stubborn ulcer, through which even bones and joints may be exposed. In these cases, as well as in other deep ulcers along the foot, transfer of a pedicle flap to cover the defect is the only possibility. A thick split graft may rarely be considered, and then only for shallow lesions with sufficient subcutaneous padding still present. Avellan and Johanson take a full-thickness skin graft from the dorsum of the foot if possible. Any underlying general disease should, of course, be treated first.

Smaller defects may be covered by rotation flaps from the neighborhood. Farmer uses the entire distal half of the sole for rotation (Case 125, p. 1163). Sometimes in defects at the level of the first or fifth metatarsophalangeal joint, a flap may be slid from the dorsum of the foot followed by simple suturing of the secondary defect or by skin grafting of the donor area, or the bones of the adjacent toe are sacrificed and the skin of the toe, with or without local flaps, is used for closure of the defect (Greely, Pangman, and Gurdin).

Maisels treated lesions at the back of the heel by a rotation flap based from below the calf on the medial calcaneal vessels. The operation is done in two stages. At the first operation the flap is outlined and completely raised until the medial calcaneal vessels and nerves are seen; at the second stage the flap is rotated downward leaving a narrow defect superiorly which is covered with a split skin graft.

For larger defects, flaps must be transferred from distant places. In most instances, the direct transfer of a flap from the lower extremity of the opposite side is possible with the patient in the crossed-leg position. This method, however, should be used only if awkward positioning can be avoided, that is, the joints must be freely movable to permit easy and natural crossing of the legs. The calf of the sound side may be used as a donor site in males; in females this region is unsuitable, owing to the deep and disfiguring scar, and the thigh becomes the only possible donor site (Cases 122, 123, 124, 126). The cross-leg flap method has been thoroughly discussed by Stark, Schmid and others. If a direct transfer from the other leg is impossible, an abdominal tube flap or, better still, an open-jump flap (Cannon et al., Edwards and others) must be constructed and transferred.

THE EXTREMITIES

Technique (Cross-Thigh or Cross-Leg Flap)

For details of general technique, see pages 77-87. If the flap must be made long and narrow, it is constructed as an open flap and delayed transfer is usually advisable (p. 83). If it is possible to construct a broad-based pedicle flap, it can be raised and transferred in one stage (Brown and Fryer) (Fig. 325). A broad-based pedicle flap may be constructed (at the median-posterior surface of the leg and anterior surface of the thigh, for ex-

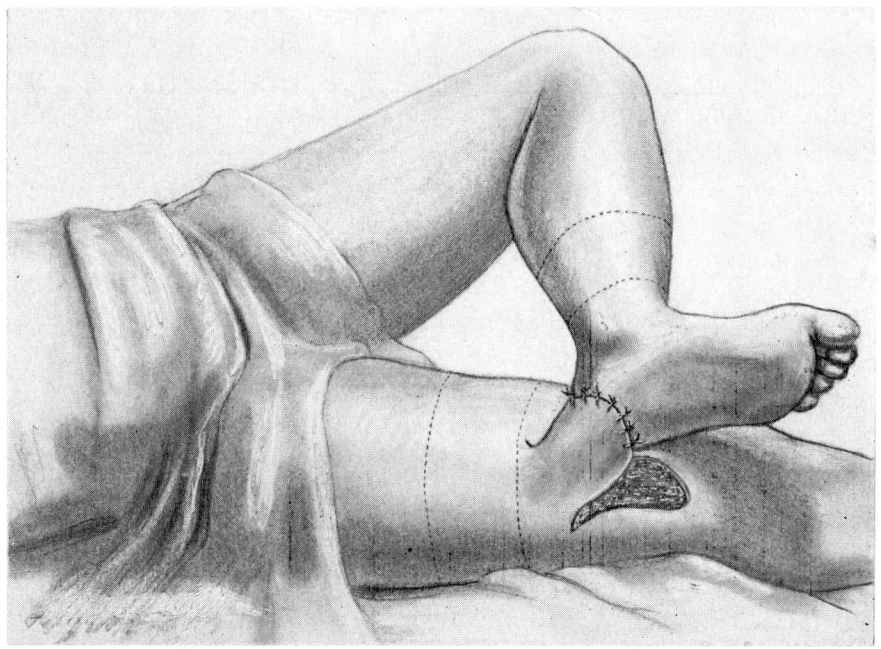

Fig. 325. Transplantation of cross-flap from right thigh to left heel. Flaps with broad pedicles can be raised and transferred in one stage; donor area is skin grafted in same stage. Dotted lines indicate pressure areas to be patted.

ample) more often than was formerly thought possible (Conway and Stark, Connelly) (cross-thigh flap). When the flap is ready to be transferred, the host area is prepared by excision until normal healthy tissue is reached. The flap at the thigh is elevated and the raw area from which the flap has been taken is covered immediately with a thick split graft, which is held in place with sutures and a pressure dressing. The legs are now crossed and the flap sutured to the defect edges with subcutaneous and skin sutures. The whole area is covered with sterile dressings. To immobilize the legs in this position, a plaster cast is applied as follows.

Immobilization of Cross-Thigh Flap: The left heel or sole is to be covered with a flap from the right thigh (Figs. 325, 326; Case 126).

720

A thick layer of felt is wrapped around the anterior surface of the right thigh above the flap bed, i.e., the area which will support the crossed left leg (Fig. 325). Another piece of felt is wrapped around the area of the head of the fibula of the right leg and beneath the heel of the same side. The whole right extremity is wrapped with rolls of Webril 4 inches wide.

A posterior, fairly thick, plaster splint (5 inches wide) is measured, rolled out on a table, dipped into water, and applied from toes to gluteal fold of the right extremity. The popliteal area is reinforced with shorter

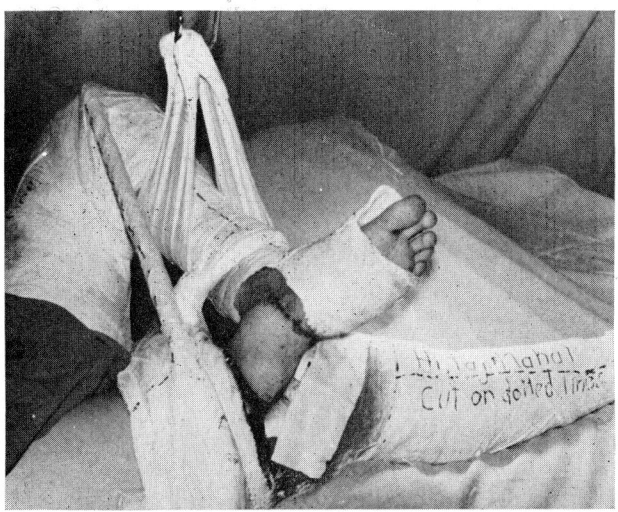

Fig. 326. Immobilization of cross-thigh flap to heel.

splints. All splints are well molded and held in place with two circular plaster-cast bandages (4 inches wide), leaving exposed the donor area at the anterior side of the right thigh. The cast is allowed to dry.

In the meantime the part of the crossed left leg which is to rest upon the cast of the other thigh is determined. In this case it is the area just above the malleolus (Fig. 325). A fairly thick layer of felt is wrapped around this area, another piece of felt is laid upon the flexed knee joint, and a roll of Webril (4 inches wide) is wrapped around the forefoot, leg and thigh, leaving the heel exposed. An anterior plaster-cast splint (5 inches wide) is measured, rolled out on the table, dipped into water and applied from toes to the upper part of the thigh. It is held in place with two circular plaster bandages (4 inches wide), leaving the heel exposed.

The most important part of the cast is now prepared, namely, the supporting link between the casts of the crossed extremities. In this example the two areas to be linked with each other are the supramalleolar area of the crossed left leg and the right thigh above the flap bed. This is best done with a plaster-cast splint of medium thickness 3 inches wide (its length measured previously by a piece of Webril) which is looped around the supramalleolar area of the left leg, and twisted once around itself (or twice or even three times depending upon the distance of the space between the two casts). The ends of the loops are separated and spread and laid upon the cast of the right thigh. One assistant now holds both legs the proper distance from each other. Another assistant lifts the donor leg while a circular plaster bandage is wrapped around the area where the two ends of the loop are lying upon the cast. To support the position of the two legs further a plaster bar is made by molding a plaster bandage in the form of a bar. Each end is left open; one end is laid upon the lateral part of the cast of the right thigh, the other end upon the flexed left knee joint area. Another circular bandage is applied to hold the open ends at the donor extremity and the flexed knee joint in place. After the cast is dry the patient is transferred into his bed, which is equipped with an overhead traction in order to support the crossed leg, as demonstrated in Figure 326. If the ankle (Case 122, p. 1158) or the anterior part of the leg (Case 124, p. 1162) is the recipient area and the thigh of the other leg the donor area, two links between the casts of the crossed extremities must be made.

Immobilization of Cross-Leg Flap: The flap is raised from the antero-median or lateral side of the leg of one side to be transplanted to the foot of the other side. The foregoing principles of applying the plaster cast are the same, but selection of the pressure area for proper padding differs.

After-Treatment

The flap is gradually severed after ten to fourteen days, using the clamp technique described on page 85; after its final separation, the cast is removed (see also p. 80). Adjustment of the free end of the flap, however, should be delayed for another week.

Other donor areas are the lateral side of the leg (for foot ulcer) and the median half of the calf, occasionally the posterior side of the leg (compare with Case 123, p. 1160). The choice depends upon the position in which the patient is comfortable. The pedicle is based proximally or distally. This is governed entirely by the location of the lesion. In females, as already mentioned, the resulting deep scar of the donor area at the leg may be objectionable; hence, the thigh may be preferable. If the cross-leg flap method cannot be used owing to the size of the defect, a tube flap from the chest via the wrist may be possible (see Fig. 46). If none of the skin-transplantation methods is possible and the defect is small and suitably located (anterior half of sole), Dickson's procedure, as he uses it for excision of plantar warts, is recommended. It consists of removal of a V-shaped section of the foot, including a wide excision of the lesion, with corresponding toe and metatarsal bone.

Technique (Dickson)

A wide, elliptical incision is made around the plantar wart, extending between the webs of both sides of the toe to be removed and over the dorsum. The metatarsal is exposed subperiosteally, with reflection of the intrinsic muscles. The extensor and flexor tendons are cut, and the metatarsal bone is removed near its base by bone-cutting forceps. The adjoining metatarsals are sutured together with chromic catgut through the capsule of the metatarsophalangeal joints, thus obliterating the space made by the removal of the bone, and closure of the skin follows.

DEFORMITIES

CICATRICIAL CONTRACTURES

Dermatogenous or desmogenous contractures are caused by the destruction of the surface and deeper parts of the surface tissue, as after extensive burns; less often they are congenital from amniotic furrows (see p. 187). The traumatic contractures usually occur at the flexor surface of the extremities or at the junction of limb and trunk. In the majority of cases, much can be done by early skin grafting to avoid them. There are, however, instances where a skin-graft operation is contraindicated because of the patient's impaired general condition or because large grafts are not available or fail to take. In such cases, proper immobilization of the affected limb may counteract the contracting forces during the waiting period. When the knee or elbow joint is involved, the extremity is immobilized on a molded plaster-cast splint. Plantar flexion of the foot at the ankle joint can be avoided by placing a wooden box at the foot of the bed so that the patient can brace the injured foot against the box, or a molded plaster-cast splint that includes the foot may be applied. Contractures of the axilla are difficult to counteract. The arm should be placed in right-angular abduction, and kept in this position with the aid of pillows. These measures should not, however, cause pain or undue discomfort.

If, in spite of all these measures, a contracture starts to develop, nothing should be done forcibly to overcome it unless the patient is ready for operation. Blair and Brown and their associates, as well as Koch and others, have pointed out that a raw surface in the flexor region of joints often decreases in size not so much by the overgrowth of epithelium from the periphery of the wound as by the drawing in of the adjacent tissues. If the process is permitted to take place without interference, healing goes on rapidly. If, on the contrary, the contracting joint is irritated by repeated forceful dressings, there will be a greater production of fibrous tissue, followed by more extensive shrinkage; if the extremity is forcefully stretched under anesthesia and fixed in this position, wide fissures are opened in the granulating wound, with the possibility of infection, delay of healing, and production of larger and denser scar tissue. What really is needed in such a case is the early covering of the raw surface with a skin graft, regardless of the degree of contracture. After healing has taken place, proper physical therapy should be instituted to lessen the contracture. Further operative procedures, however, may become necessary to overcome a remaining deformity.

To correct a contracture, several procedures or a combination of various procedures are available. If the contracture is caused by web formation and the surrounding skin is pliable, one or several Z-operations provide the procedure of choice. In contractures due to broad dense scars, the latter are incised or excised, the contracture is reduced, and the resulting defect is covered either with a skin graft or with local or distant flaps. The profession is indebted to J. B. Brown for having perfected the technique of skin grafting to such a degree that it has become the method of choice in the majority of contractures where a flap formerly was considered indicated.

Axilla

Z-Operation (Case 109, p. 1135)

Indication for this operation arises when the contracture is due to binding webs and the surrounding skin is pliable. Sometimes the web is so long as to necessitate several Zs. Sometimes the arm is bound to the chest by several webs, which all have to be broken up. For technique of the Z-operation, see page 185.

Use of Graft (Cases 111-115, pp. 1138-1145)

This method is indicated whenever the contracting scar is broad. During the repair vessels and nerves do not need to be exposed or, if exposed, can be covered by surrounding fat tissue. The contracture is released with a transverse relaxation incision through the entire thickness of the scar. Excision of the scar is rarely necessary. The incision should not be made through the center of the scar but near the chest wall. This will shift the defect rather toward the chest below the axilla. The arm is now forcibly abducted and all cicatricial bands as they represent themselves in the wound are incised or excised. The surgeon soon reaches the vena axillaris. Abduction should now be carried out cautiously. Stretching of the vein can be facilitated by ligating and separating some of its branches coming from the chest wall. The other contents of the axilla should not be exposed. The musculus pectoralis major, as well as the musculus latissimus dorsi, may become an obstacle, resisting reduction of the contracture. In most cases, the muscles can be stretched. Stretching may be facilitated by separation of some of the fibrosed fibers running within the muscle substance. They can be easily palpated while the arm is held in abduction. Incision of the free borders or severance of the insertion of the muscles is rarely necessary.

The defect, which is diamond shaped, is now prepared for skin grafting. Hollow spaces, as those beneath the pectoral muscle, are obliterated by tacking the axillary fat tissue to the free border of the muscle. Vessels and nerves, if exposed, must be covered with surrounding fat tissue. From the thick wound edges, a wedge-shaped piece of the dense fibrotic subcutaneous tissue should be excised. The now overhanging skin edges either are turned downward and sutured to the base of the wound or, if they are pliable, are turned outward and folded over so that skin comes to lie upon skin. The wound edges are held in this position with a few sutures (Cases 111, 112, pp. 1138, 1139). Blair recommended this procedure for the purpose of increasing the size of the graft bed, to compensate for contraction following the grafting operation.

The area is now ready to be grafted. The graft of choice is the thick split graft. Full-thickness grafts have less chance of "take," owing to irregularity of the graft bed and difficulty with complete immobilization. Preferably, the graft should be removed in one piece. It must be sutured carefully to the wound edges and anchored with basting sutures to the bottom of the wound. To facilitate this, the author has found the following steps helpful: The graft is first sutured to the anterior wound edges; it is now lifted up; under direct vision, the anchoring basting sutures are led through the graft and the depth of the wound. This not only facilitates accurate stitching but avoids injury to such important structures as the vena axillaris. Another row of similar sutures may be necessary along the deep posterior boundary of the axilla. Finally, the graft is sutured to the remaining wound edges.

The usual pressure dressing is applied after numerous stabholes have been made in the graft. It may also be possible to tie the skin sutures which have been left long over the mechanic's waste (p. 36). The arm is held in abduction by fastening the hand to the head of the bed and supporting the arm with pillows.

The dressing is changed aften ten days; active exercises should be undertaken after the third postoperative week. One of the simplest is exercise on the swing. If, in spite of active and passive exercises, the contracture should recur to some degree, another skin-graft operation should be performed.

Variation: There are cases of contracture where a strip of normal or at least pliable skin is left in the depth of the axilla. In these cases, the relaxation incision is not carried through the axilla but long the median border of the pliable skin portion; that is, along the chest wall (Burton) (Case 115, p. 1144 [right axilla]). If the arm is forcibly abducted, the skin—partly by dissection and partly by being pushed laterally—moves upward and is held in the new position with sutures, or it may be turned outward, as just discussed. The remaining defect at the chest wall is skin grafted, as also described in the foregoing.

Use of Flap

In those cases of extensive contracture in which the binding scar consists of heavy fibrous tissue, necessitating partial excision of the scar and exposure of vessels and nerves to overcome the contracture without available fat tissue to cover these structures, transplantation of a flap for covering the defect becomes indicated. Another indication for the use of a flap is previous failure to correct the contracture by the free-graft method. The flap is preferably taken from the neighborhood (chest or back), and, as a rule, needs to be made so long that delayed transfer becomes necessary (Case 115, p. 1144 [left axilla]). Occasionally, a flap can be rotated from the immediate neighborhood into the defect in one stage and secondary defect, consisting of the original flap bed, can be skin grafted (Case 114, p. 1142). Two flaps may be needed. Davis suggests raising one from the front and the other from the back, the free ends being sutured together.

Prevention of Contractures after Radical Removal of Breast

A popular incision in radical operations for cancer of the breast is the elliptical incision around the diseased breast and its longitudinal extension upward along the lateral border of the musculus pectoralis major. It is this latter part of the incision which in a certain number of cases causes later limitation of motion of the arm in the shoulder joint. After removal of the pectoral muscles, the incision—or rather the resulting scar—comes to lie across the axilla. If this scar contracts, it becomes a bridle scar or a binding web. In extensive cases, the contracture can be corrected by a Z-operation.

726

To counteract the possibility of a contracture by a binding web, it seems logical to perform the Z-operation with formation and interposition of two triangular flaps at the time of the first operation. This can be done by additional incisions to the original longitudinal incision. The objects of such a procedure would be (1) to interrupt a longitudinal direction of the original incision and to change it into a transverse or oblique course, and (2) to increase its length. The condition could now be compared physically to an accordion.

The same result can be achieved with a much simpler procedure, by changing the straight course of the longitudinal incision into a spiral form. The course of the incision is marked out preoperatively with one of the aniline dyes. One third of the spiral should lie anteriorly to the border of the musculus pectoralis major, two thirds posteriorly to it in the axilla.

There are two precautions to observe: (1) to avoid making the spiral cut too steep and too high; (2) to mark two opposite points at the extreme parts of the curves with a drop of methylene blue injected percutaneously. This will later facilitate correct adjustment of the wound edges.

Elbow Joint

The underlying principles in repairing flexor contractures of the elbow joint are the same as those previously described. If a Z-plastic procedure is possible, partial or even complete relief can be achieved. In some instances, a combination of the Z-operation and skin grafting will lead to success. In extensive contractures, particularly those of long standing, the contracted biceps and the involvement of the joint structures may offer a major obstacle to reducing the contractures. When opening the contracture, great care should be taken not to injure main vessels or nerves and not to expose tendons. If it is found impossible to relieve the contracture completely without exposing or endangering those structures, one should be satisfied with a temporary partial success, that is, to skin graft the defect, encase the extremity in a plaster cast, and repeat the procedure after healing has taken place. The first cast should not be changed for at least two weeks unless there is evidence of infection.

In those extensive cases in which exposure of the contents of the cubital region and tendon lengthening must be anticipated, the use of a flap becomes primarily the method of choice. A direct transfer of the flap can be planned if it is possible to raise the flap from the lateral chest region on the same side. The direction of the flap is transverse, the pedicle (compare with Case 120, p. 1154) located anteriorly opposite the contracted joint. Alternately, the flap can be taken from a more distant region and then transported by way of the wrist of the other arm. Such a flap should be tubed (Case 116, p. 1146).

If lengthening of the biceps tendon becomes necessary, the Z-method is effective. However, in a few instances, the contracture of the biceps is so extensive that even the Z-operation is insufficient to permit complete reduction. If such is the case, one should not hesitate to sever the biceps tendon and either transfer its insertion to a position higher up or permit the tendon to retract without suturing (Case 116, p. 1146). It is amazing that the lifting power of the affected arm is hardly impaired.

In cases where almost the entire joint region is enveloped in a large, thick, contracted scar, a relaxation procedure—such as later described in the discussion on contractures of the hip joint—should be given a trial.

WRIST

Contractures of the wrist can involve the extensor side as well as the flexor side and are, as a rule, associated with contractures of the fingers. They are repaired by the use of grafts or flaps, the proper choice depending entirely on whether or not the tendons must be exposed during the dissection. The binding scar should be carefully dissected from the underlying tendons, while the latter are gradually stretched. If possible, a thin layer of scar should remain on the tendons; this makes the use of a thick split graft or even of a full-thickness graft possible. If the contracture cannot be overcome without wide exposure of the tendons, one abandons further dissection, proceeding with skin grafting of the raw area and planning subsequent similar repair work (see foregoing discussion). Such a plan of gradual repair is particularly advisable in cases where the tendons have been found too tight. Sometimes freeing the tendons is completed in the first operation. Then, however, the use of free grafts cannot be considered. A flap is now indicated. The usual type is the open abdominal flap. A flap is also indicated in cases which need later repair work of tendons. Immobilization of the grafted area should include the fingers, and is performed as described on page 810. Sometimes in a flexion contracture of the wrist of long standing, the carpal bones become subluxated dorsally and resist dorsal extension after release of the contracting forces on the flexor side. It then becomes advisable to remove the proximal row of the carpal bones and arthrodese the wrist in the position of function (see p. 907).

HIP JOINT

Flexion contracture of the hip joint can be almost always corrected with the use of grafts. The general technique is similar to that described in the former discussions. Old, extensive, contracted, thick, and adherent burn scars, which may involve thighs, pubic region, and abdominal wall, are troublesome and difficult to correct. It would be inadvisable to remove the whole scar, for it would be impossible to obtain sufficient skin with which to cover the defect. To relieve these large, thick scars, Davis' relaxation procedure is a good one. The contracted region is put on a stretch, and the most binding area or areas are located and marked out. The scar is divided completely through its full depth until normal tissue is reached. Sometimes radiating incisions from the tight margins are necessary to complete the relaxation. If, after the incisions are made, the scar is found to be very thick, excision of a wedge-shaped slice of the deeper layer is advisable, so that the thinned surface edges may be drawn downward and attached to the normal base by a few sutures. The defects are now covered with split skin grafts. After application of a proper pressure dressing, the leg is supported by pillows and sand bags and thus semi-immobilized. If the flexion deformity could not be overcome in one stage, the leg is placed under some sort of traction, on a Braun-Böhler type of splint, for instance. Subsequent relaxation and skin grafting are performed after the wounds have healed.

In extreme and rigid cases, one of the relaxation incisions should be made over the spina iliaca anterior superior; after incision of the scar, a tenotomy of the musculus sartorius, musculus tensor fasciae latae, and the fascia lata should be performed directly below the spina. In adductor deformity, the relaxation incision is laid over the adductor region close below the pubic bone, and the musculus adductor longus and musculus gracilis are tenotomied. The defects are covered with skin grafts.

Knee Joint

The principles in correcting contracture of the knee joint are similar to those already enunciated. Flaps are rarely needed. If needed, they are taken from the opposite thigh or transferred from the opposite thoraco-epigastric region by way of the wrist of the same side. The relaxation incision is led transversely through the most binding area. Care should be taken not to expose the popliteal contents, particularly the tendons. If the contracture cannot be overcome in one stage, the defect is skin grafted, the extremity encased in a plaster cast, and one or more similar procedures performed subsequently. The first plaster cast should not be changed for at least two weeks unless there is evidence of infection.

In this way, most of the contractures, even the extensive ones, can be repaired. There are, however, cases where the contractures can be overcome in the longitudinal direction, but the result is spoiled by a posterior subluxation of the tibia due to shortness of the posterior ligaments (Case 110, p. 1136). O'Donaghue recommends application of horizontal and vertical traction to the legs. In extensive cases, however, traction alone is not successful. The author has been able to reduce the subluxation, as evidenced clinically and roentgenologically; when traction was removed, however, the subluxation recurred within a few days. Hence, it is recommended that the subluxation be reduced under traction, followed by application of a plaster cast with incorporation of the pins. The cast should be applied while the leg is suspended in traction. The pins and the anterior half of the cast are removed after two weeks, while the posterior half is kept to be applied during the night. Active exercises are instituted. Resistance exercises have been found particularly valuable: placing one sandbag beneath the leg, another upon the thigh, and then instituting active motion of the knee. Walking is also permitted.

In contractures due to extensive, heavy, thick scars, relaxation incisions as previously described are of great benefit. In rare instances where the contracted flexor muscles present the main obstacle, tenotomy of the latter should be performed. The tenotomy should be made oblique. Before one tenotomizes the biceps, the peroneal nerve, running mediad and close to the tendon, should be exposed and held away. The deep portion of the biceps insertion should be left behind to avoid separation of the important ligamentum collaterale fibulare. The tendon of the musculus semitendinosus, musculus semimembranosus, and musculus gracilis are tenotomized on the median side. In reducing these extreme contractures, one should avoid a posterior subluxation of the tibia by overstretching the contracted posterior ligaments and should be satisfied with a temporary partial success.

Ankle Joint

Extensor deformities (dorsiflexion) are treated like those of the wrist. Moderate flexor deformities (plantar flexion) are treated by gradually stretching the Achilles tendon and replacing the binding scar by skin grafts. The leg is encased in a plaster cast after each procedure. Severe flexor deformities are the most difficult to handle. Generally speaking, the gradual-relaxation procedure just described is the most satisfactory, although time consuming. If the contracted Achilles tendon is found to be the main obstacle, requiring lengthening, the problems mount. Lengthening of the tendon should go hand in hand with replacement of the covering scar. Simple skin grafting after wide exposure of the tendon cannot be entertained. Hence, the entire scar should be excised prior to the tendon lengthening and replaced by a flap, preferably one taken from the other extremity (compare with Case 122, p. 1158; Fig. 326,

p. 721). After the flap is healed in place, the tendon is exposed and lengthened. (For technique of tendon lengthening, see Figs. 327, 328.) The contracted posterior ligaments and capsule of the ankle joint may need relaxation incisions; care must be taken not to injure the tibial vessels and nerve.

LYMPHEDEMA (ELEPHANTIASIS)

Acquired Lymphedema

The so-called "idiopathic elephantiasis" (elephantiasis arabum) is an acquired lymphedema, and may involve legs, arms, genitalia, or face. It is preceded by lymphedema, which may be due to the removal of infected or carcinomatous lymph glands or to an increase of lymph flow such as is seen after thrombophlebitis or in association with varicose veins. The endemic form of elephantiasis, rare in this country but not infrequent in the tropics, is caused by the Wuchereria bancrofti (Filaria sanguinis-hominis) or other species of filaria.

It is of importance to differentiate between venous and lympatic lymphedema. Larson and co-workers and Lewis and Smith have described in detail the diagnostic measures for determining the primary defect in lymphatic lymphedema. The causes and treatment of the venous lymphedema have already been described on page 713. The underlying pathology of lymphatic lymphedema is characterized by two main features: the enlargement of the lymph vessels and a chronic inflammatory fibrosis of the derma and the subcutaneous tissue. The important fact is that the superficial lymph system alone is involved, even in advanced cases, and this system is definitely separated from the deep lymphatic system by the aponeurosis covering the muscles. Kondoleon, with an idea of connecting these two systems by removing a large amount of the aponeurosis, modified Lanz's method and devised an operation which has been popularized in this country and improved by Sistrunk. The operation consists of removing a large amount of skin and subcutaneous tissue, together with the fasciae. The operation has lost popularity since many failures have been reported because the theory of establishing a communication of the superficial and deep lymph systems by this operation is no longer tenable.

A new method has been described by Thompson for connecting the superficial and deep lymphatic systems. He removes the outer layer of the skin of certain portions of the extremity—the skin of the lateral side of the entire arm, for instance. The remainder of the skin is elevated as a dermal flap. The tissues between the flap and the muscles are excised; the muscles are separated and the dermal flap is placed into this cleft and held in the deep compartment with retention sutures. Burying the deepithelia-

731

lized skin portion is completed by suturing the free margin of the anterior skin to the posterior limit of the denuded area of the flap. A second stage procedure is performed on the other side of the extremity three months later. Thompson has demonstrated remarkable softening of tissues and lessening of edema. He has recently summarized his experience in a well-documented treatise.

In very extensive cases one may resort to a radical type of operation which was originally devised by Macey in 1940, and modified by Poth. It consists of the removal of the affected skin and subcutaneous tissue of the entire leg, with the exception of the toes, the sole of the foot, and a small strip over the Achilles tendon. The raw surface is covered with thick split skin grafts followed by application of a pressure dressing and immobilization in a plaster cast for seven days. Good results from this operation have been reported by Blocker, Farina, Kirschner, Schuchardt, Scriba, Gibson and Tough, and others. As a preoperative measure, it is advisable to keep the patient in bed two weeks with the leg elevated and firmly bandaged to reduce the edema as much as possible. Every source of infection should be checked. Daily tub baths and thorough cleansing of the leg with soap and water are of benefit.

Congenital Elephantiasis (Milroy's Disease)

In 1892, Milroy described a hereditary form of lymphedema. This disease is characterized by its familial incidence, lymphedema, and elephantiasic enlargement of the extremities, usually of the lower extremities. As a rule, both sides are involved. Unilateral involvement, however, and negative family history have been reported (personal communication from Dr. Fred Hartmann). There is no evidence of lymphatic obstruction or of fibrosis. The cause is unknown. For this type of elephantiasis, operative procedures are of no avail, as the author can confirm from personal experience. The treatment consists of the use of supportive dressings, such as elastic bandages or rubber stockings, and massage to control the edema.

BIBLIOGRAPHY

ANNING, S. T.: *Leg Ulcers; Their Causes and Treatment.* Little, Brown & Co., Boston, 1955.

AVELLAN, L., and JOHANSON, B.: *Hyperkeratosis of scars in the weight-bearing areas of the foot.* Acta Chir. Scand., 131:269, 1966.
Full thickness skin graft from the dorsum of the foot to its weight-bearing areas. Acta Chir. Scand., Excerptum Vol. 126:497, 1963.

SKIN, SUBCUTANEOUS TISSUE, AND THE FASCIAE

BARROW, D. W.: *The Clinic Management of Varicose Veins.* P. B. Hoeber, Inc., New York, 1948.

BLAIR, V. P., BROWN, J. B., and HAMM, W. G.: *The release of axillary and brachial scar fixation.* Surg. Gynec. Obstet., 56:790, 1933.

BLOCKER, T. G.: *Surgical treatment of elephantiasis.* Plast. Reconstr. Surg., 4:407, 1949.

BROWN, J. B., BYARS, L. T., and BLAIR, V. P.: *A study of ulcerations of the lower extremity and their repair with thick split skin grafts.* Surg. Gynec. Obstet., 63:331, 1936.

BROWN, J. B., and CANNON, B.: *The repair of surface defects of the foot.* Ann. Surg., 120:417, 1944.

BURTON, T. F.: *Brachiothoracic adhesions.* Surg. Gynec. Obstet., 70:938, 1940.

CAMPBELL, W. C.: *Operative Orthopedics.* C. V. Mosby Co., St. Louis, 1939.

CANNON, B., ET AL.: *The use of open jump flaps in lower extremity repairs.* Plast. Reconstr. Surg., 2:336, 1947.

CARPENTER, E. B.: *Clinical experiences with chlorophyll preparations: with particular reference to chronic osteomyelitis and chronic ulcers.* Amer. J. Surg., 77:167, 1949.

CONVERSE, J. M.: *Plastic repair of the extremities by non-tubulated pedicle skin flaps.* J. Bone Joint Surg., 30A:163, 1948.

CONWAY, H., and STARK, R. B.: *Soft tissue coverage for injuries to the foot and leg.* Ann. Surg., 143:371, 1956.

DAVIS, J. S.: *Arm chest adhesions.* J. Bone Joint Surg., 6:167, 1924.
Use of relaxation incisions when dealing with scars. Penn. Med. J., 41:565, 1938.

DAVIS, J. S., and KITLOWSKI, E. A.: *The theory and practical use of the Z incision for the relief of scar contractures.* Ann. Surg., 109:1001, 1939.

DEMING, E. G.: *An alternative to cross-leg pedicle flap.* Plast. Reconstr. Surg., 17:399, 1956.

DICKSON, F. D., and DIVELY, R. L.: *Functional Disorders of the Foot; Their Diagnosis and Treatment.* J. B. Lippincott, Philadelphia, 1944.

DOMINGO, LUCCA R.: *Surgical treatment of lymphoedema of the lower extremities.* Plast. Reconstr. Surg., 19:488, 1957.

DuVRIES, H. L.: *Surgery of the Foot.* C. V. Mosby Co., St. Louis, 1959.
Surgery of the Foot. In collaboration with Members of the Faculty of the Univ. of Calif. School of Med., San Francisco. Henry Kimpton, London, 1965.

EDWARDS, S.: *Evaluation of the open jump flap for lower extremity soft tissue repair.* Ann. Surg., 128:1131, 1948.

FARINA, R.: *Elephantiasis of the lower limbs.* Plast. Reconstr. Surg., 8:430, 1951.

FOLEY, W. T.: *The treatment of edema of the arm.* Surg. Gynec. Obstet., 93:568, 1951.

GHORMLEY, R. K., and OVERTON, L. M.: *The surgical treatment of severe forms of lymphedema (elephantiasis) of the extremities.* Surg. Gynec. Obstet., 61:83, 1935.

733

THE EXTREMITIES

GIBSON, T., and TOUGH, J. S.: *The surgical correction of chronic lymphoedema of the legs.* Brit. J. Plast. Surg., 7:195, 1954.

HAMM, W. G., and KITE, J. H.: *The relief of contractures of the knee following extensive burns.* South. Surgeon, 10:795, 1941.

HARRISON, S.: *Fractures of the tibia complicated by skin loss.* Brit. J. Plast. Surg., 21:262, 1968.

JACOBSSON, S., and NETTELBLAD, S. C.: *Surgical treatment of lymphoedema. Three cases of giant lymphoedema. of the lower limb.* Acta Chir. Scand., 122:187-196, 1961.

KEYSSER: *Zur operativen Behandlung der Elephantiasis.* Deutsche Ztschr. f. Chir., 203-204:356, 1927.

KIRSCHNER, H., SCHUCHARDT, K., SCRIBA, K.: *Zur Chirurgischen Behandlung und Pathology der Elephantiasis der unteren Extremitäten.* Der Chirurg., 26:512, 1955.

KOCH, S. L.: *Burn contractures of the axilla.* S. Clin. N. Amer., 14:751, 1934.

KONDOLEON, E.: *Die Operative Behandlung der Elephantiastischen Odeme.* Zentralbl. f. Chir., 39:1022, 1912; 50:443, 912, 1923.

LAKE, N. C.: *The Foot.* William Wood Co., Baltimore, 1943.

LANZ, O.: *Eröffnung neuer Abfuhrwege bei Stauung im Bauch und untern Extremitäten.* Zentralbl. f. Chir., 38:153, 1911.

LARSON, D. L., COERS, C. R., DOYLE, J. E., RAPPERPORT, A .S., KLOEHN, R., and LEWIS, S. R.: *Lymphedema of the lower extremity.* Plast. Reconstr. Surg., 38:293, 1966.

LEWIN, P.: *The Foot and Ankle*, 4th ed. Lea and Febiger, Philadelphia, 1959.

LEWIS, S. R., and SMITH, J. R.: *Lymphedema. In Reconstructive and Plastic Surgery*, edited by John M. Converse. W. B. Saunders, Philadelphia, 1964.

LEXER, E.: *Lehrbuch der Allgemeinen Chirurgie.* F. Enke, Stuttgart, 1934.

LINTON, R. R.: *The post-thrombotic ulceration of the lower extremity: Its etiology and surgical treatment.* Ann. Surg., 138:415, 1953.

MACEY, H. B.: *A surgical procedure for lymphedema of the extremities.* J. Bone Joint Surg., 30A:339, 1948.

MAISELS, D. O.: *Repairs of the heel.* Brit. J. Plast. Surg., 14:117, 1961.

MAY, H.: *Correction of cicatricial contractures of axilla, elbow joint and knee.* S. Clin. N. Amer., 1945, p. 1229.
The surgical treatment of intractable plantar warts. Surg. Clin. N. Amer., 31:607, 1951.

McKEE, D. M., and EDGERTON, M. T.: *The surgical treatment of lymphedema of the lower extremities.* Plast. Reconstr. Surg., 23:480, 1959.

MELENEY, F. L.: *Zinc peroxide in the treatment of micro-aerophilic and anaerobic infections.* Ann. Surg., 101:997, 1935.
Treatise on Surgical Infections. Oxford University Press, New York, 1948.
Present role of zinc peroxide in treatment of surgical infections. JAMA, 149:1450, 1952.

734

SKIN, SUBCUTANEOUS TISSUE, AND THE FASCIAE

MELENEY, F. L., and HARVEY, H. D.: *The combined use of zinc peroxide and sulfanilamide in the treatment of chronic undermining burrowing ulcers due to the micro-aerophilic hemolytic streptococcus.* Ann. Surg., 110:1067, 1939.

MENENDEZ, C. V.: *Ulcers of the Leg; Cause and Treatment.* Charles C Thomas, Springfield, 1967.

MILROY, W. F.: *Chronic hereditary edema: Milroy's disease.* JAMA, 91:1172, 1928.

MORTON, D. T.: *The Human Foot.* Columbia University Press, New York, 1935.

O'DONOGHUE, D. H.: *A method of application of skeletal traction for treatment of contracture of the knee.* Southern Med. J., 32:1023, 1939.

OWENS, N., and BETHEA, H.: *Further consideration of the surgical management of chronic varicose ulcers.* Plast. Reconstr. Surg., 3:633, 1948.

PEER, L. A., SHAHGHOLI, M., WALKER, J. C., and MANCUSI-UNGARO, A.: *Modified operation for lymphedema of the leg and arm.* Plast. Reconstr. Surg., 14:347, 1954.

POTH, E. J., BARNES, S. R., and ROSS, J. T.: *A new operation for elephantiasis.* Surg. Gynec. Obstet., 84:642, 1947.

RUTTER, A. G.: *Chronic ulcer of the leg in young subjects.* Surg. Gynec. Obstet., 98:291, 1954.

SCHEDEL, F.: *Beitrag zur Behandlung von dermatogenen Kontrakturen.* Der Chirurg., 23:18, 1952.

SCHMID, M. A.: *Plastic repair of heel defect (Zur plastischen Deckung von Fersendefekten).* Langenbeck's Arch. u Deut. Zschr., 1958, 288:256.

SIGG, K.: *Varicose Veins, Leg Ulcer and Thrombosis. New Methods in the Nonoperative Treatment.* Basel, Springer-Verlag, Berlin, 1958.

SISTRUNK, W. E.: *Contribution to plastic surgery (the Kondoleon operation for elephantiasis).* Ann. Surg., 85:185, 1927.

SMITH, J. W., and CONWAY, H.: *Selection of appropriate surgical procedures in lymphedema.* Plast. Reconstr. Surg., 30:10, 1962.

SNYDER, G. B., and EDGERTON, M. T.: *The principle of the island neurovascular flap in the management of ulcerated anesthetic weightbearing areas of the lower extremity.* Plast. Reconstr. Surg., 36:519, 1965.

STEINDLER, A.: *Orthopedic Operations.* Charles C Thomas, Springfield, 1943.

SUNDELL, B.: *Repair of the soft tissues of the plantar foot and the heel.* Acta Chir. Scand., 124:552, 1962.

THOMPSON, N.: *Surgical treatment of chronic lymphoedema of the lower limb. With preliminary report of new operation.* Brit. Med. J. 2:1567, 1962.
The surgical treatment of chronic lymphedema of the extremities. Surg. Clin. N. Amer., 47:445, 1967.

WEBSTER, G. V., PETERSON, R. A., and STEIN, H. L.: *Dermal overgrafting of the leg.* J. Bone Joint Surg., 40A:796, 1958.

WINKLER, E.: *The treatment of desmogenous finger contractures.* Klin. Med. (Wien.) 10:277, 1955.

735

THE MUSCLES AND TENDONS 22

TRAUMATIC DEFECTS

HERNIA OF MUSCLES

THERE are three types of muscle hernia: congenital, traumatic, and idiopathic. The traumatic type is the most common. The subcutaneous tear of a muscle fascia is due to sudden, forceful contraction of the muscle. The rent in the fascia can be palpated when the muscle is relaxed. The muscle herniates through the tear upon contraction. Operative closure of the fascial rent is rarely necessary. The suture is carried out with cross-stitches to achieve firmer hold of the fascial wound edges. In large hernias, removal of some of the protruding muscle substance is necessary before closure of the fascia can be achieved or else a dermal graft must be used (see p. 45).

RUPTURE OF MUSCLES AND TENDONS

The tear of a muscle may be complete or incomplete, and may involve the belly, the musculotendinous junction, or the tendon. The lightning-like severe pain, followed by loss of function, is characteristic. In complete ruptures a cleft can be felt, which effuses after formation of a hematoma. Incomplete ruptures present a diffuse, painful swelling of the affected muscle, due to hemorrhagic infiltration. Incomplete ruptures are treated by firmly bandaging and immobilizing the affected part for two

737

weeks, followed by massage and active-motion exercise. Complete ruptures require operative repair. This chapter will describe only the repair of those muscle ruptures with which the general plastic surgeon occasionally will have to deal.

RUPTURE OF MUSCULUS QUADRICEPS FEMORIS

The site of the rupture may be above, below, or through the patella. Inability to extend the leg actively and the presence of a gap above the patella are typical signs of suprapatellar ruptures; upward shift of the patella, with inability to extend the leg, is characteristic of infrapatellar ruptures. A gap within the patella with inability to extend the leg is a diagnostic sign of fracture of the patella. The rupture or fracture of the patella may be complete or incomplete. In either case, operative repair is indicated. Even in incomplete tears, the operation offers quicker and better end results, as aptly pointed out by Conway.

Technique (Suprapatellar Ruptures)

An S-shaped incision is made, starting from the median border of the patella, upward along the median boundary of the musculotendinous portion of the quadriceps for a distance well above the site of the rupture (Conway, Scuderi). Skin, subcutaneous tissue, and fascia are severed. After exposure of the rupture, it is determined whether or not the tear includes the joint capsule. If the joint is entered, the next step consists of closure of the synovial membrane. Then follows closure of the rent of the quadriceps tendon or, in ruptures higher up, of the muscle itself, with several wire mattress sutures. McLaughlin supports these sutures by internal fixation with the removable traction suture after Bunnell. In those tears close to the superior edge of the patella, it may be necessary to anchor sutures through drill holes through the patella. In late cases, all cicatricial tissue must be removed before the structures are united with mattress sutures. Overlapping the suture line with a dermal graft is advisable to strengthen the suture and to bridge any existing gap. The graft is taken from the upper lateral thigh or gluteal region of the same side. It is sutured with anchoring stitches upon the tendon above and below the suture line. In some cases in which the union is very weak, the graft should be cut sufficiently broad that it can be wrapped around the entire tendon anteriorly and posteriorly.

After-Treatment

The extremity is immobilized in a plaster cast, from below the pubic region to the toes, for three weeks during which time quadriceps exercises are taught and encouraged. At the end of that time, the cast is replaced by a shorter one reaching from midthigh to below the calf. Walking is permitted six weeks after the operation. The cast is removed; massage and active-motion exercises are instituted.

Technique (Infrapatellar Ruptures)

From a median S-shaped incision (p. 738), the site of the rupture is exposed. In the majority of cases it involves the patellar or tibial insertion of the tendon, rarely the midportion. In ruptures close to the patella, wire mattress sutures anchored through drill holes through the patella are most satisfactory. In ruptures near the insertion of the tendon at the tibia, the following procedures are recommended: If the tibial tubercle is avulsed, it is returned to its original site and fastened in place with a straight nail. If the rupture is just above the insertion, a medium-sized stainless-steel wire is placed, like a mattress suture, through the tendon and through the tibia by way of a transverse canal drilled posteriorly to (beneath) the tubercle. In late cases of infrapatellar rupture, the use of dermal transplants, as previously described, may become necessary.

After-treatment is as in suprapatellar ruptures.

Rupture of Tendo Calcaneus

The usual site of rupture of the tendo calcaneus (the Achilles tendon) is either at or near the insertion of the tendon at the calcaneus or at the junction of tendon and muscle. If it occurs at the point of insertion, the bone, as a rule, becomes avulsed. In ruptures of the tendon itself, the tendon generally is frayed. A distinction must be made between fresh and old ruptures. Immediate repair of fresh ruptures presents less difficulties than delayed repair of old defects, since contracture of the calf muscle is not encountered in fresh ruptures. This subject has been discussed extensively by Arner and Lindholm.

There is a recent trend to treat fresh ruptures as well as older unhealed ones conservatively—by immobilization of the foot in equinus position in a below-the-knee plaster cast for four weeks, followed by application of a walking cast with the foot in semi-equinus position for another four weeks (Lea et al., Gillies and Chalmers). In a case of a delayed rupture after an electrical burn around the heel, when the rupture occurred just before a cross-thigh flap was applied (Fig. 326, p. 721), the author followed the above treatment which resulted in firm healing of the tendon. In wide defects of older tendon ruptures, however, operative treatment is the only choice.

Technique

From an incision along the lateral border of the tendon, the wound edges are reflected and the site of the rupture exposed; the frayed wound edges of the tendon are excised as sparingly as possible and the tendon stumps sutured together. McLaughlin supports these sutures by internal fixation with the removable traction suture after Bunnell. If the tendon is much frayed the suture should be reinforced with an overlapping dermal graft (p. 45) which is sutured with anchoring stitches upon the tendon above and below the suture line. The graft is taken from the upper lateral thigh or gluteal region of the same side. In some cases in which the union is very weak the graft should be cut sufficiently broad that it can be wrapped around the entire tendon anteriorly and posteriorly. In older cases, scar tissue may have bridged the gap; hence, the tendon may be too long. This necessitates shortening of the tendon according to the method described on page 743. If it is too short the gap may be bridged according to a technique depicted in Figure 329 (Christensen), or according to Bosworth with tendon flaps taken from the raphe of the tendo Achilles and the posterior surface of the calf muscle. The author prefers bridging the gap with a dermal graft (p. 45). In cases with avulsion of bone, the avulsed bone is anchored in place with a wire suture. The wire is passed transversely through the tendon, above the avulsed piece of bone, and then through a canal drilled through the calcaneus beneath the site of avulsion. A small incision on the median side of the calcaneus is necessary to lead the wire the proper way.

After-Treatment

After closure of the wound, the extremity is encased in a plaster cast. The foot should be in position that will keep the suture line relaxed (equinus position). The cast remains in place for six weeks. The patient is then permitted weightbearing.

Open Injuries of Tendons

The treatment of severed tendons is discussed on page 847.

DYSFUNCTIONS

In addition to many other causes, dysfunctions of joints may be caused by tendons which are either too short or too long. In some cases tendon lengthening or shortening may suffice to overcome the dysfunction.

740

THE MUSCLES AND TENDONS

LENGTHENING OF TENDONS

Tendons are lengthened either subcutaneously or by the open method. The latter is preferable in the majority of cases. The open lengthening is performed in one of three ways: by lateral or frontal Z-method or by hinging a tendon flap.

Technique (Z-Method) (Figs. 327-328)

The tendon is divided in its entire length either in the sagittal plane (Bayer) (Fig. 327) or in the frontal plane (Fig. 328) with a Z-incision.

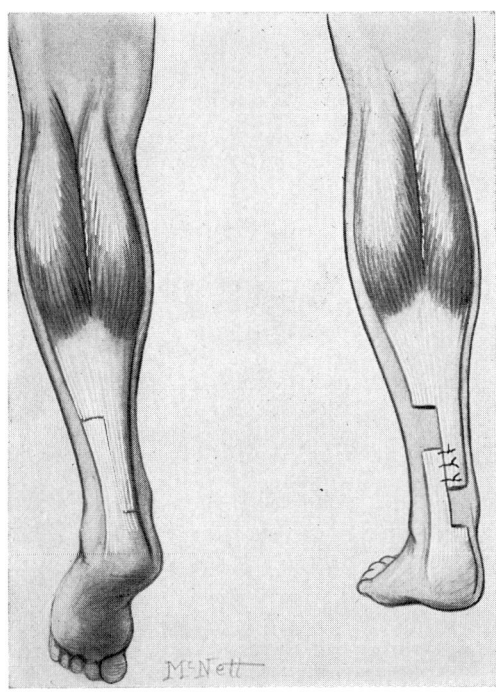

Fig. 327. Lengthening of Achilles tendon. *Left:* Z-like division of tendon in sagittal plane. *Right:* After lengthening and suturing.

After lengthening of the tendon, the tendon stumps are sutured together. The frontal lengthening has the advantage of creating two broad tendon flaps, which provide more satisfactory and firmer coaptation.

Technique (Flap Method) (Figs. 329-330)

Plastic lengthening of one tendon stump to bridge a tendon defect can be performed by using a flap formed in such a way that it can be hinged and connected with the other tendon stump. In broad tendons (quadriceps tendon), two such flaps may be formed and hinged.

741

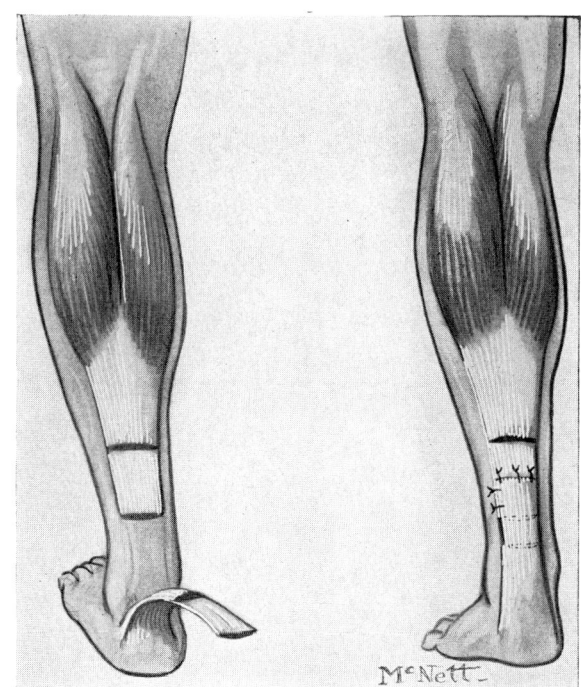

Fig. 328. Lengthening of Achilles tendon. *Left:* Z-like division of tendon in frontal plane. *Right:* After lengthening and suturing.

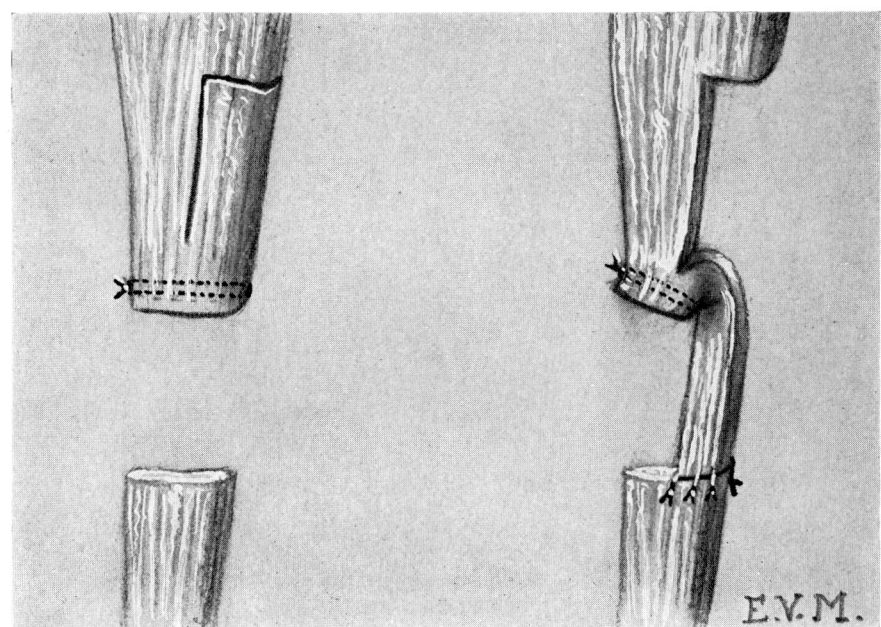

Fig. 329. Lengthening of tendon by flap method. *Right:* After hinging of flap and suturing.

THE MUSCLES AND TENDONS

After-Treatment

Immobilization of the extremity from three to four weeks is advisable if the Z-method has been used, from five to six weeks if the flap method has been used.

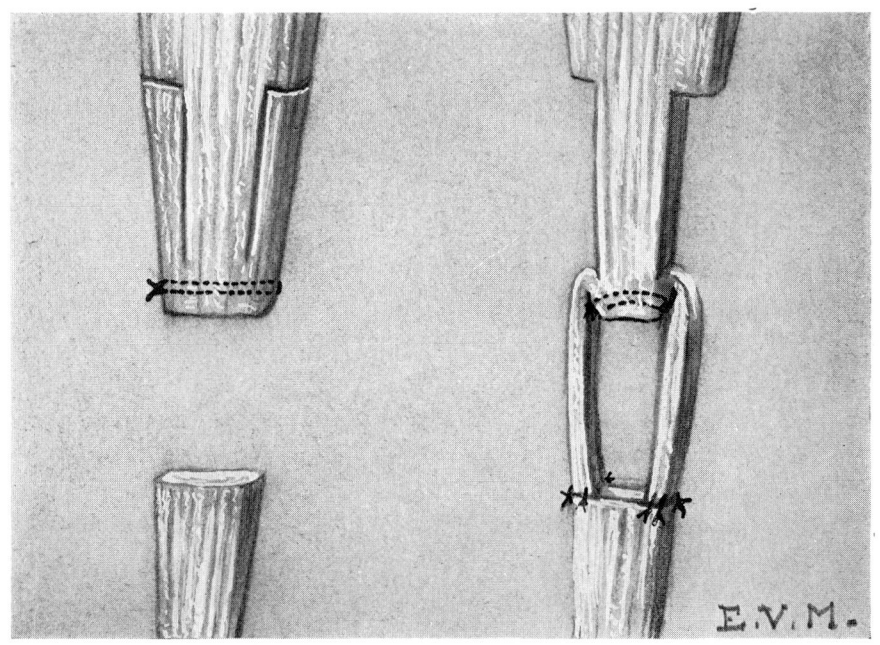

Fig. 330. Lengthening of tendon by bilateral flap method. *Right:* After hinging of flaps and suturing.

SHORTENING OF TENDONS

A tendon can be shortened according to the Z-incision (see the foregoing), followed by excision of a proper-sized piece from each tendon stump and tendon suture. Another way is the pleating method, in which the tendon is lifted with a single-pronged retractor. The tendon loop, so formed, is sutured together and to the tendon itself (Haas) (Fig. 331).

TRANSPOSITION OF TENDONS

Tendons are transposed for the purpose of transferring the action of a functioning muscle to a paralyzed muscle. The pioneer work in this field of surgery was done by Nicoladoni, Drobnik, Lange, Goldwaith, Parrish, Milliken, Codivilla, Vulpius, Biesalski and Mayer, and others.

743

THE EXTREMITIES

Most of these operations belong to the orthopedic field, and hence will not be discussed in detail. (Reference is made to an excellent treatise on this subject by Witt.) The general principles, however, are outlined, since the general reconstructive surgeon is occasionally confronted with these problems, such as in restoration of function after facial palsies and of the function of hand and fingers after palsies of one or more nerves of the arm.

Operative Indications

These are correction of a functional imbalance of a joint caused (1) by a paralysis of one muscle or group of muscles or (2) by an over-

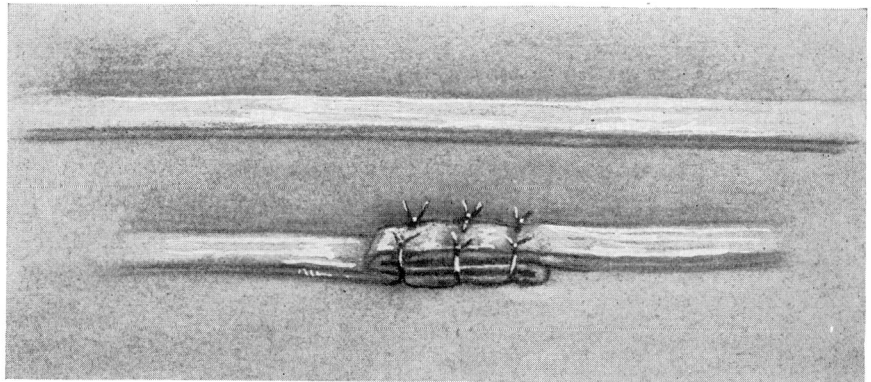

Fig. 331. Shortening of tendon by pleating. *Lower:* After suturing tendon loop together and to tendon itself.

action of muscles. In the former case (palsies due to nerve injuries and poliomyelitis), the transposition aims at the replacement of the lost function and avoidance of a deformity. In the latter case (spastic paralysis), it attempts to achieve a balanced redistribution of forces by overcoming the disharmony between too much and too little.

Technique

A great number of operations have been worked out since the introduction of the method by Nicoladoni. The principle of the method is to attach a functioning tendon to a paralyzed tendon. The ways of attaching the donor and receiver tendons are manifold. We distinguish between a descending and an ascending method (Vulpius). In the *descending method*, the tendon of the selected functioning muscle is severed and transferred to the paralyzed muscle. In the *ascending method*, the tendon

744

of the paralyzed muscle is severed and transferred to the tendon of the selected functioning muscle. Hence, in the ascending method the original action of the functioning muscle is not disturbed, but some of its function is transferred to replace the paralyzed muscle. Therefore this method has advantages over the descending method; however, for technical reasons it can rarely be employed.

The descending method is more versatile; it offers three possibilities: (1) The tendon of the functioning muscle is transferred and fastened to the tendon of the paralyzed muscle (Vulpius). (2) The tendon of the functioning muscle is fastened to the periosteum at or near the insertion of the tendon of the paralyzed muscle (Lange, Codivilla). (3) One may use the so-called "physiological method," by which the paralyzed tendon is severed near its insertion, pulled out of its sheath, and replaced by the functioning tendon, which is inserted through the empty sheath (Biesalski and Mayer).

Any of these methods should be carefully planned and worked out. A thorough electrical examination should be the first step to obtain a clear picture of the quantitative and qualitative extent of the muscle damage. Proper selection of the muscle or muscles to be transferred is the next step. The muscle to be transferred must have sufficient power. It should be a muscle which, after its transfer, will not cause functional imbalance at its original site. It should have a tendon which permits rerouting in the shortest and straightest way and which allows transfer through a tendon sheath or through tissue, with satisfactory gliding conditions. It is also important that the transferred tendon be under normal physiological tension after its insertion.

BIBLIOGRAPHY

ARNER, O., and LINDHOLM, A.: *Subcutaneous rupture of the Achilles tendon.* Acta Chir. Scand., Suppl. 239, 1959.

BATE, T. H.: *Subcutaneous rupture of tendo Achilles.* Arch. Surg., 62:14, 1951.

BAYER, V.: *Sehnenverkürzung.* Zentralbl. f. Orthop., 6:308, 1912.

BIESALSKI, K., and MAYER, L.: *Die physiologische, Sehnenverpflanzung.* F. Springer, Berlin, 1916.

BOSWORTH, D. M.: *Repair of defects in the tendo Achilles.* J. Bone Joint Surg., 38A-111, 1956.

CHRISTENSEN, I. B.: *Rupture of the Achilles tendon; 57 Cases.* Acta Chir. Scand., 106:50, 1953.

745

THE EXTREMITIES

CODIVILLA: *Sui trapianti tendinei nella pratica ortopedica.* Arch. di ortop., 1899, No. 4.

CODMAN, E. A.: The Shoulder. Boston, 1934.

CONWAY, F. M.: *Rupture of the quadriceps tendon.* Amer. J. Surg., 50:3, 1940.

DEPALMA, A. F.: *Diseases of the Knee.* J. B. Lippincott, Philadelphia, 1954.

DROBNIK, T.: *Ueber die Behandlung der Kinderlähmung mit Funktionsteilung und-übertragung.* Deutsche Ztschr. f. Chir., 43:473, 1896.

GILLIES, H., and CHALMERS, J.: *The management of fresh ruptures of the tendo Achilles.* J. Bone Joint Surg., 52A:337, 1970.

GOLDWAITH, F.: *The Direct Transplantation of Muscles.* Trans. Amer. Orthop. Assoc. 1897, Vol. 10.

GRANEY, C. M.: *Bilateral rupture of quadriceps femoris tendons with six years' interval between injuries.* Amer. J. Surg., 61:112, 1943.

HAAS, J.: *Konservative und Operative Orthopädie.* J. Springer, Vienna, 1934.

LANGE, F.: *Ueber die periostale Sehnenüberpflanzung.* Münchn. med. Wchnschr., 1900, No. 15.

MARSH, H. O., ANDERSON, H. P., and PLIEGO, O.: *Patellectomy: Repair by quadriceps tenoplasty.* Amer. Surgeon 24:273, 1958.

MAYER, L.: *The physiological method of tendon transplantation.* Surg. Gynec. Obstet., 22:182, 298, 472, 1916.

McLAUGHLIN, H. L.: *Repair of major tendon ruptures by buried removable suture.* Amer. J. Surg., 74:758, 1947.

MILLIKEN, S. E.: *Tendon grafting for infantile paralysis: a reply.* Med. Rec., 49: 133, 1896.

NICOLADONI: *Über den pes calcaneus.* Wien. med. Press., 1881, p. 46.

PARRISH, B. F.: *A new operation for paralytic talipes valgus and the annunciation of a new surgical principle.* New York State J. Med., 56:402, 1892.

SCUDERI, C.: *Ruptures of the quadriceps tendon.* Amer. J. Surg., 95:626, 1958.

SCUDERI, C., and SCHREY, E. L.: *Ruptures of the quadriceps tendon: Study of 14 tendon ruptures.* Arch. Surg., 61:42, 1950.

SIMON, H. E., and SACCHET, H. A.: *Muscle hernias of the leg: Review of literature and report of twelve cases.* Amer. J. Surg., 67:87, 1945.

von BRANDIS, H. J.: *Über Subcutane Muskelrisse.* Deutsche Ztschr. f. Chirurgie, 253:639, 1940.

VULPIUS, O.: *Die Sehnenüberpflanzung und ihre Verwertung in der Behandlung der Lähmungen.* Veit. u. Co., Leipzig, 1902.

WAUGH, R. L., HATHCOCK, T. A., and ELLIOTT, J. L.: *Ruptures of muscles and tendons.* Surgery, 25:370, 1949.

WITT, A. N.: *Sehnenverletzungen und Sehnen-Muskel-Transplantationen.* von J. F. Bergmann, München, 1953.

THE MOTOR NERVES   23

OPEN INJURIES

A NERVE IS severed either completely or incompletely, depending upon the type of injury. If it is severed completely or its substance interrupted and replaced by scar tissue, as seen after a severe crushing injury, certain degenerative processes set in before regeneration and healing can occur. Immediately after trauma the injured nerve undergoes traumatic degeneration, which is followed two to four days later by secondary (paralytic) (Wallerian) degeneration of the entire peripheral-nerve segment. Much later, the nerve becomes regenerated through complicated processes. The secondary degeneration of the periphral segment starts with disintegration of the myelin sheath which surrounds the axis cylinders (neurofibrillae). It is soon followed by degeneration of the axis cylinders themselves, which break up into fragments and granules. Regenerative processes of the proximal end go hand in hand with these degenerative processes: The nuclei of the neurilemma (sheath of Schwann), surrounding the myelin sheath, enlarge and multiply, forming protoplasmic bands. It is still problematic whether these cell formations actually form the axis cylinder or are only an advance protection for the newly formed neurofibrillae. Nevertheless, they play an important part in the regenerative process. The young neurofibrillae appear first at the central stump. With the help of the advancing protoplasmic bands, they invade the peripheral segment. According to one theory, they gradually grow through the entire peripheral segment; according to another, they connect themselves with less differentiated cell groups which have formed in the peripheral segment. No matter which theory is right, it is generally agreed that the Schwann cells form the all-important bridge by which outgrowing axons are conducted to the peripheral stump. The rate of regeneration is estimated to be from 1 to 3 mm. a day. For detailed information, the work of Waller, Ziegler, Marchand, Ranvier, Spielmeyer, Dean Lewis, Loyal Davis, Kirk, Gutmann, Young, Seddon, Bateman, Nigst, Mumenthaler and Schliak and others may be referred to (see also Bibliography, p. 755). Healing of a nerve, however, can occur only if the regenerative processes are undisturbed. If, owing to infection or destruction, the continuity remains disrupted or becomes so, the central nerve stump becomes bulbous and forms a neuroma, while the peripheral segment atrophies and undergoes fibrotic changes followed by muscle atrophy, trophic skin changes, and reflex disorders.

The diagnosis depends more upon the loss of motor than of sensory function. The faradic and galvanic responses are also of importance, both of which gradually subside within the first twelve days, and finally disappear. The galvanic response, however, recurs in a reverse way later (two weeks later), until the respective muscles have atrophied (reaction of degeneration). Of greater value in assessing motor function, however, is electromyography, which records the minute electrical changes that occur when muscles contract. This is done by means of small needle electrodes inserted directly into the muscle. Vasomotor trophic disturbances and causalgia may also be of diagnostic value. Highett introduced nerve blocking in diagnosis of certain peripheral nerve lesions. (For detailed study, among others, see monographs of Groff, Haymaker, Seletz, Davis, Bateman, Nigst, Mumenthaler and Schliak.)

TREATMENT

In every case of open nerve injury the question arises as to whether to undertake primary or secondary nerve suturing. Vast experience of the last war taught that results after secondary nerve suturing are better than they are after primary repair (Sperling and Woodhall, Zachary and Holmes, Seddon's unrivaled experience with nerve injuries in the British Army, and others). Grantham et al., however, leave this question open. In war wounds the local damage to the nerve ends is, in most cases, extensive and the chances of performing adequate excision of the damaged nerve trunk and adequate epineural suturing at the primary operation are not good. Hence, early secondary suturing (also called delayed primary repair) becomes more reliable (Woodhall and Beebe, Nigst, Bateman). The nerve ends are approached only at the time of the wound excision and brought together with two stitches placed to prevent rotation of the stumps. The optimum time of suturing of the divided nerve is considered to be from three to four weeks after wound healing. Seddon emphasizes that the nerve suture should never be performed without adequate resection of the stumps and without adequate mobilization of the nerve. In primary repair of a badly contused wound one will be reluctant to embark on wide exposure of the main nerve stump. Also, the all-important nerve sheaths through which the sutures are laid may be too delicate and frayed to hold the sutures, while, after a few weeks' waiting, the sheath is thicker and firmer due to epineural fibrosis. Furthermore, this second operation can be carried out through incisions of election which will permit adequate mobilization of the nerve stumps and preparation of a suitable bed for the nerve. These are the main arguments in favor of delayed primary repair.

In civilian practice, however, in cases in which the nerve has been injured by sharp instrumentation and the wound is not infected and not badly contused, the nerve stumps do not need much resection and mobilization repair should be carried out immediately.

Unless early primary repair is performed, the preoperative treatment is of utmost importance. The nerve injury results in a paralysis of a muscle or muscle group. Unless the affected limb is properly splinted and exercised, an irreparable functional damage will result from shortening of the unprotected antagonist and eventual contracture, and from lymphedema with transformation of stagnated lymphocytes into fibroplasts which deposit collagen throughout the soft tissues. Hence, the extremities should be elevated in widespread paralysis, or properly splinted in partial paralysis, and every defective joint should be put through a full range of passive motion exercises several times daily (see also page 752, *After-Treatment*).

Technique (Primary Suture)

Under general anesthesia with a pneumatic tourniquet applied (see also p. 849) and an electric stimulator available, the severed nerve is exposed. If necessary the wound is enlarged to facilitate exposure. The nerve segments should be handled with the greatest care. The ends are freshened with a razor knife, not with scissors, until normal-looking nerve bundles are encountered. Obtaining an exact coaptation of the nerve ends is the next step, so that the corresponding fasciculi are opposite each other.

749

Small vessels visible in the epineurium in either section may be helpful in obtaining proper coaptation. To avoid displacement three interrupted stay sutures are placed through the epineurium of both ends. Fine silk is the best suture material and is used on a round curved atraumatic needle. Sutures with wires offer no special merit. The same is true with the plasma clot suture, which is of value only in nerve grafting. The wound edges to be sutured are those of the epineurium, not of the nerve substance. The wound edges are everted, not inverted. The sutures are interrupted and snugly approximate the nerve stumps, so that the opposing fasciculi are in close contact. It is advisable to place a few radiopaque sutures in some manner near the ends of the nerve so that a subsequent roentgenogram will yield information concerning the presence or absence of disruption of the suture line. After completion of the suturing, the nerve is placed into neighborhood muscle tissue or, if none is available, it is surrounded by a flap or graft of fat tissue. Routinely wrapping the suture line in tantalum foil (Spurling and Woodhall) has not proven of discernible advantage (Seddon, Kirklin, et al.). Surrounding the sutured nerve with a millipore membrane (Campbell and Bassett, Böhler, Schaaf) appears promising in preventing adhesions and neuroma formations.

Secondary repair is carried out either as an early secondary repair in cases where the division of the nerve was diagnosed during the primary wound treatment but primary nerve suture was delayed, for reasons explained above, or as a late secondary repair where the anatomical state of the nerve had not been disclosed during the wound treatment or, if recognized, repair had been delayed with the hope that spontaneous recovery would occur. While in the former case suture of the nerve is carried out as soon as the wound has healed (three to four weeks after the accident), in the latter case it is delayed somewhat. It is undeniable that the repair of a severed nerve is a matter of some urgency, but, as yet, the degree of urgency is not known. Foerster, drawing from his vast experience of nerve injuries in the German army during World War I, advised waiting for a period of four to six months before exploring the injured area, since such a delay appeared not to be harmful and intervention within that period might entail an unnecessary operation in those cases where the continuity of the nerve offered an excellent prospect of useful spontaneous recovery. His experience was augmented during World War II by Zachary, Seddon and others. Spurling and Woodhall, et al., Nigst, Bateman and others urge a policy of very early secondary suture (four to six weeks after the accident). Kirklin et al. state that suture of a divided nerve within three months after injury gives superior results. Nerves which have been sutured after three months, but not more than nine months, show a reasonable amount of recovery. If exploration must

750

be delayed, physiotherapy is carried out in the meantime as outlined on page 752. Also, revision of excessive scarring of the skin and subcutaneous tissue is performed; this may entail transplantation of a pedicled flap.

Technique (Secondary Nerve Suture)

Under general anesthesia, with a pneumatic tourniquet applied and a nerve stimulator at hand, a longitudinal incision is made over the injured site. The incision, which should be adequate, should be spiral rather than straight and bayonet over flexor region of the joints to counteract any possibility of contracture. The old scar is included in the incision, but excision of this scar is delayed if adherence to the underlying nerve is suspected, until the nerve is explored in normal surroundings; there the nerve is dissected free toward the scar. It is better to dissect the scar away from the nerve than to grasp the nerve and free it from the scar tissue. Should the nerve be completely divided, the bulbous neuroma which in the meantime has formed is excised in thin serial sections with a razor blade. The excision should be as sparing as possible in the proximal neuroma, but should be sufficient to expose normal-looking nerve substance. In the distal neuroma the resection should be more generous, if the nerve lesion was due to a severe injury, since serious intrafascicular collaginization which cannot be detected with certainty by the naked eye may be present. An obstacle to the performance of a neat suture can be the retraction of the sheath after section and protrusion of the nerve bundles. Seddon overcomes this difficulty by circumcision of the sheath, followed by section of the bundles at the level to which the margin of the sheath retracts. The pneumatic tourniquet is now deflated and thorough hemostasis performed. The tourniquet then is reinflated and remains so until the dressing is applied (see also p. 849). The nerve stumps are sutured together as already described on page 750. The nerve is then surrounded by healthy tissue or, if excision of all surrounding scar has been impossible, the scarred surface is folded on itself and obliterated by sutures. It may be helpful, prior to this, to surround the suture line with a millipore membrane (Campbell and Bassett, Böhler, Schaaf). The wound is sutured in layers. If the wound is near or within the flexion crease of joints, it should be closed at its extremities before the nerve is sutured. This reduces to a minimum the awkward part of the wound suture and manipulation of the limb (Seddon).

Complications of Repair

If after resection of the neuroma a wide gap should result which makes direct approximation of the nerve stumps impossible or insecure, the nerve should be extensively mobilized from its bed. This inevitably requires separation of the nerve from the surrounding blood supply. However, this separation does not endanger the viability of the proximal stump since the longitudinal blood supply is profuse; it may, however, be harmful to the distal stump. Extensive mobilization should be limited to the central stump. Should this maneuver be insufficient to permit easy approximation of the stumps, the course of the nerve can be shortened either by rerouting the ulnar nerve from its position behind the median condyle of the elbow joint or by flexion of joints that lie in the path of the nerve (Naffziger, Platt, Babcock). (In rerouting the ulnar nerve the author agrees with Grantham and Pollard. The ulnar nerve should not be placed beneath the detached flexor group of muscles, but the transposition should begin in the midforearm and the nerve passed through a hiatus in the deep fascia and into a subcutaneous position.) The extremity is encased in a plaster cast which is replaced after three weeks by a cast that is hinged at the joint and has incorporated a screw turnbuckle. The limb is then straightened at the rate of 10 to 12 degrees a week. There is, however, a physiological limitation to overcoming nerve gaps this way, as has been brought out by Highett and co-workers, Zachary, Grantham et al. Roughly, it can be said that any suture requiring more than 90 degrees flexion of a joint may result in failure. A more reliable method should then be employed, i.e., nerve grafting (p. 58) or, in rare instances (defect of ulnar and median nerves), nerve anastomosis between the proximal stump of one nerve (ulnar) to the distal stump of another (St. Clair, Nigst, Oakey, Seddon) (see p. 61). Only rarely is one justified in resecting a piece of bone (oblique or stepladder section, followed by internal fixation) unless the local condition invites such procedure (nonunion of the humerus and co-existing radial palsy).

After-Treatment

The injured extremity is encased in a plaster cast or placed on another suitable splint. The paralyzed muscles should be in a position of relaxation to overcome the action of the functioning antagonists. The splint should be removable so that after the union of the nerve stumps physical and occupational therapy can be carried out; otherwise, prolonged immobilization would lead to stiffness of joints. Bunnell's so-called "active splinting" has lessened this danger (p. 815). In uncomplicated cases—that is, without tendon or bone injuries—physiotherapy is started on the seventh postoperative day, consisting of massage and galvanic exercises of the paralyzed muscles. If it is inadvisable to remove the cast, windows should be cut over the paralyzed muscles and daily galvanic stimulation applied. On the fourteenth postoperative day, passive motion exercises are added consisting of transient stretching of the paralyzed muscles. These exercises are carried out daily after temporary removal of the splint. Between the exercises, the patient is urged to move all those joints which are not necessarily immobilized. Occupational therapy is added to the physical therapy. Exercises are designed to re-educate the muscles to their normal coordinated function by carpeting, leatherwork, weaving, etc. These exercises should become more vigorous with the advancement of recovery. This is the time to stress synergic actions as well as dissociated movements of paralyzed muscles. The splint can be discarded at this stage of recovery.

Re-exploration of the sutured nerve should be performed if signs of regeneration are absent. Hence, *signs of regeneration* should be discussed here. The first evidence of success is the return of sensory function; this sign, however, may be deceptive, owing to innervation from the neighborhood. The next evidence is return of the reaction of degeneration (galvanic response in reverse) and, later, return of a normal response of nerve and muscles to galvanic and faradic stimuli. Of more importance, however, in assessing regeneration are electromyographic studies, which demonstrate motor action before voluntary power can be observed clinically. The final evidence of success is return of active motility in the form of feeble contraction which gradually increases. The interval between operation and return of function differs with various nerves and locations of lesions. As a rule, sensitivity returns after two to four weeks; function, after six weeks. The final result, however, can be estimated only at a much later date—months and years after repair. If signs and symptoms of regeneration are lacking for longer than three months, the site of the lesion should be re-explored and neurolysis should be performed (see below), with removal of any source of pressure or with resuturing of the nerve if the first suture has given way.

SUBCUTANEOUS INJURIES

Subcutaneous nerve injuries consist of palsies from pressure, stretching, or tearing. The mildest form of pressure palsy is that from unfavorable positions of the extremities during sleep. It is transitory. Palsies due to pressure of nerves during anesthesia (radial-nerve palsy from pressure of the edge of the table, plexus palsy after extreme abduction of the arm) take longer for recovery (three months). The same is true with palsies resulting from tourniquet pressure or from dressings which are too tight. Palsies from pressure caused by cicatricial tissue and callus develop gradually, and may be permanent unless released by neurolysis.

Palsies due to overstretching of the nerves (after fractures and dislocations) may be either transitory or permanent.

Palsies due to tearing are permanent, unless repaired.

THE EXTREMITIES

The diagnosis depends upon the disturbed function and the location of the lesion (see p. 748).

As already discussed on page 750 the treatment of subcutaneous nerve injuries is conservative at first. The injured limb is immobilized for one week and then treated with electric stimuli and massage, as already outlined. If conservative measures fail to obtain results within four to six weeks (electromyographic studies are valuable in assessing the damage), an operation is indicated, since successes with conservative methods become doubtful and the results of operative treatment less promising after this time.

Exploration

The site of the suspected lesion is widely exposed. The involved nerve or nerves are located and, if severed, are sutured as previously described. If the nerve is not severed but found irregular in its outline, it means either that the nerve bundles are destroyed and replaced by scar tissue or that they are intact but the nerve sheath is the seat of cicatricial changes. To prove the destruction or integrity of the nerve fibers, the sheath is freely opened and the nerve bundles exposed by endoneurolysis (hersage) (see following paragraph). As a matter of fact, endoneurolysis is also indicated in cases where the nerve looks normal but definite clinical evidence of nerve interruption exists. If endoneurolysis shows the nerve bundles destroyed and replaced by scar tissue, the treatment is the same as for secondary nerve suture (p. 751). If the bundles are intact, neurolysis is sufficient.

Neurolysis

Neurolysis is a sort of decompression treatment. The nerve is freely exposed by dissecting all scar tissue or callus away or removing foreign bodies. The epineurium is incised at the site of the lesion to relieve any tension and to reveal the condition of the nerve bundles. If simple incision of the epineurium does not expose a clear picture of the situation, endoneurolysis, or hersage, should be added, that is, the nerve fibers are separated from each other by incisions in the long axis of the nerve. If the bundles are intact, the nerve is now placed into a newly prepared bed of normal soft tissue (muscle tissue or fat tissue of the neighborhood, pulled together beneath the nerve), and the wound is closed. If part of the bundles is replaced by scar tissue, the scar is carefully excised without injuring the normal fasciculi. After excision of the scar, one may be able to suture the resected nerve ends together with preservation of the intact bundles.

The after-treatment is the same as that described on page 752.

754

BIBLIOGRAPHY

BABCOCK, W. W.: *A standard technique for operations on peripheral nerves with especial reference to closure of large gaps.* Surg. Gynec. Obstet., 45:364, 1927.

BACSICH, P.: *An extensive accumulation of biographical data.* Transplant. Bull., 1:211, 1954.

BATEMAN, J. E.: *Trauma to Nerves in Limbs.* W. B. Saunders, Philadelphia, 1962.

BJÖRKSTEN, G.: *Suture of war injuries to peripheral nerves. Clinical studies of results.* Acta Chir. Scand. (Suppl. 119) p. 7, 1947.

BODECHTEL, G., KRANTZUN, K., and KAZMEIER, F.: *Grundriss der Traumatischen Peripheren Nervenschädigungen.* Geo. Thieme, Stuttgart.

BÖHLER, J.: *Nervennaht und homoioplastische Nerventransplantation mit millipore-Umscheidung.* Langenbeck's Arch. f. Chir., 301:900, 1962.

BOWDEN, R. E. M.: *Peripheral Nerve Injuries.* H. K. Lewis & Co., Ltd., London, 1958.

BUNNELL, S.: *Surgery of the nerves of the hand.* Surg. Gynec. Obstet., 44:445, 1927.

BUNNELL, S., and BOYES, J. H.: *Nerve graft.* Amer. J. Surg., 44:64, 1939.

CAMPBELL, J. B., and BASSETT, C. A. L.: *Microfilter sheaths in peripheral nerve surgery.* J. Trauma, 1:139, 1961.

DANDY, W.: *A method of restoring nerves requiring resection.* JAMA, 122:35, 1943.

DAVIS, L., PERRETT, G., HILLER, F., and CARROL, W.: *Experimental studies of peripheral nerve injuries. A study of recovery of function following repair, end to end suture, and nerve grafts.* Surg. Gynec. Obstet., 80:35, 1945.

DAVIS, L.: *Methods of nerve repair.* Surg. Clin. N. Amer., 27:117, (Feb.) 1947.

DAVIS, L. E.: *The Principles of Neurological Surgery,* 4th Ed. Lea & Febiger, Philadelphia, 1953.

FOERSTER, O.: *Handbuch der Neurologie.* Julius Springer, Berlin, 1929.

FREEMAN, B. S.: *Adhesive neural anastomosis.* Plastic Reconstr. Surg., 35:167, 1965.

GRANTHAM, E. G., POLLARD, C., and BRABSON, J. A.: *Peripheral nerve surgery.* Ann. Surg., 127:696, 1948.
Peripheral nerve surgery: Results of 281 cases followed six to twenty-four months. Ann. Surg., 134:145, 1951.

GROFF, R. A., and HOUTZ, S. J.: *Manual of Diagnosis and Management of Peripheral Nerve Injuries.* J. B. Lippincott, Philadelphia, 1945.

GUTMANN, E., and YOUNG, J. Z.: J. Anat., London 78:15, 1944.

HAYMAKER, W., and WOODHALL, B.: *Peripheral Nerve Injuries: Principles of Diagnosis.* W. B. Saunders, Philadelphia, 1945.

HIGHETT, W. B.: *Splintage of peripheral nerve injuries.* Lancet, 1:555, 1942. J. Neurol. Psychiatrie, 5:101, 1942.

THE EXTREMITIES

HIGHETT, W. B., and SANDERS, F. K.: *The effects of stretching nerves after suture.* Brit. J. Surg., 30:355, 1943.

KIRKLIN, J. W., MURPHEY, F., and BERKSON, J.: *Suture of peripheral nerves.* Surg. Gynec. Obstet., 88:719, 1949.

LEWIS, D.: *Peripheral Nerves.* In LEWIS: *System of Surgery.* W. F. Prior Co., Hagerstown, Md., 1929, Vol. 3, Chap. 6.

LEWIS, D., and KIRK, E. G.: *Regeneration in peripheral nerves, an experimental study.* Bull. Johns Hopkins Hosp., 28:71, 1917.

LYONS, W. R., and WOODHALL, B.: *Atlas of Nerve Injuries.* W. B. Saunders, Philadelphia, 1948.

MARCHAND, F.: *Der Prozess der Wundheilung.* Deutsche Chir., 1901.

MASSIE, W. K., and ECKER, A.: *Internal fixation of bone and neurorrhaphy. Combined lesions of radial nerves and humerus fractures.* Bone Joint Surg., 29:977, 1947.

MUMENTHALER, M., and SCHLIACK, H.: *Läsionen peripherer Nerven. Diagnostik und Therapie (Peripheral Nerve Lesions. Diagnosis and Therapy.)* Georg Thieme Verlag. 1965.

NAFFZIGER, H. C.: *Methods to secure end to end sutures of peripheral nerves.* Surg. Gynec. Obstet., 32:139, 1921.

NIGST, H.: *Die Chirurgie der Peripheren Nerven.* Georg Thieme Verlag, Stuttgart 1955.
Freie Nerventransplantationen und Cortison. Basel, Benno Schwabe, 1957.
Operative Behandlungsmöglichkeiten bei Erkrankungen und frischen Verletzungen peripherer Nerven. Langenbeck's Arch. f. Chir., 301:855, 1962.

PLATT, H.: *The Surgery of Peripheral Nerve Injuries.* Humberton Lecture, 1921, Bristol.

SANDERS, F. K.: Brain, 65:281, 1942.

SANDERS, F. K., and YOUNG, J. Z.: J. Anat., London, 76:143, 1942.

SCHAAF, F.: *Tubulisation von Nervennähten Vorläufige Mitteilung uber Erfahrungen mit dem Millipore-Filter.* Langenbeck's Arch. f. Chir., 301:905, 1962.

SEDDON, H. J.: *The use of autogenous grafts for the repair of large gaps in peripheral nerves.* Brit. J. Surg., 35:151, 1947.
War injuries of peripheral nerves. War Surgery Supplement No. 2, Wounds of the Extremities. Brit. J. Surg., 36:325, 1949.
Peripheral Nerve Injuries. (Privy Council, Medical Research Council Special Report Series. No. 282) London, Her Majesty's Stationery Office, 1954.

SELETZ, E.: *Surgery of Peripheral Nerves.* Charles C Thomas, Springfield, 1951.

SPIELMEYER, W.: *Degeneration und Regeneration am peripherischen Nerven.* Handb. d. normal u. pathol. Physiologie, 9:285, 1929.

SPURLING, R. G.: *Peripheral nerve injuries in European theater of operations.* JAMA, 123:1011, 1945.

SPURLING, R. G., and WOODHALL, B.: *Experiences with early nerve surgery in peripheral nerve injuries.* Ann. Surg., 123:731, 1946.

756

THE MOTOR NERVES

STRUPPLER, A.: *Das Elektromyogramm in der Beurteilung peripherer Nerven-verletzungen.* Arch. f. klin. Chir. 301:885, 1962.

TARLOV, I. M., DENSLOW, C., SWARZ, S., and PINELES, D.: *Plasma clot of nerves, experimental technic.* Arch. Surg., 47:44, 1943.
How long should an extremity be immobilized after nerve suture? Ann. Surg., 126: 366, 1947.
The Plasma Clot Sutures of Peripheral Nerves and Nerve Roots. Charles C Thomas, Springfield, 1950.

WOODHALL, B.: *Peripheral nerve injury.* Surg. Clin. N. Amer., 34:1147, 1954.

WOODHALL, B., ET AL.: *Peripheral Nerve Regeneration.* Government Printing Office, Washington, D. C., 1957.

WOODHALL, B., and BEEBE, G. W.: *Peripheral Nerve Regeneration. A Follow-up Study of 3,656 World War II Injuries.* U. S. Government Printing Office, Washington, D. C., 1956.

YOUNG, J. Z., and MEDAWAR, P. B.: *Fibrin sutures of peripheral nerves.* Lancet, 2:126, 1940.

YOUNG, J. Z.: Physiol. Rev., 22:318, 1942.

ZACHARY, R. B., and HOLMES, W.: *Primary suture of nerves.* Surg. Gynec. Obstet., 82:632, 1946.

ZIEGLER, P.: *Untersuchungen über die Regeneration des Achsenzylinders durch-trennter peripheren Nerven.* Arch. f. klin. Chir., 51:796, 1896.

THE BLOOD VESSELS

24

REPARATIVE surgery of the blood vessels belongs to the surgeon trained in this field. However, for the sake of information to the general plastic surgeon, treatment of open injuries to blood vessels and of aneurysms is outlined and discussed.

OPEN INJURIES

Pathology, Symptoms, Signs

In open injuries of the blood vessels (cut, stab, or bullet wounds; extensive crush injuries), the veins, being attached to the fascia, are more often involved than the arteries, which are more mobile and stronger and hence dodge more easily. If only the outer wall of a vessel is injured—from tangential blows, for instance—such a wound heals ordinarily without consequences; only in rare instances may an aneurysm develop. Penetrating wounds of the vessels, however, are followed by more severe consequences, of which hemorrhage is the most outstanding sign. In the case of a vein, the wound may heal spontaneously under development of a thrombus, while the blood escaping from an arterial wound may bury a cavity into the surrounding hematoma (false aneurysm). If vein and artery are injured and the respective openings are in apposition, an arteriovenous aneurysm may form; a large hematoma may be absent, owing to the suction effect of the vein.

759

THE EXTREMITIES

If a vessel is severed with a sharp cutting instrument, the lumen gapes—that of the vein more than that of the contractile artery. If a vessel is severed by blunt forces (torsion), the intima and tunica media roll in, and the adventitia may elongate and thin out like a piece of glass after it is heated and pulled apart. Hence, a hemorrhage may be absent even if large vessels are involved.

The diagnosis of open injuries of the vessels is not difficult unless the most important sign—the hemorrhage—is absent. If large hematomas and small wounds are present, the nature of the vessel injury is difficult to diagnose. If the peripheral pulse is absent, a complete separation or thrombosis of the artery can be assumed. If pulsation is present but less distinct than on the other side, and systolic murmurs are noticeable over the site of the injury and peripheral to it, a lateral penetration of the vessel is most likely. If the murmur is also noticeable centrad to the injury, the injury must have resulted in a communicating wound of artery and vein, with the arterial blood flowing into the vein.

Treatment

The treatment of vessel injuries with hemorrhages consists of emergency hemostasis, final—or definitive—hemostasis, and measures to replace the lost blood.

Emergency Hemostasis: This is best obtained by a pressure dressing or by correct application of a tourniquet. The tourniquet may remain in place for one hour; if the emergency status is to last longer than one hour, the tourniquet should be loosened and then reapplied. In regions where application of a tourniquet or pressure dressing is impossible, digital pressure against the artery centrad to the injury stops the bleeding. With the second and third fingers of the left hand, upon which the thumb of the right hand is pressed, the arteria femoralis is pressed against the horizontal ramus of the pubic bone, the arteria subclavia against the first rib, the arteria carotis communis against the transverse processes of the cervical spine, the abdominal aorta with the whole fist against the lumbar vertebrae. The surrounding wound is now covered with a clean emergency dressing and the extremity splinted.

Final, or Definitive, Hemostasis: After the patient has arrived in the operating room, the clothing is cut away, the wound area is surgically prepared, the injured vessel or vessels are clamped with vessel clamps (see below), and the tourniquet is removed. If the injured vessels cannot be found, they are located by using an anatomic surgical approach regardless of the location of the wound. Before approaching the site of arterial injury directly it is advisable to establish proximal vascular control by passing a tape around the artery. An exposure of the artery and vein should also

760

THE BLOOD VESSELS

be undertaken in those cases with small wounds and large hematomas. The repair after removal of the hematoma is much easier and more effective than the later repair of the aneurysm which may result from such an injury.

The treatment of the wound itself is done after completion of the arterial repair.

The question now arises as to the best treatment of the injured artery for the individual case—ligation or suture. Ligation used to be the method of choice. Because of the great strides that have been made recently in the field of vascular surgery, the suture method is now more often employed, with greater benefit to the patient than was heretofore thought possible. Ziperman's statistics show a decrease of the amputation rate by this method from 40.3 per cent (World War II) to 17.9 per cent (Korean War). Jahnke, Seeley, Howard, Hughes, Spencer and Grewe report similar good results, i.e., achievements just short of the miraculous. Kremer, Hughes, Morton et al., Eufinger and Vollmar have discussed this subject in detail.

Ligation: Ligation is a simple procedure. With the clamps already applied to the transversely severed ends of the vessel, the vessel is pulled forward, dissected free for a short distance, and ligated. In lateral wounds, the ligature is applied above and below the wound, while the part between is resected.

Ligation is the method of choice for vessels which, if ligated, will not cause any serious damage or in cases of hemorrhage from larger vessels which are not controllable by other means. In these cases, ligation of the accompanying vein is advised because clinical and experimental experience has shown that this decreases the chance of gangrene, as first demonstrated by V. Oppel (Heidreich, Brooks, Johnson, Kirtley and Wilson, and others). The explanation is not altogether clear. It seems that ligation of the accompanying vein decreases the rapidity of the venous return, thus maintaining a proper balance between the arterial and venous systems. The blood which flows in reduced amount through the arterial collaterals remains longer in the extremity, thus providing better nutrition. It also raises the tone of the smaller arteries, thus stimulating collateral circulation. Opinions concerning the beneficial effect of venous ligations differ, however (Makins). DeBakey and Simeone, Mason and Brown, from vast experience with battle casualties in World War II, Ziperman with those of the Korean War, Cullen et al., and others came to the conclusion that ligation of the concomitant vein furnishes no protection whatever against the development of gangrene after acute arterial occlusion and ligation in battle casualties.

Blood-Vessel Suture: Suturing of vessels was introduced about 1900 (Murphy, Gluck, Carrel, Guthrie, Stich, and others) (see also p. 51). Its

761

advantages, however, were not really appreciated until much later, during World War I (Goodman, Bier, von Haberer, and others). The introduction of anticoagulants, sympathetic nerve block to relieve arterial spasm, the use of vascular grafts, and the development of special instruments, such as toothed bulldog and Potts serrated clamps to control bleeding without injury to the wall of the blood vessel, have added tremendously to the development of vascular surgery and to the success of the vessel suture in particular, which offers the greatest hope of survival of the limb.

The success of the suture depends, among other factors, upon the suture material. Fine silk or nylon thread is used on the fine round, straight, or curved needles. The thread is attached to the end of the needle, the so-called "atraumatic suture." These arterial sutures are obtained from surgical supply houses. Exposure of the injured vessel is performed as previously described. It should be emphasized that exposure must be adequate; control of the artery above the site of the injury either by tourniquet or by temporary tape ligation through a separate incision should be considered; if for this purpose the subclavian artery must be exposed a segment of the clavicle should be removed with Gigli saw (this piece of bone does not need to be replaced later). Following the wound excision drapes, gowns, gloves, and instruments are changed, the ends of artery are clamped a few centimeters above and below the laceration with artery clamps and the tourniquet is released. Ligation and separation of a few of its branches may facilitate mobilization of the vessel. Some of the damaged adventitia is now trimmed off. This not only removes a source of infection but provides also a sort of periarterial sympathectomy, aiding in interrupting spastic sympathetic reflexes and thus preventing arterial spasm (see p. 764). All clots should be expressed from the proximal artery. The distal end should be perfused with a dilute heparin solution and any clots should be removed by flushing the distal end with saline solution through a Fogarty catheter. In suturing the vessel, Carrel's technique is generally accepted as simple and effective. Nonsuture anastomosis, judging from DeBakey's experience, apparently reveals no better results, and does not shorten the operating time. Its principle consists of approximating intima to intima. If the vessel is severed transversely, three traction sutures, penetrating the entire wall of the vessel stumps, are placed evenly about 1.5 mm. ($\frac{1}{16}$ inch) from the wound edges (Fig. 332, B). In tying these sutures, it is important to evert the vessel wall so that intima comes to lie on intima. If traction is now applied to these stay sutures, the circumference of the vessel is changed into a triangle, thus facilitating suturing and approximation. The remainder of the wound is closed with a continuous overhand stitch. The continuous suture commences at the site of one of the stay sutures. The latter is kept under traction by the operator's left hand, while the other one in front of it is held by an assistant. The suture penetrates the entire thickness of the vessel wall under eversion of the intima. After one third of the suture is completed, the operator takes the traction suture from the assistant, and the assistant takes the third suture; after the second third is completed, the operator takes the third traction suture while the assistant holds the first one. The blood stream is now gradually released by opening the clamps. Oozing from the stitch canals is checked by gentle pressure with moist gauze. If there is still some bleeding, one or two interrupted sutures will control the hemorrhage.

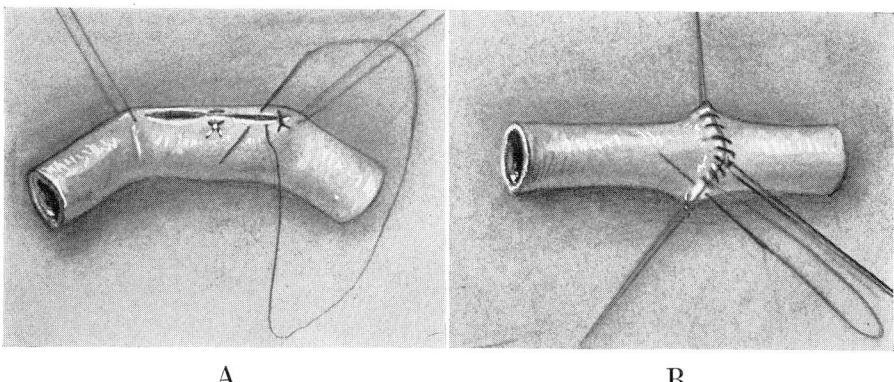

A   B

Fig. 332. *A:* Suture of lateral wound of artery. A traction suture is placed at each end. A mattress suture, through all layers of wall under eversion of wound edges, is placed at middle of wound. Remainder of wound is closed with continuous, everting overhand stitch. *B:* Suture of transverse wound of artery. Round circumference of vessel is changed into triangle with three traction sutures placed at equal distance through entire wall of vessel stumps. In tying these sutures, vessel wall is everted so that intima comes to lie upon intima. Remainder of wound is closed with continuous, everting overhand stitch.

In cases where the wound edges are under tension, it is more advisable to use a mattress suture under eversion of the intima (Dorrance) (Fig. 27) than to suture with a simple overhand stitch.

In lateral wounds, the principle of closure is the same as described, that is, placement of a traction suture at each end of the rent, eversion of the intima of the wound edges, and their approximation by a continuous suture. Eversion of the intima can be facilitated by placing a mattress suture through all layers of the vessel at the middle of the wound before starting the continuous suture (Fig. 332, *A*). If lateral closure would result in constriction (which would occur in actual defects of the wall) application of a venous or Teflon patch graft becomes necessary.

763

THE EXTREMITIES

In incomplete transverse wounds in which more than half of the circumference is involved, it is advisable to sever the vessel completely and to perform an end-to-end suture.

If the vessel's sound edges cannot be united without tension or there is an actual defect of the artery, and if wound conditions permit, the defect should be bridged with a reversed vein graft, which is taken from adjacent veins, the internal diameter of which approximates that of the injured vessel (v. saphena or cephalica) or an homologous arterial graft (p. 53). The concomitant vein, however, should not be used. Plastic tubes, such as Tuffier's, Mustard's, Hufnagel's, Donovan's, have been used to bridge the defect, but are now superseded by flexible prostheses of plastic fabric p. 52).

The peripheral pulse usually returns quickly. In some cases there is, however, a slow return. This is thought to be due to arterial spasm from vasoconstrictor reflexes which originate in the sympathetic nerve fibers of the adventitia at the site of the injury. To relieve this spasm, removal of the adventitia from the wound edges before suturing them (see the foregoing) is of advantage. Others recommend injection of 2 cc. of 2 per cent procaine solution into the adventitia above and below the laceration.

A thorough wound excision is now performed, the repaired vessels are well covered with soft tissue, the wound is sutured or left open to drain (p. 129). The extremity is immobilized on a molded plaster-cast splint or wooden splint. The position of an extremity after ligation of vessels is of importance. Elevation of the extremity above the heart level accentuates the ischemia by forcing the blood flow to overcome the amount of gravity pull created by the degree of elevation above the level of the heart. Hence, the extremity should be elevated at heart level or preferably in a slight dependent position (DeBakey).

A sympathetic nerve block by paravertebral injection of procaine to counteract arterial spasm may be necessary (p. 762). Anticoagulants have not been found necessary (Ziperman, Hughes, Spencer and Grewe); they may cause bleeding of the entire wound. Blood and plasma expanders should be available to combat shock and to replace blood. In addition, antibiotic therapy is instituted.

ANEURYSM

ARTERIAL ANEURYSM

As already mentioned, the following procedures obviously do not belong in the realm of the general plastic surgeon but are included for his general information.

764

THE BLOOD VESSELS

Pathology, Symptoms, Signs

Arterial aneurysm is a circumscribed enlargement of an artery of congenital or acquired origin. It is due either to weakness of the entire vessel wall or to bulging of certain layers: herniation of the intima through a rent of the tunica media; bulging of the adventitia after destruction of the intima and tunica media (from atheromatous ulcers, for instance). This form of aneurysm is called "aneurysma verum." Another form of aneurysm is the false aneurysm, aneurysma spurium, which is caused by a laceration or rupture of an artery. The blood stream, escaping from the injured vessel, burrows a cavity into the surrounding tissues. The peripheral parts of this pulsating hematoma coagulate. The coagulum is gradually invaded by fibrous tissue; thus a fibrous capsule is formed. The artery itself is not enlarged. The anatomical picture of both types of aneurysm naturally differ in many respects: In a true aneurysm, the artery is enlarged; the wall is thin, endothelial lined, and slightly adherent. In a false aneurysm, the arterial wall is not enlarged; the aneurysmal wall is thick, cicatricial, and adherent. The clinical picture is the same. In the beginning, symptoms and findings may be indistinct; later, however, after a tumor becomes palpable and visible, a typical clinical picture develops which is characterized by a pulsating and compressible tumor and by crepitation with the pulsation and association of a systolic bruit and thrill. All these signs disappear upon compression of the afferent artery. The peripheral pulse, as compared with the other site, is weaker and delayed; edema, claudication, neuralgia, ulceration, and palsies may be present. Angiography can be of great help to verify the diagnosis and outline the extent of the aneurysm and collaterals.

Treatment

In most instances, the treatment is operative. The majority of opinions favor late operation to allow formation of an adequate collateral circulation. The adequacy of the latter can be tested by the Matas method, which Gage describes as follows:

> A Martin rubber bandage is applied from the toes or fingers to a point just above the aneurysm. The Matas compressor is now applied to the main artery above the rubber bandage. The compressor is screwed down until the main artery is obliterated. The Martin rubber bandage is now removed. One must be absolutely certain that the compressor does not slip. The foot or hand immediately after the removal of the rubber bandage has a cadaveric color. The blanched toes or fingers are now carefully watched for the return of a pink color. The time interval between the removal of the rubber bandage and the return of color determines the presence of an adequate or inadequate collateral circulation. If the time interval is over three minutes, the collateral circulation is inadequate.

765

THE EXTREMITIES

Shumacker, who has considerable experience with the Mattas test, considers it superior to all other preoperative methods of study. He modified it slightly by producing ischemia with a sphygomanometric cuff and arterial compression by digital pressure.

Development of Collateral Circulation: Whenever there is some doubt of the adequacy of the collateral circulation, the latter should be improved. The simplest method is to delay the operation because the aneurysm itself is a powerful stimulus. Passive vascular exercises (Shumacker) and temporary occlusion of the afferent artery by digital pressure or the use of the Matas compressor, ten to twenty minutes several times daily, are efficient. Sympathetic nerve block or even sympathectomy is recommended as the "physiologic" method (I. M. Gage and A. Ochsner). Rarely may one have to resort to gradual occlusion of the artery by metallic bands (Halsted, Matas) or by an hourglass-shaped rubber band (J. C. Owings).

Operation: Ligation of the artery above and below the aneurysm, with or without removal of the aneurysmal sac, is the classical method practiced for many centuries. The basic principles are still in vogue. The so-called "ideal" method, consisting of extirpation of the aneurysm and restoration of the continuity of the affected artery either by lateral suture or preferably direct end-to-end suture (Murphy), or by bridging the defect with a vessel graft (p. 51), heretofore considered only in exceptional cases, is now favored as a desirable objective (Hughes, Jahnke, Seeley, Creech). It is especially applicable in young people; in older people with degenerative diseases of the vessel walls it may be contraindicated. It is more and more becoming the method of choice in the treatment of aneurysms of the aorta (DeBakey et al.), the popliteal artery (Seeley et al.), carotid artery, etc. Nevertheless, these reconstructive methods cannot be applied or counted upon to function in every case. Hence, a sufficient collateral circulation must be assured preoperatively.

Ligation of the artery above and below the aneurysm, with removal of the sac, is known as the "operation of Purmann" (1680). The operation is difficult, and may interfere with the neighboring structures and impair collateral circulation. Ligation of the artery above and below the aneurysm, with incision of the sac, is known as the "operation of Antyllus" (fourth century A.D. or earlier). The disadvantage of this operation is the remaining sac, which has to be obliterated, ordinarily by packing. Its advantage is that it does not interfere with surrounding tissues and structures or the collateral circulation. The greatest improvement in the surgery of aneurysm is the operation of Matas (1888) who, as in the operation of Antyllus, leaves the sac behind but obliterates it with a so-called "endoaneurysmorrhaphy." Matas devised three types of endo-

766

aneurysmorrhaphy: obliterative, restorative, and reconstructive. Of those three methods the obliterative type is the most effective one.

OBLITERATIVE ENDOANEURYSMORRHAPHY (Fig. 333): This type is indicated for the majority of cases, particularly for those in which there are two main openings in the sac and these openings are some distance apart.

Hemostasis: Circulation of the limb is controlled, preferably with a tourniquet. If, owing to the situation of the aneurysm, a tourniquet cannot be applied, vessel clamps are used.

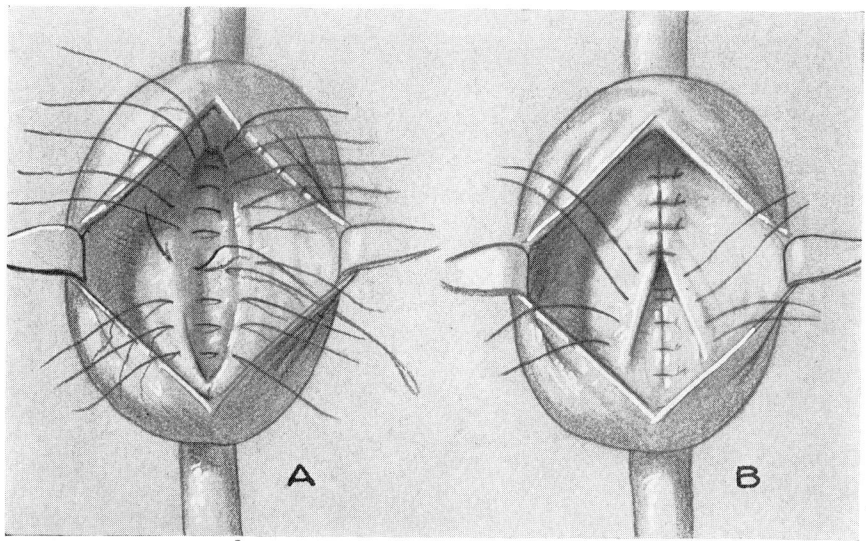

Fig. 333. Obliterative endoaneurysmorrhaphy (Matas). *A:* Aneurysm with two main openings in sac, both some distance apart. Obliteration of sac by rows of Lembert-type sutures obliterating space between arterial openings. *B:* Second row of sutures buries first one in same fashion.

Incision: From a longitudinal incision (over the joints, the bayonet incision, as recommended by Shumacker, is advisable), the sac is exposed. If a tourniquet is not used, the artery leading to and from the aneurysm is dissected free, and the clamps are applied. The sac is now incised with a longitudinal incision from one end to the other. All blood clots are evacuated and the interior of the sac exposed by retracting the wound edges. In the fusiform type of aneurysm, two large openings are found, usually at the bottom of the sac, separated by an intervening space, frequently marked by a shallow groove, which represents the continuation of the floor of the parent artery. A search should now be made for more openings derived from collaterals.

THE EXTREMITIES

Obliteration: The openings of the main artery, as well as of the collaterals, are thoroughly closed with sutures. The circulation is now released to find out whether all openings have been closed. Obliteration of the sac by rows of Lembert-type sutures follows. The first row obliterates the space between the arterial openings. A second row of sutures buries the first one in the same fashion. A large surface of the sac is thus brought into apposition. The closing of the remaining aneurysmal space is now readily accomplished by turning the wound edges of the sac into the interior of the cavity and tacking and holding them in contact with the bottom and sides of the sac with mattress or simple sutures. The skin is now closed without drainage.

As already mentioned, revival of vascular grafts in the 1940s led to return of the so-called "ideal" method of surgical treatment of an aneurysm, consisting of excision of the sac and restoration of the continuity of the artery by means of a vascular graft. It has become the method of choice for aortic aneurysm. The difficulties with this method, however, are due to attempts to remove the sac, which are time consuming. There is also the possibility of injury to important adjacent structures (inferior vena cava for instance). To save time and prevent injury to these structures, Creech modified Matas' endoaneurysmorrhaphy and, as in the case of an abdominal aneurysm, applies intravascular sutures to the intercostal and lumbar branches, then divides the aortal ends within the sac and bridges the defect with a knitted dacron prosthesis. Upon completion of the anastomoses, any redundant part of the anterior portion of the sac is trimmed away; the posterior wall is left behind.

After-Treatment: The limb is dressed without undue pressure and immobilized. It is only slightly elevated. The patient is allowed to be up and around after ten to fourteen days.

ARTERIOVENOUS ANEURYSM

Pathology, Symptoms, Signs

The arteriovenous aneurysm or fistula (Hunter's aneurysma per anastomosin, 1784) is a communication between an artery and a vein. It is seldom congenital (reviewed in detail by Cross, Glover, Simeone and Oldenburg). In the majority of cases, it is due to stab and gunshot wounds, penetrating artery and vein at opposite places (v. Bramann, v. Bergmann, Bier, Makins). The communication may be intimate; if such is the case, the wall of the vein opposite the fistula is bulging (aneurysmal varix), rarely the wall of the artery. In other instances, the arterial and venous openings may be apart from each other, separated by a hematoma which

768

gradually develops into an aneurysmal sac, thus establishing a communication between artery and vein (varicose aneurysm) (Fig. 334). Although the majority of the abnormal arteriovenous communications are acquired, some are congenital; cases with single communications have been described. Reid and others consider circoid aneurysms, pulsating angiomas, and racemose aneurysms as arteriovenous communications, not as tumors.

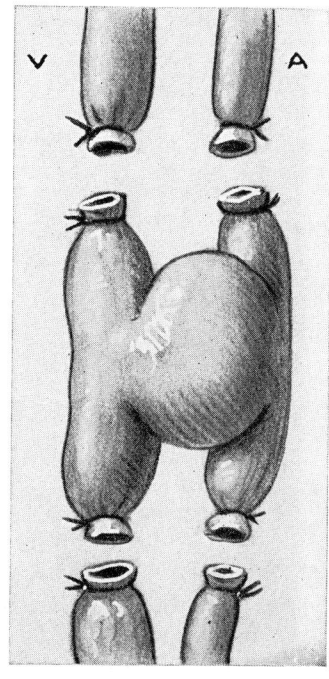

Fig. 334. Arteriovenous aneurysm. Quadruple ligation of artery and vein. Excision of involved vessels, together with fistula between ligatures.

The clinical picture, with the exception of the pulsating compressible tumor, differs in every respect from that of the arterial aneurysm, since the arterial blood is diverted into the vein, causing grave consequences. The effects produced by the arteriovenous fistula are local, regional, and systemic (Pemberton).

The pulsation not only is confined to the tumor, but can also be noticed peripherally and centrally in the vein. Stasis in the dependent veins is evident, owing to interference with the venous circulation. Edema and varicose enlargement of the subcutaneous veins are common. Pulsation of the subcutaneous veins may be visible and palpable wherever there are larger connections between the deep and superficial system (arm, for instance). The venous blood contains oxygen and is red, compared with the venous blood of the other side. Trophic disturbances, atrophies, ulcers, and necrosis are not infrequent. Upon auscultation, a long bruit and thrill are noticeable, particularly over the fistula but also peripherad and, what is an important diagnostic phenomenon, centrad as well. Another differential diagnostic point is that the bruit is continuously audible, roaring during systole, diminishing and becoming softer at diastole, unlike the bruit of the arterial aneurysma which is intermittent. In addition there may be slowing of pulse and rising of blood pressure on digital closure of the artery proximal to the lesion. This never occurs in the presence of a simple arterial aneurysm, since the total blood volume is not increased (Holman).

Owing to the fact that arterial blood enters the vein and is carried back to lungs and heart, less arterial blood reaches the periphery. This may cause cardiovascular disturbances (dyspnea, tachycardia, dilatation of the heart), as well as compensatory phenomena. Holman could demonstrate an increased blood volume and minute volume output of the heart. When compensation takes place, blood pressure rises and the pulse rate decreases. Cardiac hypertrophy takes place as the result of the increased blood flowing through the heart per unit of time, while the dilatation of the heart is part of the general dilatation of the vessels necessary to handle the increased volume of blood flowing through the circuit of heart, artery, fistula, and veins. X-ray of the heart and arteriography are essential.

Treatment

The operation should be performed under local anesthesia without the use of a tourniquet, since the involved vessels and their collaterals are identified better when filled. Quadruple ligature was the method of choice in the treatment of arteriovenous fistulae but is being gradually replaced by methods which preserve or restore the continuity of the affected artery (Freeman, Jahnke, Holman, Shumacker, Matheson, Seeley, Hughes, etc.). The modern immediate repair of injured vessels, including potential arteriovenous fistulae as outlined in the preceding chapters, has reduced the late development of arteriovenous fistulae. If they do develop, delayed operations consisting of restoration of arterial continuity should be the desirable objective, at least for arteriovenous fistulae of major vessels. Excision of the damaged vessel wall and end-to-end anastomosis give better results than transverse and longitudinal suturing of arterial rents. This excision should not be limited to the obviously damaged segment only but should include 1 cm. (⅖ inch) of apparently normal vessel wall at each end of the divided artery. When vessels cannot be united without tension a vessel graft should be employed (p. 51). Quadruple ligation should be considered as second choice. From a longitudinal bayonet incision (transverse incision at the neck), the involved artery and vein are exposed and ligated above and below the aneurysm. The aneurysm is now dissected free from the

770

surrounding tissue; the collaterals emptying into the aneurysm are ligated and severed; finally, the segment of artery and vein, together with the fistula, is excised between the quadruple ligature (Fig. 334).

Alternative Methods: If excision is hazardous, owing to inaccessibility or adherence to important structures, a quadruple ligation should be performed, possibly with division of the artery proximal to the aneurysm. Obliteration of the aneurysmal sac with mattress sutures may be added (Reid).

For after-treatment, see page 768.

BIBLIOGRAPHY

ALLEN, E. V., BARKER, N. W., and HINES, E. A.: *Peripheral Vascular Diseases,* 3rd Ed. W. B. Saunders, Philadelphia, 1962.

BACTYNER, K.: *Uber die Chirurgie der Arterienverletzungen und die Frage der Ventransplantation.* Chirurg., 17-18:345, 1947.

v. BERGMANN, E.: *Zur Kasuistik des arteriell venösen traumatischen Aneurysma.* Arch. f. klin. Chir., 69:515, 1903.

BIER, A.: *Abstracts of the Most Important Papers by German Surgeons (1914-1918)* . British War Office Medical Research Committee, 1918, Vol. 1, p. 402. (See also Franz.)

BIGGER, I. A.: *Aneurysms, Arteriovenous Aneurysms.* In J. SHELTON HORSLEY: *Operative Surgery.* C. V. Mosby Co., St. Louis, 1940, Vol. 1, p. 135.

BLAKEMORE, A. H.: *Restorative endoaneurysmorrhaphy by vein graft inlay.* Ann. Surg., 126:841, 1947.

BRADHAM, R. R., BUXTON, J. T., and STALLWORTH, J. M.: *Arterial injury of the lower extremity.* Surg. Gynec. Obstet., 118:995, 1964.

v. BRAMANN: *Das arteriell-venöse Aneurysma.* Arch. f. klin. Chir., 33:1, 1886.

BROOKS, B., JOHNSON, G. S., and KIRTLEY, J. A., JR.: *Simultaneous vein ligation: an experimental study of the effect of ligation of concomitant vein on the incidence of gangrene following arterial obstruction.* Surg. Gynec. Obstet., 59:496, 1934.

CARREL, A.: *Surgery of the Blood Vessels.* Bull. Johns Hopkins Hosp., 1907.

CREECH, O.: *Endo-aneurysmorrhaphy and treatment of aortic aneurysm.* Ann. Surg., 164:935, 1966.

CROSS, F. S., GLOVER, D. M., SIMEONE, F. A., and OLDENBURG, F. A.: *Congenital arteriovenous aneurysms.* Ann. Surg. 148:649, 1958.

CULLEN, M. L., ET. AL.: *Studies on the effects of concomitant venous ligation in arterial (acute) occlusion.* Surg. Gynec. Obstet., 89:722, 1949.

DeBAKEY, M. E., and SIMEONE, F. A.: *Battle injuries of the arteries in World War II, an analysis of 2471 cases.* Ann. Surg., 123:534, 1946.

THE EXTREMITIES

DE TAKATS, G.: *Vascular Surgery.* W. B. Saunders, Philadelphia, 1959.
Aneurysms, general considerations. Angiology 5:173, 1954.

DONAVAN, T. J.: *Uses of plastic tubes in reparative surgery of battle to injuries to arteries with and without intra-arterial heparin administration.* Ann. Surg., 130: 1024, 1949.

EUFINGER, H.: *Akute Chirurgie der Arterien.* Ferdinand Enke Verlag, Stuttgart, 1961.

FERGUSON, I. A., BYRD, W. M., and McAFEE, D. K.: *Experiences in the management of arterial injuries.* Ann. Surg., 153:980, 1961.

FRANZ: *Lehrbuch der Kriegschirurgie.* J. Springer, Berlin, 1936.

FREEMAN, N. E.: *Burns, Shock, Wound Healing, and Vascular Injuries. Military Surgical Manuals.* National Research Council. W. B. Saunders, Philadelphia, 1943.
Arterial repair in the treatment of aneurysms and arteriovenous fistulae. Ann. Surg., 124:888, 1946.
Acute arterial injuries. JAMA, 139:1125, 1949.

FREEMAN, N. E., WYLIE, E. J., and GILFILLAN, R. S.: *Regional heparinization in vascular surgery.* Surg. Gynec. Obstet., 90:406, 1950.

GAGE, I. M.: *The technical simplicity of the Matas endoaneurysmorrhaphy.* Ann. Surg., 119:468, 1944.

GAGE, I. M., and OCHSNER, A.: *The prevention of ischemic gangrene following surgical operations upon the major peripheral arteries by chemical section of the cervico-dorsal and lumbar sympathetics.* Ann. Surg., 112:938, 1940.

GOODMAN, C.: *Blood vessel suture, its use instead of the ligature in war surgery.* Amer. J. Surg., 60:196, 1943.

GUTHRIE, C. C.: *Blood Vessel Surgery and Its Applications.* Longman, Green & Co., New York, 1912.

v. HABERER, H.: *Weitere Erfahrungen über Kriegsaneurysm mit besonderer Berücksichtigung der Gefässnaht.* Wien. klin. Wchnschr., 28:435, 471, 1915.

HALSE, T.: *Heparin und Heparinoide Dicumarol.* S. Hirzel, Stuttgart, 1950.

HALSTED, W. S.: *Partial, progressive, and complete occlusion of the aorta and other large arteries in the dog by means of the metal band.* J. Exper. Med., 11:375, 1909.
The effect of ligation of common iliac artery on the circulation and function of the lower extremity. Bull. Johns Hopkins Hosp., 23:191, 1912.

HARRISON, J. H.: *Synthetic materials as vascular prostheses: III. Long term studies on grafts of nylon, dacron, orlon and teflon replacing large blood vessels.* Surg. Gynec. Obstet., 108:433, 1959.

HEIDRICH, L.: *Ueber Ursache und Häufigkeit der Nekrose bei Ligaturen grosser Gefässtämme.* Beitr. z. klin. Chir., 124:607, 1921.

HERRMANN, L. G., and REID, M. R.: *The management of arteriovenous aneurysm in the extremities.* Amer. J. Surg., 44:17, 1939.

HOLMAN, E.: *Arteriovenous Aneurysm.* The Macmillan Company, New York, 1937.

THE BLOOD VESSELS

Clinical and experimental observations on arteriovenous fistulae. Ann. Surg., 112:840, 1940.
Arteriovenous fistula. Ann. Surg., 122:214, 1945.
Fundamental principles governing the care of traumatic arteriovenous aneurysm. Angiology, 5:145, 1954.
New Concepts in Surgery of the Vascular System. Charles C Thomas, Springfield, 1955.

HUFNAGEL, C. A.: *The use of rigid and flexible artery prosthesis for arterial replacement.* Surgery, 37:165, 1955.

HUGHES, C. W.: *The primary repair of wounds of major arteries.* Ann. Surg., 141:297, 1955.
Vascular surgery in the armed forces. Mil. Med. 124:30, 1959.

HUGHES, C. W., and BOWERS, W. F.: *Traumatic Lesions of Peripheral Vessels.* Charles C Thomas, Springfield, 1961.

JAHNKE, E. J., JR., and SEELEY, S. F.: *Acute vascular injuries in the Korean War.* Ann. Surg., 138:158, 1953.

JAHNKE, E. J., JR., and HOWARD, J. M.: *Primary repair of major arterial injuries.* Arch. Surg., 66:646, 1953.

KREMER, K.: *Chirurgie der Arterien.* Georg Thieme Verlag, Stuttgart, 1959.

KREMER, K., VOLKMANN, E., FRANCKE, D., and SUCHOWSKY, G.: *The problem of transplantation of blood vessels: Experimental studies of autoplastic vein transplantation.* Langenbeck's Arch. u. Deut. Ztchr. Chir. 277:471, 1953.

LANDIS, E. M., and GIBBON, J. A., JR.: *Effects of alternating suction and pressure on the blood flow to the lower extremities.* J. Clin. Invest., 12:925, 1933.

LERICHE, R.: *Les maladies des ligatures moyens de les prévenir et de les traiter.* Presse méd., 1:41, 1940.

LILLY, G. D.: *The management of aneurysms of the lower extremities.* Surgery, 123:601, 1946.

LIPPMAN, H. I.: *Intra-arterial priscoline therapy for peripheral vascular disturbances.* Angiology, 3:69, 1952.

MAKINS, G. H.: *Gunshot Injuries to the Blood Vessels.* John Wright & Sons, Ltd., Bristol, 1919; American edition, William Wood, New York, 1919.

MASON BROWN, J. J.: *War injuries of the peripheral arteries. War Surgery Supplement No. 2. Wounds of Extremities.* Brit. J. Surg., 36:354, 1949.

MATAS, A.: *An operation for the radical cure of aneurysm based upon arteriorrhaphy.* Ann. Surg., 37:161, 1903.
Experiences and observations on the treatment of arteriovenous aneurysm by the intrasaccular method of suture (endoaneurysmorrhaphy with special reference to the transvenous route). Ann. Surg., 71:403, 1920.
Military Surgery of the Vascular System, Keen's Surgery Supplementary. 7:713-819, W. B. Saunders, Philadelphia, 1921.
Personal experiences in vascular surgery. Ann. Surg., 112:802, 1940.

McSWAIN, B., and DIVELEY, W.: *Arterial aneurysms.* Ann. Surg., 132:214, 1950.

MORTON, J. H., SOUTHGATE, W. A., and DEWEESE, J. A.: *Arterial injuries of the extremities.* Surg. Gynec. Obstet., 123:611, 1966.

THE EXTREMITIES

MOSZKOWICZ: *Wie vermindern wir die Gefahr der Gangrän nach Aneurysma-Operationen.* Beitr. z. klin. Chir., 97:569, 1915.

MURPHY, J. B.: *Resection of arteries and veins injured in continuity, end to end, suture, experimental and clinical research.* Med. Rec., 51:73, 1897.

MUSTARD, W. T.: *Technic of immediate restoration of vascular continuity after arterial wounds.* Ann. Surg., 126:46, 1946.

OCHSNER, A.: *Indications and technique for the interruption of impulses transversing the lumbar sympathetic ganglia.* Surg. Clin. N. Amer., 23:1318, 1943.

v. OPPEL, W. A.: *Reduzierter Blutkreislauf.* Trans. Intern. Cong. Med., London, 1913, p. 189.

OWINGS, J. C.: *Quoted by R. Matas in discussion of H. E. Pearse's Paper.* Ann. Surg., 112:935, 1940.

PATMAN, R. D., POULOS, E., and SHIRES, G. T.: *The management of civilian arterial injuries.* Surg. Gynec. Obstet., 118:725, 1964.

PEARSE, H. E.: *Experimental studies on the gradual occlusion of large arteries.* Ann. Surg., 112:923, 1940.

PEMBERTON, J. deJ., and BLACK, B. M.: *Surgical treatment of acquired aneurysm and arteriovenous fistula of peripheral vessels: Review of sixty-seven cases.* Surg. Gynec. Obstet., 77:462, 1943.

PENICK, R. M.: *The treatment of traumatic arteriovenous aneurysm.* Surg. Clin. N. Amer., 23:1377, 1943.

POTTS, W.: *A new clamp for surgical division of the patent ductus.* Quart. Bull. Northwestern Univ. Med. School., 22:321, 1948.

PRATT, G. H.: *Surgical Management of Vascular Diseases.* Lea & Febiger, Philadelphia, 1949.

REID, M. R.: *Studies on abnormal arteriovenous communications, acquired and congenital.* Arch. Surg., 10:601, 1925; 10:996, 1925; 11:25, 1925; 11:237, 1925.

REID, M. R., and ANDRUS, W. D.: *Surgery of the Arteries. In: Nelson Looseleaf Surgery.* Thomas Nelson & Sons, New York, 1927, Vol. 1, p. 733.

SEELEY, S. F., HUGHES, C. W., JAHNKE, M. C., and JAHNKE, E. J.: *Surgery of the popliteal artery.* Ann. Surg., 138:712, 1953.

SHUMACKER, H. B.: *Incisions in surgery of aneurysms.* Ann. Surg., 124:586, 1946.
Tests for and means of improving the collateral circulation in cases of aneurysm and arterio-venous fistula of the extremities. Angiology, 5:167, 1954.
The problem of maintaining the continuity of the artery in the surgery of aneurysms and arteriovenous fistulae. Ann. Surg., 127:193, 1948.

SHUMACKER, H. B., CARTER, V. L.: *Tests for collateral circulation in the extremities.* Arch. Surg., 53:359, 1946.

SPENCER, F. C., and GREWE, R. V.: *The management of arterial injuries in battle casualties.* Ann. Surg., 141:304, 1955.

STICH, R., MAKKAS, M., and DOWMAN, C. E.: *Beiträge zur Gefässchirurgie; cirkuläre Arteriennaht und Gefässtransplantationen.* Beitr. z. klin. Chir., 53:113, 1907.

774

THE BLOOD VESSELS

THOMASON, J. R., and MORETZ, W. H.: *Continuous lumbar paravertebral sympathetic block maintained by fractional instillation of procaine.* Surg., Gynec. Obstet., 89:447, 1949.

VOLLMAR, J.: *Reconstructive Chirurgie der Arterien.* Georg Thieme Verlag, Stuttgart, 1967.

WARREN, R.: *Procedures in Vascular Surgery.* Little Brown and Co., Boston, 1960.

WHITAKER, W. G., DURDEN, W. F., and FERGUSON, I. A.: *Acute Arterial Injuries.* Surg., Gynec. Obstet., 99:1, 1954.

WILSON, W. C.: *Occlusion of the main artery and main vein of a limb.* Brit. J. Surg., 20:393, 1933.

ZIPERMAN, H. H.: *Acute arterial injuries in the Korean War.* Ann. Surg., 139:1, 1954.

THE BONE
STRUCTURES 25

OF THE defects of bones, only the acquired ones will be discussed in a general way.

GENERAL DIRECTIONS

Acquired defects of bones are due to ununited fractures or to actual loss of bone from injuries (traumatic or operative) or infection. In either case, transplantation of bone grafts offers a good chance to bring about union. The success of the operation depends a great deal upon the local condition found and the technique used. In nonunion with a narrow cleft in which the surrounding tissues are healthy, the chances of regeneration of the graft are much better than in wide defects, particularly those with cicatricial changes of the surrounding soft parts.

The regeneration of a bone graft, like that of any other graft, depends upon the rapid re-establishment of its interrupted blood supply. Hence, any scar tissue surrounding the graft, any hematoma separating the graft from the surrounding tissue, or any infection is likely to lead to poor operative results. The second important factor in regeneration is the osteogenic force of the host bone and of the graft itself. The graft always dies, at least most of it, but it becomes revivified and regenerated by ingrowth of osteoblasts derived from the host bone and periosteum less than by its own surviving osteoblasts. The osteoblasts accompany the ingrowing vessels (see p. 66). Hence, a broad intimate contact between graft, host bone, and periosteum is of utmost importance.

THE EXTREMITIES

General Rules

Needless to say, the operation should not be performed in the presence of even the slightest infection. As a matter of fact, if the bone defect has been due to infection (osteomyelitis), bone grafting should be delayed for at least three months after the last fistula has closed. Prophylactic use of antibiotics is also indicated in an operation in such a case.

Any extensive destruction of the covering skin must be replaced by skin flaps prior to the bone-grafting operation. As a matter of fact, spontaneous healing of nonunions of the tibia after replacement of the overlying scars with a pedicle flap has been observed by the author. Zachariae reported several such cases. In carrying out the bone-grafting operation, thorough hemostasis is essential. A tourniquet should not be applied, to prevent postoperative hematomas. All cicatricial tissue should be removed and replaced by healthy tissue from the surroundings. This may be difficult at times, but in most instances it can be achieved by sliding muscle tissue into the defect. Sclerotic, atrophic bone ends must be removed, no matter how wide the resulting defect, until bleeding bone is encountered. Whenever the periosteum of the host area is destroyed, a periosteum-covered graft should be used, since the periosteum is not only a protection against fibrous erosion but also a bone regenerative membrane.

Technique

Exposure of Host Bone: The operation, after the usual aseptic precautions, starts with the preparation of the host bone. The incision through the skin is curved so that the subsequent scar will not encroach upon the graft. The incision penetrates through all layers of the soft tissue, including the periosteum down to the bone. The bone itself is exposed subperiosteally by stripping the periosteal soft-tissue cuff away with a periosteal elevator. In other words, it is important to leave the periosteum, if it is present, attached to the soft tissues and not to the bone, since its blood supply is mainly derived from the surrounding soft tissues. The importance of the periosteum has been previously stressed. (For proper incisions for adequate exposure, see Henry, Nicola.)

Preparation of Host Bone: The host bone is now prepared for reception of the graft. There are various ways to do this. Whenever possible, the author prefers the one demonstrated in Figure 335, *left.* So, for instance, in a case of simple nonunion where the cleft is small and the bone stumps are healthy and bleeding, the outer cortex of the bone is removed in a staircase manner with an electric saw and chisels well above and below the cleft, until the medullary cavity is freely exposed (see p. 70). Exposure of the

778

medullary cavity opens up a vascular bed and frees the medullary osteo-genetic forces—both essential factors for a quick vascularization and re-generation of the graft. The posterior halves of the cortex remain in place, as well as the posterior part of the thin disk of scar tissue, furnish-ing a firm connection. Four wires of stainless steel to be used later for fixation of the graft are now looped around the bone with a ligature car-rier, two above and two below the cleft. Fixation of the graft with screws may be preferable to wire fixation (Fig. 335, *right*). The whole wound is covered with wet gauze.

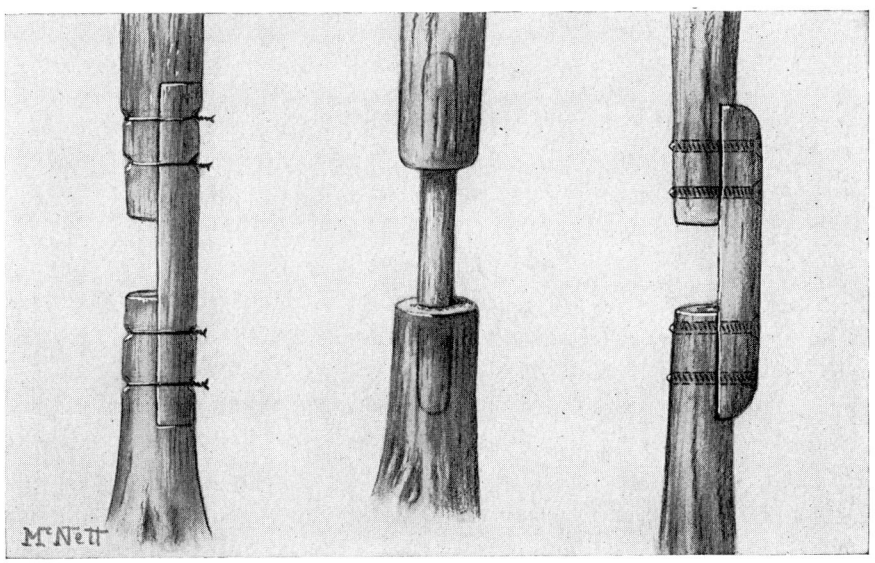

Fig. 335. Various ways of fitting and fixing bone grafts to host bone.

Transplantation and Fixation of Graft: The bone graft is now re-moved (from the anterior surface of the tibia, for instance) (for technique, see p. 70). If two operating teams are available, the graft may be removed at the same time the graft bed is prepared. If the periosteum of the graft bed is destroyed, the tibia graft should be removed, covered with its periosteum. The graft should be a full-thickness cortical graft; in other words, its posterior surface should be lined with the medullary endos-teum. The graft is made to fit into the graft bed, with its medullary side against the medullary surface of the host bone and fastened in place by twisting the four wires firmly around it. To prevent slipping of the wires, graft and cortex are notched with a rongeur, as demonstrated in the draw-ing (Fig. 335, *left*). The wires may be twisted with a special twister, but may also be firmly twisted with ordinary pliers by pushing the bone away with the thumb of the left hand while pulling and twisting the crossed wire ends at the same time with the right hand. If vitallium screws are used for fixation of the graft, the graft is held in place with a bone clamp while three holes are drilled above and below the cleft through graft and posterior cortex of the host bone. The drill used for this procedure should be thinner than the selected screws. The screws are then inserted through the drill holes and should be long enough to penetrate the opposite cortex of the host bone. After fixation of the graft, the soft tissues are sutured firmly around the graft so that they are in intimate contact with it. To facilitate closure of the periosteum-soft tissue cuff it may be advisable to make longitudinal slits through the periosteum opposite the graft (Bishop et al.). Closure of the skin follows.

Since the introduction of the intramedullary nail by Küntcher an excellent method of fixation may be provided for certain cases of grafting of the long bones. Its advantages for fixation of the femur and the humerus are particularly striking. D'Aubigné immobilizes the extremity after such a procedure for only one month.

In case of nonunion with a wide cleft or an actual defect of bone, all scar tissue between the bone stumps must be removed. If the bone stumps are sclerotic and avascular, they must be resected until bleeding bone is encountered. The bone stumps are now brought into alignment and prepared as described in the foregoing. To facilitate this, it may become necessary to lift the bone stumps out of the wound with a special bone clamp. This can be done, to a certain extent, without disturbing the circulation of the bone, since each bone stump ordinarily has a well-developed collateral circulation through the epiphyseal and metaphyseal vessels. The adjustment and fixation of the full-thickness cortical graft is the same as that previously described.

After-Treatment

The extremity is immobilized in an unpadded split plaster cast. The immobilization must be complete; hence, the cast must include the joints proximal and distal to the grafted bone. The place from which the graft was taken is sutured and dressed in such a way that the dead space at the site of removal is obliterated by placing a longitudinally folded compress of gauze upon the skin over the donor area. A dressing pad is applied; moderate pressure is applied by a circular bandage. If a thick graft was taken, the donor leg should be encased in an unpadded plaster cast for four weeks. If the tibia, unfortunately, should have been fractured during the removal of the graft, the leg should remain immobilized for eight weeks.

780

THE BONE STRUCTURES

A bone graft passes through three phases before it becomes an organic unit (see p. 75): (1) the stage during which the graft is dead; (2) the stage of transformation into living tissue (the osseous tissue condenses, the surface becomes smooth, and organic fusion occurs between graft and host bone); (3) the stage of functional adaptation in form and increased strength of the graft to its mechanical requirements, whereby the graft becomes thinner or thicker according to the functional demand. Hence, the important principle of the after-treatment is absolute immobilization of the grafted limb during the first and second stages of regeneration, that is, from two to five months. It is during those stages that the graft has the least resistance, not only to rough handling but also to minor influences, especially when the latter are ever present. Therefore, fractures or formation of fissures are the consequence of too-early mobilization. Thus, the grafted limb must remain immobilized until the roentgenogram shows good fusion between graft and host bone. If infection should occur, the graft need not be removed immediately for it may happen that, in spite of pus formation, the entire graft or parts of it heal.

Alternative Methods

Massive Onlay Graft (Henderson-Campbell): The principle is demonstrated in Figure 335, *right.* The medullary cavity is not opened. The anterior rounded surface of the cortices above and below the cleft are shaved off with a chisel until a flat surface is created; a full-thickness cortical graft from the tibia is removed and placed with its medullary side against the prepared surface of the cortices. It is held in place with a bone clamp and fastened with vitallium screws. In addition, cancellous spongy bone taken from the donor bone and scrapings or shavings from the host bone are placed about the site of the cleft and the margins of contact between bone graft and fragments.

Inlay Graft (Albee): With a twin-bladed, circular motor saw, a full-thickness piece of cortex of sufficient size is removed from above and below the cleft. A slightly wider but otherwise identically shaped graft, corresponding in length to the entire length of the gutter, is removed from the tibia and driven into and fastened firmly to the gutter with vitallium screws.

Sliding Graft: In suitable cases—mostly the tibia when the cleft is small and the adjacent bone stump healthy, vascular, and of sufficient length—a sliding inlay graft (Albee) or massive sliding graft (Gill) can be used.

Bone-Pegging (Fig. 335, *center*): This has been a popular method, popular because of its simplicity. The destruction of medullary tissue, resulting from driving the peg into the medullary cavity, has often caused failures. Hence, a bone peg should be used only in exceptional cases, that is, in regions where the peg is driven through cancellous bone and not through the medullary cavity—for instance, in bridging nonunions of the neck of the femur, of the naviculare of the wrist, of the internal malleolus, of the head of the humerus, of the upper condyle of the tibia.

Interposition of Cancellous Bone Blocks: Nicoll advocates the use of a solid block of cancellous bone which is interposed between the ends of the host fragments and must be tight fitting. It is held in this position by internal fixation with a metal plate.

Bone Chips: See page 74.

DEFORMITIES

Only the deformities of the shaft of the bones will be discussed in a general way; most of these operations belong to the orthopedic field. Those deformities which are caused by rickets or malunions after fracture are amenable to correction, while those caused by osteomyelitis, syphilis, and otitis fibroid cannot be attacked owing to the massive thickening of the bone.

DIAPHYSIS

In severe deformities of the diaphysis, a simple osteotomy through the height of the convexity, followed by proper alignment of the shaft and immobilization in a plaster cast, is sufficient. In more severe cases, a wedge-shaped osteotomy (the base of the wedge over the convexity), with removal of a piece of bone of proper width, or a curved osteotomy, permitting rotation of the fragments in the plane of the curvature, or multiple simple osteotomies through the convex side of the shaft are required to straighten the deformed shaft. In selecting the site of the artificial fracture line, the height of the convexity should not be the only guide. If possible, the shaft should not be osteotomized through the entrance canal of the nutrient artery, which may be demonstrable by x-ray examination.

METAPHYSIS AND EPIPHYSIS

Deformities of the metaphysis and epiphysis resulting in genu varum are of rachitic origin or are osteodystrophies from endocrine or unknown disturbances (Blount) or traumatic premature closure of a portion of the epiphyseal cartilage plate (Abbott and Gill). Others develop after fractures or infections.

782

In genu valgum the seat of the deformity is ordinarily found in the distal metaphysis (part between the epiphysis and shaft) of the femur. The typical appearance of the deformity is the abduction and slight inward rotation of the leg, causing the so-called "knock-knee." The correction is by means of an osteotomy through the median side of the lower metaphysis of the femur, followed by proper alignment of the fragments. McEven osteotomizes only the median side and fractures the lateral side manually in greenstick fashion, thus avoiding lateral displacement of the fragment.

In genu varum the deformity usually occurs at the upper metaphysis (part between upper epiphysis and shaft) of the tibia. The deformity is overcome by an osteotomy through the curved part of the tibia through the lateral and anterior cortex in a plane parallel to that of the knee joint. The remaining part of the cortex is fractured manually in greenstick fashion while the deformity is corrected. Prior to this step, however, a subperiosteal osteotomy of the fibula is performed with the costotome or chisel. The fragments are brought into alignment, the wounds are closed, and the leg is encased in a plaster cast from toes to midthigh. After four weeks this cast is changed to a walking cast, which is worn until firm union becomes demonstrated in the x-ray picture.

BIBLIOGRAPHY

ALBEE, F. H.: *Bone Graft Surgery.* W. B. Saunders, Philadelphia, 1915.
Principles of the treatment of nonunion of fracture. Surg. Gynec. Obstet., 51:289, 1930.

ARMSTRONG, J. R.: *Bone Grafting in the Treatment of Fractures.* Williams and Wilkins, Baltimore, 1945.

BANKS, S. W., and LAUFMAN, H.: *An Atlas of Surgical Exposures of the Extremities.* W. B. Saunders, Philadelphia, 1953.

BERGMANN, E.: *The role of aseptic bone necrosis in hip lesions.* Amer. J. Surg., 63:219, 1944.

BIER, A.: *Ueber Knochenregeneration, über Pseudarthrosen, und über Knochentransplantate.* Arch. f. klin. Chir., 127:13, 1923.

BISHOP, W. A., STAUFFER, R. C., and SWENSON, A. L.: *Bone grafts. An end-result study of the healing time.* J. Bone Joint Surg., 29:961, 1947.

BLOUNT, W. P.: *Tibia vara, osteochondrosis deformans tibiae.* J. Bone Joint Surg., 19:1, 1937.

BÖHLER, L.: *Die Technik der Knochenbruchbehandlung 12-13th Ed.* Wilhelm Maudrich, Wein, 1951. 5th English Ed., Grune and Stratton, New York, 1956.

CAMPBELL, W. C.: *Treatment of ununited fractures.* Amer. J. Surg., 37:1, 1923.
Operative Orthopedics. C. V. Mosby Co., St. Louis, 1939.

THE EXTREMITIES

CAMPBELL, W. C., and BOYD, H. B.: *Fixation of onlay bone grafts by means of vitallium screws in the treatment of ununited fractures.* Amer. J. Surg., 51:748, 1941.

CARLING, SIR. E. R., and OSS, J. P.: Brit. Surg. Practice, 3:225, 1948.

DARRACH, W.: *Surgical approaches for surgery of the extremities.* Amer. J. Surg., 67:237, 1945.

D'AUBIGNÉ, R. M.: *Surgical treatment of non-union of long bones.* J. Bone Joint Surg., 31A:256, 1949.

HENDERSON, M. S.: *Nonunion in fractures. The massive bone graft.* JAMA, 81:463, 1923.
The massive bone graft in ununited fractures. JAMA, 107:1104, 1936.

HENRY, A. K.: *Exposure of long bones and other surgical methods.* John Wright & Sons, Ltd., Bristol, 1927.
Extensile Exposure. Williams & Wilkins, Baltimore, 1957.

LEXER, E.: *Die Verwendung der freien Knochenplastik.* Chir. Kongr. Verhandl., 1908, II, p. 188. *Zwanzig Jahre Transplantationsforschung in der Chirurgie.* Arch. f. klin. Chir., 138:25, 1925.

MAY, H.: *Anzeigstellung zer Behandlungsart der Pseudarthrosen der langen Röhren Knochen.* Deutsche Ztschr. f. Chir., 239:184, 1933.
Regeneration of bone transplants. Ann. Surg., 106:441, 1937.
The regeneration of joint transplants and intracapsular fragments. Ann. Surg., 116:297, 1942.
Double fractures and double non-unions of the shaft of the tibia. Amer. J. Surg., 75:796, 1948.

MOORE, J. R.: *Bridging of bone defects in compound wounds.* J. Bone Joint Surg., 26:455, 1944.
Osteotomy-osteoclasis. J. Bone Joint Surg., 29:119, 1947.

MOSELEY, H. F.: *Shoulder Lesions.* Paul B. Hoeber, Inc., New York, 1953.
The Atlas of Musculo-Skeletal Exposures. J. B. Lippincott, Philadelphia, 1955.

NICOLA, T.: *Atlas of Surgical Approaches to Bones and Joints.* The Macmillan Company, New York, 1945.

NICOLL, E. A.: *The treatment of gaps in long bones by cancellous insert grafts.* J. Bone Joint Surg., 38B:70, 1956.

PHEMISTER, D. B.: *Bone growth and repair.* Ann. Surg., 102:261, 1935.

RUSSE, O.: *An Atlas of Operations for Trauma.* Wilhelm Maudrich, Wien-Bonn, 1954.

SPEED, J. S., and KNIGHT, R. A.: *Campbell's Operative Orthopaedics.* Vol. I and II, 3rd Ed. C. V. Mosby Co., St. Louis, 1956.

THOMPSON, J. E.: *Anatomical methods of approach in operations of the long bones of the extremities.* Ann. Surg., 68:309, 1918.

VENABLE, C. S.: *The Internal Fixation of Fractures.* Charles C Thomas, Springfield, 1947.

WATSON-JONES, R.: *Fractures and Joint Injuries.* Vol. 2, 4th Ed. Williams and Wilkins, Baltimore, 1955.

ZACHARIAE, L.: *Tibial pseudarthroses treated by cross-leg flap.* Acta Chir. Scand., 124:557, 1962.

THE
ARTICULATIONS   26

REPARATIVE and reconstructive surgery of the joints has a wide field of application. A detailed description of the whole subject would be far beyond the scope of this book, particularly since much of this surgery belongs to the orthopedic field. Only arthroplasty and joint transplantations have been selected for short general discussion in this chapter.

ARTHROPLASTY

The first attempts at mobilizing ankylosed joints were made at the end of the last century. Helferich (1894) is given the credit for having performed the first arthroplasty in the modern sense; he mobilized an ankylosed mandibular joint, and interposed a muscle flap from the temporal muscle. Murphy (1905), however, must be given credit for having popularized this method; he transferred the principle of the flap interposition to other joints. Lexer (1906) simplified the method by using, instead of a flap, a free graft of fat tissue, while Payr and Putti became advocates of the fascial graft. They were followed in this country by Baer, Henderson, MacAusland, and Campbell. Smith-Petersen, although preceded by others in the use of foreign material, introduced vitallium cups in arthroplasties of the hip joint. Soon, other types of foreign material were advocated, such as radiotransparent cups of methacrylate resin (Harmon and others), cellophane (Wheeldon, McKeever). Buxton, in his monograph, deals with this subject from most points of view and with authority.

785

THE EXTREMITIES

Arthroplasty consists in severance of the synostosis, formation of articular surfaces, and interposition of tissue which prevents recurrence of the ankylosis and allows the articular surfaces to glide against each other.

Technique

The joint is opened with an incision which permits adequate exposure without interfering with future function (Henry, Nicola). The important ligaments are left intact or severed from their insertion near the bone in such a way that they can be reattached subsequently. If the ankylosis is due to fibrous adhesions, the latter are severed. The cicatricial joint capsule is removed as thoroughly as possible. The joint surfaces are now freshened with chisel or saw, whereby normal contours should be imitated. In bony ankylosis, the synostosis is severed, at the level of the joint cleft, with chisel or saw or burr. The joint surfaces are modeled until a sufficiently wide cleft is created. A graft of fascia lata and fat tissue is removed from the lateroposterior surfaces of the thigh (see p. 48). The fascial surface of the graft is placed upon one of the raw bony surfaces and sutured in place. (For the use of foreign-body material for interposition, see above and also p. 586.) Closure of the wound in layers follows.

After-Treatment

The extremity is immobilized in a plaster cast for two to four weeks. The cast is then removed temporarily and physical therapy is given daily under expert supervision, starting with massage and active-motion exercises. The cast may be entirely discarded after another week, and passive-motion exercises are added. Active- and passive-motion exercises should go hand in hand. Passive-motion exercises should not be forced beyond tissue tolerance. Upon evidence of exertion (pain, tenderness, hyperemia, swelling), the limb must be immobilized and all physical therapy interrupted until active symptoms have subsided.

TRANSPLANTATION OF JOINTS

In discussing joint transplantation, it is important to distinguish between transplantation of an entire joint and transplantation of half a joint. Lexer (1907) was the first to perform transplantation of an entire joint. This startling operation, mostly performed for replacement of ankylosed joints, was soon given up by its originator and replaced by simpler operations, namely, arthroplasty. Nevertheless, of the twenty-three cases in which Lexer performed such homologous transplantation, twelve cases resulted in healing of the transplant, and mobility remained

786

for a number of years. Later, however, mobility decreased and became painful, owing to extensive arthritic changes from subarticular break-down of the subchondral cancellous bone. Two of these patients—the transplant for one was taken from an executed criminal—were followed for fourteen and sixteen years, respectively. Entin et al., Erdelyi and others experimented recently with autogenous whole joint transplantations and met with the same failures. Even in homologous half-joint transplanta-tions, where only one epiphysis is transplanted, the success seems to be only temporary. More promising are autogenous half-joint transplantations.

The author has reported an experiment where he took out entire radii in dogs and returned them to their original places. Thus, transplanta-tion of bones was combined with transplantation of epiphyses (see Fig. 29). The roentgenological and histological examinations revealed complete re-generation of the bony, as well as of the cartilaginous, parts of the graft after the initial degeneration.

The author has also reported on the regeneration of joint transplants in human beings; for the literature on this subject, the reader is referred to these articles and to the articles of Herndon and Chase.

Hence, transplantation of half a joint, particularly if performed autogenously, can be considered an established procedure. The aim of the procedure is the replacement of half a joint, as a rule together with part of the bone. In short medullated bones, it is possible to replace the bone together with the two joint surfaces. If possible, the joint capsule and the periosteum of the host area should be left behind. If both must be removed, the graft should be taken without capsule but covered with peri-osteum.

AUTOGENOUS TRANSPLANTATION OF HALF A JOINT

This operation is possible only for joints in which the replacement can be made with an epiphysis which can be removed without causing damage. Hence, the source is limited. As a rule, one of the phalanges of the toes, the fourth or fifth metatarsal bone (Fig. 260), and the upper part of the fibula are the available graft sources (Fig. 33, p. 72). Only replacement of the radial part of the wrist joint with the upper part of the fibula will be described here. Replacement of metacarpal heads and shafts with corresponding metatarsal bones is described elsewhere (p. 934).

Technique

The distal part of the radius is exposed from an incision, as outlined in Figure 336 between the abductor pollicis longus and extensor pollicis brevis which are retracted toward the extensor side, and the extensor carpi

787

THE EXTREMITIES

radialis longus and brevis which are retracted to the volar side; the brachio-radialis tendon is split at the epiphysis. With a Gigli saw, the shaft of the radius is severed at a predetermined level. By pulling the distal fragment out of the wound, the remaining adherent soft tissues are severed. The ligaments and joint capsule are dissected away from the radial epiphysis, and the diseased bone is removed. Thorough hemostasis follows.

Transplantation of Fibular Graft: The proximal part of the fibula is removed, as depicted in Figure 33. It is placed in the prepared graft bed so that the head of the fibula replaces the radial epiphysis. Only after the

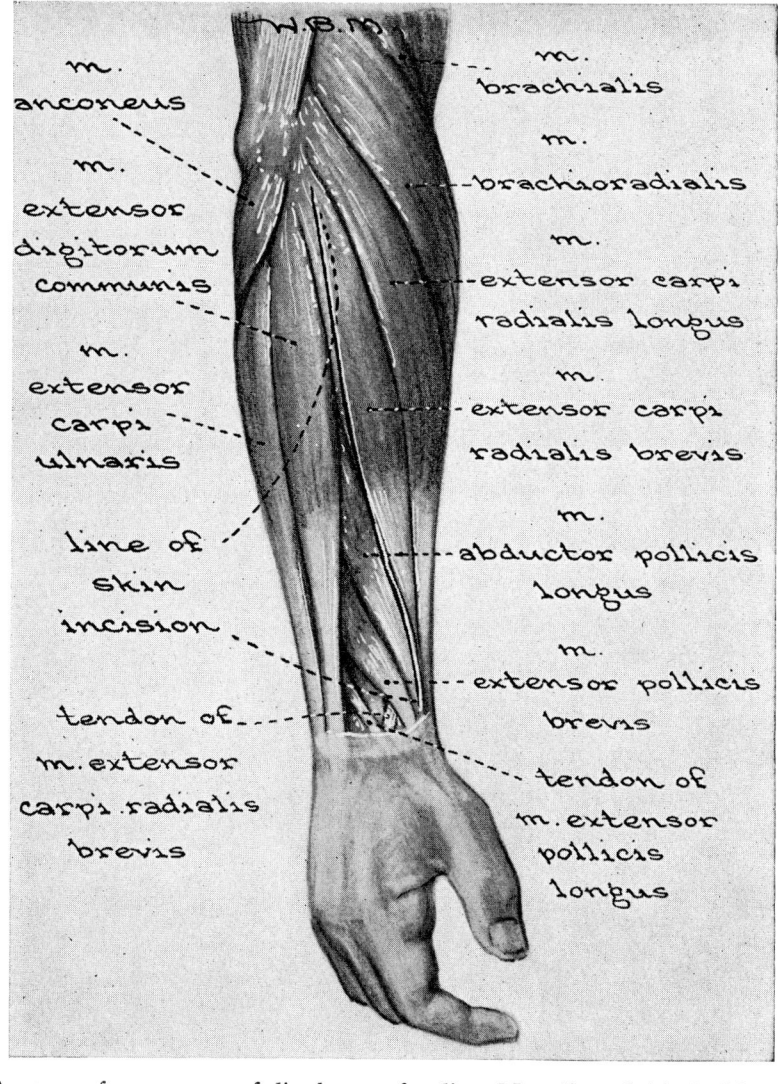

Fig. 336. Anatomy for exposure of distal part of radius. Note line of skin incision.

788

articular surface fits snugly into the joint, the shaft of the fibula and of the proximal part of the radius are shaped in a staircase manner, similar to that in Figure 335, left. Both bones are fastened together with two stainless-steel wires or screws.

After-Treatment

A plaster cast is applied from the knuckles to the upper arm, with the elbow joint in 90-degree flexion, and the forearm is kept in midposition between pronation and supination. The arm should remain immobilized for at least three months. A light leather brace is then applied, and is removed daily for bathing the arm and cautious active-motion exercises during the bath. Rotary movements of the forearm, however, should be avoided. The brace is discarded only after there is evidence of firm fusion and regeneration of the graft (five to six months postoperatively).

HETEROLOGOUS TRANSPLANTATION OF A JOINT

This method recently has become popular in replacement of the femoral head and neck (half joint transplantation) as introduced by the Judet brothers, of Paris. It has less often been used in other joints (shoulders, etc.). It is a precise operation demanding careful selection of the patient, points which have been extremely well stressed by the Judet brothers in their book. There are various types of prosthesis available made of various materials. It would be beyond the scope of this discussion to go into details. The reader is referred to the publications of Judet, Thompson, and D'Aubigné.

Recently attempts have been made to replace entire joints with foreign body substances, such as acrylic or vitallium prostheses. Mac-Ausland reported a case of an entire knee joint replacement by a vitallium prosthesis. Half and entire finger joints have been replaced with such protheses (Flatt, p. 934). This new approach to the problem of mobilization of a joint is very stimulating but still in the pioneering stage.

BIBLIOGRAPHY

ADAMS, J. C.: *A Reconsideration of cup anthroplasty of the hip.* J. Bone Joint Surg., 32B:183, 1950.

AUFRANC, O. E.: *Constructive hip surgery with the vitallium mold. A report on 1,000 cases of arthroplasty of the hip over a fifteen-year period.* J. Bone Joint Surg., 39A:237, 1957.

BÖHLER, L.: *Die Technik der Knochenbruchbehandlung 12-13th Ed.* Wilhelm Maudrich, Wien, 1951, 1957, 5th English Ed., Grune & Stratton, New York, 1956.

THE EXTREMITIES

BURMAN, M., and ABRAHAMSON, R. H.: *The use of plastics in reconstructive surgery. Lucite in arthroplasty.* Mil. Surgeon, 93:405, 1943.

BUXTON, St.J.: *Arthroplasty.* J. B. Lippincott, Philadelphia, 1955.

CAMPBELL, W. C.: *The present status of artroplasty.* Surg. Gynec. Obstet., 41: 843, 1925.
Campbell's Operative Orthopaedics. Edited by A. H. Crenshaw, M.D., 4th Ed., Vols. I and II. C. V. Mosby Co., St. Louis, 1963.

D'AUBIGNÉ, R. M., and POSTEL, M.: *Functional results of hip arthroplasty with acrylic prosthesis.* J. Bone Joint Surg., 36A:489, 1954.

DEBEYRÉ, J., and DOLIVEUX, P.: *Les Arthroplasties de la Hanche (Etudes critiques a propos de 200 cas operés).* Editions Médicales, Flammarion, Paris, 1954.

ENTIN, M., ALGER, J. R., and BAIRD, R. M.: *Experimental and clinical transplantation of autogenous whole joints.* J. Bone Joint Surg., 44A:1518, 1962.

ERDELYI, R.: *Experimental autotransplantation of small joints.* Plast. Reconstr. Surg., 31:129, 1963.
Reconstruction of ankylosed finger joints by means of transplantation of joints from the foot. Plast. Reconstr. Surg., 31:140, 1963.

HARMON, P. H.: *Arthroplasty of the hip for osteoarthritis utilizing foreign body cups of plastic.* Surg. Gynec. Obstet., 76:347, 1943.

HELFERICH, H.: *Ein neues Operations-verfahren zur Heilung der knöchernen Kiefergelenksankylose.* Verhandl. d. deutsch. Gesellsch. f. Chir., 3:504, 1894.

HENDERSON, M. S.: *What are the real results of arthroplasty?* Amer. J. Orthop. Surg., 16:30, 1918.

HENRY, A. K.: *Exposure of Long Bones and Other Surgical Methods.* William Wood & Co., New York, 1927.
Extensile Exposure. Williams & Wilkins, Baltimore, 1957.

HERNDON, C. H., and CHASE, S. W.: *Experimental studies in the transplantation of whole joints.* J. Bone Joint Surg., 34A:564, 1952.
The fate of massive autogenous and homogenous bone grafts including articular surfaces. Surg. Gynec. Obstet., 98:273, 1954.

JUDET, R., and JUDET, J.: *Technic and results with the acrylic femoral head prosthesis.* J. Bone, Joint Surg., 34B:173, 1952.

JUDET, J., et al.: *Resection—Reconstruction of the Hip; Arthroplasty with an Acrylic Prosthesis.* K. I. Nissen, Edinburgh, Livingston, 1954.

KOCHER, T.: *Text-book of Operative Surgery.* Adams, Charles Black, London, 1903.

LAMBERT, C. H., et al.: *Symposium on femoral-head replacement prostheses. Based on the report of the Committee for the study of Femoral-Head Replacement Prostheses.* J. Bone Joint Surg., 38A:407, 1956.

LAW, W. A.: *Vitallium mould arthroplasty of the hip joint.* J. Bone Joint Surg., 30B:76, 1948.

LEXER, E.: *Das Beweglichmachen versteifter Gelenke mit und ohne Gewebs-zwischenlagerung.* Zentralbl. f. Chir., p. 1, 1917.
Joint transplantations and arthroplasty. Surg. Gynec. Obstet., 40:782, 1925.

790

THE ARTICULATIONS

MacAUSLAND, W. R.: *The mobilization of elbow by free fascia transplantation, with report of thirty-one cases.* Surg. Gynec. Obstet., 33:223, 1921.
Total replacement of the knee joint by a prosthesis. Surg. Gynec. Obstet., 104:579, 1957.

MacAUSLAND, W. R., and MacAUSLAND, A. R.: *The Mobilization of Ankylosed Joints by Arthroplasty.* Lea & Febiger, Philadelphia, 1929.

MAY, H.: *The regeneration of bone transplants.* Ann. Surg., 106:441, 1937.
The regeneration of joint transplants and intracapsular fragments. Ann. Surg., 116:297, 1942.

MOSELEY, H. F.: *Shoulder Lesions.* Paul B. Hoeber, Inc., 1955.
The Atlas of Musculoskeletal Exposures. J. B. Lippincott, Philadelphia, 1955.

MURPHY, J. B.: *Ankylosis, arthroplasty.* JAMA, 44:1573, 1905.
Arthoplasty. Ann. Surg. 57:593, 1913.

NICOLA, T.: *Atlas of Surgical Approaches to Bones and Joints.* The Macmillan Company, New York, 1945.

PAYR, E.: *Gelenksteifen und Gelenkplastik.* J. Springer, Berlin, 1934.

PUTTI, V.: *Arthroplasty.* J. Orthop. Surg., 3:421, 1921.

RUSSE, O.: *An Atlas of Operations for Trauma.* Wilhelm Maudrich, Wien-Bonn, 1954.

SHEPHERD, M. M.: *A review of 650 hip arthroplasty operations.* J. Bone Joint Surg., 36B:567, 1954.

SMITH-PETERSEN, N. M.: *Arthroplasty of the hip; a new method.* J. Bone Joint Surg., 21:269, 1939.
Evolution of mould arthroplasty of the hip joint. J. Bone Joint Surg., 30B:59, 1948.
Approach to and exposure of the hip joint for mould arthroplasty. J. Bone Joint Surg., 31A:40, 1949.

SPEED, J. S., and KNIGHT, R. A.: *Campbell's Operative Orthopaedics.* Vols. I and II, 3rd Ed., C. V. Mosby Co., St. Louis, 1956.

THOMPSON, F. R.: *Two and a half years' experience with vitallium intramedullary hip prosthesis.* J. Bone Joint Surg., 36A:489, 1954.

THOMPSON, J. E.: *Anatomical methods of approach in operations on the long bones of the extremities.* Ann. Surg., 68:309, 1918.

VENABLE, C. S., and STUCK, W. G.: *The effects on bone of the presence of metals, based on electrolysis, an experimental study.* Ann. Surg., 105:917, 1937.

WATSON-JONES, R.: *Fractures and Joint Injuries,* 4th Ed. Williams & Wilkins, Baltimore, 1955.

WILSON, P. D., and McKEEVER, D. C.: *Symposium on femoral-head replacement prostheses. Based on the report of the Committee for the Study of Femoral-Head Replacement Prostheses.* J. Bone Joint Surg., 38A:407, 1956.

Section Two
The Hand

INTRODUCTORY
ASPECTS   *27*
OF THE HAND

O<small>UR</small> present time, sometimes called the "mechanized age," accounts for a great number of injuries and infections of the hand. It is estimated that in industry more than one third of all accidents involve the hands. Loss of parts or of the whole hand, either actual or functional, means in most cases a decrease in the earning capacity of the victim. Hence, the responsibility of the surgeon who takes care of a patient with an injured or infected hand is great. Unfortunately, it is not uncommon that many lesions of the hand are treated by young, surgically inexperienced physicians; often an intern sutures a lacerated tendon in an inadequately equipped outpatient department without any assistance and with results which are far from satisfactory. Perhaps a fresh surface defect is left to granulate, with the result that possible reconstruction is delayed while immediate transfer of a graft or flap would have saved the patient valuable time. Again, an infection may be opened inadequately or with an incorrect incision, resulting in extension of the infection and possible loss of function. These are only a few examples of the consequences of inexperienced surgery.

A great impetus to the development of hand surgery was brought about by World War II. In his stimulating and vividly written survey of fifty years' progress in surgery of the hand, Michael L. Mason, of Chicago, summed up by saying:

THE EXTREMITIES

"At the beginning of the second World War the Surgeon General (Kirk) requested Sterling Bunnell to supervise the handling of hand surgery in the Army. Bunnell expended a great amount of time and energy in this task and accomplished some excellent results. Various centers were established in Army hospitals throughout the country and to these patients with hand injuries were funnelled after their return from overseas. In each installation Bunnell undertook the tremendous task of training by precept and example young surgeons in the reconstructive procedures and technic of hand surgery. It was a huge job well done and gave a significant impetus to the development of hand surgery throughout the country. The young men whom he trained, along with certain others long interested in this field, formed the nucleus for the development of the American Society for Surgery of the Hand. Similar organizations in England and Sweden, and a special division in the French Society of Plastic Surgeons attest to the world-wide interest in surgery of the hand. . . . From a somewhat neglected field, turned over to the most junior man on the service, it now demands the attention of some of our best surgeons."

The progress of surgery of the hand is based on the improvement and refinement of older methods and the introduction of new and valuable therapeutic adjuncts. Of the pioneers in this field, those particularly to be mentioned are Kanavel, Bunnell, Koch, Mason, Mayer, Lexer, and Iselin. The author has referred to them extensively as well as to many other outstanding surgeons in this field, here and abroad, and wishes to acknowledge his indebtedness for their invaluable help.

The general principles of reparative surgery of the hand do not differ from those applied to other parts of the extremities, but, since the hand is the most useful member of the body, those principles need amplification and specification.

The following chapters are based on anatomical units as were the former ones: namely, the skin, subcutaneous tissue, and the fasciae; the muscles, tendons, nerves, and blood vessels; and the bones and joints. In addition, there are discussions of the hand in toto (neoplasty of fingers, cineplasty, and congenital deformities).

796

SKIN, SUBCUTANEOUS TISSUE, AND THE FASCIAE

28

DEFECTS

IN MOST cases, defects are accidental, less often due to pathological conditions such as tumors.

WOUNDS

The treatment of wounds has been described in detail on page 125. Following injuries, the hand is particularly susceptible to the development of complications leading to serious disability. For this reason, it is important to protect the freshly injured hand most carefully against such complications as infection, additional tissue damage, and stiffening. This protection is best afforded by noninterference with the wound, cleanliness of the surrounding areas, and the application of sterile protective dressings. The definitive treatment of an open hand injury should be performed only if adequate facilities for the purpose are available, such as aseptic surgical technique, adequate anesthesia, proper instruments, sufficient assistants, good lighting, and a bloodless operative field. A proper evaluation of the extent of the injury should be made at this stage. After this is done and while the wound remains covered with sterile compresses, a wide area is given a thorough cleansing, consisting of shaving and then scrubbing with soap and water. Flynn's procedure is as follows:

797

THE EXTREMITIES

Two surgeons are scrubbed. The dressing is removed and the wound covered by a sterile gauze pad. Surgeon A, with gloved hands, shaves the injured extremity from elbow to fingertips. He then rescrubs. A new sterile gauze pad is now placed over the wound, and Surgeon B with gloved hands scrubs the extremity from elbow to fingertips with a pHiso-derm, G-11, solution. Gauze pads—not brushes—are used for scrubbing. The wound is constantly protected by the sterile gauze pad during the cleansing. The scrubbing is performed for ten minutes, by the clock. With dirty and greasy skin, the scrubbing is performed for twenty minutes. The skin is then washed with saline solution, and Surgeon B rescrubs. Irrigation of the wound is now performed by Surgeon A. The injured part is placed on a sterile modified Bryant irrigating pan, so that irrigation may be performed under sterile conditions. From 2 to 20 liters of isotonic saline solution are used, depending upon the type, location, size, depth, and contamination of the wound. Surgeon A rescrubs. The skin from elbow to fingertips is now prepared by Surgeon B, with ether and aqueous Zephiran. Colored solutions are never used. The wound is protected with a sterile gauze pad so that no chemical enters the wound. The wound is draped, and Surgeon B rescrubs. Débridement and reconstruction are then performed.

General or local anesthesia may be used, depending upon the size and extent of the wound. In many cases, a pneumatic tourniquet must be applied (see p. 849).

The therapeutical principles as applied to wounds of the hand are the same as those for other wounds (p. 125), and can be summarized: conversion of the contaminated wound into a clean wound; primary closure of the wound, if it is treated within the first twelve hours; open surgical drainage, if the wound is treated later; secondary closure on the fourth day (see p. 130). The contaminated wound is changed into a clean wound by excision of the ragged wound edges and of devitalized tissue; tissue that can be preserved should not be sacrificed. This is particularly true in wounds with avulsion of skin if the skin flap is viable. The wound is closed with a few interrupted sutures. If large parts of skin have had to be sacrificed or are missing, the defect is primarily covered by skin sliding or by skin transplants, as described later. If the wound is infected, it is only débrided and not excised, and open surgical drainage is applied as outlined in greater detail on page 134. Hyaluronidase, which tends to prevent swelling, is injected subcutaneously: 150 units for each finger, 300 units for the base of the thumb and as high as 800 units for the palm. In either case, a moderate pressure dressing is applied, and the extremity is splinted with the wrist in cocked-up position, the fingers in semiflexion, and the thumb in semiflexion, abduction, and opposition.

A useful splint for this purpose is the simple universal hand splint developed by Mason and Allen. Flat splinting of the hand or any of the digits must be avoided at all times. The arm is elevated either on a pillow or in a sling. Tetanus antitoxin and antibiotics are administered.

For complicated compound wounds, the treatment should be preceded by a diagnosis and estimation of injuries to important structures. Those injured should be treated accordingly, as outlined later under the appropriate headings.

There have recently been trends to delay the primary closure. Iselin treats all of his compound hand injuries with "urgence avec opération différée" (deferred urgency): the surrounding area is cleansed, hemostasis is done if necessary, severed tissue is removed, and then the wound is dressed. The dressings are changed daily, while the definitive treatment including reconstructive measures is deferred up to three to five days. Iselin reasons that after this time the patient's general condition is improved, infection and edema are combatted, the line of demarcation is established and the patient can now be operated on under optimum technical conditions; in an emergency situation this may not be the case. Although these reasons are sound, and others—notably Scharitzer and Zubecki of Germany and Burkhalter and co-workers during the Vietnam war—have proven the rationality of this treatment in a large number of cases, most surgeons will hesitate to apply the treatment routinely until more widespread experience has been gained.

If a wound has resulted in a defect of the covering tissue, the defect should be covered with a skin graft or a pedunculated flap immediately following excision of dead tissue, unless the wound is grossly infected. This procedure not only shortens the healing period but also counteracts functional disabilities and deformities. If the defect is left to granulate scar tissue will develop, which may cause irreparable damage. Indications for the use of the different types of skin transplants are outlined in the following discussions.

BURNS

For general treatment of burns see page 156. The popular methods of local burn treatment are the pressure dressing or the exposure treatment (see 160). Although the exposure treatment seems to be preferred at the present time, it is not the ideal treatment for all burns; it is particularly unsuitable for treatment of burns of the hand. A burn of the hand causes an edema which involves not only the skin but the underlying fascia, tendons and ligaments, favoring stiffness and contracture. There is no way of preventing edema with the exposure treatment; hence, even strong advocates do not advise exposure when treating burns of the hand. The pressure dressing minimizes development of edema and also permits immobilization of the hand in the position of function. These are two important factors which counteract stiffness and contracture.

The treatment of the burned area starts with proper cleansing. Oil and grease, if used as a first-aid treatment, are removed with ether. The area surrounding the burn is cleansed with a pHisoderm, G-11, solution while the burned area itself is gently wiped with saline solution. (For details see foregoing chapter, p. 798). Blisters are not opened since they form a fine protection for regeneration of the epithelium. The entire area is rinsed with saline solution, dried and covered smoothly with vaseline gauze. Each finger is wrapped separately. A layer of flat moist dressing gauze and a bulky layer of fluffed gauze which is held in place with an elastic bandage are then applied. The hand is immobilized in the position of function (see p. 811): the wrist in cocked-up position, fingers semiflexed, and thumb in abduction and opposition. Immobilization can frequently be achieved by molding the moist gauze firmly around the fingers, hand, and wrist, thus omitting an immobilizing splint. The arm is held elevated. If the burn is of third degree and circumferential there may be potential danger of constriction, causing ischemia of the fingers. Decompression by means of relaxation incisions through the burned skin of palm and dorsum of the hand and the lateral sides of the fingers may safeguard adequate circulation.

The first dressing is changed on the tenth day unless there is evidence of infection. From then on the dressings are changed daily and consist of moist saline dressings. Loosened eschar is gently cut away with scissors. A daily arm bath in saline solution, permitting active exercises of fingers and hand, is also recommended. If the eschar has not come off completely on the eighteenth day, it is excised under light anesthesia, followed by application of alternate Dakin's solution and saline dressings for two or three days to hasten elimination of any remaining dead tissue and to prepare the granulations for skin grafting (Case 134, p. 1176).

Skin grafting is carried out as soon as possible. The raw surface is covered with a thick split skin graft. It is advisable to remove the skin graft in one piece to avoid unnecessary scarring. The graft is tailored by cutting it over fingers and hand to conform to the burned area. A bulky pressure dressing is applied over it. Over the fingers the dressing may be held in place by tying the sutures, which had been left long, over it, care being taken to keep the hand in the position of function. Unless there is evidence of infection the dressing is changed on the seventh day, sutures are removed, and a moist (saline) gauze dressing is applied; from the tenth day the dressings are changed daily and the arm is placed in a hand bath of warm saline solution for active exercises. Alternate moist and ointment dressings are applied until the graft has become an organic unit. Occupational therapy may also be needed (Case 134, p. 1176).

By maintaining immobilization of the hand in the position of function and by early skin grafting of the raw areas it is possible to prevent or at least to counteract contractures. If contractures have developed they present some of the most difficult problems in reconstruction surgery. This topic is discussed in detail on page 810.

For treatment of electrical burns see page 167.

DEFECTS OF FINGERTIPS

This very frequent injury is often treated expectantly, in the hope that the wound will granulate and heal. If the defect is only superficial, not exposing the phalanx, the resulting scar may be of good quality. Nevertheless, the healing process is much shortened and the surface more adequately protected if primarily covered with a skin graft (Reed and Harcourt, McCarroll, Sternberg). In those traumatic defects which result in exposure of the bone, Gatewood and Jones recommend the transfer of a flap from the palm—a simple and highly effective procedure. It provides skin which is similar to that lost. The cosmetic effect in one of the author's patients was such that the site of the former injury escaped the scrutinizing eyes of three medical examiners. It provides an adequate padding; it shortens the healing period; it makes amputation of the phalanx unnecessary.

Technique

The hand is prepared in the usual way and the finger is anesthetized by blocking the digital nerves at the proximal phalanx. Procaine, 2 per cent, is used without epinephrine. (The latter may cause gangrene of the finger.) The devitalized tissue is excised. If bone is not exposed, the defect is covered with a full-thickness graft which is taken from the cubital region of the elbow joint of the same side. The graft is sutured in place. The sutures are left long, a small pad of mechanic's waste is applied, and the sutures are knotted over the pad. If bone is exposed, the finger is bent so that the defect touches the palm, leaving a bloodstained pattern on it. A flap of suitable width and length is outlined with an aniline dye. The flap is constructed so that the pedicle comes to lie proximally. The important creases of the hand should not be crossed. The donor area is anesthetized, and the flap containing a sufficient amount of subcutaneous fat tissue is raised. After hemostasis, the injured finger is bent and the peripheral end of the flap sutured to the dorsal wound edge of the finger, that is, to the nail bed and also to the lateral edges (Case 128, p. 1167). If a long flap is required, the circulation may be insufficient; hence, transfer of the flap should be delayed for one week by returning the flap to its original site. (In the vast majority of cases, delay is not necessary since the blood supply is abundant; however, a sufficient amount of subcutaneous fat must be left on the flap.) After the flap is sutured to the finger, the finger is immobilized with adhesive strips, which are passed through an alcohol flame (Case 128, p. 1167). The underlying wound is covered with petrolatum gauze; a gauze dressing is applied over the immobilized finger, leaving the other fingers free. The wound is inspected two days later; the immobilizing adhesive strips may need reinforcement. Ten days after the operation, the adhesive strips are removed, and the base of the flap is incised from each side under local anesthesia, thus narrowing the pedicle. This step is followed by reapplication of the adhesive strips. On the twelfth postoperative day the pedicle is severed completely, and the flap is adjusted to the finger on the fourteenth day. This is done by means of a wedge-shaped excision of the raw surface of flap and finger and suturing of the wound edges. The raw area at the palm is left to granulate and heals quickly. In none of the author's numerous cases did this area require skin grafting or skin sliding.

If the defect involves the volar surface of the terminal phalanx, the flap is constructed so that it opens up laterad or mediad. Such a flap may also be used for small volar defects of the middle phalanx. In some cases in which the palmar flap is not applicable, the cross-finger flap may be possible (Cronin) (see below). The cross-finger flap is also suitable for amputation stumps at any level. This subject has been thoroughly discussed by Tempest, Horn, Curtis and Hoskins. Hueston closes guillotine stump defects of fingers by rotating broad-based flaps from the volar surface of the finger and skin grafting the secondary defect.

A very simple method of closing fingertip defects by utilizing small triangular flaps from the immediate neighborhood was originally demonstrated by Kutler and popularized by Fisher. In the early 1940s Kutler of Cleveland practiced the conventional closure of fingertip defects by shortening the finger and covering the stump with a local volar flap. This required removal of lateral "dog-ears." In one case he preserved the dog-ears, mobilized them, and moved them over the stump for closure. Fisher describes the method as follows: The fingertip is débrided, and the uneven edges of soft tissue and bone are trimmed (Fig. 337, *a*, *b*). Two triangular flaps are developed, one on each side of the finger, by sharply incising through the skin, with the apex of each flap directed proximally and centered in the midlateral line on either side of the finger. The flaps should not be

802

too large, each side measuring approximately one-quarter of an inch in length and the base about the same length or slightly less. Each flap is further developed by incising the skin deeper toward the nail bed and toward the volar pulp, as shown in Figure 337, *c*. The flap of pulp tissue should not be pinched or clamped with thumb forceps or hemostats, as this could impair its vascularity. A small skin hook is placed in the pulp

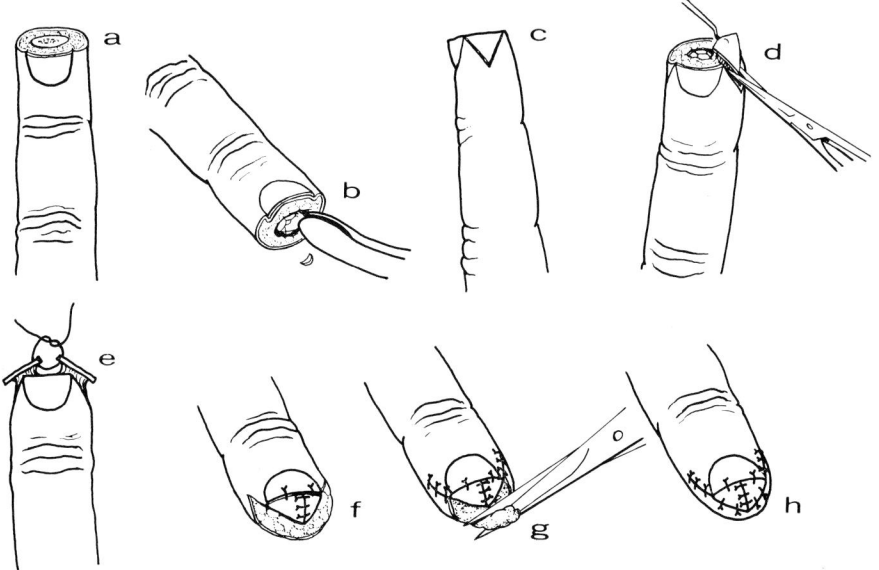

Fig. 337. The Kutler method of repair of finger-tip amputation. *a:* The uneven edges of the amputated finger tip are debrided and smoothed. *b:* The sharp corners of the amputated phalanx are rounded to provide a normal contour and to prevent impingement upon the pulp of the flaps as they are sutured together. *c:* The triangular flaps are developed by incising the skin as shown in the diagram which depicts the lateral side of the finger. *d:* The flaps are mobilized by using small plastic scissors at the apex, dividing just the amount of pulp necessary, while traction is applied at the base of the flap with a skin hook, to permit displacement of the flap distally over the tip of the phalanx. *e:* The two flaps are sutured together. *f:* The flaps are sutured in the remaining nailbed. *g:* Some of the pulp usually has to be excised before completing the closure. *h:* The completed closure is shown. (R. H. Fisher: J. Bone Joint Surg.)

toward the base of the flap and used to apply light tension in a distal direction. A pair of small scissors is used to divide just the amount of pulp at the apex of each flap necessary to free the flap so that it can be mobilized toward the tip of the finger (Fig. 337, *d*). It is not desirable nor is it necessary to divide any of the pulp toward the distal margin or base of each triangular flap. Usually not more than 50 per cent of the thickness of the proximal part of the pulp need be severed before it is possible to move

803

each flap toward the tip of the finger and to suture them together. It is very important as stated above (Fig. 337, *b*) to round off and to reshape the sharp corners of the amputated distal phalanx to simulate the normal rounded tuft and to avoid pressure on the pedicles of the two triangular flaps as they are sutured together. The bases of the two small flaps are approximated with three interrupted 00000 Dermalon sutures (Fig. 337, *e*) and then the dorsal margins of each flap are sutured to the remaining nail or nail bed (Fig. 337, *f*). This leaves fish-mouth defects on each side of the finger tip which can be closed with sutures. It is usually necessary to trim some of the excess pulp (Fig. 337, *g*) prior to suturing the volar portion of the skin of the pulp to the triangular flaps (Fig. 337, *h*).

A restoration of a fingertip is incomplete unless sensory perception is restored also. The importance of tactile gnosis has been repeatedly stressed by Moberg of Sweden, who has devised several critical tests for evaluation and to whose work we owe much in this respect. The two fingers especially requiring critical sensation are the thumb and the opposing index finger. It was Moberg (1955) who first suggested transfer of a neurovascular skin island flap from a less critical portion of the hand to restore tactile gnosis to the thumb or index finger, a procedure which was carried out by Littler and by Tubiana and Duparc in 1960 and was enthusiastically endorsed by Frackelton and Teasley, Sullivan and associates and others, but less enthusiastically by Murray and co-workers. Zrubecky has published an interesting monograph on the subject of tactile gnosis of the hand. The donor area is usually the ulnar side of the middle or ring finger or radial side of the little finger where loss of sensation is less important. Winsten selects the donor site first but starts the actual dissection in the palm.

Technique (Fig. 338)

The donor site on the ulnar side of the third (or fourth or, seldom, the fifth) finger is selected and outlined according to a pattern made of the size of the ulnar-volar side of the tip of the thumb. The line of incision is marked on the ulnar lateral side of the finger continuing in a spiral way in the palm (Fig. 338, *A*). The first incision is made in the palm and the common digital artery and nerve of the neurovascular pedicle are isolated. Mobilization of this pedicle requires ligation and separation of the branch artery to the fourth finger (Fig. 338, *B*) and careful splitting of the digital nerve proximally in the palm. The incision is then carried to the base to the outlined island of skin. The neurovascular bundle with its skin island is now dissected free. The scar or the asensitive area of pulp of the thumb is excised. If the skin is normal it can be used as a graft to cover the surface defect of the third finger; otherwise a full-thickness skin graft must be used for this purpose. A subcutaneous tunnel is now made (Fig. 338, *B*) from the midpoint of the palm to the base of the defect to be repaired. Torsion of the neurovascular pedicle must be avoided. An alternative method is a continuous incision instead of tunneling. The palmar incision would then have to be continued in a spiral way to the midlateral (ulnar) portion of the base of the thumb. When a wide defect is to be covered, turning the island flap upon itself at the natural flexion crease (Fig. 338 insert) will not compromise the circulation of the distal portion of the flap. The skin-grafted area at the third finger is

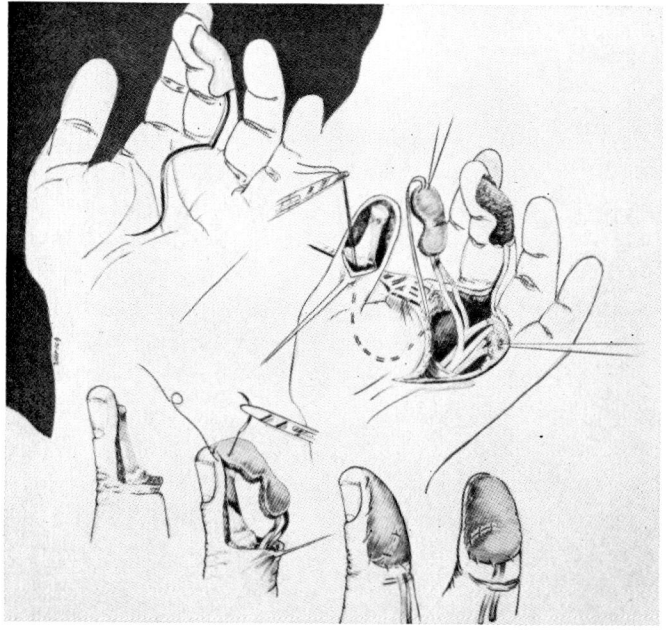

Fig. 338. *A:* Neurovascular island flap on ulnar side of midfinger and palmar incision. *B:* Dissected flap with neurovascular pedicle. Common digital nerve is split from bifurcation back into palm; branch of the common digital artery is divided. Dotted lines on thumb signify subcutaneous tunnel through which flap is drawn. *Insert:* In larger defects flap is drawn upon itself to cover digital stump pad. (J. Winsten: New Eng. J. Med.)

covered with the usual pressure dressing (see p. 801) and a light pressure dressing is applied to palm and thumb for five days. There is always a certain degree of cyanosis in the island flap following the operation which gradually subsides within a few days.

Sensory rehabilitation of the thumb can also be provided by utilizing dorsal skin of the index finger or the web between index and thumb which is supplied by the superficial radial nerve, either in the form of a neurovascular island flap (Holevich, Wilson) or by transfer of a cross-finger flap (Ardao quoted by Adams, Horton and Crawford).

LARGE DEFECTS OF DORSAL OR VOLAR SURFACE OF FINGERS

The indications for a graft or a flap are as mentioned in the foregoing, that is, a thick split graft is used if no tendons (naked tendons without tendon sheath) and no bones are exposed. If those structures are exposed, a free graft will not take. Hence, the defect must be covered with a flap.

If the defect is small, a flap from the immediate neighborhood should be raised. Several useful methods are available, notably the sliding flap from the same finger (Lewin) and the cross-finger flap (Cronin). These methods are mainly applicable to defects on the volar surface of the finger. This subject has been thoroughly discussed by Tempest, by Horn, by Curtis and by Hoskins. Lewin elevates a single-pedicle flap (pedicled proximally) from the dorsolateral finger surface; a layer of soft tissue should be left behind to cover the neurovascular bundle and the dorsal aponeurosis. The flap is rotated into the defect and resulting secondary defect covered with a full-thickness graft.

A more versatile method is the cross-finger flap (Cronin). For example, a defect of the volar side of the index finger is covered with a flap which is raised from the dorsoradial side of the third finger and pedicled volarward without injuring the digital vessels and nerves. It is hinged volarward and sutured into the defect of the index finger. The donor area at the third finger is skin grafted. The flap can usually be transplanted without delayed stages. A light plaster splint is used for immobilization. Kislov and Kelly immobilize the fingers by drilling a Kirschner wire through two adjacent phalanges. The flap is gradually severed from its pedicle after twelve to seventeen days.

For large dorsal defects, if local flaps cannot be used, the pocket flap from the abdomen is recommended (p. 86; Cases 127, 131, pp. 1166, 1172). For volar defects, a single-pedicle flap can be constructed from the same or the opposite side of the abdomen (Cases 129, 133, pp. 1168, 1175). The flap should be cut as thinly as possible, without, however, endangering its blood supply. The donor site can be closed primarily by undercutting the wound edges and by skin shifting. To counteract shrinkage, the flap should be made one-third larger than required. (For immobilization, see p. 808.)

Another donor area to be recommended is the forearm or upper arm of the opposite side. The injured hand is laid upon the opposite arm, and both are immobilized. Means of closing the donor site and counteracting shrinkage are the same as just described for the single-pedicle abdominal flap. Reid, McCash, and others have demonstrated the versatility of this technique. If the forearm must be held strongly supinated, a heavy Kirschner wire is drilled into radius and ulna and left in place until the flap is severed from its pedicle (Howard quoted by Bunnell) (Fig. 339).

LARGE DEFECTS OF DORSAL OR VOLAR SURFACE OF HAND

The causes of large surface defects of the hand are manifold. Crushing injuries, avulsion of the skin, and severe burns are the common causes; less common are defects from removal of tumors or from other pathological conditions. Again, it is emphasized that these defects should be covered as early as possible. If the injury has resulted in loss of the covering tissue from avulsion of the skin, for instance, without exposure of important subfascial structures, the contaminated wound is converted into a clean wound (see p. 798) and the raw surface covered with a thick split graft. It is advisable to remove the graft in one piece to avoid unnecessary scarring.

In all cases where tendons and other important structures are exposed or will need replacement in the future, transfer of a pedunculated flap is the only choice. The flap is usually raised from the same or less often from the opposite side of the abdomen or lower chest, very rarely from the median part of the thigh. The tube flap, being a more complicated method, is not needed for most surface defects of the hand. The larger pocket flap may also be of limited use. In addition to having unquestionable advantages, it has many drawbacks. The tremendous raw surface of the donor site, which after the flap is raised and sutured to the hand comes to lie beneath the latter, causes a great deal of drainage and is a constant threat of infection. Primary closure of the donor wound by skin shifting or skin grafting has been unsuccessful in the author's hands. Hence, a large pocket flap should be used only rarely, and may be indicated for large transverse defects comprising the entire dorsum of the hand (Case 132, p. 1174).

In all cases in which only a part of the dorsal or volar surface is denuded, a pocket flap is contraindicated, since large parts of the flap—those lying on the uninjured skin of the hand—are not needed. They also add another source of irritation and possible infection to the large raw surface of the donor wound. In these cases, and they are the majority, the author prefers the open single-pedicle flap. The abdominal flap is used for dorsal defects as well as for volar defects. If the forearm must be held strongly supinated, a heavy Kirschner wire is drilled into radius and ulna and left in place until the flap is severed from its pedicle (Howard quoted by Bunnell) (Fig. 339). For defects at the ulnar side of the dorsum of the hand, the flap should be pedicled in the lower portion (Cases 130, 131, pp. 1170, 1172); for defects at the radial side of the dorsum (Fig. 340; Case 140, p. 1182) and the palmar surface (Fig. 339) in the upper portion. This position of the pedicle has some bearing upon circulation of the flaps. The venous return is better in a flap with an inferior—that is, dependent—pedicle and vice versa. Hence, the circulation is more adequate in a flap with a lower rather than with an upper pedicle. This raises the question of immediate or delayed transfer of the flap. If the pedicle of the flap can be made broad—and this can be done often—the flap can be transferred immediately. If the pedicle must be narrow, transfer must be delayed (see p. 83). If delaying becomes necessary in a traumatic defect, the wound of the hand is covered temporarily with sterile dressings or, if a long interval is expected, a split skin graft is used or a "biological dressing"; a moderate pressure dressing and a splint are applied. If there is no evidence of infection, the dressing is left in place for one week. It is then changed and the arm placed in a warm hand bath, and active finger exercises are instituted while the hand is in the water. This process should be repeated every day and the splint reapplied each time. Whenever the flap is ready for transfer (for details, see p. 83) it is raised, and if the circulation remains adequate it is transferred. Prior to the transfer of the flap, however, the abdominal donor wound is skin grafted. If the flap is too bulky, some fat is excised from its raw surface. The flap is sutured to the defect of the hand after the granulations of the wound have been sliced down to their yellow vascular base, or after excision of the skin graft if such had been employed. The suturing should be done as accurately as possible, particularly if the webs between the fingers need covering. The arm is now immobilized to the abdomen in a plaster cast.

Technique (Immobilization of Left Forearm to Abdomen)
(Figs. 339, 340)

If the patient is under general anesthesia he is propped up and held in this position by one assistant who places the flexed elbow joint on the table and supports the back of the patient with his hyperflexed hand; another helper holds the left arm of the patient in position and a third holds the right arm abducted while the anesthetist holds the head. One strip of felt 6 to 8 inches wide is laid longitudinally against the left loin and lateral side of chest. Another piece 5 inches wide is laid over either the left or the right shoulder. A roll of Webril 5 inches wide is wrapped around the lower part of the chest and around the left or right shoulder. A plaster bandage 4 inches wide is wrapped in the same manner as the Webril. The patient is placed in supine position.

The cast must be allowed to dry. A strip of felt 4 inches wide is then wrapped around the forearm and held with adhesive strips. A piece of Webril is used for measuring the length of a loop around the forearm

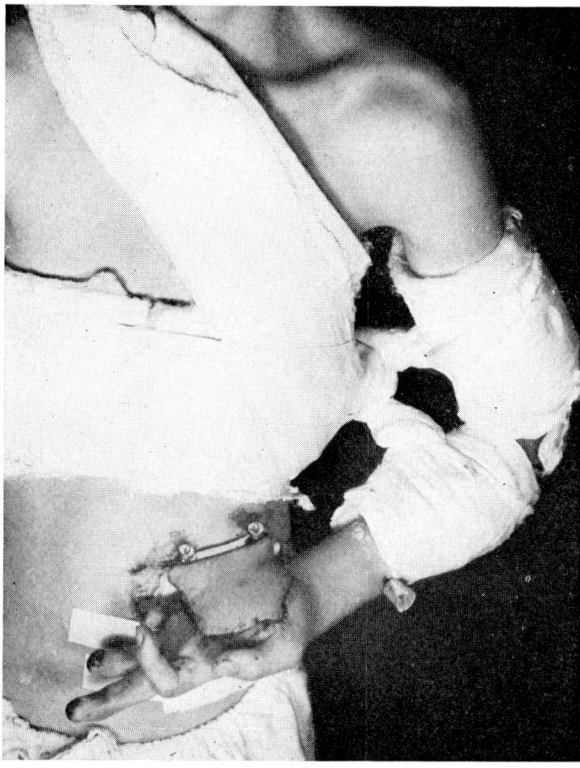

Fig. 339. Immobilization of hand to same side of abdomen. Shoulder plaster strap over opposite shoulder. Clamp applied to pedicle for gradual separation. Kirschner wire covered with a cork through radius and ulna to keep arm in pronation.

to be twisted once—as a figure-of-8—or several times, depending upon the distance of the forearm from the chest; one free end of the loop is placed on the front part of the chest cast and one on the back. The Webril loop is then untwisted. A dry plaster bandage 3 inches wide is rolled out to make a layer using the Webril for measurement. This is immersed in water and wrapped around the forearm and twisted as the Webril had been twisted, one or several times. One free end is laid upon the anterior part of the chest cast and the other around the posterior one. The patient

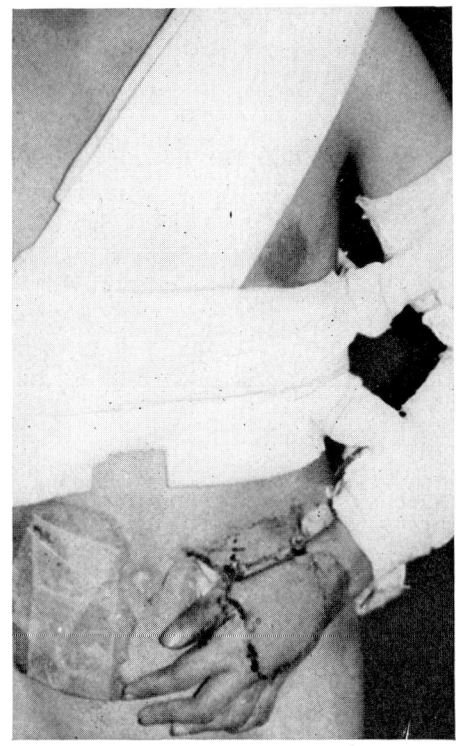

Fig. 340. Immobilization of hand to same side of abdomen. Shoulder plaster strap over shoulder of same side. Clamp applied to pedicle for gradual separation.

is again elevated to a half-sitting position and a plaster bandage 4 inches wide is wrapped around the chest part of the cast to incorporate the free ends of the loop. The patient is replaced in the supine position while an assistant holds the arm to the abdomen so that the flap is not under tension. After this part of the cast has dried, a similar procedure to hold the upper arm immobilized to the chest part of the cast is performed.

After-Treatment

See page 80. (Cases 130, 131, 140, pp. 1170, 1172, 1182.)

DEFORMITIES

CICATRICIAL CONTRACTURES

Cicatricial contractures are more often due to burns than infections. They present some of the most difficult problems in reconstructive surgery. These problems increase with the depth of the scar. While in other parts of the body a second-degree burn, as a rule, does not cause any

810

functional damage, in the hand, particularly at the dorsum, it is quite frequently followed by severe contractures. In a second-degree burn, the deep layer of skin remains undamaged. Ordinarily, epithelium regenerates from this area and covers the raw surface. Occasionally in the hand however, particularly at the dorsum, the deep layer of skin does not regenerate epithelium but develops an irregular hypertrophic or keloid-like contracting scar. Infection plays a role, but even without infection such a scar can develop. The contracture of the skin soon causes a secondary contracture of the deep fascia, tendon, joint capsules, and ligaments. Of these structures, the contractures of the collateral ligaments of the metacarpophalangeal joints are most disastrous. When the metacarpophalangeal joints are in extension or hyperextension, the collateral ligaments are maximally relaxed. Prolonged immobilization in hyperextension of the fingers or fixation of the joints in this position from dermatogenous or desmogenous contractures causes a rapid shortening of the collateral ligaments, which prevents a normal rotation of the phalangeal joint over the head of the metacarpal bone (Case 136, p. 1178). It also causes a contracture of the posterior part of the joint capsule, upsets the normal action of the interosseous and lumbrical muscles, and increases the pull of the flexor tendons, causing a flexion of the interphalangeal joints and the well-known picture of claw hand (Bodenham). Such a contracture can readily be prevented by immobilizing the hand in the position of function (Kanavel, Koch, Mason, Bunnell), that is, flexion of the metacarpophalangeal joints, midflexion of the interphalangeal joints, and extension (cocked-up position) of the wrist. The best way to counteract contractures, however, is by active-motion exercises in a warm saline bath. Hence, immobilization should be discarded temporarily or permanently as soon as possible.

This claw contracture is also termed the "intrinsic-minus" hand (Bunnell), since it is due to a complete loss of action of the intrinsic muscles as one sees it also after median-nerve and ulnar-nerve palsies. From this sort of contracture, one must distinguish the "intrinsic-plus" hand, or intrinsic contracture of the hand, which has been recognized as an entity and was first reported as such by Bunnell, Doherty and Curtis. This contracture, which is due to ischemia, fibrosis, or spasm of the intrinsic system, gives the impression that the intrinsic muscles are acting to a much greater degree than normal, i.e., the metacarpophalangeal joints are strongly flexed, the first interphalangeal joints are in full extension, and the distal joints may be in slight flexion. This intrinsic contracture, however, is only rarely associated with contracture of the skin. Curtis described the various tests and treatment. A good description of the condition and treatment by the Littler "release" operation is also given by Harris and Riordan.

THE EXTREMITIES

In a third-degree burn, the superficial fascia may act as a barrier. On the dorsum of the hand, however, skin and superficial fascia are thin; hence, in penetrating burns, the superficial fascia is very likely to be destroyed. This results in exposure of the tendons and, at the dorsum of the fingers, exposure of the interphalangeal joints. Contractures develop early. Those of the web and interphalangeal joints are the most serious. On the volar side, skin and fascia are thicker. Hence, the deeper structures are less often involved. However, if the tough palmar fascia is destroyed and the tendon sheaths, the powerful flexor tendons, and other fascial or tendon structures are exposed and contractures develop, the latter are much more difficult to overcome than those at the dorsum.

The principle in correcting these contractures consists of excision of the entire scar, reduction of the contracture, and closure of the defect with a graft or a flap. It has been the experience of a number of surgeons (Blair, Brown, Koch, Garlock, Padgett, MacCollum, Conway, Dufourmentel, Tierny, Krömer, Greeley, May, Matev and Holevich) that grafts can more often be used than previously thought possible. Brown states that grafts have given satisfactory results in a high percentage of patients and in many where the use of a pedicle flap might have been thought necessary. The application of a skin graft may require more time at one operation, but the total amount of work may be much less. A free graft, however, can be used only if the tendons, bones, and joints do not need to be exposed. If they must be exposed or need later reconstruction, the transfer of a flap is the only choice (Case 140, p. 1182).

Technique (Contracture of Dorsum of Hand)
(Cases 135, 136, pp. 1177, 1178)

The operation is performed under general anesthesia, the operating field prepared in the usual way with soap, water, and alcohol, and a blood-pressure cuff inflated to obtain a bloodless field (see p. 849). The entire scar is outlined with an incision; it is important that every bit of scar tissue should be removed, and hence that the outlining incision should run within normal tissue. At the finger webs, the incision must usually be carried to the flexor side.

The depth of the incision depends upon the depth of the scar tissue. As explained previously, in a second-degree burn the cicatricial changes primarily involve the skin. Hence, the incision should penetrate just through the skin and reach the space between the skin and superficial fascia. The subcutaneous veins are in this space; care should be taken not to injure them. Excision of the cicatricial skin is performed at the level of the veins (Case 135, p. 1177). In third-degree burns, in which the superficial fascia is destroyed and replaced by scar tissue, excision of the scar tissue is performed at the level of the deeper structures, but care should be taken not to expose the tendons if the use of a free skin graft is considered. To avoid exposure of the tendons, the scar tissue over the tendons is removed in layers and the tendon is gradually stretched by cross cutting the covering tissue in numerous places until full flexion can be reached. If the collateral ligaments of the metacarpophalangeal joints are contracted and have caused hyperextension fixed deformity of the metacarpophalangeal joints, it is most difficult to overcome the contracture merely by simple stretching. Invariably the ligaments have to be severed from their insertion at the metacarpal heads. This is best done according to the technique of Bunnell. The tendon of the interosseous muscle is identified and retracted away, exposing the joint capsule between the tendons of the long extensor and the interosseous muscles. By moving the joint, the thickened collateral ligaments are found. The ulnar ligament is then completely excised; the radial ligament may be left behind (p. 885). However, the capsule of the joint should not be incised, particularly not transversely, since this would lead to subluxation of the joint. Fowler points out a few obstacles that may still be in the way of joint rotation. If by flexing the proximal phalanx the interphalangeal joints extend, this is an indication that the extensor tendon is caught in scar tissue, and this must be corrected. If the joint opens like a book, instead of the phalanx gliding around the metacarpal head, the base of the phalanx is being blocked by adhesion of the anterior capsule to the metacarpal head. If this is the case, the anterior capsule should be explored and reflected from the metacarpal head with a probe or dural elevator.

If the proximal interphalangeal joints are contracted they are released according to Curtis' method (p. 816). If the dissection lasts longer than ninety minutes, the blood-pressure cuffs should be deflated temporarily and then reinflated. After dissection is completed, the blood-pressure cuff is deflated and thorough hemostasis instituted. The cuff is then reinflated.

The volar side of the forearm and hand is placed on a sterile, well-padded splint (wire-mesh splint or aluminum). The splint is bent until the fingers are in semiflexion. The wrist is slightly extended. The arm is immobilized on the splint by bandaging the wrist. The fingers are kept in semiflexion and abduction, either by simple bandaging or by wire traction applied through the bone of the terminal phalanx; the wires are fastened to the end of the splint (compare with Fig. 342). The simplest way of applying wire traction through the bone of the terminal phalanx is as follows: A thin Kirschner wire is drilled through the bone and cut; rubber bands or thin stainless-steel wires are fastened to the ends of the Kirschner wire; the ends of the latter are bent acutely to prevent slipping of the elastic bands or wires.

The defect is covered with a thick split thickness graft. A large split graft is removed with the dermatome. The entire sheet of graft is laid upon the raw surface. Between the fingers, the graft is incised longitudinally with straight scissors; thus, individual extensions are formed for each finger and finger web. The graft is sutured in place as accurately as possible, and the usual pressure dressing is applied. A more efficient but more time-consuming way of applying the pressure dressing is by leaving the sutures, which hold the graft in place, long to tie them over the mechanic's waste of the pressure dressing. To avoid confusion by too many sutures, it is good to complete the dressing over one finger before suturing the graft to the other finger.

If the contracture cannot be overcome without wide exposure of the tendons, then the following possibilities of repair are available. Either one proceeds with excision of the cicatricial tissue as far as possible without exposure of tendons, covers the defect with a skin graft, and plans subsequent similar repair work (such gradual repair work is particularly advisable where the tendons have been found too tight), or, if tendons or deeper structures must be exposed, the transfer of a flap becomes necessary (Case 140, p. 1182).

After-Treatment

Dressings and sutures are removed ten days after the operation. The pressure dressing is reapplied and should remain applied for another eleven days. Dressings, splint, and traction wires are then removed. If the pressure dressing is removed too early, particularly if motility is allowed prematurely, an acute swelling of the hand may occur, causing a delay or uncertainty of return of function.

Particularly valuable are composition exercises: tying of knots; double motions, such as gripping a square mallet handle and using the mallet; pressing spring plungers; turning square- or round-headed screws against elastic resistance; cutting with spring scissors An intriguing method of "homework" is the use of the so-called "Bouncing Putty," which is an elastic plastic material; it usually fascinates the patient, thus stimulating his digital activity.*

In a number of cases, however, splints must be reapplied between the exercises to prevent recurrence of the contracture. Some of these splints

---

* "Bouncing Putty" is made by General Electric Company and distributed by S. R. Gittens, 1620 Callowhill Street, Philadelphia, Pa. 19130.

must be especially constructed, with incorporation of elastic appliances, to hold the tissues on a mild stretch until they grow longer. Such appliances should be easily adjustable and should not cause pain. An ingenious innovation is the so-called "active splinting" of the hand as introduced by Bunnell. He found that a spring or elastic splinting is more efficient than unyielding splinting. Rigid splinting makes rigid hands. In splinting with springs or elastic, the joints are never strained to excess, nor are they immobilized. Active splinting is physiological splinting. The hands work continuously against the spring or elastic, and with

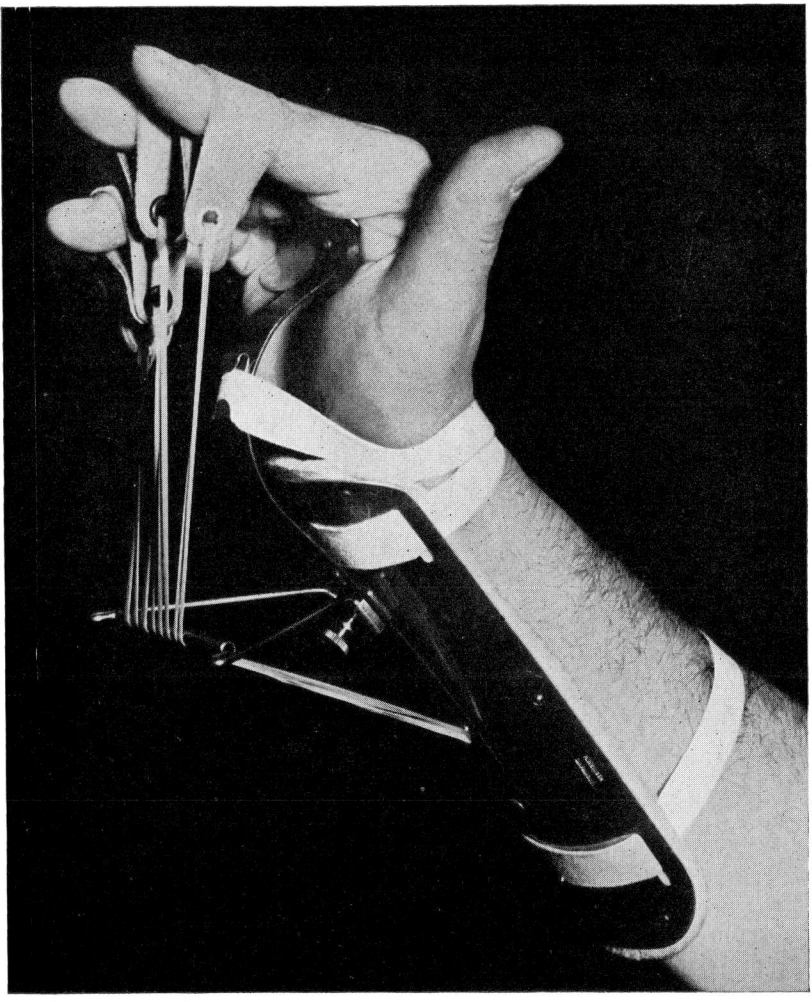

Fig. 341. *A:* Cock-up splint of flat spring steel or piano wire for dorsal flexion of wrist. It has an outrigger over which metal tube is slipped to act as roller. Outrigger gives desired direction of pull of rubbers to fingers. (Bunnell.)

815

these springs they are usually exercised. Bunnell states, "By this system you splint to mobilize, not to immobilize. It is functional splinting" (Figs. 341, *A-D*). Peacock has demonstrated many varieties of this sort of splint. Nearly all of them can be readily made in the hospital workshop. Bruner has added valuable information.

If the contracture is unyielding, forced motion may be attempted under anesthesia and the gained improvement in position maintained until the traumatic reaction is over.

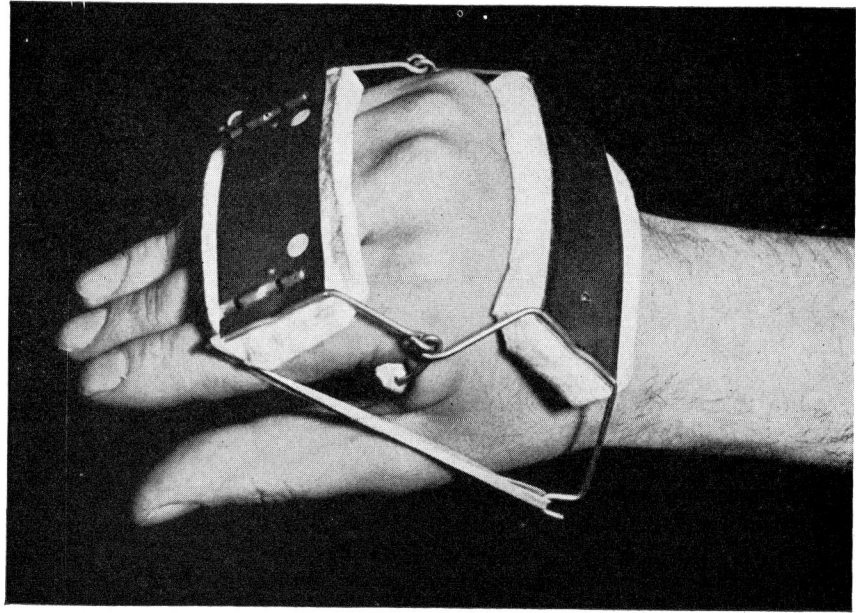

Fig. 341. *B:* Knuckle bender (Bunnell) to flex and exercise proximal joints of fingers. Splint has three padded points of pressure activated by rubber bands, with pivots corresponding to axes of joint. Rubber on back of thumb helps to oppose it.

Alternative Method: If a flap instead of a graft is to be used, the method of covering the defect is similar to that described on page 83.

In those cases in which the clawing of the fingers is due mainly to contracture of the ligamentous structures and less to contracture of the skin, repair is best performed according to the joint release method after Curtis. This technique has many followers but few have achieved the success of its originator. Adamson after a visit with Curtis stated that much of the success seems to be related to Curtis' very meticulous, carefully planned and thoughtful operative technique, clear exposure of the ligaments and a few (dental) special instruments. Being acquainted with this operation only from Curtis' article and personal communication with him, I know of no way to describe it better than to report Adamson's account after he had seen it performed by Ray Curtis (letter, published by the American Society for Surgery of the Hand).

Technique (Joint Release after R. Curtis)

The interphalangeal joint is approached from a linear and longitudinal dorsal incision extending from just beyond the metacarpophalangeal joint distally almost to the distal IP joint. By sharp dissection and coagulation of minute bleeding areas, the skin flaps are reflected laterally down

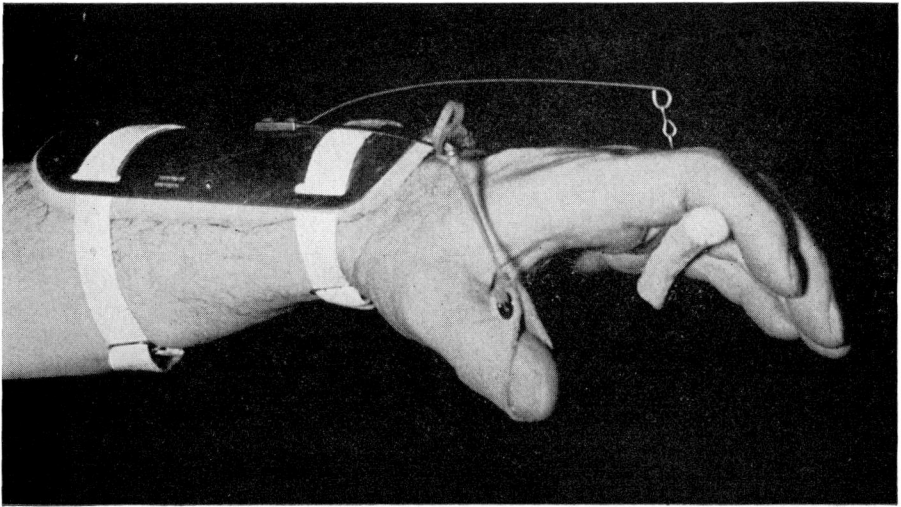

Fig. 341. *C:* Splint for radial palsy (Thomas) to furnish muscle balance. Spring wire which holds thumb is very light.

to almost the level of the flexor tendon sheath. Cleland's ligaments are clearly defined and preserved initially. A layer of deep fascia over the lateral and median sides of the joint, the transverse retinocular ligaments, are exposed. The fascial cuff is preserved in order to maintain stability of the joint after the collateral ligaments have been excised. It is not easy to dissect out the proximal and distal margins of these ligaments on either side of the proximal interphalangeal joints. Curtis frequently incises the margins so as to develop an appropriate plane to get beneath this ligament. An anatomical dissecting probe can be easily passed beneath this ligament in the plane overlying the collateral ligament of the joint. A total resection of the collateral ligament is performed by inserting the scalpel parallel to the bony insertion and proximal from the bony insertion of the collateral

817

ligament and actually cutting off the collateral ligament at its insertion in a tangential fashion. This dissection is carried distally or proximally depending upon the way one approaches the ligament and on the opposite lip of the joint; they are dissected from the bony attachment and removed in one piece.

The same procedure is performed on the other side of the joint. Now a little discoid dental probe is slipped beneath the common extensor mechanism and passed dorsally all along its course. Using the angled

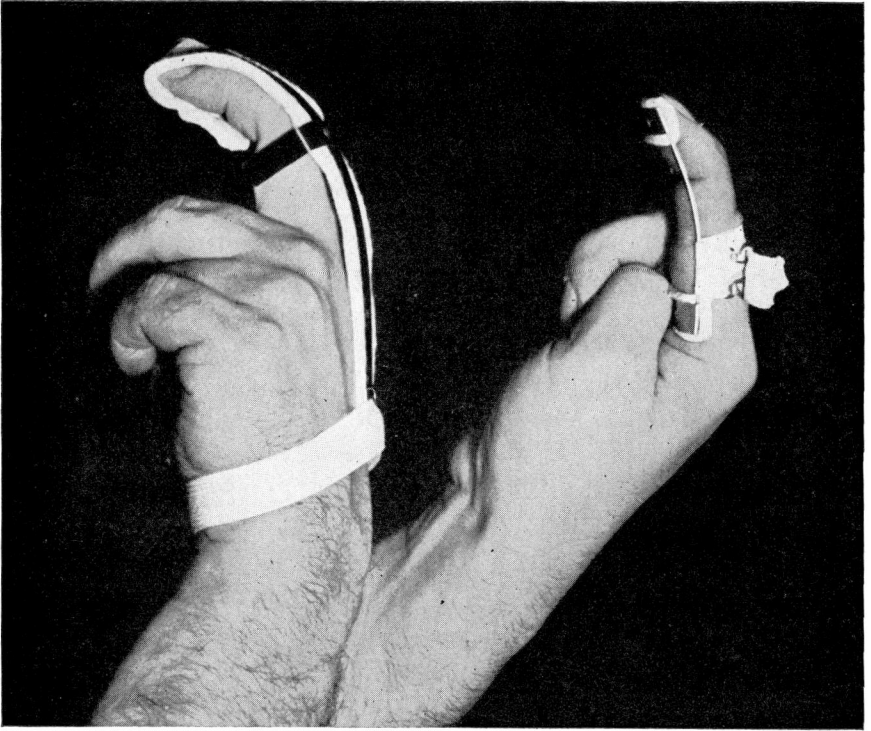

Fig. 341.   *D: Left:* Simple splint of clock spring to extend fingers. *Right:* Safety-pin splint of spring wire to straighten fingers.

portion of this instrument the dorsal capsule of the PIP joint is punctured completely along the top so that any adhesions or shortening that has occurred in the dorsal capsule will be freed. The same instrument is slipped into the joint—this may be facilitated by letting the assistant distract the joint—and the volar plate is freed bluntly from possible adhesions.

The secret of the operation is to release all those structures which are tight to such a degree that the finger drops passively into flexion with

818

ease. A bulky pressure dressing is applied for three days with the finger joints in light flexion. It is then replaced with a small volar splint to support the wrist and slight active motion several times daily is started. In addition light rubber-band traction is applied to gradually bring about complete flexion of the finger; at times traction of extensions is necessary for proper balancing.

Technique (*Contractures of Volar Surface of Hand*)

The procedure is similar to that described for contractures of the dorsum. The dissection is more difficult than that on the dorsal side, particularly at the side of the fingers. Great care must be exercised not to injure the digital vessels and nerves. Stretching of the fingers should be cautious and gradual; cross cutting the covering of the tendons and separating the lateral ligaments of the interphalangeal joint facilitate stretching. After completion of the dissection and hemostasis, the arm is placed on a sterile well-padded wooden splint. The places where the knuckles and the interphalangeal joint come to lie should be particularly well padded (with rubber sponge) to avoid pressure ulcers and exposure of the dorsal joint surface. Hand and fingers are fastened as previously described.

If a skin graft can be used to cover the raw surface, and it can in most cases, a thick split graft or full-thickness graft is available. The author has used both with equally good results. The application of the thick split graft is simpler and the donor area heals faster. The technique of application has been described (Fig. 342). For application of the special pressure dressing, see page 814.

The after-treatment is similar to that described on page 814.

Alternative Method: If a flap instead of a graft is to be used, the method of covering the defect is similar to that described on page 83.

Technique (*Contracture of Thumb*)

Adduction contracture of the thumb may not only cripple the action of the thumb but also block flexion of the fingers. If the contracture involves the skin only, a vertical relaxation incision is made through the contracted web. This incision, however, should be made sufficiently deep toward palm and dorsum to make the resulting dorsal and volar scar V-shaped, thus counteracting recontracture. The contracture is released by abducting the thumb, and the raw surface is skin grafted. Deeper contractures, however, require excision of all deep contracted structures, i.e., first dorsal interosseous muscle and part of the adductor and palmar fascia. If release of the soft tissue contracture does not release the contracture of the thumb, Goldner and Clippinger overcome the fixation at the base of the thumb by excision of the greater multangular bone; in case of traumatic arthritis, they include excision of a portion of the base of the first metacarpal bone. Closure of the raw surface in such a case invariably requires transfer of an abdominal flap. While the flap or graft is healing, abduction of the thumb can be temporarily maintained with a bent Kirschner wire drilled through the dorsal surface of the first and second metacarpal bones or by a unit of the Roger-Anderson extraskeletal fixation splint (see p. 553).

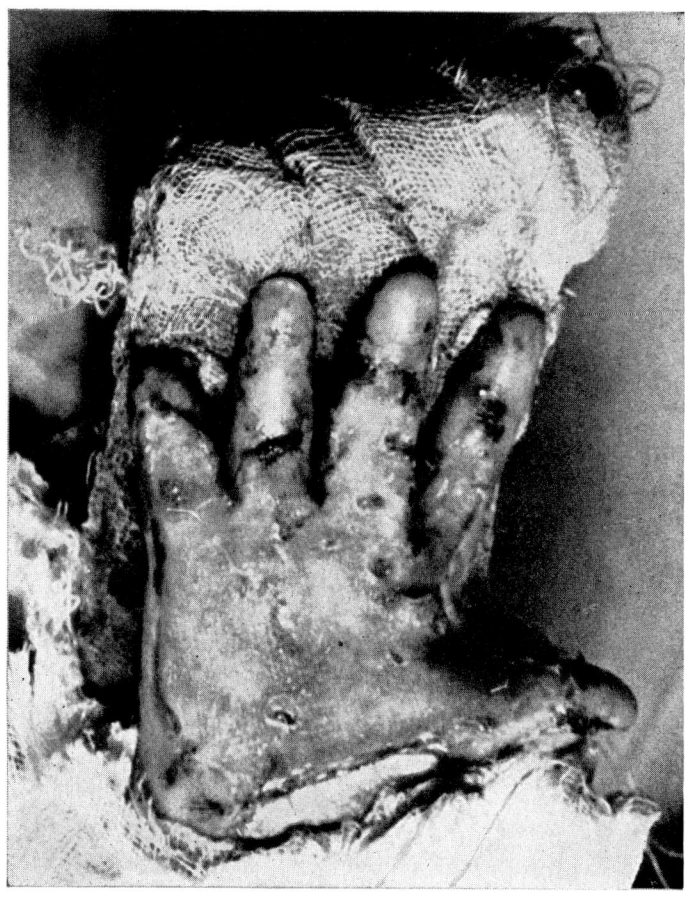

Fig. 342. Way of immobilizing hand and fingers after release of contractures. This child had cicatricial contracture of all fingers. Contracting scar was excised, denuding palm and volar surface of fingers. Contracted tendons were stretched without opening tendon sheaths. Hand was placed on sterile, well-padded wooden splint. Forearm and wrist were bandaged to splint. Wire traction was applied through bone of each finger (p. 813). The wires were fastened to end of splint, keeping fingers in extension and abduction. Thumb was held against bandage roll in abduction. Raw surface was then skin grafted. Figure depicts hand ten days after operation following removal of first dressing and of sutures. Graft took well.

In rarer cases, in which abduction is difficult to maintain, transplantation of a bone strut may be subsequently required (see p. 901) (Case 139, p. 1181).

CONTRACTURE OF PALMAR APONEUROSIS (DUPUYTREN'S CONTRACTURE)

Contracture of the palmar aponeurosis, known as "Dupuytren's contracture," must be classed among diseases of unknown origin, in spite of many attempts to explain it. A tremendous amount of literature dealing with this topic has accumulated in the past ten years—more than for any other single subject in plastic and reconstructive surgery—which presents many diverging concepts about its etiology and pathology. More light, however, has been shed upon this phenomenon since important advances in the studies of the growth and metabolism of connective tissue have increased our knowledge of changes in response to metabolic fluctuation, injury and disease. It now has become evident that the pathological changes of the palmar fascia and the resulting contracture cannot be considered any longer as local but, rather, must be thought of as part of a systemic disease of the fibrous tissue. Contributing factors, such as trauma and a curious association between Dupuytren's contracture and epilepsy, must be mentioned (Lund, Skoog). A congenital predisposition is also unquestionable. It would go far beyond the scope of this book to discuss the subject in detail, and I refer the reader to the excellent treatises of McIndoe, Skoog, Larsen, Posch, Luck, Hueston, Tubiana, Kostek and many others listed in the Bibliography.

The disease progresses gradually involving not only the palmar part of the aponeurosis but its extensions to the fourth and fifth fingers, less often to other fingers, very rarely to the thumb. The superficial palmar fascia (see Fig. 345) is the continuation of the palmaris longus muscle. It fans triangularly across the palm with extension into the fingers, forming the superficial digital fascia. The entire aponeurosis consists of longitudinal bands, which in the palm are connected with each other by transverse bands (*17* and *19* in Fig. 345). In the palm, innumerable minute fibrous fasciculi extend from the palmar aponeurosis to the skin. These hold the skin close to the underlying palmar aponeurosis, permitting comparatively little sliding movement of one upon the other. These thread-like fibrous strands divide the subcutaneous fat into small, irregular masses. Numerous minute blood vessels pass through this subcutaneous tissue to the derma. In Dupuytren's contracture, hypertrophy and hyperplasia of this fibrous tissue result in ultimate displacement of the fat masses and partial obliteration of the blood vessels, thereby interfering markedly with the nutrition of the

821

skin. In the distal part of the palm, septa extend from the deep aspect of the palmar aponeurosis to the deep transverse palmar ligament, forming the sides of annular fibrous canals for the passage of the ensheathed flexor tendons and lumbrical muscles as well as of the blood vessel and nerves. If these septa are contracted they may interfere with the proper function of the fingers.

It is generally agreed that the only effective treatment of Dupuytren's contracture is surgery. Nonoperative treatment, such as irradiation or vitamin E (Richards, King) or cortisone (Baxter et al., Zachariae), is disappointing. However, not all cases of Dupuytren's contracture require

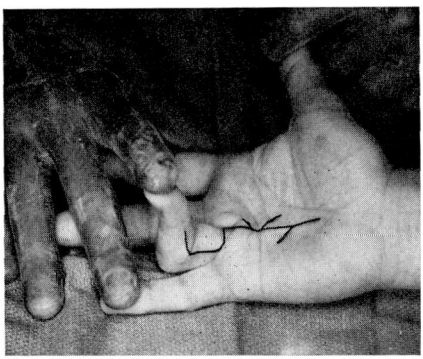

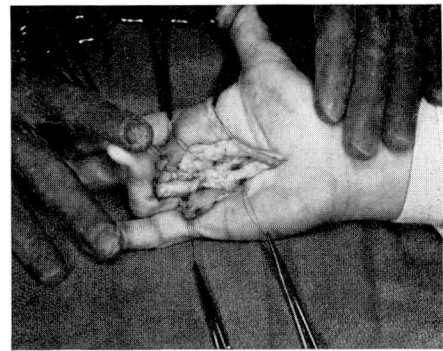

Fig. 343. *A:* Dupuytren's contracture mainly of ring finger; contracting bands also radiating into third and fifth fingers. Lines of incisions are marked out; lines for multiple Z-plasty also indicated.

B: Skin is dissected away from underlying contracted fascial band.

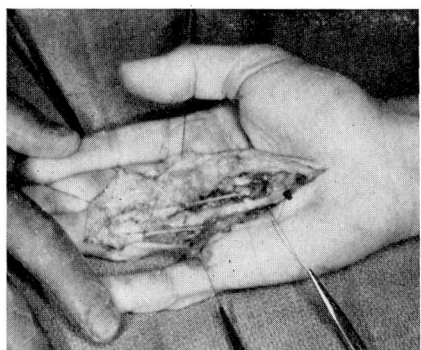

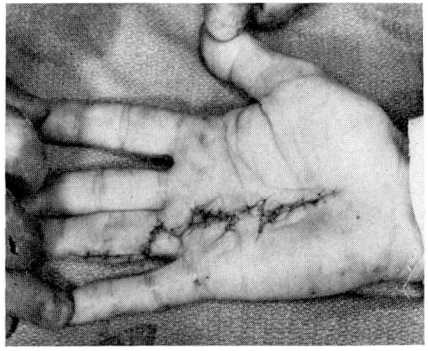

C: Contracting fascial bands have been dissected away from underlying digital nerves and vessels and flexor tendon sheath; interconnecting bands to third and fifth finger also removed; contracture is overcome.

D: Wounds are sutured after Z-plasties in palm and base of finger.

surgery; operation is necessary only for those patients in whom the disease progresses to the point of developing actual contractures of the finger, where those of the interphalangeal joints are more important than those of the metacarpophalangeal joint. One should not wait until such contractures are fully developed because of the likelihood of contractures of the collateral ligaments and secondary joint changes which may be irreparable. When operative treatment is decided upon, a question arises as to the type of operation: fasciotomy, partial fasciectomy or total fasciectomy. The simplest of these is either blind subcutaneous or open fasciotomy. Blind fasciotomy has a strong advocate in Luck, but it is risky since the neurovascular structures cannot be clearly visualized; open method, performed from small transverse incisions, is safer. We restrict this method, however, to cases where a more extensive operation is contraindicated. This leaves limited or total fasciectomy as the preferred treatment. For many years the operation of choice was total fasciectomy with or without skin grafting, for the following reasons.

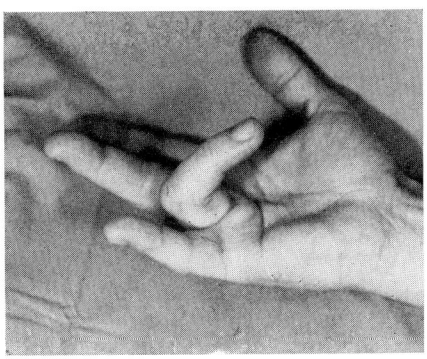

E

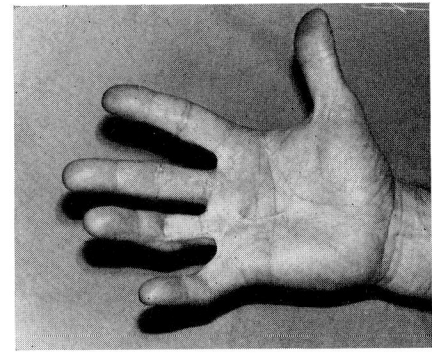

F

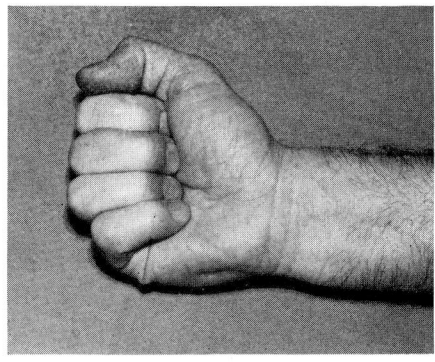

G

E, F, G: Pre- and postoperative result.

823

THE EXTREMITIES

The peculiar pathological process in Dupuytren's contracture is not confined to the palmar fascia, although this is the primary seat. The nodules and the shrinkage of the skin over the diseased fascia and the not infrequent recurrence of the contracture in the skin, even after thorough removal of the underlying fascia, are definite proof of this statement. These findings led Lexer (his work was published by his pupil Janssen in 1902) to remove not only the entire fascia but also the involved skin. Macroscopic and microscopic examinations of removed specimens clearly reveal that the palmar fascia is intimately connected with the skin and also with the underlying tendons and tendon sheaths by dense fascial extensions.

In recent years, however, there has been a revival of interest in a less extensive method, i.e., partial fasciectomy (Hamlin, Conway, Wakefield, Hueston, Nigst, Milesi and others). This has a lower morbidity in that it produces fewer hematomas, less edema of the hand, and less joint stiffness of the uninvolved fingers; therefore the convalescent period is considerably shortened. Also, it has become evident that radical fasciectomy is not a sure method to avoid recurrences. I had been an advocate of the radical method for many years, but experience with partial fasciectomy has convinced me of the great advantages of the latter technique. I restrict it, however, to cases where only one or two rays are involved, and follow largely the method of Hueston.

Technique (Hueston) (Fig. 343)

Under general or brachial block anesthesia and with the tourniquet applied, a midlateral incision is made at the involved finger and from here straight over the web-like band into the palm. The underlying contracting band is exposed further by dissecting away the skin flaps. This may be difficult where the skin is intimately adherent to the contracted palmar fascia. One must develop a plane between the derma and the fascia and create skin flaps which are raised until the limits of the palpably affected areas are defined. The contracted fascial band is severed proximally. Under vertical traction on the fascial band the superficial palmar arch and neurovascular bundles are exposed. The fascia is dissected away from these structures; this includes the fascial extension which connects the fascia with the underlying tendon sheath. The dissection is carried out along the entire length of the incision into the finger. It is even possible with this incision to clear the interconnecting bands over two adjacent sheaths and if neighboring fingers are involved to remove the respective contracting bands in the palm; the respective fingers, however, must be exposed from separate midlateral incisions. The tourniquet is released for hemostasis and then reinflated. After the finger has been straightened, Z-flaps are lined out in

824

proper areas to lengthen the skin. They may be outlined before the longitudinal incision is made but may need rearrangement after extension of the finger. After the flaps have been cut they are interchanged and the wound is sutured. If a Z-plasty is not sufficient to straighten the finger, one should not hesitate to close the defect with a skin graft. A pressure dressing and then a posterior molded plaster-cast splint are applied. The forearm is kept elevated for two days. When the patient is up and around, the arm is elevated in a sling. The dressing is changed after one week and active finger exercises are encouraged (p. 814).

In cases which are more extensive and involve more than two rays, total fasciectomy, without or with skin grafting, is the operation of choice. Lexer was the first to advocate this radical operation with routine excision of the involved skin of the palm and skin grafting. There is no doubt that his operation is still the best where the involved skin is so adherent that dissecting it away from the underlying fascia would leave it so thin as to endanger its blood supply or where the contracture is so severe that the fingers after dissection cannot be straightened out without leaving a surface defect, but there are cases where skin grafting is not needed.

Radical Fasciectomy without Skin Grafting: If skin grafting is not anticipated, a long transverse incision is made in the distal palmar crease (McIndoe, Skoog, Mason, Weckesser, Shaw) and the skin is carefully dissected away from the underlying palmar fascia. A vertical incision following the curve of the thenar crease of the palm may be necessary to reach the insertion of the fascia to the palmaris tendon, where dissection of the fascia from the underlying structures is started. The fascia is removed completely from the thenar to the hypothenar eminence. The excision must also include the fascial extension which connects the fascia with the underlying tendons and tendon sheaths. This must be carried out with great care to avoid injuries to the digital nerves and vessels. The tendon sheaths should not be opened. The fingers are approached from separated incisions for removal of the contracted fascia. A midlateral incision along the side of the digit will be adequate if the contracture is limited to one side of the finger. If both sides of the finger are involved Z-incisions in the skin overlying the proximal phalanx of the digit give good exposure of the underlying fascia (McIndoe, Skoog). Transposition of the flaps at the time of wound closure promotes lengthening of the contracted skin. The operation is performed in a bloodless field (p. 849). After dissection is completed the tourniquet is deflated and after hemostasis it is reinflated. The wound is closed; a large compression dressing and a posterior molded plaster-cast splint, with the fingers as straight as possible in the metacarpophalangeal joints, are applied; only then is the tourniquet deflated. The arm is kept elevated for two days, and when the patient is out of bed the arm is supported above shoulder level. McIndoe uses one small rubber drain inserted on the ulnar edge of the wound. McFarlane and Jamieson use suction tubes inserted into the palm through the second and fourth web spaces. I have used the latter method but not routinely because of occasional impairment of suction from cloaking of the small holes of the tubes. Suction is continued for three to five days. The dressing is changed after ten to fourteen days and daily hand baths and active and passive motion exercises are instituted (p. 814).

If invasion of the Dupuytren's nodules into the skin is widespread and contracture is extensive, a radical excision of the palmar fascia together with the involved skin (which is replaced with a skin graft) as recommended by Lexer is the method of choice.

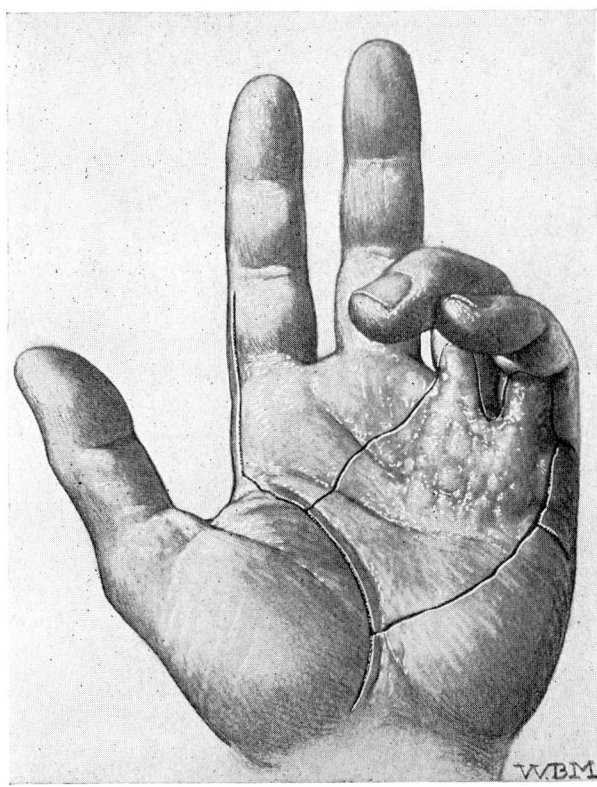

Fig. 344. *A:* Repair of Dupuytren's contracture of palmar aponeurosis (Lexer). Incision starts over origin of palmar fascia, proceeds along main longitudinal crease, crosses transverse creases at radial side of palm, and ends over radial side of index finger. The diseased part of skin is circumscribed by another incision while small transverse incision is added at ulnar side.

826

SKIN, SUBCUTANEOUS TISSUE, AND THE FASCIAE

Technique *(Lexer)* (Fig. 344) (Cases 141, 142)

In a bloodless field (p. 849) the incision starts over the origin of the palmar fascia, proceeds along the main longitudinal palmar crease, crosses the transverse creases at the radial side of the palm, and ends over the radial side of the base of the index finger. The diseased part of the skin is circumscribed by another incision, while a small transverse incision is added at the ulnar side to facilitate exposure. The skin and subcutaneous tissue of the thenar and hypothenar region are dissected away from the palmar fascia. The same is done with the healthy skin of the radial and distal parts of the palm. Thus, four flaps of skin and subcutaneous tissue are

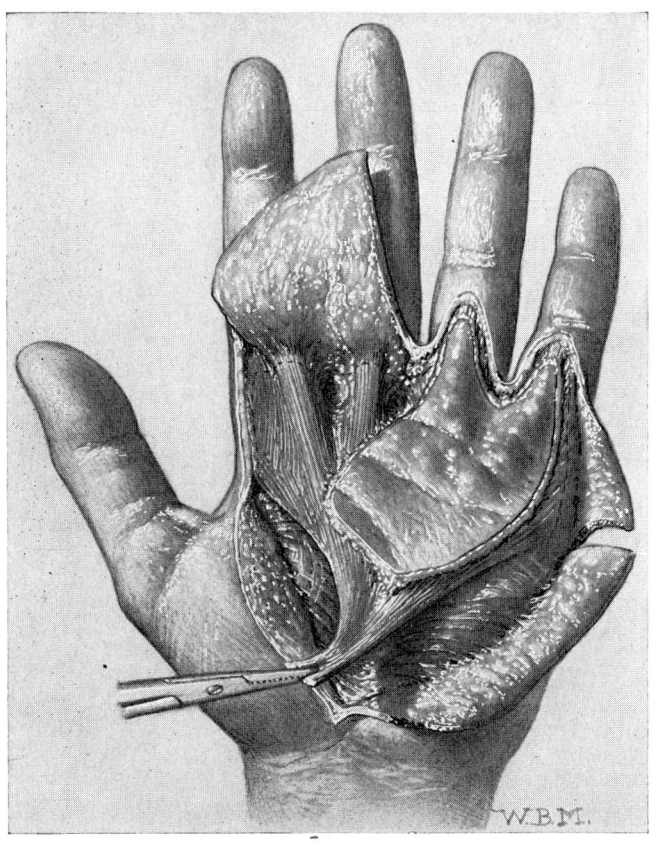

Fig. 344. *B:* Skin and subcutaneous tissue of thenar and hypothenar region are dissected away from palmar fascia. Same is done with healthy skin of radial and distal parts of palm. The four skin flaps are reflected, exposing entire palmar fascia and leaving island-like diseased part of skin in connection with fascia. Palmar fascia is severed from tendon and entirely excised. Dotted line indicates distal lines of excision.

formed which, if lifted up, expose the entire palmar fascia and leave the island-like diseased part of the skin in connection with the fascia.

The fascia is then severed from its tendon. Under constant vertical traction, the entire fascia is excised. The excision must be radical; it must include the fascial extension over the thenar region and the extension to the second, third, fourth, and fifth fingers; it must also include the fascial extensions which connect the fascia with the underlying tendons and tendon sheaths, and the diseased skin island. The dissection is tedious, and should be carried out with great care to avoid injury to the digital nerves and vessels. The tendon sheaths should not be opened.

The blood-pressure cuff is now deflated. Obtaining thorough hemostasis is the next step. The blood-pressure cuff is reinflated and remains in place until the pressure dressing is applied. Forearm, hand, and fingers are immobilized in a previously prepared, well-padded splint. The four

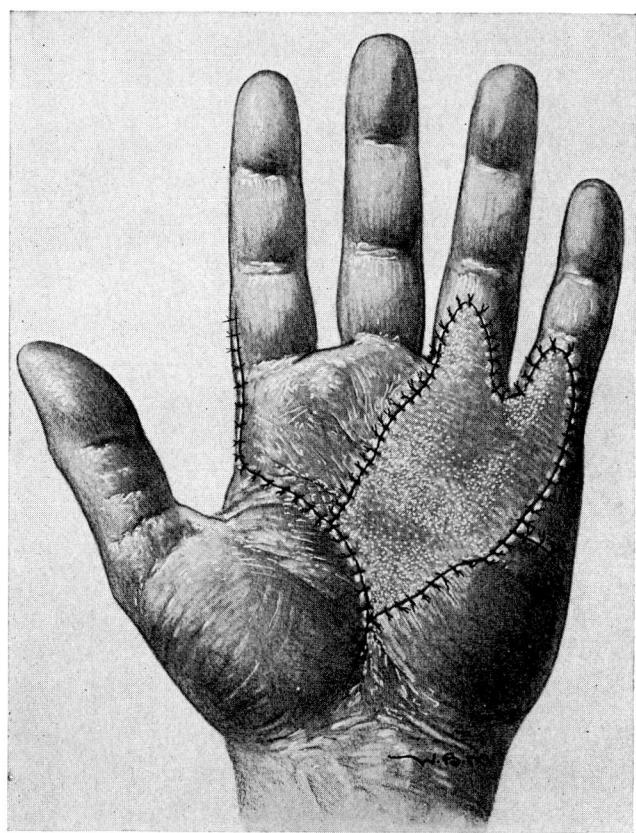

Fig. 344. C: The skin flaps are returned and defects covered with full-thickness graft.

skin flaps are returned. The defect left from excision of the diseased skin is covered with a full-thickness or thick split skin graft. The usual pressure dressing is now applied.

Von Seemen and independently Bruner describe a technique whereby the palmar defect is covered with a sliding flap from the ulnar side of the dorsum of the hand.

After-Treatment

The dressing is changed on the tenth postoperative day. The splint is temporarily removed two weeks after the operation. From then on, the treatment is similar to that described on page 814.

SYNDACTYLISM

Syndactylism is a deformity which shows hereditary tendencies and association with other congenital deformities (Murphy, Snedecor). It occurs in various forms and degrees, from the simple web of skin joining the fingers to the fibrous or complete cartilaginous or osseous fusion. In the latter case, fused tendons, tendon sheaths, digital vessels, and nerves may also be found. Fused fingers can be severed only by operation. The question of the best time to operate will arise. If the operation is performed early in life, the newly formed web has a tendency to move distally with the growth of the fingers; the chances are that another operation will have to be performed later. Hence, the operation should not be performed before the age of six, possibly later. The only indication for early operation is if the deformity should cause a distortion or contracture of the joints, which happens not infrequently.

What type of operation should be performed? There are a number of cleverly devised methods which aim to sever the skin between the fingers in such a way as to establish local flaps with which to cover the raw surfaces. For all practical purposes, however, one can safely say that none of these procedures is adequate; some may even be harmful (Case 137, p. 1179). One exception, however, is that of Zeller, which in incomplete cases may be applicable. The reason is that after the fingers are severed the raw surfaces are so large that there is not enough local tissue available to close the defects. Any attempt to stretch the available tissue will inevitably lead to skin necrosis. The resulting scar tissue may cause distortion and contracture of the fingers, which is exceedingly difficult to overcome even if operated on again. The aim of the operation is to sever the interdigital fusion sufficiently to permit normal abduction of the fingers and to cover all raw surfaces with normal covering tissue. Kanavel, in his outstanding monograph "Congenital Malformations of the Hand," emphasizes that digital vessels and nerves should not be injured, that two sides of the same finger should not be operated upon at the same sitting. It may happen, particularly in more extensive cases, that two fingers, along their fused portion, are supplied by only one digital artery. Hence, if in complete syndactylism all fingers were severed at the same time, partial or complete necrosis of some or all of the fingers may result. Hence, the fusion between thumb and index finger and third and fourth fingers can be safely severed in one sitting. After establishment of a sufficient collateral circulation (several months later), the remaining fused parts between the index, third, fourth, and fifth fingers are severed. In those extensive cases in which bones, joints, and tendons are fused, severance of the fused structures is inadvisable if the two fingers function effectively as one and the severance would result in loss of function of one.

Technique (Case 143, p. 1186)

The fusion between two fingers is severed longitudinally without injury to the digital arteries and nerves. The dorsal and volar longitudinal incisions, however, should not be made straight but Z- or S-shaped, as recommended by J. Webster, Cronin and others, to counteract secondary contractures along the scars. The separation should be carried as proximally as possible until the division of the digital arteries is reached on the volar side, while on the dorsal side the separation should reach even farther proximally. Thus, the floor of the web is oblique, its obliquity sloping from palm to dorsum. After complete hemostasis, a full-thickness graft is removed and cut according to pattern and applied as accurately as possible. The commissure at the base of the finger should be well covered, keeping in mind its obliquity. A pressure dressing is applied with incorporation of mechanic's waste cotton between the fingers. The sutures, which have been left long, are tied over it. Immobilization on a molded plaster-cast splint follows.

Alternative Method (Case 144, p. 1187): In cases in which the fused portion of the skin at the base of the web is redundant, a dorsal triangular flap of skin and subcutaneous tissue can be formed—after the suggestion of Zeller—to cover the floor of the commissure. The base of the flap is at the level of the metacarpophalangeal joints, its tip at the level of the proximal interphalangeal joint. The fusion is then severed as described. The flap is laid upon the floor of the cleft between the fingers and its tip sutured to the skin of the volar side. The remaining raw surfaces are covered with skin grafts as previously described.

830

SKIN, SUBCUTANEOUS TISSUE, AND THE FASCIAE

After-Treatment

Splint, dressing, and sutures are removed eight days after operation. From the tenth day on, the dressings are changed daily, the hand is placed in a warm hand bath, and active finger motions are instituted.

BIBLIOGRAPHY

ADAMSON, J. E., HORTON, CH. E., CRAWFORD, H. H.: *Sensory rehabilitation of the injured thumb.* Plast. Reconstr. Surg., 40:53, 1967.

ARCARI, F. A., LARSEN, R. D., and POSCH, J. L.: *Injuries to the hand from homemade rockets.* Amer. J. Surg., 97:471, 1959.

BARCLAY, T. L.: *Edema following operation for Dupuytren's contracture.* Plast. Reconstr. Surg., 23:348, 1959.
The late results of finger-tip injuries. Brit. J. Plast. Surg., 7:34, 1955.

BAXTER, H., ET AL.: *Cortisone therapy in Dupuytren's contracture.* Plast. Reconstruct. Surg., 9:261, 1952.

BLAIR, V. P., and BROWN, J. B.: *The use and uses of large split skin grafts of intermediate thickness.* Surg. Gynec. Obstet., 49:82, 1929.

BODENHAM, D. C.: *Restoration of function in burnt hands.* Lancet, 1:298, 1943.

BOJSEN MOLLER, J., PERS, M., and SCHMIDT, A.: *Finger-tip injuries: Late results.* Acta Chir. Scand., 122:177-183, 1961.

Bouncing Putty. J. Indust. Hyg. Toxicol., 306:332, 1948.

BRODY, G. S., CLOUTIER, A. M., and WOOLHOUSE, F. M.: *The finger tip injury—an assessment of management.* Plast. Reconstr. Surg., 26:80, 1960.

BROWN, J. B.: *The repair of surface defects of the hand.* Ann. Surg., 107:952, 1938.

BRUNER, J. M.: *Problems of postoperative position and motion in surgery of the hand.* J. Bone Joint Surg., 35A:355, 1953.
The use of dorsal skin flap for the coverage of palmar defects after aponeurectomy for Dupuytren's contracture. Plast. Reconstr. Surg., 4:559, 1949.

BUCK-GRAMCKO, D.: *Plastisch-chirurgische Behandlung von Narbenkontrakturen der Hand.* Münchener Medizinische Wochenschrift, 104:311 and 358, 1962.
Wiederherstellung der Sensibilität bei Teilverlust des Daumens. Langenbeck's Arch. und Deutsche Zeitschrift f. Chir., 299:99, 1961.

BUNNELL, S. T.: *Active splinting of the hand.* J. Bone Joint Surg., 28:732, 1946.

BURKHALTER, Lt. Col. WM. E., BUTLER, B., METZ, Col. W., and OMER, Col. GEORGE: *Experiences with delayed primary closure of war wounds of the hand in Viet Nam.* J. Bone Joint Surg., 50A:945, 1968.

BÜRKLE DE LA CAMP, H.: *Behandlung der Dupuytren'schen Kontraktur im jugendlichen Alter.* Med. Welt, 1939.

CANNON, B.: *Open grafting on raw surfaces of the hand.* J. Bone Joint Surg., 49-2:79, 1958. (Abstr. Plast. Reconstr. Surg., 21:332, 1958.)

831

THE EXTREMITIES

CANNON, B., and GRAHAM, W. C.: *Plastic and reconstructive surgery of the hand.* Mil. Surgeon, 97:137, 1945.

CARSTENSEN, E.: *Begutachtung und Wiederherstellung von Hand—Nerven-verletzungen.* Langenbeck's Arch. klin. Chir., Bd 306, 33, 1964.

CLARKSON, P.: *The care of open injuries of the hand and fingers with special reference to the treatment of traumatic amputations.* J. Bone Joint Surg., 37A:521, 1955.
The radical fasciectomy operation for Dupuytren's disease: A condemnation. Brit. J. Plast. Surg., 16:273, 1963.

CLARKSON, P., and PELLY, A.: *The General and Plastic Surgery of the Hand.* F. A. Davis, Philadelphia, 1962.

CONWAY, H., STARK, R. B., and NIETO-CANO, G.: *The arterial vascularization of pedicles.* Plast. Reconstr. Surg., 12:348, 1953.

CRONIN, T. D.: *The cross-finger flap—A new method of repair.* Amer. J. Surg., 17:419, 1951.

CURTIS, R. M.: *Capsulectomy of the interphalangeal joints of the fingers.* J. Bone Joint Surg., 36A:1219, 1954.
Cross-finger pedicle flap in hand surgery. Ann. Surg., 145:650, 1957.

DAVIS, J. E.: *On surgery of Dupuytren's contracture.* Plastic Reconstr. Surg., 36:277, 1965.

DELBET, J. P., and WALLICH, E.: *The cross-arm flap in surgery of the hand (La place du "cross-arm-flap" dans la chirurgie de la main).* Ann. Chir. Plast., 9:159, 1964.

DEMING, E. G.: *Y-V advancement pedicles in surgery for Dupuytren's contracture.* Plast. Reconstr. Surg., 29:581, 1962.

DOUGLAS, B. L.: *Successful replacement of completely avulsed portions of fingers as composite grafts.* Plast. Reconstr. Surg., 23:213, 1959.

DUBEN, W.: *Zur Chirurgie der Hand.* Der Chirurg, 24:61, 1953.

DUFOURMENTEL, L.: *La Practique des Greffes Libres des paen totale.* Bull. et. mém. Soc. d. chirurgiens de Paris, 29:306, 1937.

DUPUYTREN, BAREN (1833): *Clinical Lectures on Surgery,* translated by A. S. Doane. Boston, Carter, Hendee & Co.

EARLY, P. F.: *Population studies in Dupuytren's contracture.* J. Bone Joint Surg., 44B:602, 1962.

EBSKOV, B., and ZACHARIAE, L.: *Surgical methods in syndactylism.* Acta Chir. Scand., 131:258, 1966.

EINARSSON, G.: *On treatment of Dupuptren's contracture.* Acta Chir. Scand., 93:1, 1946.

ENDER, J., KROTSCHECK, H., and SIMON-WEIDNER, R.: *Die Chirurgie der Handverletzungen.* Springer-Verlag, Wien, 1956.

FISHER, R. H.: *The Kutler method of repair of finger-tip amputations.* J. Bone Joint Surg., 49A:317, 1967.

FLATT, A. E.: *Care of Minor Hand Injuries.* C. V. Mosby, St. Louis, 1959.

SKIN, SUBCUTANEOUS TISSUE, AND THE FASCIAE

FLYNN, F. E.: *Compound wounds of the hand.* Ann. Surg., 135:500, 1952.

FOWLER, S. B.: *Mobilization of metacarpophalangeal joints, anthroplasty, and capsulotomy.* J. Bone Joint Surg., 29:193, 1947.

FRACKELTON, W. H., and TEASLEY, J. L.: *Neurovascular island pedicle— extension in usage.* J. Bone Joint Surg., 44A:1069, 1962.

FREEHAFTER, A. A., and STRONG, J. M.: *The treatment of Dupuytren's contracture by partial fasciectomy.* J. Bone Joint Surg., 45A:1208, 1963.

GARLOCK, J. H.: *The full thickness skin graft; its field of applicability and technical considerations.* Ann. Surg., 97:259, 1933.

GATÉ, P. A., and DELEVZE, R.: *The surgical treatment of deep burns of the hand.* Ann. Chir. Plast., 6:211, 1961.

GATEWOOD, A.: *A plastic repair of finger defect without hospitalization.* JAMA, 87:1479, 1926.

GEISSENDÖRFER: *Finger Kuppen Plastik.* Zentralbl. f. Chir., 70:1107, 1943.

GEORG, H.: *Kritische Betrachtungen zur aufgeschobenen Primarversorgung von Handverletzungen; Indikation und Ergebnisse.* Langenbeck's Arch. f. klin. Chir., 306:157, 1964.

GIRDWOOD, W.: *Hyperextension fixed deformity of the metacarpophalangeal joints.* In PENN, JACK (Editor): *Brenthurst Papers.* Witwatersrand University Press, Johannesburg, 1944.

GOLDNER, J. L., and CLIPPINGER, F. W.: *Excision of the greater multangular bone in mobilization of the thumb.* J. Bone Joint Surg., 40A:957, 1958.

GORDON, S.: *Dupuytren's contracture. The significance of various factors in its etiology.* Ann. Surg., 140:683, 1954.

GORDON, S., and ANDERSON, W.: *Dupuytren's contracture following injury.* Brit. J. Plast. Surg., 14:129, 1961.

GOTTLIEB, O., and MATHIESEN, F. R.: *Thenar flaps and cross-finger flaps (A preliminary analysis of 28 cases).* Acta Chir. Scand., 122:166-176, 1961.

GREELEY, P. W.: *Plastic repair of extensor hand contractures following deep second degree burns.* Surgery, 15:173, 1944.

HAMLIN, E.: *Limited excision of Dupuytren's contracture.* Ann. Surg., 155:454, 1962.

HARRIS, C., and RIORDAN, D. C.: *Intrinsic contracture in the hand and its surgical treatment.* J. Bone Joint Surg., 36A:10, 1954.

HOLEVICH, J.: *A new method of restoring sensibility to the thumb.* J. Bone Joint Surg., 45B:496, 1963.

HORNE, J. S.: *The use of full-thickness hand skin flaps in the reconstruction of injured fingers.* Plast. Reconstr. Surg., 7:463, 1951.

HOSKINS, H. D.: *The versatile cross-finger pedicle flap.* J. Bone Joint Surg., 42A:261, 1960.

HUESTON, J. T.: *Dupuytren's contracture.* Williams & Wilkins, Baltimore, 1964. *Local flap repair of finger-tip injuries.* Plast. Reconstr. Surg., 37:349, 1966.

THE EXTREMITIES

Limited fasciectomy for Dupuytren's contracture. Plast. Reconstr. Surg., 27:569, 1961.

Recurrent Dupuytren's contracture. Plast. Reconstr. Surg., 31:66, 1963.

Dupuytren's contracture: The trend to conservatism. Ann. Roy. Coll. Surg., 36:134, 1964.

HUNTER, JAMES M.: *Salvage of the burned hand.* Surg. Clin. N. Amer., 47, No. 5, Oct., 1967.

ISELIN, M.: *Chirurgie de la Main (Surgery of the Hand),* 2nd Edition. Paris, Masson et Cie, 1955.

Aufgeschobene Dringlichkeit bei der Wundversorgung. Arch. f. klin. Chir., 301:91, 1962.

Atlas de Technique Operatoire de Chirurgie de la Main. Publisher Editions Medicales, Flammarion, Paris, 1958.

JAMES, J. I. P., TUBIANA, R.: *La maladie de Dupuytren.* Rev. Chir. Orthop., 38:352, 1952.

JONES, F. W.: *The Principles of Anatomy as Seen in the Hand.* Williams & Wilkins, Baltimore, 1943.

JONES, R. A.: *A method for closing a traumatic defect of a finger tip.* Amer. J. Surg., 55:326, 1942.

KANAVEL, A. B.: *Congenital malformations of the hands.* Arch. Surg., 25:1-53, 282, 320, 1932.

KETTELKAMP, D. B., and FLATT, A. E.: *An evaluation of syndactylia repair.* Surg. Gynec. Obstet., 113:471, 1961.

KING, R. A.: *Vitamin E therapy in Dupuytren's contracture. Examination of the claim that Vitamin E therapy is successful.* J. Bone Joint Surg. 31B:443, 1949.

KISLOV, R., and KELLY, A. P.: *Cross-finger flaps in digital injuries, with notes on Kirschner wire fixation.* Plast. Reconstr. Surg., 25:312, 1960.

KOCH, S. G.: *The transplantation of skin and subcutaneous tissue to the hand.* Surg. Gynec. Obstet., 72:1, 157, 1941.

KOSTEIK, T.: *Die Dupuytren'sche Kontraktur unter besonderer Berücksichtigung der Atiologie in mesenchympathologischer Sicht.* Vorträge aus der Plastischen Chirurgie, Vol. 72, Ferdinand Enke, Verlag, Stuttgart W., 1965.

KRÖMER, K.: *Die Verletzte Hand.* H. Maudrich, Wien, 1945.

KUTLER, WM.: *A new method for finger tip amputation.* JAMA, 133:29, 1947.

LARSEN, R. D., and POSCH, J. L.: *Dupuytren's contracture. With special reference to pathology.* J. Bone Joint Surg., 40A:773, 1958.

Dupuytren's contracture. Surg. Gynec. Obstet., 115:1, 1962.

LARSEN, R. D., TAKAGISHI, N., and POSCH, J. L.: *The pathogenesis of Dupuytren's contracture.* J. Bone Joint Surg., 42A:993, 1960.

LEWIN, M. L.: *Digital flap.* Plast. Reconstr. Surg., 7:46, 1951.

LEXER, E.: *Die gesamte Wiederherstellungs Chirurgie.* J. A. Barth, Leipzig, 1931. *Under* JANSSEN: Arch. f. klin. Chir., 67:761, 1902.

LITTLER, W.: *Neurovascular skin island transfer in reconstructive hand surgery.* Trans. Int. Cong. Plast. Surg., London, 1959.

834

SKIN, SUBCUTANEOUS TISSUE, AND THE FASCIAE

LUCK, J. V.: *Dupuytren's contracture—A new concept of the pathogenesis correlated with surgical management.*" J. Bone Joint Surg., 41A:635, 1959.

MacCOLLUM, D. W.: *Burns of the hand.* JAMA, 116:2371, 1941.

MANNERFELT, L.: *Evaluation of functional sensation of skin grafts in the hand area.* Brit. J. Plast. Surg. 15:136, 1962.

MATEV, I., and HOLEVICH, Y.: *Surgical treatment of scar contractures of the hand and fingers following burns.* Acta Chir. Plast., 4:152, 1962.

MAY, H.: *Closure of surface defects of the hand.* Penn. Med. J., Nov. 1945.
Repair of cicatricial and Dupuytren's contractures of the hand. Plast. Reconstr. Surg., 3:439, 1948.
Behandlung von Verbrennungen und Verbrennungskontrakturen der Hand. Langenbeck's Arch. und Deutsche Zeitschrift f. Chir., Band 302, Heft 1 (1962) Springer Verlag, Berlin.

McCARROLL, H. R.: *Immediate application of free full-thickness skin graft for traumatic amputations of the finger.* J. Bone Joint Surg., 26:489, 1944.

McCASH, C. R.: *Cross-arm bridge flaps in the repair of flexion contractures of the fingers.* Brit. J. Plast. Surg., 9:25, 1956.

McFARLANE, R. M.: *The use of continuous suction after operation for Dupuytren's contracture.* Brit. J. Plast. Surg., 11:301, 1959.

McFARLANE, R. M., and STROMBERG, W. B.: *Resurfacing of the thumb following major skin loss.* J. Bone Joint Surg., 44A:1365, 1962.

McFARLANE, R. M., and JAMIESON, W. G.: *Dupuytren's contracture (the management of one hundred patients)* J. Bone Joint Surg., 48A:1095, 1966.

McINDOE, A., BEAR, R. L.: *Surgical management of Dupuytren's contracture.* Amer. J. Surg., 25:197, 1958.

MOBERG, E.: *Transfer of sensation.* J. Bone Joint Surg., 37A:305, 1955.
Objective methods for determination of the functional value of sensibility in the hand. J. Bone Joint Surg., 40B:454, 1958.

MURPHY, D. P.: *The duplications of congenital malformations in brothers and sisters and among other relatives.* Surg. Gynec. Ostet., 113:443, 1936.

MURRAY, J. F., ORD, J. V. R., and GAVELIN, G. E.: *The neurovascular island pedicle flap.* J. Bone Joint Surg., 49A:1285, 1967.

NICHOLS, H. M.: *Manual of Hand Injuries.* Year Book Publishers, Inc., Chicago, 1955.

NIGST, H.: *Zu den Resultaten nach operativen Behandlung der Dupuytren'schen Kontraktur.* Hand chirurgie, 2:100, 1969.

PADGETT, E. C.: *Calibrated intermediate skin grafts.* Surg. Gynec. Obstet., 69: 779, 1939.

PEACOCK, E. E.: *Dynamic splinting for the prevention and correction of hand deformities. A simple and inexpensive method.* J. Bone Joint Surg., 34A:789, 1952.

PENN, J.: *Brenhurst Papers.* Witwatersrand University Press, Johannesburg, 1944.

PIERCE, G. W., and O'CONNOR, G. B.: *Pedicle flap patterns for hand reconstruction.* Surg. Gynec. Obstet., 65:523, 1937.
Repair of the burned hand. Surgery, 15:153, 1944.

835

THE EXTREMITIES

POSCH, J. L., and WELLER, C. N.: *Mangle and severe wringer injuries of the hand in children.* J. Bone Joint Surg., 36A:57, 1954.

RANK, B. K., WAKEFIELD, A. R., and HUESTON, J. T.: *Surgery of Repair as Applied to Hand Injuries.* 3rd ed. Williams & Wilkins, Baltimore, 1968. Livingstone, Edinburgh, 1953.

REED, J. V., and HARCOURT, A. K.: *Immediate full-thickness grafts to finger tips.* Surg. Gynec. Obstet., 68:925, 1939.

REID, D. A. C.: *Experience of a hand surgery service.* Brit. J. Plast. Surg., 9:11, 1956.

RICHARDS, H. J.: *Dupuytren's contracture treated with Vitamin E.* Brit. Med. J., 1:1328, 1952.

ROBINS, R. H. C.: *Injuries and Infections of the Hand.* Williams & Wilkins, Baltimore, 1961.

ROSS, J. A., and ANNAN, J. H.: *Dupuytren's contractures: A clinical review.* Ann. Surg., 134:186, 1951.

SCHARITZER, E.: *Die organisatorische Bedeutung der "aufgeschobenen Dringlichkeit" in der Unfall-Chirurgie.* Hefte zur Unfallheilkunde, 1962.

SCHINK, W.: *Operative treatment of Dupuytren's contracture (Das operative Vorgehen bei der Dupuytrenschen Kontraktur).* Chir. Praxis, 1962, 6:195.

SEDDON, H. J.: *L'Ischemie de Volkmann: Une Nouvelle Etude de Son Traitement.* Rev. Chir. Orthop., 46:149, 1960.

v. SEEMEN, H.: *Operat. d. Palmarkontraktur,* Dtsch. Z. Chir., 246, 1936, *Dupuytrenschen Kontraktur,* Bay. Chir. Tag, 1951.

SHAW, M. H., BARCLAY, T. L.: *Dupuytren's Contracture—The Results of Radical Fasciectomy.* Trans. Int. Soc. Plast. Surg. Williams & Wilkins, Baltimore, 1957.

SHIH-JENG, K., HSIEN-WEN, S., SHIH-YING, L., and HSIN KUANG, H.: *The reparative treatment of severe dorsal contracture of burned hands.* Chin. Med. J., 83:358, 1964.

SHIH-JENG, K., HSIN-KUANG, H., KUANG-CHAO, K., YI-CH'UN, L., and SHIH-YING, L.: *The technique of split thickness skin grafting in the repair of contractures of burned hands.* Chin. Med. J., 83:343, 1964.

SKOOG, T.: *Dupuytren's contraction with special reference to aetiology and improved surgical treatment, etc.* Acta Chir. Scand., 96: Suppl., 139, 1948.
The pathogenesis and etiology of Dupuytren's contracture. Plast. Reconstr. Surg., 31:258, 1963.
Syndactyly. A clinical report on repair. Acta Chir. Scand., 130:537, 1966.
Dupuytren's contracture: Pathogenesis and surgical treatment. Surg. Clin. N. Amer., 47:433, 1967.

SNEDECOR, S. T., and HARRYMAN, W. K.: *Surgical problems in hereditary polydactylism and syndactylism.* J. Med. Soc. New Jersey, 1940.

SOUQUET, R., and CHAN-CHOLLE, A. R.: *Plaies de la Main.* Paris, G., and Cie, 1959.

SKIN, SUBCUTANEOUS TISSUE, AND THE FASCIAE

STENBERG, G.: *Full thickness grafts in finger tip injuries.* Acta Chir. Scand., 99:435, 1950.

STURMAN, M. J., and DURAN, R. J.: *Late results of finger-tip injuries.* J. Bone Joint Surg., 45A:289, 1963.

SULLIVAN, J. G., KELLEHER, J. C., BAIBAK, G. J., DEAN, R. K., and PINKNER, L. D.: *The primary application of an island pedicle flap in thumb and index finger injuries.* Plast. Reconstr. Surg., 39:488, 1967.

TANZER, R. D.: *Dupuytren's contracture.* New Eng. J. Med., 246:807, 1952.

TEMPEST, M. N.: *Cross finger flaps in the treatment of injuries to the finger tip.* Plast. Reconstr. Surg., 9:205, 1952.

TENNISON, C. W., and AZZATO, N. M.: *Use of the chest flap for resurfacing defects of the hand, wrist, and forearm.* J. Int. Coll. Surg., 34:521, 1960.

TIERNY, A.: *Free full-thickness skin grafts.* Gaz. méd. de France, 49:795, 1937.

TUBIANA, R.: *Prognosis and treatment of Dupuytren's contracture.* J. Bone Joint Surg., 37A:1155, 1955.
Rev. Chir. Orthop. 50:311, 1964.

TUBIANA, R., DUPARC, J., and MOREAU, C.: *Restoration of sensation to the hand by heterodigital neurovascular skin pedicle graft (Restauration de la sensibilite au niveau de la main par transfert d'un transplant cutane heterodigital muni de son pedicule vasculo-nerveux).* Rev. Chir. Orthop., Paris, 1960, 46:163.

TUBIANA, R., STACK, H. G., HAKSTIAN, R. W.: *Restoration of prehension after severe mutilations of the hand.* J. Bone Joint Surg., 48B:455, 1966.

TUBIANA, R., THOMINE, J. M., and BROWN, S.: *Complications in surgery of Dupuytren's contracture.* Plast. Reconstr. Surg., 39:603, 1967.

TUBIANA, R., and DUPARC, J.: *Un procede nouveau de reconstruction d'un pouce sensible (Rapport de R. Merle d'Aubigne)* Mem. Acad. Chir., 86:264, 1960.

WANG, M. K. H., MACOMBER, W. B., STEIN, A., RAJPAL, R., and HOFFERNAN, A.: *Dupuytren's contracture.* Plast. Reconstr. Surg., 25:323, 1960.

WARREN, R. F.: *The pathology of Dupuytren's contracture.* Brit. J. Plast. Surg., 6:324, 1953.

WECKESSER, E. C.: *Results of wide excision of palmar fascia for Dupuytren's contracture.* Ann. Surg., 160:1007, 1964.

WINSTEN, J.: *Island flap for finger injuries.* New Eng. J. Med., 268:124, 1963.

ZACHARIAE, L., and ZACHARIAE, F.: *Hydrocortisone acetate in the treatment of Dupuytren's contraction and allied conditions.* Acta Chir. Scand., 109:421, 1955.

ZRUBECKY, G.: *Derzeitige Grenzen bei der Planmassigen Versorgung Schwerer Handverletzungen.* Journal Hefte zur Unfallheilkunde Vol. 83, 1965, Springer Verlag, Berlin.
Wiederherstellung des normalen Hautgefuhles nach irreparablen Nervenschaden. Arch. f. klin. Chir., 301:888, 1962.
Die Hand, das Tastorgan des Menschen. Stuttgart, Ferdinand Enke, 1960.

THE MUSCLES, TENDONS, NERVES, AND BLOOD VESSELS

29

It is customary to discuss the surgery of the muscles and tendons separately from that of the nerves and blood vessels. This distinction, however, is abandoned to simplify the discussion, since the anatomical and functional relationships of these structures are particularly close in the hand.

ANATOMY

DEEP PALMAR STRUCTURES

The bulk of the deep palmar structures lies beneath the palmar aponeurosis within the three main spaces: thenar space, middle palmar space, and hypothenar space (Figs. 345, 346, 347).

Thenar Space (Figs. 346, 347)

This contains the short muscles of the thumb: the musculus abductor pollicis brevis, flexor pollicis brevis, adductor pollicis, opponens pollicis, and the tendon of the flexor pollicis longus. The superficial ramus of the arteria radialis, which branches off to form the arcus volaris superficialis, lies upon these muscles, while the deep ramus for the formation of the arcus volaris profundus enters the bottom of the thenar space between the first and second metacarpal bones. The innervation of the musculus abductor pollicis brevis, opponens pollicis, and part of the short flexor is provided by the nervus medianus, while the other part of the short flexor and the adductor is supplied by the nervus ulnaris.

Middle Palmar Space (Figs. 346, 347, 348)

The superficial part of the space directly beneath the palmar aponeurosis comprises the arcus volaris superficialis (arteria ulnaris and small branch of arteria radialis) and the nervus medianus with its digital branches beneath it. The middle layer contains the tendons of the long flexor muscles, their gliding structures, and the musculi lumbricales. The latter originate from the deep flexor tendons. The deep part of the space contains the arcus volaris profundus, which, in contradistinction to the superficial arcus, is formed by a strong branch of the arteria radialis and a small branch of the arteria ulnaris. It also contains the deep branch of the nervus ulnaris.

Hypothenar Space (Figs. 346, 347)

This embodies the three short muscles of the fifth finger: the musculus abductor digiti quinti, flexor digiti quinti, and opponens digiti quinti; it also contains the strong ramus superficialis of the arteria ulnaris (for the formation of the arcus volaris superficialis) and the ramus superficialis of the nervus ulnaris. The deep branches of the same artery and nerve are deeply embedded between the short abductor and flexor muscles of the fifth finger.

The arterial pattern of the hand varies a great deal; however, I refer the reader to the interesting anatomical studies of Coleman and Anson.

FLEXOR TENDONS AND MUSCLES

The flexor tendons of the five fingers enter the deep volar spaces of the hand after having passed through the canalis carpi (Figs. 346, 347, 348). In the canal, they lie close together in two layers. The tendons of the deep flexors lie one by one in normal sequence; the tendons of the superficial flexors, however, superimpose two by two. The radial group of the superficial tendons is covered by the nervus medianus.

All these structures are confined to the canal by two covering membranes, the ligamentum carpi volare and the ligamentum carpi transversum (also called the "anterior annular ligament"). The ligamentum carpi volare is a continuation of the fascia antibrachii; above the wrist,

840

it forms a transverse fascia, which passes over into the ligamentum carpi transversum. In addition to the flexor tendons, it covers the ulnar artery and nerve as both emerge to cross over the ligamentum carpi transversum. The latter is a tough fibrous band which crosses the arch formed by the carpal bones and connects the os naviculare and os multangulum majus on the radial side with the os pisiforme and os hamatum on the ulnar side. The ulnar nerve and artery cross the ligament on the radial side of the os pisiforme to dip beneath the palmar fascia. On the radial side the ligament is crossed by the superficial volar branch of the radial artery, which helps to form the arcus volaris superficialis.

Bursae (Figs. 346, 348)

The tendons of the musculi flexorum digitorum communium are invested in the carpal canal by a common synovial sheath (ulnar bursa). The latter commences just proximal to the ligamentum carpi transversum and stops in the middle of the palm, with the exception of the fifth finger. Here, in most cases, the synovial bursa becomes continuous with the tendon sheath of this finger. The long flexor tendon of the thumb has a separate sheath (radial bursa), which commences just proximal to the ligamentum carpi transversum and reaches to the second phalanx. In about half of the cases, this bursa communicates with the ulnar bursa. Distally, the two flexor tendons of each finger are surrounded by a similar synovial sheath, which starts at the level of the heads of the metacarpal bones and reaches to the third phalanx of each finger. The tendons, on their way through the digital sheath, are bridged by strong fibrous ligaments, ligamenta vaginalia, which insert at the proximal and middle phalanx on each side. These so-called "pulleys" confine the tendons in the bed. Their action is supported by other, less strong, ligaments over the joints (ligamenta cruciata and ligamenta annularia). The long flexor tendon of the thumb has only one vaginal ligament opposite the proximal phalanx.

Insertion of Tendons (Fig. 349)

In the proximal part of each digital sheath, the two flexor tendons are superimposed. At the level of the proximal phalanx, the superficial flexor tendon divides into two slips, through which the deep flexor tendon passes. These slips are inserted into the sides of the middle phalanx at its base, while the deep flexor tendon is inserted into the base of the distal phalanx. The tendon of the musculus flexor pollicis longus passes alone through the osteoaponeurotic canal and is inserted into the base of the terminal phalanx. Before insertion to the phalanges, each tendon connects itself with the bone by fine fibrous filaments, called "vincula tendinum."

THE EXTREMITIES

Musculi Lumbricales (Figs. 346, 348)

The musculi lumbricales are situated between the deep flexor tendons, from which they originate, and form the base for the digital nerves and vessels. They pass toward the dorsal side of the finger, and insert into the tendinous expansion of the musculus extensor digitorum communis (Fig. 353). Their action is to flex the proximal phalanges and to extend the middle and distal phalanges of the second to fifth fingers, together with the musculi interossei forming the intrinsic muscle system of the hand. Its function is described on pages 844-845.

Musculi Interossei (*Volar Group; for Dorsal Group, see p. 843*)

These form the deepest layer of muscles, and are situated in the interspaces of the metacarpal bones. They originate at their lateral surfaces and, like the former muscles, insert into the tendinous expansion of the musculus extensor digitorum communis. Their function is to support the action of the lumbrical muscles, with which they form the intrinsic system of the hand (see pp. 844-845), and to adduct the proximal phalanges of the second, fourth, and fifth fingers toward the middle finger. They are all supplied by the ulnar nerve.

DORSAL STRUCTURES

Fascia Dorsalis (Fig. 350)

The extensor tendons are covered by a veil of tough connective tissue, the deep dorsal fascia, upon which the subcutaneous veins and the cutaneous branches of the nervus radialis and the nervus ulnaris are resting. The dorsal fascia is connected proximally with the deep fascia of the forearm and distally with the dorsal aponeurosis of the fingers.

Ligamentum Carpi Dorsale (Figs. 350, 351)

At the level of the wrist the fascia becomes thick and tough, forming the ligamentum carpi dorsale (posterior annular ligament). Laterally the ligament is attached to the facies radialis and processus styloideus radii, medially to the processus styloideus ulnae and the ulnar border of the carpus. Septal partitions connect the ligament with the dorsal surface of radius and ulna, forming six tunnels for the passage of the extensor tendons and their sheaths.

Tendons and Muscles of Middle Portion of Hand (Figs. 351, 352)

After the extensor tendons have passed the osteofascial spaces beneath the ligamentum carpi dorsale, they divide into an ulnar and a

842

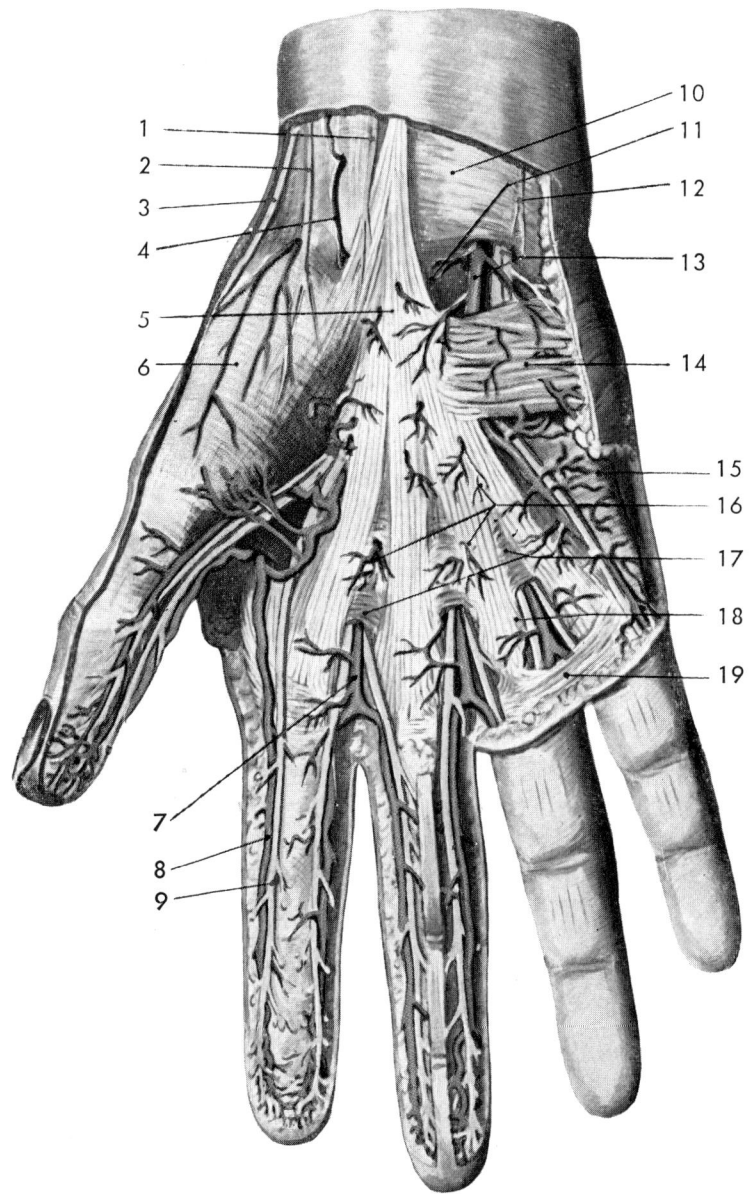

Fig. 345. Aponeurosis and extrafascial structures of palm. (R. von Lanz and W. Wachsmuth: Praktische Anatomie. Julius Springer, Berlin.)

1: Ramus palmaris nervus medianus. *2:* Nervus cutaneus antibrachii lateralis (terminal branch). *3:* Ramus superficialis nervus radialis. *4:* Ramus volaris superficialis arteria radialis. *5:* Aponeurosis palmaris with tendon of musculus palmaris longus. *6:* Fascia of thenar eminence. *7:* Arteria digitalis volaris communis. *8:* Arteria digitalis volaris propria. *9:* Nervus digitalis volaris proprius.

10: Ligamentum carpi volare. *11:* Ligamentum carpi transversum. *12:* Ramus palmaris nervus ulnaris. *13:* Arteria ulnaris and nervus ulnaris. *14:* Musculus palmaris brevis. *15:* Fascia of hypothenar eminence. *16:* Rami cutanei of nervus digitalis volaris communis. *17:* Fasciculi transversi. *18:* Retinacula. *19:* Ligamenta basium.

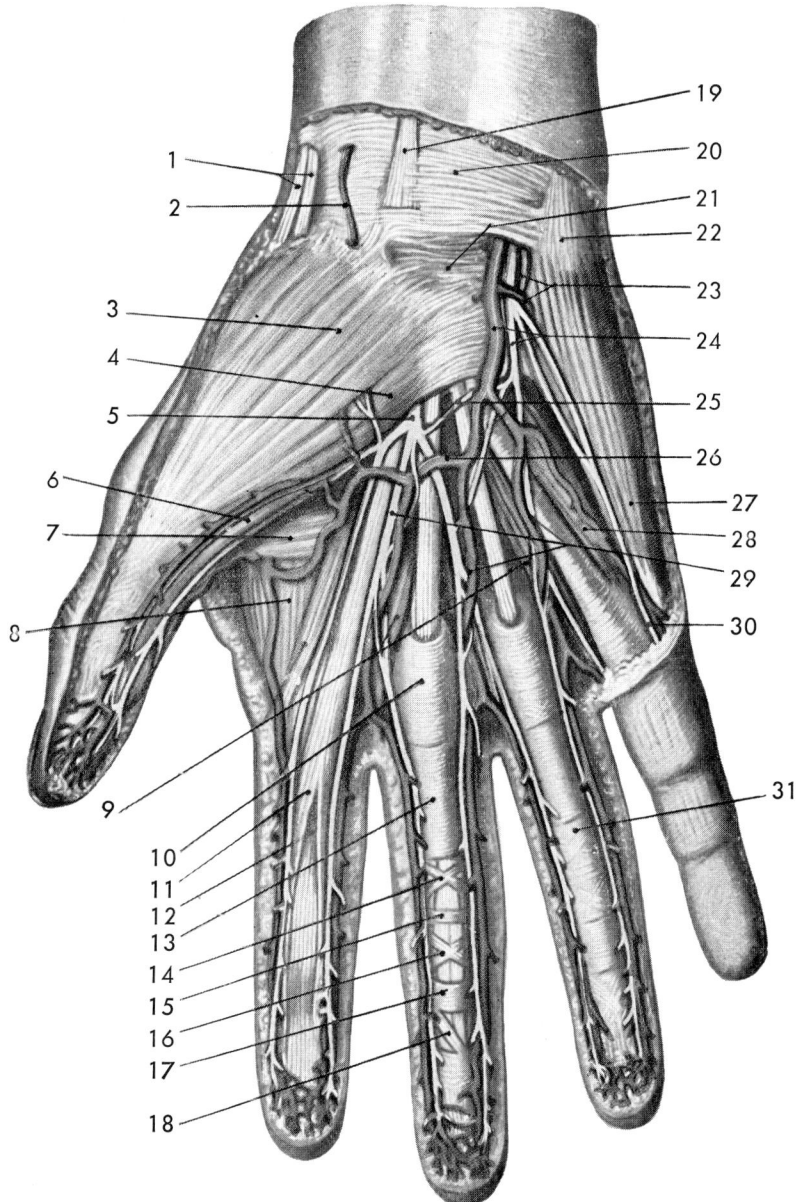

Fig. 346. Superficial arcus volaris. Palmar fasciae removed; tendon sheath of index finger removed; ligamenta vaginalia, annularia, and cruciata of middle finger depicted. (R. von Lanz and W. Wachsmuth: Praktische Anatomie. Julius Springer, Berlin.) 1: Tendon of the musculus abductor pollicis longus and musculus extensor pollicis brevis. 2: Ramus volaris superficialis arteria radialis. 3: Musculus abductor pollicis brevis. 4: Musculus flexor pollicis brevis, caput superficiale. 5: Nervus medianus. 6: Tendon sheath of musculus flexor pollicis longus. 7: Musculus adductor pollicis. 8: Musculus interosseus dorsalis I. 9: Musculi lumbricales I-IV.

10: Ligamentum vaginale accessorium. 11: Musculus flexor digitorum sublimis (perforatus). 12: Musculus flexor digitorum profundus (perforans). 13: Ligamentum vaginale I. 14: Ligamentum cruciatum. 15: Ligamentum annulare. 16: Ligamentum cruciatum. 17: Ligamentum vaginale II. 18: Ligamentum obliquum. 19: Tendon of musculus palmaris longus (severed).

20: Ligamentum carpi volare. 21: Ligamentum carpi transversum. 22: Os pisiforme. 23: Ramus profundus nervus ulnaris and arteria ulnaris. 24: Ramus superficialis nervus ulnaris and arteria ulnaris. 25: Rami anastomotici nervus ulnaris with nervus medianus. 26: Arcus volaris superficialis. 27: Musculus abductor digiti quinti. 28: Musculus flexor digiti quinti brevis. 29: Arteriae and nervi digitalis volares communes. 30: Arteria and nervus digitalis volaris proprius. 31: Tendon sheath of ring finger (intact).

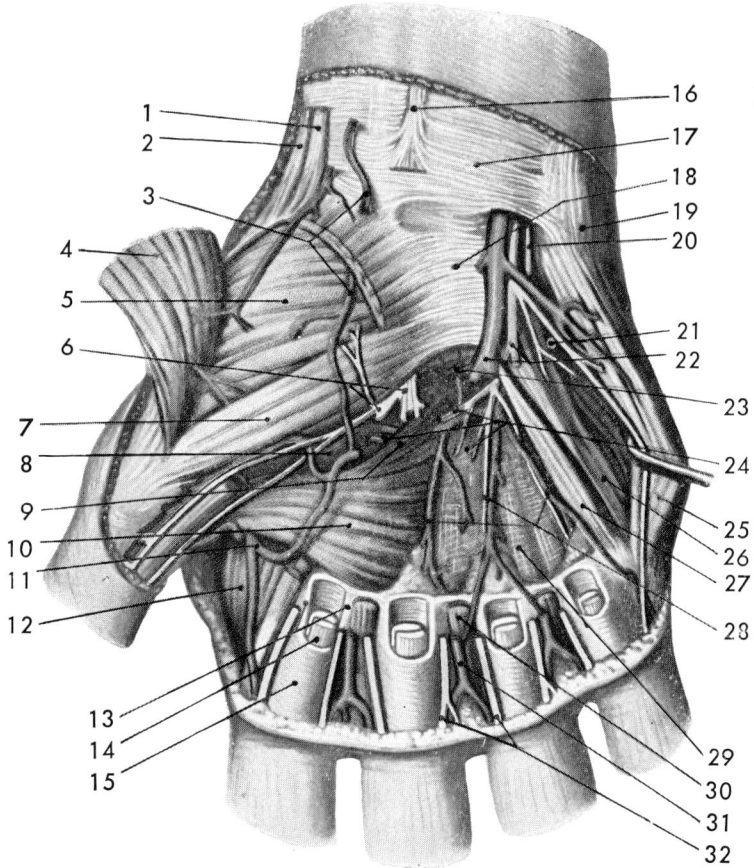

Fig. 347. Deep arcus volaris and deep palmar fasciae muscles and thenar and hypothenar regions. Palmar aponeurosis, superficial arcus volaris, and tendons removed. (R. von Lanz and W. Wachsmuth: Praktische Anatomie. Julius Springer, Berlin.) *1:* Tendon of musculus abductor pollicis longus. *2:* Tendon of musculus extensor pollicis brevis. *3:* Ramus volaris superficialis arteria radialis. *4:* Musculus abductor pollicis brevis (severed). *5:* Musculus opponens pollicis. *6:* Nervus medianus with branches to muscles of thumb. *7:* Musculus flexor pollicis brevis, caput superficiale. *8:* Musculus flexor brevis, caput profundum. *9:* Musculus adductor pollicis, caput obliquum.

10: Musculus adductor pollicis, caput transversum. *11:* Anastomosis of arcus volaris superficialis to arteria metacarpea volaris I. *12:* Musculus interosseus dorsalis I. *13:* Ligamenta capitulorum transversa. *14:* Tendons of musculus flexor digitorum (severed). *15:* Ligamentum vaginale I. *16:* Tendon of musculus palmaris longus (severed). *17:* Ligamentum carpi volare. *18:* Ligamentum carpi transversum. *19:* Os pisiforme.

20: Ramus profundus nervus ulnaris. *21:* Ramus profundus arteria ulnaris. *22:* Ramus superficialis nervus ulnaris and arteria ulnaris (severed). *23:* Tendons of musculus flexor digitorum in carpal canal (severed). *24:* Arcus volaris profundus and ramus profundus nervus ulnaris with muscle branches. *25:* Musculus abductor digiti quinti. *26:* Musculus opponens digiti quinti. *27:* Musculus flexor digiti quinti brevis. *28:* Arteriae metacarpea volares and articular branches of ramus profundus nervus ulnaris. *29:* Fascia palmaris profunda.

30: Musculi lumbricales III (severed). *31:* Arteria digitalis communis (severed). *32:* Nervi and arteria digitales volares proprii.

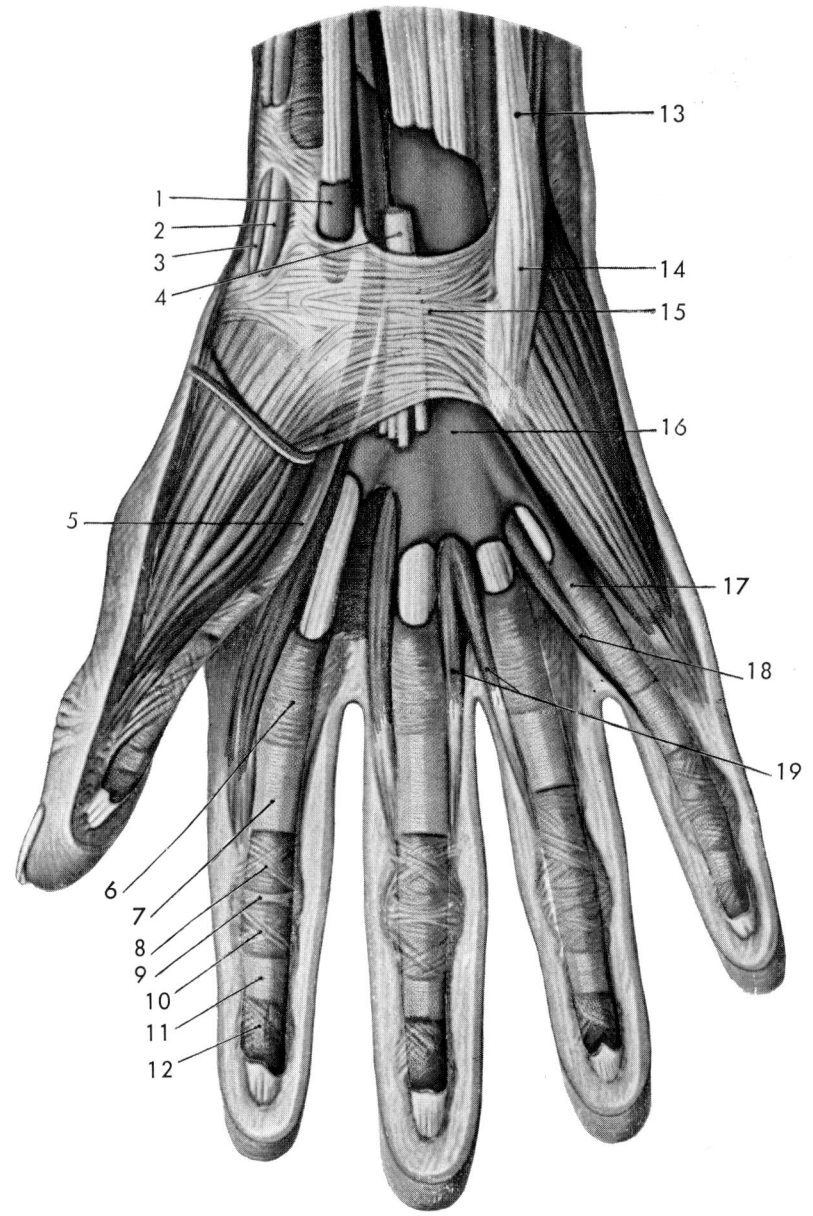

Fig. 348. Gliding apparatus of flexor tendons. Tendon sheaths filled with blue rubbery mass. Ligamentum carpi volare removed. (R. von Lanz and W. Wachsmuth:
Praktische Anatomie. Julius Springer, Berlin.)

1: Musculus flexor carpi radialis. *2:* Musculus abductor pollicis longus. *3:* Musculus
extensor pollicis brevis. *4:* Nervus medianus. *5:* Tendon sheath of musculus flexor
pollicis longus. *6:* Ligamentum vaginale accessorium. *7:* Ligamentum vaginale I.
8: Ligamentum cruciatum. *9:* Ligamentum annulare.
10: Ligamentum cruciatum. *11:* Ligamentum vaginale II. *12:* Ligamentum cruciatum. *13:* Musculus flexor carpi ulnaris. *14:* Os pisiforme. *15:* Ligamentum carpi
transversum. *16:* Common tendon sheath of musculus flexor digitorum. *17:* Tendon
sheath of flexor tendons of little finger continuous with common tendon sheath in
wrist. *18:* Musculus lumbricalis IV. *19:* Musculus lumbricalis III (insertion also at
middle finger, exceptional case).

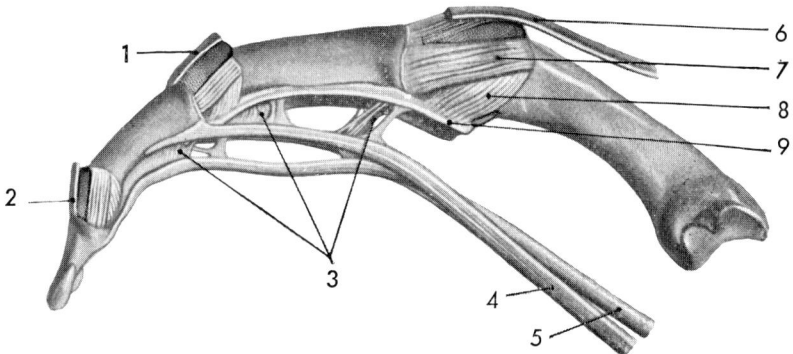

Fig. 349. Capsules and auxiliary ligaments of finger joints. Vincula tendinea. Ulnar side of middle finger. Joints filled with blue rubbery mass. (R. von Lanz and W. Wachsmuth: Praktische Anatomie. Julius Springer, Berlin.)
Articulatio interphalangea proximalis. *1:* Middle slip of aponeurosis dorsalis.
Articulatio interphalangea distalis. *2:* Lateral slip of aponeurosis dorsalis. *3:* Vincula tendinea. *4:* Tendon of musculus flexor digitorum sublimis. *5:* Tendon of musculus flexor digitorum profundus.
Articulatio metacarpophalangea. *6:* Aponeurosis dorsalis. *7:* Ligamentum collaterale. *8:* Ligamentum collaterale accessorium. *9:* Fibrocartilago volaris.

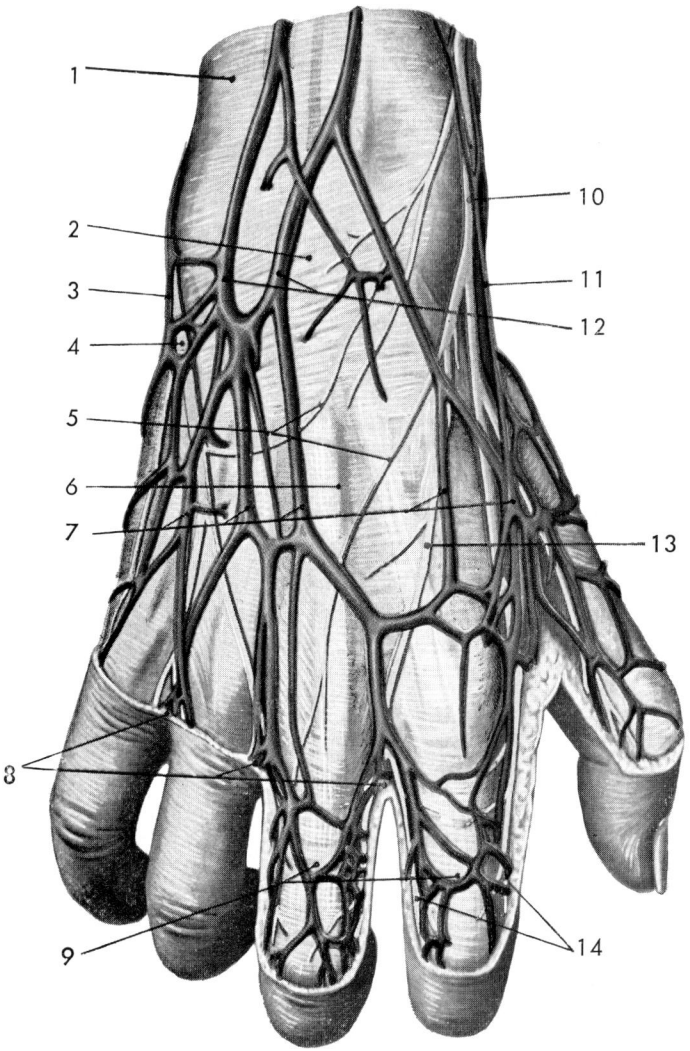

Fig. 350. Veins, skin, nerves, and superficial fasciae of dorsum of hand. (R. von
Lanz and W. Wachsmuth: Praktische Anatomie. Julius Springer, Berlin.)
1: Fascia antibrachii. *2:* Ligamentum carpi dorsale. *3:* Vena salvatella. *4:* Ramus
dorsalis nervus ulnaris. *5:* Rami anastomotici. *6:* Fasci dorsalis superficialis. *7:*
Venae metacarpeae dorsales. *8:* Venae intercapitulares. *9:* Arcus venosi digitalis.
10: Ramus superficialis nervus radialis. *11:* Vena cephalica pollicis. *12:* Venae
cephalicae accessoriae. *13:* Nervus digitalis communis dorsalis. *14:* Nervi digitales
dorsales proprii.

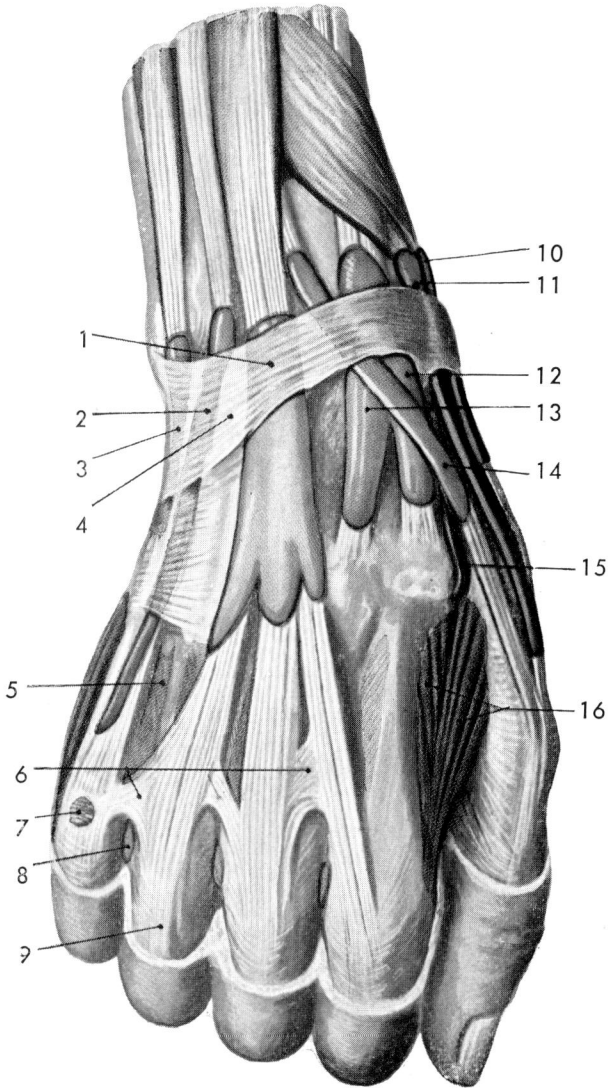

Fig. 351. Extensor tendons, tendon sheaths, and bursae dorsum of hand. Tendon sheaths and bursae filled with blue rubbery mass. (R. von Lanz and Wachsmuth: Praktische Anatomie. Julius Springer, Berlin.)

Ulnar group of tendon sheaths. *Fourth space.* 1: Musculus extensor digitorum communis, musculus extensor indicis proprius.

Fifth space. 2: Musculus extensor digiti quinti proprius.

Sixth space. 3: Musculus extensor carpi ulnaris. 4: Ligamentum carpi dorsale. 5: Fascia dorsalis profunda. 6: Juncturae tendinea. 7: Bursa mucosa subcutanea metacarpophalangea dorsalis. 8: Bursa mucosa intermetacarpophalangea. 9: Aponeurosis dorsalis.

Radial group of tendon sheaths. *First space.* 10: Musculus abductor pollicis longus. 11: Musculus extensor pollicis brevis.

Second space. 12: Musculus extensor carpi radialis longus. 13: Musculus extensor carpi radialis brevis.

Third space. 14: Musculus extensor pollicis longus. 15: Arteria radialis. 16: Musculus interosseus dorsalis I.

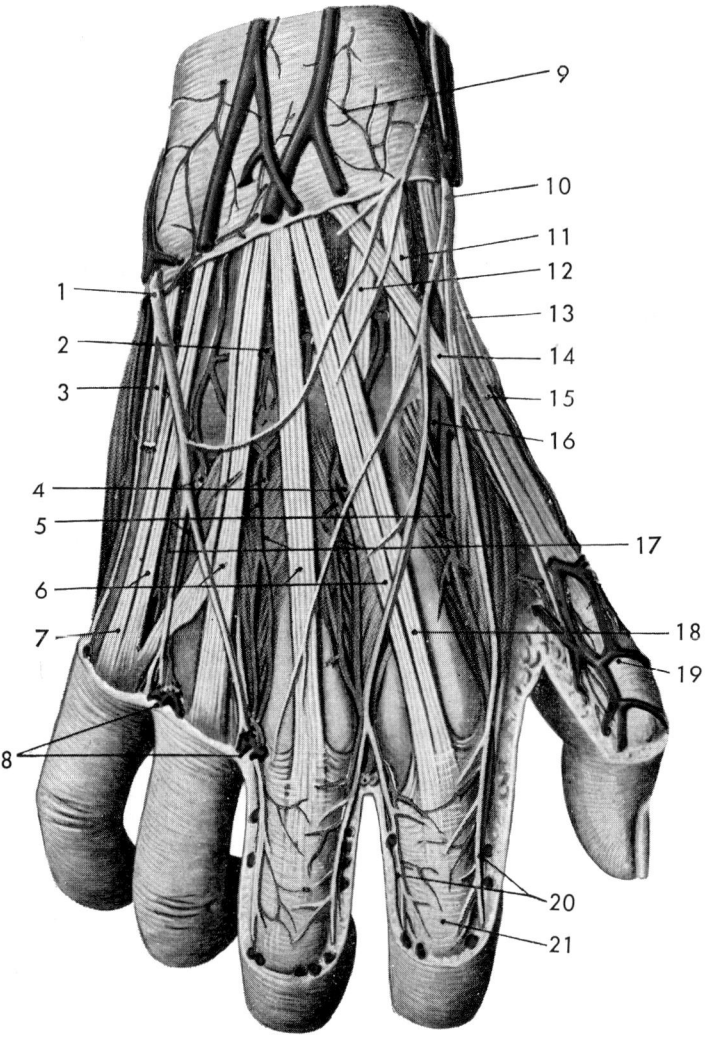

Fig. 352. Deep layer of dorsum of hand. Subcutaneous veins, superficial fasciae, and juncturae tendinea are removed. Distal junctura (IV/V) is trimmed distally and displaced proximally and radially to expose spatium interosseum IV. (R. von Lanz and W. Wachsmuth: Praktische Anatomie. Julius Springer, Berlin.)

1: Ramus dorsalis nervus ulnaris. *2:* Ramus carpeus dorsalis. *3:* Tendon of musculus extensor carpi ulnaris. *4:* Rami perforantes. *5:* Arteriae metacarpeae dorsales. *6:* Tendons of musculus extensor digitorum communis. *7:* Tendon of musculus extensor digiti quinti proprius. *8:* Venae intercapitulares. *9:* Rete arteriosum carpeum dorsale.

10: Ramus superficialis nervus radialis. *11:* Musculus extensor carpi radialis longus. *12:* Musculus extensor carpi radialis brevis. *13:* Musculus abductor pollicis longus. *14:* Musculus extensor pollicis longus. *15:* Musculus extensor pollicis brevis. *16:* Arteria radialis. *17:* Musculi interossei dorsales. *18:* Tendon of musculus extensor indicis proprius. *19:* Rete venosum dorsale pollicis. *20:* Arteriae and nervi digitales dorsales proprii. *21:* Aponeurosis dorsalis.

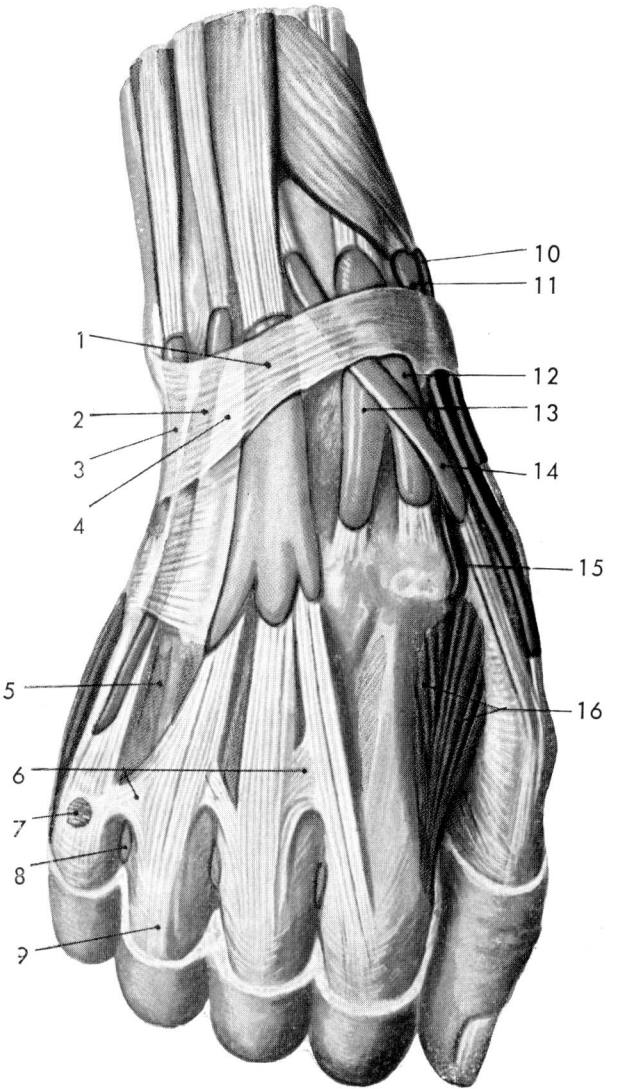

Fig. 351. Extensor tendons, tendon sheaths, and bursae dorsum of hand. Tendon sheaths and bursae filled with blue rubbery mass. (R. von Lanz and Wachsmuth: Praktische Anatomie. Julius Springer, Berlin.)

Ulnar group of tendon sheaths. *Fourth space*. 1: Musculus extensor digitorum communis, musculus extensor indicis proprius.

Fifth space. 2: Musculus extensor digiti quinti proprius.

Sixth space. 3: Musculus extensor carpi ulnaris. 4: Ligamentum carpi dorsale. 5: Fascia dorsalis profunda. 6: Juncturae tendinea. 7: Bursa mucosa subcutanea metacarpophalangea dorsalis. 8: Bursa mucosa intermetacarpophalangea. 9: Aponeurosis dorsalis.

Radial group of tendon sheaths. *First space.* 10: Musculus abductor pollicis longus. 11: Musculus extensor pollicis brevis.

Second space. 12: Musculus extensor carpi radialis longus. 13: Musculus extensor carpi radialis brevis.

Third space. 14: Musculus extensor pollicis longus. 15: Arteria radialis. 16: Musculus interosseus dorsalis I.

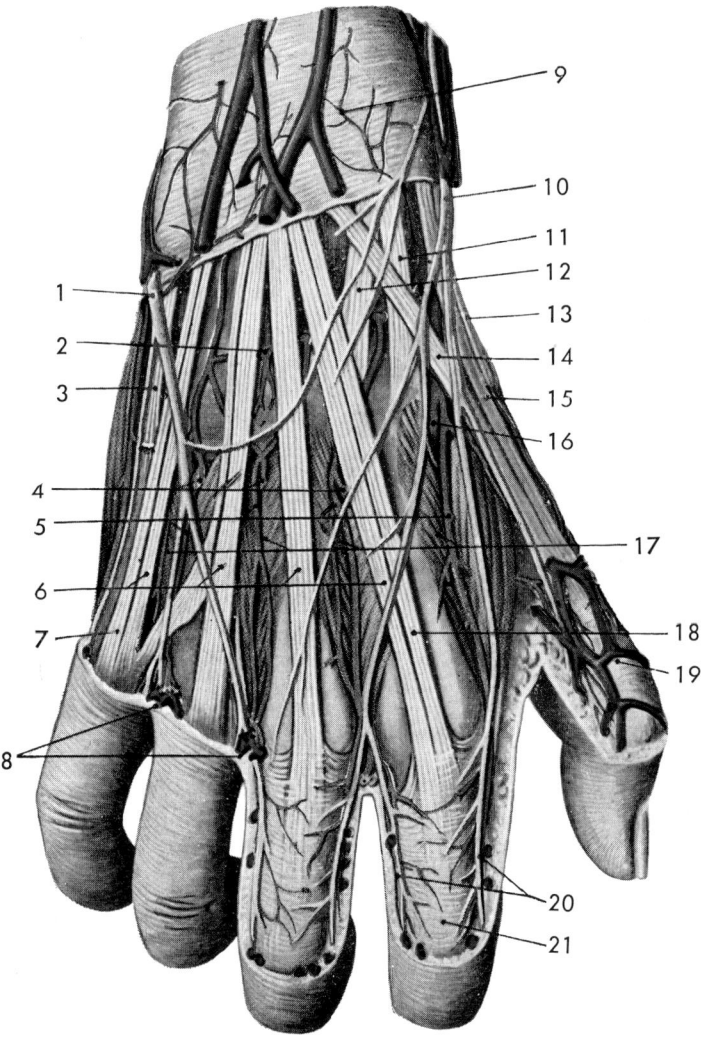

Fig. 352. Deep layer of dorsum of hand. Subcutaneous veins, superficial fasciae, and juncturae tendinea are removed. Distal junctura (IV/V) is trimmed distally and displaced proximally and radially to expose spatium interosseum IV. (R. von Lanz and W. Wachsmuth: Praktische Anatomie. Julius Springer, Berlin.)

1: Ramus dorsalis nervus ulnaris. *2:* Ramus carpeus dorsalis. *3:* Tendon of musculus extensor carpi ulnaris. *4:* Rami perforantes. *5:* Arteriae metacarpeae dorsales. *6:* Tendons of musculus extensor digitorum communis. *7:* Tendon of musculus extensor digiti quinti proprius. *8:* Venae intercapitulares. *9:* Rete arteriosum carpeum dorsale.

10: Ramus superficialis nervus radialis. *11:* Musculus extensor carpi radialis longus. *12:* Musculus extensor carpi radialis brevis. *13:* Musculus abductor pollicis longus. *14:* Musculus extensor pollicis longus. *15:* Musculus extensor pollicis brevis. *16:* Arteria radialis. *17:* Musculi interossei dorsales. *18:* Tendon of musculus extensor indicis proprius. *19:* Rete venosum dorsale pollicis. *20:* Arteriae and nervi digitales dorsales proprii. *21:* Aponeurosis dorsalis.

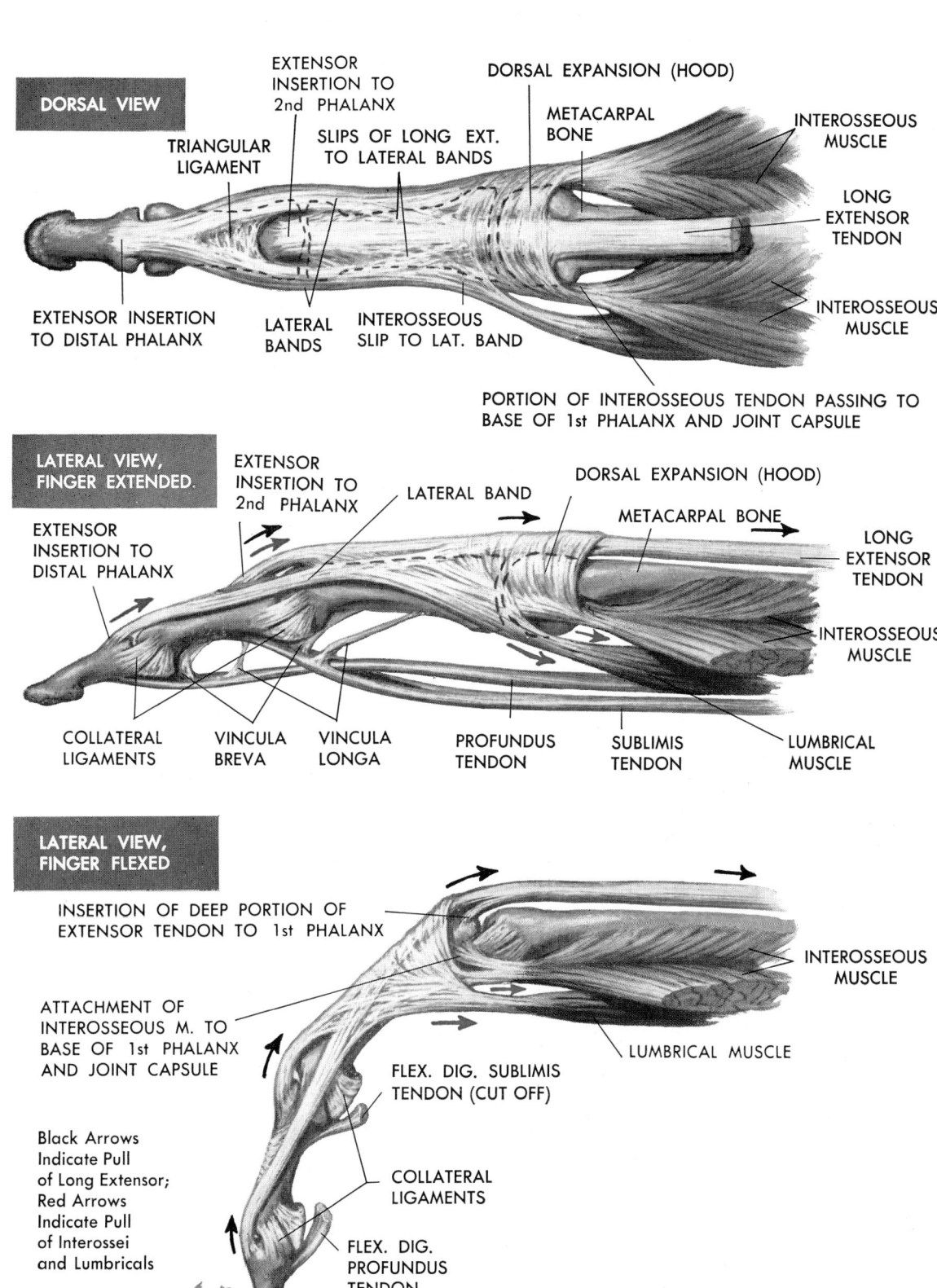

DORSAL VIEW

EXTENSOR INSERTION TO 2nd PHALANX

DORSAL EXPANSION (HOOD)

TRIANGULAR LIGAMENT

METACARPAL BONE

SLIPS OF LONG EXT. TO LATERAL BANDS

INTEROSSEOUS MUSCLE

LONG EXTENSOR TENDON

EXTENSOR INSERTION TO DISTAL PHALANX

LATERAL BANDS

INTEROSSEOUS SLIP TO LAT. BAND

INTEROSSEOUS MUSCLE

PORTION OF INTEROSSEOUS TENDON PASSING TO BASE OF 1st PHALANX AND JOINT CAPSULE

LATERAL VIEW, FINGER EXTENDED.

EXTENSOR INSERTION TO 2nd PHALANX

LATERAL BAND

DORSAL EXPANSION (HOOD)

METACARPAL BONE

EXTENSOR INSERTION TO DISTAL PHALANX

LONG EXTENSOR TENDON

INTEROSSEOUS MUSCLE

COLLATERAL LIGAMENTS

VINCULA BREVA

VINCULA LONGA

PROFUNDUS TENDON

SUBLIMIS TENDON

LUMBRICAL MUSCLE

LATERAL VIEW, FINGER FLEXED

INSERTION OF DEEP PORTION OF EXTENSOR TENDON TO 1st PHALANX

INTEROSSEOUS MUSCLE

ATTACHMENT OF INTEROSSEOUS M. TO BASE OF 1st PHALANX AND JOINT CAPSULE

LUMBRICAL MUSCLE

FLEX. DIG. SUBLIMIS TENDON (CUT OFF)

Black Arrows Indicate Pull of Long Extensor; Red Arrows Indicate Pull of Interossei and Lumbricals

COLLATERAL LIGAMENTS

FLEX. DIG. PROFUNDUS TENDON (CUT OFF)

F. Netter M.D.

©CIBA

Fig. 353. Anatomy and display of function and synergic-stabilizing action of the intrinsic system. (E. W. Lampe, Ciba Clinical Symposia.)

radial group. The ulnar group fans out over the middle part of the hand to the second to fifth fingers, while the radial group passes to the radial side of the midhand and the thumb, forming the tabatière anatomique, which contains the arteria radialis and the ramus superficialis nervus radialis. There are altogether six extensor tendons for the second, third, fourth, and fifth fingers; one tendon for the third and fourth fingers; and two each for the second and fifth fingers. Near the metacarpophalangeal joints, the tendons are connected with each other by fibrous bands, the juncturae tendinum.

Beneath the extensor tendons are found the four musculi interossei dorsales, which arise from the metacarpal bones and which are inserted in a way similar to that of the volar group (see Fig. 353). While the volar group adducts the second, fourth, and fifth fingers toward the third finger, the dorsal group abducts them. The musculi interossei dorsales also aid the action of the musculi lumbricales in flexing the fingers in the metacarpophalangeal joints and extending the fingers in the interphalangeal joints. Together, the interossei and lumbricales form the intrinsic system of the hand (see pp. 844-845). The interossei dorsales are innervated by the deep palmar branch of the ulnar nerve.

Digital Insertion of Tendons (Fig. 353)

After having crossed the metacarpophalangeal joint, each extensor tendon flattens out to form an aponeurosis over the proximal phalanx, which is intimately connected with the capsule and lateral ligaments of the metacarpophalangeal joint. The extensor tendon also inserts into the dorsum of the proximal phalanx. By means of this insertion, the tendon can carry out two functions: first, to extend the proximal phalanx to extension and hyperextension; second, to stabilize the metacarpophalangeal joints so that the intrinsic muscles (lumbricales and interossei) not only can extend the middle and distal phalanges but also are able to give lateral movements to the fingers. Over the first interphalangeal joint, the dorsal aponeurosis splits into three slips: the central slip, fused with the joint capsule, is inserted to the base of the middle phalanx; the two lateral slips, after having received the insertions of the musculi lumbricales and musculi interossei, converge to fuse with the capsule of the terminal joint and to attach to the base of the terminal phalanx.

Intrinsic Muscles of Fingers

The lumbricales and the interossei make up the intrinsic-muscle system of the hand—the most important structure for the stabilization of the hand and fingers. Textbooks commonly give an accurate description of the anatomy, but fail to consider the synergic balancing function. Among

843

other investigators, Sterling Bunnell and his co-workers Howard and Pratt have advanced our knowledge of the function of the intrinsic system, which has been described in a stimulating review by Eyler, Markee, and E. W. Lampe.

The intrinsic muscles act in coordination. Together with the long extensor tendon they exert a synergic balancing function which permits a variety of finger motions. The difference in action is made possible by a remarkable mechanism at the base of the finger in the form of a thin, sliding aponeurotic sleeve ("hood"), which with transverse fibers connects the conjoined lumbrical-interosseus tendons with the extensor tendon over the dorsum of the proximal phalanx. The aponeurotic sling can be shifted forward and backward with the extensor tendon, acting like a gear shift. By means of this mechanism, the intrinsic muscles can stabilize the metacarpophalangeal joints in flexion so that the long extensor can extend the interphalangeal joints. By means of this same device, the long extensor tendons can stabilize the metacarpophalangeal joints in extension so that the intrinsic muscles can give lateral motion and can extend the interphalangeal joints. This synergic action improves the ability of the long extensors to extend the interphalangeal joints when the metacarpophalangeal joints are flexed, as well as that of the intrinsic muscles to extend the interphalangeal joints when the metacarpophalangeal joints are extended.

The following description of the synergic-stabilizing action of the intrinsic system in collaboration with the extensor tendon is taken from E. W. Lampe (Fig. 353): "A central slip inserts into the dorsum of the proximal end of the middle phalanx. Two lateral tendinous slips unite with the tendons of the lumbrical and interosseus muscles and continue distally to the proximal end of the dorsum of the terminal phalanx for insertion. Despite the insertions of the extensor digitorum communis into the middle and terminal phalanges, this muscle can extend these two phalanges only very slightly, if at all, when the proximal phalanges are in extension. This occurs because so much of each of the extensor digitorum communis tendons is inserted into the dorsum of the proximal phalanges that when the muscle contracts most of its power is concentrated in extending the proximal phalanges.

"Furthermore, this firm anchoring of the tendons to the proximal phalanges permits but little extension of the middle and terminal phalanges by the extensor communis when the proximal phalanges are in the extended position. The arrows in [Figure 353] show how the tendons of the lumbrical muscles and interosseous muscles, especially the volar interossei, inserted into the lateral slips of the extensor digitorum communis, are able to do most of the extending of the middle and terminal phalanges when the proximal phalanges are extended. The situation changes, however, as soon as the extensor digitorum communis relaxes sufficiently to permit the flexors digitorum sublimis and profundus to begin flexing the middle and terminal phalanges. Simultaneously, this causes the extensor communis 'hood' to be pulled distally away from the metacarpophalangeal joint just enough so that when the lumbricales and interossei contract they then flex the proximal phalanges. In fact, the important flexors of the proximal phalanges are the lumbrical and interosseous muscles.

"It seems almost paradoxical to have these intrinsic muscles flex the proximal phalanges and extend the middle and terminal phalanges. But a study of [Figure 353] will show that if the dorsal expansion or 'hood' is pulled proximally to the metacarpophalangeal joint (this occurs when the extensor digitorum communis has extended the proximal phalanges), contraction of the lumbricales and interossei extends the middle and terminal phalanges. On the other hand, when the 'hood' is pulled distal to the metacarpophalangeal joint (this occurs with the synergic relaxation of the extensor digitorum communis and flexion of the digitorum sublimis and profundus), contraction of the lumbricales and interossei results in flexion of the proximal phalanges. Now when the fingers are flexed (for example, 45 degrees), the extensor digitorum communis, via its lateral slips, takes over about half the control of the extension of the middle and terminal phalanges; and when the fingers are three-fourths flexed, the extensor digitorum communis assumes full control in the extension of these phalanges.

"The interosseous muscles gain partial insertion not only into the lateral aspects of the proximal ends of the proximal phalanges but also into the lateral aspects of the capsules of the metacarpophalangeal joints. It is these insertions which enable the ulnar-nerve-controlled interossei to spread and approximate the fingers."

PHYSIOLOGY AND REGENERATION OF TENDONS AND TENDON GRAFTS

The function of a tendon is to transmit the contractile force of the muscle (its physiology has been described in classic treatises by Bielsalski and Mayer and by L. Mayer). For proper functioning the gliding mechanism of a tendon is of the utmost importance. The tendon is surrounded on all sides by a loose fatty meshwork of tissue which is rich in elastic fibers, enabling the tendon to glide to and fro. This tissue is termed "paratenon." The tendon sheath is a closed sac, containing fluid. It is found wherever the tendon changes its direction and serves as a fluid buffer to diminish friction of that joint. The sheath consists of a parietal and a visceral layer. Both layers are connected with each other by the mesotenon, which carries the nutrient vessels and nerves (Colville, Callison and Wink). Other blood vessels supply the tendon proper which are derived from the muscular tendinous juncture and the osteotendinous insertion. According to the extensive research studies of Peacock and the fine vascular injection studies of Smith, however, these vessels nourish only the proximal and distal third of the tendon, i.e., they do not anastomose. Hence, the middle third or even a larger segment of the tendon depends upon extrinsic sources for vascular nourishment. When a tendon is freed during surgery, the mesenteric source of its blood supply is interrupted. The greater part of the tendon then functions like a free graft until new vessels develop to restore its circulation. If this does not happen, scar tissue will envelop the tendon and lead to adhesions. Disastrous as adhesions are from the standpoint of function they are beneficial in supplying extrinsic blood supply to the tendon. Shielding the tendon by mechanical barriers to prevent adhesions is apt to lead to necrosis of the tendon with eventual disintegration of collagen bundles. This is particularly true in a tendon graft, which always should be transplanted with its paratenon so that the latter can find access to the surrounding vessels and can maintain the extrinsic blood supply and gliding mechanism of the graft.

The healing of a tendon and the tendon graft have been extensively studied by Allan and Mason, Mason and Shearon, Iselin, Skoog and Persson, Peacock, Lindsay and McDougall, Flynn, Wilson, Child and Graham, and others. Quoting Lindsay, a tendon is composed of three elements: collagen, ground substance and fibroblasts. The fibroblasts are variably shaped cells capable of ameboid movement and responsible for the production of both collagen and ground substance. Divided tendons and free tendon grafts exhibit collagenous fiber changes, hypercellularity, and adhesion formation during the process of healing. The origin of the new cells is still controversial. It seems, however, that the fibroblasts responsible for the repair come from the outside and form at the site of the anastomosis a connective tissue callus; this is the proliferative stage of the healing process and lasts about two weeks. It is followed by the formative stage, during which the fibrous tissue cells become oriented and mature and are gradually converted into tendon. Hence, it seems that adhesions are part of the physiological process in tendon healing.

The regeneration of a tendon graft occurs from the stumps of the host. Whether the whole graft survives and through revascularization a

846

gradual reconstitution or replacement of the original collagen occurs (Lindsay and McDougall, Mason and Shearon), or whether the transplant undergoes necrosis and acts as a strut along which it is replaced by tenoblasts from the stumps of the host (Flynn, Child and Graham) or by cells which infiltrate from the paratenon (Skoog and Persson), are questions which are still controversial. There is no doubt, however, that the graft ultimately becomes regenerated to function as a normal tendon.

DIVISION OF TENDONS AND NERVES

OPEN INJURIES

General Rules and Technique

Diagnosis

Whenever a wound occurs in the hand, an exact anatomical test should be made for possible injuries of tendons and nerves. Inability to flex the terminal phalanx indicates a division of the profundus tendon. Partial disability to flex the proximal interphalangeal joint indicates a division of the sublimis tendon. Inability to flex the terminal and proximal interphalangeal joints indicates a division of both flexor tendons. Inability to flex the terminal joint of the thumb indicates a division of the musculus flexor pollicis longus. On the dorsal side, the diagnosis may be less easy, owing to the support the extensor tendons receive from the lumbrical and interosseous muscles (Fig. 353). Furthermore, the fibrous bands, the juncturae tendinum (Fig. 351), connecting the extensor tendons with each other may be strong enough to transmit the function of an uninjured tendon to its injured neighbor.

With each tendon injury there is a possibility of nerve injury. Hence, preoperative tests should be made. However, it must be remembered that the muscle bellies of the long flexors and extensors are innervated in the forearm. Therefore, testing intrinsic muscles of the hand and sensation is of value. Loss of sensation of the fifth finger and the ulnar half of the fourth finger, loss of abduction and adduction of the completely extended fingers, and loss of adduction of the thumb—that is, an inability to make a perfect O between thumb and index finger or to hold a piece of paper firmly between these fingers—indicate injury to the ulnar nerve. Loss of sensation of the palmar surface of the thumb, index, and middle fingers and of the radial half of the fourth finger, together with the inability to rotate the thumb to face the fingers (opposition), indicates injury to the median nerve. Loss of sensation of the radial half of the dorsum of the hand is the sign of injury to the superficial branch of the radial nerve.

However, it has been found that the usual tests for pain with pin-prick and for touch with cotton wool are inadequate when one wishes to get information about the functional value of hand sensitivity. The examination must instead aim to determine the complex sensory function that gives the grip "sight." The term "tactile gnosis" has been coined for this quality by Moberg, to whom we are indebted for recent investigations on this subject. He described three clinical methods by which the quality can be tested: the two-point discrimination test, the picking-up test and the Ninhydrin printing test. He considers the latter as the only objective test since it is based on the fact that the sweat glands of the skin cease to function when their nerve supply from the sympathetic nervous system is blocked. Zrubecky has published a monograph on this subject (see also p. 804).

In older cases in which the injury has resulted in disability of flexion of the fingers, the degree of impairment of flexion should always be recorded. Boyes offers a simple way of measuring. He states: "In order to flex the interphalangeal joints of the finger completely, the deep flexor tendon must make an excursion of three-fourths of an inch in the proximal segment of the finger and one and three-eighths inches in the palm. If this excursion is limited, the tip of the finger fails to touch the distal crease of the palm. The measurement of this distance, the lack of flexion to the distal crease, thus becomes an easily recorded and readily understood index of the results of flexor-tendon action in the fingers. Function of the long flexor tendon of the thumb is measured by the degrees of flexion of the interphalangeal joint."

Primary versus Secondary Repair of Tendons and Nerves

There is no question that the prognosis is better for the functional result after a primary than after a secondary tendon and nerve repair; there is also no question that the prognosis is poor for secondary repairs following failure of a primary one. Hence, in any open tendon and nerve injury, the surgeon is confronted with the question of whether to repair tendons and nerves primarily or simply to close the wound and delay the tendon and nerve repair until after the wound has healed. In coming to the right decision the time factor must be taken into consideration, although this is no longer as important as it once was. Other factors to be considered are: degree of contamination, type of wound, location of injury, condition of the patient, operative facilities available, experience of the surgeon. Immediate repair of divided tendons and nerves (except for tendons severed within the flexor sheaths where as a rule repair work must be delayed; see p. 853) can be undertaken (1) if the wound is clean and made by sharp instruments, such as glass or knives, (2) if the emergency dressing was carried out aseptically, and (3) if the patient is seen within a few hours after the accident. Some authors place the time limit from two to six hours, others up to twelve or even twenty-four hours following the accident. The writer prefers to suture tendons and nerves up to eight hours following the accident. If the wound is soiled or contused or the patient is seen after the eight-hour limit, the wound is excised and closed, but the repair of tendons and nerves is delayed until the wound has healed, usually after three to four weeks. Infected wounds, however, are left open, and tendons and nerves should not be repaired until at least six months have elapsed since the healing of the wound. Since the introduction of antibiotics, the time interval can be shortened to three months.

General Technique

The author follows the general and now classical rules of Bunnell, Koch and Mason (Peacock and Hartrampf published a fine collective review on the repair of flexor tendons of the hand; for more and recent references the reader is referred to the Bibliography of this section). The operative field is cleansed aseptically (p. 798). The operation is performed under general or brachial block anesthesia. A blood-pressure cuff is applied and inflated to obtain a bloodless field. Before inflation, the arm is elevated and held elevated for five minutes. The cuff is then pumped to a pressure of 280 mm. of mercury. This pressure may be maintained as long as necessary to complete the dissection. It is then lowered to enable the surgeon to ligate the bleeders. When all bleeders have been ligated, the arm is again elevated for five minutes and the cuff is reinflated to 280 mm. of mercury and kept inflated until the operation is completed and the pressure dressing is applied. In primary repairs, the wound edges should be excised as sparingly as possible. If additional incisions are necessary for locating retracted tendons, the location of the incisions is of the utmost importance. At the fingers, lateral incisions (Fig. 354, A) or bayonet incisions (Fig. 354, B) are the best. Unless long, the lateral incisions should be made opposite the joints, where there are no pulleys. In the palm, the incision should not cross a flexion crease at right angles; it should be parallel to the creases. In the wrist, the incision should be transverse. If the original wound is to be enlarged, the additional incisions should be planned so that the foregoing rules are obeyed; furthermore, the line of tendon repair is overlaid by a flap of skin and subcutaneous tissue and not by the line of skin suture. So, for instance, the incision of finger and palm may be combined in suitable places (Fig. 354, A). At the wrist, a transverse incision can be enlarged by

849

adding secondary longitudinal incisions on each side, resulting in a bayonet-form incision (Figs. 354, *A, B*). On the dorsum, the incisions are similar to those on the volar surface. If, instead of elective incisions, the surgeon is confronted with an already present wound or scar and the wound must be enlarged, compromise incisions must be made, which should be outlined according to the aforementioned principles.

The handling of tendons and nerves should be as gentle as possible. These structures should remain exposed only a short time. They should

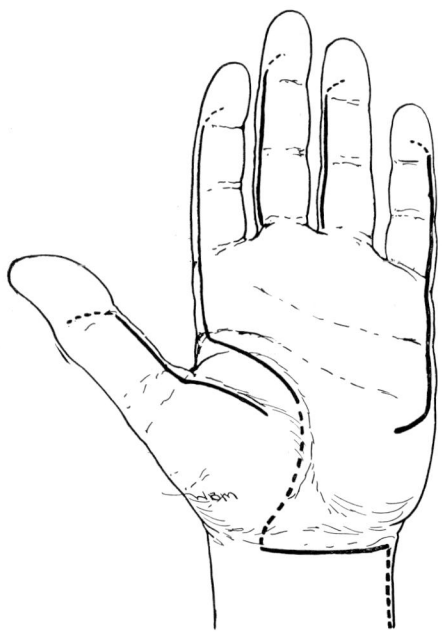

Fig. 354. *A:* Correct incision in hand. At fingers, lateral incisions are best. In palm, incisions should be parallel with creases; in wrist, they should be transverse. Dotted lines indicate additional extensions and combinations. (H. May: Surg. Obstet. Gynec.)

be covered with moist gauze. They should not be grasped with rough instruments. If grasped, only their divided ends should be clamped with a mosquito forceps, and no more should be traumatized than the part to be sacrificed. There are a great variety of tendon sutures. Those which the author has used are depicted in Figures 355, *A, B*, 356. For suture material, fine twisted silk (No. 6) or stainless-steel wire (No. 35) is recommended on a straight needle. Each piece is tested in advance to assure sufficient strength. Severed nerves are treated with a similar atraumatic technique and sutured as described on page 748.

MUSCLES, TENDONS, NERVES, AND BLOOD VESSELS

PRIMARY REPAIR OF SEVERED TENDONS AND NERVES

Volar Side of Wrist and Forearm

As an example, Case 145, page 1188 is cited. In this case, the examination revealed division of the median and ulnar nerves and of the superficial and deep tendons of second, third, fourth, and fifth fingers, of the musculus flexor carpi radialis, flexor carpi ulnaris, and of the ulnar artery just above the wrist.

Step 1: After excision of the wound edges, the original wound may need enlargement (Figs. 354, *A*, *B*). The nerves are exposed first. The

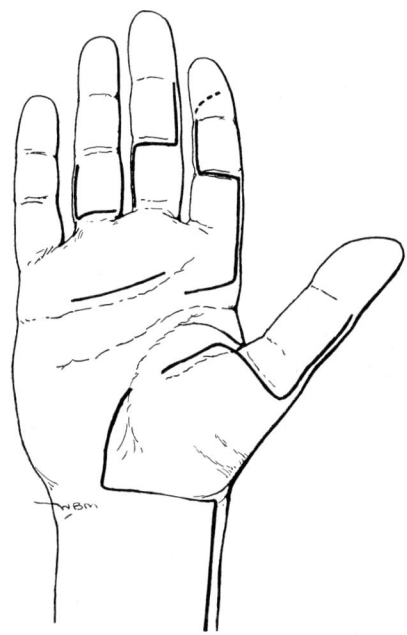

Fig. 354. *B:* Bayonet incisions in hand (Mason). (H. May: Surg. Gynec. Obstet.)

proximal end of the median nerve is located. It is found at the level of the divided musculus palmaris longus tendon as the most superficial structure. Higher up in the forearm, it dips between the superficial and deep flexor tendons. The distal end is found beneath the ligamentum carpi transversum, which should be divided longitudinally over the nerve. The nerve could not be distinguished from the surrounding tendons were it not for its dull gray color (the tendons are shiny and glistening) with the appearance of nerve bundles on transverse section. The extreme tips of the nerve stumps are transfixed with a mosquito forceps and the nerve ends wrapped in moist gauze. Location of the divided ulnar nerve follows.

851

THE EXTREMITIES

The proximal end is in close proximity to the ulnar artery and vein, covered by the musculus flexor carpi ulnaris. Ulnar artery and vein, if divided, should be ligated at this point. The distal end of the nerve is found, unlike the median nerve, upon the ligamentum carpi transversum covered only by the ligamentum carpi volare (Fig. 346). If the division is more distal where the ulnar nerve splits up into superficial and deep branches, both branches must be located and secured.

Step 2: The stumps of the divided tendons are now located. The proximal ends may have retracted considerably. Unless it is possible to

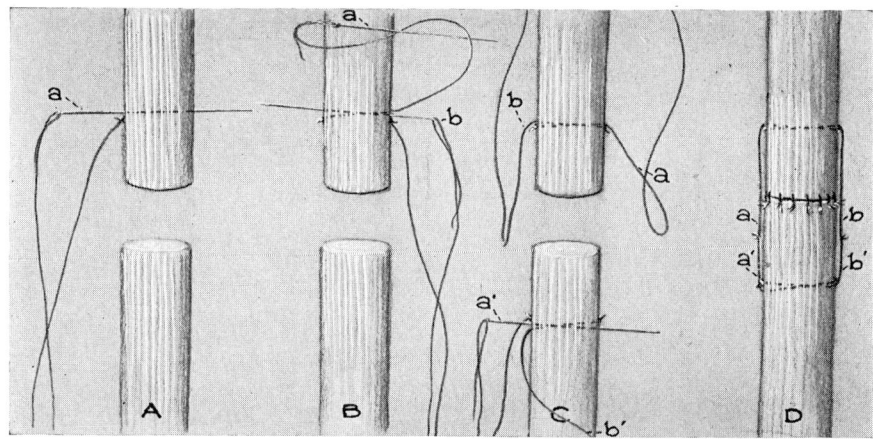

Fig. 355. *A:* Tendon suture (Mason). Small bundle of peripheral tendon fibers is caught with a suture about 1 cm. (⅜ inch) above tendon end. Short end of suture is cut. Long end of suture is passed through tendon with needle to come out on opposite side at level of about 0.5 cm (³⁄₁₆ inch) higher than level of knot. Second suture is tied about small bundle of peripheral tendon fibers just below point of emergence of first suture. Short end of suture is cut; long end of suture is passed with needle through tendon so as to come out on opposite side directly above knot of first suture. Similar sutures are placed in opposite stump and tendons approximated by tying corresponding sutures. A few coaptation sutures are placed to coapt tendon stumps end to end.

make them appear in the wound by bending the forearm or milking the muscles, the incision is enlarged according to the foregoing principles. First the superficial tendons are secured with mosquito hemostats, then the deep tendons. All stumps are covered with moist gauze. The distal tendon stumps, if retracted, ordinarily reappear in the wound when fingers and wrist are flexed; otherwise, the carpal ligament is severed.

Step 3: Suture of the tendons is carried out first by uniting the corresponding tendon stumps. This is followed by suture of the nerves (see also p. 749) and closure of the subcutaneous tissue and the skin with a

852

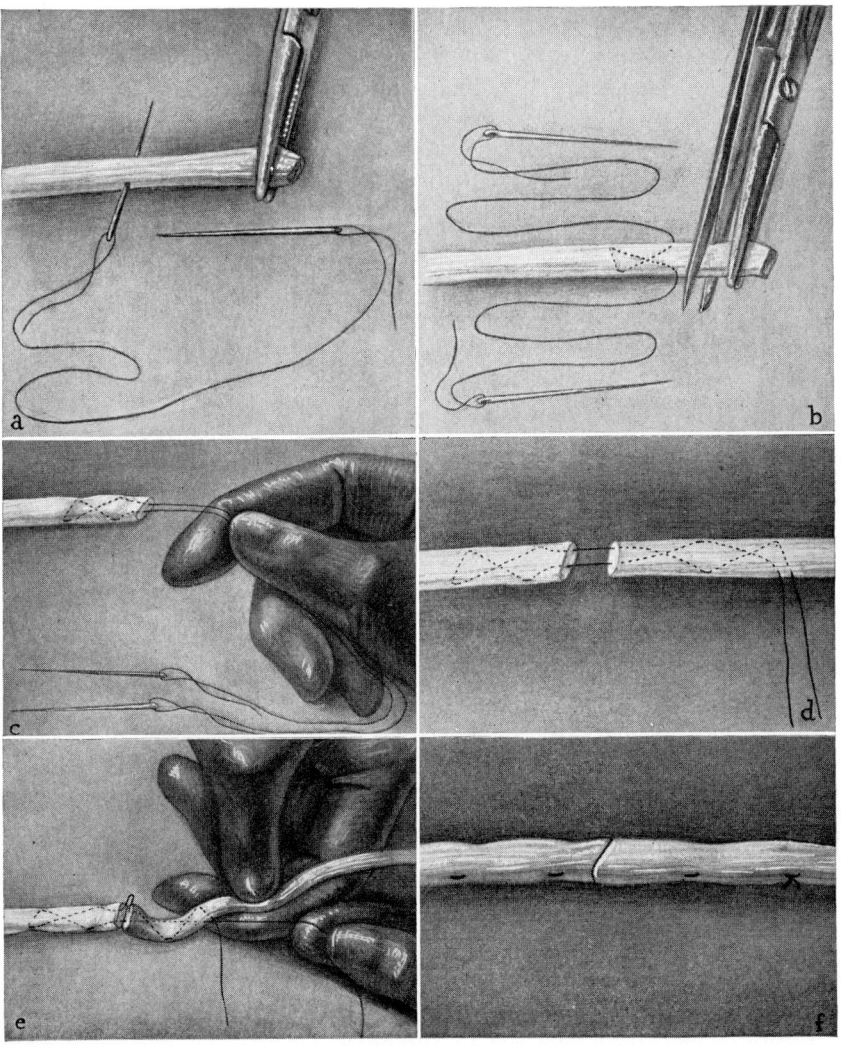

Fig. 355. *B:* Tendon suture (Bunnell). *a, b:* Silk sutures are placed transversely in tendon from two to four times, emerging through end. *c:* All slack is drawn out. *d:* Suture is continued similarly up other tendon. Both ends are brought out at same side. In placing last strand in second tendon end, needle must not spear other threads or they will not slip. By keeping on separate sides of tendon, this is avoided; better, both needles may be thrust through tendon simultaneously. *e:* One of the silk strands is now pulled straight and taut, and second end is slid down over it until it pushes against first tendon end. Then second silk strand is to be drawn straight and taut until it also has slipped through tendon. *f:* There is but one knot. When tied, it sinks into tendon, and it is placed where it receives least strain, since knots are the weakest parts of a tendon suture.

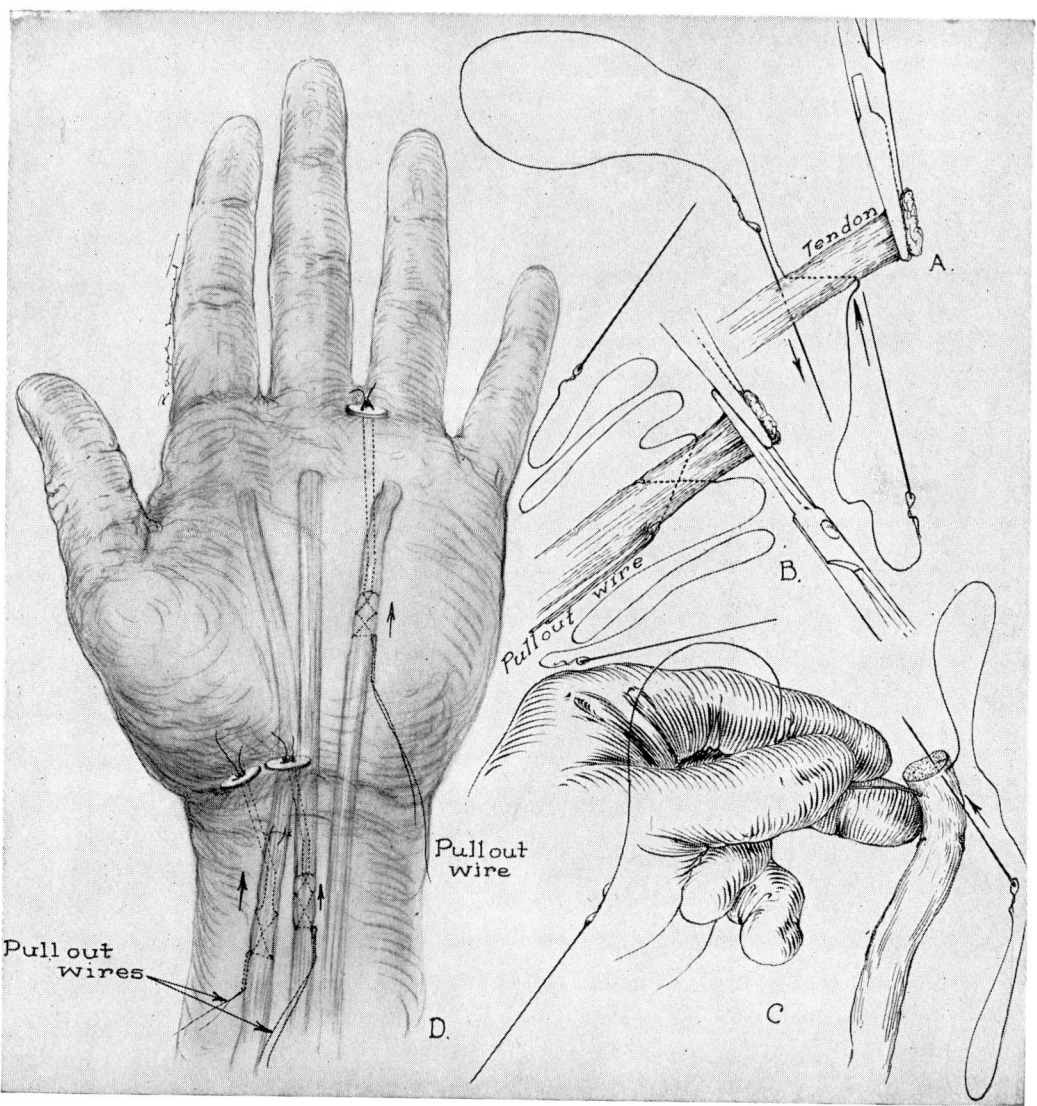

Fig. 356. Suturing tendons with removable stainless-steel wire. Each suture has a pull-out wire with which the main wire can be removed after three weeks. In the hand are three types of suture: The first one is end-to-end suture (D, middle and ring finger); second one is called "suture at a distance" because it is remote from the juncture to avoid causing adhesions (D, index finger); the third one is tendon to bone (compare with Figs. 359, C; 360). The pull-out wire may be twisted to avoid catching tissue in its loop. (S. Bunnell: Surgery of the Hand, J. B. Lippincott.)

few interrupted sutures. It is not necessary to suture the carpal ligament. If the division of the tendons occurs within the carpal tunnel, only the profundi are sutured in order to avoid crowding of sutures within a narrow space.

Palm

Step 1. EXPOSURE OF DIVIDED PALMAR NERVES: To find the delicate nerve trunks, it may become necessary to enlarge the original wound.

Step 2. LOCATING TENDON STUMPS: The proximal stumps, particularly the stump of the musculus flexor pollicis longus, gliding in a separate sheath, are apt to contract considerably, and may be found above the wrist. The distal stumps retract to a lesser degree—unless the finger was bent at the time of the accident—and ordinarily appear in the wound if the corresponding finger is flexed. They are secured with a mosquito hemostat. To locate the proximal stumps, small separate incisions should be made where one expects to find them. These incisions should be parallel to the creases of the palm and transverse over the wrist. Injury to the palmar nerves should be avoided at the site of these incisions. The nerves should be exposed before locating the tendons. The same is true at the wrist. So, for instance, the retracted proximal segment of the musculus flexor pollicis longus has usually retracted so far that a separate transverse incision over the wrist is necessary to find it. Before one locates the tendon, however, the median nerve should be exposed and safeguarded. After this precaution, the tendon segment is pulled out of the proximal wound and the very tip grasped with a mosquito forceps. A temporary guide suture is passed through the tip and tied. The ends of the suture are left long. To pull the proximal stumps peripherally into the original wound, the opening of the proximal tendon canal in the original wound is located. A probe, with eye first, is inserted through the opening and passed in a retrograde manner through the canal until it appears in the proximal wound. The author has found the retrograde way more helpful than passing the probe from proximal to distal. The temporary silk sutures are threaded into the eye of the probe and the probe is withdrawn, pulling the proximal tendon stump into the original wound (compare with Fig. 359, B.

Step 3: Suture of the nerves follows. This is a more difficult task than at the wrist, particularly if the separation happens to be at a place where the palmar trunk divides into small branches. Bunnell advises gathering the branches by a circular suture and suturing them en masse to the main trunk. The tendons are united in the usual way. If sublimis and profundus tendons are divided, Koch and Mason doubt the wisdom of having two lines of sutures at the same level in close approximation. To prevent ad-

855

herence to one another, they advise laying the lumbrical muscle between the two tendons at the line of suture, and holding it in place by one or two fine sutures. Closure of the wounds follows.

Volar Side of Fingers

In this region, primary repair should be attempted only under the most favorable circumstances. The slightest infection or irritation following repair will cause scar formation within the sheath and adherence of the tendon to the sheath, so that not only is the immediate result spoiled but also secondary repair becomes more difficult and handicapped. However, excellent functional results have been reported after sacrificing the sublimis tendon and primary suture of the profundus tendon by highly skilled hand surgeons (Mason and Koch, Siler, Hauge, Harrison, Verdan, Kelly, Rank and Wakefield). Almost all of those surgeons admit that the indications for primary repair are limited: the patient must be operated on within two hours after the injury, the wound must have been inflicted by a sharp cutting instrument, and it must have been dressed aseptically (Mason and Koch). Hence, although primary suturing of the profundus tendon has been successful, the consensus of most experienced hand surgeons (Bunnell, Littler, Iselin, Boyes, Pulvertaft, Frackelton, Posch, Graham, Flynn, Lindsay, Peacock and others) appears to be that unless rather rigid criteria have been fulfilled for selection of patients and unless the surgeon is exceptionally well qualified simple closure of the soft-tissue wound—including repair of the digital nerves if they have been lacerated—followed by tendon grafting several weeks later (p. 864) will be likely to give the highest incidence of good results.

Although the tendon division may occur at any point along the volar surface of the finger, the most common site is at the level of the web. At this level, there are three tendons within the sheath—the two slips of the sublimis tendon and the long flexor tendon passing between the slips. If sublimis and profundus tendons are divided, and if the exceptional primary repair is considered, it is generally agreed that only the profundus tendon should be united. If the sublimis tendon is sutured also, a considerable mass of sutures is brought together in a small space, causing adhesions and preventing the profundus tendon from its action on the terminal phalanx.

Step 1. EXPOSURE OF INJURED DIGITAL NERVES: Lengthening of the wound is usually necessary (see Figs. 354, *A, B*). The nerve stumps are located and held away.

Step 2: The digital tendon stumps are now located. They may reappear if the finger is flexed. The proximal stump of the profundus tendon, however, has usually retracted, and is located from an additional incision

856

within the palm or at the wrist (flexor pollicis longus). It is secured and guided through the original wound, as described previously.

Step 3: If the laceration is at the level of the proximal phalanx, the stumps of the sublimis tendon are excised distally; the proximal stump has usually retracted. The stumps of the profundus tendon are now sutured together. To follow Mason's advice, the fibrous tendon sheath is excised over the area of repair for a distance of about 0.6 cm. (¼ inch) proximal and distal to the suture line. Thus, the line of suture comes to lie directly against fatty subcutaneous tissue with less likelihood of adhesions. Suture of the divided nerve follows. If the laceration has occurred at the level of the middle phalanx beyond the insertion of the slips of the sublimis tendon, the profundus tendon is repaired in a similar way. The tendon suture, however, may become difficult if the distal stump is short. Here again, the part of the tendon sheath overlying the area of repair should be excised. The wound is closed with interrupted sutures.

Let is be stated again, however, that primary repair of both tendons severed within the flexor sheath should be considered very rarely and only under the most favorable circumstances. In the vast majority of cases, it is much safer to close the wound with a few sutures and wait until it has healed—this usually takes from three to four weeks—and then perform a secondary repair consisting of tendon grafting as described in detail on page 862 (primary tendon grafting is still in the experimental stage). In a division of the pollicis longus, which is the only tendon in its sheath, this rule may be relaxed to a certain degree but only if the division occurs distal to the metacarpophalangeal joint. Proximal to it the tendon is in close relation to sensory and motor branches of the median nerve which have usually escaped injury. If primary repair is undertaken in this region, damage to these structures is possible and would be greater than the loss of tendon function (Pulvertaft). The rule may also be relaxed and primary repair of the profundus tendon be done in children under four years of age (Wakefield). There are other exceptions to the rule: for instance, should the division of the profundus tendon occur within the extreme proximal or extreme distal part of the sheath, then it may be possible to place the tendon sutures outside the sheath through tendon advancement—as advised by Cutler and Mueller, and referred to by Littler, Nichols—and primary repair becomes feasible. For example, the profundus tendon, if severed within the distal ½ inch, can be advanced and sutured to the distal phalanx (for technique, see p. 868). The distal portion of the tendon sheath, with the exception of the annular ligament, should be excised. More will be said about secondary repair of the divided profundus tendon distal to the sublimis slips (p. 862). Primary repair is also feasible when sublimis and profundus tendons are divided near the proximal portion of the sheath.

857

In such a case, the sublimis tendon is sacrificed and the proximal profundus stump is shortened, so that the tendon suture of the profundus stumps is advanced proximally and comes to lie outside the sheath. In addition the proximal part of the sheath is removed. A ½-inch shortening of the profundus tendon is usually compensated for later by stretching of its muscle belly.

For after-treatment see page 874.

Dorsum of Hand (Case 146, p. 1190)

Severance of extensor tendons most often occurs over the dorsum of the wrist, less often over the metacarpus and over the knuckles of the digital joints. In tendon injuries over the wrist, the most common injury is division of the extensor digitorum communis, together with the extensor indicis proprius, being invested in the same compartment of and beneath the ligamentum carpi dorsale. In injuries over the radial side of the wrist, the whole radial group, consisting of the abductor pollicis longus and both extensors of thumb and wrist, may be injured or only the lateral group (abductor pollicis longus and extensor pollicis brevis) or the median group singly. Severance of the ulnar group of extensors (extensor digiti quinti proprius and extensor carpi ulnaris) without injury to other tendons is rare. Characteristic of dorsal tendon injuries over the wrist is marked retraction of the proximal as well as of the distal ends. In separations over the metacarpus, retraction of the distal segment is less marked, particularly if only a single group is divided. The fibers of the junctura tendinum (Fig. 351) not only prevent retraction but, as already mentioned, may also be strong enough to transmit the function of an uninjured tendon to its injured neighbor. Over the knuckles, injury of the extensor tendon (dorsal fascia) without severance of the joint capsule is rare.

In repairing severed dorsal tendons, the same rules are applicable as for repairing volar tendons. The original wound frequently must be enlarged. The next step is location of severed nerves if there is clinical evidence of their involvement. The stumps of the severed tendons are located and the corresponding stumps sutured together with the usual tendon sutures. Over the knuckles, the rents in the extensor fascia and the underlying joint capsule are united with simple interrupted sutures. The divided nerves are finally sutured and the wound closed in layers. For after-treatment see page 874.

SECONDARY REPAIR OF SEVERED TENDONS AND NERVES

Secondary repair of severed tendons and nerves becomes necessary if, owing to the foregoing conditions of the wound or elapse of time limit, primary repair has been omitted; secondary repair is also indicated in those cases in which a primary repair attempt has been unsuccessful. As already mentioned, in a so-called "clean case" secondary repair work can be undertaken from three to four weeks after the wound has healed. If the wound was or has become infected, the operation should be postponed until at least three months have elapsed since healing of the wound. Penicillin should be administered preoperatively and postoperatively. The problems involved in secondary repair work are far more difficult to deal with than those in primary repair, owing to adhesions and retraction of the severed tendons. Quite often, retraction is of such a degree as to make an approximation of the corresponding tendon ends impossible; hence, the surgeon must resort to tendon grafting to bridge the gap. Surface defects or dense scarring of the skin require transfer of flap prior to tendon grafting (see Cases 140, 157, pp. 1182, 1204). One should not forget that stiff joints which cannot be moved passively are strict contraindications to any tendon repair unless mobilization is possible, either by physiotherapy or by operation. In every case of secondary tendon repair, it is advisable to prepare thigh and foot preoperatively in case either a tendon or fat graft is required.

Wrist and Forearm (Case 147, p. 1192)

The incision to expose the field must often include the previous scar. If possible, the involved area is widely exposed by incisions as outlined in Figures 354, *A, B*. The next step consists of locating the severed stumps of the median and ulnar nerves, if there is clinical evidence of their involvement, and of the divided tendons. This is done in a way similar to that already described. The surrounding adhesions should be divided with the knife until the tendons can be drawn into the wound. The surrounding scar tissue should be thoroughly excised until good tissue is left. If adhesions have formed within the digital sheaths, preventing flexion of the fingers or independent function of the profundus tendon when pulling at the distal tendon stumps, one may be able to break them up by forceful pulling on the distal tendon segments. If this procedure does not succeed, Koch and Mason advise making an anterolateral incision in each finger and freeing the tendon from the surrounding tissue by sharp dissection. The firmest adhesions are usually found at the point of bifurcation of the sublimis where the profundus tendon passes between the two slips of the sublimis tendon and the proximal end of the digital sheath opposite the metacarpophalangeal joint. If the adhesions are too dense the sublimis tendons should be excised (see p. 896). Under flexion of fingers, wrist, and elbow joint, one will ordinarily succeed in approximating the corresponding tendon and nerve stumps and uniting them with sutures in the usual

THE EXTREMITIES

way. (For secondary suture of nerves, see also p. 751.) However, only the profundus tendons should be sutured. If sublimis and profundus tendons are sutured there is a likelihood of adhesions between the two tendon groups. This will prevent the longer acting profundus tendon from flexing the terminal joint. If all tendons are matted together at the site of division, and separation becomes difficult, one may separate the superficial and deep groups en masse and unite them as if dealing with single tendons. If healthy, clean-cut tendon ends cannot be approximated, one may be able to use their fibrous tissue extensions, which are found bridging the gap between the retracted tendon stumps, and to unite them side by side. If the latter method does not succeed in uniting the tendons, tendon grafts taken from the long extensors of the toes are utilized to bridge the defect. (For variation of technique of tendon grafting en masse, see Case 157, p. 1204.)

In the presence of dense cicatricial tissue around the lines of tendon and nerve suture, thin layers of fat grafts are removed from the deep fat layer, lying like a veil directly upon the fascia lata of the thigh, and are interposed between the bottom of the carpal tunnel and deep flexors, between deep and superficial flexors, and around the sutured nerves.

Then follow closure of the subcutaneous tissue (it is not necessary to suture the carpal ligament) and closure of the skin.

Palm

The incision, as a rule, has to include the scar of the original injury, and may need extension according to aforementioned principles (see Figs. 354 *A, B*). The area should be widely exposed and—unlike primary repairs—subcutaneous dissection through small incisions avoided. The divided nerves are located first, particularly the motor branch of the median nerve to the thenar muscles.

Locating the stumps of the divided tendons is the next step. Frequently, they have retracted considerably, particularly the proximal stump of the dividend pollicis longus, which glides in a separate tendon sheath. In dissecting the tendon stumps free from the surrounding scar tissue, the layer of areolar tissue surounding the tendon (paratenon) should be preserved to provide better gliding. If it is possible to approximate the tendon stump without undue tension, the ends are united in the ordinary way. If the suture is under tension, tension may be relaxed by myotomy of the corresponding muscle belly above the wrist (after Blum): From a small transverse incision above the wrist, the corresponding muscle is identified and delivered into the wound by passing a forceps beneath it; the tendon, while joining the muscle belly, is here superficial; the tendon, together with some of the muscle substance, is divided, permitting relaxation of the tendon distal to this point. If the division happens to be close to the digital sheath or even within the digital sheath, only the profundus tendon is united, and the ends of the sublimis tendon are excised for reasons mentioned previously (p. 860). For technique see page 896. If the suture happens to be within a tendon sheath (pollicis longus), a section of the overlying sheath is excised, as has been described (p. 857). To prevent adhesions of the tendons with surrounding tissue, if the latter is cicatricial, interposition of a fat graft may be necessary (for source of graft, see end of paragraph). A fat graft is also placed between the tendons if sublimis and profundus have been severed and repaired and the suture line happens to be on the same level; it may be possible to suture together two neighboring lumbrical muscles between the suture lines. If in doubt as to the wisdom of suturing both tendons with the suture lines superimposing, one should not hesitate to excise the distal end of the sublimis tendon. If direct union of the tendon segments is impossible because of rigid contraction of the muscles or because tendons have sloughed away or become cicatricial, necessitating excision, one must resort to tendon grafting or tendon transfer to bridge the intervening gap. Thus, if both tendons, the sublimis and profundus, are divided, the distal end of the sublimis is excised while the proximal end is used as a free graft. To bridge the gap in the profundus tendon, the graft, after it is placed between the segments of the profundus tendon, should be under moderate tension. To follow Koch's advice, the hand should be flexed in the wrist to an angle of 120 to 110 degrees and the fingers semiflexed at the metacarpophalangeal joints to an angle of 120 degrees. The width of the resulting gap of the profundus tendon is measured and this distance marked off on the proximal segment of the flexor sublimis. The latter tendon is severed at that point and excised. The excised part is laid between the ends of the profundus tendon and fastened to them with the usual tendon suture. If a sublimis tendon is not available for grafting, the tendon of the palmaris longus or a long extensor of a toe may be utilized. In using any of these tendon grafts, one should not forget that a graft will become adherent unless a proper gliding mechanism is provided. Hence, whenever a tendon graft is removed, the dissection should be performed in such a way as to leave the paratenon, or gliding tissue (see p. 50), intact; this is elastic fat tissue surrounding any tendon in the straight part of its course. If it cannot be preserved, it is replaced by a graft of elastic areolar fat tissue, which is found lying as a thin layer upon the fascia lata or beneath it in the interspace between fascia lata and muscle fascia (p. 870).

Rarely one must resort to transfer of a tendon from an uninjured finger (Mayer). So, for instance, the sublimis tendon of an uninjured index finger can be divided at a proper level and used to replace the divided flexor profundus tendon of the third finger. Although sacrificing a sublimis tendon does not cause a serious disability, it does hamper the flexion of the involved finger to a certain degree; this constitutes the disadvantage of the method.

After the tendons are repaired, the nerves are sutured together. Whenever the separation happens to be at a place where the palmar trunk divides into small branches, Bunnell advises gathering the branches by a circular suture and suturing them en masse to the main trunk. Closure of the wound follows.

Volar Side of Fingers

The repair work in this region varies with the site of the injury.

Division of the Profundus Tendon Distal to the Insertion of the Sublimis Tendon: There are four possibilities of dealing with this injury:

Primary suture or advancement of the proximal tendon stump is possible provided that the site of the division is within ½ inch of the distal flexion crease of the finger. This has already been discussed on page 857.

Tenodesis is most often indicated for laborers in whom the injury is too proximal for primary suture and who need to be able to return to work as soon as possible—a stable tip being their only functional requirement (Pulvertaft). The disadvantage of this method is that with the passage of time the tenodesis tends to stretch and elongate so that the initial partial flexion becomes straight. Arthrodesis may then become necessary. I perform the tenodesis after Oakey (personal communication) whereby the distal profundus tendon stump is armed with a pull-out wire suture, as described on page 869, and pulled through a bone canal which is drilled through the middle phalanx or, in case of the thumb, through the middle of the first phalanx; the wire is fastened over a button on the dorsal skin. The distal interphalangeal joint should be pulled in 35- to 45-degree flexion. In addition the terminal joint is immobilized with an intramedullary pin, which is buried beneath the skin (Fig. 357; Cases 150, 151, pp. 1197, 1198). Thus external immobilization is not needed.

Arthrodesis is unquestionably the more reliable procedure to hold the terminal joint in semiflexion. If fusion has occurred, the joint can no longer straighten out. However, it takes some time (up to three months) before a stable fusion is established. The procedure is simple (for technique see p. 901); external immobilization is unnecessary if cross wiring of the joint is used.

Tendon grafting may become necessary for division of the index profundis and the long finger when the conditions are favorable and the patient demands that the procedure be done (Pulvertaft). It is also done in the ring and little fingers for patients with special occupations, such as musicians. If the profundus tendon is replaced with a graft—a small-caliber graft such as the palmaris tendon or toe extensor should be used—the sublimis tendon should not be sacrificed (Littler) unless it is damaged. If the space between the sublimis slips is not passable, Bell recommends laying the graft upon the sublimis; otherwise it is threaded through the space between the slips. The tendon sheath should be removed except for the

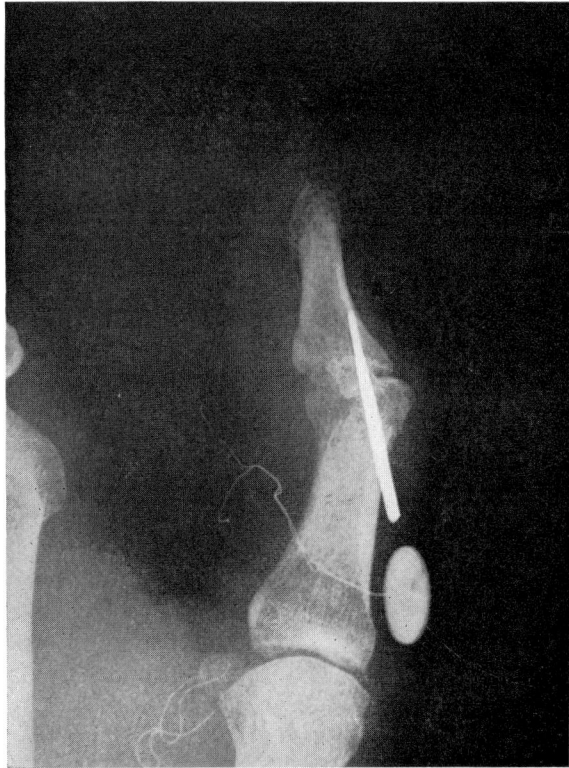

Fig. 357. Division of flexor pollicis longus. Tenodesis of distal stump to hold terminal phalanx in position of function. With pull-out wire tendon is pulled into drill canal of first phalanx. Immobilization of terminal joint with intramedullary pin.

retention of pulleys over the proximal and middle phalanges. Jaffe and Weckesser report favorable results with this method, and Goldner and Conrad recommend it strongly for the digit of a growing child or young adult in carefully selected cases. For technique see page 864.

Division of Both Flexor Tendons: In secondary repair of this injury almost all authorities agree that the sublimis tendon should be sacrificed

THE EXTREMITIES

and the profundus tendon be replaced with a full-length graft—provided that all finger joints have full passive mobility (Figs. 359, *A-C;* Cases 149, 152, 153, pp. 1196, 1199). The site of the injury is exposed first with an adequate incision (Figs. 354, *A, B*). If the digital nerves are divided, their segments should be located. The distal tendon stumps are approached first. The empty sheath has usually collapsed and its walls have become adherent. It is opened by an incision close to its attachment to the bone. If possible its "floor" (Koch) should be preserved while the "roof" usually must be excised except for a narrow proximal and distal pulley (annular ligament) to prevent bow stringing. If, however, the entire fibrous sheath must be excised, one annular ligament (the proximal one) will need reconstruction as described later. The distal tendon stump or stumps are then approached and carefully dissected free. If the division has occurred over the proximal phalanx, three tendon segments must be looked for: the two slips of the sublimis tendon and the profundus tendon as it passes through the latter. The distal tendon stump or stumps are excised, i.e., the sublimis slips are severed just beyond the proximal interphalangeal joint while a short stump of the profundus tendon is left at the terminal phalanx to be used later for anchorage of the graft. Two points of caution might be inserted here. Tubiana advises leaving one sublimis slip longer than the other and fastening it to the lateral side of the middle phalanx to prevent hyperextension of the first interphalangeal joint. In reference to excision of the distal profundus stump, the author advises the surgeon not to leave this stump too long, since it may become adherent to the distal end of the middle phalanx, either causing a flexion contracture of the terminal joint or preventing the graft from acting on the terminal phalanx. The next step consists of exposing the proximal tendon stumps, which usually have retracted into the palm or wrist (in the case of the flexor pollicis longus). They are located from a separate incision in the palm or over the wrist (the possibilities of proper lengthening are outlined in Figs. 354, *B;* 355, *A*). The tendons are freed from scar tissue and pulled into the wound. The range of motion should be checked by traction, because it is futile to extend a severely contracted flexor muscle with a graft and expect sufficient amplitude for full-finger flexion.

A tendon graft is taken. Small-caliber grafts are preferable. Thin grafts regenerate more quickly, cause fewer adhesions and are less constricted by the rigid annular ligaments than thick grafts.

Source of Graft: The palmaris longus tendon makes a good graft. It is pulled through a separate transverse incision in the palm and forearm. Second choice is one of the long extensor tendons of the toes, which are surrounded by gliding tissue. To preserve the latter the tendon is exposed from a longitudinal curved incision along the dorsum of the foot. The

864

little toe does not possess a second extensor tendon; hence its extensor tendon should not be used as a graft. The plantaris tendon has been recommended by Pulvertaft, Brand, White. As a last resort the sublimis of a damaged finger may be taken as a graft. This makes a poor graft because the thickness of the tendon is a handicap to its nourishment (see also p. 50).

The plantaris tendon is frequently used when a long tendon graft is needed (see p. 903). The plantaris muscle with its long slender tendon is inconstant; it is absent only in a small percentage (7 per cent) of human beings. Its use in hand surgery has been suggested by several authors,

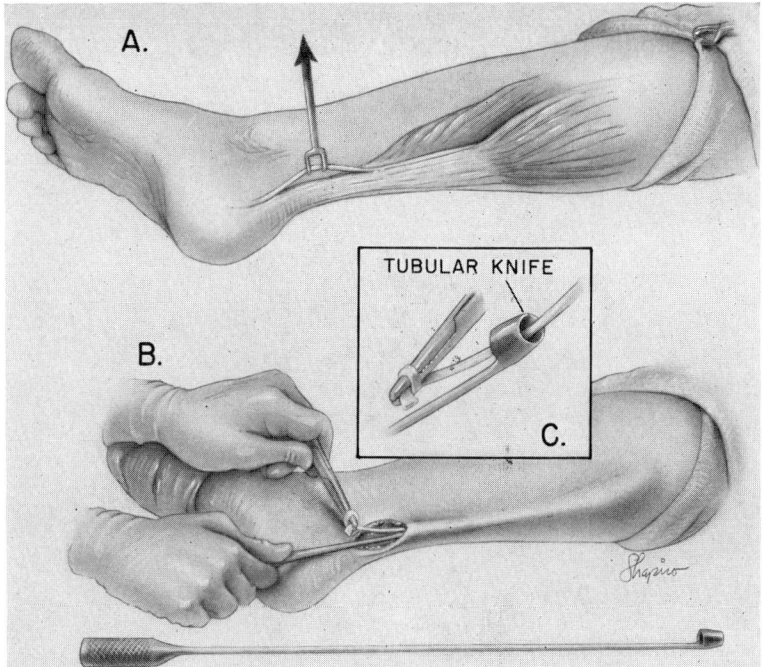

Fig. 358. Removal of plantaris tendon with tendon stripper. (W. L. White: Plast. Reconstr. Surg.)

notably by Brand and White. Its removal became much facilitated after Brand devised a light tendon stripper with a cutting edge. To obtain the plantaris tendon White recommends the following procedure:

Technique (Removal of Plantaris Tendon) (Fig. 358): An incision 1 inch long is made on the median aspect of the Achilles tendon about 1 inch proximal to its insertion into the os calcis. The incision is made deeply to expose the tendon by cutting through the areolar tissue and the paratenon. By means of a small hemostat the tissue is opened and the Achilles tendon exposed, so that with the aid of retractors the plantaris tendon may

865

be located. It may be found in one of several locations from the antero-medial to the posteromedial aspect of the Achilles tendon. The plantaris is a slender strand of isolated tendon which may be drawn upward or downward without comparable movement of the Achilles tendon. If the structure isolated exposes denuded tendon beneath its fibers and if traction causes gross movement of Achilles tendon, it is likely that an accessory slip of the Achilles tendon has been isolated. The tendon of the plantaris should be cut near its insertion into the os calcis. The tendon end is passed through the loop of the Brand tendon stripper and grasped securely with a Kocher clamp. The clamp is turned one full turn to wind up the tendon and permit a secure grasp. The tendon stripper is then forced up the leg keeping the knee fully extended and held to pervent flexion. It will pass easily first on the median side then higher up into the popliteal area until

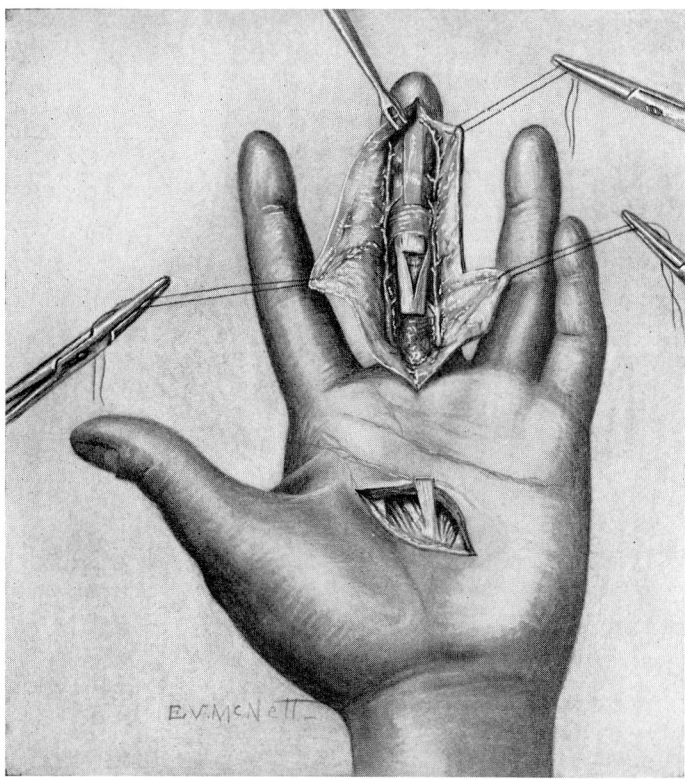

Fig. 359. *A:* Division of flexor tendons of third finger within tendon sheath. Exposure from bayonet incision; proximal annular ligament is missing; from palmar incision profundus tendon is exposed and shortened to near insertion points of lumbricale muscles; proximal sublimis stump has retracted proximally.

866

it meets resistance at the fleshy belly at about 8 to 12 inches. At this point the tubular opening is filled with muscle which prevents the cutting edge from inflicting injury to the adjacent structures. The stripper is forced further, and the tendon will pull free and can be withdrawn with a portion of its muscle attached. There is little bleeding. The wound is closed with sutures. The patient is permitted to walk the following day.

The graft is now tunneled through the palm, as demonstrated in Figure 359, *B*, and anchored to the terminal phalanx. This is done in one of two ways, depending upon whether or not a distal profundus stump is present.

FIRST METHOD: If there is no distal profundus stump at the terminal phalanx preserved, for instance, after subcutaneous rupture of the tendon, Koch's method of sliding the graft around the terminal phalanx is excellent. A sharply curved aneurysm needle is passed around the terminal phalanx; the anchoring wires of the graft are threaded through the eye

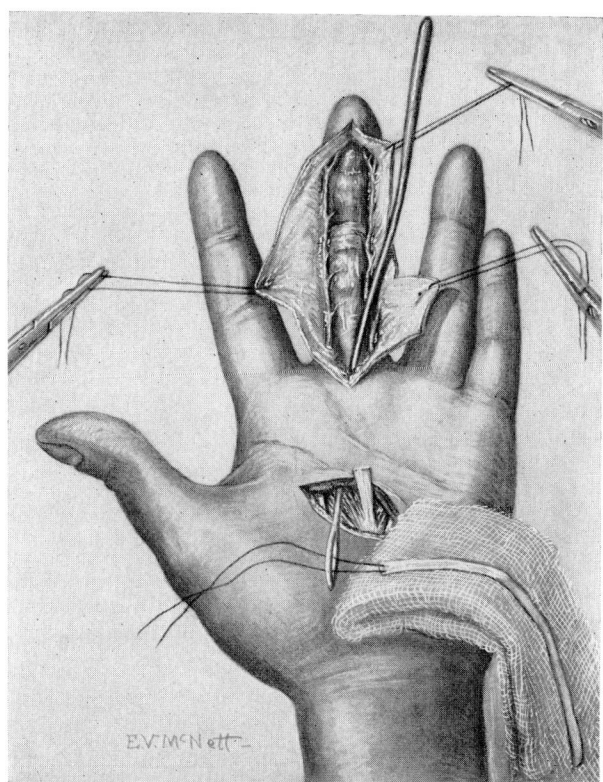

Fig. 359. *B:* Tendon graft (long extensor tendon of third toe) being led through palmar incision into finger wound.

of the needle; needle and graft are withdrawn. The graft is then united on the volar surface of the phalanx by an end-to-side suture.

SECOND METHOD: In those cases where a stump of profundus tendon is left at the terminal phalanx, the writer has advised a modification of the Bunnell method (Figs. 359, C; 360). The profundus stump is shortened to a point just distal to the terminal joint. (For reasons explained on p. 864, it should not bridge the terminal joint.) This short stump is split in half. A hole is drilled through the terminal phalanx just beyond the split (Fig. 360). The hole must be large enough to allow the tendon graft to pass

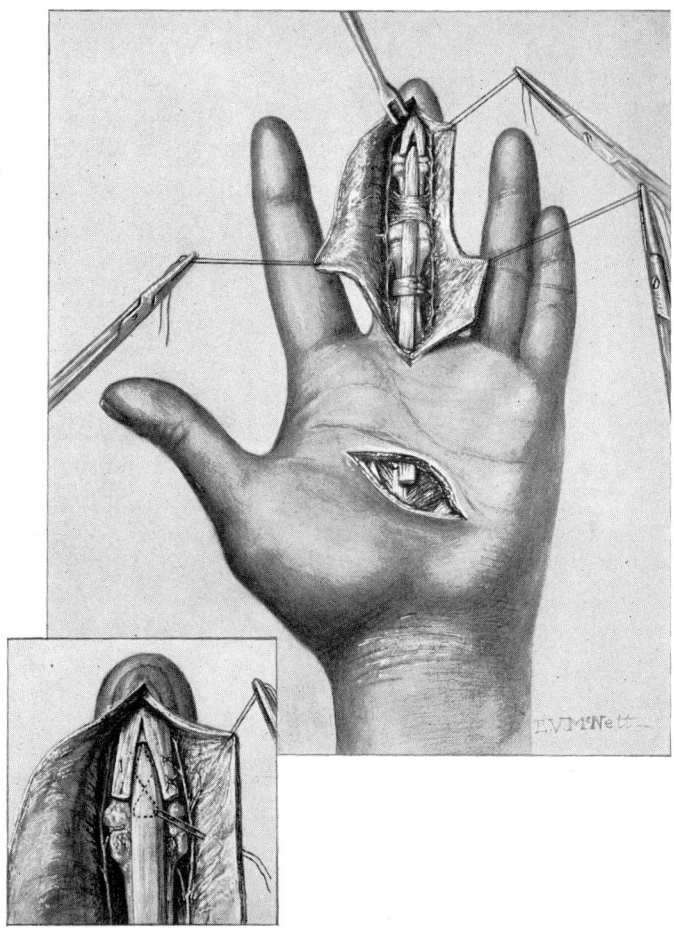

Fig. 359. C: Fixation of tendon graft to terminal phalanx through drill hole in between slips of split distal end of profundus tendon; graft is armed with pull-out wire (see insert, also Figs. 356, 360); additional fixation with mattress sutures through profundus slips and tendon graft; proximal annular ligament replaced with another tendon graft.

snugly through it. The canal is drilled obliquely to—but not through—the nail. The tendon graft is armed with Bunnell's "pull-out" wire (Figs. 356; 359, C). A fine stainless-steel wire (No. 35), with a needle on each end, is sewed in mattress-suture fashion crisscrossing the terminal 0.5 cm. ($\frac{3}{16}$ inch) of the graft. To remove the wire later, a second wire is threaded through the proximal loop of the suture wire. Both ends of this wire are threaded together on a curved or straight needle and brought out through the skin proximal to the tendon insertion and left there. This is the pull-out wire. The two needles of the suture wire are passed through the bony canal and through the nail, thus pulling the distal part of the graft into the bony canal. The two ends of the suture wire are tied to a small role of gauze or to a rubber button. The terminal end of the tendon graft thus comes to lie within the bone and between the two slips of the profundus stump, to which it is sutured with one or two mattress sutures

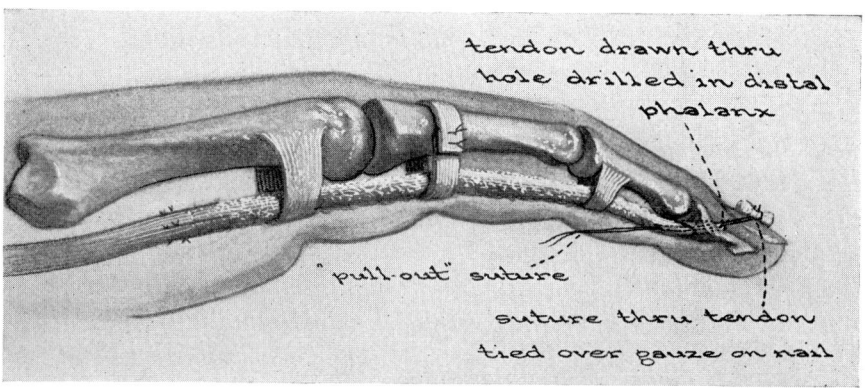

Fig. 360. Grafting of flexor tendon and reconstruction of annular ligament (Bunnell). Loose areolar fat tissue is wrapped around tendon graft to provide gliding tissue. Distal end of graft is fastened directly to bone. Hole is made through terminal phalanx large enough to allow tendon graft to pass snugly through it. Canal is drilled obliquely from proximal part of volar surface of bone, distal to but not through the nail. The holding suture of graft is made removable from outside. Fine, stainless-steel wire needle on each end is followed in crisscross fashion through end of graft. To remove wire three weeks later, second wire is threaded through proximal loop of suture wire, and then its two ends are threaded together on straight needle and led proximad out through skin and left there. This is pull-out wire. Two needles of the suture wire are passed through bone canal and through nail, thus pulling distal part of graft into bony canal. Two ends of suture wire are tied over small roll of gauze or rubber button. Annular ligament is constructed with piece of tendon graft that is passed around phalanx with sharply curved aneurysm needle. Ends of new annular ligament are overlapped and sutured together. Suture would come to lie at side of bone and not over tendon. Proximal end of tendon graft is sutured to proximal end of profundus tendon. (H. May: Surg. Gynec. Obstet.)

of fine silk (Fig. 359, *C, insert*). Thus, a bony and tendinous anchorage of the graft is achieved. (The wire suture is removed after four weeks.)

In those cases in which owing to excision or destruction of the tendon sheath the annular ligaments are absent, a new annular ligament must be reconstructed to hold the tendon in place over the volar surface of the finger. This is done, according to Bunnell's plan, as follows (Figs. 359, *C*; 360): Another tendon graft, available from the sources already mentioned (long extensor tendon of second, third, fourth toe), is passed around the proximal phalanx with a sharply curved aneurysm needle. The tip of the aneurysm needle is kept in close contact with the bone so as not to include any of the digital vessels or nerves or the extensor tendon. The ends of the new annular ligament are overlapped and sutured together. The suture should come to lie at the side of the bone and not over the tendon. Another good method is applicable if one of the sublimis slips is available and fairly long and free of adhesions. It then should not be sacrificed in the first phase of the operation but utilized at this stage. The slip is laid across and over the graft and sutured to the other side of the proximal phalanx.

The next step is suture of the divided digital nerves with fine silk on an atraumatic needle. At this point, the use of a fat tissue graft should be mentioned. Such a graft becomes necessary in extensive cicatrization or exposure of bone. To prevent adhesions between the tendon graft and bone, a slippery piece of fat tissue—removed from the thin areolar veil-like fat layer immediately overlying the fascia lata (see p. 51)—is interposed. These delicate tissues are awkward to suture in place, but the following makes it easy (Bunnell): The fat graft is spread between tendon and bone; each corner is tied to a thread of 000 plain catgut carried with a straight needle. The needle is passed lateral to the phalanx to emerge at the dorsal surface of the finger where the opposite sutures are tied to each other. After a few days, the sutures will pull out. Closure of the finger wound in layers follows. Koch points out that it is a real advantage to be able to close the incision in the finger while the finger is still extended and before the suture of the graft to profundus stump in the palm is carried out. It is a difficult task to close an incision extending along the greater part of the finger while the finger is supported in flexion and while one is attempting to avoid tension on a newly sutured tendon.

After the finger wound is closed, the proximal end of the graft is attached to the proximal tendon segment. The question of whether only the profundus tendon or both profundus and sublimis tendons should be utilized to empower the graft has been frequently discussed. It appears that most surgeons select the profundus tendon while the sublimis tendon is cut short in the palmar incision. I weave the graft through the pro-

870

fundus tendon after Koch, Mason, Allen, Bell and add as a refinement a "fish-mouth" opening in the very end of the profundus tendon to achieve a smooth incorporation of the graft. I use 0000 silk as suture material and hold the profundus tendon temporarily transfixed with a straight needle until the anastomosis is completed. The tendon junction should come to lie at the origin of the lumbricale at the profundus stump so that this muscle may be used for covering the junction (Mason). In the thumb the graft is sutured to the musculotendinous origin of the flexor pollicis longus at the wrist (Case 149, p. 1196). Since this procedure requires a rather long graft, a plantaris tendon graft (p. 865) should be chosen. Before the proximal flexor stump is withdrawn through the wrist incision, it is armed with a wire. This same wire will lead the graft from the wrst incision into the finger. The graft should be under moderate tension. To follow Koch's advice, with the hand flexed at the wrist to an angle of from 120 to 110 degrees, with the fingers semiflexed at the metacarpophalangeal joints to an angle of 120 degrees, the ends to be united should come together at normal tendon tension. If the flexor pollicis longus is the involved tendon, the amount of tension is that resulting from supporting the thumb in semiflexion at an angle of 120 degrees at interphalangeal and metacarpo-phalangeal joints and the hand in semiflexion at the wrist at an angle of 135 degrees.

The remaining wound or wounds are closed in layers and a volumi-nous pressure dressing is applied; hand and forearm are immobilized with a molded dorsal plaster-cast splint. The forearm is kept elevated at all times until the immobilization is removed (see After-Treatment, p. 874).

At this point, it should be noted that a tendon-grafting operation, tedious as it is, should not be carried out in a finger which has no sensa-tion; if no return of sensation by repair of the digital nerves can be hoped for, there is a tendency for the patient to use another finger with normal sensation in preference to the one which has been grafted.

Reviews and follow-up examinations of large series of cases of flexor tendon grafting have been reported on by many surgeons mentioned throughout this chapter, with good results in from 70 to 80 per cent of the cases.

Dorsum of Hand

If proper splinting of the hand was carried out after primary repair of the original wound, it not infrequently occurs that an extensor tendon wound heals in the meantime, resulting in perfect function.

If, however, a secondary tendon repair becomes necessary, the pro-cedure is as follows: The segments of the divided tendons are exposed from the scar of the former injury. Lengthening the incision or making addi-

871

tional incisions—over the wrist, for instance—may be necessary for locating the retracted proximal segment (see also Primary Repair of Severed Tendons and Nerves). The tendons are carefully dissected free from surrounding scar tissue and, if sufficiently mobilized, can ordinarily be brought together without undue tension. The corresponding ends are fastened together with the usual tendon suture. If the proximal stumps were located from a separate incision, the subcutaneous tissue between the incisions is tunneled and the proximal tendon segment pulled through (compare with Fig. 359, B).

If a gap exists between the segments owing to contraction of the muscle bellies or to destruction of the proximal segment, the gap should be bridged with a tendon graft (Cases 140, 154, 155, pp. 1182, 1201, 1202). The graft source is the palmaris tendon, a long extensor tendon of a toe. (For technique, see p. 864 and following.) The insertion of extensor-tendon grafts should be quite tight, as tight as the neighboring tendon is. The metacarpophalangeal joint should be in 175-degree flexion, with the interphalangeal joints in semiflexion. If the gap happens to be in the extensor tendon of the third finger, Mayer proposes transferring one of the two extensors of the index finger to the third finger through a subcutaneous tunnel and fastening it there to the distal tendon segment. If the gap happens to be over the middle phalanx of a finger, the defect ordinarily does not need to be bridged. The extensor tendon divides here into three slips (see p. 843). It rarely happens that all three slips are missing, and it is the author's experience that the two lateral slips or even one of them is sufficient to carry on most of the function; there may be a moderate limitation of extension of the terminal phalanx left, which, however, does not hamper the function of the hand seriously unless the lateral slips dislocate and need to be repaired (method outlined on p. 879). For repair of tendon tears over the proximal or distal interphalangeal joints, see page 879 and page 876 respectively.

Nerves, if severed, are repaired after the tendons are sutured. The wound is now closed in layers.

The Use and Purpose of Artificial Tendon Grafts

Artificial tendons of various materials have been used by numerous investigators (Mayer, Thatcher, Hunter, Carroll and Barrett, Gaisford, Hanna and Richardson, Herzog, Geldmacher) as substitutes for lost tendons but seldom have they proved successful as functioning grafts. The best results seem to be those of Hunter with silicone rods and of Peacock and Madden and of Seiffert with human cadaver grafts. Artificial grafts have, however, been of value in forming false tendon sheaths around

872

themselves (Schink, Böhler, Pieper, Buck-Gramcko, Mittelmeier); this favors the gliding of an autogenous graft after removal of the artificial one. All authors stress that this method should be considered only as an adjunct in the care of those injured hands in which there is little hope of obtaining reasonable function by the ordinary methods. Gaisford, Hanna and Richardson after much experience with this procedure have endorsed it enthusiastically and describe it as follows: "The profundus tendon is removed distally near its attachment to the distal phalanx and proximally in the palm as far as indicated by the injury. The tendon sheath is excised with only narrow bands left to provide pulleys. A solid rod of silicone rubber is inserted into the area previously occupied by the profundus tendon. If the sublimis tendon is intact it is not disturbed. The silicone is secured to the distal cut end of the profundus tendon with 0000 black silk sutures. This prevents the silicone from drifting proximally, thus alowing the space to scar shut. . . . The rod should not be attached proximally as contraction of the profundus tendon can separate the rod from the distal profundus stump. The diameter of the rod chosen for insertion is usually slightly smaller than the diameter of the excised tendon. The rods that we use measure 3 mm. in diameter. The proximal end of the rod is overlapped for one inch along side of the cut end of the proximal profundus tendon and the hand is closed.

"A false sheath of scar promptly forms around the silicone and does not adhere to it. There is no clinically demonstrable adverse tissue reaction to the foreign implant. Active and passive movement of the finger joints is begun approximately five days postoperative. We have elected to do autogenous free tendon grafting on these hands three months after inserting the rods. Several tendon grafts have been inserted less than two months following the initial silicone implant and the fingers have shown noticeably more stiffness than the ones done after three months transfer. It is therefore advised that the three-month interval should not be shortened. . . . In this second procedure a short incision is made in the palm and the proximal end of the profundus tendon and the end of the rod are located. A second short midlateral distal finger incision is made and the distal profundus tendon and rod are found. A tendon is then obtained for grafting. The end of the tendon graft is sutured to the distal end of the rod and with no difficulty pulled through the sheath which is formed around the rod. This tendon is then managed as in any routine tendon grafting operation by attaching it distally and proximally in an acceptable fashion and by closing the two short incisions. The hand is ordinarily kept in plaster cast for two to three weeks."

THE EXTREMITIES

The healing process of a tendon wound has already been discussed on page 846. This process can be summarized as passing through two stages: the proliferative and the formative. The first stage lasts about two weeks. During this time, the tendon stumps become united by a connective-tissue callus, which is then gradually converted into tendon. Mason and Allen, who did considerable experimental work on this subject, came to the conclusion that function during the first phase did not accelerate the development of the tendon callus. On the contrary, early function appeared to be harmful insofar as it caused more reaction of the surrounding tissue and weakening of the union. Later, however, after the first callus was formed, restricted use of the tendon caused but slight irritation with rapid increase in tensile strength of the union.

It is the common belief among surgeons that motion, if started early, will prevent the adhesion of tendons. However, according to the foregoing findings and the clinical experience of most hand surgeons, the opposite seems to be the case. It would seem to be substantiated that early motion, restricted or unrestricted, favors adhesions. Iselin, however, who has admirably described the healing process of a tendon wound in the recent edition of his book, and Pulvertaft believe otherwise. Nevertheless, it can be said that adhesions are due not only to irritation of the surrounding tissue but also to disturbance of the vascularization of the tendon. This is a factor which should be pointed out strongly. The bulk of the blood supply of a tendon outside its sheath is derived from the paratenon, or gliding mechanism, which is in intimate contact with the surrounding tissue. It is only natural that a tendon operation causes some disturbance of the local circulation, since it is almost inevitable to leave the intimate connection of the paratenon and surrounding tissue undisturbed. If, however, the involved tendon is adequately immobilized, the interrupted blood supply of paratenon and tendon will become reestablished. Early motion may disturb vascularization, leading to necrosis of the gliding mechanism and formation of adhesions.

Hence, it is advisable to immobilize a repaired tendon for three weeks. The author prefers the molded plaster-cast splint to any other kind. The hand is placed in such a position that the suture lines are free or under a minimum of tension. If flexor tendons are severed, the maximum flexion should be at the wrist and the metacarpophalangeal joints. The interphalangeal joints should be slightly flexed. The thumb is held flexed in abduction and facing the fingers. If extensor tendons are involved, maximum extension should be at the wrist and the metacarpophalangeal joints. If the thumb is involved, it is held extended and

874

abducted. Without removal of the immobilizing splint, the dressings are changed on the eighth postoperative day, and the sutures are removed. Splint and dressings are removed on the twenty-first postoperative day, and motion should be started gradually; the healed tendon is not subjected to full activity for at least two more weeks. After repair of the extensor tendons, it is wise for the patient to wear the splint overnight during these two weeks; during sleep the hand is clenched, causing a strain on the repaired tendons. Forearm and hand are placed daily in a warm saline bath and active motion exercises encouraged from the third week. Two weeks later, local heat (baking, warm-water bath, whirlpool bath), massage, and passive exercises are added to the active exercises. One of the author's patients developed a simple but effective splint for exercising those joints having limited motion, while arresting motility of those joints that move freely. The method is clearly depicted in Figure 361. Since this splint was introduced, some of the author's patients have regained full motility of the fingers without needing other forms of physical therapy. In addition to physical therapy, occupational therapy is of great importance (p. 814—After-Treatment).

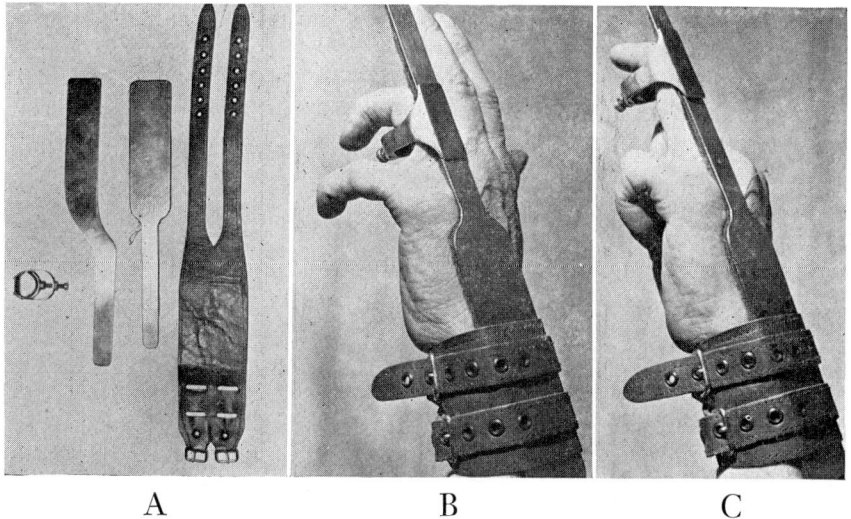

| A | B | C |

Fig. 361. *A:* Finger splint which permits independent active exercises of interphalangeal joints of fingers. *B:* Splint in use. Flexor profundus tendon of fourth finger was replaced by tendon graft. When active exercises were instituted without splint, patient mainly moved joint which was movable before operation, namely, metacarpophalangeal joint. To force other joints to active exercises, splint is applied, clamp is slipped over finger and splint, holding the metacarpophalangeal joint immobilized. Patient now moves first interphalangeal joint. *C:* Clamp immobilizing middle phalanx. Patient can now exercise terminal joint. (H. May: Surg. Gynec. Obstet.)

THE EXTREMITIES

If severed nerves were sutured at the time of the tendon repair, the antagonists of the paralyzed muscles must be kept from contracting by intensive passive motion exercises under supervision, that is, the affected muscles must be kept continually relaxed until signs of regeneration are evident; otherwise, the paralyzed muscles would be overstretched by the uninjured antagonists, resulting in delay of regeneration and in contractures. If the patient fails to cooperate, continuation of splinting may be necessary. The splint, however, should be removed temporarily every day for these exercises and electric treatment of the paralyzed muscles (see also p. 752).

Complications

Occasionally after tendon grafting, the flexor grafts attached to the terminal phalanx of the finger may pull loose. If this is the case, immediate regrafting gives gratifying results. Sometimes a patient is reluctant to exercise the repaired tendons on account of pain. Daily median- and ulnar-nerve blocks promote flexion in the anesthetized finger. Should the tendons become adherent, tenolysis should be performed after six to eight weeks. Tenolysis is carried out either (1) with a tendon stripper from an incision over the wrist, followed immediately by active finger exercises (median- and ulnar-nerve blocks may be helpful) or (2) by exposing the tendon and, after tenolysis, wrapping the tendon in fat tissue (for source, see p. 50). Formation of a false tendon sheath before inserting another graft is recommended in certain cases and described on page 872.

SUBCUTANEOUS INJURIES OF TENDONS

Subcutaneous ruptures of tendons follow direct or indirect trauma or are due to preexistent pathological processes. In the majority of cases, the extensor tendons are involved; the flexor tendons, less often.

RUPTURE OF EXTENSOR TENDONS

RUPTURE AT TERMINAL JOINT

The cause is usually a severe blow, which results in flexion of the extended distal phalanx. The most common seat is a tear of the dorsal aponeurosis at its insertion into the distal phalanx, usually with avulsion of bone. The distal phalanx is flexed, and cannot be extended actively (so-called "mallet" or "baseball" finger).

876

The extensor apparatus over the distal finger joint is formed by the fused parts of the lateral slips, which, as extensions of the interosseous and lumbrical muscles, converge over the middle phalanx and insert into the joint capsule (Hauck) (see Fig. 353). Hence, over the terminal joint, the extensor apparatus forms the main part of the joint capsule (Duncan). Its undersurface is lined with synovial membrane.

There are two main types of mallet finger (Duncan): (1) Here, the tendon insertion of the dorsal margin of the base of the terminal phalanx is avulsed with a piece of bone—this can be diagnosed by x-ray examination. (2) This is the nonfracture type, in which the tendon is ruptured from its base at the terminal phalanx or at a more proximal level (Fig. 362). Regardless of the level of the rupture, there is always some damage to the joint capsule.

The prognosis of functional recovery after repair of a mallet finger is good only if treatment is applied within ten days after the accident. It becomes progressively worse later on. Stark, Boyes and Wilson however after a carefully conducted follow-up study of a large number of cases seem to contradict this statement. The treatment of choice during the first ten days is closed manipulation to restore the continuity of ruptured or avulsed tendon. To achieve this, the terminal joint must be held in hyperextension; to make up for the retraction of the lateral bands, the middle joint must be in moderate flexion. The finger should be rigidly splinted in this position. Thumb and finger are pinched together to maintain the position (middle finger joint not too acutely flexed!). Then, narrow wet strips of plaster of Paris are applied to the volar surface of the finger, with cross-strips placed across the dorsum just proximal to the joints (Smillie, Bunnell). Pratt recently devised an ingenious method (Fig. 362). Under digital nerve block, a Kirschner wire (0.045 inch) is drilled through the tip of the finger and the hyperextended phalanx and terminal joint; with the proximal interphalangeal joint held in 60-degree flexion, the wire should then come to lie anterior to the middle phalanx and is drilled into the first phalanx. Pratt claims that if the point of the wire emerges centrally on the dorsum of the middle third of the proximal phalanx, the wire will have missed the flexor tendons. Hence, the proximal interphalangeal joint should not be flexed too acutely. The wire is then withdrawn until its point is just palpable beneath the skin of the dorsum of the proximal phalanx. The distal end is cut off just beneath the skin of the finger. The wire is withdrawn after four weeks. Note two precautions: First, the terminal joint should not be held in extreme hyperextension because of danger of necrosis of the dorsal skin. One can notice the blanching of the skin of the hyperextended joint on one's own finger.

THE EXTREMITIES

Secondly, if the intramedullary pin was placed in the wrong direction, do not remove this wire but use it as a guide to insert a second wire.

Amongst others Casscells and Strange have experienced occasional distressing, painful limitations of motions in the proximal interphalangeal joint after using Pratt's method. Hence, they recommend placing the Kirschner wire only through the hyperextended distal joint, the proximal joint being maintained in 60 degrees of flexion by means of a

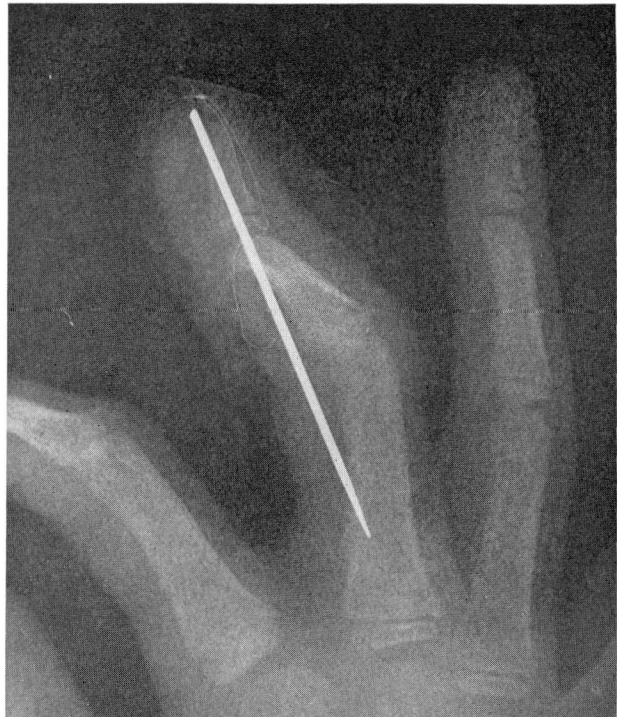

Fig. 362.   Mallet finger: Repair of extensor tendon with pull-out wire and insertion of intramedullary pin to splint terminal joint in extension and proximal interphalangeal joint in slight flexion.

plaster cast. The author places the pin only into but not through the proximal phalanx (Fig. 362). Stark, Boyes and Wilson warn against using this method at all. Pratt himself no longer uses it routinely and employs it only in operative cases.

In late cases, operative repair should be given a chance if the patient is anxious to have the deformity overcome and is aware of the possibility of failure.

878

MUSCLES, TENDONS, NERVES, AND BLOOD VESSELS

Technique

The joint is exposed from an L-shaped incision, the short arm of the L running just proximal and parallel to the base of the nail, the long arm at the posterolateral surface of the finger. After reflection of the skin flap, the site of the rupture is exposed. If a piece of bone is attached to the avulsed tendon, a wire stitch is inserted into the end of the tendon close to the dorsal margin of the fragment. The wire is then inserted through the terminal phalanx just beneath the site of avulsion, by drilling a cutting edge needle through it, and tied. In the nonfracture type, there is always some damage to the synovial reflection over the articular head of the middle phalanx. The extensor tendon becomes firmly adherent to the neck of the middle phalanx, preventing the extensor tendon from acting on the terminal phalanx. Hence, the tendon must be completely mobilized. If it is not frayed and ruptured from its insertion near the terminal phalanx, it is fastened with a pull-out wire (see p. 869) to the terminal phalanx. The wire is led dorsally to the fingernail and tied to its rim (Fig. 362). Insertion of a fat graft (see p. 51) between tendon and bone and joint may be advisable to counteract adhesions. If the tendon is ruptured farther distally or is frayed and must be excised, the gap is bridged with a tendon graft from the long extensor tendon of one of the toes (see p. 864). Ample gliding tissue should remain attached to the graft. The graft is sutured in place with a proximal and distal pull-out wire. The placing of the wire sutures is facilitated by inserting them with the graft in situ. Closure of the skin follows.

After-Treatment

The finger is immobilized as described (p. 877). Splinting is removed after four weeks and physiotherapy instituted.

RUPTURE OF DORSAL APONEUROSIS OVER FIRST INTERPHALANGEAL JOINT

This rupture of the dorsal aponeurosis may be defined as a tear of its central slip. (The functional anatomy of the extensor mechanism of the finger has been described on p. 844.) The extensor tendon over the dorsum of the finger forms three slips (Fig. 353): a middle one, which is inserted to the joint capsule of the first interphalangeal joint and the base of the middle phalanx; and two lateral slips, which pass laterally to each side of the first interphalangeal joints, converge over the middle phalanx, and insert to the joint capsule of the second interphalangeal joint and the base of the distal phalanx. The interosseous and lumbrical muscles fuse with the lateral

879

slips. The function of the dorsal aponeurosis has been extensively studied by Hauck, whose experiments and observations were confirmed by Mason, Landsmeer, and Littler. If, owing to a direct or indirect blow, the dorsal aponeurosis ruptures over the first interphalangeal joint, the middle slip becomes detached from its insertion at the base of the middle phalanx and pulls away proximally; the two lateral slips of the aponeurosis become disengaged and move from the dorsum laterally to a volar position. The volar dislocation is increased by the pull of the lumbrical and interosseous muscles. The joint protrudes between the displaced lateral slips, as through a buttonhole. This so-called boutonnière deformity consists of extension or hyperextension of the distal interphalangeal and the metacarpophalangeal joints and flexion of the proximal interphalangeal joint (Case 156, p. 1203).

There are numerous operative techniques described to overcome this deformity. All however attest to the unpredictable results of any approach. The author has lately followed a method suggested by Fowler and recently described by Mateo. The functional result in five recent cases was most satisfying.

Technique (Fig. 363; Case 156, p. 1203)

The dorsum of the middle phalanx of the finger is exposed from a double bayonet incision whereby a rectangular skin flap is formed (Fig. 363, *A*). One lateral slip is divided level with the middle of the middle phalanx (the one on the left of Fig. 363, *B*), the other one more distally. The proximal ends are mobilized up to and proximal to the first interphalangeal joint to dislodge them from their volar position. The proximal part of the first slip is passed through a horizontal slit in the distal stump of the divided middle slip, i.e., the insertion of the middle slip at the base of the middle phalanx. With the proximal interphalangeal joint held in extension the band is sutured to the central slip and the periosteum of the dorsum of the middle phalanx. The proximal stump of the second band is led across the dorsum of the middle phalanx and is sutured to the distal stump of the first slip with the distal joint held in extension. Thus the extensor mechanism of the proximal interphalangeal joint is restored and the lateral slips are lengthened to overcome the hyperextension of the distal joint. In involvement of the index or little finger the ulnar or radial bands are divided respectively and the proximal ends used for suturing to the insertion of the middle slip. It may not become necessary to divide the other bands if through division of the first bands the hyperextension of the terminal joint can be overcome. The finger is immobilized on an aluminum splint for three weeks with the metacarpophalangeal joint held in 45-degree flexion and the interphalangeal joints in extension.

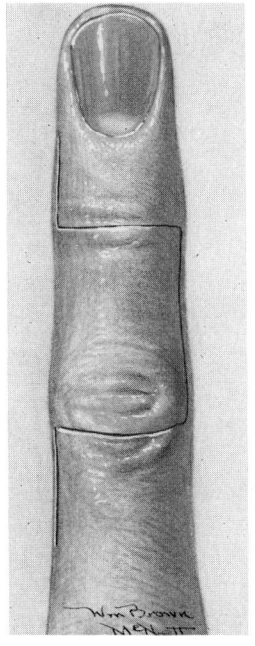

A

Fig. 363. Repair of boutonnière deformity after Fowler. *A:* Double bayonet incision on dorsum of finger lined out. (Redrawn from I. Mateo.) *B:* One lateral slip (left) is divided in level of middle phalanx, the other one more distally. The proximal part of the first (left) slip is passed through a horizontal slip in the distal stump of the divided middle slip and sutured to the center slip and the periosteum. The proximal stump of the second slip is being led across the dorsum of middle phalanx to be sutured to the distal stump of the first slip. *C:* All slips are sutured together.

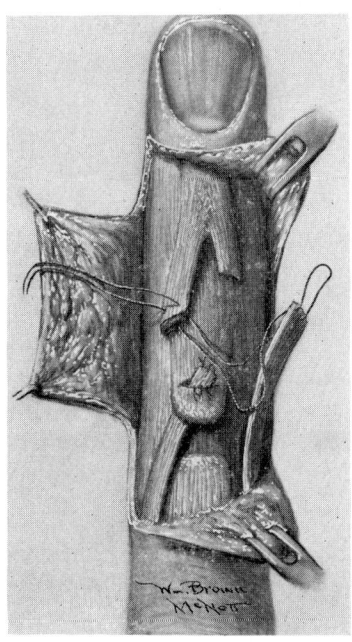

B

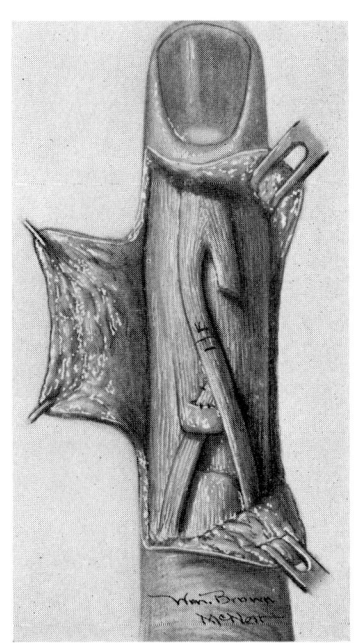

C

THE EXTREMITIES

Dolphin recommends a simple tenotomy of the extensor tendon over the middle phalanx just distal to the triangular ligament in boutonnière deformities of long standing. He claims that appearance and function of the finger improve greatly if hyperextension of the distal joint can be relieved and active flexion of this joint regained.

RUPTURE OF EXTENSOR POLLICIS LONGUS TENDON

According to the references in the literature (Hauck, Mason, Broder, Smith, Calberg, Delmotte, Stehman and Van Gaver and others), it is doubtful whether a normal tendon ever ruptures. Usually preexistent pathological conditions (after fracture of the radius, for instance, or after tenovaginitis, known as "drummer's palsy") weaken the tendon and lead to spontaneous rupture. The deformity is typical: inability to extend the acutely flexed terminal joint and the less acutely flexed metacarpophalangeal joint and impairment of abduction and adduction of the thumb. Treatment is operative.

Technique (Compare with Case 155, p. 1202)

From a longitudinal incision in the tabatière anatomique, the tendon stumps of the long extensor are located. This may be difficult, since the tendon glides in a sheath, and is apt to contract considerably. For the same reason, establishment of direct union after mobilization of the tendon segments may become impossible. Shortening of the distance by rerouting the tendon from its normal course in the groove of the crista radii to a course over the styloid process may facilitate direct union. If this is impossible, Smith recommends suturing the distal end of the extensor pollicis longus end-to-side to the tendon of the extensor carpi radialis longus. Following this, the tendon of the extensor pollicis brevis is freed from the styloid groove and is drawn over to it and sutured side-to-side. If the distal end of the long extensor is too short or much of it must be sacrificed because the tendon is cicatricial or frayed, one must resort to the use of a tendon graft.

Galberg, Delmotte, Stehman and Van Gaver seem to have overcome the above-mentioned difficulties by transferring the extensor indicis proporius tendon. They state that it can be cut to the correct length, runs in the same direction, and is not essential to extension of the index finger. The extensor digitorum communis alone suffices. Three incisions are used. The extensor indicis proprius is severed in the distal second metacarpal area. It is the more internal of the two index extensors. The distal portion of the extensor indicis proprius is sutured with wire to its mate, the extensor digitorum communis. An incision is made on the dorsum of the

882

wrist over the site of the rupture, the tendons are visualized, and the extensor indicis proprius is pulled back and out. A third incision is made over the distal first metacarpal, well distal from the degenerated portion of the torn extensor pollicis longus, which is excised; the extensor indicis proprius is threaded through the extensor tunnel and sutured to the distal healthy portion of the extensor pollicis longus. The degree of tension on this anastomosis must be such that it holds the distal phalanx of the thumb extended but permits easy passive flexion of this phalanx.

After-Treatment

The thumb is immobilized on a plaster-cast splint in extension and abduction for three weeks (if a tendon graft was used, for four weeks). Physical therapy is then instituted.

RUPTURE OF FLEXOR TENDONS

Traumatic subcutaneous rupture of a normal flexor tendon is rare (Case 153, p. 1200). Only a few cases have been reported (Mason). The treatment does not differ from primary or secondary tendon repair.

DYSFUNCTION OF MUSCLES, TENDONS AND NERVES

CONTRACTURES AND ADHESIONS OF TENDONS

The repair of contractures of tendons has been discussed previously (see pp. 810, 812, 819; see also p. 860 for tendon lengthening by myotomy).

Tenolysis has been discussed under Secondary Repair of Severed Tendons and Nerves (pp. 858 et seq.); (see also p. 51 for the use of fat-tissue grafts).

TRIGGER, OR SNAPPING, FINGER

The characteristic sign is the jerking of the finger. When the flexed fingers are extended, the involved finger extends only to a certain point; upon forced extension, however, the finger snaps into complete extension. This phenomenon may also be noticed upon flexion. Often the help of the other hand is necessary to move the finger over the critical point. The condition is more common among females than males, and is found more often in the middle finger than the thumb or other fingers (Hiller). The underlying cause is a hindrance which prevents the tendon from gliding freely in its sheath. The hindrance may be in the sheath or in the tendon. The sheath may be reduced in caliber (inflammatory changes, hypertrophic villi, fibromas of the sheath, duplications) or the tendon may be enlarged. The local enlargement of the tendon is usually nodular (fibroma, tear of the tendon), the nodule passing with difficulty through the opposite pulley or most often through the tight ring at the proximal end of the tendon sheath in the palm.

Treatment

Conservative measures should be tried first: hydrocortisone injection, immobilization of the finger in extended position for several weeks, followed by local heat application, massage, and active exercises. If this treatment is of no avail, a simple operation is indicated.

Technique: Under local anesthesia the affected tendon is exposed from an incision within the distal palmar crease. With a pair of fine straight scissors the ring and the proximal part of the tendon sheath are severed and opened up. The patient is then instructed to flex and to extend the finger. Should there still be a hindrance the incision is extended but care should be taken not to incise the pulley in its entire length, since this would favor forward displacement of the tendon upon flexion.

After-Treatment: After closure of the wound, the patient is permitted to move the finger immediately.

WRITER'S CRAMP

According to Benedict, a spastic and a paralytic form of writer's cramp may be distinguished. In the spastic form, clonic and tonic cramps appear most frequently in the thumb and index finger, forcing the fingers into flexion. The paralytic form, according to Steindler, manifests itself as a sensation of fatigue of arm and hand, making it impossible to use the hand in writing. In some cases, a tremor of the entire hand is noted, which may increase and make writing impossible. These forms are characterized by the fact that the trouble appears only when an attempt has been made to write or soon after the beginning of writing, with no symptoms in the intervals.

Treatment

The treatment consists of massage around the muscles of the extremity, particularly those of the hand. Specially constructed braces

884

should be worn while holding the pen. The action between thumb and index finger may be eliminated, for instance, by the use of a bracelet encircling these fingers (Cazenave and Zabludowski) or the patient may be given a ring or ball for the palm of the hand, to which the pen is attached, the fingers pressing against the ball.

DYSFUNCTION OF NEUROGENIC ORIGIN

Four examples are selected for discussion: dysfunction following irreparable traumatic paralysis of (1) the nervus ulnaris, (2) the nervus medianus, (3) the nervus ulnaris and nervus medianus combined, and (4) the nervus radialis. The extent of the dysfunction depends much upon the level of the nerve injury. Severance of the radial nerve at the level of the wrist, for example, mainly causes loss of sensation, while that of the ulnar and median nerves at the same level is followed by sensory and motor disturbances. The latter involve only the intrinsic muscles of the hand because the long flexors are supplied at a much higher level.

We are indebted to the pioneer work of Sterling Bunnell, among others, for the progress of surgery of the intrinsic muscles of the hand. He summarizes the motor disturbances following paralysis of the intrinsic muscles as follows: With loss of action of the intrinsic muscles, the thumb cannot oppose or adduct. It lies to the side of the hand. The carpal and metacarpal arches are flat and the fingers are clawed (intrinsic minus hand, p. 811). They cannot simultaneously flex in their proximal joints and extend in their distal two joints, and are practically devoid of lateral motion. The hand has lost its skill and finer movements (Case 147, p. 1192).

If the three nerves are severed higher up in the forearm or above the elbow joint, paralysis of the long flexors and extensors and other muscles are added, which will be described in more detail. In cases where repair of the nerves is no longer possible, much of the imbalance can be corrected by tendon transfer and tendon transplantation.

Certain fundamental requirements for a satisfactory tendon transfer must be mentioned. Prior to the transfer, special effort must be made either to overcome an established contracture of the fingers and hand or to prevent contracture by counteracting the pull of the antagonists. Excision of the collateral ligaments in an effort to overcome hyperextension contracture of the metacarpophalangeal joints in interosseus muscle paralysis may further cripple the hand because severance of both collateral ligaments tends to throw the fingers into marked ulnar deviation. Hence, the collateral ligaments on the radial side should be left intact if possible; enough relaxation can often be achieved to permit flexion without undue loss of stability (see p. 813). Furthermore, a satisfactory and functioning

885

muscle and tendon should be available for transplantation, and scar tissue in the path of the transplant should be excised. Flap transplantation to cover the resulting defect may become necessary.

In addition to tendon transfer, anthrodesis must be mentioned as a useful adjunct, especially when there are not enough tendons available to stabilize certain joints in the position of function. As a rule, a proximal joint must be stabilized to permit the tendons on the distal joints to function (arthrodesis of base of thumb, of metacarpophalangeal joints, or any joint of any digit). A wrist arthrodesis in 30-degree dorsoflexion gives but little disability; in addition, out of six wrist muscles, some could be made available to act on the digits.

Dysfunction after Irreparable Paralysis of Nervus Ulnaris

The ulnar nerve supplies the musculus flexor carpi ulnaris, flexor digitorum profundus of the fourth and fifth fingers, the musculi interossei (three palmar and four dorsal), the musculi lumbricales of the fourth and fifth fingers, the ulnar half of the flexor pollicis brevis, the adductor pollicis, and the muscles of the hypothenar eminence.

The deformity following low ulnar-nerve palsy is usually referred to as "clawhand" (Duchenne) or intrinsic minus hand (Bunnell, p. 811) and is beautifully described by Littler, Bunnell, and Kaplan. Normally the lumbricales, acting through the common extensor tendon, cause flexion of the first phalanx and extension of the last two phalanges (Fig. 353). As a matter of fact they are the prime flexors of the metacarpophalangeal joints. When these muscles are paralyzed, the antagonistic muscles act, causing hyperextension of the first phalanx and partial flexion of the last two phalanges (compare with Case 147, p. 1192).

The palmar interossei muscles adduct the fingers toward the middle finger, while the dorsal interossei abduct from the same finger. As a result of paralysis of the interossei, the fingers can no longer be adducted or abducted. Abduction of the little finger is impossible. All the symptoms from loss of function of the interossei are more pronounced in the fourth and fifth fingers than in the second and third, for in these the lumbricales still function (see also p. 893) being supplied by the median nerve.

As to how all this comes about, the following points need to be stressed. The long flexors flex the metacarpophalangeal joints only after the intrinsic muscles have stabilized the metacarpophalangeal joints; if these joints are in hyperextension—and in intrinsic palsy the metacarpophalangeal joints retain a powerful extensor in the extensor digitorum—the long flexors flex only the terminal joints. As far as extension of these joints is concerned, the interphalangeal joints can be extended by the

886

intrinsic muscles acting through the lateral band (Fig. 353). They can also be extended by the long extensors provided, however, the intrinsic muscles stabilize the metacarpophalangeal joints. Thus in intrinsic palsy the interphalangeal joints have no prime extensor and the metacarpophalangeal joints no prime flexor. The secondary extensors and flexors can be put to action, however, if the metacarpophalangeal joints are stabilized and thus prevented from moving into hyperextension.

In ulnar-nerve paralysis, the adductors of the thumb are also paralyzed. Two signs are of particular interest (Bunnell): The patient cannot make a perfect O with the thumb and index finger, since the abductor (first interosseus) of the index finger and the adductor of the thumb, which are necessary antagonists to give a firm pinch, are paralyzed and the pinch between them is weak. A paper held between the thumb and index finger can easily be withdrawn. Another sign is the inability to scrape the extended thumb across the palm and bases of the fingers to the ulnar side of the hand.

In high lesions of the ulnar nerve, aside from the dysfunctions just described, the tendons of the musculus flexor digitorum profundus of the fourth and fifth fingers are paralyzed. Flexion of the terminal phalanges of these fingers is impossible.

In ulnar paralysis, the object of treatment is the correction of the claw deformity of the fifth and fourth fingers, less often of the third finger, restoration of adduction to the thumb, and correction of the curvature of the carpal and metacarpal arches. Claw deformity of the fingers after an ulnar-nerve lesion, however, may be so little that surgery may not be warranted. Further, if the long flexors are functioning—and they do in distal lesions of the ulnar nerve since only the intrinsic system is paralyzed—and good opposition of the thumb is present, restoration of the adduction power of the thumb may not be warranted either.

In most hands, the middle and terminal phalanges can be extended by the long extensor tendons, if hyperextension of the metacarpophalangeal joints is prevented. This function is lost when the intrinsic muscles, which stabilize the metacarpophalangeal joints, are paralyzed. To overcome the claw deformity of the fourth and fifth fingers in ulnar palsy, the metacarpophalangeal joints must be stabilized in semiflexion. This can be done either by transfer of the sublimis tendon of the involved finger through the lumbrical canals into the lateral bands of the extensor mechanism (Fig. 364), as devised by Stiles (1922) and modified and improved by Bunnell (1942), or by the use of an extensor of the fingers (Fowler, 1949) or an extensor of the wrist elongated by tendon graft (Brand, 1954) to replace the lumbricale muscle. It can also be done by an arthrodesis of the metacarpophalangeal joint. The Bunnell technique was the most popular, but Riordan and Brand's extensive experience with the Fowler principle in using extensor tendons instead of a flexor tendon to replace the paralyzed intrinsic system in the treatment of the paralytic hand in leprosy has proved its value.

Brand pointed out that the sublimis transfer was successful in many of his five hundred and sixty-four cases (fingers), but due to the fact that a very powerful muscle—the sublimis—is used to replace a very small muscle it became in numerous later cases the source of its greatest weakness. It produced the opposite deformity—intrinsic overaction. The reason for this is that the prime flexor of the proximal interphalangeal joint is removed and used as an extensor of the same joint. It seems that a finger with intrinsic paralysis cannot really spare its flexor sublimis and that, in the absence of this muscle as a flexor, it is too powerful to be used as an extensor.

Brand formulated several indications and rules: In all cases in which there is a significant contracture at the proximal interphalangeal joint and in which the contracture cannot be fully overcome before operation, the sublimis transfer is the operation of choice. Its powerful corrective effect may produce results that are better than could be predicted from the limited preoperative range of movement. In stable hands with low range of passive hyperextension of the interphalangeal joints a sublimis transfer under moderate tension will usually give a good result, although an operation which avoids the removal of the sublimis tendon would give a stronger and more useful hand.

For hypermobile, flexible fingers the sublimis transfer is contra-indicated. For this type of hand better results will be achieved by Fowler's operation or by the four-tailed graft from the extensor carpi radialis brevis (after Brand) referred to later (p. 903).

Technique (Bunnell) (Compare with Fig. 364)

Restoration of Muscle Balance in Claw Deformity of Fourth Finger Due to Ulnar-Nerve Palsy Caused by Low Lesions: From a bilateral dorsolateral incision along the proximal third of the fourth finger, the slips of the sublimis tendon are located; through a nick in the tendon sheath directly opposite the first interphalangeal joint, the sublimis tendon is severed. An incision is now made in the palm parallel to or within the proximal transverse flexion crease. The severed sublimis tendon is withdrawn (the chiasm of Camper may hinder withdrawal, and if so must be divided). With the back of the knife, the slips are slit further apart for about 3 cm. (1¾₁₆ inches) or longer. The ends of the slips are crisscrossed with a thin wire suture, which acts as a guide. A probe is now passed from the palmar incision through the lumbrical canal. The wire of the corre-

888

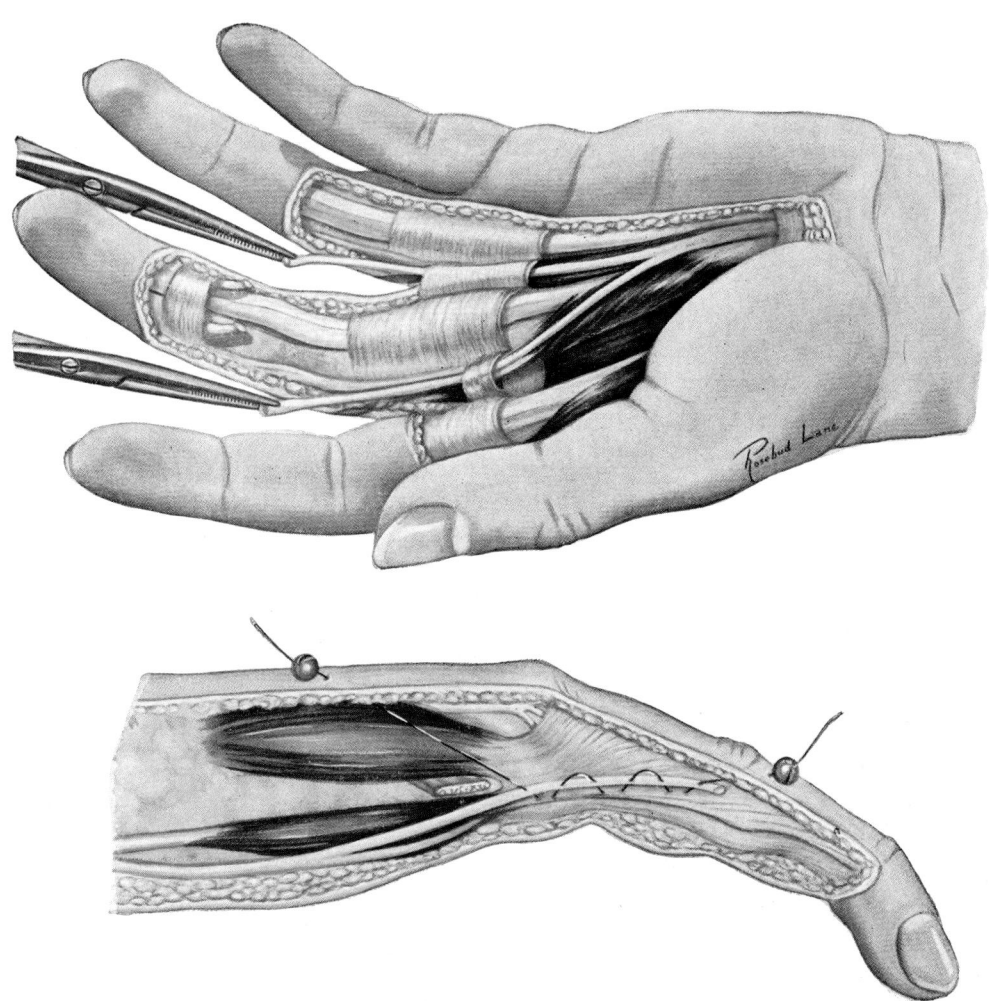

Fig. 364. Operation to restore normal balance in fingers in claw hand from paralysis of interosseus and lumbricalis muscles. The tendon of each flexor digitorum sublimis is split, transferred through a lumbrical canal and fastened to a lateral band of a dorsal aponeurosis by a removable stainless-steel wire either by the pull-out stitch or the running suture method. (S. Bunnell: Surgery of the Hand, J. B. Lippincott.)

sponding sublimis slip is threaded through the eye of the probe and with-drawn through the finger incision; a similar procedure is performed with the other slip. (The retrograde way may however be easier.) The transverse fibers and lateral band of the extensor mechanism (see Fig. 353) are located in the finger wound. The metacarpophalangeal joint and wrist are semiflexed, and the sublimis slip is led through the transverse fibers and lateral band to the dorsal surface of the lateral band. The contiguous surfaces of the lateral band and sublimis slip are scraped to favor adhesions between the two structures. Both are now fastened to-gether either by a removable running wire suture (after Bunnell) or with five silk sutures. The same procedure is performed on the other side of the finger, followed by closure of the wound and application of a dorsal molded plaster-cast splint for three weeks.

In case of claw deformity of the fifth finger, the sublimis slips of this finger are used to overcome the muscle imbalance. Here, however, it is sufficient to anchor both slips together on the radial side of the finger.

Technique (Brand)

Brand follows Fowler's principle and uses an extensor, the extensor carpi radialis longus, extended by a many-tailed free tendon graft (plantaris tendon) to stabilize the metacarpophalangeal joints and to activate the paralyzed intrinsic system. At first he passed the grafts from the dorsum to the palmar side anterior to the deep transverse metacarpal ligament to the fingers. In his last four hundred cases (fingers) however (personal communication), he chose the anterior route via the carpal tunnel. He found re-education after operation much easier and prefers this modifica-tion. The operation is similar as to the one described for combined low ulnar and median lesions, and I refer the reader to the details of the operation on page 903.

Technique

In High Lesions of Ulnar Nerve: In lesions of the ulnar nerve above its branches to the flexor profundus of the fourth and fifth fingers, the sublimis of the third finger—if a sublimis transfer is considered— must be used, since sacrificing the sublimis tendon of the fourth and fifth fingers in which the flexor profundus muscles are paralyzed would only add markedly to the dysfunction. One slip of the sublimis tendon of the third finger goes to the radial side of the ring finger and one to the radial side of the fifth finger. The results, however, are not as good as when the sublimis tendon of the involved finger is transplanted to the extensor mechanism of the same finger (Luckey and McPherson). Therefore the use of the exten-

889

sor carpi radialis longus extended by strips of tendon graft as described above and in detail on page 903 is preferable.

If the second to the fifth fingers are clawed, as in combined lesions of the ulnar and median nerves, the technique described on page 903 should be followed.

Paralysis of the first interosseus muscle, or abductor of the index finger, as caused by ulnar or local lesions, may result in weakness of opposition or inability to pinch between thumb and index finger. The patient is unable to make a perfect O with thumb and index finger, since the abductor of the index finger and adductor of the thumb are necessary antagonists for a strong pinch. The index finger is pushed by the thumb into ulnar deviation. To furnish abduction of the index finger, Bunnell transfers the index proprius tendon, Graham the sublimis tendon of the ring finger, and Bruner the tendon of the extensor pollicis brevis. The author has found Bruner's method most satisfactory, particularly in combined ulnar- and median-nerve lesions.

Technique (Bruner)

Restoration of Abduction of Index Finger: A transverse incision is made over the dorsal surface of the metacarpophalangeal joint of the thumb. The tendon of the short extensor muscle is severed at its insertion into the base of the proximal phalanx, and care is taken to preserve all possible length. A second short incision is made over the proximal end of the "anatomical snuffbox," avoiding injury to the radial nerve. The short extensor tendon of the thumb is freed and withdrawn through this incision. A third short incision is made at the radial side of the index finger near the metacarpophalangeal joint at the insertion of the first dorsal interosseus muscle. The end of the tendon of the short extensor muscle of the thumb is crisscrossed with a wire suture of thin stainless steel. A probe is passed retrograde from the incision at the index finger subcutaneously beneath the tendon of the long extensor of the thumb to escape through the incision made over the wrist. The wire is now threaded through the probe and withdrawn through the incision at the index finger. The surface of the tendon of the short extensor is roughened and then woven back and forth through the tendinous portion of the first dorsal interosseus muscle near its insertion. Fixation is obtained by means of a single pull-out wire (after Bunnell, compare with Fig. 364) or with fine silk sutures. The wounds are then sutured.

After-Treatment

Hand and forearm are placed on an anterior molded plaster-cast splint, with extension of plaster to hold the metacarpophalangeal joint of

890

the index finger in slight abduction. Mobilization is removed after three weeks, and active motion exercises are instituted.

In a few patients, the extensor pollicis brevis is absent. If this is the case, a sublimis tendon—possibly of the fourth finger, otherwise of the third or index finger—should be utilized for restoring the abduction of the index finger, as devised by Graham and Riordan. The severed sublimis tendon is withdrawn from a transverse incision at the wrist and rerouted, without acute angulation, around the radial side of the forearm, subcutaneously behind the thumb over the anatomical snuffbox to the insertion of the first dorsal interosseus muscle. Fixation and after-treatment are described above.

Restoration of the adductor power of the thumb, as already pointed out, may not be warranted if the long flexors are functioning and good opposition of the thumb is present or can be restored, as in combined lesions of ulnar and median nerves. If restoration of adduction of thumb and little finger and of the carpal and metacarpal arches becomes necessary, Bunnell's tendon T-operation is the choice (Fig. 365). It consists of one free tendon graft spanning across the palm behind the flexor tendons from the base of the proximal phalanx of the thumb to the neck of the metacarpal of the little finger. One of the long flexor tendons of the forearm, such as the sublimis or palmaris longus, is attached by a loop to the center of the cross-tendon, thus forming a T. On flexion of the muscle, the T is drawn to a Y, drawing the thumb and fifth metacarpal toward each other and restoring the arches. The cross-member lies in soft movable tissue behind the profundus tendons, and can be drawn proximally without resistance.

Technique (Bunnell) (Fig. 365)

Restoration of Adduction of Thumb: The fifth metacarpal is exposed in its ulnar volar aspect just proximal to its head. One end of the tendon graft (one of the long extensor tendons of the toes, see p. 864) to be used as cross-tendon is fastened to it under a chipped flake of bone (Fig. 365, B). It is anchored with a thin wire suture, to which a pull-out wire is attached, as described on page 869. The tendon wire escapes through the skin of the back of the hand over the dorsoradial aspect of the fifth metacarpal, and is tied over a button. The pull-out wire is placed on the opposite side. The palm is now opened by an incision paralleling the longitudinal crease. The flexor tendons are visualized through this incision. With a suture carrier (see Fig. 61), the other end of the tendon graft is passed across through the palm behind the flexor tendons, and is made to emerge through a small lateral incision over the ulnar aspect of the base of the proximal phalanx of the thumb. Here it is fastened in a manner similar to that described on page 869 and depicted in Figure 360; the wires are passed through the phalanx and thumb and tied over a button. The pull-out wire is placed on the opposite side. The tendon should be slack when the hand is fully spread, since grafts shrink a little. From the mid-palm incision, either the tendon of the musculus palmaris longus, with its prolongation of palmar fascia, or a sublimis tendon—one, of course, which

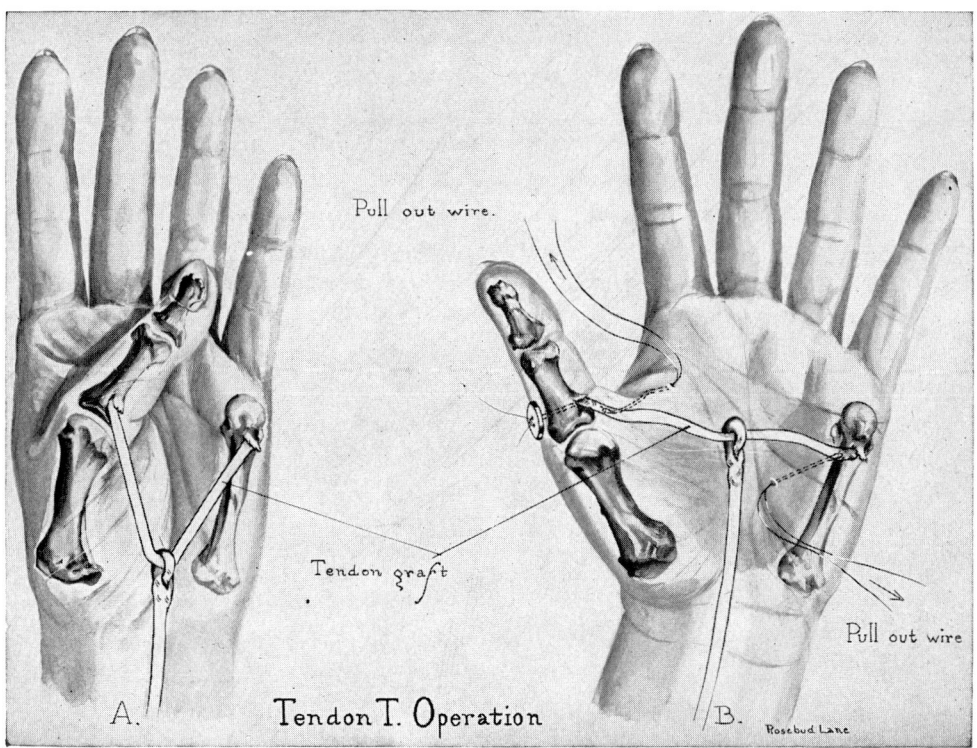

Fig. 365. Restoration of adduction of thumb (Bunnell). In T-operation, one free tendon graft spans palm behind flexor tendons from base of proximal phalanx of thumb to neck of metacarpal bone of little finger. One of the long flexor tendons of forearm (palmaris longus or flexor sublimis) is attached by loop to center of cross-tendon, thus forming a T. On flexion of muscle, the T is drawn to a Y, thus adducting thumb and restoring arches. (S. Bunnell: Surgery of the Hand. J. B. Lippincott.)

has not been used in the first step of the operation (see foregoing remarks on claw deformity)—is severed at the proper level and then looped around the center of the cross-tendon, embedding it in and suturing it to itself; one stitch is placed to keep it from sliding along the cross-tendon. The wounds are closed.

MUSCLES, TENDONS, NERVES, AND BLOOD VESSELS

Littler's suggestion of utilizing a sublimis tendon, if such is available, to restore the palmar and thumb arches is a good modification of the Bunnell T-operation. The sublimis tendon is severed near its insertion, withdrawn through an incision in the palm, and split in two strands. One strand is attached to the adductor pollicis insertion and the other to the base of the proximal phalanx of the little finger on its ulnar aspect. This procedure simulates the tendon T-operation of Bunnell or the entire tendon may be sutured only to the adductor insertion of the thumb.

After-Treatment

Forearm and hand are immobilized on a dorsal molded plaster-cast splint for three weeks. Immobilization is then discarded, sutures and wires are removed, and physiotherapy is instituted.

DYSFUNCTION AFTER IRREPARABLE PARALYSIS OF NERVUS MEDIANUS

The median nerve supplies the musculus flexor digitorum sublimis and musculus digitorum profundus of the second and third fingers, the musculus pronator teres and pronator quadratus, the musculus flexor carpi radialis and flexor pollicis longus, the musculus abductor pollicis brevis, the radial head of the flexor pollicis brevis, the musculus opponens pollicis, and the two radial musculi lumbricales. The disability following division of the median nerve is not great, even if the median nerve is severed in the cubital region, since its motor branches enter the long flexors high in the arm. The greatest disability is due to loss of opposition of the thumb with the other fingers and loss of sensation (see also p. 885). Atrophy of the thenar eminences usually develops early and is striking. The thumb can no longer be rotated to face the fingers. The pincer-like action of the thumb, resulting from its opposition with the other fingers, adds much to the efficiency of the hand. The thumb to be in true opposition must be opposite the fingers—that is, the pulp of the thumb must face that of the fingers—and the thumbnail must be parallel to the volar surface of the fingers. If this function is lost from irreparable nerve damage, it can be restored by tendon transplantation (compare with Cases 148, 157, pp. 1194, 1204).

Bunnell stresses that two essential principles must be adhered to: direction of pull and correct insertion of the tendon graft to give pronation. Quoting Bunnell:

1. The tendon from its insertion in the thumb should pass subcutaneously in the direction of the pisiform bone so that it will pull the thumb in the correct direction and the insertion of the tendon should be on the dorsoulnar aspect of the base of the proximal phalanx of the thumb, so as to restore the pronatory component.

2. To make the tendon pull toward the pisiform bone either a tendon pulley is constructed there or the tendon is looped around the distal part of the tendon of the flexor carpi ulnaris. There will then be a similar arrangement to that found anatomically in the omohyoid or the tensor veli palatini muscles.

Bunnell offers a varied choice in the selection of muscle and tendon and the reconstruction of the pulley, depending on which are available or advantageous in the particular case of reconstruction.

For motor power, the musculus flexor carpi ulnaris, the musculus palmaris longus, the musculus flexor digitorum sublimis of the ring finger or any other available long flexor muscle may be used.

In regard to tendons, various combinations are depicted in Figure 366.

For the construction of a pulley at the pisiform bone, a free tendon graft, either from the palmaris longus or from any other available tendon, may be looped through the short muscle and tendon attachment to the pisiform bone and sutured to itself, so that it forms a circle 2 cm. (¾ inch) in diameter. The sutured junction is then slipped around until it is within the muscle. Another method of making a pulley is to use one half of the thickness of the flexor carpi ulnaris tendon, severing one of the halves high and suturing this free end to the ligament of the pisiform bone to complete the loop. Similarly, the tendon of the musculus palmaris longus may be severed 4 cm. (1⅝ inches) above its insertion and made to act as a loop or pulley by suturing it into the pisiform ligamentous tissue, leaving its original insertion intact. Instead of constructing a pulley, one may pass the tendon used around the flexor carpi ulnaris tendon and on to its insertion in the phalanx of the thumb.

Incisions, if possible, should be made along skin-tension lines. They should, however, not directly overlie tendons after rerouting. Finding the proper plane of rerouting is important. This plane lies just superficial to the palmar fascia, and should be deep enough in respect to the skin itself so that the tendon does not become adherent to overlying skin.

The most useful variations will be described in detail. Among others, Kirklin and Thomas, Luckey and McPherson, Royle, Thompson, Littler, Riordan, Phalen and Miller, Brand and Tubiana, have contributed much to the success of the original methods.

The procedure of choice, since it is the most physiological method, becomes possible if a sublimis tendon, preferably of the fourth finger, is available for activation. The tendon is rerouted through a pulley at the pisiform bone, subcutaneously to the dorsal aspect of the proximal phalanx of the thumb, and fastened to the abductor pollicis brevis. Normally, this muscle is the most important one of the thenar group. By virtue of its insertion into the lateral part of the base of the proximal

894

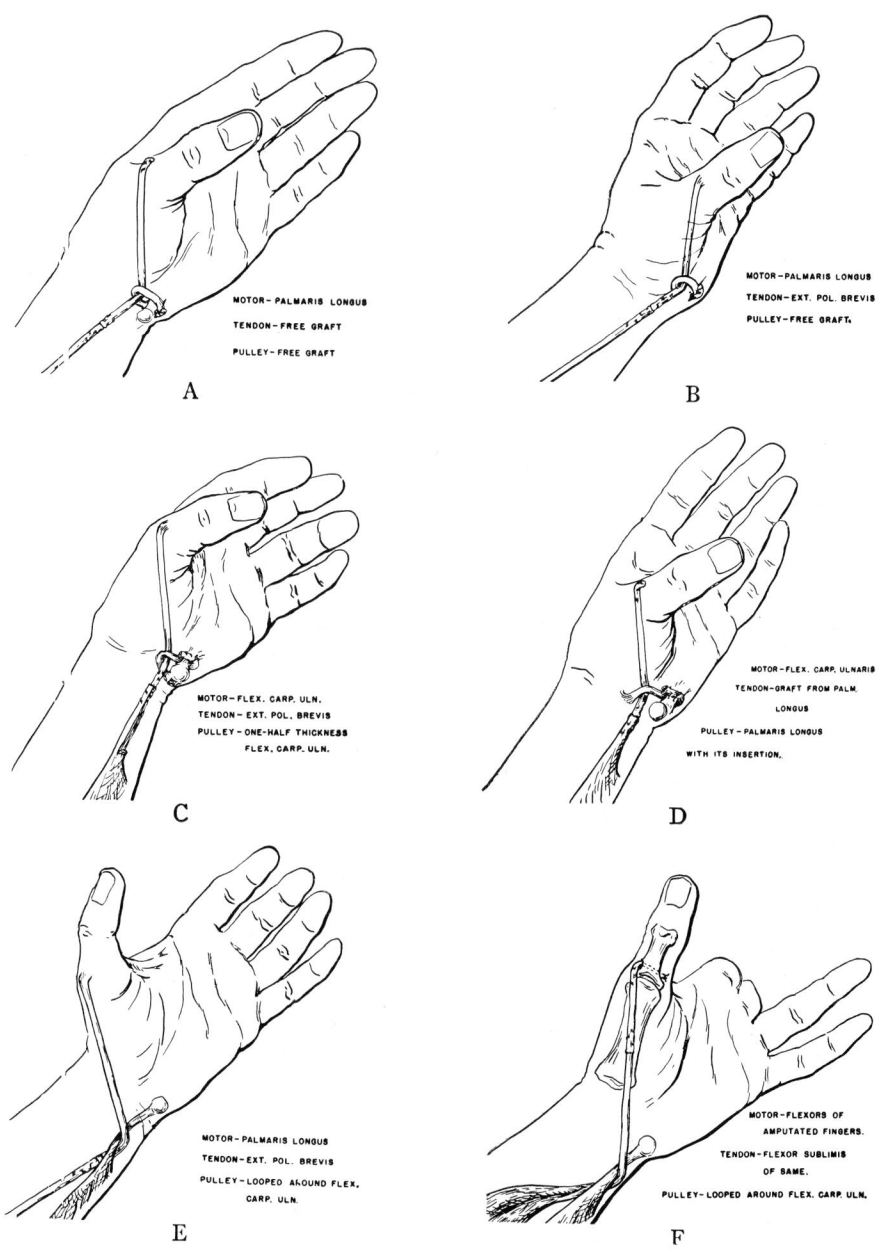

Fig. 366. Restoration of opposition of thumb (Bunnell). Various combinations of motor power, tendon transfer, and construction of pulley. (S. Bunnell: Surgery of the Hand. J. B. Lippincott.)

phalanx of the thumb and into the long extensor tendon, the abductor pollicis brevis can stabilize the metacarpophalangeal joint in abduction, flexion, and pronation, and can assist extension of the terminal phalanx —the essential functional components of opposition. Hence, good results are obtained by suturing one slip of the transferred sublimis tendon to the tendinous insertion of the paralyzed abductor pollicis brevis (Littler), the other one into the long extensor for additional stabilization (Riordan).

Technique (Use of Sublimis Tendon) (Fig. 367)

From an incision just distal and parallel to the volar crease of the metacarpophalangeal joint of the fourth finger, a short transverse incision is made through the flexor sheath, and the slips of the sublimis tendon are isolated. The finger is then flexed in the first interphalangeal joint, and the slips are severed. From a transverse incision over the insertion of the flexor carpi ulnaris, the latter is isolated. From the same incision, the severed sublimis tendon is withdrawn (the chiasm of Camper may hinder withdrawal, and if so must be divided). It is now passed beneath, around, and over the flexor carpi ulnaris tendon. This is the simplest and most satisfactory pulley. The flexor carpi ulnaris tendon should not be mobilized during this procedure, for this would allow it to bow radially. If the flexor carpi ulnaris is not available as a pulley, a pulley must be constructed from a free tendon graft, either from the palmaris longus tendon or from one of the toe extensor tendons (Fig. 366, A-D). The graft is looped around the short tendon attachment distal to the pisiform bone and sutured to itself so that it forms a circle 2 cm. ($1\frac{3}{16}$ inch) in diameter. The sutured junction is then slipped around so that it will not be in contact with the transferred sublimis tendon. An inverted hockey-stick incision is made on the dorsoradial side of the thumb, starting just proximal to the distal joint and ending on the radial side proximal to the metacarpophalangeal joint. A fascia carrier (Fig. 61) (or uterine-packing forceps) is inserted through this part of the incision and pushed subcutaneously through the incision at the wrist. The sublimis tendon slips are crisscrossed with a fine-wire suture of stainless steel; the wire is threaded through the eye of the fascia carrier and withdrawn through the incision at the thumb. The tendon is led through a slit in the fascia overlying the abductor muscle. One slip of the tendon is threaded through the loose ligaments between the abductor tendon and the bone. The other slip is led beneath the extensor pollicis longus tendon, which is perforated about 1 cm. ($\frac{3}{8}$ inch) distal to the metacarpophalangeal joint, and through this perforation the slip is slung dorsally over the tendon to be united with the first slip (Fig. 367). Brand extended this procedure by splitting the sublimis tendon farther and attaching one slip to the ulnar side of the metacarpophalangeal joint. The other slip is passed beneath the tendinous portion of the paralyzed abductor pollicis brevis and is then fixed to the extensor pollicis brevis at the proximal phalangeal level. When pulled snugly, an additional stitch to fix the transferred slip to the abductor pollicis brevis will maintain its position. This forms a yoke around the metacarpophalangeal joint with the first slip providing an extra element of rotational opposition. All wounds are then closed.

After-Treatment

The thumb must be immobilized in the position of abduction and opposition and slight flexion of the metacarpophalangeal joint; this is best achieved by taping the opposed tips of the thumb and the fifth finger

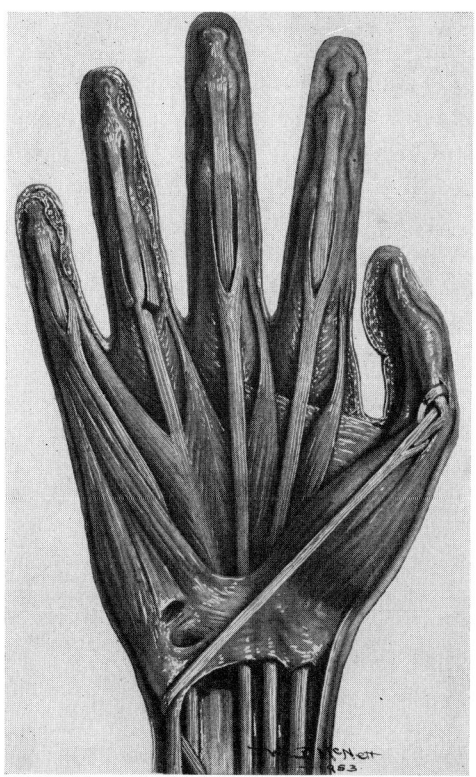

Fig. 367. Sublimis tendon transfer (of fourth finger) to restore opposition of thumb in irreparable median nerve palsy. Flexor carpi ulnaris is used as pulley. One slip of sublimis tendon is threaded through loose ligaments between abductor tendon and bone, i.e., proximal to metacarpophalangeal joint. The other slip is led beneath the extensor pollicis longus tendon and through a perforation of the same, 2 cm. (0.79 inches) distal to the metacarpophalangeal joint; it is then slung dorsally around the tendon to be united with the other slip, either end to end with one of the usual tendon sutures or by overlapping the ends of the slips.

together, thus holding them in correct position while a dorsal molded plaster-cast splint is applied. The latter must include the slightly flexed wrist, the knuckles, and the entire thumb. The other fingers are left free, and should be moved as soon as patient is awake. The immobilization is removed after twenty-one days. Semi-immobilization is then applied by adhesive rubber-band traction, which pulls the proximal phalanx of the thumb toward the pisiform bone. It is explained to the patient which tendon has been rerouted as the motor tendon, and he is urged to practice with this tendon. After one week, the adhesive traction is removed, and the patient is allowed to move the wrist.

In some cases, extensive scarring on the volar side of the wrist may make the Bunnel type of opponens transfer difficult. As already stated in the discussion of the Bunnell procedure, the motor tendon is rerouted proximal to the transverse ligament, and some sort of pulley in the repair of the pisiform bone is employed. In modifying Royle's operation, Thompson withdraws the sublimis tendon through a longitudinal incision at the radial side of the hypothenar eminence in the palm, in other words, distal to the transverse carpal ligament. He then reroutes the tendon subcutaneously across the palm to the thumb. In this instance, the palmar fascia, around which the tendon is rerouted, acts as a pulley. This procedure is preferred if the wrist and forearm are scarred, since all transfer can be performed in normal tissue without entering scarred areas.

If one of the sublimis tendons is not available, the next best method is the use of the flexor carpi ulnaris as motor power, a pulley of one half thickness of the flexor carpi ulnaris tendon at the pisiform bone, and the extensor pollicis brevis tendon as a means of prolonging the motor power.

Technique (Flexor Carpi Ulnaris to Ext. Pollicis Brevis) (Fig. 366)

From a curved incision ulnar to the insertion of the flexor carpi ulnaris of the pisiform bone, the flexor carpi ulnaris tendon is located. It is split in half, beginning at the pisiform bone. The ulnar half is severed proximally and is used to make the pulley; the latter should have a circle of 2 cm. ($1\frac{3}{16}$ inch) and the loop should be formed so that the outer surface of the tendon slip forms the inner circumference of the circle to prevent adhesions within the pulley. The free end is sutured to the ligament of the pisiform bone. The radial half of the carpi ulnaris tendon is severed from the pisiform bone to be used as the active tendon.

The insertion of the extensor pollicis brevis tendon is located from a small curved incision over the radial aspect of the metacarpophalangeal joint. Through another incision over the radial aspect of the wrist, the musculotendinous junction of the musculus extensor pollicis brevis is located and the tendon severed at that point. The tendon is now withdrawn through the distal incision of the thumb and guided with a fascia carrier (Fig. 61) or uterine-packing forceps through this incision subcutaneously toward the pisiform bone. The free end of the tendon is looped through the pulley; with the thumb in abduction and opposition, this free end is sutured to the flexor carpi ulnaris tendon by interweaving or by end-to-end suturing.

After-Treatment (See p. 897)

When this method is used, a few technical details are of importance, and they have been aptly pointed out by Kirklin and Thomas. First, an accurate localizing and recognition of the extensor pollicis tendon are necessary. In a few patients, the tendon is absent. If this is so, the prolongation must be made with a free graft either from the palmaris longus or from one of the extensor tendons of the foot. The free end of the graft is attached to the thumb, as shown in Figure 366, D. If the tendon is present, it must be dissected out in such a manner that when it is pulled upon in the direction of the pisiform bone it produces satisfactory opposition of the thumb. If it is dissected too far distally across the metacarpophalangeal joint of the thumb, it will markedly flex this joint, and this is undesirable. In a few instances, if the tendon is not dissected far enough distally, it will hyperextend this joint. Therefore, dissection must be carried out to just such a point that the desired rotation and opposition are obtained without either of the aforementioned undesirable actions. Occasionally also, a slip connecting this tendon to the extensor pollicis longus must be severed so that it does not exert an extending action on the distal phalanx. In some cases, despite severance of all connections to the long extensor tendon of the thumb, the extensor pollicis brevis continues to extend the distal phalanx. In these situations, it is probably best not to utilize this tendon but to use a free tendon graft for prolongation of the motor power.

Instead of the flexor carpi ulnaris, the palmaris longus or the extensor carpi ulnaris may be used as motor muscles. If the palmaris longus is used, the flexor carpi ulnaris tendon will serve as a pulley. If the extensor carpi ulnaris is used, no pulley is necessary. The direction of pull after rerouting from the extensor side to the flexor side is toward the pisiform bone. There are numerous other methods available to restore opposition. Henderson demonstrated that any of the wrist extensors or the brachioradialis can be used as motor (Case 157, p. 1204.) Littler preceded by Huber and by Nichols transferred the ulnar innervated abductor digiti quinti on its neurovascular pedicle to serve as an effective substitute for the abductor pollicis to restore thumb opposition.

THE EXTREMITIES

In these lesions, in addition to restoring opposition of the thumb, the flexor action of thumb, index finger, and middle finger must be restored. The flexor pollicis brevis, however, is often supplied by the ulnar nerve, and may therefore be spared in complete median palsy (Highet, Rowntree). Stiles and Forrester recommend transferring the extensor pollicis brevis to the flexor pollicis longus, splitting the extensor carpi radialis longus in two, and transferring it to the profundus tendons of index and third fingers (see also p. 902). If the extensors are not available, Forrester recommends the following procedure: From an L-shaped incision along the flexor creases of the wrist and the radial side of the forearm, the flexor pollicis longus tendon and the profundus tendons of the second and third fingers are severed proximally and inserted through buttonholes into the profundus tendons of the fourth and fifth fingers (in a way similar to that depicted in Fig. 372). Opposition of thumb is restored as described in the foregoing discussions.

BONE AND JOINT OPERATIONS TO RESTORE OPPOSITION OF THUMB

Whenever rotation of the thumb is markedly restricted from ankylosis of the joints or contracture, or tendon transfer cannot be performed to restore active opposition of the thumb, rotation osteotomies, arthrodesis, arthroplasty, excision of the greater multangular bone and the bone-bloc operations are good methods to hold the thumb permanently in the position of function.

Arthrodesis

If the carpometacarpal joint of the thumb is cicatricially contracted while the surrounding soft tissues are not contracted, arthrodesis of this joint with the thumb in abduction and opposition is performed. The joint is exposed from the radial side, the articular surfaces are removed with burr and chisel, and the thumb is placed in the position of function. This position is temporarily maintained best by fastening the pulps of the first three digits together with one stainless-steel suture. A groove is chiseled into both articular bones and a matchstick-size inlay bone graft placed across the joint. The bone graft is taken with chisels from the subcutaneous border of the ulna or tibia. For better stabilization, a short Kirschner wire is drilled into the marrow through the proximal half of the first metacarpal and the greater multangulum; greater stabilization can be achieved by cross-pinning the first and second metacarpals (com-

900

pare with Case 160, p. 1208); all wires are placed subcutaneously. A cast is applied with the hand in the position of function.

Goldner and Clippinger are opposed to arthrodesis. They achieve better functional results from excision of the greater multangular bone with portions of the first, second or both first and second metacarpals, an operation which is similar to an arthroplasty. Littler and Eaton however came out recently in defense of arthrodesis after long-term analysis of their cases.

If, aside from the contracture of the first carpometacarpal joint, the surrounding soft tissues are rigidly contracted, the bone-bloc operation has a better chance to overcome the deformity (see below).

If the first carpometacarpal joint is obliterated by bony fusion, a metacarpal osteotomy is performed (see below).

If the first metacarpophalangeal joint or the terminal joint of the thumb are contracted in malposition, arthrodesis of these joints is indicated. After removal of the articular surfaces from a longitudinal, dorsal, tendon-splitting incision, the joint surfaces are brought into 25-degree flexion; they are held together by an inlay bone graft (except in the terminal joint) (bone graft to be taken from subcutaneous border of ulna or tibia) and an intramedullary cross-pinning of the joint by a short, subcutaneously placed Kirschner wire (compare with Fig. 370). This is followed by immobilization with a dorsal molded plaster-cast splint for about four to six weeks (see also p. 932).

Osteotomy

When the carpometacarpal joint is fused in malposition of the thumb, osteotomy is performed through the proximal third of the first metacarpal from a dorsoradial incision. The thumb is rotated into opposition. A small wedge of bone may need removal to permit smooth fitting of the fragments. The latter are held together by intramedullary cross-pinning of the fracture line, by cross-pinning the first two metacarpals (compare with Case 160, p. 1208), and by immobilization in a plaster cast for about four to six weeks.

Intermetacarpal Bone Grafting (Case 139, p. 1181)

This operation, first devised by Foerster and later elaborated on by Thompson, Brooks, and others, is indicated in permanent paralysis of abduction and opponens muscles for which tendon transplantation to restore active opposition cannot be performed, in spastic cases with adduction contracture, or in post-traumatic and postinfection cases with rigid scar contracture. Prior to the bone-grafting operation, any fixed adduction contracture, particularly of the skin, must be overcome. Stripping of the contracted adductor and interosseous muscles and removing of all scar tissue in the cleft and the cicatricial web may necessitate transplantation of an abdominal flap as a preliminary step. If this is not necessary, the operation is performed in one stage. The bone graft, taken from the crest of the ilium and wedge shaped, is inserted through an incision along the web. If the muscles in the web are contracted they are stripped or excised, and the bone graft is driven between the first two metacarpals (Frackelton). The opposing bone surfaces of the latter should be roughened with a chisel prior to the wedging. The thumb is placed in the position of function. This is best achieved by temporarily fastening the pulps of the first three digits together with one stainless-steel suture. The bone graft is held in place with a Kirschner wire drilled from a small incision over the radial side of the first metacarpal through the latter and bone graft into the second metacarpal. The wire, cut flush with the bone and the wound edges, is sutured over it. Plaster-cast immobilization is not necessary.

Dysfunction after Irreparable Paralysis of Nervus Medianus and Nervus Ulnaris

COMBINED IRREPARABLE MEDIAN AND ULNAR LESIONS AT WRIST LEVEL

The dysfunction following a combined injury of median and ulnar nerves at the level of the wrist is mainly from loss of sensation and of function of the intrinsic system. This is because the long flexors are supplied at a much higher level. Loss of sensation and early pulp atrophy are severe disabilities in themselves. They become aggravated by clawing of the fingers, by loss of opposition of the thumb, and by finger extension. The thumb lies at the side of the hand; it can neither oppose nor adduct. The fingers are hyperextended in the metacarpophalangeal joints and flexed in the interphalangeal joints ("intrinsic minus hand," p. 811). They cannot simultaneously flex in their metacarpophalangeal joints and extend in the interphalangeal joints; they have no lateral motion. The carpal and metacarpal arches are flat, the thenar region is atrophied, and the dorsal aspect of the thumb web is hollow (Case 147, 148, pp. 1192, 1194; p. 885).

The motor dysfunction can be much improved by tendon transfer (see also p. 887). It is again pointed out that contracture must be absent or overcome. Opposition of the thumb is restored as already described. If a sublimis tendon is available, it is used as a motor (see p. 896); otherwise, one may use the flexor carpi ulnaris (see p. 898). The bone-bloc operation and arthrodeses are indicated (see pp. 900-901) only in rigid ad-

duction contractures. Abduction of the index finger is preferably overcome by transfer of the extensor pollicis brevis. A sublimis tendon should
not be used for this purpose; such tendons are better used for restoring thumb opposition and intrinsic action. The paralyzed intrinsic
system is activated by utilizing the sublimis tendons: sublimis 2, both
slips for index finger; sublimis 3, for third and fourth fingers; sublimis 5,
both slips for fifth finger; sublimis 4, for opposition of thumb. The
tendons are withdrawn at the wrist (the chiasm of Camper may hinder
withdrawal, and if so must be divided). The slips are split further apart
with the back of the knife, then passed from the wrist through the lumbrical canals and fastened to the dorsal aponeurosis and lateral bands of the
fingers, with the wrist dorsiflexed 45 degrees and metacarpophalangeal
joints flexed (Littler, Brand) (see also p. 888 and Fig. 364). The strands are
fastened on the radial sides of the fingers, except for the index finger, where
an abductor transfer is necessary. In this case, the sublimis strand is not
passed through the lumbrical canal but sutured to the lateral band on the
ulnar side of the index finger, where it serves to adduct and flex the metacarpophalangeal joint and to assist in extension of the interphalangeal joints.
Even one sublimis tendon with each slip split in two may suffice for transfer
to the four fingers (compare with Case 148, p. 1194).

It has already been pointed out that in many cases it is better to use
an extensor (Fowler, 1949) instead of a flexor to stabilize the motor carpophalangeal joints, for reasons explained on page 887. Riordan and Brand's
extensive experience in leprosy cases with the Fowler principle has proved
its value. Brand has formulated several indications and rules (p. 888) as to
when to use a sublimis or an extensor transfer. According to a recent
personal communication he prefers, whenever possible, rerouting the extensor carpi radialis longus to the anterior side of the forearm; he extends
it by a many-tailed free tendon graft (plantaris tendon) which is passed
deep through the carpal tunnel to the fingers.

Technique (Brand) (Figs. 368, 369)

The extensor carpi radialis longus is divided at the distal end of
the radius through a short transverse incision. It is withdrawn halfway
up the forearm through a transverse incision. It is then tunneled deep to
the brachioradialis to the anterior side of the forearm and withdrawn
through a short transverse incision, 3 inches proximal to the wrist, and
laid on wet gauze. The tendon is slit open along a natural place of cleavage
and is opened out and unrolled. The plantaris tendon is used as a tendon
graft (see p. 865) and incorporated within the unrolled extensor carpi radialis longus tendon as depicted in Figure 368. The plantaris tendon which
had been doubled upon itself at first is now quadrupled by splitting the

end of each half. The tunneling forceps or fascia carrier (Fig. 61) is introduced through a midpalmar incision and passed deep along the bottom of the carpal tunnel. From this point each strand of graft is passed separately on to each finger. This is done as follows: each strand is crisscrossed with a thin wire suture which acts as a guide. A dorsolateral incision is made in the proximal segment of the radial side of the fingers, except for the index finger where on the radial side an abduction transfer is necessary;

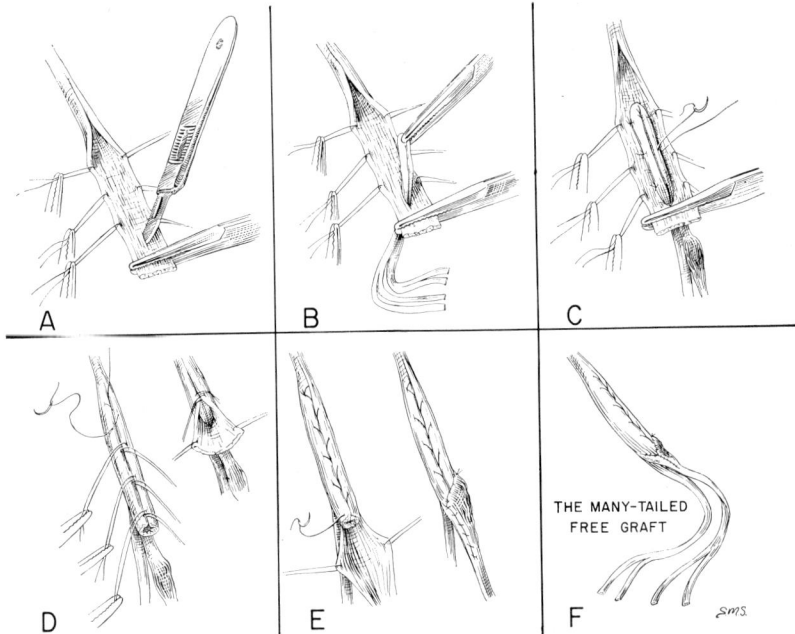

Fig. 368. Insertion of plantaris tendon graft into motor tendon. *A:* Perforation of the opened extensor carpi radialis longus tendon. *B:* Insertion of the doubled-up plantaris tendon. *C:* Fixation of the plantaris tendon by small sutures. *D:* Closure of the extensor carpi radialis longus tendon by running suture. *E:* Spreading the fibers of the plantaris tendon to close over the stump of the extensor carpi radialis longus. *F:* The many-tailed graft with the tendon ends split. The point of juncture is covered with paratenon from the plantaris. (W. L. White: Surg. Clin. N. Amer.)

here the incision is made on the ulnar side. The lumbricale tendon and lateral band of each finger are identified and the fascia carrier is now passed from this point into the palm. A strand of tendon graft is grasped and withdrawn into the finger. The first tendon attachment is to the ulnar band of the index finger. The transfer slip is woven into the lateral band of the dorsal expansion and sutured with a running wire suture or silk sutures. The next finger to be sutured is the fifth where the slip is led to the dorsum of the middle phalanx and sutured to the extensor apparatus; suture of the intermediate fingers, then the third and fourth fingers

(Fig. 369), follows. The tension chosen is such that the tendons are completely relaxed when the wrist is dorsiflexed 45 degrees, the metacarpophalangeal joints are flexed to 70 degrees and the interphalangeal joints are straight. This position is maintained in a light plaster cast for three weeks. Restoration of abduction of the index finger by means of transfer of the extensor pollicis brevis (p. 890) can be carried out in the same operation. Restoration of thumb opposition, however, requires another stage.

If there is marked hyperextension of the metacarpophalangeal joint of the thumb, adduction must also be restored (see p. 891).

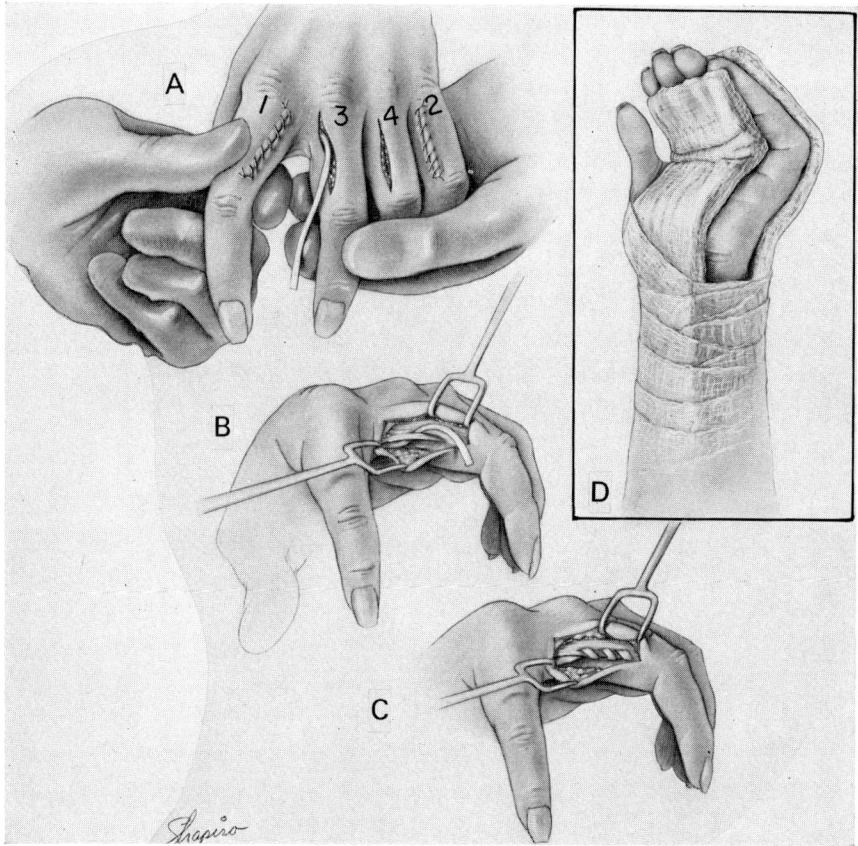

Fig. 369. *A:* Pattern of distribution of the tendon ends of the plantaris graft (Fig. 368) and their course. The first tendon attachment is that to the index finger into its ulnar lateral band. Next the attachment to the radial lateral band of the little finger is fixed to balance the transfer. Subsequently the middle and ring finger slips are inserted into the radial lateral bands. This order of insertion, seen in *A,* provides balanced movement. *B* and *C* illustrate the method of weaving the transfer flips into the lateral bands of the dorsal expansion, *D* the type of plaster splint immobilization used to maintain extension of the wrist and flexion of the metacarpal joints. (W. L. White: Surg. Clin. N. Amer.)

THE EXTREMITIES

High combined lesions of median and ulnar nerves cause a severely disabled hand. Aside from lack of sensitivity, which in itself is a great handicap, the intrinsic and long flexor muscles are paralyzed. Even if function of all long flexors could be restored, without the intrinsic muscles they are useless from the point of view of function. Yet some usefulness can be restored to the hand by transfer of extensor tendons to the flexors of the hand. To permit use of all extensor tendons, the wrist should be fused (for technique, see p. 907). Arthrodesis of the metacarpophalangeal joints may also be considered (p. 900). However, before the wrist is fused, the opponens transfer (utilizing the extensor carpi ulnaris as motor; see p. 899) should be carried out first, so that relaxation of the transferred tendon by wrist flexion may be obtained. The rest of the reconstructive program is undertaken after the wrist fusion. Various methods of extensor transfer are available (Stiles and Forrester, Brown, Bunnell, Foerster, Luckey and McPherson, Phalen, and Miller).

Luckey and McPherson suggest the following combination: The tendon of the musculus brachioradialis is transferred to the flexor pollicis longus. The tendon of the extensor carpi radialis longus is severed close to its insertion, freed well up into the forearm, rerouted subcutaneously on the volar aspect of the wrist, and inserted into the flexor digitorum profundus tendon of the index finger. The extensor carpi radialis brevis is rerouted in a similar way and inserted through buttonholes into the flexor digitorum profundus of long, ring, and little fingers. Digital balance can be achieved by Fowler's proprii extensor transfers. All reroutings are made in similar ways, namely, severance of tendons from their inserting points (through a small transverse incision), withdrawal of the tendons higher up in the forearm (through small transverse incisions), and rerouting and reinsertion of the tendon (through a transverse incision in the wrist). To restore opposition of the thumb, the extensor carpi ulnaris is rerouted and either inserted to the extensor pollicis brevis or lengthened by a free graft, as described on pages 898 and 899. As already mentioned, the opponens transfer is the first stage of the reconstructive program, fusion of the wrist the second stage, and the rest of the transfers the third stage.

The transplants should be under proper tension. According to Luckey and McPherson, the tension should permit the proximal two joints to extend to about 140 to 150 degrees at the time of transplantation and permit the distal joint to extend to about 160 degrees. If the tension is too great, there will be excessive clawing, and the thumb and fingers will not come together in a functional position. On the other hand, excessive length will allow complete extension, but will not permit enough flexion for a satisfactory grasp.

ARTHRODESIS OF WRIST

During the foregoing reconstructive program, primary arthrodesis of the wrist is essential. Arthrodesis permits the subsequent borrowing of the extensors of the wrist (extensor carpi ulnaris; extensor carpi radialis, longus, and brevis) for transplantation into the flexors of the digits. In most methods of arthrodesing the wrist, the carporadial joint is fused— usually with bone grafts (Abbott et al., Campbell and Keokarn)—while the carpometacarpal joints are not fused, thus adding strength to the grasp of the hand. To shorten the healing process by avoiding bone grafting, Robinson and Kayfetz have developed a method which consists of resecting the proximal row of carpal bones, with fixation of the capitate to the radius by means of a screw. In this way, viable cancellous bones, with an intact blood supply, are opposed to one another, and the internal fixation provides a positive means of maintaining position. Cancellous grafts are used to reinforce the fusion, but healing is not dependent upon any grafted bones. In twelve arthrodeses, all successful, the average immobilization time was eight weeks. The author has found this method particularly useful in contracted wristdrop, where the contracture could not be overcome by simple stretching.

Technique (Robinson and Kayfetz) (Fig. 370)

Starting over the dorsal aspect of the distal third of the ulna, a bayonet incision is made over the wrist. After retraction of the skin and subcutaneous tissue, the dorsal carpal ligament is incised. The extensor tendons are then retracted, and the dorsal aspect of the wrist is exposed.

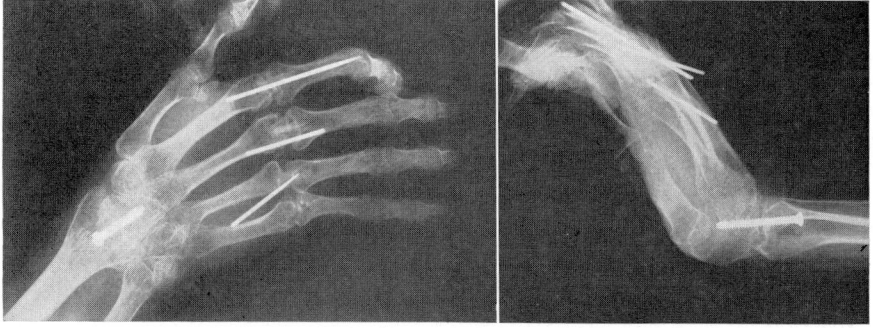

Fig. 370. Arthrodesis of wrist and metacarpophalangeal joints of fingers in patient with irreparable median and radial palsy. Wrist fusion done first (after Robinson-Kayfetz), followed by fusion of metacarpophalangeal joints (see p. 932) three months later. Pins gradually worked themselves out. Screw was removed after nine months. This roentgenogram shows result seven months after wrist fusion (four months after metacarpophalangeal joint fusion).

907

The capsule is incised and the navicular, lunate, and multangular bones are completely removed. Sometimes it may be difficult to identify the bone area without undue dissection. In these cases, the removal of a thin layer of bone and periosteum from the dorsal aspect of the radius and the carpal bones, in one piece, with a broad, thin osteotome is advised. Following this, the various carpal bones are easily identified. A thin layer of bone and periosteum may be replaced at the end of the operation. Next, the articular surfaces of the radius, capitate, and hamate bones are removed with a chisel and gouge, until a surface of cancellous bone can be seen. A small, shallow depression is gouged into the distal surface of the radius to accommodate the head of the capitate. The radial side of the incision is retracted, and the lateral aspect of the radial styloid is exposed 1.5 cm. (⅝ inch) from its tip. A drill is run through the styloid into the depression made for the head of the capitate, followed by the insertion of a stainless-steel or vitallium screw, 3 to 3.8 cm. (1¼ to 1½ inches) long. When the tip of the screw appears on the bottom of the depression in the end of the radius, the head of the capitate is forced into the depression. The screw can then be driven into the capitate without prior drilling of the bone. One precaution should be observed: The screw should not be placed too far on the palmar side, but must be sufficiently angulated dorsally to obtain a good bite on the capitate. While the screw should be long enough to hold firmly in the capitate, it must not cross the carpometacarpal joint. After firm fixation and proper position have been accomplished, chips of cancellous bone taken from the removed proximal row are now placed about the fusion site to round out the bony mass and to reinforce the fusion. Care should be taken not to extend the bony mass on the dorsum, where it might interfere with the function of the extensor tendons.

After-Treatment

After closure of the wound, a plaster-of-paris cast is applied, extending from the upper arm to the tips of the fingers and the thumb, with the elbow held at a right angle and the forearm to midprone position. The wrist is fixed in dorsal angulation of 20 to 30 degrees, or such that the opposed thumb is in line with the forearm. To this, about 20 degrees of deviation of the wrist toward the ulnar side is added. This combination approximates the normal clenched-fist position in which the grip is strongest. The cast is carefully molded and cut over the back of the wrist and forearm to allow for swelling. At the end of three weeks, a second, short plaster cast, extending from just below the elbow to the metacarpophalangeal joints, is applied. The position of the wrist is checked carefully at this time.

908

DYSFUNCTION AFTER IRREPARABLE PARALYSIS OF NERVUS RADIALIS

The deformity following palsy of the radial nerve is typical. The nervus radialis supplies the extensors of the hand and fingers. Hence, palsy of this nerve causes the hand, if the forearm is held horizontally, to drop. The extensor tendons are maximally stretched in this position, and cannot be stretched (relaxed) further if an attempt is made to close the hand to a fist. This prevents the flexors from fully functioning. If, however, the hand is held in dorsal flexion (cocked up) in the wrist, the flexors regain their full range of function. Hence, the object of reconstruction should be twofold: (1) restoration of dorsal flexion of the wrist; (2) restoration of extension of the fingers.

Dorsal flexion of the wrist can be achieved in various ways. Steindler and Abbott fixed the wrist in position of extension by arthrodesis, Perthes by tenodesis. Either method produces a permanent cocked-up position, which complicates the operation and is not felt to be an advantage by the patient. However, it may be indicated in paralysis of long duration with secondary contracture of the wrist. In most cases, transfer of tendons without tenodesis is sufficient to stabilize the wrist well; furthermore, it permits flexion in the wrist, and the operation is less complicated. Consequently, tendon transfer is preferable.

Robert Jones's principles of tendon transfer are still widely used today, consisting of transfer of the flexor carpi ulnaris tendon to the extensor communis tendons of the fingers, of the pronator teres to the extensor carpi radialis longus and brevis, and of the flexor carpi radialis to the extensors and abductors of the thumb. A similar method was advocated by McMurray, Stoffel, and by Billington in the United States (Figs. 371, 372). Starr (1922) was the first to suggest leaving one wrist flexor in its original place. In a careful analysis of a large series of tendon transplantations performed for radial palsy during World War II in England, Zachary brought out this very important point again, and Scuderi, and Young and Lowe, in this country, concur. A transplanted muscle, like any other, has only a limited range of action; if, owing to absence of an antagonist on the flexor side of the wrist, the length of contraction of the fibers is used up in extending the wrist, there will be little left to extend the digits. Scuderi, after analysis of his large series of World War II cases, brought out another important point, namely, that the flexor carpi ulnaris muscle is capable of extending the wrist and all the fingers, if properly sutured under the correct amount of tension. The author concurs. Scuderi also stresses that transplantation of a single tendon into the extensor pollicis longus is far more efficient than transplantation of a single tendon into the extensor and abductor of the thumb

909

or thumb and index finger. He therefore makes five points: (1) The palmaris longus tendon is transplanted into the severed extensor pollicis longus tendon. (2) The flexor carpi ulnaris is transferred into the extensor tendons of the second, third, fourth, and fifth fingers; the flexor carpi ulnaris must be sutured at a 45-degree angle to the long axis of the extensor tendons so that the anastomosis to the extensor tendon of the second finger is about 2 cm. (¾ inch) distal to the anastomosis to the extensor tendon of the fifth finger. (3) The action of the flexor carpi radialis into one of the thumb tendons is advocated only if the palmaris longus tendon is absent. (4) The transplanted tendon must exert its pull in as straight a line as possible from the origin of the muscle to the insertion of the recipient tendons. (5) Preoperative physical therapy must be carried out until complete range of motion is possible in the interphalangeal and metacarpophalangeal joints of the finger.

Technique (Scuderi) (Figs. 371, 372; Case 158, p. 1206)

Before the operation, a volar splint of sheet metal (aluminum) should be prepared to hold the wrist in full hyperextension, the fingers in extension, and the thumb in full abduction. The splint is sterilized and may be applied during the operation, thus replacing an assistant.

With the wrist held in extension, the insertions of the palmaris longus and flexor carpi ulnaris are easily identified. Short longitudinal incisions are made over the insertion points, and the isolated tendons are cut free. When the cut tendon is pulled gently, its proximal portion can be palpated in the forearm, 15 to 17 cm. (6 to 8 inches) proximally; then through individual, short longitudinal incisions, each tendon is exposed.

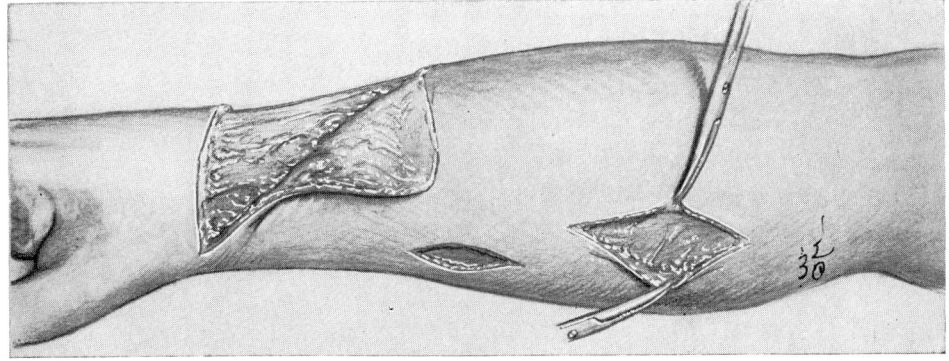

Fig. 371. Tendon transfer in paralysis of nervus radialis (Billington). An L-shaped incision is made over dorsum of wrist. Dissection of triangular skin flap. Two incisions are made on radial side: proximal incision, for exposure of pronator teres tendon; distal incision, for exposure of flexor carpi radialis.

910

The tendon of the palmaris longus is withdrawn through the proximal incision. The flexor carpi ulnaris has a very low attachment of muscle fibers, which usually reach far down toward the insertion of the tendon. They should be sheared off from the tendon up to a point 7.5 cm. (3 inches) above the wrist to permit better suturing to the recipient tendons and to provide better gliding. This tendon is then withdrawn through the proximal incision.

The forearm is now pronated. In the "anatomical snuffbox," the extensor pollicis longus is located from a longitudinal incision radial to the tendon. The dorsal carpal ligament is severed over the tendon; the tendon is severed as far proximally as possible. With a Kelly forceps, a

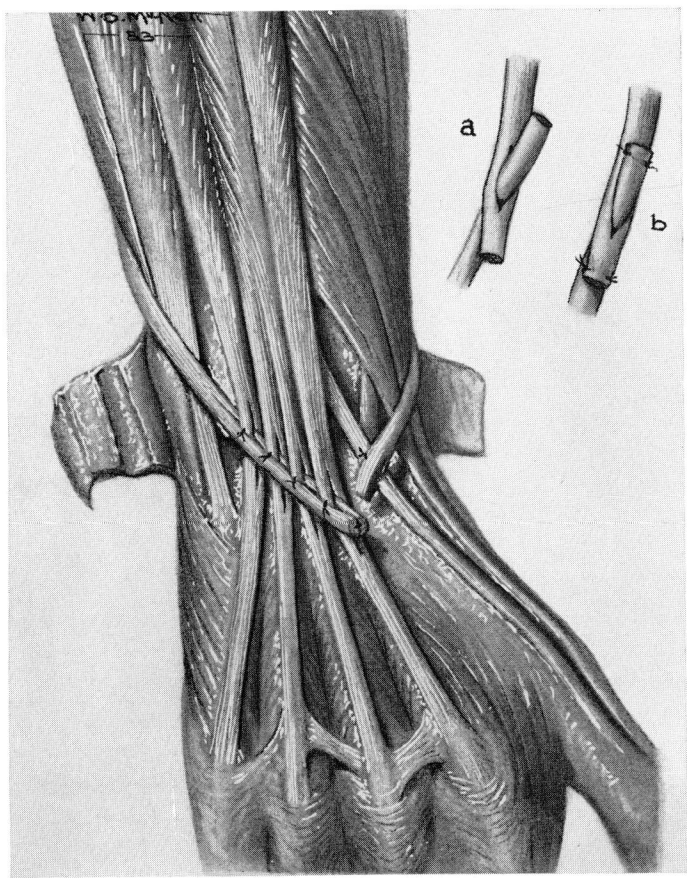

Fig. 372. Tendon transfer in irreparable radial palsy, after Scuderi. Transfer of palmaris tendon to extensor pollicis longus and transfer of flexor carpi ulnaris tendon to extensors of second to fifth fingers. Insert shows alternate way of tendon attachment of palmaris tendon and thumb extensor by "buttonhole" technique.

911

tunnel is made between the incision in the "snuffbox" and the proximal incision of the palmaris longus. The tunnel must be in a straight line with the palmaris longus tendon and the extended and abducted thumb, and must come to lie between the subcutaneous fat tissue and the fascia of the forearm. The palmaris longus tendon is withdrawn through this tunnel.

A transverse incision is made over the dorsum of the wrist, and the common extensor tendons of the fingers are exposed. The ligamentum carpi dorsale is excised over the tendons. (Absence of this ligament does not cause a functional handicap!) A straight tunnel is made to connect the wrist incision with the proximal incision of the flexor carpi ulnaris tendon. The latter is then withdrawn through the wrist incision. All wounds on the flexor side of the forearm are closed.

The palmaris longus is anastomosed with the extensor pollicis longus tendon, the thumb being held in extension and abduction, and in a straight line with the palmaris tendon. For tendon attachment, the buttonhole technique or a similar one is used. The wound is closed.

The flexor carpi ulnaris tendon is anastomosed with the common extensor tendons of the fingers. The latter and the wrist are held in extension (seldom will a radial transplant be too tight!). The anastomosis is oblique, the tendon suture to the little finger being 1.5 cm. ($\frac{5}{8}$ inch) proximal to the suture to the tendon of the index finger. The recipient tendons are buttonholed at the desired level. The transferred flexor carpi ulnaris tendon is slit longitudinally, and half is drawn through the recipient tendons with a Kelly forceps. Two interrupted silk sutures are used to fix each tendon. The other half of the tendon is laid over the recipient tendons and held in place with only two silk sutures at the proximal and distal ends of the anastomosis. The wound is closed in layers: first the subcutaneous fat tissue, then the skin edges.

After-Treatment

The previously prepared aluminum splint is firmly bandaged in place. If such a splint is not available, a volar plaster-cast splint is applied, reaching from the tips of the fingers, with the fingers slightly flexed in the proximal interphalangeal joints, to the elbow joint. Immobilization is removed after three weeks and physical therapy begun.

If the palmaris longus is absent, the flexor carpi radialis is rerouted subcutaneously and anastomosed with the extensor pollicis longus, followed by transfer of the flexor carpi ulnaris to the common extensors of the fingers (Fig. 373). In this case, the wrist is deprived of both flexors. This has certain disadvantages, as mentioned previously. To stabilize the

912

wrist, it may then be of advantage to transplant one or two sublimis tendons into the wrist, as suggested by Bickel (after Luckey and McPherson).

If the flexor carpi ulnaris is not sufficient to extend wrist and fingers, the pronator teres may be transplanted subsequently into the extensor

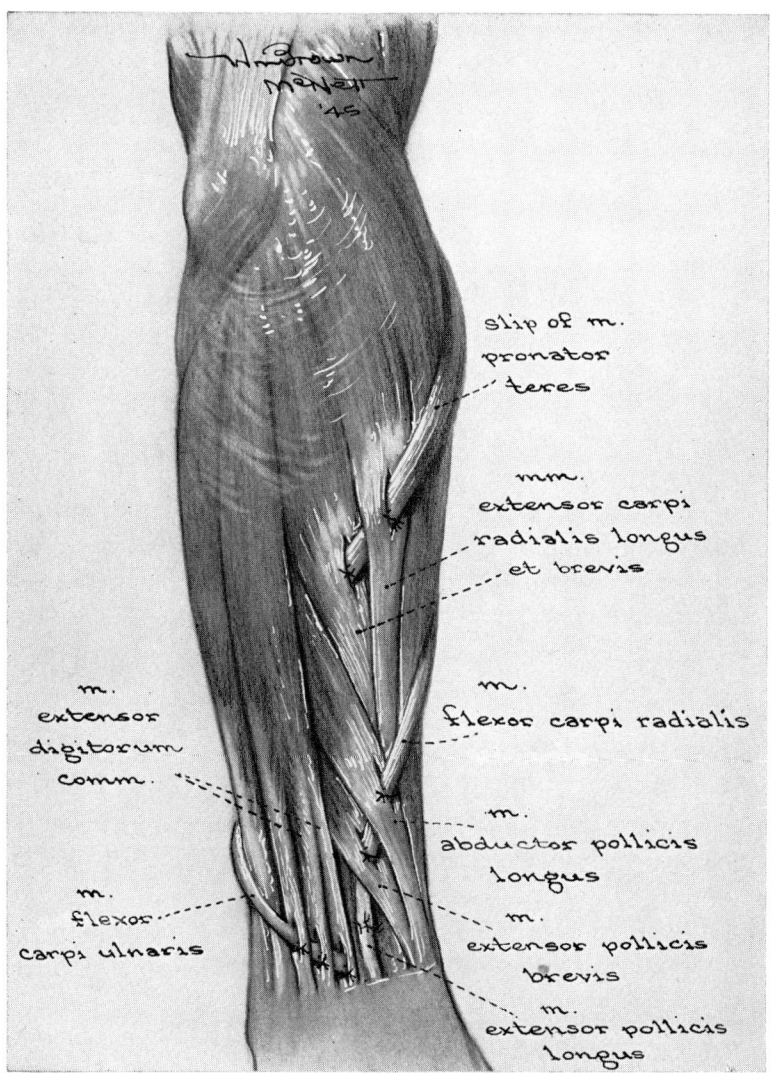

Fig. 373. Rerouted flexor carpi ulnaris tendon is drawn through buttonholes in extensor digiti quinti and extensor digitorum tendons and fastened to them. Rerouted pronator radii teres tendon is inserted into tendon of extensor carpi radialis longus and brevis. Rerouted tendon of flexor carpi radialis is drawn through buttonholes of abductor pollicis longus and extensor pollicis brevis tendons and sutured end to end to severed extensor pollicis longus tendon in case of absence of the palmaris tendon.

913

carpi radialis longus and brevis (after Jones and Billington) (see Fig. 372). Saikku advises separating the pronator completely from its whole insertion.

Arthrodesis of the wrist in extension should be the last resort. It should be reserved for those patients with long-standing secondary contractures of the wrist. (For technique, see p. 907.)

VESSELS

Reparative surgery of the vessels of the hand is essentially the same as described previously (Chapter 24, p. 759). A few points, however, may be emphasized. Suture of a torn vessel will hardly be required, since the hand has abundant vascular anastomoses and therefore a good collateral circulation. Ligation of the injured vessel is the method of choice.

The lesions that require reparative surgery are arterial aneurysm and arteriovenous fistula; the former is of traumatic origin, the latter quite often congenital. The symptoms do not differ from those of aneurysms in other parts of the extremities (see p. 764). The congenital type results from failure of differentiation of the common embryonic anlage into artery and vein (Reid and others). Extensive reviews of the subject were presented by Seeger, Horton, Allen, Barker, Hines and Curtis, Castro-Farinas and Riviera-Lopez. In Horton's series of thirty-four cases, seventeen involved the arm and hands. In some patients, signs and symptoms were present at birth; in others, they were noted much later. The involved extremity is usually larger in circumference and length than the other side, and the superficial veins are dilated. There is increase of heat from arterialization of the venous blood, and blood removed from a superficial vein proximal to the fistula shows the bright red color of arterial blood (compare with the blood of a similar vein of the other extremity) and greater oxygen saturation. Arteriography can be of great help in establishing the diagnosis and the site of the lesion; as Allen, Barker, and Hines point out, however, interpretation of the arteriogram may be difficult when small vessels are involved or the fistulas are small. From 20 to 30 cc. of contrast material (Diodrast) are injected under local anesthesia into the brachial artery, just above the lacertus fibrosus.

Treatment

It is unfortunate that in cases of arteriovenous fistulas of the hand or of the finger the arteriovenous communications are numerous. Hence, in the majority of cases, it is impossible to save the finger. Amputation seems to be the only solution, particularly if bone is involved. There is only one exception: If, in a rare case, only one side of the finger is involved and the artery on this side can be ligated, the other artery may be sufficient to keep the finger alive. Injection of the superficial veins with sclerosing solutions may be given a trial before amputation is considered, although one must be aware that this may produce necrosis of functioning parts. One other method, which has been suggested recently, is compression by rubber bandages. Pressure of the superficial veins makes it more difficult for the blood to flow from the artery into the vein, and thus encourages the blood to pursue a normal course.

BIBLIOGRAPHY

ABBOTT, L. C., SAUNDERS, J. B., DeC. M., and BOST, F. C.: *Arthrodesis of the wrist with use of cancellous bone.* J. Bone Joint Surg., 24:883, 1942.

ADAMSON, J. E., and WILSON, J. N.: *The history of flexor-tendon grafting.* J. Bone Joint Surg., 43A:709, 1961.

ALLEN, E. V., BARKER, N. W., HINES, JR., E. A.: *Peripheral Vascular Diseases.* W. B. Saunders, Philadelphia, 1946.

ALLEN, H. S.: *Flexor-tendon grafting to the hand.* Ann. Surg., 63:362, 1951.

ALTMAN, C. H., and TROTT, R. H.: *Muscle transplantation for paralysis of the radial nerve.* J. Bone Joint Surg., 28:440, 1946.

BARNES, R., BACSICH, P., WYBURN, G. M., and KERR, A. S.: *A study of the fate of nerve homografts in man.* Brit. J. Surg., 34, 34, 1946.

BAUER, K. H.: *Methods of repair of radial palsy.* Der Chirurg., 17:272, 1946.

BELL, J. L., MASON, M. L., NOCH, S. L., and STROMBERG, W. B.: *Injuries to flexor tendons of the hand in children.* J. Bone Joint Surg., 40A:1220, 1958.

BIESALSKI, K., and MAYER, L.: *Die physiologische Sehnenverpflanzung.* F. Springer, Berlin, 1916.

BILLINGTON, R. W.: *Tendon transplantation for musculospiral (radial) nerve injury.* J. Bone Joint Surg., 20:538, 1922.

BLUM, L.: *The use of myotomy in the repair of divided flexor tendons.* Ann. Surg., 116:461, 1942.

BÖHLER, J.: *Behandlung von Sehnenverletzungen.* Klin. Med. (Wien), 18:71, 1963.

BOYES, J. H.: *Flexor-tendon grafts in the fingers and thumb. An evaluation of end results.* J. Bone Joint Surg., 32A:489, 1950.
Why tendon repair? Editorial. J. Bone Joint Surg., 41A:577, 1959.

BOYES, J. H., WILSON, J. N., and SMITH, J. W.: *Flexor-tendon ruptures in the forearm and hand.* J. Bone Joint Surg., 42A:637, 1960.

915

THE EXTREMITIES

BRAND, P. W.: *Tendon grafting*. J. Bone Joint Surg., 40B:618, 1958 and 43B:444, 1961.
Paralytic claw hand. J. Bone Joint Surg., 40B:618, 1958.
Leprosy in Theory and Practice. John Wright and Sons, Bristol, 1959.

BROOKS, D. M.: *Inter-metacarpal bone graft for thenar paralysis*. J. Bone Joint Surg., 31B:511, 1949.

BRUNER, J. M.: *Tendon Transfer to restore abduction of the index finger using the extensor pollicis brevis*. Plast. Reconstr. Surg., 3:197, 1948.
Problems of postoperative position and motion in surgery of the hand. J. Bone Joint Surg., 35A:355, 1953.

BUCK-GRAMCKO, D.: *Probleme bei der Behandlung der Beugesehnenverletzungen der Hand*. Chir. Praxis, 11:577, 1967.

BUNNELL, S.: *An essential in reconstructive surgery, atraumatic technique*. Calif. State J. Med., 19:204, 1921.
Surgery of nerves of hand. Surg. Gynec. Obstet., 45:136, 1927.
Reconstructive surgery of hand. Surg. Gynec. Obstet., 39:259, 1924.
Surgery of Tendons. In LEWIS: *Practice of Surgery*. W. F. Prior Co., Inc., Hagerstown, 1927.
Opposition of thumb. J. Bone Joint Surg., 20:269, 1938.
Primary repair of severed tendons. Amer. J. Surg., 47:502, 1940.
Surgery of intrinsic muscles of hand other than those producing opposition of thumb. J. Bone Joint Surg., 24:1, 1942.
Surgery of the Hand. J. B. Lippincott, Philadelphia, 1944, and 3rd Ed., 1956.
Tendon transfers in the hand and forearm. Amer. Acad. Orthop. Surg. Instruct. Course Lectures, Vol. VI (1949).
Ischaemic contracture, local, in the hand. J. Bone Joint., Surg., 35A:88, 1953.

BUNNELL, S., HOWARD, L. D., and PRATT, D. R.: *Mallet finger. Classification and methods of treatment*. J. Surg., 93:573, 1957.

BÜRKLE DE LA CAMP: *Neuzeitliche Fragen der operativen Handchirurgie*. Archiv fur Klinische Chirurgie, 287:489, 1957.

BYRNE, J. J.: *The Hand: Its Anatomy and Diseases*. Blackwell Scientific Publications, Oxford, 1959.
The Hand: Its Anatomy and Diseases. Charles C Thomas, Springfield, 1959.

CALBERG, G., DELMOTTE, S., STEHMAN, M., and VAN GAVER, P.: *Rupture du tendon long extenseur du pouce apres fracture du poignet*. Acta orthop. beg., 27:493, 1961.

CAMPBELL, C. J., and KEOKARN, T.: *Total and subtotal arthrodesis of the wrist, inlay technique*. J. Bone Joint Surg., 46A:1520, 1964.

CARROLL, R. E., and BASSETT, C. A. L.: *Formation of tendon sheath by silicone rod implant*. Bull. Dow Corning Center Aid Med. Res., 6:5, No. 2, April 1964.

CARSTMA, N.: *The effect of cortisone on the formation of tendon adhesions and on tendon healing; an experimental investigation in the rabbit*. Acta Chir. Scand. Suppl., 182, 1953.

CASSCELLS, S. W., and STRANGE, T. B.: *Intramedullary wire fixation of mallet-finger*. J. Bone Joint Surg., 39A:521, 1957.

CASTRO-FARINAS, E., and RIVERA-LOPEZ, R.: *Arteriovenous fistulas of the hand. (Fistulas arteriovenosas de la mano)*. Angiologica, 12:200, 1960.

MUSCLES, TENDONS, NERVES, AND BLOOD VESSELS

CLARKSON, P., and PELLY, A.: *The General and Plastic Surgery of the Hand.* F. A. Davis, Phila., 1962.

COLEMAN, S. S., and ANSON, B. J.: *Arterial patterns in the hand based upon a study of 650 specimens.* Surg. Gynec. Obstet., 113:409, 1961.

COLVILLE, J., CALLISON, T. R., and WHITE, W. L.: *Role of paratenon in tendon blood supply.* Plast. Reconstr. Surg., 43:53, 1969.

COUCH, J. H.: *Surgery of the Hand.* Univ. of Toronto Press, 1939.

CURTIS, R.: *Congenital arteriovenous fistulae of the hand.* J. Bone Joint Surg., 35A:917, 1953.

CUTLER, C. W.: *The Hand, Its Disabilities and Diseases.* W. B. Saunders, Philadelphia, 1942.

DOLPHIN, J. A.: *Extensor tenotomy for chronic boutonnière deformity of the finger.* J. Bone Joint Surg., 47A: 161, 1965.

DUCHENNE, G. B. A. (1867): *Physiologie des Mouvements.* English edition translated by E. B. Kaplan, W. B. Saunders, Philadelphia, 1959.
Physiologie des mouvements démontrée a l'aide de l'expérimentation électrique et de l'observation clinique et applicable à l'étude des paralysies et des déformations. J. B. Baillière et Fils, Paris, 1867.

DUNCAN, J. McK.: *Trauma of the hand.* Brit. J. Surg., 35:397, 1948.

DUPARC, J.: *Plaies des Tendons, des Nerfs et des Vaisseaux de la Face Anterioure du Poignet.* Revue de Chirurgie Orthopedique, 46:215, 1960.

ENDER, J., KROTSCHECK, H., and SIMON-WEIDNER, R.: *Die Chirurgie der Handverletzungen.* Springer-Verlag Wien, 1956.

ENTIN, M. A.: *Repair of extensor mechanism of the hand.* Surg. Clin. N. Amer., 40:275, 1960.
Reconstruction of congenital abnormalities of the upper extremities. J. Bone Joint Surg., 41A:681, June 1959.

EYLER, D. L., and MARKEE, J. E.: *The anatomy and function of the intrinsic musculature of the fingers.* J. Bone Joint Surg., 36A:1, 1954.

FLATT, A. E.: *Care of Minor Hand Injuries.* C. V. Mosely, St. Louis, 1959.

FLYNN, J. E.: *Compound wounds of the hand.* Ann. Surg., 135:500, 1952.

FLYNN, J. E., WILSON, J. T., CHILD, C. G., and GRAHAM, J. H.: *Heterogenous and autogenous-tendon transplants.* J. Bone Joint Surgery, 42A:91, 1960.

FOERSTER, O.: *Handbruch der Neurologie.* J. Springer, Berlin, 1929, p. 2.
Value of orthopedic fixation operations in nerve disease; compensation for combined serratus-trapezius paralysis by fixation of scapula to ribs with silver wire; compensation for thenar paralysis by fixation of first metacarpal in flexed position by a bone implant between first and second metacarpals. Acta Chir. Scand., 67:351, 1930.

FOWLER, S. B.: *The management of tendon injuries.* Editorial. J. Bone Joint Surg., 41A:579, 1959.

FURLONG, R.: *Injuries of the Hand.* Little, Brown & Company, Boston, 1957.

THE EXTREMITIES

GAFFNEY, C. J., HERSHEY, F. B., and ALLEN, W. E., Jr.: *Arteriography of the upper extremity*. Surg. Gynec. Obstet., 106:63, 1958.

GAISFORD, J. C., HANNA, D. C., and RICHARDSON, G. S.: *Tendon grafting: A suggested technique*. Plast. Reconstr. Surg., 38:302, 1966.

GELDMACHER, J.: *Freie zweizeitige beugeschnentraus plantation handchirurgie*. 3:109, 1969.

GEORG, H.: *Indikation und Technik bei der Versorgung schwerer Hand- und Fingerverletzungen*. Archiv für Klinische Chirurgie, 287:508, 1957.

GILLIES, SIR. H.: *Autograft of amputated digit, a suggested operation*. Lancet, i, 1002, 1940.

GILLIES, SIR. H., and CUTHBERT, J. B.: *Operation for Pollicization of the Index Finger*. In Medical Annual, p. 262. John Wright & Sons Ltd., Bristol, 1943.

GLASSER, S. T.: *Principles of Peripheral Vascular Surgery*. F. A. Davis, Philadelphia, 1959.

GOLDNER, J. L., and IRWIN, C. E.: *An analysis of paralytic thumb deformities*. J. Bone Joint Surg., 32A:627, 1950.

GOLDNER, J. L., and CLIPPINGER, F. W.: *Excision of the greater multangular bone as an adjunct to mobilization of the thumb*. J. Bone Joint Surg., 41A:609, 1959.

GOLDNER, J. L., and CONRAD, R. W.: *Tendon grafting of the flexor profundus in the presence of a completely or partially intact flexor sublimus*. J. Bone Joint Surg., 51A:527, 1968.

GRAHAM, W. C.: *Flexor tendon grafts to the finger and thumb*. J. Bone Joint Surg., 29:553, 1947.

GRAHAM, W. C., BROWN, J. B., CANNON, B., RIORDAN, C. D.: *Transposition of fingers in severe injuries of the hand*. J. Bone Joint Surg., 29:998, 1947.

GRAHAM, W. C., and RIORDAN, D.: *Sublimis transplant to restore abduction of index finger*. Plast. Reconstr. Surg., 2:459, 1947.

GUNTER, G. S.: *Traumatic avulsion of the insertion of flexor digitorum profundus*. Aust. New Zeal. J. Surg., 30:1, 1960.

HANDFIELD-JONES, R. M.: *Surgery of the Hand*. Williams & Wilkins, Baltimore, 2nd Ed., 1946.

HARMER, T. W.: *Tendon suture*. Boston Med. Surg. J., 177:808, 1917.
Traumatic lesion of the nerves of the wrist and hand. Amer. J. Surg., 47:517, 1940.

HARRISON, S. H.: *Repair of digital flexor tendon injuries in the hand*. Brit. J. Plast. Surg., 14:211, 1961.
Primary flexor tendon grafts. Brit. J. Plast. Surg., 11:106, 1958.

HAUCK, G.: *Die Ruptur der Dorsalaponeurose am ersten Interphalangealgelenk, zugleich ein Beitrag zur Anatomie und Physiologie der Dorsal-aponeurose*. Arch. f. klin. Chir., 123:197, 1923.
Ueber die Ruptur der Extensor-pollicis-longus—Sehne nach typischem Radiusbruch und ihre operative Behandlung. Arch. f. klin. Chir., 124:81, 1923.

HENDERSON, E. D.: *Transfer of wrist extensors and brachioradialis to restore opposition of the thumb*. J. Bone Joint Surg., 44A:513, 1962.

918

MUSCLES, TENDONS, NERVES, AND BLOOD VESSELS

HERZOG, KARL HEINZ: *Sehnenkonservierung und -Transplantation (Preservation and Transplantation of Tendon)*. 1965 Jena: Gustav Fischer Verlag.

HIGHET, W. B.: *Procaine nerve block in the investigation of peripheral nerve injuries.* J. Neurol. Psychiat., 5:101, 1942.

HILLER, A.: *Ueber den schnellenden Finger.* Ztschr. f. orthop. Chir., 20:48, 1908.

HOHMANN, G.: *Hand und Arm.* Y. F. Bergmann, München, 1949.

HORTON, B. T.: *Some medical aspects of congenital arteriovenous fistula: Report of thirty-eight cases.* Proc. Staff Meet., Mayo Clin., 9:460, 1934.

HUGHES, N. C., and MOORE, F. T.: *A preliminary report on the use of a local flap and peg bone graft for lengthening a short thumb.* Brit. J. Plast. Surg., 3:34, 1951.

HUNTER, J.: *Artificial tendons, early development and application.* Amer. J. Surg., 109:325, 1965.

ISELIN, M.: *Chirurgie de la main.* Masson, Paris, 1933; 2nd Ed. 1955.
Atlas de Technique Operatoire. Chirurgie de la Main. Publisher Editions Medicales, Flammarion, Paris, 1958.
Gegenwärtiger Stand des Behandlungs-problems der verletzten Beugesehnen. Arch. f. klin. Chir., 287:533, 1957.

ISELIN, M., and ISELIN, F.: *Traite de Chirurgie de la Main.* Editions Medicales, Flammarion, Paris, 1967.

JACOBS, B., THOMPSON, T. C.: *Opposition of the thumb and its restoration.* J. Bone Joint Surg., 42A:1015, 1960.

JAFFE, S., WECKESSER, E.: *Profundus tendon grafting with the sublimis intact.* J. Bone Joint Surg., 49A:1298, 1967.

JENNINGS, E. R., ET AL.: *A new technique in primary tendon repair.* Surg. Gynec. Obstet., 95:597, 1952.

JONES, F. W.: *Principles of Anatomy as Seen in the Hand.* The Blakiston Co., Philadelphia, 1920.

JONES, R.: *Notes on Military Orthopaedics.* Cassel & Co., London, 1917.

KANAVEL, A. B.: *Infections of the Hand.* Lea & Febiger, Philadelphia, 1939.

KAPLAN, E. B.: *Anatomy of the Hand.* J. B. Lippincott, Philadelphia, 1953.
Functional and Surgical Anatomy of the Hand, 2nd ed. J. B. Lippincott, Philadelphia, 1965.

KIRKLIN, J. W., and THOMAS, C. G., JR.: *Opponens transplant: An analysis of the methods employed and results obtained in 75 cases.* Surg. Gynec. Obstet., 86:213, 1948.

KELLY, A. P.: *Primary tendon repairs. A study of 789 consecutive tendon severances.* J. Bone Joint Surg., 41A:581, 1959.

KOCH, S. L.: *Injuries of the parieties and extremities.* Surg. Gynec. Obstet., 76:1, 189, 1943.
Complicated contractures of the hand. Their treatment by freeing fibrosed tendons and replacing destroyed tendons by grafts. Ann. Surg., 98:546, 1933.
Division of the flexor tendons within the digital sheath. Surg. Gynec. Obstet., 78:9, 1944.

919

THE EXTREMITIES

Four splints of value in the treatment of disabilities of the hand. Surg. Gynec. Obstet., 48:416, 1929.
Injuries of the hand. Northwest. Univ. Bull., Med. School, Chicago, 19:265, 1945.

KOCH, S. L., and MASON, M. L.: *Division of the nerves and tendons of the hand.* Surg. Gynec. 56:1, 1933.
Purposeful splinting following injuries of the hand. Surg. Gynec. Obstet., 68:1, 1939.

KRÖMER, K.: *Die Verletzte Hand.* W. Maudrich, Wien, 1945.

LAMPE, E. W.: *Surgical anatomy of the hand.* Ciba Clin. Symp., Vol. 3:8, Dec. 1951.

LANDSMEER, J. M. F.: *Anatomical and functional investigation on the articulation of the human fingers.* Acta Anat. Suppl. 24, 1955.
The anatomy of the dorsal aponeurosis of the human finger and its functional significance. Anat. Rec., 104:41-44, 1967.

LEWIS, D.: *Peripheral nerves.* In LEWIS: *Practice of Surgery.* W. F. Prior Co., Hagerstown, 1943, Vol. 3, Chap. 6.

LEXER, E.: *Die gesamte Wiederherstellungs-chirurgie.* J. A. Barth, Leipzig, 1930.
Die Verwertung der freien Schnentransplantation. Arch. f. klin. Chir., 98:818-852, 1912.

LINDSAY, W., and McDOUGALL, E. P.: *Direct digital flexor tendon repair.* Plast. Reconstr. Surg., 26:613, 1960.
Digital flexor tendons: An experimental study. Part III. The fate of autogenous digital flexor tendon grafts. Brit. J. Plastic Surg., 13:293, 1961.

LINDSAY, W., and THOMSON, H. G.: *Digital flexor tendons: An experimental study.* Brit. J. Plast. Surg., 12:289, 1960.

LINDSAY, W. K., and BIRCH, J. R.: *The fibroblast in flexor tendon healing.* Plast. Reconstr. Surg., 34:223, 1964.

LITTLER, J. W.: *Free tendon grafts in secondary flexor tendon repair.* Amer. J. Surg., 74:315, 1947.
Tendon transfers and arthrodeses in combined median and ulnar nerve paralysis. J. Bone Joint Surg., 31A:225, 1949.

LITTLER, J. W., and COOLEY, S. G. E.: *Opposition of the thumb and its restoration by abductor digiti quinti transfer.* J. Bone Joint Surg., 45:1389, 1963.
Congenital dysplasia of the thumb: Reconstruction using the index finger. Paper presented at the nineteenth annual meeting, Amer. Soc. Surg. of Hand, Jan. 17th, 1964, Chicago, Ill.
The finger extensor mechanism. Surg. Clin. N. Amer., 47:415, 1967.

MASON, M. L.: *Primary and secondary tendon suture.* Surg. Gynec. Obstet., 70:393, 1940.
Rupture of tendons of the hand. Surg. Gynec. Obstet., 50:611, 1930.
The treatment of open wounds of the hand. Surg. Clin. N. Amer., Feb. 1948, page 4.
Fifty years' progress in surgery of the hand. Surg. Gynec. Obstet., 101:541, 1955.
Primary tendon repair. Editorial. J. Bone Joint Surg., 41A:575, 1959.

MASON, M. L., and ALLEN, H. S.: *Rate of healing of tendons. Experimental study of tensile strength.* Ann. Surg., 113:424, 1941.

MASON, M. L., and SHEARON, C. G.: *The process of tendon repair. An experimental study of tendon suture and tendon graft.* Arch. Surg., 25:615-692, 1932.

MUSCLES, TENDONS, NERVES, AND BLOOD VESSELS

MASON BROWN, J. J.: *War injuries of the peripheral arteries.* Brit. J. Surg., 36:354, 1949.

MATEV, I.: *Transposition of the lateral slips of the aponeurosis in treatment of long-standing "boutonniere deformity" of the fingers.* Brit. J. Plast. Surg., 17:281, 1964.

MAY, H.: *Tendon transplantation in the hand.* Surg. Gynec. Obstet., 83:631, 1946. *Reparative surgery of severed tendons and nerves of the hand.* Surg. Clin. N. Amer. Dec. 1947, page 1474. *Chirurgie der Offenen Sehnen-und Nervendurchtrennungen der Hand, Einschliesslich Anwendung der Freien Sehnentransplantation.* Langenbeck's Arch. u. Dtsch. Z. Chir., Bd. 277, S. 599-610 (1954). *Freie Sehnenverpflanzung bei Verletzung der Fingersehenen.* Langenbeck's Archiv und Deutche Zeitschrift für Chirurgie, 279, April 1954.

MAYER, L.: *The physiological method of tendon transplantation,* Surg. Gynec. Obstet., 22:182, 298, 472, 1916. *Physiological method of tendon transplantation.* Surg. Gynec. Obstet., 33:528, 1921. *Repair of severed tendons.* Amer. J. Surg., 42:714, 1938. *Surgery of Tendons.* In LEWIS: *Practice of Surgery.* W. F. Prior Co., Hagerstown, 1943, Vol. 3, Chap. 5.

MAYER, L., and RANSOHOFF, N.: *Reconstruction of digital tendon sheath; contribution to physiological method of repair of damaged finger tendons.* J. Bone Joint Surg., 18: 607, 1936.

McCORMACK, R. M., DEMUTH, R. J., and KINDLING, P. H.: *Flexor-tendon grafts in the less-than-optimum situation.* J. Bone Joint Surg., 44A:1360, 1962.

McMURRAY, T. P.: *Transplantation in gunshot injuries of nerves.* J. Orthop. Surg., 1919.

MILLESI, H.: *Zur Technik der freien Sehnentransplantation.* Langenbeck's Arch. klin. Chir., 309:40, 1965.

MITTELMEIER, H.: *Experimentelle Untersuchungen zur Pathologie und Verhütungen posttraumatischer Sehnenverwachsungen. Heft 73 der Hefte zur Unfallheilkunde.* Springer-Verlag, Berlin-Göttingen-Heidelberg, 1963.

MOBERG, E.: *Aspects of sensation in reconstructive surgery of the upper extremity.* J. Bone Joint Surg., 46A:817, 1964. *Transfer of sensation.* J. Bone Joint Surg., 37A:305, 1955.

MOBERG, E., and RATHKE, F. W.: *Dringliche Handchirurgie.* G. Thieme, Stuttgart, 1964.

MOREL-FATIO, D.: *Acute injuries of the tendons of the hand.* Rev. Chir. Orthop., Paris, 46:179, 1960.

NICHOLS, H. M.: *A discussion of tendon repair.* Ann. Surg., 129:223, 1949. *Repair of extensor-tendon insertions in the finger.* J. Bone Joint Surg., 33A:836, 1951. Manual of Hand Injuries. Year Book Publishers, Inc., Chicago, 1955.

NIGST, H.: *Ergebnisse der Sehnenplastiken an der Hand.* Langenbeck's Arch. klin. Chir., 299:122-125, 1961.

NUSSBAUM, J. W. (Quoted by FOERSTER): *Handbuch der Neurologie.* 1929, p. 1631.

THE EXTREMITIES

PEACOCK, E. E., JR.: *A study of the circulation in normal tendons and healing grafts.* Ann. Surg., 149:415, 1959.
Fundamental aspects of wound healing relating to the restoration of gliding function after tendon repair. Surg. Gynec. Obstet., 119:241, 1964.

PEACOCK, E. E., and HARTRAMPF, C. R.: *The repair of flexor tendons in the Hand.* Int. Abstr. Surg., 113:411, 1961.

PEACOCK, E. E., MADDEN, J. W.: *Human composite flexor allografts.* Amer. Surg., 166:624, 1967.

PERTHES, G.: *Ueber Sehnenoperationen bei irreperabler Radialislähmung, nebst Studien über die Sehnenverpflanzung und Tenodese im allgemeinen.* Bruns' Beitr. z. klin. Chir., 113:289-368, 1918.
Die funktionellen Ergebnisse der Sehnenoperation bei irreperapler (sic) Radialislähmung. Klin. Wchnschr., 1:127-129, 1922.

PHALEN, G. S., and MILLER, R. C.: *The transfer of wrist extensor muscles to restore or reinforce flexion power of the fingers and opposition of the thumb.* J. Bone Joint Surg., 29:993, 1947.

PIEPER, W.: *Neuere Operationstechniken in der Beugesehnenchirurgie. Chirurgia plastica et reconstructiva, 6.* Springer-Verlag, Berlin-Heidelberg-New York, 1969.

POSCH, J. L., WALKER, P. J., and MILLER, H.: *Treatment of ruptured tendons of the hand and wrist.* Amer. J. Surg., 91:669, 1956.

POSCH, J. L.: *Primary tenorrhaphies and tendon grafting procedures in hand injuries.* Arch. Surg., 73:609, 1956.

POTENZA, A. D.: *Tendon healing within the flexor digital sheath in the dog.* J. Bone Joint Surg., 44A:49, 1962.

PRATT, D. R.: *Internal splint for closed and open treatment of injuries of the extensor tendon at the distal joint of the finger.* J. Bone Joint Surg., 34A:785, 1952.

PULVERTAFT, R. G.: *Tendon grafts for flexor tendon injuries in the fingers and thumb.* J. Bone Joint Surg., 38B:175, 1956.
The treatment of profundus division by free tendon graft. J. Bone Joint Surg., 42A:1363, 1960.
Reparative surgery of flexor tendon injuries in the hand. J. Bone Joint Surg., 36B:689, 1954.
Tendon grafts for flexor tendon injuries in fingers and thumb. J. Bone Joint Surg., 38B:175, 1956.

RANK, B. K., WAKEFIELD, A. R., and HUESTON, J. T.: *Surgery of Repair as Applied to Hand Injuries,* 3rd ed. Williams & Wilkins, Baltimore, 1968.

RECHT, P.: *Frische Nervenverletzungen an der Hand (Mit 5 Textabbildungen).* Arch. f. klin. Chir., 287:538, 1957.

REID, M. R.: *Abnormal arteriovenous communications, acquired and congenital.* Arch. Surg., 10:997, 1925; and 11:25 and 237, 1925.

REINHARDT, F. E.: *Ueber den Ansatz der Musculi Lumbricales an der Hand des Menschen.* Anat. Anz. 20:129, 1901.

RIORDAN, D.: *Tendon transplantation in median nerve and ulnar nerve paralysis.* J. Bone Joint Surg., 35A:312, 1953.

ROBINSON, R. F., and KAYFETZ, D. O.: *Arthrodesis of the wrist.* J. Bone Joint Surg., 34A:64, 1952.

ROGINS, R. H. C.: *Injuries and Infections of the Hand.* Williams & Wilkins, Baltimore, 1961.

ROWNTREE, T.: *Anomalous innervation of the muscles of the hand.* J. Bone Joint Surg., 31B:505, 1949.

ROYLE, N. D.: *An operation for paralysis of the intrinsic muscles of the thumb.* JAMA, 111:612, 1938.

SAIKKU, L. A.: *Tendon transplantation for radial paralysis; factors influencing results.* Acta Chir. Scand. Suppl. 132, Vol. 96, 1947.

SCHARIZER, E.: *Erfahrungen und Engebnisse nach 367 Beugeschnenoperationen.* Handchirurgie, 2:92, 1969.

SCHINK, W.: *Die Wiederherstellungschirurgie verletzter Hände.* Chirurg., 36:211, 1965.
Die Behandlung frischer Sehnenverletzungen. Zbl. Chir., 93:62, 1968.

SCUDERI, C.: *Tendon transplants for irreparable radial nerve paralysis.* Surg. Gynec. Obstet., 88:643, 1949.

SEDDON, H. J.: *Nerve grafting.* J. Bone Joint Surg., 45B:447, 1963.

SEEGER, S. J.: *Congenital arteriovenous anastomoses.* Surgery, 3:264, 1938.

SEIFFERT, K. E.: *Biologische Grundlagen der Homologen Transplantation Konservierter Bindegewebe. Hefte zur Unfallheilkunde. Beihefte zur Monatsschrift fur Unfallheilkunde Versicherungs, Versorgungsund Verkehrsmedizin.* Heft 93. Springer-Verlag/Berlin Heidelberg, New York, 1967.

SHAFFER, J. M., and CLEVELAND, F.: *Delayed suture of sensory nerves of the hand.* Ann. Surg., 131:556, 1950.

SILER, V. E.: *Primary tenorrhaphy of the flexor tendons in the hand.* J. Bone Joint Surg., 32A:218, 1950.

SKOOG, T., PERSSON, B.: *An experimental study of the early healing of tendons.* Plast. Reconstr. Surg., 13:384, 1959.

SMITH, J.: *The blood supply of tendons with injury and repair.* J. Bone Joint Surg., 47A:631, 1965.

SMITH, F. M.: *Late rupture of the extensor pollicis longus following Colles's fracture.* J. Bone Joint Surg., 28:49, 1946.

SOUQUET, R., and CHANCHOLLE, A. R.: *Plaies de la Main.* G. Dein et Cie., Paris, 1959. (Brit. J. Surg., July 1959).

STACK, H. G.: *Muscle function in the fingers.* J. Bone Joint Surg., 44B:899, 1962.

STARK, H. H., BOYES, J. H., and WILSON, J. N.: *Mallet finger.* J. Bone Joint Surg., 44A:1061, 1962.

STEINDLER, A.: *Reconstructive Surgery of the Upper Extremity.* D. Appleton & Co., New York, 1923.
Orthopedic Operations. Charles C Thomas, Springfield, 1943.
The Traumatic Deformities and Disabilities of the Upper Extremity. Charles C Thomas, Springfield, 1946.

THE EXTREMITIES

STILES, H. T., FORRESTER-BROWN, M. F.: *Treatment of Injuries of the Peripheral Spinal Nerves.* H. Frowde, London, 1922.

STRANGE, F. G. St. C.: *An operation for nerve pedicle grafting.* Brit. J. Surg., 34:423, 1947.

STROMBERG, W. B., McFARLANE, R. M., BELL, J. L., KOCH, S. L., and MASON, M. L.: *Injury of the median and ulnar nerve.* J. Bone Joint Surg., 43A:717, 1961.

STRUPPLER, V., and WITT, N.: *Erster Teil. Verletzungen und Widerherstellung der Oberen Extremitaten Einschliesslich der Hand. Neue Deutsche Chirurgie, Band 68.* Ferdinand Enke, Verlag, Stuttgart, 1961.

THATCHER, H. V.: *Use of stainless steel rods to canalize flexor tendon sheaths.* Southern. Med. J., 32:13, 1939.

THOMPSON, C. F.: *Fusion of metacarpals of thumb and index finger to maintain functional position of the thumb.* J. Bone Joint Surg., 24:907, 1942.

TUBIANA, R.: *Flexor tendon grafts of the fingers and thumb.* Rev. Chir. Orthop., Paris, 46:191, 1960.
Incisions and technics in tendon grafting. Amer. J. Surg., 109:339, 1965.
Greffes des Tendons Flechisseurs des Doigts et du Pouce. Technique et Resultats. Rev. Chir. Orthop., 46:191, 1960.
Anatomic and physiologic basis for the surgical treatment of paralyses of the hand. J. Bone Joint Surg., 51A:643, 1968.

VERDAN, C. E.: *Primary repair of flexor tendons.* J. Bone Joint Surg., 42A:647, 1960.
Chirurgie Reparatrice et Fonctionnelle des Tendons de la Main. Scientifique Francaise, 1952.

VERSACI, A. D.: *Tendon transfers in ulnar nerve injuries.* Plast. Reconstr. Surg., 26:500, 1960.

WAKEFIELD, A.: *The management of flexor tendon injuries.* Surg. Clin. N. Amer., 40:267, 1960.

WATSON, A. B.: *Some remarks on the repair of flexor tendons in the hand with particular reference to the technique of free grafting.* Brit. J. Surg., 43:35, 1955-56.

WHITE, W. L.: *Restoration of function of tendon transfers.* Surg. Clin. N. Amer., 40:427, 1960.
The unique, accessible and useful plantaris tendon. Plast. Reconstr. Surg., 25:133, 1960.

WILLIAMS, S. B.: *New dynamic concepts in the grafting of flexor tendons.* Plast. Reconstr. Surg., 36:377, 1965.

WINSTEN, J.: *Island flap to restore sterognosis in hand injuries.* New Eng. Med. J., 268:124, 1963.

WITT, A. N.: *Die Wiederherstellungsoperationen bei irreparablen Nervenlähmungen der oberen Extremität.* Arch. f. klin. Chir., 301:962, 1962.
Berlin: Funktionsverbessernde Eingriffe an den Fingergelenken (Mit 6 Textabbildungen), Arch. f. Klin. Chir., 287:541, 1957.

MUSCLES, TENDONS, NERVES, AND BLOOD VESSELS

YOUNG, H. H., and LOWE, G. H., Jr.: *Tendon transfer operation for irreparable paralysis of the radial nerve; long term follow-up of patients.* Surg. Gynec. Obstet., 84:1100, 1948.

ZACHARY, R. B.: *Tendon transplantation for radial paralysis.* Brit. J. Surg., 33:358, 1946.

ZRUBECKY, G.: *Derzeitige Grenzen bei der Planmassigen Versorgung Schwerer Handverletzungen.* Journal Hefte Zur Unfallheilkunde, Vol. 83, 1965.
Ergebnisse von 82 plastischen Beugesehnenoperationen nach einer Durchtrennung im Niemandsland. Arch. orthop. Unfallchir., 53:93, 1961.
Probleme bei der Wiederherstellung durchtrennter Beugesehnen im Niemandsland der Finger. Jahrbuch Wiederherstellungschirurgie und Traumatologie, Band 9. S. Karger, Basel-New York, 1967.

THE BONES
AND
ARTICULATIONS

30

THE BONES

DEFECTS (TRAUMATIC)

CONCERNING the traumatic defects amenable to treatment, there are non-union of the os naviculare (scaphoid bone) and nonunion of the meta-carpal bones and phalanges. (For replacement of an entire metacarpal bone or phalanx, see p. 934. For congenital defects, see p. 979.)

NONUNION OF OS NAVICULARE

A fairly large percentage of fractures of the carpal scaphoid bone result in nonunion. The cause is mainly an anatomical one. In fractures of other bones—with few exceptions—the periosteum plays an important role in the formation of callus. Most of the surface of the scaphoid, how-ever, consists of articular cartilage, leaving little room for active osteo-genetic periosteum. Hence, its viability and regenerative power depend entirely upon its intramedullary circulation. From clinical and experi-mental experiences (Watson-Jones, Obletz, and Halbstein), it is known that in about one third of the cases most of these vessels enter the bone on the distal (lateral) aspect of the bone and in the constricted mid-portion, leaving the proximal (median) half supplied by the branches of the main vessels so that this part is rather poorly vascularized (Speed)

927

(see also Bibliography under May). If, in such a case, a fracture occurs within the proximal half of the scaphoid or through the waist of the bone where the center vessels enter, rupturing their trunks, the proximal half of the scaphoid is cut off from its circulation and dies (Fig. 374). In this respect, it resembles the central fragment of the neck of the femur in a true intracapsular fracture (Fig. 374). The only way in which the necrotic fragment can become regenerated is by ingrowth of vessels and osteoblasts from the live part. To assure this, absolute prolonged immobilization must be carried out until the x-ray picture reveals complete regeneration. If nonunion should develop and the median fragment remains necrotic, excision of the fragment may be considered. (Waugh and Reuling have suggested the entire replacement of the os naviculare by a vitallium replica.) If, however, the x-ray picture reveals nonunion and both fragments are alive (after a fracture through line *a*, for example), a

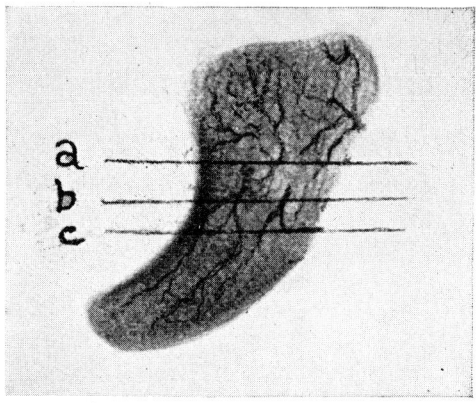

Fig. 374. Right carpal scaphoid bone. Representation of its vessels (compare with Fig. 29) and relation between fracture lines and these vessels (Böhler and Schneck). In fracture through *a*, both fragments remain alive; fracture through *b* and *c* will cause necrosis of median (proximal) fragment.

bone-pegging operation has a good chance of uniting the fragments. The author has preferred an autogenous tibial bone peg as a graft (Case 159, p. 1207). Nyga and Bougert use homogenous bone pegs which, because of their slow regeneration, provide a long stabilization for the fragments. Barnard and Stubbins point out that the removal of the radial styloid process does not interfere with a normally functioning wrist joint, and its removal simplifies the surgical approach; the removed bone can be used as a graft. A recent presentation by Stubbins of a long-term follow-up examination of his patients, all successfully healed after this technique, is impressive. Mazet and Hohl prefer styloidectomy combined with a bone graft of the Murray type.

Technique (Case 159, p. 1207)

After the application of a pneumatic tourniquet (see p. 849), a curved incision is made on the radial surface of the wrist joint, extending about 3.2 cm. (1¼ inches) upward and downward from the radial styloid. The incision is curved toward the volar surface of the wrist, and the convexity should reach the tendon of the musculus abductor pollicis longus. The superficial radial nerve should be exposed and then retracted ulnarward. The deep fascia and the dorsal carpal ligament are divided longitudinally, exposing the extensor pollicis brevis and abductor pollicis longus tendons. These tendons are retracted toward the volar side, together with the radial artery, while the tendon of the musculus extensor pollicis longus is retracted ulnad (see Figs. 351, 352). The periosteum over the styloid process is then incised in the long axis, together with the capsule of the wrist joint, which at this point is largely the radial collateral ligament. The process is then freed subperiosteally of all soft tissue and removed with an oblique osteotome. The starting point should be 1.5 cm. (⅝ inch) up the radial shaft in order to obtain a sufficiently large fragment to be re-shaped. Upon removal of the process, the navicular bone will be found to lie directly in the wound; in most instances, the fracture will be visible. The tuberosity of the navicular can then be exposed easily with avoidance of its dorsal arterial supply. After the most prominent areas of the tuberosity have been cleared, a small nick is made in the bone with rongeurs, in order to provide for countersinking of the graft and prevention of bone proliferation, which might interfere with abduction of the wrist. With a small drill (⁵⁄₁₆ inch), a hole is drilled beginning at the neck of the tuberosity, through the proximal fragments, across the fracture line, and into the distal fragment, care being taken not to perforate the semilunar facet of the scaphoid. A picture by portable x-ray equipment is taken to evaluate the position of the drill. If the position is correct, a bone peg is shaped from the removed styloid process or the subcutaneous border of ulna or tibia. It is then driven into the drill canal. Again, an x-ray picture of the scaphoid should be taken to evaluate the position of the graft. If the graft is found in correct position, bridging both fragments, only then should the projection of the graft be cut at the entrance of the drill canal. If this had been done before the x-ray examination, one would have been deprived of the possibility of removing the graft to correct its position if such were warranted. The radial collateral ligament is sutured over the raw surface of the radius and the wound closed in layers.

After-Treatment

The hand is supported in a circular plaster cast in cock-up position, with the thumb in abduction, for eight weeks. After removal of the cast, an x-ray picture is taken for evidence of union of the fragments. If it is satisfactory, physical therapy is instituted. Should union be delayed, immobilization of the wrist for another four weeks is advisable.

NONUNION OF METACARPAL BONES AND PHALANGES

Nonunion of these bones may cause pain and dysfunction, particularly if the fragments are displaced. Bridging the defect with a bone graft offers a good chance for establishing bony union (Murray).

Technique

Nonunion of Metacarpal Near Head of Bone: The bone is exposed from a dorsal incision. The extensor tendons are mobilized and retracted. The distal head fragment is usually displaced toward the palm; it is mobilized and, after removal of all scar tissue between the fragments, the latter are brought into alignment. A thin cortical bone graft is removed from the subcutaneous border of ulna or tibia, and driven into the proximal fragment. A hole is now drilled into the distal fragment and the latter fitted over the distal part of the bone peg.

If the fragments cannot be separated and retracted sufficiently to fit the distal fragment over the bone peg, the author recommends the following procedure: The bone graft (peg) is fitted first into the distal (head) fragment. A graft bed is prepared in the proximal fragment by removing the dorsal part of the cortex until the medullary cavity is exposed. The proximal portion of the bone graft is laid upon the proximal fragment and held in place with two thin wires slung around the bone.

Nonunion of Shaft of Metacarpal Bone (after Armstrong): From a dorsal incision, the extensor tendons are retracted and the affected metacarpal bone exposed by a longitudinal incision through its periosteum. The bone ends are exposed subperiosteally and cleared of fibrous tissue, and the fracture is reduced. With a double saw, adjusted so that the outer surface of the blades are 0.5 cm. ($\frac{3}{16}$ inch) apart, a graft bed about 3.8 cm. ($1\frac{1}{2}$ inches) long is cut on the dorsal aspect of the bone. A cortical graft is removed from the tibia with a double saw, adjusted so that the inner surfaces of the blades are just over 0.5 cm. ($\frac{3}{16}$ inch) apart.

930

This graft is inserted into the graft bed, and should fit very closely. It is driven in with a punch until its cortical surface is flush with the cortex of the host bone. If the graft fits closely, no other fixation is necessary. Otherwise, Kirschner wires are drilled through the affected and neighboring metacarpal bones (see the following discussion).

Defects of Shaft of Metacarpal Bones (after Littler): In any of these cases, the overlying skin may be cicatricial, and may need replacement. If later tendon work is planned, it will be necessary for the skin to be replaced by a well-padded abdominal flap (compare with Case 162, p. 1211). The metacarpal defect is exposed from a longitudinal incision. All fibrous tissue between the fragments must be removed radically. In most cases, the proximal fragment must be sacrificed as far as the base, where it is resected with an osteotome with an angle of approximately 30 degrees. With traction on the finger, the defect between the metacarpal fragments is measured and a graft, measuring at least 1.3 cm. (½ inch) longer than the estimated defect, is taken from the upper end of the tibia. A dowel is fastened at one end of the graft and, with a circular saw, the other end is cut obliquely at an angle of 30 degrees. The dowel end of the graft is inserted into the medullary end of the cavity at the distal fragment; at the proximal end, the graft is pressed into the metacarpal or carpal recess. Compression of the graft between the two fragments is sufficient to hold it in place at the base. Should additional fixation be required, it can be obtained by the use of Kirschner wires drilled either longitudinally from the carpal bones into the graft or transversely to transfix the graft between two normal metacarpal bones (Cases 160, 162, pp. 1208, 1211). The wounds are then carefully sutured.

Defects of Several Metacarpal Bones (after Bruner): If the shafts of several metacarpal bones are missing, a full-thickness iliac bone graft (see p. 938) in interposed en bloc and held transfixed with Kirschner wires. A tendon defect, which may exist simultaneously, should be bridged later, after the bone graft has healed.

Nonunion of Phalanges: The bone is exposed from a lateral incision and the bone graft inserted in a manner similar to that described for nonunion of the metacarpal bone near the head of the bone.

After-Treatment

A plaster cast is applied in the position of function. About twelve days later, the cast is changed, sutures are removed, and a new cast applied immobilizing the wrist and the proximal phalanx of the grafted metacarpal. This cast remains for about two months.

THE EXTREMITIES

DEFORMITIES (TRAUMATIC)

Traumatic deformities of the metacarpal bones or the phalanges are the result of malunion after fractures. Such a deformity rarely causes dysfunction of a degree such as to handicap the patient. Open reduction, after osteotomy of the bone, however, is indicated in some cases. Internal fixation by bone grafting (see Nonunion of Metacarpal Bones, p. 930) or wiring may be necessary, in addition to external immobilization. A good method of fixation is by drilling Kirschner wires through the affected and neighboring metacarpal bones (Snedecor) (compare with Cases 160, 162, pp. 1208, 1211). (For congenital deformities, see p. 979.)

THE ARTICULATIONS

ARTHRODESIS

Arthrodesis of the digital joints is a helpful procedure for stabilization of the joints in certain irreparable nerve lesions or contractures, and for correction of position in joints fused in malposition, rarely for relief of arthritic lesions. The joints to be arthrodesed are the metacarpophalangeal joints; less often is there an indication for fusing the interphalangeal joints.

Technique (See Fig. 370)

Metacarpophalangeal Joint: From a U-shaped skin incision with the pedicle distally and a dorsal tendon-splitting incision, the joint capsule is incised longitudinally. The articular surfaces are demoved with a gauged chisel. With a V-shaped chisel, a groove is carved on the dorsal surfaces of the bones for reception of the bone onlay graft. The latter is removed from the lateral surface of the ulna of the same arm or from the anterior edge of the tibia. The joint is flexed in the position of function, i.e., semiflexion in the metacarpophalangeal joints of the second to fifth fingers, while the metacarpophalangeal joint of the thumb is flexed so that the tip of the thumb and the other fingers can be apposed. A short Kirschner wire is drilled through the bones across the joint surfaces well anterior to the graft bed. The bone graft is now placed into the previously prepared graft bed. The capsule is closed over the graft, and this is followed by suture of the split extensor tendon and the skin. A dorsal molded plaster-cast splint is applied from the forearm to the arthrodesed finger, with the wrist in cocked-up position.

932

THE BONES AND ARTICULATIONS

Interphalangeal Joint: The interphalangeal joints are exposed from a distally curved incision. The joint surfaces are removed with a burr so that the bone surfaces will fit together in the position of function. Two Kirschner wires are drilled across the joint surfaces and buried subcutaneously. Splinting with an aluminum splint is necessary for about two weeks. (Compare with Case 148, p. 1194.)

After-Treatment

The cast is temporarily removed on the tenth day for removal of the sutures. It is then reapplied for at least eight weeks, until there is roentgenological and clinical evidence of sufficient fusion.

ARTHROPLASTY

Arthroplasty of an ankylosed finger joint is rarely performed because the operation is not often successful: ankylosis is apt to recur, since the tendons, owing to long inactivity, have contracted and instability is difficult to control. In some selected cases, however, the operation may be warranted. It is indicated only for the metacarpophalangeal joint, except for that of the thumb. The surrounding skin must be in good condition, and the muscles and tendons must be functioning well.

Technique (Campbell)

The ankylosed joint is exposed through a 5-cm. (2-inch) longitudinal incision on the dorsal surface of the joint. The extensor tendon is either held laterally or split longitudinally and retracted. The joint region is exposed. The ankylosis of the joint is broken up with a small-gauge chisel and the ends of the bone remodeled, the head of the proximal part being smoothed to present a rounded convex surface which conforms to a concavity created in the articular surface of the base of the distal part. A thin strip of fascia lata of appropriate size is removed from the thigh, folded over the proximal head, and held by a purse-string suture. The remaining portion of fascia is reflected over the distal joint surface and stitched in place to form a double lining of the articular surfaces. The wound is closed in layers.

After-Treatment

The finger is placed in semiflexion on a dorsal molded plaster-cast splint. After three weeks, the splint is removed and active exercises are instituted, followed by passive exercises one week later.

933

THE EXTREMITIES

TRANSPLANTATION OF JOINTS

Transplantation of autogenous whole joints is still in the experimental stage (Entin, Alger and Baird, Erdelyi) although some success has been achieved by Erdelyi on reconstructing ankylosed finger joints by means of transplantation of joints from the foot. Homogenous whole-joint transplantation is doomed to eventual failure as demonstrated by Lexer. Much more successful are the vitallium prostheses which were ingeniously devised by Adrian Flatt for replacement of joints in the rheumatoid arthritis. Transplantation of half joints, however, consisting of the joint surface and the adjacent bone, leads to total regeneration of the graft (May) (p. 787), hence is feasible and practical. It is indicated for replacement of metacarpal bones after removal of the same in badly comminuted fractures or for benign tumors (enchondroma), low-grade malignant tumors, or those malignant tumors which are still confined to the bone itself. Replacement is indicated in order to preserve the finger and its motility.

In traumatic cases, preliminary operations may be necessary: Any missing skin must be replaced with a well-padded flap prior to the transplantation; all destroyed tissue—this includes bone also—and all scar tissue must be removed. The missing metacarpal cannot be replaced during the flap transfer. This, however, would inevitably cause the digital phalanges to retract into the defect. To prevent this, the first phalanx must be suspended temporarily with the aid of a Kirschner wire drilled horizontally through the neighboring phalanges, the wire coming to lie just beneath the digital webs. At the entrance the wire is cut, and the small entrance incision is closed (see Case 162, p. 1211). After all wounds have healed, the metacarpal defect is replaced with a metatarsal graft. Graham and Riordan use the fourth and fifth metatarsals as a graft, since they are functionally less important than the others; they prefer the fifth because it has caused less impairment to the foot than removal of any other one. The author agrees with this from his own experience.

Technique (Case 162, p. 1211)

From a dorsal longitudinal or other suitable incision, the bone is exposed by holding the extensor tendon laterally. The diseased or damaged metacarpal should be removed, leaving the base and as much of the shaft as possible. The entire joint capsule should be removed. The shaft of the metacarpal is cut in such a manner that a close approximation with the transplanted metatarsal will be possible. The metatarsal bone, preferably the fifth, is removed with a Gigli saw. Care should be taken that the periosteum remains intact. The bone graft is then inserted into the defect and held in place with a Kirschner wire, which is drilled from the proximal

934

portion of the metacarpal bone through the center of the transplanted metatarsal. Another Kirschner wire is then inserted through the proximal heads of the neighboring metacarpals and the head of the transplanted metatarsal. Graham and Riordan advise fixing the extensor tendon to the proximal end of the proximal phalanx to prevent anterior subluxation of the phalanx. The exposed bone surface should be covered with fat tissue or soft tissue to prevent adhesions of the extensor tendons (see Case 160, p. 1208, in which part of the subcutaneous tissue of the flap was used for this purpose). All wounds are then closed.

After-Treatment
The hand is splinted in full extension for three weeks. Active and passive mobilization is then instituted. After the bone graft has completely healed in place, which is usually the case after about four months, the transverse wire is removed. The longitudinal one is left in place. It may happen that in traumatic cases the intrinsic system is damaged; a sublimis transplant may then be necessary to replace the damaged intrinsic muscles, as described on page 888. To obtain a stable joint, the restoration of intrinsic function is absolutely necessary.

BIBLIOGRAPHY

ARMSTRONG, J. R.: *Bone Graft in the Treatment of Fractures.* Williams & Wilkins, Baltimore, 1945.

BARNARD, L., and STUBBINS, S. G.: *Styloidectomy of the radius in the surgical treatment of non-union of the carpal navicular.* J. Bone Joint Surg., 30A:98, 1948.

BARR, J. S., ET AL.: *Fracture of the carpal navicular (scaphoid) bone.* J. Bone Joint Surg., 35A:609, 1953.

BÖHLER, L.: *Die Technik der Knockenbruchbehandlung.* 12-13 Edit. Wilhelm Maudrich, Wien, 1951, 1957; 5th English Ed. Grune and Stratton, New York, 1956.

BRUNER, J. M.: *Use of single iliac bone graft to replace multiple metacarpal loss in subtotal injuries of the hand.* J. Bone Joint Surg., 39A:44, 1957.

CAMPBELL, W. C.: *Operative Orthopedics.* C. V. Mosby Co., St. Louis, 1939.

CARROLL, R. E., and TABER, T. H.: *Digital arthoplasty of the proximal interphalangeal joint.* J. Bone Joint Surg., 36A:912, 1954.

CAUCHOIX, S., HAUTIER, S., LEMOINE, A.: *Pseudarthrosis of the scaphoid (Les Pseudarthroses du Scaphoïde).* J. Chir., 94:21, 1967.

DICKINSON, J. C., and SHANNON, J. G.: *Fractures of the carpal scaphoid in the Canadian army.* Surg. Gynec. Obstet., 79:225, 1944.

ENDER, J., KROTSCHECK, H., and SIMON-WEIDNER, R.: *Die Chirurgie der Handverletzungen.* Springer-Verlag Wien, 1956.

ENTIN, M., ALGER, J. R., and BAIRD, R. M.: *Experimental and clinical transplantation of autogenous whole joints.* J. Bone Joint Surg., 44A:1518, 1962.

935

THE EXTREMITIES

ERDELYI, R.: *Experimental autotransplantation of small joints.* Plast. Reconstr. Surg., 31:129, 1963.
Reconstruction of ankylosed finger joints by means of transplantation of joints from the foot. Plast. Reconstr. Surg., 31:140, 1963.

FLATT, A. E.: *The Care of the Rheumatoid Hand.* C. V. Mosby Co., St. Louis, 1963.

FOWLER, S. B.: *Mobilization of metacarpophalangeal joints. Arthroplasty and capsulotomy.* J. Bone Joint Surg., 29:193, 1947.

GRAHAM, W. C., and RIORDAN, D. C.: *Reconstruction of a metacarpophalangeal joint with a metatarsal transplant.* J. Bone Joint Surg., 30A:848, 1948.

KRÖMER, K.: *Die Verletzte Hand.* Verlag Maudrich, Wien, 1945.

LEXER, E.: *Die freien Transplantationen.* Neue deutsche Chir. Ferd. Enke, 1919, 1924, Stuttgart, Vol. 26a, 26b.

LIEBOLT, F. L.: *The use of capsulectomy and arthroplasty for limitation of finger motion.* Surg. Gynec. Obstet., 90:103, 1950.

LITTLER, J. W.: *Metacarpal reconstruction.* J. Bone Joint Surg., 29:723, 1947.

MARCER, E.: *Trapianti articolare dal piede alla mano (Articular Transplants from Foot to Hand.)* Achr. Putti chir. org. mavim, 3:276, 1953.

MAY, H.: *The regeneration of joint transplants and intracapsular fragments.* Ann. Surg., 116:297, 1942.
The regeneration of bone transplants. Ann. Surg., 106:441, 1937.

MAZET, R., and HOHL, M.: *Fractures of the carpal navicular.* Surg. Gynec. Obstet., 45A:82, 1963.

McLAUGHLIN, H. L.: *Fracture of the carpal navicular (scaphoid) bone. Some observations based on treatment by open reduction and internal fixation.* J. Bone Joint Surg., 36A:765, 1954.

MOBERG, E.: *Fractures and ligamentous injuries of the hand and fingers.* Surg. Clin. N. Amer. 40:297, 1960.

NYGA, W., BOUGERT, H. W.: *Behandlung der Kahnbeinpseudarthrose unter besonderer Berücksichtfigung des Fremdspanes.* Handchirurgie, 1:57, 1969.

MURRAY, G.: *Bone graft for nonunion of the carpal scaphoid.* Surg. Gynec. Obstet., 60:540, 1935.
Small bone grafts of extremities. Canad. Med. Assoc. J., 48:137, 1943.
End results of bone-grafting for nonunion of the carpal naviculare. J. Bone Joint Surg., 28:749, 1946.

OBLETZ, B. E., and HALBSTEIN, B. M.: *Nonunion of fractures of the carpal navicular.* J. Bone Joint Surg., 20:769, 1930.

SNEDECOR, S. T.: *Bone surgery of the hand.* Amer. J. Surg., 72:363, 1946.

STEINDLER, A.: *Orthopedic Operations.* Charles C Thomas, Springfield, 1943.

WATSON-JONES, R.: *Fractures and Joint Injuries.* Vol. II. Williams & Wilkins, Baltimore, 1955.

WAUGH, R. L., and REULING, L.: *Ununited Fractures of Carpal Scaphoid.* Amer. J. Surg., 67:184, 1945.

THE HAND
AND FINGERS 31
IN TOTO

NEOPLASTY OF FINGERS

THE handicap following loss of fingers is severe; that from the loss of the thumb is even more so. There are various methods of repair. Each one—however ingenious—may result in failure, a possibility to be recognized by surgeon and patient before the operation. Neoplasty of the fingers has undergone many changes since World War II. Some of the older methods were found unsatisfactory and given up; others proved satisfactory but needed improvement. The replacement of digital phalanges by composite flaps was found to have only limited use. The replacement of the thumb by another finger has stood the test of time in principle, but the method has been much modified and improved. In certain cases, phalangization (using the metacarpal bones for restoring function when phalanges are missing) is still a useful device. Rotation osteotomies and the interchange of fingers have definite usefulness in limited fields, as does replacement of avulsed portions of fingers with the avulsed parts.

REPLACEMENT OF PHALANGES BY COMPOSITE FLAPS

Various methods have been devised (Schepelmann, Albee, Kallio, Greeley, Tubiana, Stack and Hackstian, Flynn and Burden, Broadbent) employing the principle of transplanting a flap from the abdomen containing a bone graft. The bone graft is incorporated into the flap either before or after the latter is transferred to the finger. Regardless of the

937

source of the graft, the danger of its absorption is always present, and the flap lacks tactile sensation. Consequently, this method should be used only if other better methods (see below) are not available.

Technique

A tube flap or open pedicle flap of suitable size and length is made at the abdomen. (Tubiana, Stack and Hackstian prefer a pectoral tube flap because it has less fat.) The flap is then transferred to the hand and united with the stump of the finger. After it has healed in place, it is severed from its pedicle and the raw peripheral surface is closed. After all edema in the flap has disappeared, the flap is opened along its seam; a bone graft is taken from the crest of the ilium (p. 70), or one of the metatarsal bones is used as graft (see p. 934). This graft is either wedged into the base of the remaining phalanx or metacarpal bone or held in apposition by intramedullary Kirschner-wire fixation. The flap may need thinning by removal of some of its subcutaneous fat tissue to permit closure around the bone graft (compare with Case 160, p. 1208).

If, with the exception of the thumb, all fingers and parts of their metacarpal bones are missing, the loss is serious, since the thumb is left with no opposing structure and hence no grasping surface. To restore a grasping surface, an open abdominal flap is made and its peripheral end sutured to the dorsal defect edge. This flap should be sufficiently long to permit folding upon itself after it is severed from its pedicle. In other words, the flap will have the shape of a mitten (Case 160, p. 1208). After it has healed in place and all edema has subsided, the flap is unfolded by incising the volar scar. A periosteum-covered bone graft is removed from the anterior surface of the tibia or crest of the ilium and shaped to proper size for horizontal placement into the flap, with the medullary side against the freshened bone stumps of the metacarpal bones; it is held in place by internal fixation with Kirschner wires. The flap is then reflected over the graft and sutured in place.

After-Treatment

The newly formed extremity is encased in a plaster cast; it should remain immobilized until the x-ray picture reveals firm union between graft and host bone.

If thumb or index finger have been reconstructed with a composite tube flap, sensitivity must also be restored. To supply normal prehension, a skin-island flap is transferred on its neurovascular bundle from the ulnar side of the palmar surface of middle or ring finger (p. 804).

For discussion of absence of all finger phalanges, see page 954.

REPLACEMENT OF AVULSED PORTIONS OF FINGERS WITH THE AVULSED PARTS (COMPOSITE GRAFTS)

Successful replacement of completely avulsed portions of fingers as composite grafts of bone, ligament, nailbed and skin has been reported by Beverly Douglas. In seventeen consecutive replants—none proximal to the distal joint—the avulsed parts were carefully replaced in exactly the same position as they were originally and only the subcutaneous tissue and skin were sutured. They were temporarily splinted and all survived. Douglas explained the results on the basis of the terminal nature of the vessels in fingers which favored prompt reestablishment of the blood flow. In subsequent experiments in monkeys Douglas was able to demonstrate survival of whole fingers as composite grafts when replaced by accurate suturing of tissue without arterial sutures, a truly stimulating piece of work.

Komatsu and Tamai recently reported a successful replacement of a completely cut-off thumb using a vascular anastomosis with microsurgical technique which had been experimentally developed by Buncke and co-workers and others.

RECONSTRUCTION OF THUMB

The thumb is our most important finger. Its loss may cripple the function of the hand severely. If this is the case, a reconstruction of the thumb becomes advisable.

ANATOMICAL CONSIDERATIONS

The thumb is the shortest of all fingers; it barely reaches the first interphalangeal joint of the index finger. The latter is not the longest finger, but has the longest metacarpal bone. The first metacarpal bone is the insertion point of numerous functionally important muscles, of which the abductor and the opponens muscle are the most important. The abductor inserts at the base of the first metacarpal bone; although the opponens muscle inserts along the entire radial surface of the bone, a metacarpal stump from 1 to 1.5 cm. ($\frac{3}{8}$ to $\frac{5}{8}$ inch) long is still sufficient for satisfactory muscle action of the opponens. Hence, it would be a serious mistake to sacrifice even the smallest metacarpal stump, primarily or secondarily. Aside from sacrificing important muscle function, the replacement at the carpometacarpal joint would be difficult. This joint, formed by the greater multangular and first metacarpal bone, is a saddle joint, permitting abduction and adduction and also rotation of the thumb.

THE EXTREMITIES

CLASSIFICATION

The choice of reconstruction depends upon the level of amputation; hence classification is based on the level of loss:

1. Amputation distal to the metacarpophalangeal joint.
2. Amputation in level of the metacarpophalangeal joint.
3. Amputation through the metacarpal leaving some intrinsic muscles.
4. Amputation at the metacarpal joint; this includes most cases of congenital absence of the thumb.

RECONSTRUCTION OF THUMB IN AMPUTATION DISTAL TO THE METACARPOPHALANGEAL JOINT

Amputation distal to the metacarpophalangeal joint generally requires nothing more than the formation of a nontender, stable tip. If enough local skin is present there will be no problem in covering the stump; otherwise skin must be provided either from distant regions as described on page 806 or if possible from local sources (Gillies, Hughes and Moore, Reid, Stefans and Kelly, Lewis). Lengthening of a short stump of the first phalanx with a bone graft may be considered (see also p. 938).

RECONSTRUCTION OF THUMB IN AMPUTATION AT THE METACARPOPHALANGEAL JOINT

Amputations just distal or through the metacarpophalangeal joint leave a stump of inadequate length. Although lengthening of the stump may be considered an operation for so-called phalangization, replacement of function of the missing phalanges of the thumb by using the metacarpal bone is simpler and effective. The method is described in detail on page 950.

RECONSTRUCTION OF THUMB THROUGH THE METACARPAL LEAVING SOME INTRINSIC MUSCLES

The most effective thumb-replacing method in this level is the substitution with another finger, called pollicization. Iselin in 1955 gave a detailed historical review of this operation. Originally the method consisted of swinging the index finger ray—or even the third finger ray after sacrificing the second ray—on a broad pedicle onto the position of the thumb (Noeske, Perthes, Bunnell, Iselin and Murat, Hülsman, Porzelt, Buzello, Tanzer and Littler). The next step consisted of transferring a finger of the same hand on a narrow skin-neurovascular bundle flap

(Lucksch, Hilgenfeldt) to the metacarpal of the thumb. Then one step further was taken by moving the pollicizing finger only on the neuro-vascular bundle. This technique was independently developed by Gosset and Littler. To Littler goes the credit of having developed this method even further and for having made it more versatile. Some historical notes are of interest.

Replacement of Thumb by Another Finger

Lucksch, in 1903, presented a patient in whom he had replaced the missing phalanges of the thumb with the phalanges of the neighboring index finger. Lucksch had severed the dorsal skin and extensor tendons over the first phalanx of the index finger, then severed the first phalanx itself and the flexor tendons; he left a volar bridge of skin, containing the volar digital arteries and nerves, intact. The finger hanging on this narrow skin flap was transferred to the stump of the thumb, and the bones were fastened with silver wires. After twelve days he severed one half of the skin bridge, and the second half after three weeks. Lucksch was the first to demonstrate that a narrow strip of skin containing only the volar digital arteries provided sufficient circulation for the finger. By severing the volar pedicle, however, he deprived the finger of its sensitivity.

Hilgenfeldt's contribution is that, while he followed Lucksch's method, he incorporated the skin-vessel-nerve pedicle permanently, thus preserving sensitivity in the finger. He published his vast experience with this technique in a monograph which is a veritable gold mine of information about this topic. Whenever possible, he uses the third finger for substitution. He argues that the index finger has greater range of abduction and adduction; it has greater usefulness and for this reason should be left in situ. He severs the dorsal skin vessels, nerve, and extensor tendons (since these vessels and nerves are less important than the volar ones), disarticulates the metacarpophalangeal joint, forms a volar skin bridge containing flexor tendons and volar digital arteries and nerves, transfers the finger upon the stump of the first metacarpal bone, and permanently incorporates the volar bridge flap. In the same or a second stage, he transfers the long flexor tendon of the thumb to the flexor tendons of the transferred finger, and thus—as the experience of his patients showed—changes the sensorial conception of touch in the transferred finger to that of a normal thumb. He operates in one stage if the tendon stump of the flexor pollicis longus can be readily located; if not, a second-stage operation is performed from four to six weeks later to unite the flexor pollicis longus with the flexor profundus of the third finger (Case 163, p. 1213).

941

THE EXTREMITIES

Littler contributed greatly to this technique by demonstrating that the pollicizing finger can be transferred on the neurovascular bundle alone without the skin bridge, thus making the method even more versatile. This method is the principle of the vascular pedicle "island" flap (page 82). Gossett, who apparently had developed a similar technique, shortened the new thumb by removing part of the distal segment. Hilgenfeldt and Littler shortened it by removing part of the first phalanx.

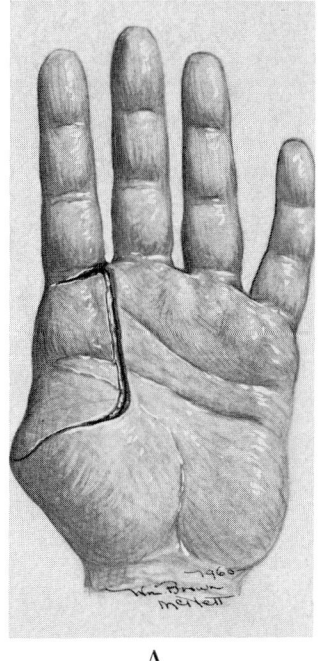
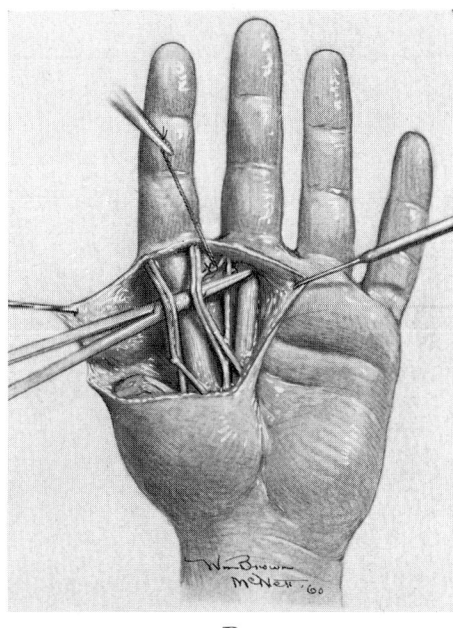

A   B

Fig. 375. *A:* Substitution of thumb with index finger. Thumb is amputated proximal to metacarpophalangeal joint. A dorsally pedicled flap is outlined between index finger and stump of first metacarpal.
B: Flap is elevated. The two neurovascular bundles are exposed. The branch of the digital artery to the third finger is being ligated.

In replacing the thumb by another finger there are certain requirements: The volar digital arteries and nerves of the replaced finger should be intact. The dorsal vessels and nerves are not important since both volar structures are sufficient to supply the dorsal skin with ample circulation and sensitivity. Tactile and thermal sensitivity alone is apparently not enough to give the patient a feeling of having a new thumb; he seems to localize the sensorial conception of touch in the replaced finger at its former site. Something else seems to be required, as reported by Hilgen-

942

feldt: A patient in whom the third finger replaced the missing thumb sensed the new thumb as a thumb only after a flexor tendon of the former thumb was attached to the flexor tendon of the transferred finger. Therefore the finger replacing the thumb should have the following qualities: It should be long enough to permit a pinch and a broad grasp, and may be shorter than the normal thumb. It is not necessary that it be mobile in all joints; however, the carpometacarpal joint must be completely mobile. There

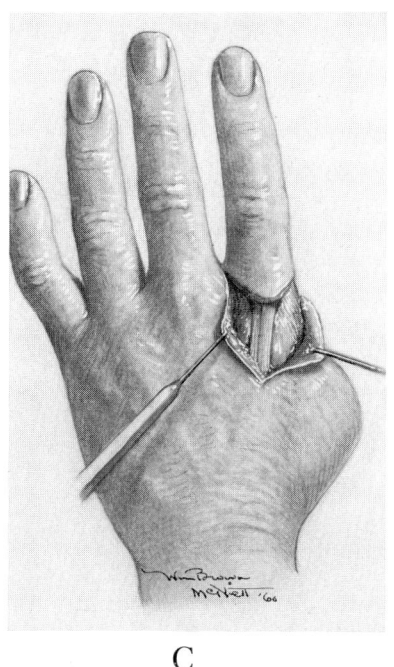 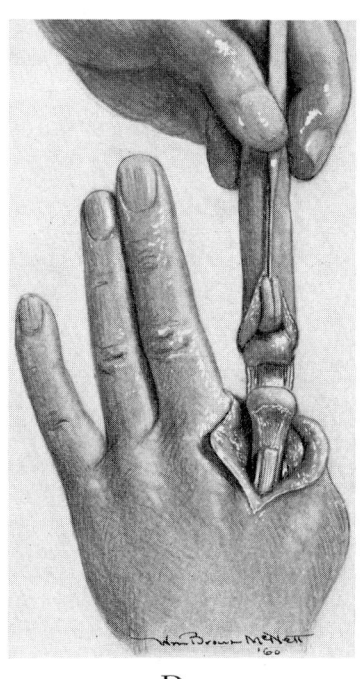

C   D

Fig. 375. C: A small dorsal triangular flap is formed with its base in level of the metacarpophalangeal joint of index finger. An encircling incision connects with the volar incision.

D: After severance of the common extensor tendon proximal to the metacarpophalangeal joint the index finger is disarticulated through the metacarpophalangeal joint and the first dorsal interosseous muscle is excised.

should be no contracture in the interdigital space, which should be deep and consist of skin with normal sensitivity. The two volar digital arteries and nerves of the replacing finger should be present. Littler, however, has succeeded in transferring a pollicizing finger on only one neurovascular bundle. If another finger is damaged in addition to the thumb, the damaged finger should be considered for replacing the thumb. Littler prefers the index finger for transfer, Hilgenfeldt the third. The fourth can also be used and even the fifth can be pollicized, as has been demonstrated (Kelleher and Sullivan, Kaplan and Plaschkes). The most important requirement is that the circulation of the pollicized finger is adequate. The following test may be helpful: A pneumatic tourniquet is applied, inflated in the usual way, and deflated after several minutes. If the finger remains anemic temporarily after the other fingers have regained normal color, the circula-

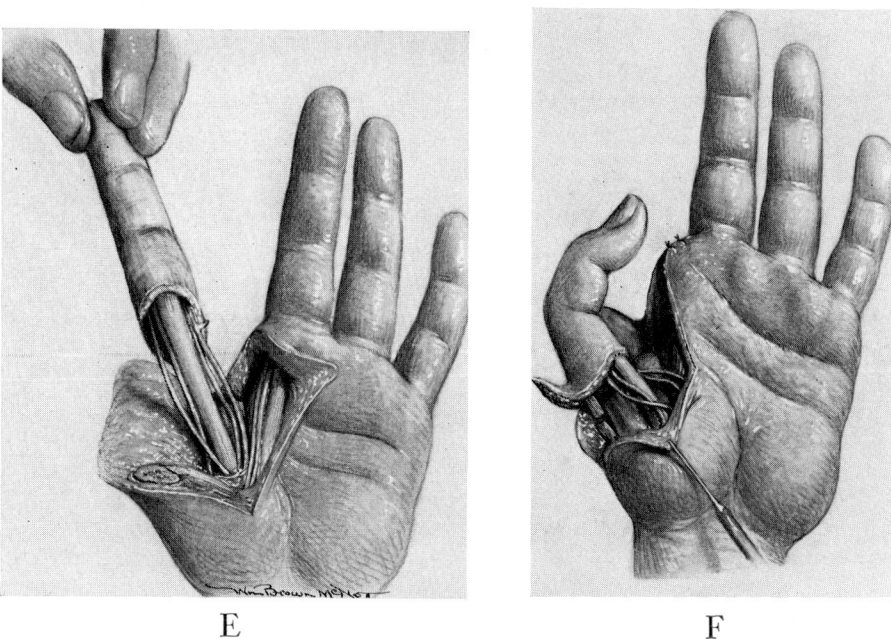

E   F

Fig. 375. *E:* The finger after division of the intermetacarpal neck ligament is hanging on neurovascular bundles and flexor tendons.
F: The index finger is rotated into opposition; the first phalanx is shortened and dovetailed into the metacarpal stump of the thumb and held with an intermedullary Kirschner wire.

tion in the anemic finger must be considered inadequate. If this is the case another finger must be used for substitution.

Technique: FIRST STAGE: Using the index finger for pollicization (Fig. 375) skin incisions are made to outline either a dorsal or volar pedicle flap for exposure and for preservation of the web. The dorsal pedicle flap as a rule yields more tissue for closure. The volar pedicle flap gives better exposure of the base of the first metacarpal and carpal area. In congenital absence of the thumb or in a case of a very short metacarpal stump the volar pedicle flap (Fig. 376, *B*) is preferable. In the case to be described the dorsal pedicle flap is chosen. It is outlined as demonstrated in Figure 375, *A*.

944

Its upper border is the volar crease of the base of the index finger; its lower border is in level of the metacarpal stump. It is dissected away from the underlying structures and from the stump of the first metacarpal after excision of the scar over it. The digital nerves are located by careful dissection, then the digital vessels. On the radial side of the index finger the lumbricale, the first dorsal interosseous and adductor muscles are exposed.

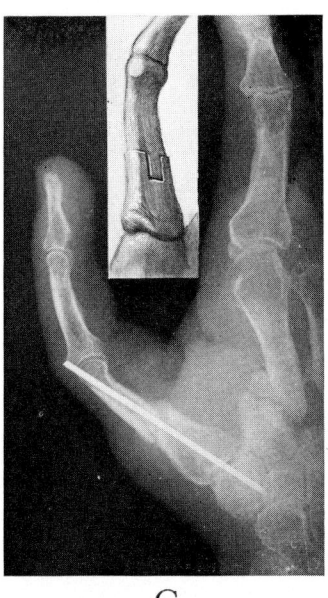

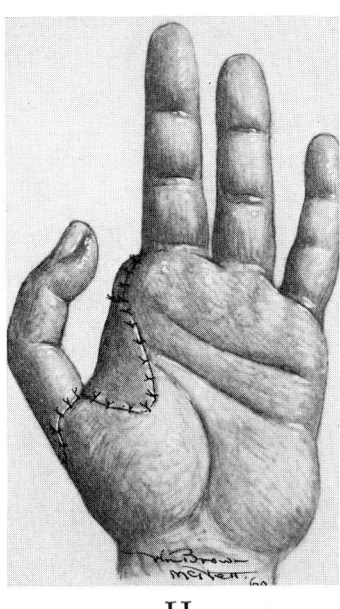

G   H

Fig. 375. *G:* Dovetailing and fixation with intramedullary Kirschner wire.
H: The extensor tendons of the index finger have been sutured to those of the thumb. The triangular dorsal flap is adjusted. The dorsal pedicle flap is swung to the volar side and sutured.

The bifurcation of the digital artery to the third finger is located—the branching occurs just proximal to the web—and this branch is ligated and severed (Fig. 375, *B*). Arteries and nerves are dissected free to the lower wound edge after the vertical septa of the palmar fascia have been divided.

The operation is now continued on the dorsal side, where a small dorsal triangular flap is formed with its base at the base of the finger. From each corner of the base an incision is made to connect with the volar finger incision. The extensor tendons are severed as proximally as possible; the junctura tendinum (Fig. 375, *B*) is also divided. The first dorsal interosseous muscle is detached from its origin at the head of the second metacarpal bone and the proximal phalanx and the muscle is excised. Then the inter-

945

metacarpal neck ligaments between the second and third metacarpal are divided. A groove director is placed between the anterior portion of the capsule of the metacarpophalangeal joint and the flexor tendons, and the finger is disarticulated at the metacarpophalangeal joint. The distal portion of the second metacarpal bone is removed.

The mobilized finger is now hanging on the flexor tendons and the neurovascular bundles. Since the entire index finger would be too long to replace the thumb, one must determine how much of the first phalanx of the index finger should be removed. The stump of the first metacarpal is left as long as possible. The shortening is done at the first phalanx of the transferred finger. The tip of the normal thumb barely extends beyond the middle of the first phalanx of the index finger; hence the first phalanx of the transferred finger should be shortened accordingly. One should, however, allow for the additional length required for the dovetailing that will hold the two bones together. The mobilized index finger is placed upon the thumb metacarpal and rotated in opposition to the remaining fingers, and the two bones are prepared for the dovetailing. The tongue is made in the first phalanx of the transferred finger, the grooving in the first meta-carpal bone (Fig. 375, G). The tongue and the groove are carved with an electric burr. The tourniquet is now released for careful hemostasis and then reinflated. A longitudinal incision is made over the first metacarpal bone to locate the tendon of the extensor pollicis longus and brevis. The two bones are now pressed into each other so that the pollicizing finger (the new thumb) is in 10-degree flexion. The bones are transfixed with a Kirschner wire. There are two ways of inserting the wire: It may be driven first through the groove and the first metacarpal stump until it appears at the dorsum of the hand and the tip is flush with the bottom of the groove; then, with the transferred finger in the proper position, the Kirschner wire is driven back into the first phalanx of the index finger. Alternately, it can be done by drilling the Kirschner wire through the tongue of the first phalanx of the index finger until it is flush with the tongue, then placing the finger in proper position and driving the Kirschner wire into the metacarpal bone. It is cut short to be buried beneath the skin (Fig. 375, G). The extensor tendon of the index finger is split longitudinally; one half is sutured to the extensor pollicis longus, the other half to the extensor pollicis brevis. The skin is then sutured on the dorsal side after excision of some of the skin to permit adjustment of the triangular dorsal flap and the index finger. The dorsal pedicle flap is swung to the volar side of the hand and all remaining wounds are closed (Fig. 375, H).

The finger is immobilized in a dorsal plaster-cast splint reaching from the forearm to the tip of the thumb, held in abduction and opposition.

946

SECOND STAGE: Two months later the flexor pollicis longus tendon is exposed from a transverse incision in the wrist. The flexor profundus of the transferred index finger is severed at the proper level and sutured to the flexor pollicis longus. The sublimis tendon is also severed and a piece is resected to readjust it to the proper length. A dorsal molded plaster-cast splint is applied for another three weeks.

VARIATIONS: Any finger of the same hand can be used for pollicization, even the little finger (Kelleher and Sullivan). The incisions for transfer of the various fingers are outlined in Figure 376, *A*. The pollicizing finger is passed between the palmar aponeurosis and the superficial volar arch. However, fingers should be used only if much of the index ray is

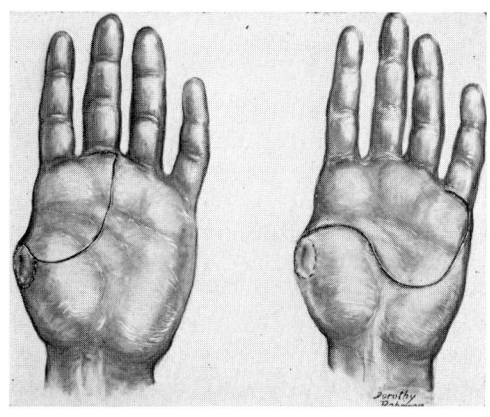

A.

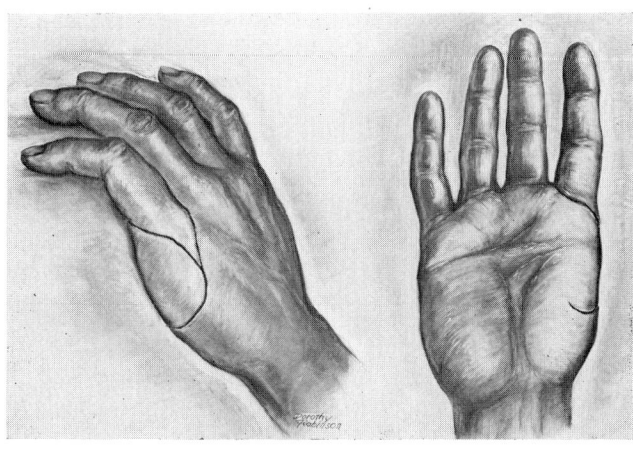

B

Fig. 376. *A:* Incisions for transfer of middle or fifth finger in pollicization. *B:* Flaps outlined for transfer of index finger and metacarpal in pollicization in total absence of thumb. Note that main flap is volar pedicled.

947

absent. If the entire index metacarpal or—even better—a stump of the first phalanx and much of the thumb metacarpal are preserved, it is better to transfer the distal part of the second metacarpal on its neurovascular bundle to lengthen the first metacarpal than to utilize another functioning finger. In this case, the tendons are left behind, unless a stump of the first phalanx is also present. Here a dorsal pedicle flap seems to provide better skin coverage for the web than does a palmar pedicle flap, as Buck-Gramcko reflects in an afterthought. However, additional coverage with skin grafts of small remaining raw surfaces may be necessary.

RECONSTRUCTION OF THE THUMB IN TOTAL ABSENCE OF THE SAME

In cases of total loss of the thumb and of congenital absence of the thumb (group 4 of classification of p. 940), the index finger is used for pollicization. In this case, a volar pedicle flap (Fig. 376, *B*) rather than a dorsal pedicle flap is used, since it affords better exposure of the carpal area.

In congenital absence of the thumb, a so-called floating thumb may be present like an appendage. Edgerton fillets it to provide additional skin for the thumb web. The flaps are outlined and raised. The neurovascular bundles are developed as described in detail above. The flexor and extensor tendons are left intact. The junctura teninum to the third finger is divided. A space is developed between the dorsal interosseous muscles, and the shaft of the second metacarpal bone is divided just beyond its base. Hilgenfeldt, Barsky, Entin and Edgerton, Snyder and Webb stress the value of saving most of the length of the metacarpal. The length of the normal adult thumb, measured from the center of the carpometacarpal joint, is only about 2 cm. longer than the index finger measured from the center of its metacarpophalangeal joint. Hence, beginning about 2 cm. proximal to the center of the index metacarpophalangeal joint, the diameter of the metacarpal shaft is reduced with an electric burr to fit into a large drill hole (equal to the reduced diameter of the metacarpal shaft) made in the deformed carpal bones on the radial side of the wrist (Edgerton, Snyder and Webb). The direction of the drill hole is determined by placing the remaining fingers in a closed-fist position with the mobilized index finger against these fingers in the position of a normal thumb when the fist is clenched. The carpus is then marked to indicate the direction and level of the drill hole. When the hole has been drilled and the metacarpal tapped into place the new thumb is checked for rotation and opposition of the pull against the long and ring finger. The index tip should be able to press against the dorsal surface of the middle phalanx of the fully flexed ring finger. Bone chips are placed about the graft base and Kirschner wires are used to secure immobilization.

948

THE HAND AND FINGERS IN TOTO

The tourniquet is released and hemostasis obtained. The skin flaps are adjusted and all wounds are sutured; additional raw surfaces along the dorsal and radial aspects of the thumb may require skin grafts for coverage. Edgerton et al. shift a bridge flap from the dorsum of the hand into the defect and skin graft the resulting flap bed. Application of a plaster cast follows. Although the long flexor and extensor tendons of the transferred index finger are quite slack at the time of the operation, they seem to shorten markedly within a few weeks and may not need to be resected later on (Reid, Edgerton et al.). Unless the metacarpophalangeal joint is only slightly mobile or deliberately fused (Entin, Littler and Cooley), tendon stabilization may be needed: The first interosseous muscle is detached and used as an abductor brevis muscle after Littler, the sublimis tendons are transferred and used for opposition or adduction, or the flexor carpi ulnaris is lengthened with the palmaris or the os pisiform after Bunnell (Schweitzer).

Reid as well as Matthews avoid this by discarding the entire distal end of the second metacarpal and fusing the proximal part of the first phalanx with the stump of the proximal part of the second metacarpal in abduction and opposition, thus creating a two-joint new thumb instead of a triphalangeal one; this seems as purposeful and less ugly. The length of the new thumb is determined by the length of the proximal second metacarpal stump. After the distal part of the second metacarpal, the meta-carpophalangeal joint and the cartilaginous epiphysis of the proximal pha-lanx are removed, Matthews reams out the proximal phalanx to receive a bone-graft peg fashioned from the discarded parts of the metacarpal shaft. The proximal stump of the index metacarpal shaft is drilled obliquely to receive the other ends of the bone peg. Bone chips are packed around this area. The hand is maintained in a plaster cast for six weeks, after which the thumb is allowed full movement except for a plaster collar around its base. A polythane splint is worn at night for three months to protect the thumb from possible injury. The disadvantage of a two-joint thumb is obvious, namely the loss of ab- and adduction. A compromise pro-cedure is that of Buck-Gramcko, whereby the head of the second meta-carpal bone is preserved. The metacarpophalangeal joint and most of the metacarpal bone are excised; the metacarpal head is fastened to a small stump of the base of the second metacarpal. To prevent hyperextension of the new thumb in the new carpometacarpal joint he rotates the metacarpal head 90 degree ulnarward. He also transfers the interossei so that the first dorsal interosseus becomes an abductor brevis and the first volar interosseus an adductor. Each interosseus tendon is fastened to the corresponding severed lateral band of the dorsal aponeurosis of the transferred index finger. He shortens the extensor tendons in the same stage. The flexor tendons gradually adjust themselves in length.

Phalangization: Replacement of Function of Missing Phalanges of Thumb by Using Metacarpal Bone

The principle of the method, first described by Huguier in 1852, is the creation of a cleft between the first metacarpal bone and the remainder of the hand, thus restoring the pincer action and grasping capacity of the hand to some degree. The method has been improved by various surgeons (Klapp, Perthes, Kallio, Pieri, Iselin, Bunnell, Kreuz,

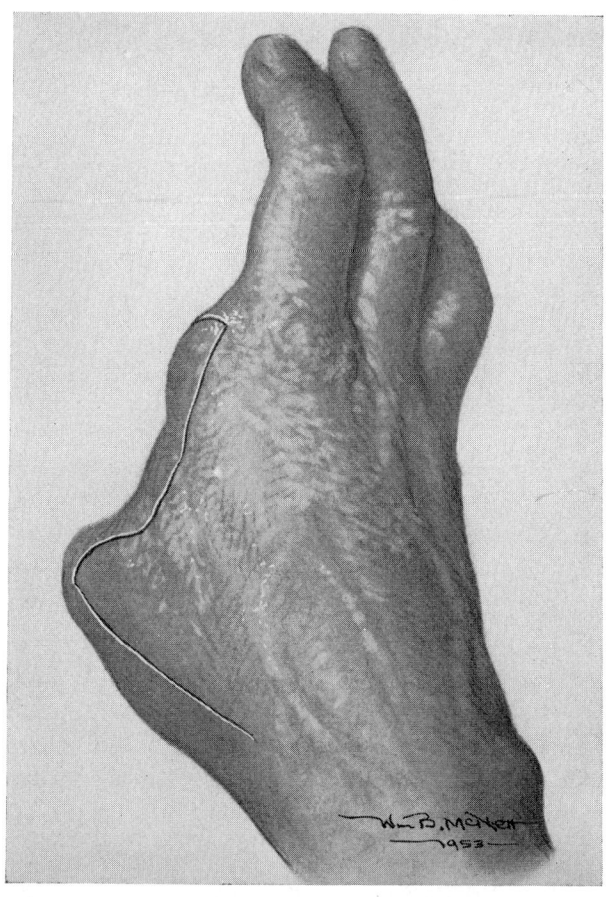

Fig. 377. Dorsal incision for phalangization of first metacarpal bone after Iselin. Incision is made over dorsum of first metacarpal bone. It then follows the web between thumb and index finger metacarpal, crosses over to palm and continues along longitudinal crease.

Brown, D'Aubigné, and others). The most recent modification comes from Hilgenfeldt, who made use of his formerly described principle of finger transfer. Phalangization is a reliable method. It can be used when the first three or four fingers or even all fingers are absent, but most of the metacarpal bones, particularly the first one, is present. It can also be used when the second to fifth fingers are present, but the thumb phalanges are absent, provided the entire thumb metacarpal is present.

To create a cleft, it is necessary to remove some of the muscles between the first and the other metacarpal bones; the first dorsal interosseous can be excised completely without subsequent impairment of function. The adductor muscle, which forms the bulk of the muscle filling the space between the first and second metacarpal bones, should be removed only partially; otherwise, the pincer action of the first metacarpal would be lost. The muscle originates along the entire length of the

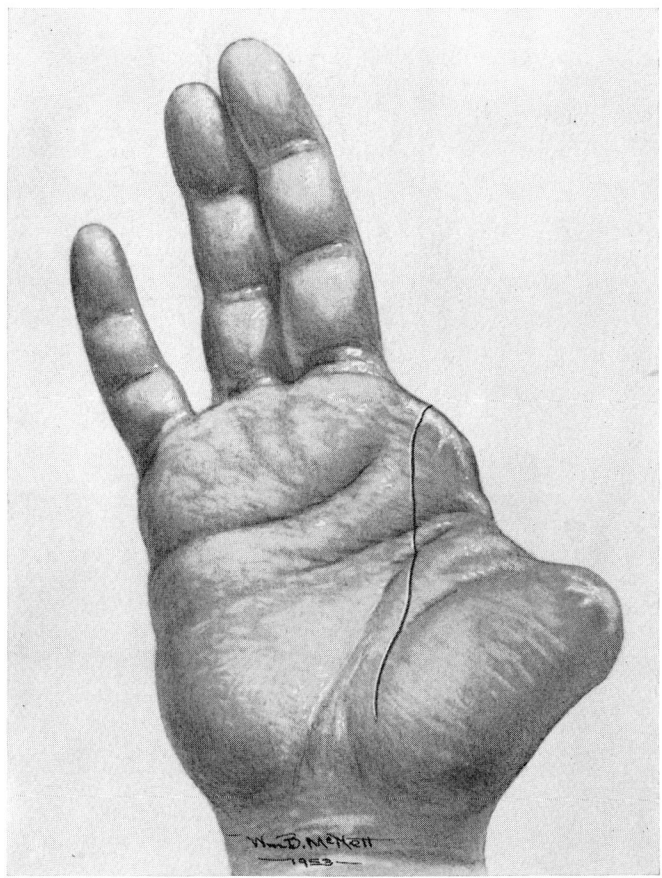

Fig. 378. Volar incision.

951

third metacarpal bone and with a smaller head at the carpal bone, and inserts at the head of the first metacarpal. In other words, it bridges the second metacarpal; hence, the second metacarpal bone can be removed without disturbing the function of the adductor muscle. To deepen the cleft, Bunnell transfers the inserting point from the head of the first metacarpal more proximally. Others incise that part of the muscle which originates along the third metacarpal bone. The author has found this latter method simple and effective. In certain cases (see p. 953) partial removal of the second metacarpal bone is advantageous to widen the cleft.

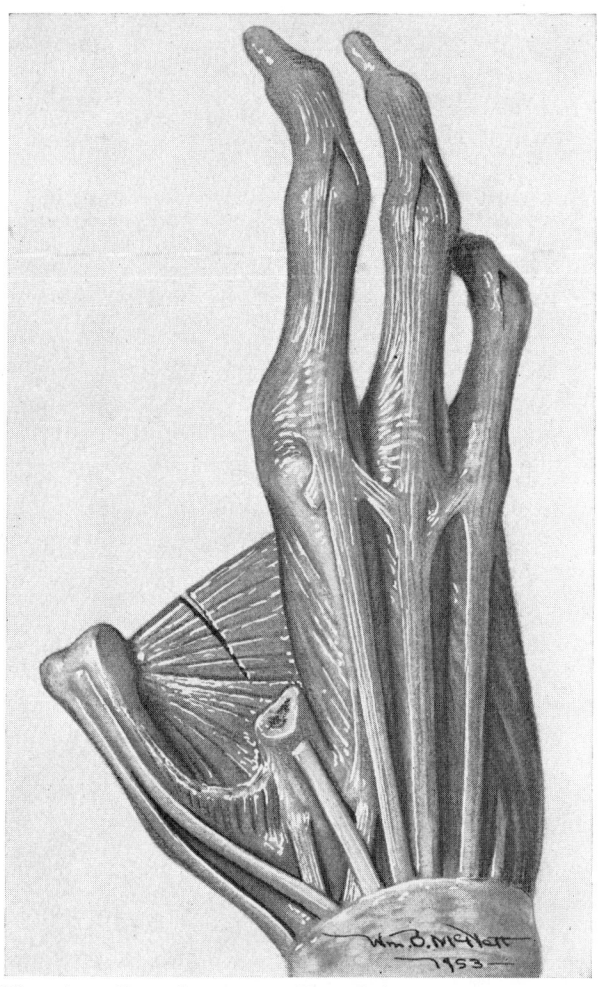

Fig. 379. Dorsal aspect. Dorsal interosseous muscle has been removed. Second metacarpal shortened to create wider cleft. Incision of distal half of abductor muscle indicated.

THE HAND AND FINGERS IN TOTO

Technique (Example: Absence of Phalanges of Thumb and Index Finger) (Figs. 377-379) (compare with Case 166, p. 1217): The incisions are outlined to form a dorsal and volar flap. In the construction of these flaps, it is well not to be too ambitious. It is preferable to make them rather short and broad than to risk necrosis of the tips. The flaps are mobilized, exposing the first dorsal interosseous and adductor pollicis muscles. The interosseous muscle is excised. The next step is the removal of the second metacarpal bone, with the exception of the base, to prevent collapse of the metacarpal arch and to preserve the insertion point of the extensor carpi radialis; care should be taken not to injure the radial artery as it crosses the interspace between the first and second metacarpal bones. The adductor pollicis muscle is now incised. It has an oblique and a transverse portion; the latter forms the bulk of the muscle. It is incised until the oblique portion of the muscle is reached; this is left intact. The incised portions of the muscle are reflected dorsally to cover the stump of the second metacarpal bone, or both portions are excised. The skin flaps are now carried around the corresponding raw surfaces and sutured to the opposite wound edges. The remaining raw surfaces are covered with a thick split skin graft. A heavily padded pressure dressing is applied.

After-Treatment: The dressing is removed after ten days, and active motion exercises are started.

Variations: If too much of the adductor muscle is incised and the pincer action of the first metacarpal bone is weakened, which has happened in one of our cases, the patient is able to rotate the thumb, but adduction resembles the action of a loose pair of scissors. Should this be the case, the grip can be tightened appreciably by transfer of one of the flexor tendons of the missing index finger or the sublimis tendon of the third finger, led dorsally to be attached to the dorsal side of the first metacarpal bone (for method of attachment, see p. 862) (Case 165, p. 1216).

It is a generally agreed-upon practice to remove the second metacarpal to widen the cleft, as described in the foregoing, in patients in whom, aside from the thumb phalanges, the phalanges of the index and third fingers are absent. In patients in whom all fingers are absent, the author's experience is that the removal of the second metacarpal is of no advantage. It narrows the hand; the patient cannot grasp larger objects owing to the absence of grasping power of the fingers, and he has difficulty in grasping smaller objects since the cleft at the bottom is too wide and cannot be closed completely. Therefore, in patients with all fingers lost at the metacarpophalangeal joints, it is better to leave the second metacarpal behind (Cases 164, 165, pp. 1215, 1216). On the other hand, in cases where the thumb is preserved but the second, third, or all fingers are missing, the second metacarpal should be removed, since the loss of grasping finer objects is outweighed by the increase of width and hence by the increase of the grasping power (Case 166, p. 1217).

If all fingers are lost and the metacarpal bones are covered with unstable scars, the latter must be replaced with a well-padded abdominal flap; the flap can be constructed so that after its severance at the time of its adjustment phalangization can be carried out in the same stage. If the flap has also to replace and form the web, the second metacarpal must be removed, since the padded flap—even if later thinned out—would fill out the grasping space. The second metacarpal bone, with the exception of its base, is removed at the time of the transfer of the flap (Case 166, p. 1217).

If the thumb metacarpal is too short, it should be lengthened with an iliac-bone graft or by utilizing part of the second metacarpal bone, if excision of the latter is contemplated(Cannon, Graham, Brown), or by the neurovascular bundle method (p. 948). The former procedure is carried out through a dorsal incision, so placed that it can be used again at the time the cleft is created. However, if the skin is too short over the first metacarpal stump, a so-called "cock-hat" flap (Lewin, Gillies) can be used to lengthen it. It is raised from a curved incision across the radial border of the hand, 2.5 cm. (1 inch) or more proximal to the tip of the stump of the first metacarpal. This flap is raised like a hood. After the metacarpal is lengthened with a bone graft, the hood of skin is placed over it, and the secondary defect on the radial side of the hand is skingrafted. The bone graft is fixed in opposition and minimal angulation, using Hilgenfeldt's dovetailing method (p. 946). Additional fixation is accomplished with the use of oblique Kirschner wires.

Hilgenfeldt lengthens the first metacarpal with part of the second metacarpal (if the phalanges of the index finger are absent) by using the underlying principles of his method of thumb substitution (p. 948).

Substitution of Toe for Thumb

This method, which is rarely applicable, was first employed by Nicoladoni. Others have followed it, and used it also for other fingers or for part of a finger (Oehlecker, Riedel, Mühsam, v. Eiselsberg, Blair, Byars, Gillies, and Young). By modifying the method, Clarkson was able in one of his cases (congenital adactylia) to substitute the toes for the fingers by a five-toe transfer. Davis, who provides a good historical background, seems to have simplified the method by transferring the toe (second toe) on a tube pedicle flap.

954

CINEPLASTY

Cineplastic operations are performed on amputation stumps of the upper extremity for the purpose of utilizing the potential and residual forces within the muscles of the stump to activate a prosthesis. In 1896, Vanghetti of Italy, in an attempt to help his countrymen who were mutilated in the first Abyssinian war, conceived the idea of cinematization of the amputation stump of the forearm. Realizing that there were still intact muscles rendered useless after the amputation, he isolated the distal tendinous parts, enclosed them with covering skin, and connected them with a specially constructed prosthesis. Others have endeavored to improve the technique.

The great credit, however, for placing the method upon a scientific basis and developing it for practical purposes goes to Sauerbruch (1915). He described the development of his ingenious thoughts in detail in his fascinating memoirs. By testing the potential power of a muscle or muscle group at various levels of the extremity, he succeeded in developing favorable combinations of muscle groups to be used for activation. He also developed the operative method and the construction of suitable prostheses. His method found many followers. Kessler did the pioneer work in the United States. For many years, he was the only person in this country to do this operation. His efforts and enthusiasm were greatly rewarded. Nissen, in collaboration with Bergmann, has published the experiences they had had with various methods of cineplasty in a well-illustrated monograph.

SKIN-MUSCLE CANALIZATION
(SAUERBRUCH'S METHOD)

While the original Sauerbruch method is still the standard, improvements have been made. Considerable work in cinematization had been done in Germany during World War II on several thousand amputees in two centers—one in Berlin under Sauerbruch, and the other in Munich under his distinguished pupil, Lebsche. To study their methods and results and to investigate the possibilities of improving the cineplastic technique and construction of artificial limbs, the United States Army sent Dr. Aldridge, accompanied by Colonel Peterson and certain engineers, to Germany after the war. As a result of their findings, the Committee on Artificial Limbs of the National Research Council began a research program on cineplasty. It started with a revival of interest in muscle physiology in relation to the mechanical needs of the prosthesis, in which Dr. Verne T. Inman and his co-workers at the University of California had been most interested, and culminated in the excellent results achieved by Colonel Spittler and his co-workers at the Cineplastic Center at Walter Reed Army Hospital. It became evident, however, that such results are possible only by integrated teamwork, as demonstrated by the extensive end-result studies of Brav, Spittler, and others. These results require proper selection of the patient, his cooperation, a well-executed operation, well-constructed prosthesis, and training in the use of the prosthesis. All those experienced with the method come to the conclusion that a patient provided with a muscle motor (cineplasty) gets better use from the prosthetic device than with the usual shoulder-strap control.

The three most important improvements over the original Sauerbruch method are: (1) a modification made by Lebsche consisting of liberating or dividing the distal insertion or attachment of the muscle through which the tunnel was placed, thus giving the muscle more strength and excursion; (2) a very much larger skin tube through which the peg is placed—the larger the tube and the peg, the less pressure there is on the skin with movement of the prosthesis; (3) the use of the biceps as a motor, whether or not the forearm stump can be utilized. The results which Lebsche and later Colonel Spittler demonstrated with this latter method were most impressive.

Selection of Muscle-Motor Sites

Of paramount importance are well-functioning muscles. Generally speaking, only those muscles should be utilized which are not needed for the movements of the stump itself. Flexor muscles are used for closing, extensor muscles for opening the artificial hand. Today, however, prostheses are constructed with a spring mechanism to be used for opening the hand; hence, construction of an extensor-muscle canal can be dispensed with. The stump itself must be in good condition and of proper length. If the stump is too short, the operation is unlikely to be successful, since the excursion of the muscle tunnel is in direct proportion to the length of the muscle through which the tube passes, and the strength of the motor is in direct proportion to the diameter of the muscle belly. Hence, the longer the stump, the better the function of the muscle motors.

In long forearm stumps, the musculus flexor sublimis, just above its musculotendinous juncture, was formerly preferred as the muscle motor. Recently, however, as already mentioned, even in long or short forearm stumps, the biceps is preferred as the muscle motor (Case 168, p. 1219), since it has more strength and excursion than the forearm flexors. Extensor motors are dispensed with.

The advantages of biceps cineplasty in the long, above-the-elbow amputation are not so apparent, and the usefulness of this procedure remains controversial.

Pectoral cineplasty has limited usefulness. It should be employed only in patients with such exceptional conditions as bilateral shoulder disarticulation; in such a patient, an additional source of prosthetic control is urgently required (Brav, Spittler, and others).

Preoperative Care

This consists chiefly of developing the strength of those muscles to be used for the cineplasty, by massaging, and by teaching the patient active use of the proper muscle groups. A patient who is willing and cooperative in carrying out these exercises will have good results. On the other hand, uncooperative patients should be excluded from the operation.

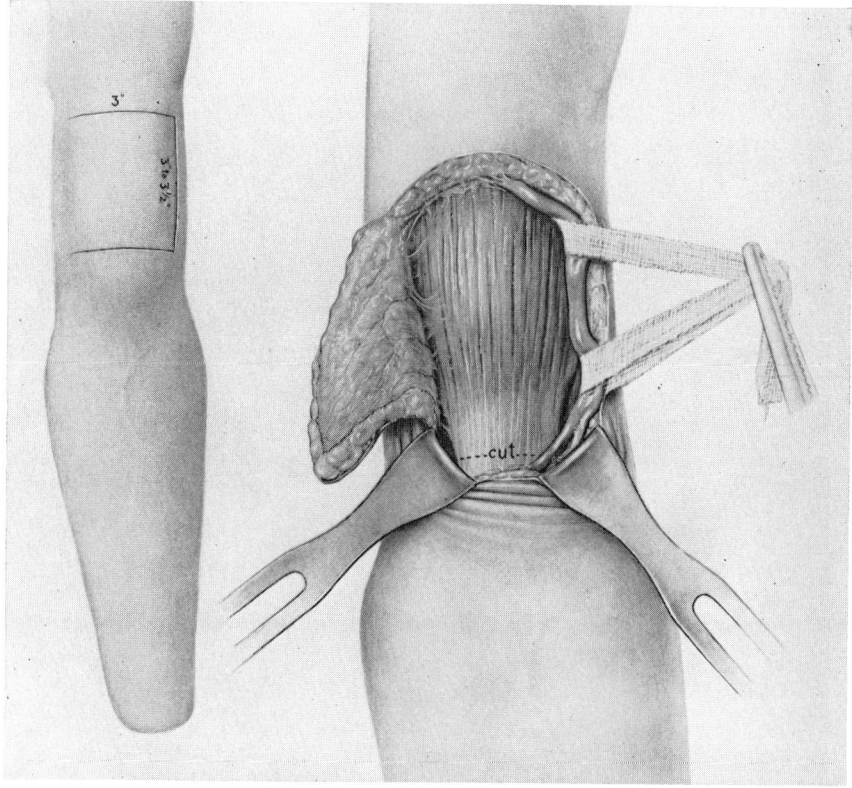

Fig. 380. Cineplasty. Construction of biceps muscle canals. To produce a tunnel with the largest diameter possible a skin flap of at least 3 inches and 3½ inches on the three sides has been outlined. Note that the skin flap contains both subcutaneous fat and deep fascia. (A. W. Spittler and I. E. Rosen: J. Bone Joint Surg.)

957

THE EXTREMITIES

Technique

Before general anesthesia is started, the proper site of the skin flaps for the skin tube is selected. Prior to the outlining of the skin flaps, the patient should contract the muscle to be used as motor. This helps the surgeon in selecting a proper site. The skin tubes should come to lie in the pass of the contracted muscles, also at right angles to the fibers of the muscle, and at a level where the muscle passes over into its tendon. The base of the flap should be toward the median side in biceps tunnels. The

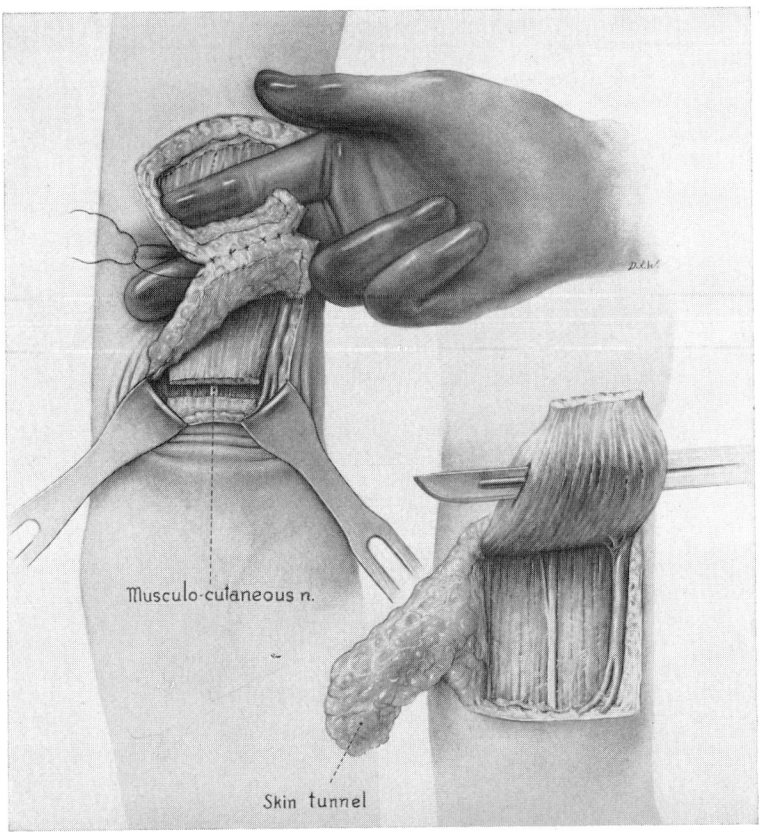

Fig. 381. Incisions are made in the muscle, and the muscle belly should be slowly and carefully dilated to avoid damage to its fibers. The skin tunnel is then drawn through the opening and the mouth of the tube is sutured to the adjacent skin. (A. W. Spittler and I. E. Rosen: J. Bone Joint Surg.)

pectoral flap should have its base toward the breast. The flap for the biceps tunnel should come to lie proximal to the distal end of the biceps muscle, with the arm held extended at the elbow joint so that the skin canal will be at a higher level than the distal end of the biceps-muscle

958

belly. The canals should be made large; hence, the rectangular skin flap should measure 7.5 by 8.8 cm. (3 by 3½ inches). The flaps are cut so that they contain subcutaneous fat tissue and deep fascia to secure an ample blood supply (Fig. 380).

Construction of Upper-Arm (Biceps-Muscle) Canal (Figs. 380-383; Case 167, p. 1218): First, the skin tube is made by everting the wound

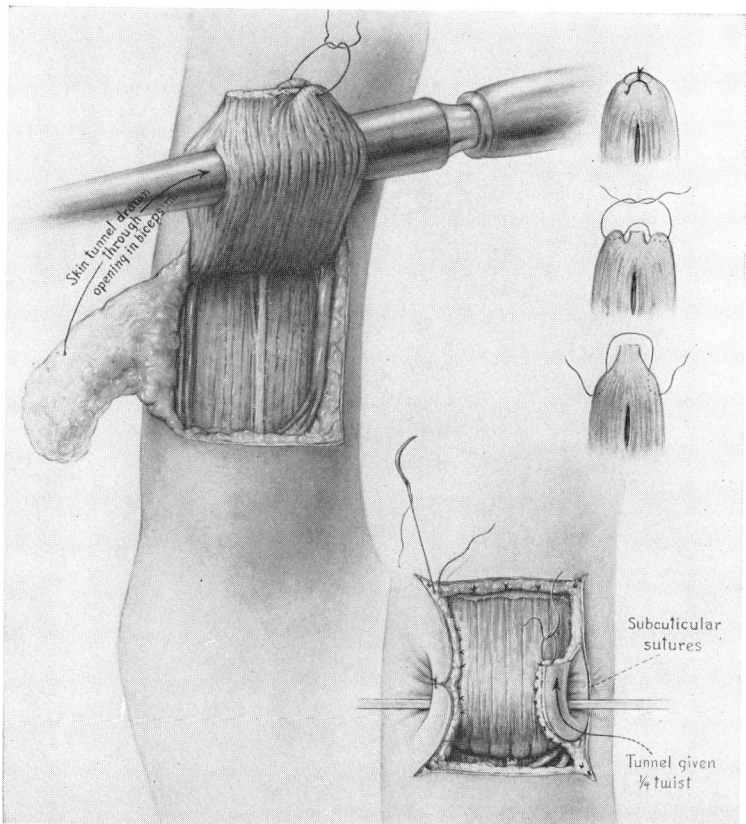

Fig. 382. The flap becomes a skin tube by reversing the flap and suturing the sides. The muscle is then liberated from its distal attachment and the surrounding fascial septa. The tendinous end should be imbricated to provide a smooth nonadherent surface. (A. W. Spittler and I. E. Rosen: J. Bone Joint Surg.)

edges of the rectangular flap. The first suture is laid through the terminal wound edges, and consists of silk or nylon (Fig. 381). The following suture, starting from the periphery toward the base of the flap, is a row of interrupted suture or a removable running percutaneous wire suture, which is laid through the skin edges to hold the tube together. The muscle is now perforated. The perforation is enlarged with a muscle dilator (rectal

959

dilators of various thickness do as well) (Fig. 382). The perforation must be made larger than the skin tube, but should not cause perforation of the muscle. The muscle should be perforated through the distal end of the muscle fibers, which is considerably distal to the skin tube. The elbow is now flexed so shift the biceps perforation proximally to the level of the skin tube. By retracting the distal wound edge, the biceps tendon and the lacertus fibrosus are severed, and the muscle is well liberated from the surrounding fascial septa. If the elbow is now extended, the biceps perforation will remain at the level of the skin canal. Before the skin tube is pulled through the muscle perforation, the tendinous end is carefully imbricated (Fig. 382), to cover the raw tendon stump. In this way, a smooth nonadherent surface is provided. The skin tube is then pulled through the perforation with the help of several traction sutures laid

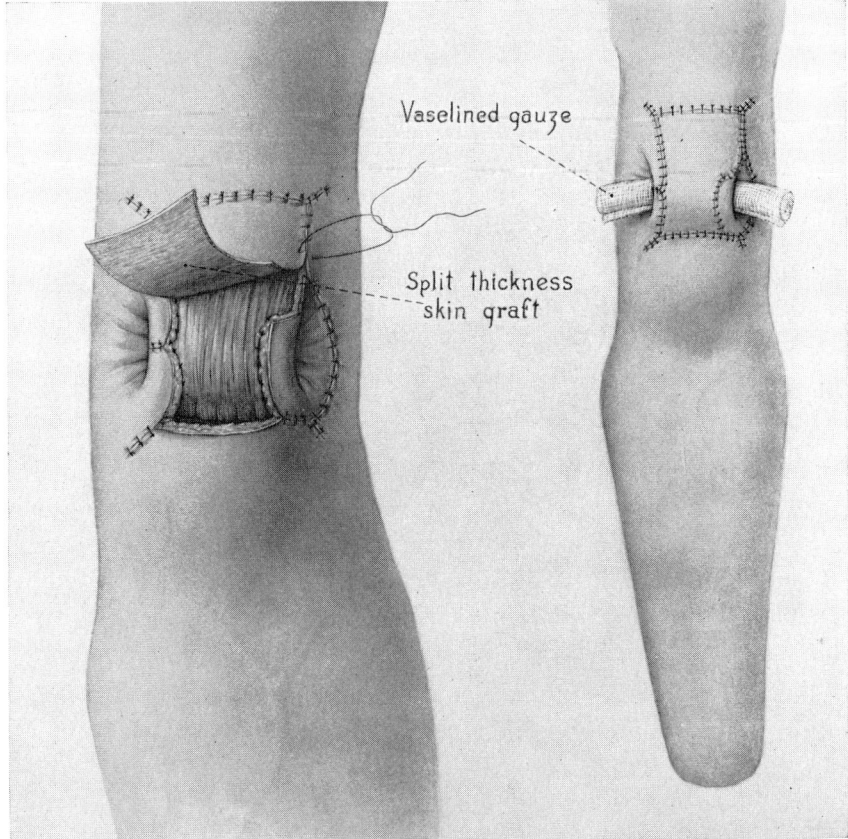

Fig. 383. A split-thickness skin graft is adequate to cover the exposed muscle surface. It should be noted that the distal end of the skin tube is well opened up over the muscle to shift the pin pressure from the suture line. (A. W. Spittler and I. E. Rosen: J. Bone Joint Surg.)

960

through the rim of the tube. To place the seam of the tube away from the pressure pull of the rod when the prosthesis is used, the traction sutures should rotate the tube so that the seam is displaced more proximally. The wound is now narrowed as much as possible with subcuticular sutures of cotton, starting with closure of the corners. If possible, the terminal part of the skin tube should project somewhat beyond the muscle, so that its very end can be opened up and spread over the muscle. This helps to cover the denuded area, and later shifts the pressure of the rod from the suture line. The rim of the proximally rotated skin tube is now sutured posteriorly to the skin edges of the wound and anteriorly to the muscle with subcuticular cotton sutures. The remainder of the raw area is covered with a thick split skin graft. A piece of tribromophenate (xeroform) gauze is drawn through the tube, and a heavily padded pressure dressing is applied.

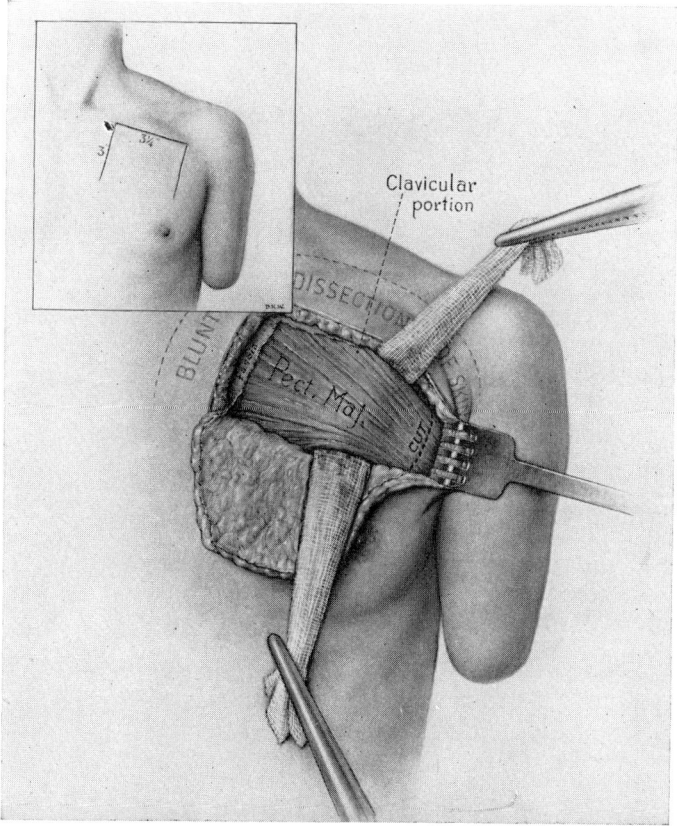

Fig. 384. Cineplasty. Construction of pectoral muscle canals. The cineplastic procedure is much the same in the preparation of pectoralis motors as it is in the creation of biceps motors. (A. W. Spittler and I. E. Rosen: J. Bone Joint Surg.)

THE EXTREMITIES

Construction of Pectoral Muscle Canal (Figs. 384-387): The general principles are the same as just described, and the details are depicted in the illustrations. It may, however, become necessary after raising the flap to make a separate incision over the anterior axillary fold to expose the insertion of the pectoral muscle. This incision, about 10 to 12 cm. (4 to

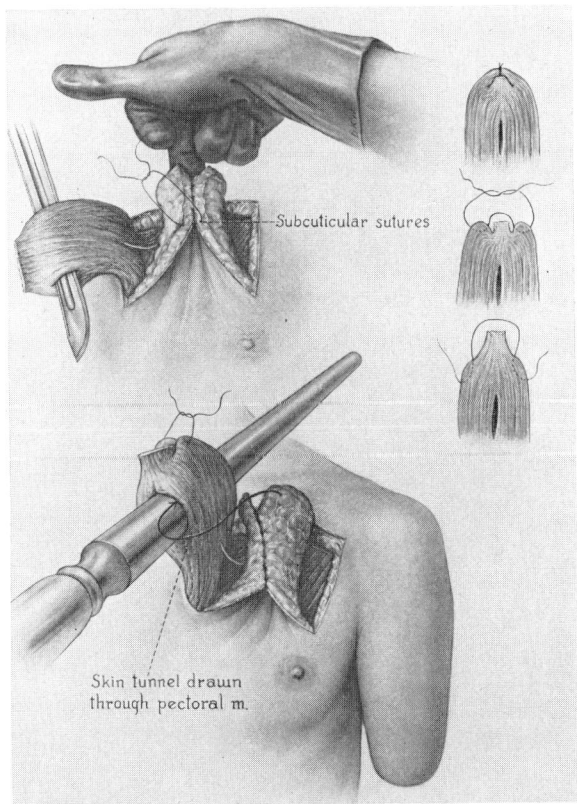

Fig. 385. A skin tunnel is created by reversing the flap and suturing the sides. Note the preparation of the tendinous end. The muscle belly is then slowly and carefully dilated to allow for the insertion of the skin tunnel. (A. W. Spittler and I. E. Rosen: J. Bone Joint Surg.)

4¾ inches) long, should be laid vertically from the center of the lateral wound edge of the donor site of the flap toward the axilla.

After-Treatment

The dressings are changed after twelve days; the sutures are removed, and molds are taken of the tunnel for the construction of the pins. The conventional ivory pins are not quite satisfactory, since they tend to slip. Spittler advises rods of acrylic plastic over a wire cable thick enough to fill the canal. The rod is curved distally on each end to keep each centered in its place. If a tunnel is slightly oblique, the end of the rod may be curved to compensate. After the first dressing, the patient is advised to do active muscle exercises with the motor muscle. After

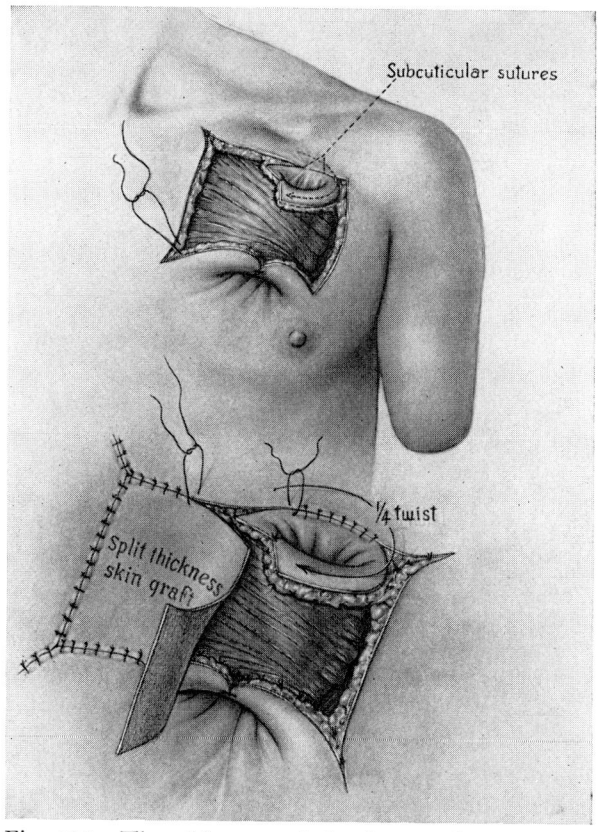

Fig. 386. The skin tunnel is drawn through the opening in the pectoralis and the mouth of the tunnel is sutured to the adjacent skin. The denuded muscle is covered with a split-thickness skin graft. (A. W. Spittler and I. E. Rosen: J. Bone Joint Surg.)

complete healing, the rod is inserted, pull is exerted on it by the patient or somebody else, and the patient performs passive motion exercises. Later, the rod is attached to a weight for hanging or horizontal pull, and the weights are increased daily. The canals are cleansed daily with applicators, using soap, water, and alcohol (no powder). A cineplasty prosthesis is fitted in the meantime. Until recently, the only one was the German type, which was very delicate and lacking in functional qualities. Improve-

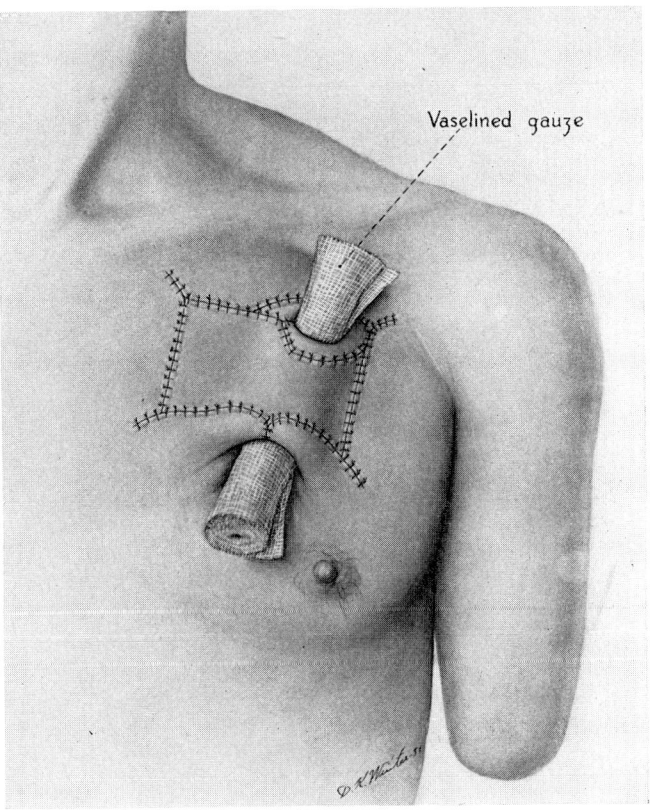

Fig. 387. A small roll of xeroform gauze is inserted in the tunnel. After ten or fourteen days, exercise is started with a forceps attached to each end of the dressing in the tunnel. (A. W. Spittler and I. E. Rosen: J. Bone Joint Surg.)

ments have now been made in this country, mainly at the Army Prosthesis Research Laboratory under Colonel Spittler and his group at the Walter Reed Army Medical Center and at the Henry Kessler Institute. There are orthopedic firms, such as Hanger, etc., which furnish adequate prostheses according to the specifications of the Prosthesis Research Laboratory.

FORCIPICATION OF FOREARM STUMP (KRUKENBERG'S METHOD)

This method consists essentially of splitting the forearm between ulna and radius and mobilizing the radius. The radius now moves independently from and against the ulna; hence, its mobility can be used in

964

a forceps-like manner to grasp things. The method can be successfully employed only in long forearm stumps. The optional length of the latter should be two thirds or one half of the forearm. Stumps which are too long are not suitable either. The best results are achieved if the distances between the tips of the branches and the opening angles are between 10 and 15 cm. (4 and 6 inches). This pincer arrangement is, although useful, a hideous thing, and patients often refuse the operation for cosmetic

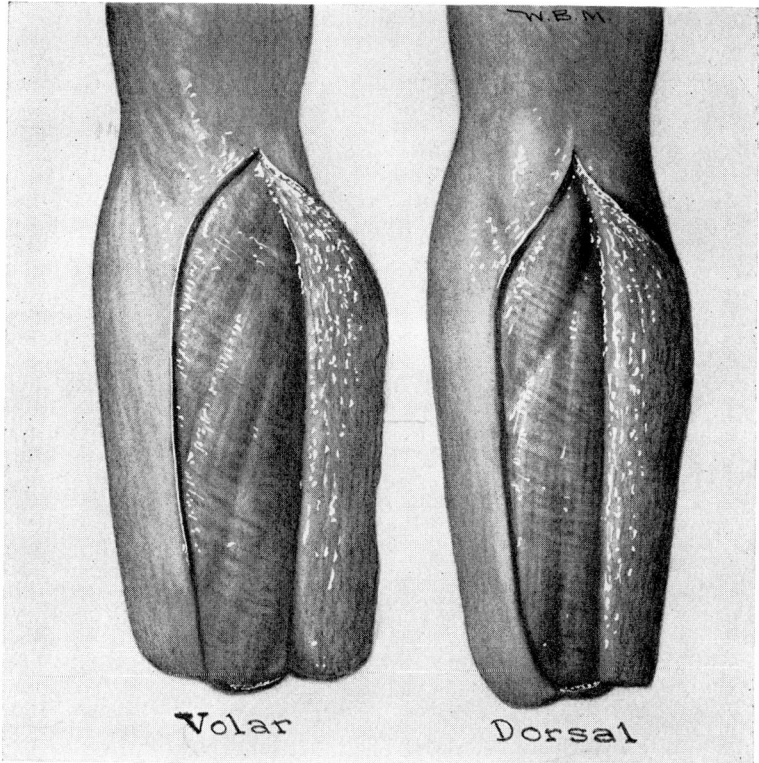

Fig. 388. Forcipication of forearm after Krukenberg-Kallio. Volar and dorsal skin flaps outlined.

reasons. For this and other reasons, the operation was not popular in this country. However, more interest has been stimulated since World War II, due mainly to the U. S. Army group under Aldridge, who had been sent to Germany to study the results of the cineplastic operations in Germany during the war, and particularly to K. E. Kallio, of Finland, who with forty-five personal cases has had the largest experience with the Krukenberg method. Kallio visited this country in 1948, and demonstrated the technique and his results with an impressive moving picture;

he later followed up the subject in an extensive article. Zanobi of Italy, Sung of China, and Boos of Germany corroborate Kallio's enthusiasm about this subject.

The forcipication of the forearm is in competition with cinematization. It has been argued that the patient has greater usefulness of the stump and a stronger grip after cineplasty than after forcipication; this, according to Kallio's experience, appears not to be true. An added advantage of forcipication is a normal sensation of the stump, so that this method becomes the method of choice in blind forearm amputees. Everybody who has experience with forcipication agrees that the best results are achieved in bilateral amputees or in those who have had one forearm amputated and the other hand badly damaged. A successful operation results in a forearm stump supplied with grasping function, a sufficient

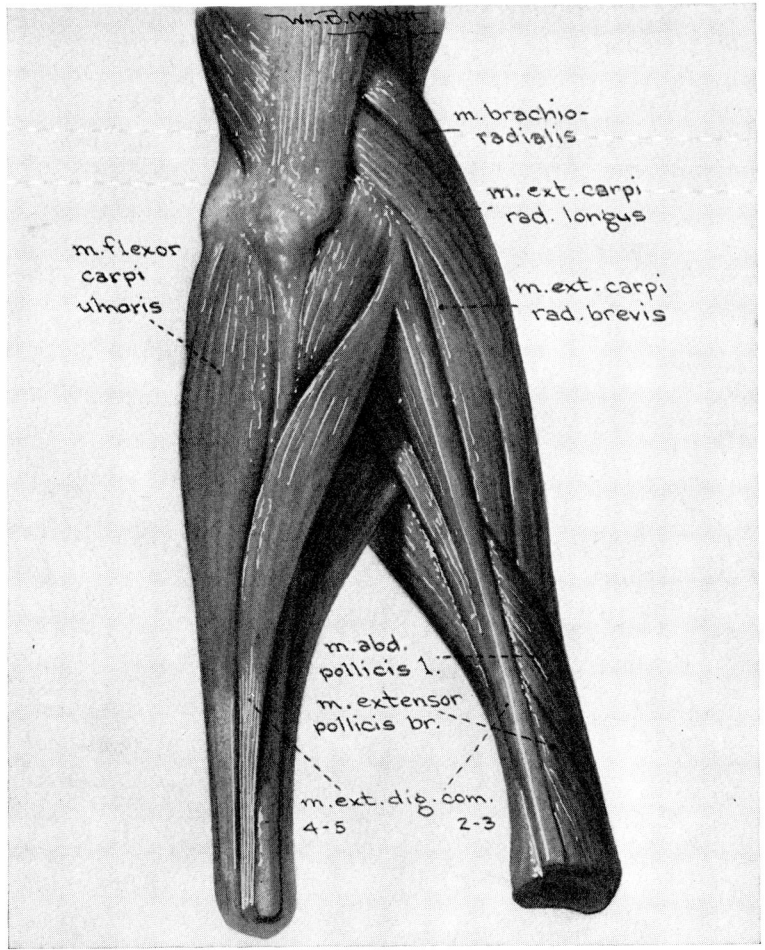

Fig. 389.   Dorsal view of split forearm.

opening angle of from about 30 to 45 degrees, a straight, hinge-like abduction and adduction when the stump is either flexed or extended, a good grasping power (about 5 to 10 kg.), a rate of motion approaching that of the normal human fingers (about 100 to 190 times a minute), a good sensation, and a good blood supply of the branches.

The operation was formerly performed in two stages. Kallio and Thompson, however, have recently advocated the use of a free skin graft to cover the raw dorsal surface of the ulna branch instead of an abdominal flap. Hence, the operation can be completed in one stage. In selected cases, the forcipication can be performed at the time of the amputation of the forearm. Kallio does not sacrifice some of the muscles, as Krukenberg originally advised; Kallio and Langenskiold devised a different way of skin incisions and development of local flaps so that the contact surfaces of the branches can be covered with local skin, and thus have normal sensation.

Technique (Figs. 388, 390; Case 168, p. 1219)

With a pneumatic tourniquet applied, a longitudinal incision is made on the dorsal aspect of the forearm along the edge of the ulna (Fig. 388). On the volar aspect, the incision is made slightly radially from the midline (Fig. 388). At the proximal end, these incisions are curved —the dorsal incision radially, the volar ulnarly. On the dorsal aspect, the skin is then mobilized slightly radially and on the volar aspect slightly ulnarly, to form two flaps of skin. The incision is then deepened on the extensor side (Fig. 389). It penetrates between the muscles so that the musculus extensor digitorum communis is divided into a radial and an ulnar part. The radial contains the tendons of the second and third finger, the ulnar the tendons of the fourth and fifth fingers. On the ulnar side are also the musculus extensor carpi ulnaris. On the radial side remain the musculus brachioradialis, musculus extensor carpi radialis (longus and brevis), and also the abductor and extensor muscles of the thumb. The incision is now continued on the flexor side (Fig. 390). The musculous flexor carpi radialis remains on the radial side; the musculus flexor digitorum sublimis and the musculus flexor digitorum profundus are divided into radial and ulnar parts. On the radial side also remains the musculus flexor pollicis longus. The main trunks of the vessels do not come in sight. The peripheral part of the median nerve is resected. The corresponding muscle groups are held together with a few sutures. The ligamentum interosseum is divided along the ulna. The arteria interossea should not be injured. When the splitting of the stump is finished, the dorsal flap is turned around the radial branch; it should be long enough to be sutured to the radial edge of the volar incision. Should this, how-ever, not be possible, the skin edges are approximated as much and as safely as possible, and the remaining raw area is skin grafted. The volar flap is too narrow to cover the entire branch, but it should have sufficient width to cover the volar aspect. The remaining dorsal raw

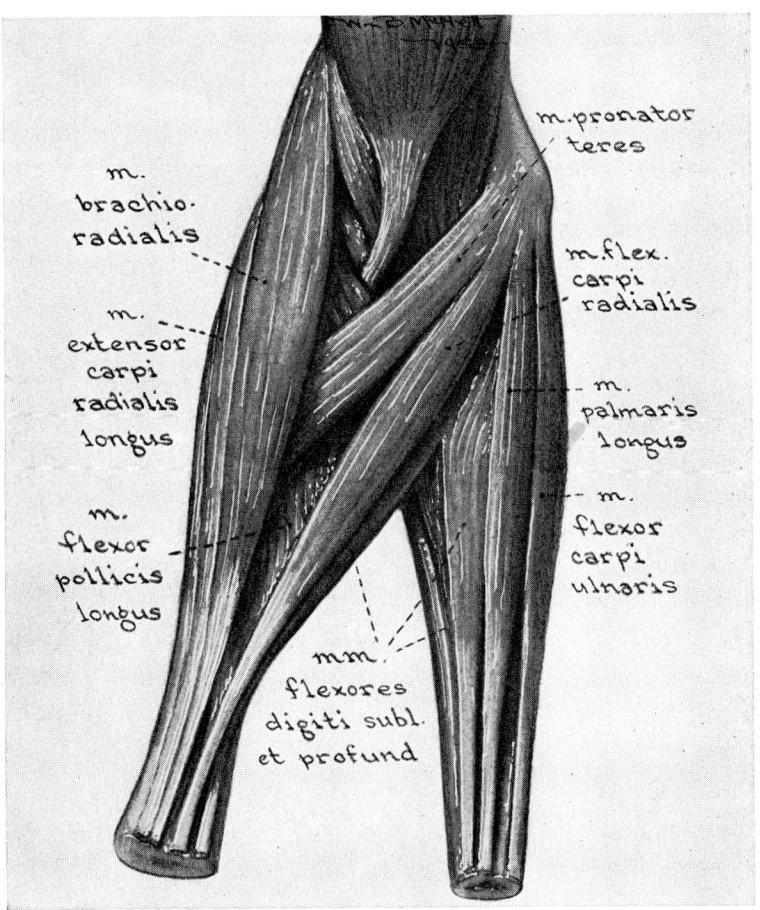

Fig. 390. Volar view of split forearm.

surface of the ulna is covered with a large thick split graft. A pressure dressing is then applied to the grafted area.

After-Treatment

The dressings are removed on the tenth postoperative day, and active exercises should be started immediately. In this operation, the fore-arm stump is cleft and formed into a kind of forceps, the radial branch of which is made to move actively against the ulnar branch. The majority of muscles, however, surrounding each branch move rather in pronation and supination than in abduction and adduction. By mere pronation and supination, objects are grasped with difficulty, since they are grasped with a twist. Hence, the exercises from the very beginning must aim at abduction and adduction; rotation must be avoided. Kallio found the following method helpful: The radial branch of the claw is grasped tightly, and the patient is asked to bend both his elbows simultaneously; experience has shown that by this motion the ulna is invariably adducted straight against the radius. The ulna is then fixed, and the patient is asked to straighten the elbow joint. To enable the patient to make good use of the hand even during the period of training, he is made to write with a pen furnished with a wedge-shaped handle of cork. His fork, knife, and spoon have special handles (Case 168, p. 1219). The patient is given a prosthesis only when the new hand is fully trained and the patient desires a prosthesis. Kallio found value in a combined prosthesis, consisting of a cosmetic hand and a detachable utility hook.

BIBLIOGRAPHY

ALDRIDGE, R. H.: *The cineplastic method in upper extremity amputations.* J. Bone Joint Surg., 30A:359, 1948.

BARSKY, A. J.: *Congenital anomalies of the hand.* J. Bone Joint Surg., 33A: 35, 1951.
Congenital Abnormalities of the Hand and their Surgical Treatment. Charles C Thomas, Springfield, 1958.
Cleft hand: Classification, incidence, and treatment. Review of the literature and report of nineteen cases. J. Bone Joint Surg., 46A:1707, 1964.
Macrodactyly. J. Bone Joint Surg., 49A:1255, 1967.
Reconstructive surgery in congenital anomalies of the hand. Surg. Clin. N. Amer., 39:449, 1959.
Restoration of thumb. Surgery, 23:227, 1948. (Year Book of Orthopedics and Traumatic Surgery, Year Book Publishers, Chicago.)

BAUER, K. H.: *Methods of repair of radial palsy.* Chirurg, 17-18:272, 1946-1947.

BLAIR, V. P., and BYARS, L. T.: *Toe to finger transplant.* Ann. Surg., 112:287, 1940.

BOOS, O.: *Die Versorgung von Einhändern.* Friedrich-Karl Schattauer-Verlag, Stuttgart, 1960.

BOWE, J. J.: *Thumb construction by index transposition.* Plast. Reconstr. Surg., 32:415, 1963.

BROADBENT, T. R., and WOOLF, R. M.: *Thumb reconstruction with continuous skin-bone pedicle graft.* Plast. Reconstr. Surg., 86:494, 1960.

THE EXTREMITIES

BRUNER, J. M.: *Use of single iliac-bone graft to replace multiple metacarpal loss in dorsal injuries of the Hand.* J. Bone Joint Surg., 39A:43, 1957.
Use of single large iliac-bone graft to replace multiple metacarpal loss. J. Bone Joint Surg., 38A:914, 1956.

BUCK-GRAMCKO, D.: *Daumenersatz aus dem zweiten, Mittelhandknochen bei Verlust des ersten und zweiten Fingers.* Langenbeck's Arch. f. klin. Chir., 306:153, 1964.
Indikation und Technik der Daumenbildung bei Aplasie und Hypoplasie. Chir. Plast. et Reconstr., 5:46, 1968, Springer-Verlag, Berlin.

BUNCKE, H. F., and SCHULZ, W. P.: *Experimental digital amputation and reimplantation.* Plast. Reconstr. Surg., 36:62, 1965.

BUNNELL, S.: *Physiological reconstruction of a thumb after total loss.* Surg. Gynec. Obstet., 52:245, 1931.
Surgery of the Hand, 3rd Ed. J. B. Lippincott, Philadelphia, 1956.

BUNNELL, S., and DEHME, E.: *Z-plasty for clinarthrosis of the wrist.* Plast. Reconstr. Surg., 16:169, 1955.

CANNON, B., GRAHAM, W. C., and BROWN, J. B.: *Restoration of grasping function following loss of all five digits.* Surgery, 25:420, 1949.

CANTY, T. J.: *New cineplastic prosthesis.* J. Bone Joint Surg., 33A:612, 1951.

CLARKSON, P.: *Reconstruction of hand digits by toe transfers.* J. Bone Joint Surg., 37A:270, 1955.

D'AUBIGNÉ, R. M., TUBIANA, R., and RAMADIER, J. O.: *Reconstruction du pouce.* Memoires de L'Academie de Chirurgie, 76:901, 1950.
The reconstruction of the thumb (reconstruction du pouce). Rev. Chir. Orthop. 38:456, 1952.

DAVIS, J. S.: *Present evaluation of the merits of the Z-plastic operation.* Plast. Reconstr. Surg., 1:26, 1946.

DAVIS, J. E.: *Toe to hand transfers (Pedochryodactyloplasty.)* Plast. Reconstr. Surg., 33:422, 1964.

DOUGLAS, B.: *Successful replacement of completely avulsed portions of fingers as composite grafts.* Plast. Reconstr. Surg., 23:213, 1959.
Union of severed arterial trunks and canalization without suture or prosthesis. Ann. Surg., 157:944, 1963.

EDGERTON, M. T., SNYDER, G. B., and WEBB, WM. L.: *Surgical treatment of congenital thumb deformities (including psychological impact of correction).* J. Bone Joint Surg., 47A:1453, 1965.

v. EISELSBERG, F.: *Ersatz des Zeigefingers.* Arch. f. klin. Chir., 61:988, 1900.

ENDER, J., KROTSCHECK, H., and SIMON-WEIDNER, R.: *Die Chirurgie der Handverletzungen.* Springer-Verlag in Wien, 1956.

ENTIN, M. A.: *Reconstruction of congenital abnormalities of the upper extremities.* J. Bone Joint Surg., 41A:681, 1959.

FLYNN, J. R., and BURDEN, C. N.: *Reconstruction of the thumb.* Arch. Surg., 85:395, 1962.

970

THE HAND AND FINGERS IN TOTO

FURLONG, R.: *Injuries to the Hand.* Little, Brown & Co., Boston, 1957.

GEORG, H.: *Kritische Betrachtungen zur aufgeschobenen Primäryersorgung von Handverletzungen; Indikation und Ergebnisse.* Langenbeck's Arch. f. Klin. Chir., 306:157, 1964.

GILLIES, H., and REID, D. A. C.: *Autograft of the amputated digit.* Brit. J. Plast. Surg., 7:388, 1955.

GILLIES, SIR. H.: *Autograft of amputated digit, a suggested operation.* Lancet, i. 1,002, 1940.

GILLIES, SIR. H., and CUTHBERT, J. B.: *Operation for Pollicization of the Index Finger.* Med. Annual, p. 262. John Wright & Sons Ltd., Bristol, 1943.

GOSSET, J.: *La Pollicisation de l'index.* J. Chir. (Paris), 65:403, 1949.

GRAHAM, W. C., BROWN, J. B., and CANNON, B.: *Elongation and digitalization of first metacarpal for restoration of function of the hand.* Arch. Surg., 61:17, 1950.

GREELEY, P. W.: *Reconstruction of the thumb.* Ann. Surg., 124:60, 1946.

HILGENFELDT, V.: *Fingerstrumpfverlängerung und Daumenbildung durch Knochenvorverpflanzung.* Handchirurgie, 1:38, 1969.
Operativer Daumenersatz und Beseitigung von Greifstörungen bei Fingerverlusten. Ferd. Enke, Stuttgart, 1950.

HUGHES, N. C., and MOORE, F. T.: *A preliminary report on the use of a local flap and peg bone graft for lengthening a short thumb.* Brit J. Plast. Surg., 3:34, 1950.

HYROOP, G. L.: *Transfer of a metacarpal, etc.* Plast. Reconstr. Surg., 4:45, 1949.

ISELIN, M.: *Chirurgie de la Main (Surgery of the Hand).* 2nd Ed. Masson et Cie, Paris, 1955.

ISELIN, M., GOSSE, L., BOUSSARD, S., and BENOIST, D.: *Atlas de Technique Operatoire.* Chirurgie de la Main. Flammarion, Paris, 1958.

ISELIN, M., and ISELIN, F.: *Traite de Chirurgie de la Main.* Medicales Flammarion, Paris, 1967.

KALLIO, K. E.: *Sur les opérations plastiques du pouce.* Acta Chir. Scand., 93:231, 1946.
Recent advance in Krukenberg's operation. Acta Chir. Scand. 97:165, 1948.

KALLIO, K. E., and THOMPSON, J. E. M.: *The use of a split thickness graft to cover the skin defect in a Krukenberg amputation.* J. Bone Joint Surg., 33A:260, 1951.

KANAVEL, A. B.: *Congenital malformations of the hand.* Arch. Surg., 25:1, 282, 1932.

KAPLAN, I., and PLASCHKES, J.: *One-stage pollicisation of little finger.* Brit. J. Plast. Surg., 13:272, 1960.

KELIKIAN, H., and BINTCLISSE, E. W.: *Functional restoration of the thumb; pollizication of the index.* Surg. Gynec. Obstet., 83:807, 1946.

KELIKIAN, H., and DOUMANIAN, A.: *Congenital anomalies of the hand.* Part I. J. Bone Joint Surg. 39A:1002, 1957. Part II. 39A:1249, 1957.

THE EXTREMITIES

KELLEHER, J. C., and SULLIVAN, J. G.: *Thumb reconstruction by fifth digit transplantation.* Plast. Reconstr. Surg., 21:470, 1958.

KESSLER, H. H.: *Cineplastic operation in rehabilitation of amputation cases.* Mil. Surgeon, 93:237, 1943.
Cineplasty. Charles C Thomas, Springfield, 1947.

KLAPP, R.: *Ueber einige kleinere plastische Operationen an Fingern und Hand.* Arch. f. klin. Chir., 118:479, 1912.

KOMATSU, S., and TAMAI, S.: *Successful replantation of a completely cut-off thumb.* Plast. Reconstr. Surg., 42:374, 1968.

KRUCKENBERG, H.: *Plastische Umwertung von Armamputations-stümpfen.* Stuttgart, 1917.

LEWIN, M. L.: *Partial reconstruction of thumb in a one-stage operation.* J. Bone Joint Surg., 35A:573, 1953.

LITTLER, J. W.: *Subtotal reconstruction of thumb.* Plast. Reconstr. Surg., 10:215, 1952.
The neurovascular pedicle method of digital transposition for reconstruction of the thumb. Plast. Reconstr. Surg., 12:303, 1953.

LITTLER, J. W., and COOLEY, G. E.: *Congenital dysplasia of the thumb: Reconstruction using the index finger.* Paper presented at the 19th Annual Meeting, Amer. Soc. Surg. of the Hand., Jan 17, 1964, Chicago, Illinois.

LUSCHK: *Daumenplastik.* Wien. klin. Wchnschr., 16:916, 1903; München. med. Wchnschr., 1916, p. 881.
Uber eine neue Methode zum Ersatz des Daumens. Verhandl. d. Deutsch. Ges. f. Chir. 1903. Teil I. 221.

MACHOL: *Beitrag zur Daumenplastik.* Beitr. z. klin. Chir., 114:181, 1919.

MARCER, E.: *Articular transplants from foot to hand (Trapianti articolare dal piede alla mano.)* Arch. Putti Chir. org. mavim., 3:276, 1953.

MATTHEWS, D.: *Congenital absence of functioning thumb.* Plast. Reconstr. Surg., 26:487, 1960.

McGREGOR, I. A., and SIMONETTA, C.: *Reconstruction of the thumb by composite bone-skin flap.* Brit. J. Plast. Surg., 17:37, 1964.

MEYERDING, H. W., and DICKSON, D. D.: *Correction of congenital deformations of the hand.* Amer. J. Surg., 54:218, 1939.

NICHOLS, H. M.: *Manual of Hand Injuries.* Year Book Publishers, Inc., Chicago, 1955.

NICOLADONI, C.: *Daumenplastik and organischer Ersatz der Fingerspitze.* Arch. f. klin. Chir., 61:606, 1900.

NISSEN, R., and BERGMANN, E.: *Cineplastic Operations on Stumps of the Upper Extremity.* Grune & Stratton, New York, 1942.

OEHLECKER, G.: *Ein Daumen durch die grosse Zehe nach Nicoladoni ersetzt.* Deutsche med. Wchnschr., 44:1207, 1919.

PORZELT, W.: *Daumenersatz aus dem verstummelten Zeigefinger unter Erhaltung der Trennungsfalte zum Mittelfinger.* Der chirurg, 1933.

972

THE HAND AND FINGERS IN TOTO

PERTHES, G.: *Ueber plastischen Daumenersatz insbesondere bei Verlust des ganzen Daumenstrahles.* Arch. f. orthop. u. Unfall-Chir., 19:199, 1921.

PIERI, G.: *Ricostruzione del pallice dal monconc della falange basale.* Chir. d. org. di movimento., 3:325, 1919.

PIERRE, M., CARCASSONNE, M., and GUASCONI, H.: *Autoplastic Reconstruction of the Thumb. (Reconstruction du pouce par la method autoplastique).* J. Chir. Par., 68:449, 1952.

PRPIC, I.: *Reconstruction of the thumb immediately after injury.* Brit. J. Plast. Surg., 17:49, 1964.

RANK, B. K., and HENDERSON, G. D.: *Cineplastic forearm amputations and prosthesis.* Surg. Gynec. Obstet., 83:373, 1946.

RANK, B. K., and WAKEFIELD, A. R.: *Surgery of Repair as Applied to Hand Injuries.* 2nd Edition. Williams & Wilkins, Baltimore, 1960.

REID, D. A. C.: *Reconstruction of the thumb.* J. Bone Joint Surg., 42B:444, 1960.

SAUERBRUCH, F.: *Die willkürlich bewegbare künstliche Hand.* Julius Springer, Berlin, 1916, 1923 (Lit).

SCHEPELMANN, E.: *Weitere Erfahrungen über Fingerplastik.* Ztschr. f. orthop. Chir., 35:827, 1916.

SNEDECOR, S. T.: *Bone surgery of the hand.* Amer. J. Surg., 72:363, 1946.

SODERBERG, L., *Repair of failing opposition of the thumb.* Acta Orthop. Scand., 22:238, 1953.

SPITTLER, A. W., and ROSEN, I. E.: *Cineplastic muscle motors for prostheses of arm amputees.* J. Bone Joint Surg., 33A:601, 1951.

STEFANI, A. E., and KELLY, A. P.: *Reconstruction of the thumb: A one-stage procedure.* Brit. J. Plast. Surg., 15:289, 1962.

STEINDLER, A.: *Reconstructive Surgery of the Upper Extremity.* D. Appleton & Co., New York, 1923.
Orthopedic Operations. Charles C Thomas, Springfield, 1943.

SUNG, R. Y.: *Experiences with the Krukenberg plastic operation.* Chin. Med. J. 75:212, 1957. (In English) Peking, China.

TANZER, R. C., and LITTLER, J. W.: *Reconstruction of the thumb.* By transposition of an adjacent digit. Plast. Reconstr. Surg., 3:533, 1948.

TUBIANA, R., STACK, H. G., and HAKSTIAN, R. W.: *Restoration of prehension after severe mutilations of the hand.* J. Bone Joint Surg., 48B:455, 1966.

VANGHETTI, G.: *Amputazione, disarticolozioni e protesi.* Florence, 1898.
Note di plastica cinematica. Dhirurgia degli Organi di Movimento, 2, 1, 1918.

YOUNG, F.: *Transplantation of toes for fingers.* Surgery, 20:117, 1946.

ZANOBI, R.: *Krukenberg-Putti amputation-plasty.* J. Bone Joint Surg., 39B:230, 1957.

CONGENITAL MALFORMATIONS OF HAND

32

N<small>UMEROUS</small> attempts have been made to classify the congenital malformations of the hand but thus far these have defied clarity. The task is made more difficult by the overlapping of some of the abnormalities. It is generally agreed that they are due to an arrest or derangement of development during the first eight weeks of intrauterine life. The causes of a great many of these lesions are unknown, in spite of elaborate theories to explain them. Abandoning complex and intricate classifications, congenital malformations of the hand may be roughly grouped into defective development (hypoplasia and aplasia) and excessive development (hyperplasia). Only a brief description of the deformities and their surgical treatment, if such is possible, will be presented. For details, authoritative publications about this subject, such as those by Kanavel, Birch-Jensen, Barsky, Kelikian and Doumanian, Patterson, Witt, Cotta and Jäger, should be consulted.

HYPOPLASIA AND APLASIA

CLUBHAND

Absence of Radius

Kanavel distinguishes four types: (1) complete absence of the radius, (2) a rudiment of the upper end with more or less of the diaphysis

THE EXTREMITIES

present, (3) a rudiment of the lower end with more or less of the diaphysis present, and (4) absence of the diaphysis.

The most common finding is complete absence of the radius or the greater part of its distal portion with radial deviation of the ulna and radial clubhand. Gegenbauer's primitive-ray theory may find support if, as so often, absence of the radius is accompanied by suppression of development of other components of the first ray, which includes radius, os naviculare, os multangulum, the first metacarpal bone, and the thumb. The ulna and other bones of the upper extremity and the shoulder girdle may also be deformed, as may other parts of the body.

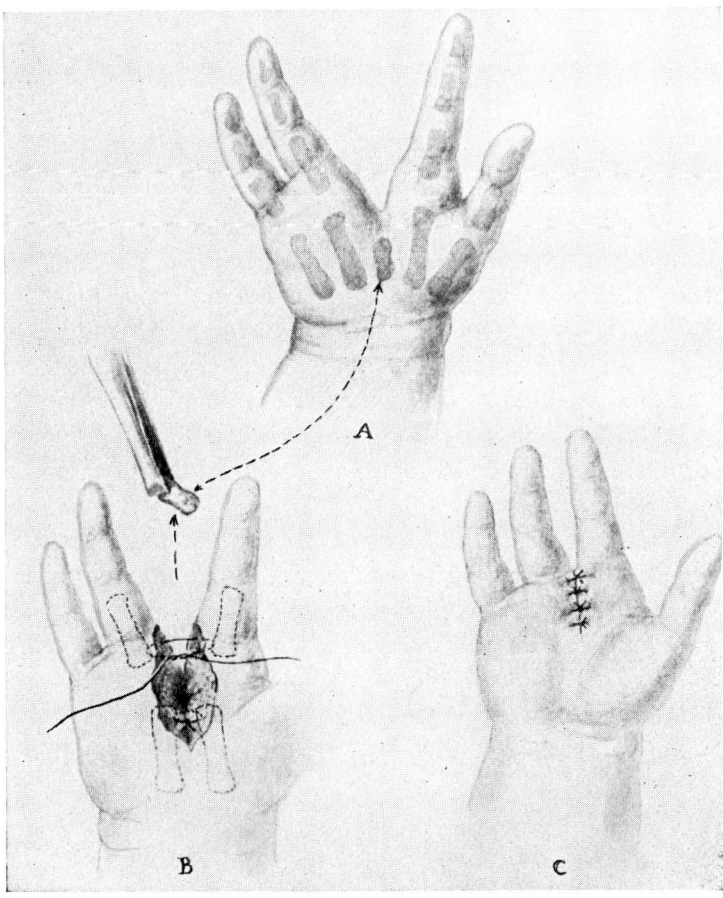

Fig. 391. Cleft hand (lobster hand). Aplasia of middle finger and parts of its metacarpal bone. Removal of metacarpal stump and approximation of radial and ulnar elements. (A. B. Kanavel: Arch. Surg.)

CONGENITAL MALFORMATIONS OF HAND

Regarding the muscular system, it is not uncommon to find absence, fibrosis, or contraction of the most radial muscle bodies. The biceps may be absent and other muscles disorientated. The radial artery is often absent, and nerves and other arteries are disorientated.

Absence of Ulna

This involves not only the ulna but, in varying degrees, the ulnar elements, with ulnar deviation of the radius and ulnar clubhand.

Treatment

If the clubhand deformity is without bone defects, tenotomies and tenoplasties, combined with Z-plasty (Bunnell and Dehne), splinting, and massage of the contracted muscle, are usually sufficient. In severe forms with bone defects, function of the arm may be improved by Z-plasty for lengthening the contracted skin (Bunnell and Dehne) and by osteoplastic

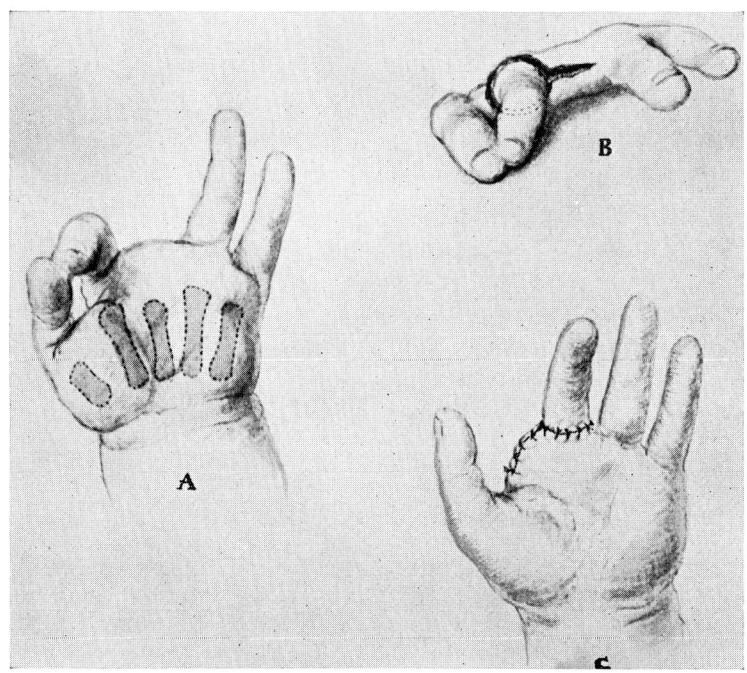

Fig. 392. Cleft hand (lobster hand). Aplasia of middle finger and syndactylism of index finger and thumb. After removal of third metacarpal bone, incision is made around base of proximal phalanx of index finger. Skin is now dissected away to form dorsal and volar flap and second metacarpal bone approximated to that of fourth finger. (A. B. Kanavel: Arch. Surg.)

977

methods, such as osteotomy, arthrodesis, and bone transplantation (methods of Romano, Bardenheuer, Steindler, Albee, Ryerson, Kanavel, and others).

ECTRODACTYLY

Barsky defines ectrodactyly as a congenital absence of one or more digits. The absence of parts of fingers he terms partial ectrodactyly. Some authors use the term in a narrower sense, to pertain to cleft or claw hand deformities (see following) or, according to Birch-Jensen, to defects of the distal phalanx alone. As a rule surgical reconstruction can provide only little functional improvement. It cannot be applied at all to restore missing parts or whole digits except in congenital absence of the thumb

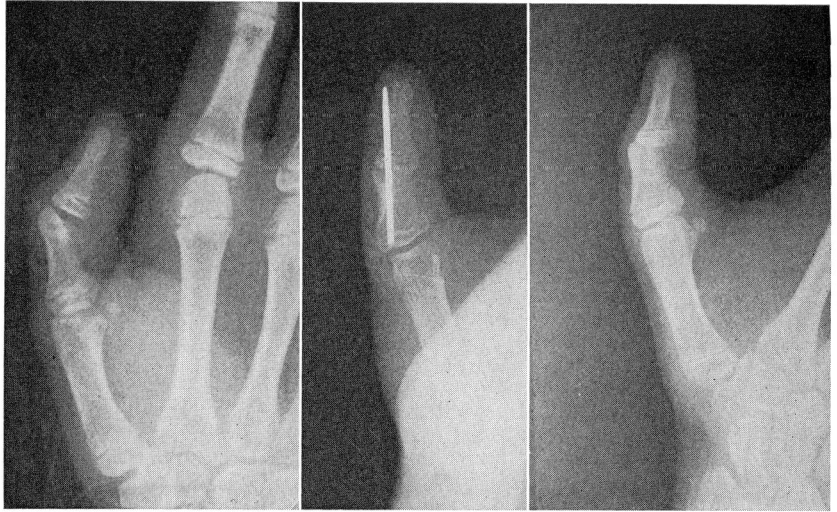

Fig. 393. Clinodactylism of thumb, repaired with arthrodesis of terminal joint in the position of function.

if the index finger is normal. In this case, the index finger can be rotated and transferred on the neurovascular bundle to replace the missing thumb (see p. 944).

Intrauterine amputations, ranging from a small part of a phalanx to the entire extremity, are conditions in which there is evidence that the missing part was present in embryonic development but that at a subsequent stage it was amputated by intrinsic or extrinsic factors. Hence strictly speaking these cases are not ectrodactyly, for in that condition there is no evidence that the digit ever existed.

978

CLEFT HAND (LOBSTER-CLAW HAND)

Strictly speaking, a cleft hand is a form of ectrodactyly (see foregoing), but as far as reconstruction is concerned it constitutes a separate entity. The simple and classic type is aplasia of the middle finger and parts of its metacarpal bones. Every degree of hypoplasia may be found, however, from this simple loss to complete loss of all medial elements with rudimentary elements of the first and fifth digits remaining alone. Associations with syndactylism, polydactylism, and other deformities have been reported. Barsky has discussed this subject from great personal experience.

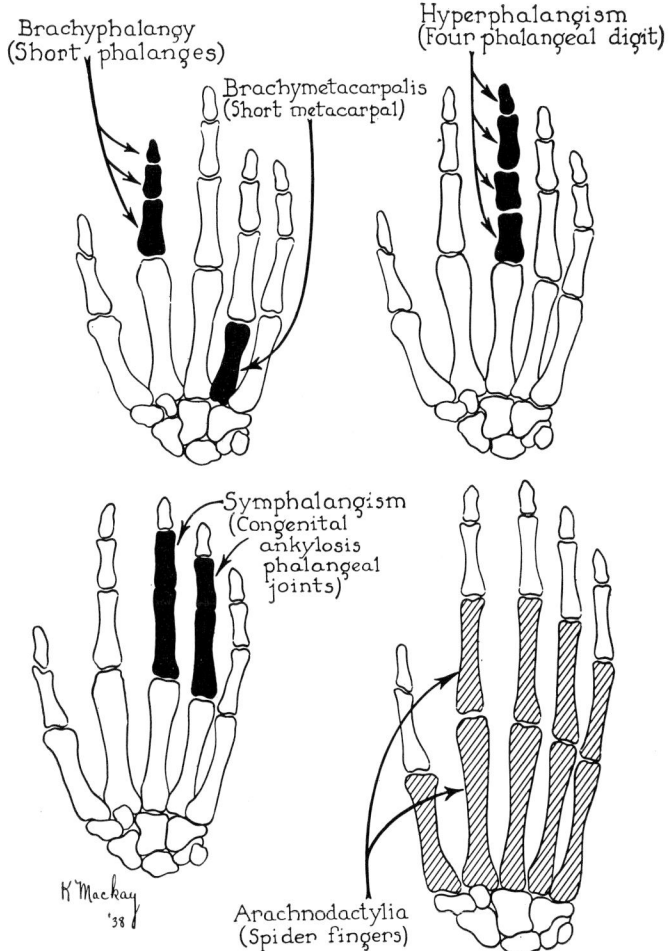

Fig. 394. Types of congenital deformities. (H. W. Myerding and D. D. Dickson: Amer. J. Surg.)

979

Technique (Figs. 391, 392) (Compare with Case 169, p. 1220)

If the deformity is associated with other malformations, the operation must be divided into several stages. If the cleft extends into the palm, a wedge-shaped incision is made extending from the proximal phalanx down through the palm. A deep dissection is then made of the metacarpal bone of the affected finger, and this is removed down to its base. The next object of the procedure is approximation of the fingers of the radial and ulnar sides (see Fig. 391). This position is maintained with slings of fascia lata around the metacarpals and proximal ends of the phalanges of

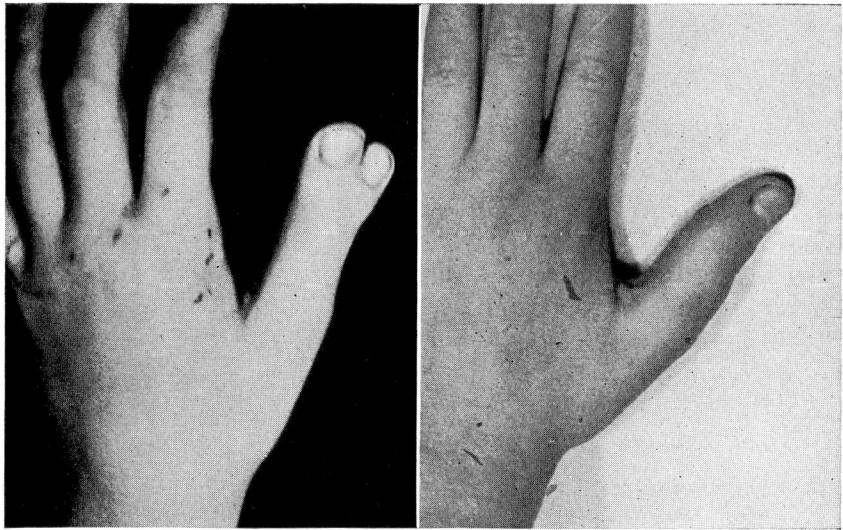

Fig. 395. Bifurcation of distal phalanx of thumb with common joint. Before and one year after removal of radial phalanx.

these fingers (Meyerding and Dickson). The wound is closed in layers. Circular adhesive strips are placed around the dressed palm and fingers to hold the bones together, and are left in place for at least three weeks.

If there is syndactylism of the index finger and thumb and the cleft is not deep, Kanavel devised a procedure for the lengthening of the web between thumb and index finger. The first part of the procedure is the same as just described. From the radial edge of the cleft, another incision is made, which passes around the base of the proximal phalanx of the index finger (see Fig. 392). The skin is now dissected away from the index finger to form dorsal and volar flaps. When the index finger with its metacarpal bone is transferred over to the ring finger, it slides between these two

980

skin flaps, thus leaving skin on the radial side of the index finger for a good web between the index finger and the thumb.

CLINODACTYLISM

This is most often found in the distal joint of the fifth finger. It is probably due to disorientation of the epiphysis, producing improper alignment of the joint surfaces and changes in the capsule which result in contracture of the joint. In early life, the condition can be corrected by proper external or internal (intramedullary pin) splinting. Later, however, surgery is the only choice, and consists of severance of contracting bands, tendon lengthening, and sometimes skin grafting and wedge osteotomies, with insertion of chips of bone to elevate the depressed joint surface. The author, however, sounds a note of warning, since in two of his cases the deformity was associated with insufficient circulatory supply to the fingers. Consequently, only in extreme cases, with definite functional handicap, should repair by surgery be attempted. This is best done by arthrodesis of the involved joint in the position of function (Fig. 393).

CONSTRICTING FURROWS

These so-called "amniotic" furrows are constricting bands consisting of fibrous tissue which may encircle the entire extremity. In the hand, as elsewhere, they may need removal, if such is possible. The multiple Z-operation is recommended. The long arm of the Z is placed within the groove; after exchange of the triangles (see Fig. 52), the groove is displaced vertically (Case 138, p. 1180).

BRACHYPHALANGISM, HYPERPHALANGISM, SYMPHALANGISM

Meyerding's illustration of these various deformities is self explanatory (Fig. 394). Surgery is rarely employed for these conditions.

SYNDACTYLISM

This deformity and its correction have been described on page 829.

POLYDACTYLISM

Polydactylism may roughly be divided into a central and a marginal form. The marginal form—that is, an extra thumb or little finger—is by far the more frequent type. The extra digit may originate from a meta-carpophalangeal joint, or there may be a bifurcation of the metacarpal bone or a partial or complete bifurcation of the phalanges. Bifurcation of the phalanges is always accompanied by syndactylism. The phalanges may be of equal (Fig. 396) or unequal size (Fig. 395).

A   B

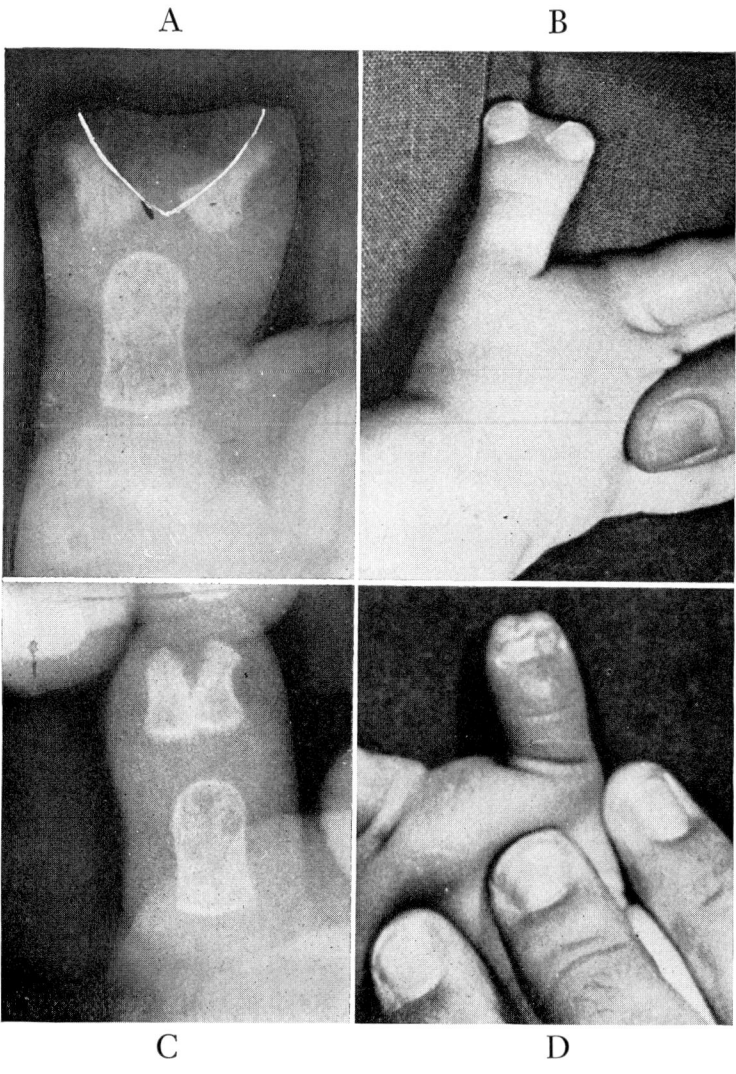

C   D

Fig. 396. *A, B:* Seven-month-old boy with bifurcation of terminal phalanx of right thumb. Both phalangeal elements are well formed. To correct deformity, V-shaped excision of median sections, together with inner (opposing halves) of phalanges, and approximation of outer halves were perfromed (Bilhaut-Cloquet procedure). *C, D:* Four months after operation; full function of joint.

Treatment

Before advisability of surgical treatment is decided, careful roentgenological and clinical studies should be made of the function and blood and nerve supply of the two digits. Nerves, blood vessels, and tendons may have atypical positions. At the thumb particularly, the intrinsic muscles of the thenar region may be atypical; removal of the extra digit may result in a flail finger, unless the tendons of the former are transferred.

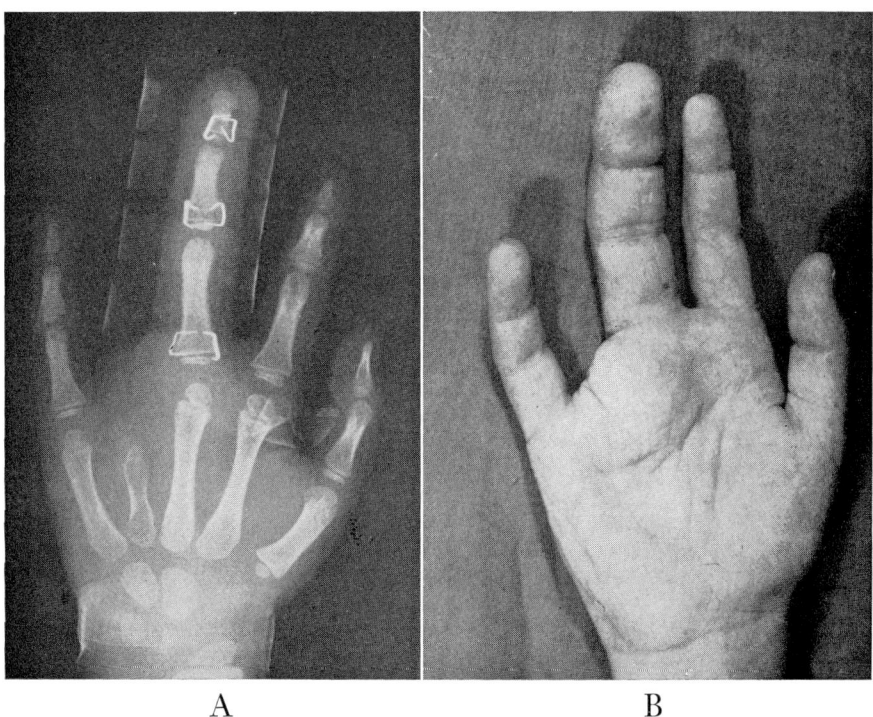

A   B

Fig. 397. *A:* Megalodactylism (giant finger): Fourth finger amputated due to rapid growth. Epiphyseal lines of third finger stapled to check growth. *B:* This picture is taken three years after roentgenogram; neither stapling nor irradiation checked growth. Finger has been amputated in the meantime due to increasing radiating pain and "embarrassment."

Hence, preservation of function should be the primary consideration. The operation is usually carried out before the child goes to school (Figs. 395, 396).

An oval incision is made at the base of the joint capsule of the extra digit, and tendons are exposed The tendons are severed and permitted to retract unless they are to be used for transfer. The joint capsule is opened and the digit disarticulated. The remainder of the capsule is

983

removed as is any abnormal bone protrusion. If an extra metacarpal bone is present, the incision is lengthened proximally until the base of the bone is reached. The bone is excised and the wound closed in layers.

In case of a bifurcation of the distal phalanx, the extra phalanx, if it is rudimentary, may be simply excised. If, however, both phalangeal elements are well formed, the Bilhaut-Cloquet procedure (Fig. 396) is advisable. This is a V-shaped excision of the median section, together with the inner (opposing) halves of the phalanges, and approximation of the outer halves. If the two phalanges are of different length, the incision must be modified to some degree.

If two functionally and anatomically abnormal thumbs are present, amputation of one of them does not necessarily improve the function and morphology of the hand, as Karchinov states. He recommends forming one thumb by making use of the existing two defective thumbs through a superposition operation.

HYPERPLASIA

MEGALODACTYLISM

This deformity appears in two forms: one due to bone growth alone, the other due to neurofibrosis. The latter, being an elephantiasic deformity, is a false form of megalodactylism, as recognized by x-ray examination. In the former, the bone overgrowth usually involves the three phalanges; the metacarpals are excluded. Barsky and Tsuge have discussed this topic recently. Barsky offers procedures to reduce the length of the phalanges. Tsuge, following McCarole's advice, partially resected the digital nerve together with the neurofibrotic tissue in the elephantiastic type with success, but amputation of such a finger may be considered after all.

In the author's experience, irradiation of the epiphyseal lines or stapling of the epiphyseal lines (Fig. 397) to stop growth has not been successful.

ARACHNODACTYLISM

This condition is well illustrated in Figure 394.

BIBLIOGRAPHY

ALBEE, F.: *Orthopedic and Reconstructive Surgery.* W. B. Saunders Co., Philadelphia, 1919.
Formation of radius, congenitally absent, condition seven years after implantation of bone graft. Ann. Surg., 87:105, 1928.

BIRCH-JENSEN, A.: *Congenital Deformities of the Upper Extremities.* Einar Munksgaard, 1949.

BLACKFIELD, H. M., and HAUSE, D. P.: *Congenital constricting bands of the extremities.* Plast. Reconstr. Surg., 8:101, 1951.

ENTIN, M. A.: *Reconstruction of congenital abnormalities of the upper extremities.* J. Bone Joint Surg., 41A:681, 1959.

KANAVEL, A. B.: *Congenital malformations of the hand.* Arch. Surg., 25:1, 282, 1932.

KARCHINOV, K.: *The treatment of polydactyly of the hand.* Brit. J. Plast. Surg., 15:362, 1962.

KELIKIAN, H., and DOUMANIAN, A.: *Congenital anomalies of the hand.* Part I, J. Bone Joint Surg., 39A:1002, 1957, Part II, 39A:1249, 1957.

MEYERDING, H. W., and DICKSON, D. D.: *Correction of congenital deformations of the hand.* Amer. J. Surg., 54:218, 1939.

MULLER, W.: *Die angeborenen Fehlbildungen der menschlichen Hand.* Leipzig, Thieme, 1937.

PATTERSON, R. J. S.: *Classification of the congenitally deformed hand.* Brit. J. Plast. Surg., 17:142, 1964.

TSUGE, K.: *Treatment of macrodactyly.* Plast. Reconstr. Surg., 39:590, 1967.

WITT, A. N., COTTA, H., and JAGER, M.: *Die angeborenen Fehlbildungen der Hand und ihre operative Behandlung. (Congenital Abnormalities of the Hand and Their Operative Treatment.)* Stuttgart, Georg Thieme Verlag, 1966.

(See also BARSKY references, page 969.)

DIVISION
FIVE
ILLUSTRATIVE
CASES

CASE

1

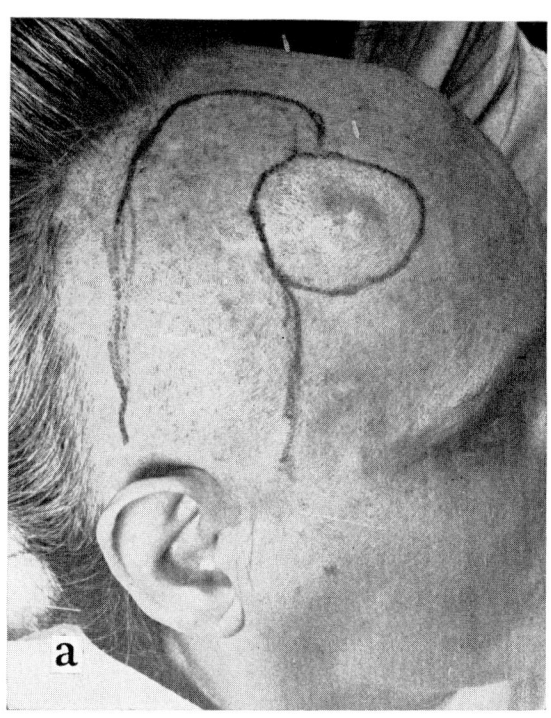

Case 1, *a:* Patient, aged sixty-five, with recurrent (colloid) carcinoma of right side of forehead. Wide excision of the tumor is marked out. A flap containing the temporal vessels to be rotated into the defect is outlined.

b: Upon operation it was found that the galea aponeurotica was not invaded. The tumor was removed with the underlying periosteum and part of the external table. The flap was rotated into the defect, care being taken to preserve the periosteum of the donor area. A thick split graft was transplanted upon the donor area.

c: Eight months after the operation. No evidence of recurrence of the tumor was noted nine years after the operation.

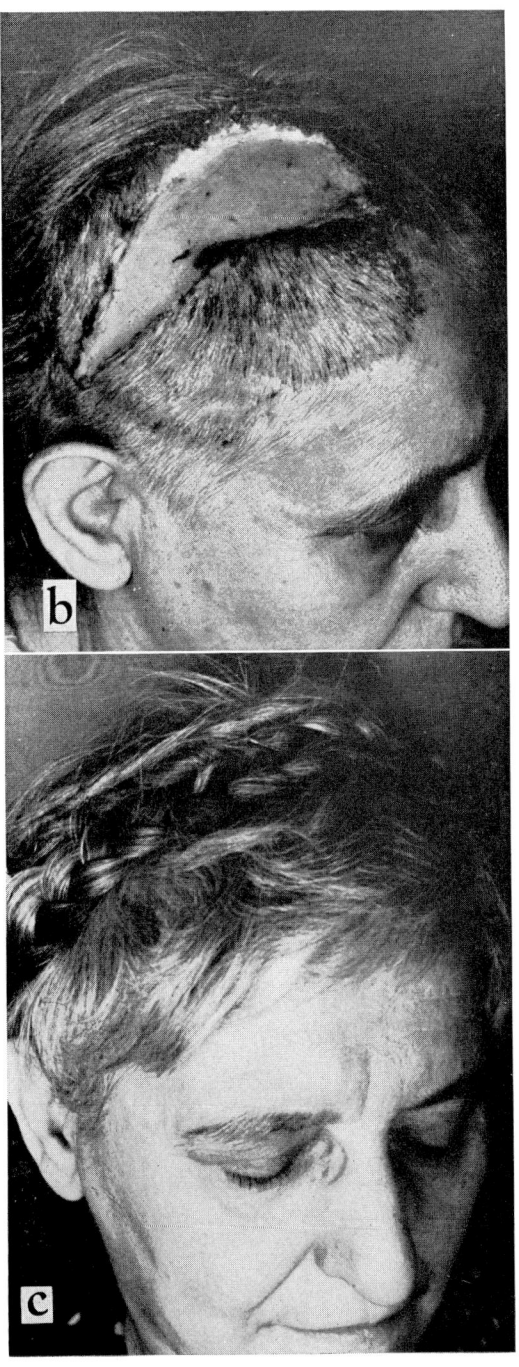

CASE
2

a

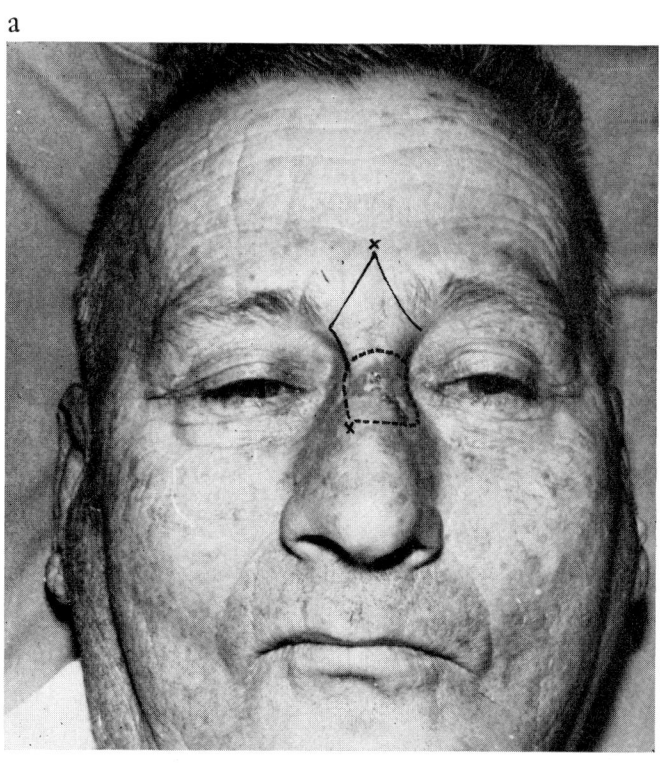

Case 2, *a:* Basal cell carcinoma at root of nose. Part to be excised marked with dotted lines. Rhomboid flap to be rotated into the defect lined out above the latter; pedicle on left side. Tip of flap x to be sutured to corner of defect marked x.

990

b

b: One week after operation.

ILLUSTRATIVE CASES

CASE
3

Case 3: Patient, aged thirty-eight, was working when flash powder exploded. Her entire face, both hands, arms, chest, and legs were burned. She was treated immediately for shock; after she had recovered from the latter, the burn areas were treated by washing with soap and water and by application of pressure dressings. The pressure dressings were removed on the twelfth day. After the third-degree burn areas sloughed off, skin-grafting operations were performed to cover the raw areas. In thirteen operations, the raw surfaces of face and upper extremities were covered, followed by repair of contractures of both axillas, both elbow joints, both wrists, and the dorsum of the right hand.

a: In the meantime, ectropion of the right lower lid, severe contracture of the neck, and microstoma had developed. The microstoma was of such degree that it was impossible to insert an endotracheal tube for administration of anesthesia. Microstoma was repaired under local anesthesia (*d*).

b: Two operations were necessary to correct the extensive contracture of the neck. The ectropion of the right lower lid was repaired with a full-thickness graft taken from the supraclavicular region. The ectropion of the lip was corrected with a full-thickness graft taken from the abdomen (see also *d, e*). She also had a partial loss of the right ala, which was repaired, according to the method of Figure 182, with a composite graft of full thickness from the anterior part of the helix of the left ear. The dotted line indicates the incision around the defect edges. The incision is placed so that a small flap is formed to be hinged inward for reception of the graft. In *c*, the size of the graft is outlined at the right ear. The graft, however, was taken from the left ear, since the left ear was already damaged.

c: After the reconstruction of the ala.

d: After the finished reconstruction, without makeup.

e: With makeup.

992

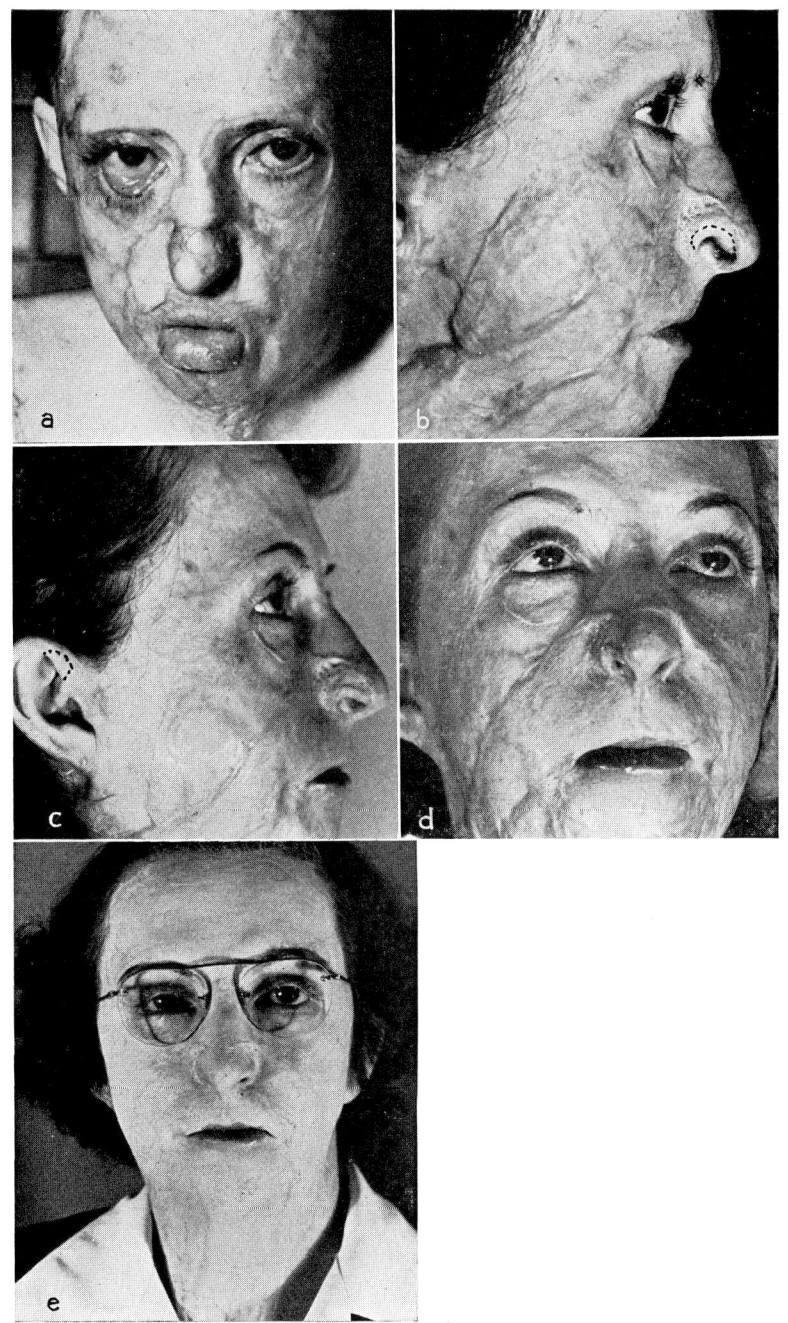

CASE

4

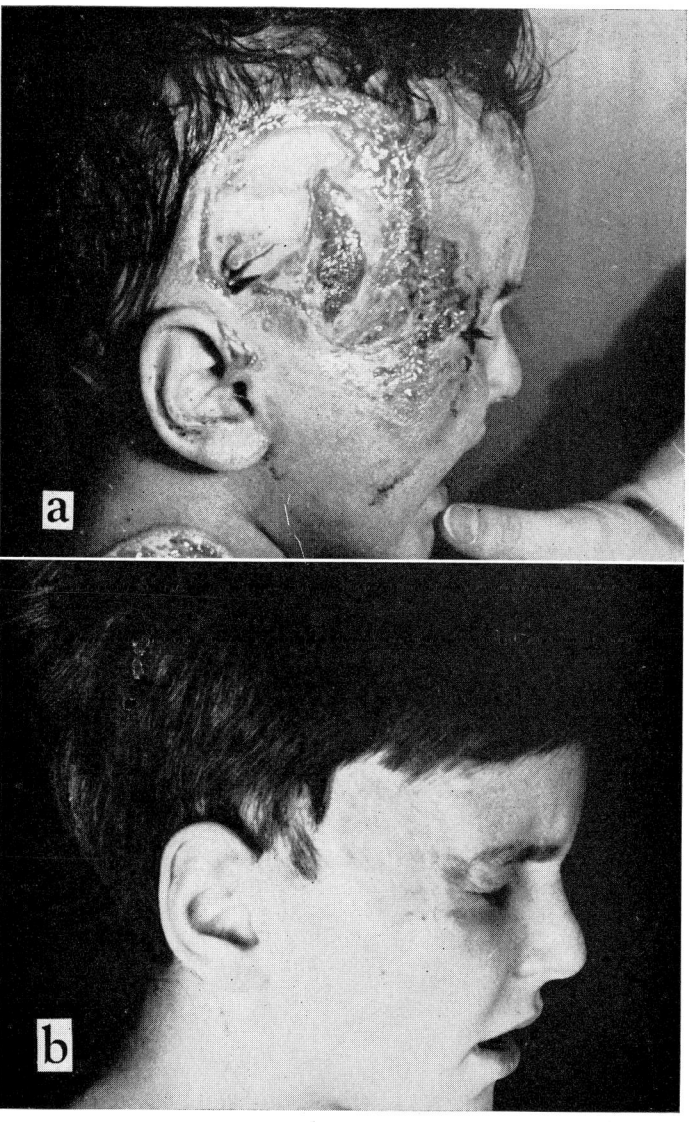

Case 4, *a:* Boy, aged four, was struck by an automobile. The accident resulted in denudation of the temporal bone and extensive surface defect of the soft tissue of the right side of the forehead.

b: The exposed bone was covered with a sliding scalp flap which was pedicled in the forehead region. The periosteum of the donor area of the flap was covered with a skin graft (compare with Case 9). The surface defect of the temporal area and forehead was covered with thick split grafts. Picture taken seven years after the operation.

CASE

5

a   b

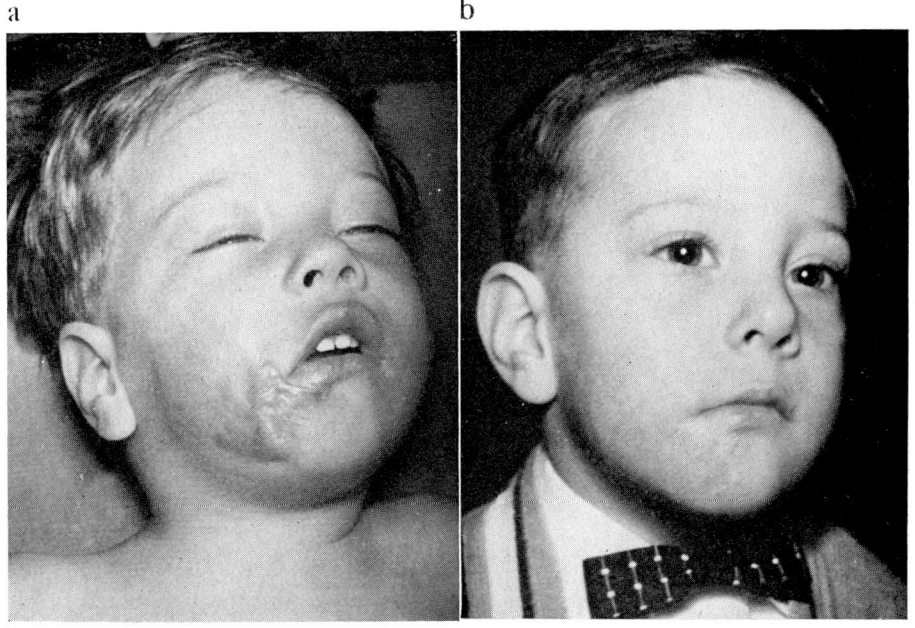

Case 5, *a:* Extensive hypertrophic scars of cheek and lips after third-degree burn; ectropion of right side of lower lip and lateral displacement and obliteration of right oral commissure.

b: After excision of all scar tissue, repair of ectropion of lip was overcome and the defect was covered with a thick split skin graft from right supraclavicular area. The obliteration of the oral commissure, however, recurred and the graft became dark brown. In a second operation the web-like scar obliterating the oral commissure was overcome with a double Z-plasty (see p. 255) and the hyperpigmentation of the graft removed by superficial dermabrasion (p. 26).

CASE

6

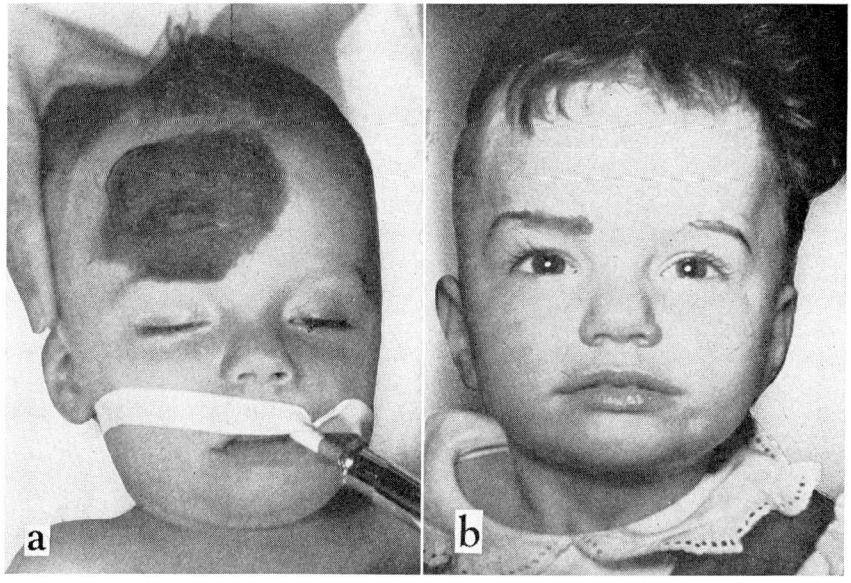

Case 6, *a:* Extensive hairy melanoma of forehead including part of the right eyebrow.

b: The tumor was excised. Excision consisted of full thickness of the skin. That part of the tumor which involved the right eyebrow was left behind to replace the missing eyebrow. Surface defect was covered with a thick split skin graft from the abdomen. Within three months post-operatively the graft changed to a brownish color. One year after the operation the surface of the graft was abraded with sand paper for removal of the superficial pigment (p. 26). Graft has assumed almost normal color since this operation. Picture taken two years after the operation.

996

CASE

7

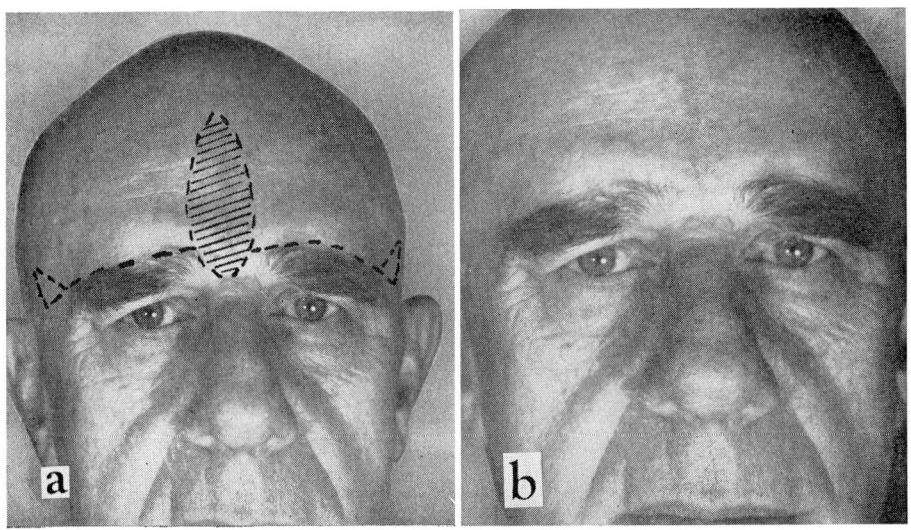

Case 7, *a:* Patient, aged sixty-two, had a basal cell carcinoma below the center of the forehead, which was treated with irradiation. The tumor recurred ten years later and was then excised and skin grafted. After four years the tumor recurred and again was excised. The tumor recurred again; the patient was then referred to the author for further treatment. A preoperative picture of the patient is not available. The involved area in the middle of the forehead and between the eyebrows is outlined in the diagram. Incisions parallel and above the eyebrows for mobilization of two forehead flaps to be rotated for closure of the defect after excision of the lesion are outlined (Fig. 13, p. 21).

b: Seven months after operation. No evidence of recurrence.

CASE
8

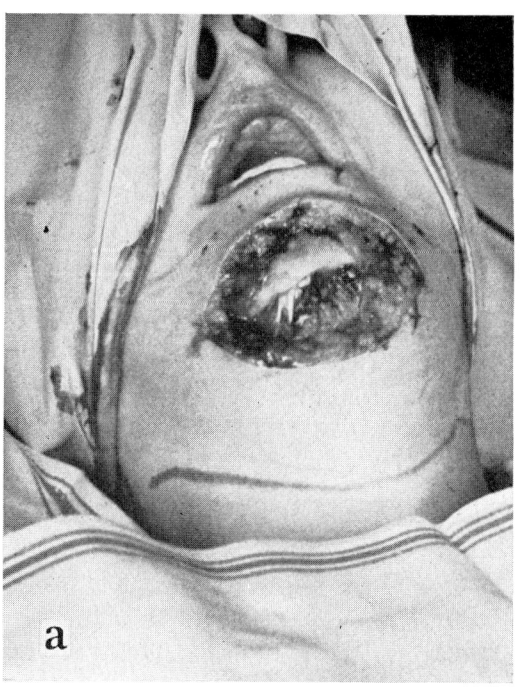

a

Case 8, *a:* In 1923 patient had 140 "light" treatments, in a beauty parlor, to the tip of the chin for removal of hair. Two years before this operation a superficial breakdown appeared in the skin. The preoperative microscopic examination of a biopsy taken from the involved part of the chin revealed a fibrosarcoma of the skin. The tumor was widely excised including the periosteum of the anterior part of the mandible. A relaxation incision in the chin-neck line is marked for the formation of a double pedicle sliding flap.

b, c: The flap was slid forward to cover the defect at the chin. The flap bed in the chin-neck line was skin grafted. No evidence of recurrence was noted four years after the operation.

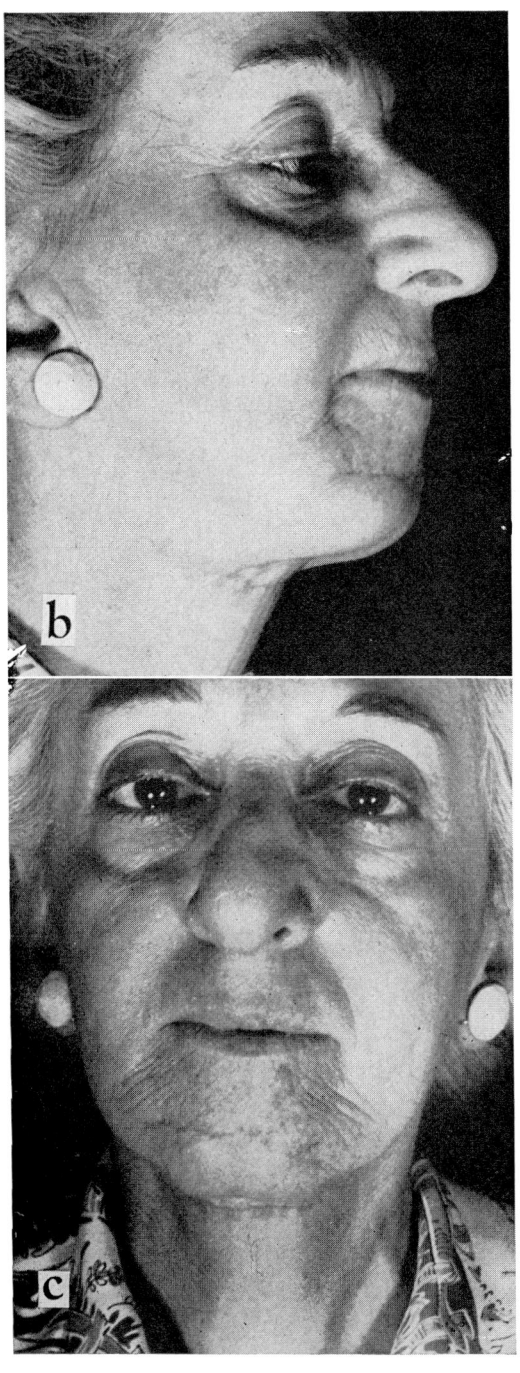

CASE
9

Case 9, *a:* Boy, aged sixteen, played on the roof of a railroad box-car; his head came in touch with an overhanging electric wire and 12,000 volts went through his body. He was unconscious for several days. He was treated for shock and severe burns of chest and left thigh. Where the scalp came in contact with the wire an area of about 8.7 cm. (3½ inches) in diameter was burned full thickness including scalp and skull bone. After both had sloughed out (three months after injury) a scalp flap was elevated. In this illustration the head is depicted resting on headrest of the operating table face downward. The peripheral end of the flap was near the forehead region, its pedicle at the occiput. The periosteum of the flap bed was left behind.

b: The flap was rotated to cover the exposed dura and the flap bed was covered with one thick split graft taken from the back.

c, d: The patient developed traumatic epileptic convulsions which occurred as frequently as three times weekly. Three months after the transplantation the flap was elevated again and sharp bone edges lying upon the dura were removed. All scar tissue between dura and skull edges was excised. A bone graft was taken from the median side of the right ilium of the pelvis, and was laid with the periosteal side upon the dura and the prepared bone edges of the skull. The bone graft was held in place with two long heavy mattress sutures of silk. The flap was then placed over the graft. One month later an infection occurred between flap and bone graft which necessitated drainage and removal of the graft. Six months later another pelvic bone graft was inserted which healed in and has become fully regenerated. The patient had had no convulsions and when seen nine years after the operation was without symptoms.

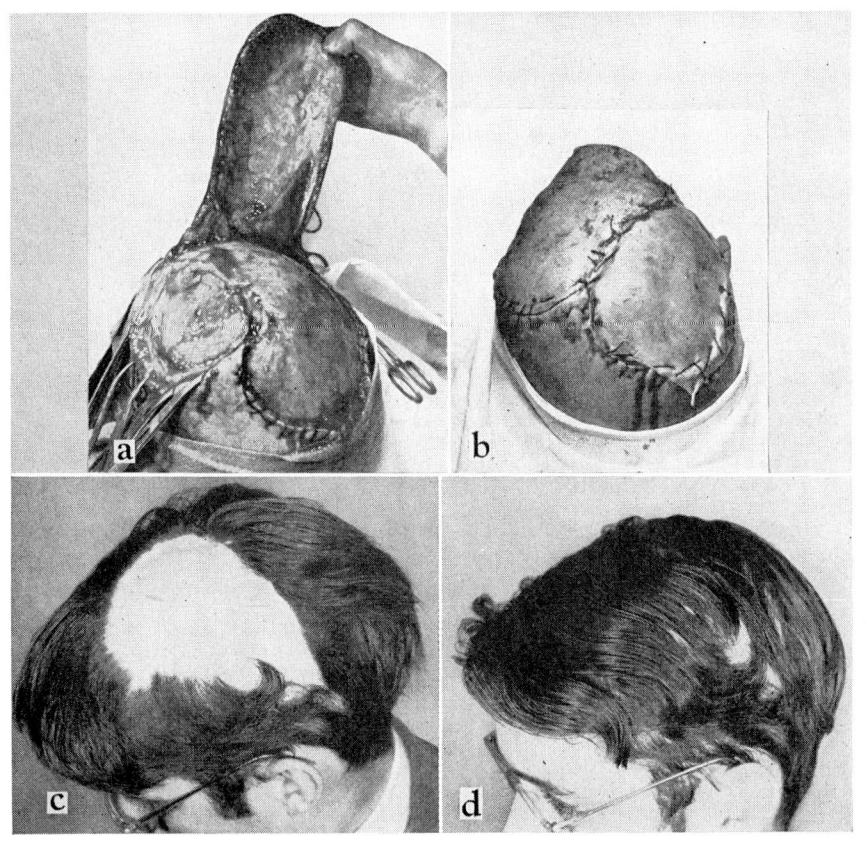

CASE
10

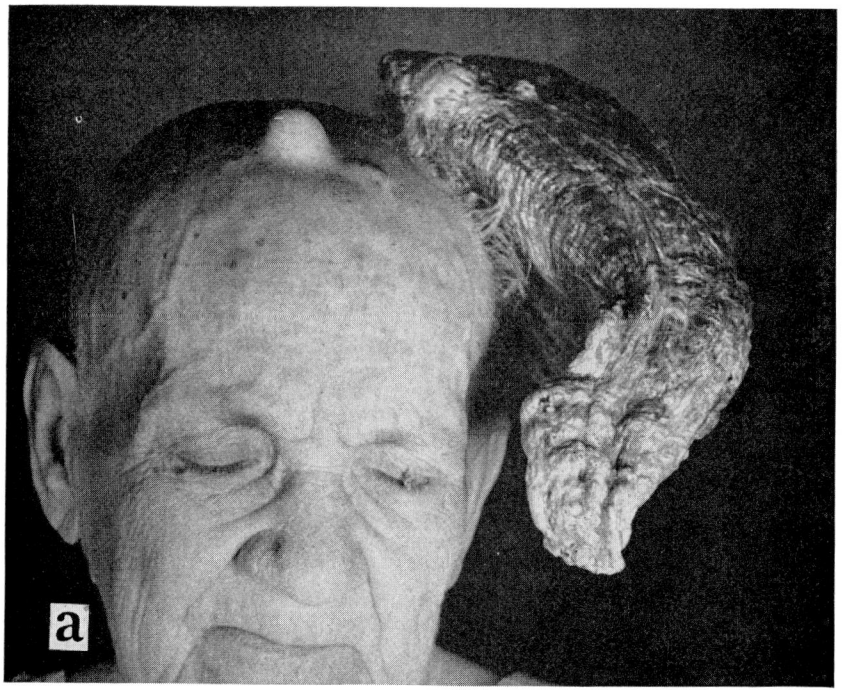

Case 10, *a:* Patient, aged eighty-three, with a large horn on the left side of the scalp. The history of this formation goes back 15 years when a sebaceous cyst was drained. The drainage continued and an ulcer developed. The ulcer grew outward and formed this large horn. Only after this mass became so heavy that it inconvenienced the patient was an operation considered.

b: Horn and outer table of skull bone were removed and a thick split graft placed upon the exposed medullary spaces of the bone. The graft took well. Microscopic examination of the tumor revealed an epidermoid carcinoma. The patient died nine years after the operation. The operated area remained closed and free of reactivation of the tumor.

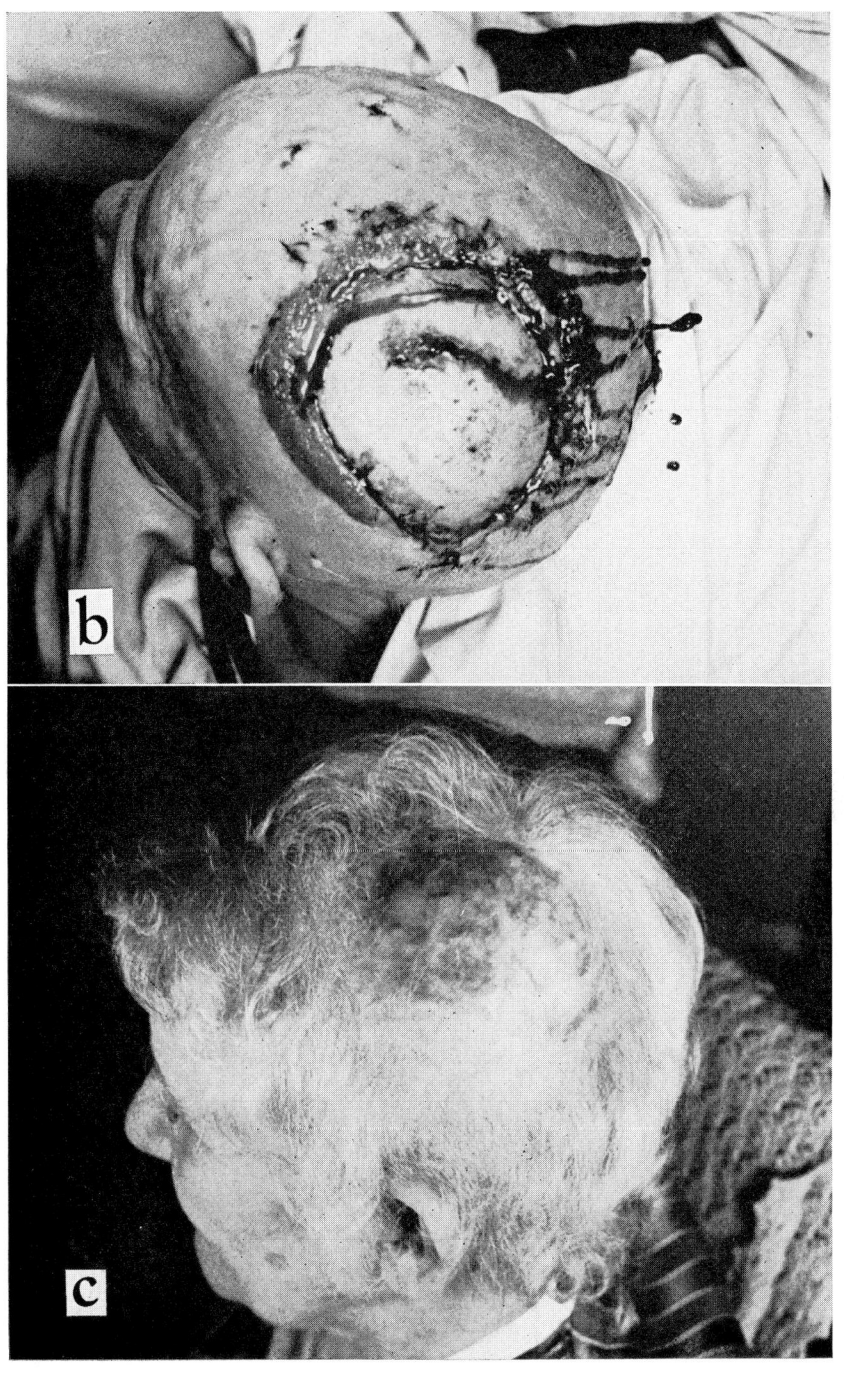

CASE
11

Case 11, *a, b:* Patient, aged twenty-one, was referred six weeks after her hair had been caught in rollers. The accident resulted in a total scalping including total loss of left ear and part of forehead skin. After shock treatment, an emergency operation was performed. The scalp which had been wrapped in clean linen was shaved and placed upon the skull. Some remaining raw areas were skin grafted. The scalp graft did not take and only small islands of other grafts remained.

c, d: In four operations the extensive raw surface was covered with split skin grafts. The missing left ear was reconstructed with a flap taken from the left forearm. The flap was tubed at its proximal pedicle and left untubed in its distal part. After several delays of transfer of the untubed part an autogenous cartilage graft was shaped and transplanted beneath the flap. Circulation of the flap became impaired in this area and part of the cartilage graft became necrotic. Four months later the remaining cartilage graft was removed and the flap transplanted to the left mastoid region. Eleven days later the flap was severed from the pedicle and after three days adjusted in place. Four months later another cartilage graft was transplanted beneath the flap at the mastoid region. Nine months later flap and cartilage graft were elevated and raw surface behind the ear was skin grafted (see Fig. 246, *A, B*). Patient wears a wig.

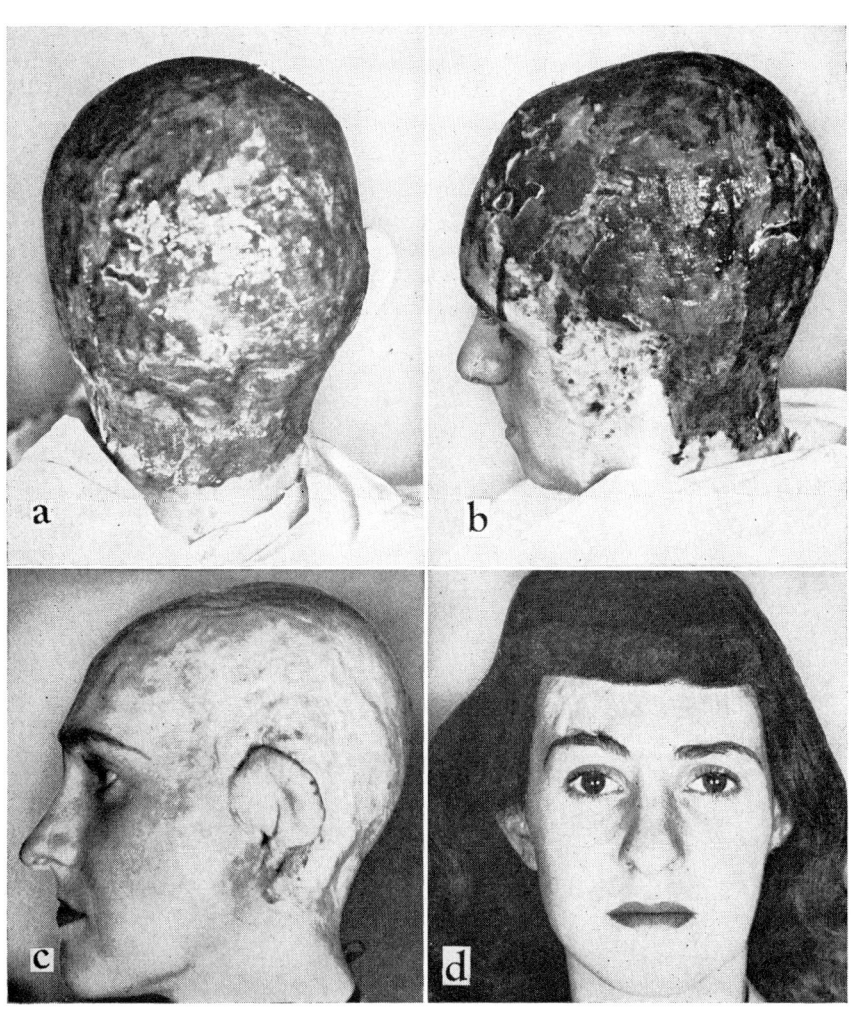

CASE
12

Case 12, *a*, *b:* Large depressed scar and partial loss of orbital rim, with displacement of right eyebrow, after compound fracture followed by osteomyelitis. The scar was excised. To rotate the lateral half of the eyebrow downward, skin and subcutaneous tissue of forehead and scalp were widely mobilized from a long sagittal incision. A fascia-lata fat graft was transplanted into the depressed area, and the wound edges were sutured together in layers.

c: Eight months after operation. *d:* Six years after operation.

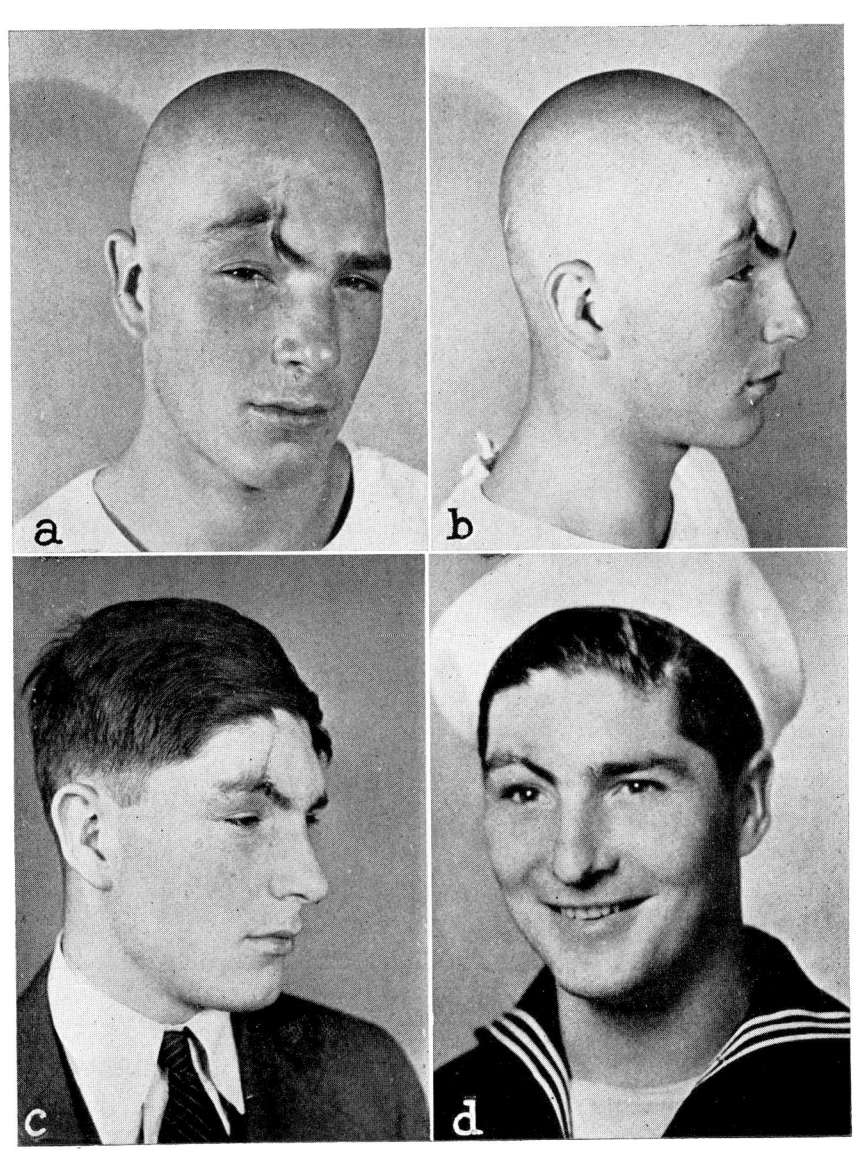

CASE
13

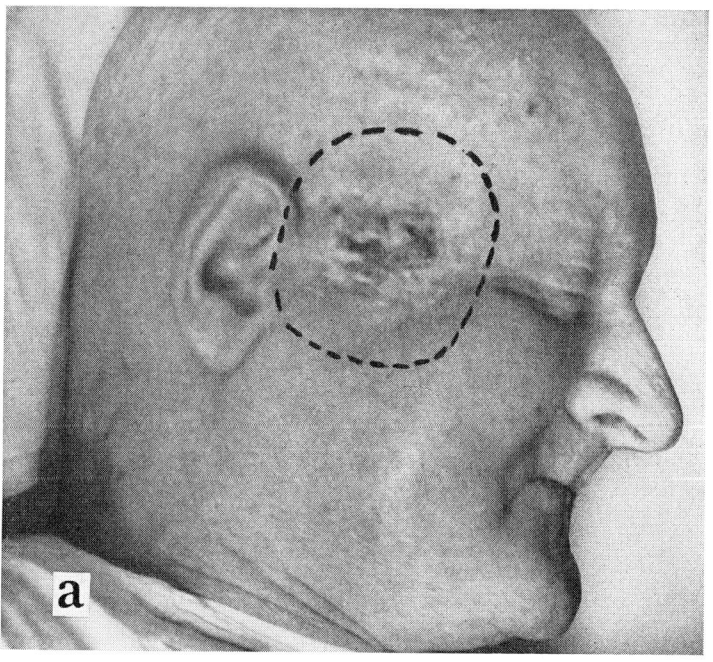

Case 13, *a:* Patient, aged sixty-one, with a basal cell carcinoma of the right temporal region which was irradiated. After initial healing the skin broke down within the irradiated area. The ulcer was approximately 3 cm. (1⅕ inches) in diameter. Microscopic examination showed ulceration and radiation effect; no tumor cells were visible. The area surrounding the ulcer showed typical evidence of x-ray damage. The base of the ulcer reached the temporal bone.

b: The area was widely excised and covered with a thick split skin graft. The upper half of the graft took while the lower half sloughed off. An open double-pedicle flap was constructed on the median surface of the right upper arm. It was elevated in stages and transferred seven weeks later. Before the flap was transplanted, the donor area at the arm was skin grafted. The arm was fastened to the forehead with adhesive strips. Clamping of the pedicle of the flap was begun ten days after the transfer. The flap was separated two weeks after the transfer, and adjusted in place ten days later. (For development of flap, see p. 83.)

c: Condition eight months after last operation.

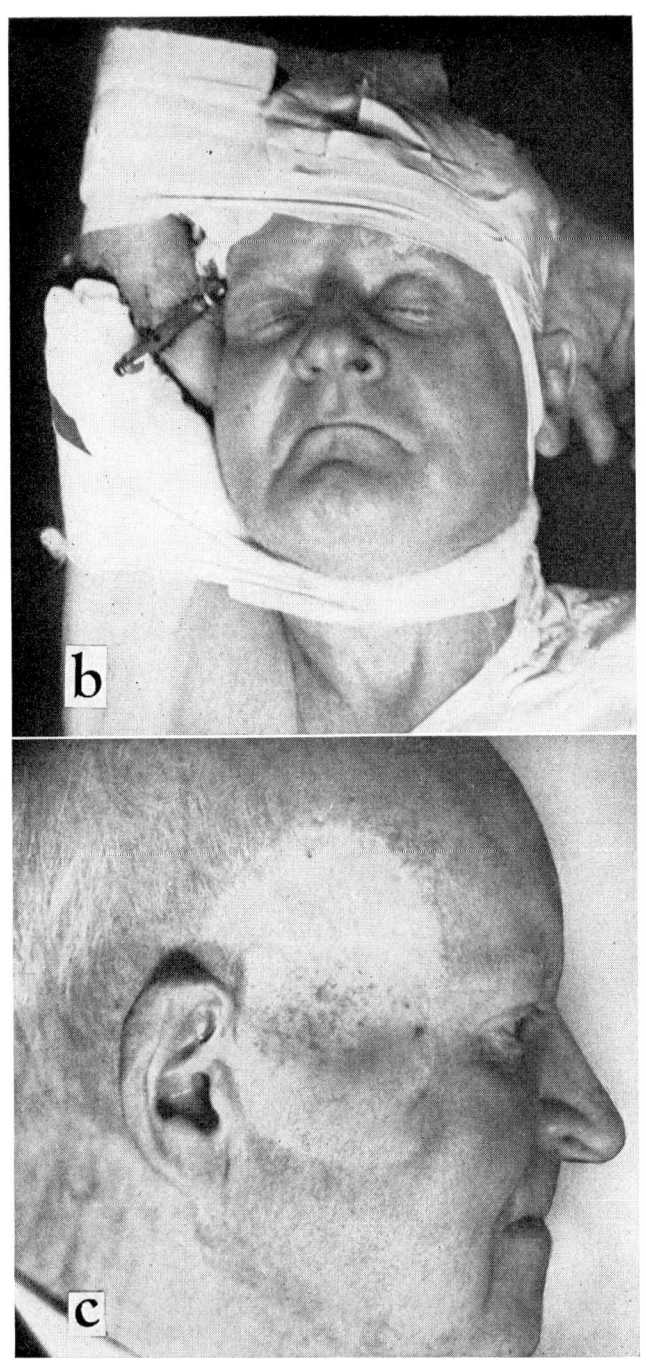

CASE

14

Case 14, *a:* Patient, aged forty-six, referred for closure of full-thickness defect of left cheek after irradiation for cancer. Frequent biopsies were negative. A cervical tube flap was constructed, reaching from the left mastoid process to the clavicle. Three weeks later, the flap was lengthened. This part of the flap was left untubed and returned to its original site. Two weeks later, it was elevated again, the peripheral pedicle narrowed from each side, and a laboratory clamp attached to the remainder of the pedicle. The pedicle was gradually crushed within five days.

b: Four weeks later, the peripheral half of the untubed part was raised and lined by folding it upon itself. The flap bed was skin grafted. Two weeks later, the entire untubed part of the flap was raised; it became cyanotic and hence was returned to its original site (see p. 97).

c: One week later, the communication of covering and lining of flap—that is, the peripheral edge of the flap—was incised. One week later, the defect edges of the cheek were denuded and freed of all scar tissue. The flap was transferred and sutured in place. Ten days later, the pedicle was gradually crushed with a laboratory clamp. This took four days, after which the flap could be severed from the pedicle and adjusted in place.

d, e: Pictures five months after last stage. (H. May: Surgery.)

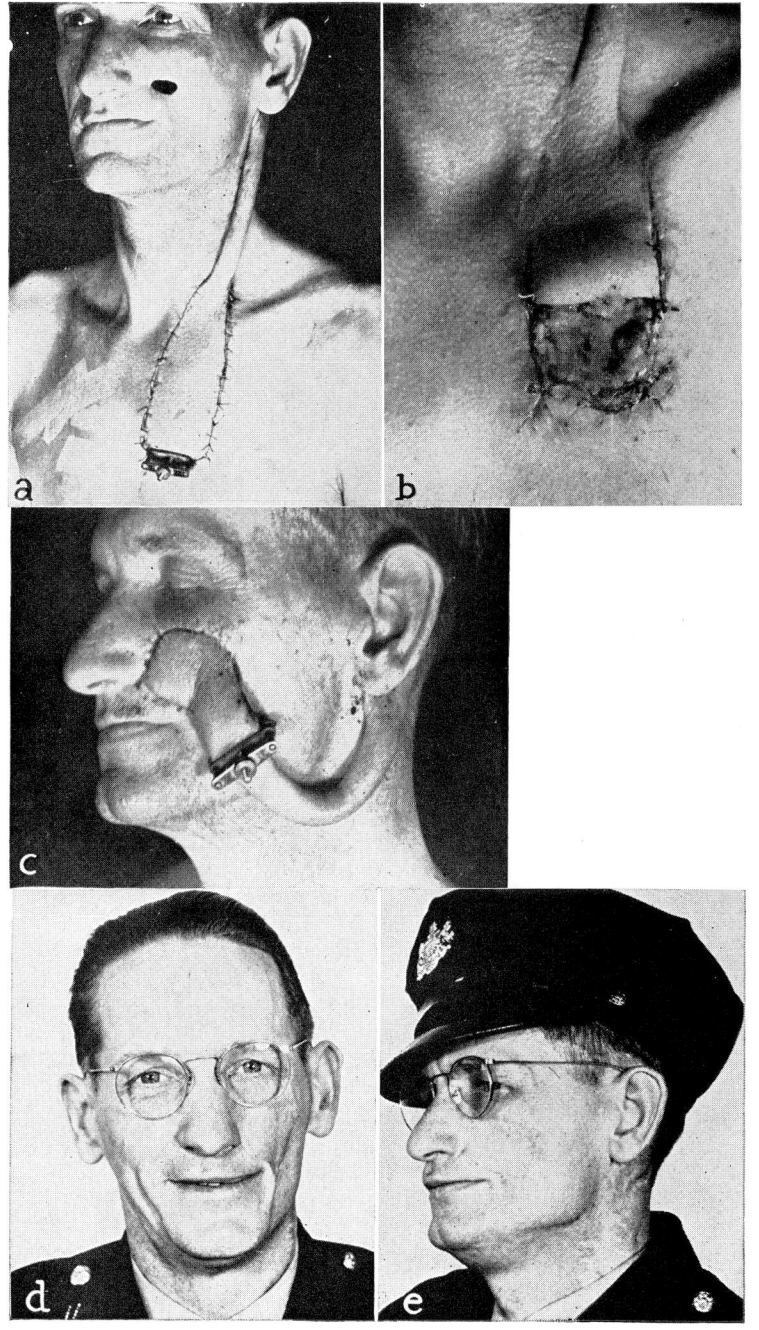

CASE
15

Case 15, *a, b:* Total right-sided facial palsy resulting from removal of malignant parotid gland. Six years later patient was referred to author for reconstruction.

c, d: A dynamic suspension operation was performed after Ragnell (p. 22). In a second stage, reconstruction of right nasolabial fold (p. 222) and lateral canthorraphy of right eyelid (p. 484) were performed. Six years after operation.

a
b

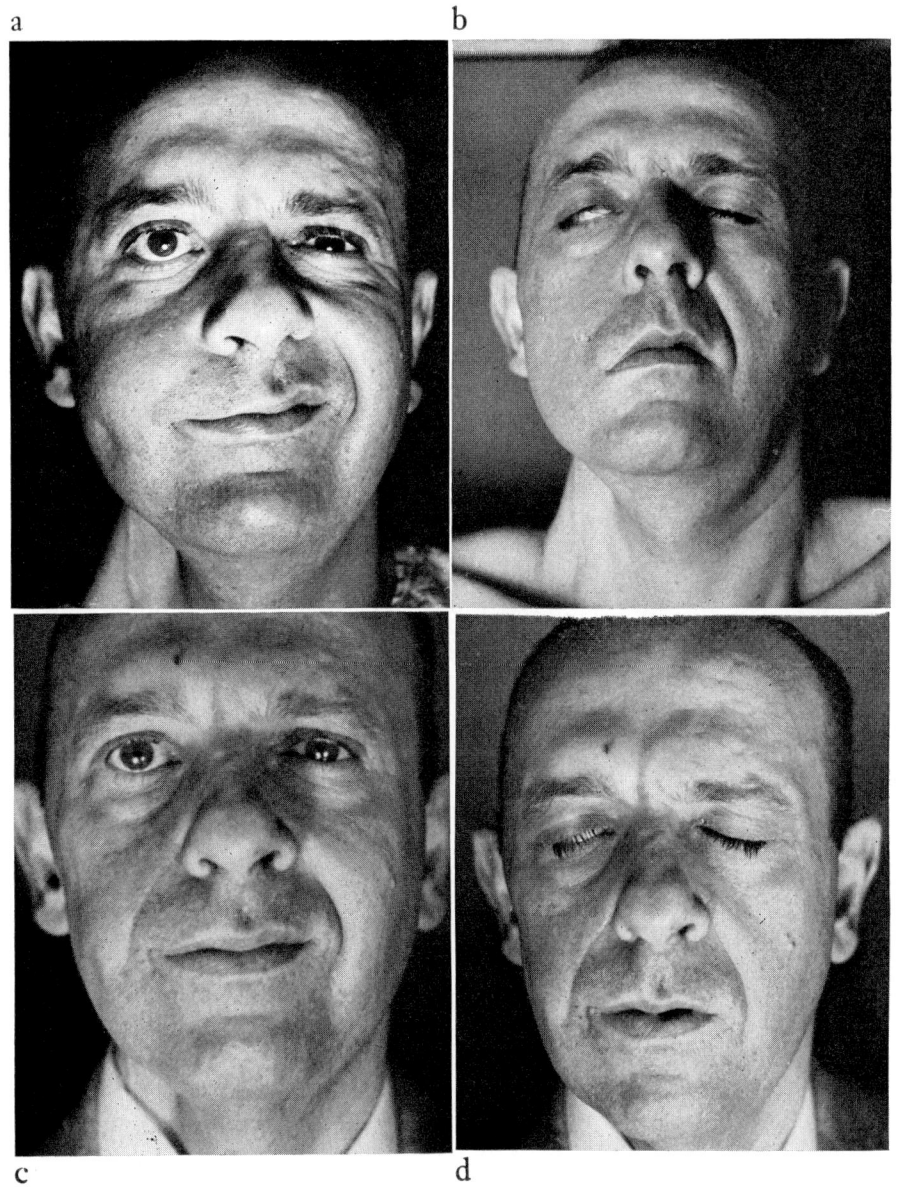

c
d

CASE
16

Case 16, *a:* Patient, aged twenty-two, gave the following history: Ten years previously a left lower molar tooth was removed under local injection with Novocain. A few hours later the anesthetic field was still present at left side of the cheek which began to look whitish. Gradually the left cheek wasted away. A few years later a whitish area appeared at the left side of her forehead and there again was wasting of tissue. Finally, the patient developed a typical picture of hemiatrophy of the left side of the face.

b: From incisions below the left side of the mandible dermal grafts which were doubled were inserted into the hemiatrophic pockets. About two weeks after the operation the cheek swelled up and aspiration revealed serum. This illustration depicts the patient eleven months after the operation.

1014

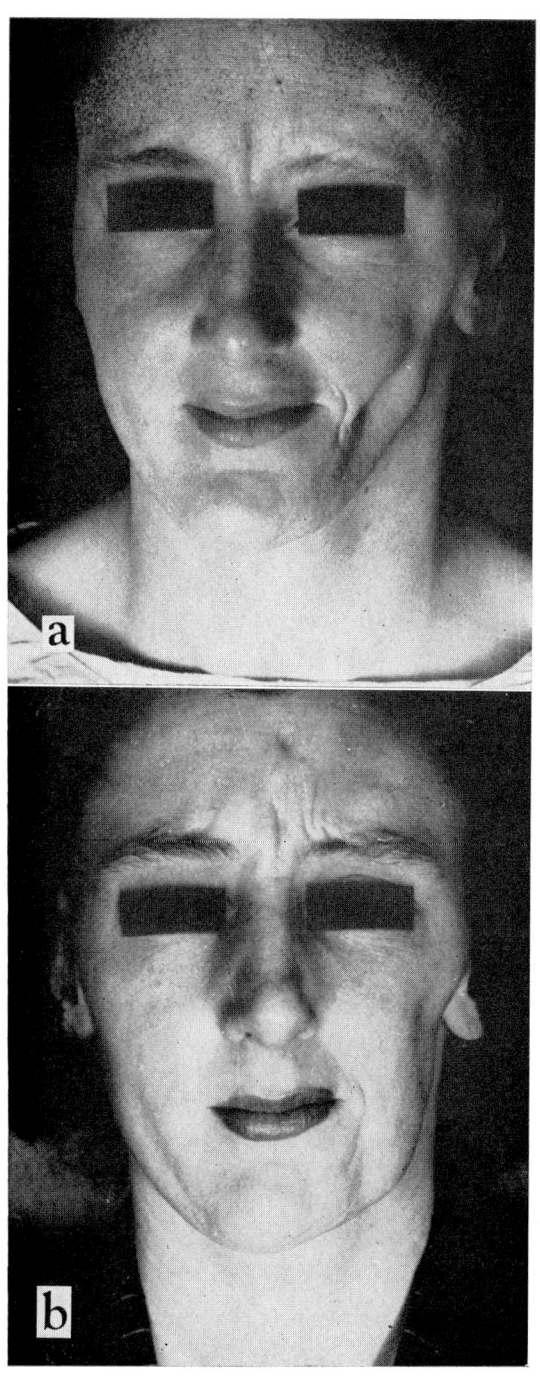

CASE
17

a   b

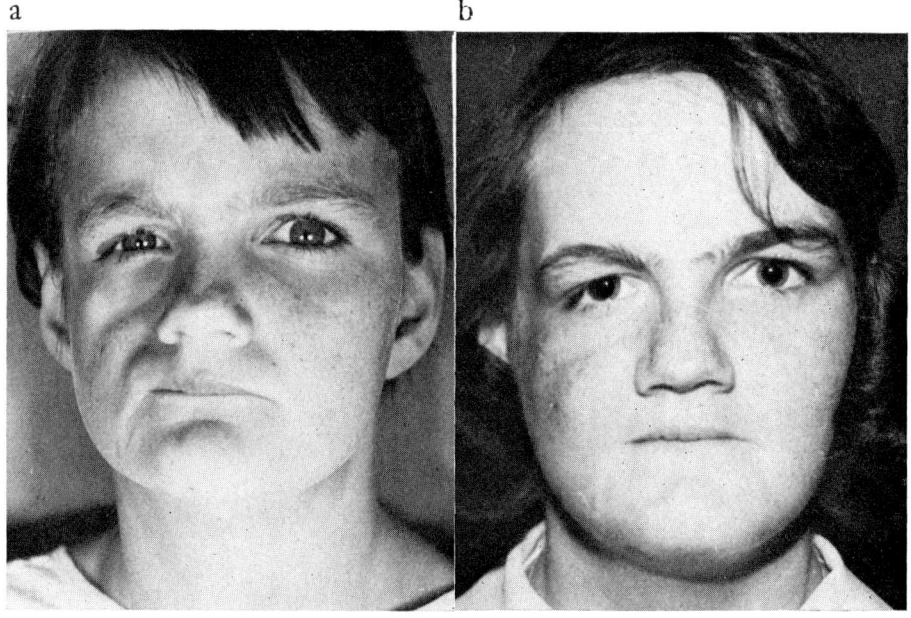

Case 17, *a:* Treacher-Collins syndrome (p. 355), right side of face: absence of orbital rim and of anterior part of zygoma and underdevelopment of right maxilla.

b: Autogenous rib cartilage grafts were inserted from an L-shaped incision along the base of the lower eyelid and lateral wall of nose. One formed the orbital rim and was fastened laterally to the stump of the zygoma. The other was laid upon the underdeveloped maxilla. In a second stage another rib cartilage graft was inserted from an intraoral incision to augment the cheek and to form the right upper alveolar ridge.

CASE
18

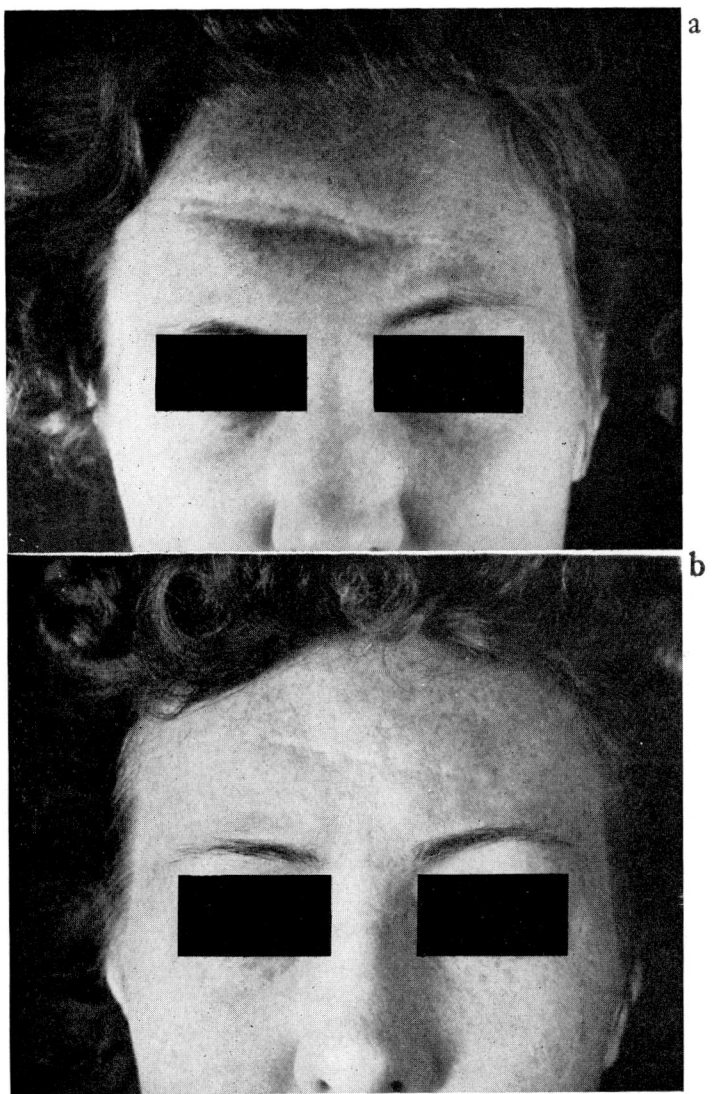

Case 18, *a:* Deep scar of forehead adherent to frontal bone.
b: After insertion of dermal graft and repair of scar.

CASE

19

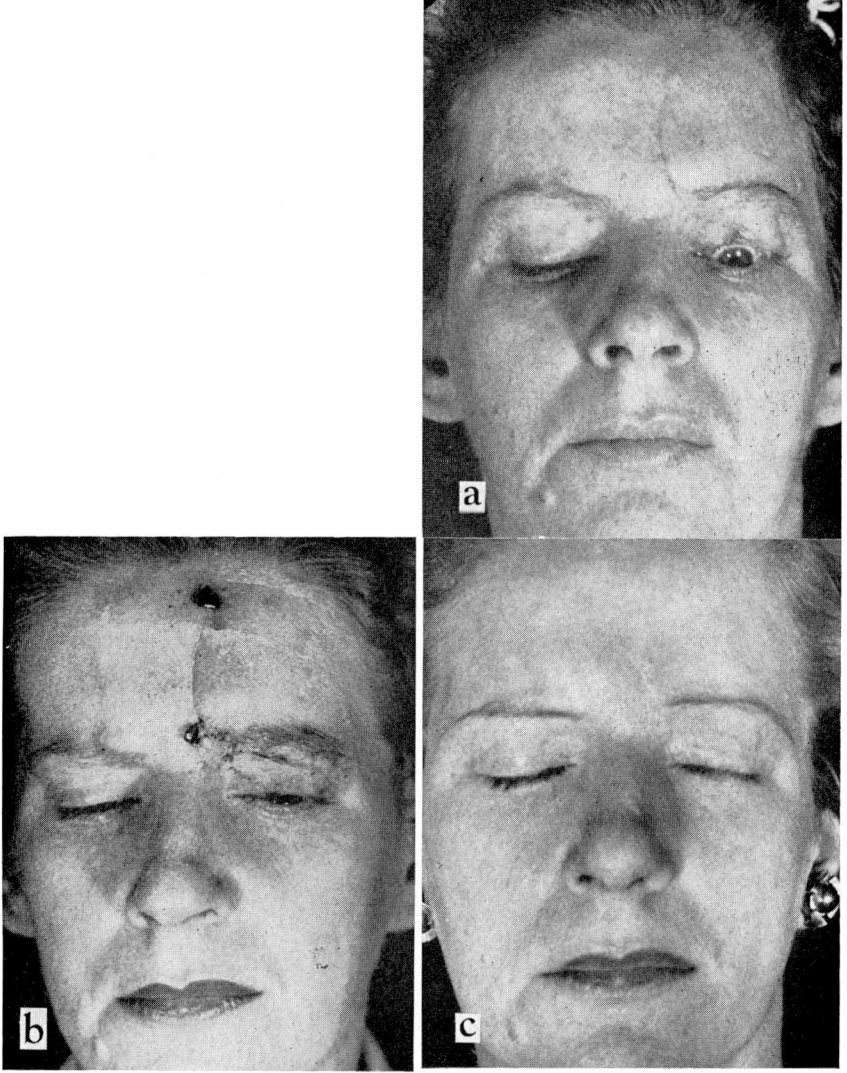

Case 19, *a:* Extensive scar of left side of forehead and left upper lid with ectropion of lid as a result of an automobile accident.

b: Excision and repair of the forehead scar with a percutaneous running wire suture. Replacement of contracting scars of left upper lid with full-thickness graft from supraclavicular region.

c: Eleven months after the operation.

1018

CASE
20

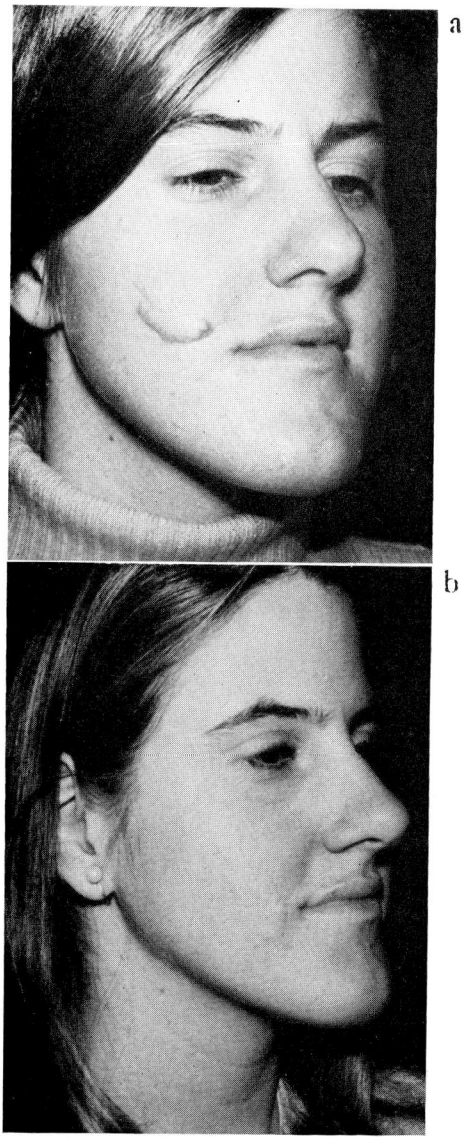

Case 20, *a:* Irregular hypertrophic scar of right cheek after automobile accident, running perpendicular to elastic lines of face.

b: One year after repair by excision and multiple W-plasty (p. 187).

CASE

21

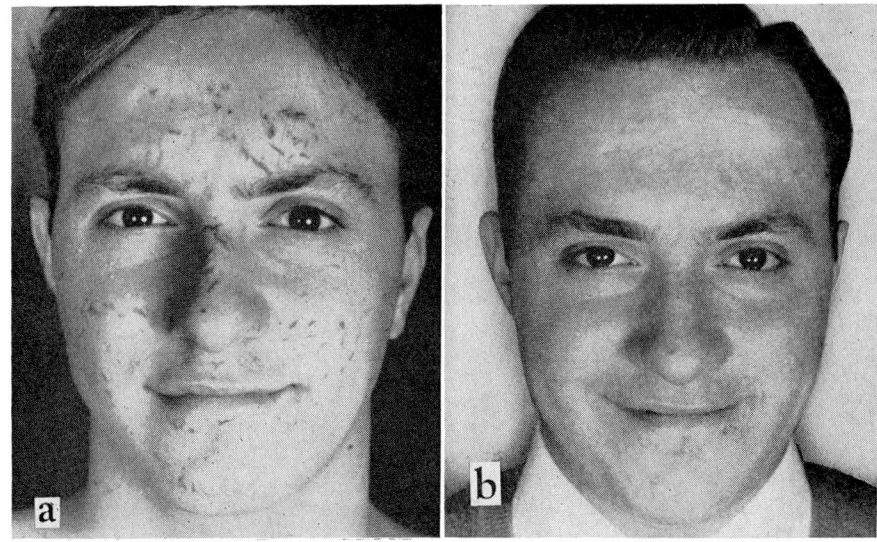

Case 21, *a:* Patient, aged nineteen, received multiple dirt-stained scars of the face in an explosion of titanium material which had a bluish color. The emergency treatment consisted of thorough cleansing and scrubbing of the skin, but it was impossible to remove the tattoo marks. Four months later thorough abrasion of the face was carried out in three stages. The forehead was operated first. Some of the deeper dirt-stained scars were excised. Four weeks later a similar procedure was performed for removal of the dirt-stained scars of the nose and right cheek, and another month later the remainder of the scars were removed.

b: The result nine months after the operation.

CASE
22

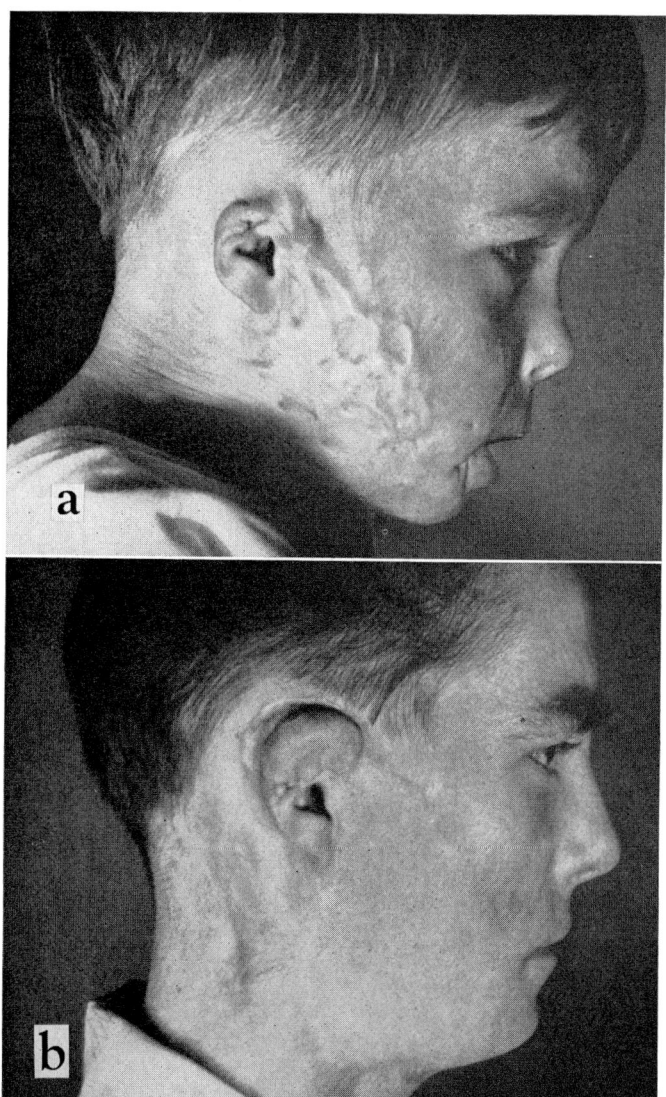

Case 22, *a:* Patient, aged seven, with a large hypertrophic scar of right side of face after second- and third-degree burns, contracting mouth.

b: The entire scar was excised, including right half of upper and lower lip, and a thick split graft was transplanted from the upper half of the chest.

The ear was reconstructed twelve years after the accident (p. 510).

CASE
23

Case 23, *a:* Small cornifying squamous-cell cancer of lower lip. Excision at lower lip and flap at upper lip marked. The width of the flap is only one half of that of the defect, in order to shorten upper and lower lip proportionately.

b: After rotation of the flap; the left commissure of the mouth is preserved; the pedicle of the flap crosses the mouth (Fig. 76, p. 254).

c, d: Three months after separation of the pedicle (Fig. 76, p. 254).

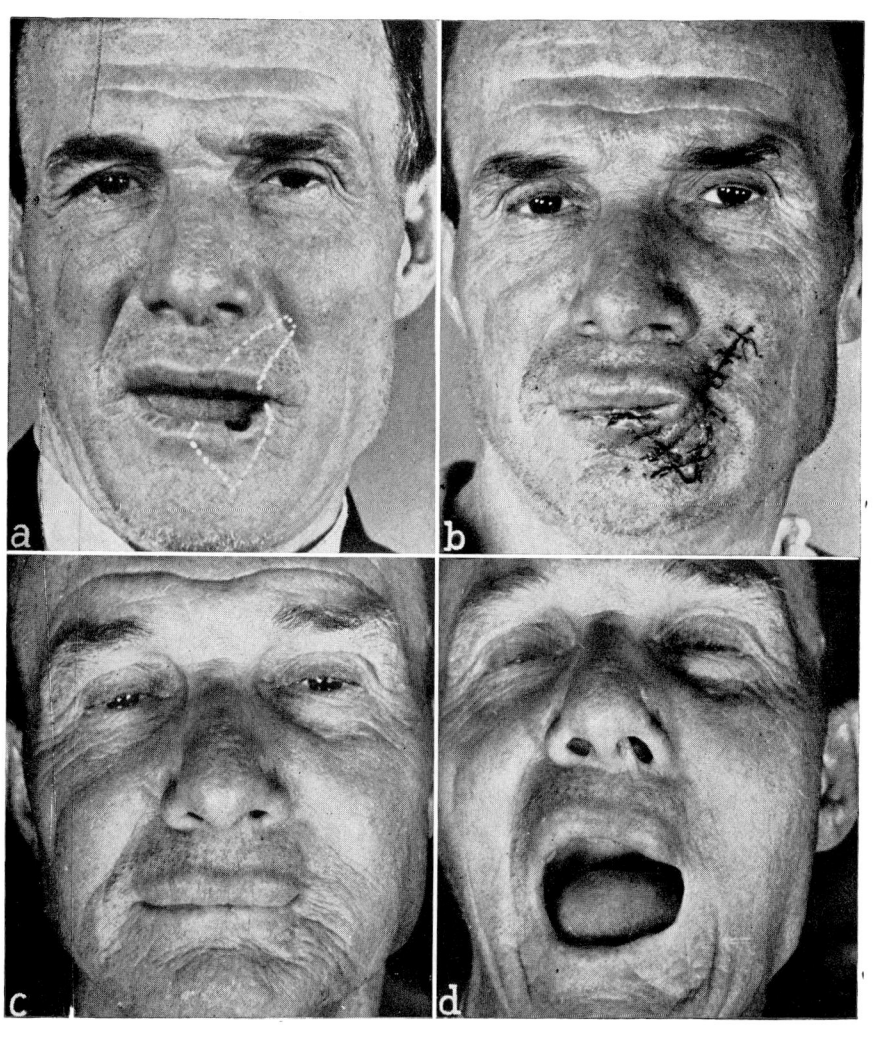

CASE

24

Case 24, *a, b:* Patient with papillomatous squamous-cell cancer inside the mouth near right commissure. Triangular excision, including upper half of commissure of mouth and parts of the adjacent cheeks, is outlined. Triangular vermilion-bordered flap at lower lip is outlined.

c: Before the flap was rotated into the defect, the latter was made smaller by closure of the lateral corner. The pedicle of the flap forms the new commissure of the mouth.

d: Four weeks after operation.

e, f: The vertical shortness at the right side of the mouth was corrected according to the method of Figure 75, page 253. No recurrence after eleven years. (H. May: Ann. Surg.)

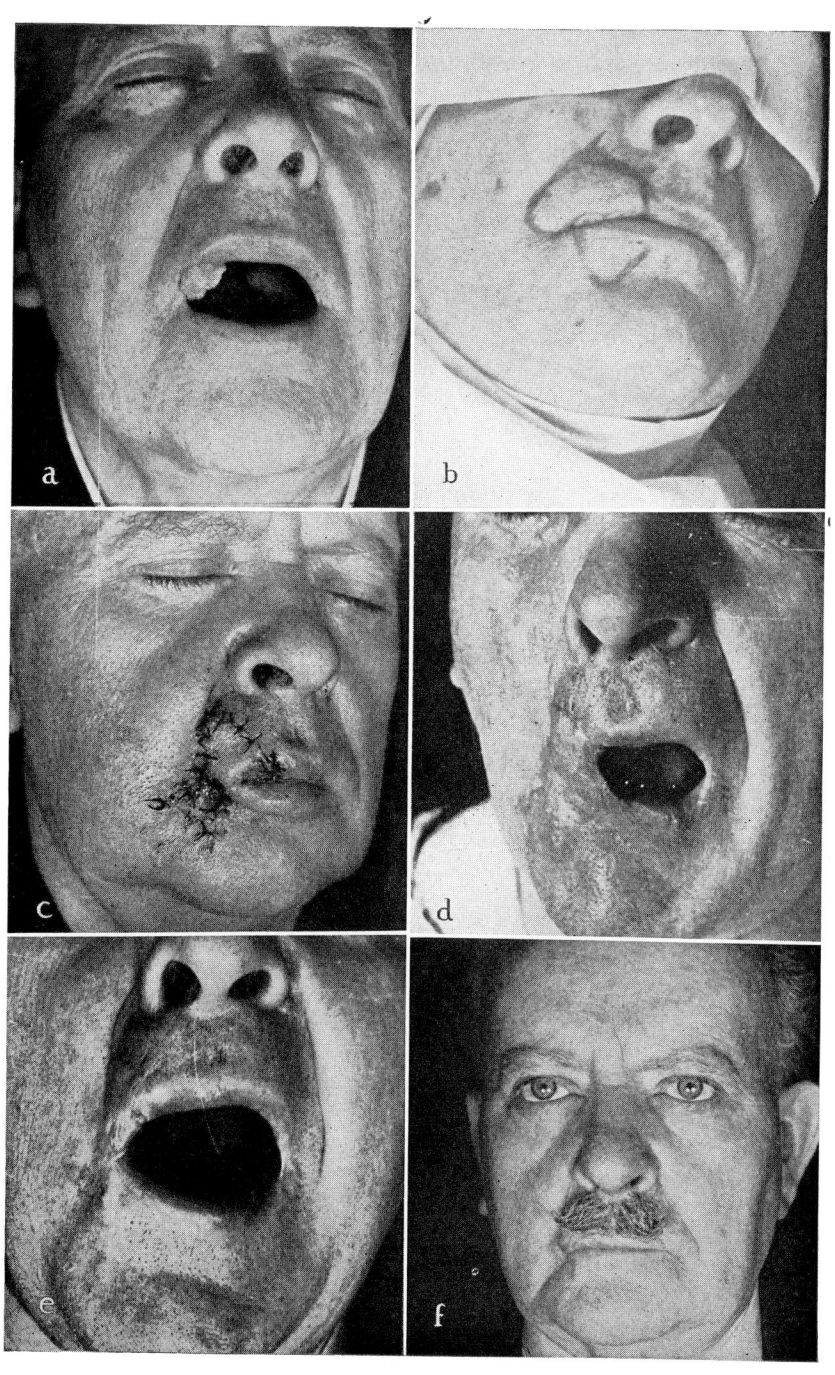

CASE

25

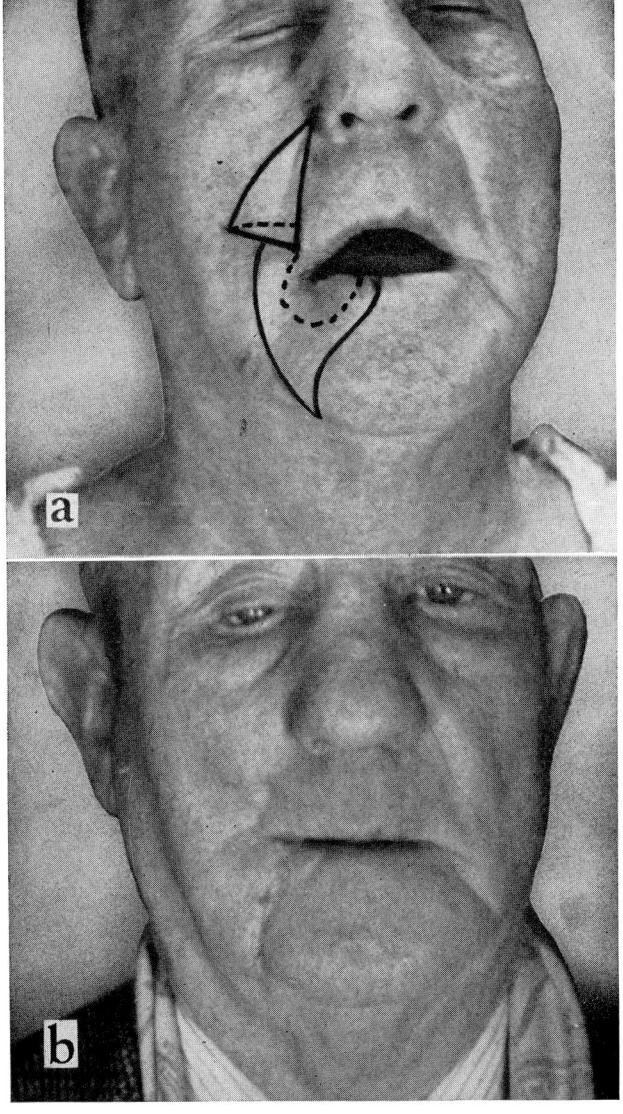

Case 25, *a:* Patient, aged seventy, with a squamous-cell carcinoma at right side of lower lip near the commissure. No evidence of metastasis. Involved area is outlined with circular dotted line. Heart-shaped excision and excision of triangle in right nasolabial fold for closure of the defect with Burow method is outlined (p. 263).

b: Six months after operation.

CASE

26

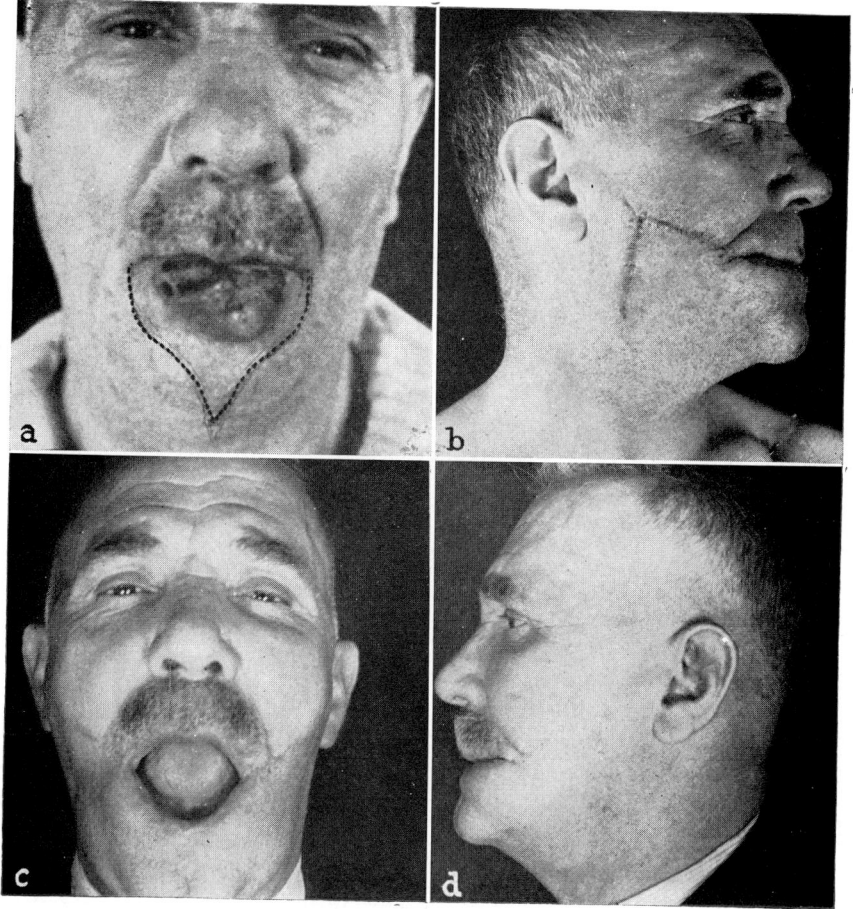

Case 26, *a:* Patient with large squamous-cell carcinoma of lower lip. No evidence of metastasis. Line of heart-shaped excision outlined. Operation according to Dieffenbach's method (Fig. 82, p. 266).

b: Same patient five days after operation. Was discharged twelve days after operation.

c, d: Same patient thirteen months after operation. No evidence of recurrence after seven years. (H. May: Surg. Gynec. Obstet.)

CASE

27

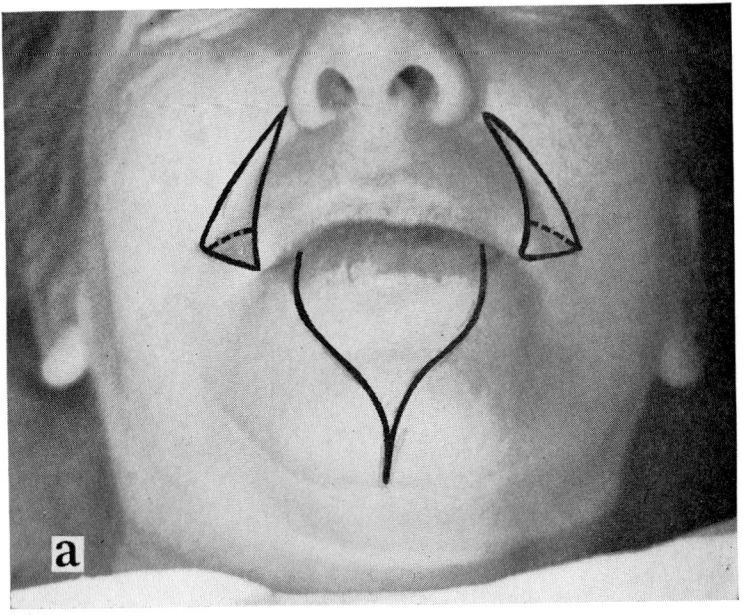

a

Case 27, *a:* Patient, aged forty-eight, with extensive hemangioma of lower lip. Heart-shaped excision of full thickness of lip and chin is outlined. Two triangles to be excised from the nasolabial region are also outlined for closure after the Burow technique. Dotted lines indicate mucous membrane triangles for formation of vermilion border of commissures.

b: After excision of tumor and nasolabial triangles. Note everted mucous membrane triangle on right side.

c: Three months after operation.

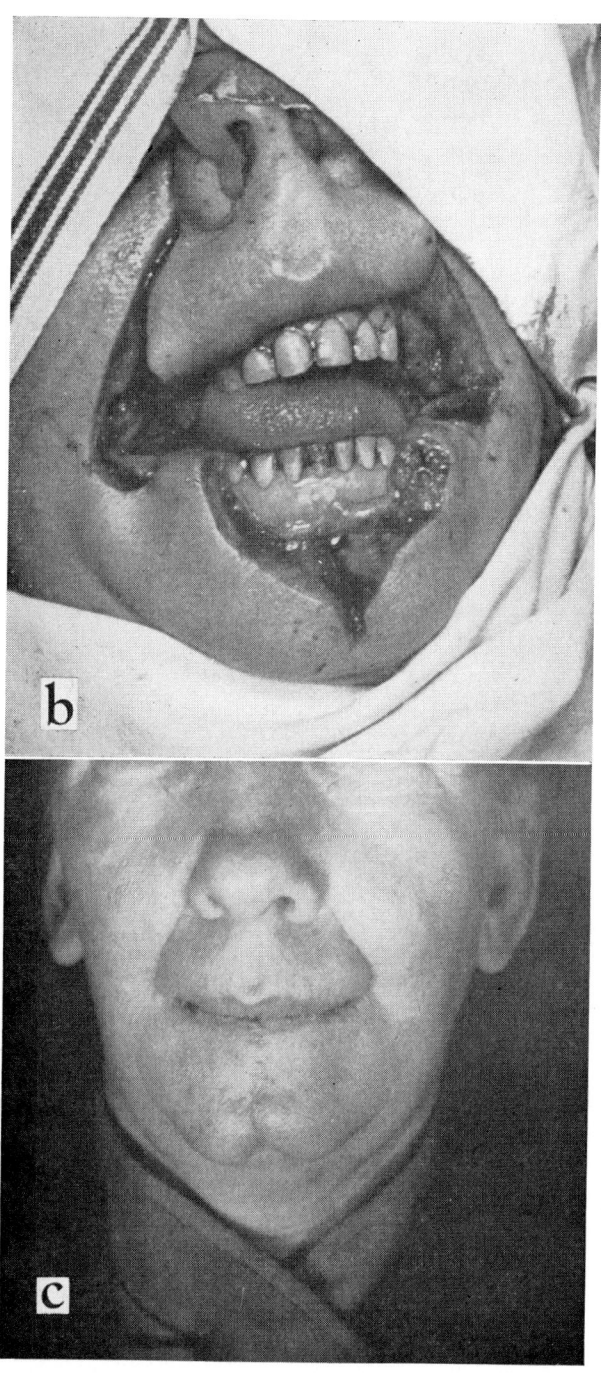

CASE
28

Case 28, *a:* Patient, aged sixty-two, had squamous-cell carcinoma, Grade II, of the lower lip, which had been treated elsewhere—first by cauterization, later by radiation. Nine months later, he was referred to the author for closure of the extensive defect, which included part of the mandible. All areas looked free of tumor, with exception of a suspected area at the bottom of the defect, but this proved to be negative on microscopic examination. There was, however, one enlarged lymph node, palpable beneath the right side of the mandible, which was freely movable. Hence, it was planned to perform a radical neck dissection. The defect's edges of soft tissue and mandible showed evidence of extensive x-ray necrosis; hence, the defect had to be enlarged until normal tissue was encountered. The shape of the defect is depicted by the heart-shaped outline of excision. The defect was closed according to the method shown in Figure 80, page 263.

b-d: Patient made an uneventful recovery. He was discharged from the hospital on the eighth postoperative day. All wounds had healed. These photographs were taken eighteen days after the operation. Twenty-one days after the operation, the submental and right submandibular glands were removed by radical dissection, as well as the right cervical glands after removal of the right sternocleidomastoid muscle and the right internal jugular vein. Patient had an uneventful recovery, and was discharged six days after the operation. No evidence of reactivation of tumors after nine years.

1030

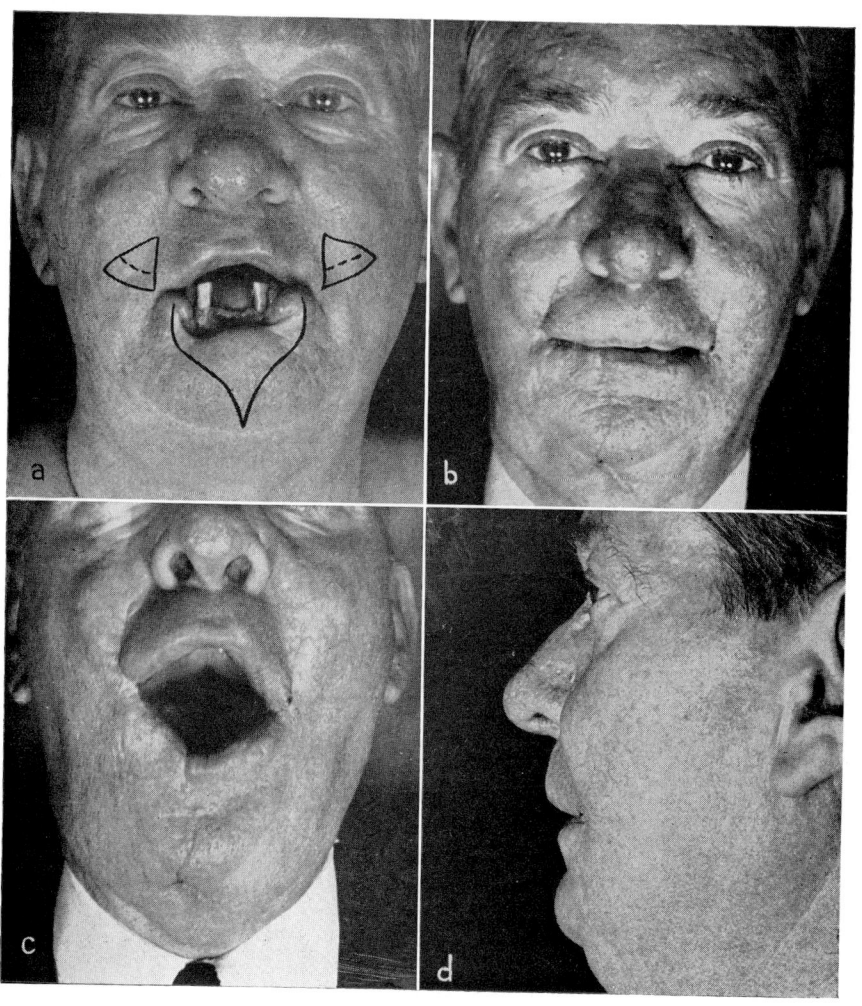

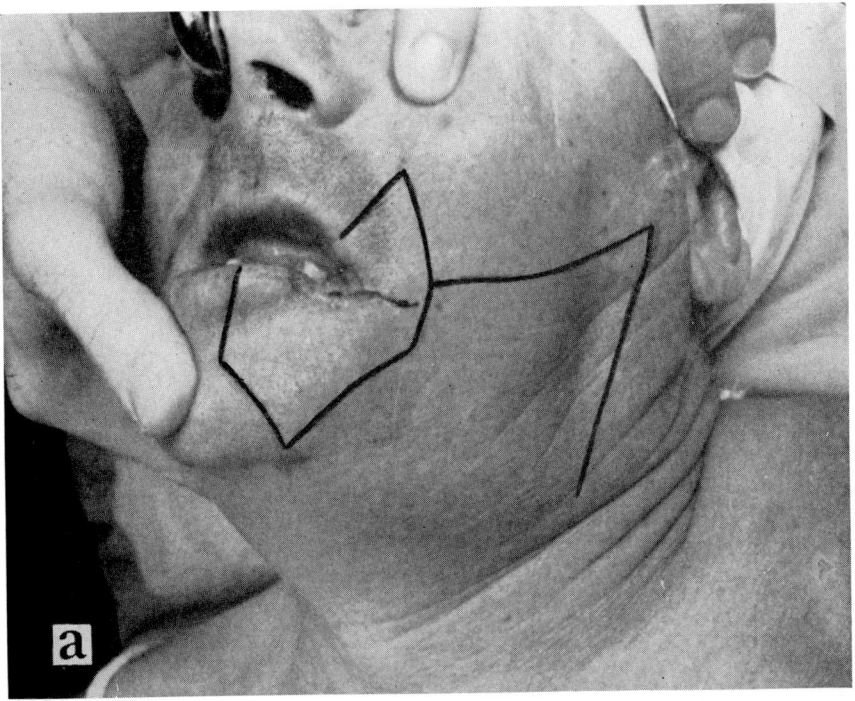

Case 29, *a:* Patient, aged forty-eight, with basal cell carcinoma of left commissure of mouth. Heart-shaped excision of lower lip and chin and adjacent cheek and excision of triangle from upper lip are marked out, together with the Dieffenbach flap for closure of the defect (Fig. 82, p. 266).

b, c: Four years after the operation there was no evidence of reactivation.

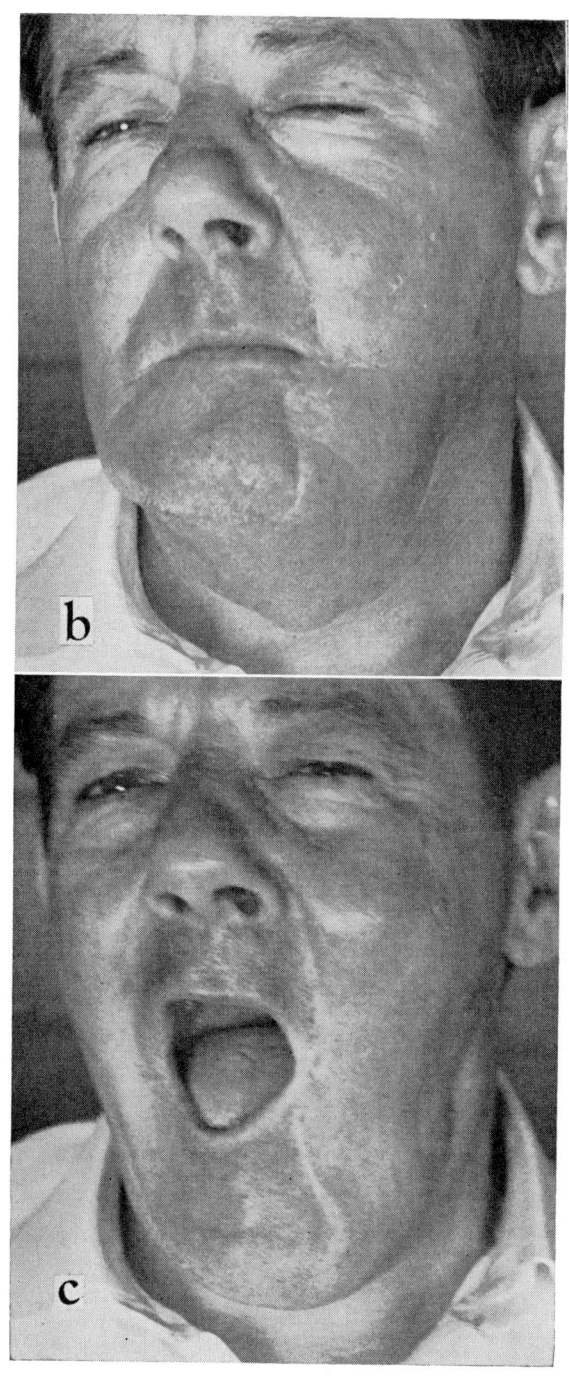

CASE
30

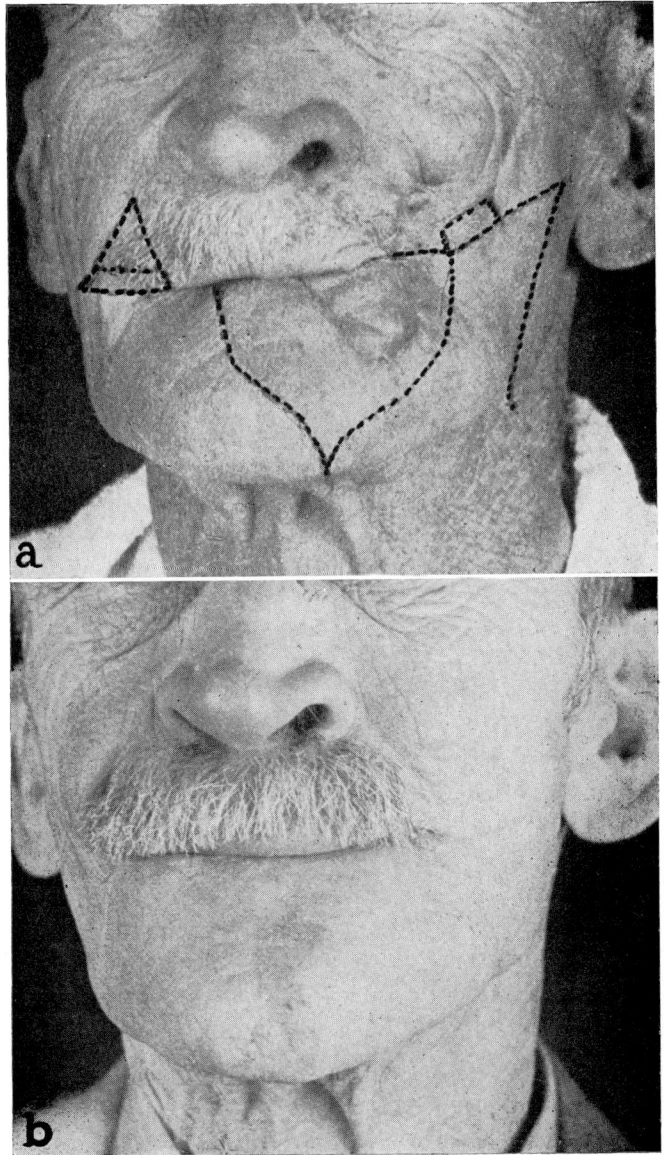

Case 30, *a:* Squamous-cell cancer of lower lip had been unsuccessfully treated with excision and Estlander rotation flap from upper lip. Hence a more radical operation was performed, Dieffenbach's method on same side and Burow's method on other side.

b: Same patient ten months after operation. He died from metastases twenty months after operation.

1034

CASE
31

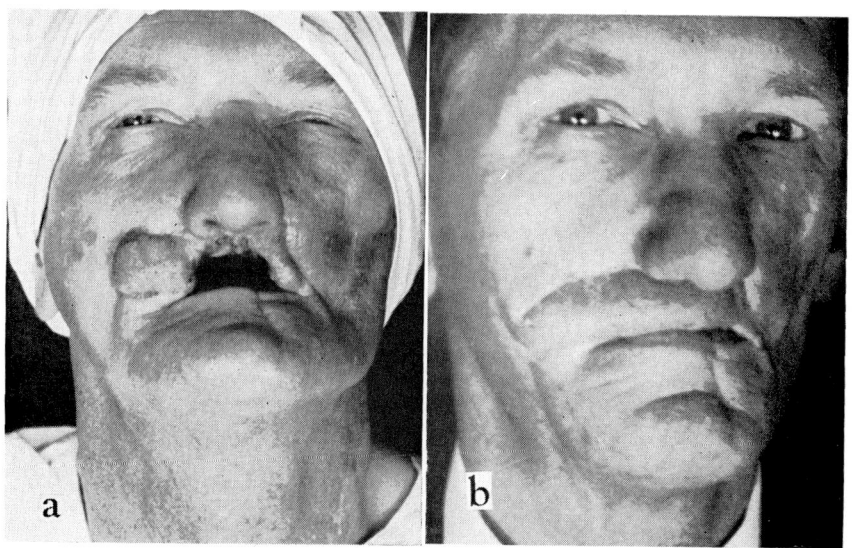

Case 31, *a:* Patient, aged fifty-two, had a basal cell carcinoma of center part of upper lip which was excised. The defect was closed with an Estlander-Abbé flap from the lower lip. The tumor, however, recurred. It was then widely excised and a turnover flap was prepared from the right side for lining of the upper lip defect after Ferris Smith (p. 256).

b: After elevation of the turnover flap the flap was depilated and turned over to form the lining of the upper lip. A cheek flap from the right side was rotated to form the outside. An oral mucous-membrane flap was rotated to resurface the raw surface of the turnover flap and to form the vermilion border. There was no recurrence of the tumor twelve years after the operation.

ILLUSTRATIVE CASES

CASE
32

Case 32, *a:* Patient, aged sixty years, with squamous-cell cancer involving almost the entire lower lip, the left angle of the mouth, and the left fourth of upper lip. Owing to extent of the lesion, radiation was contraindicated. There was no evidence of metastasis. The lines of excision are outlined.

b: After excision of the diseased tissues.

c: The defect was closed with a bilateral composite cheek flap according to the method shown in Figure 82. Formation and mobilization of the left composite cheek flap. The defect of the upper lip was closed by simple skin sliding. The patient was discharged from the hospital two weeks after the operation.

d, e: Five months after operation. No reactivation or metastasis nine years after operation.

1036

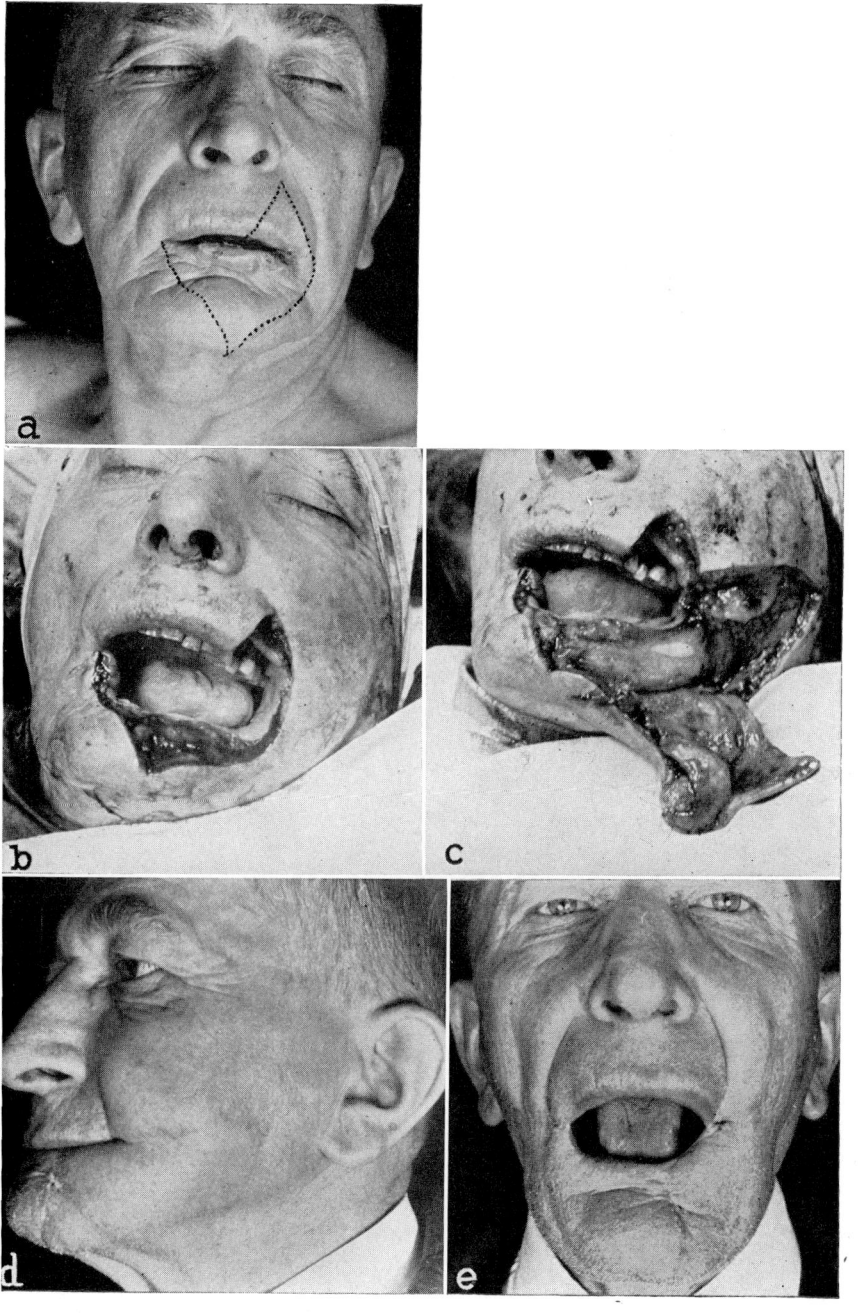

CASE
33

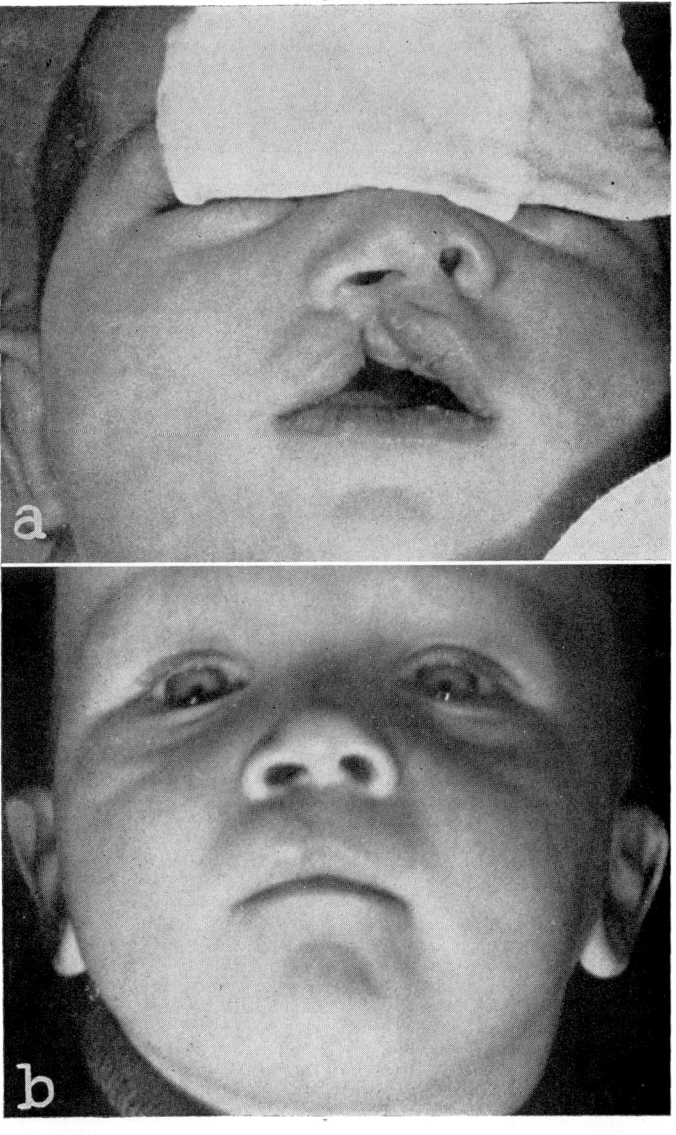

Case 33, *a:* Complete cleft lip and cleft of alveolar process. Operation seven weeks after birth.

b: Eighteen months after operation.

CASE
34

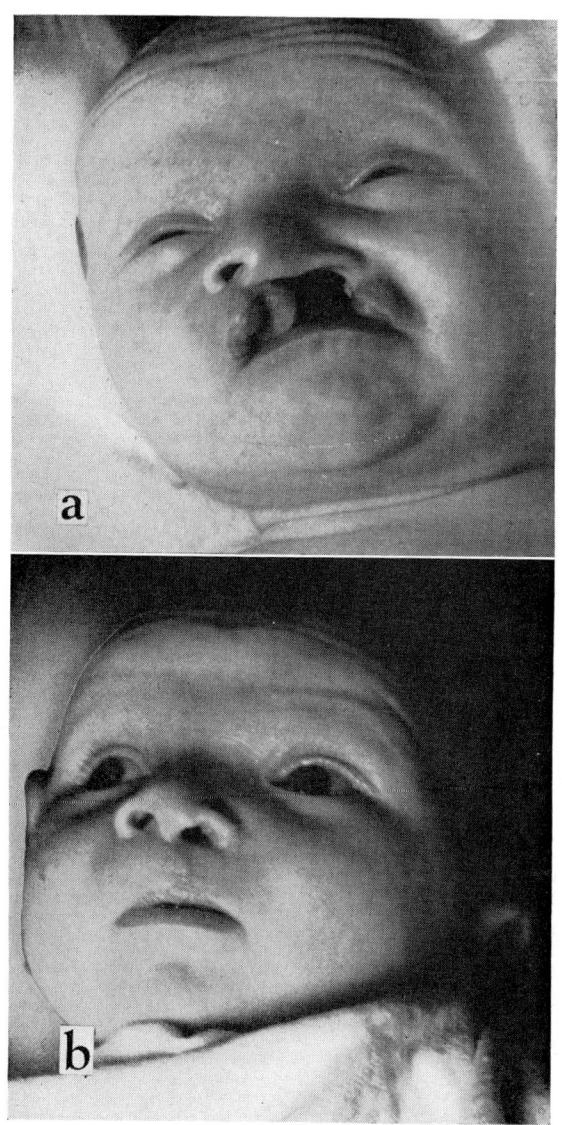

Case 34, *a, b:* Extensive through-and-through cleft lip and palate. Closure of lip cleft, formation of nostril, and bridging of the cleft in the alveolar process when child was six weeks of age. Axhausen-LeMesurier technique. Closure of palatal cleft at the age of two years.

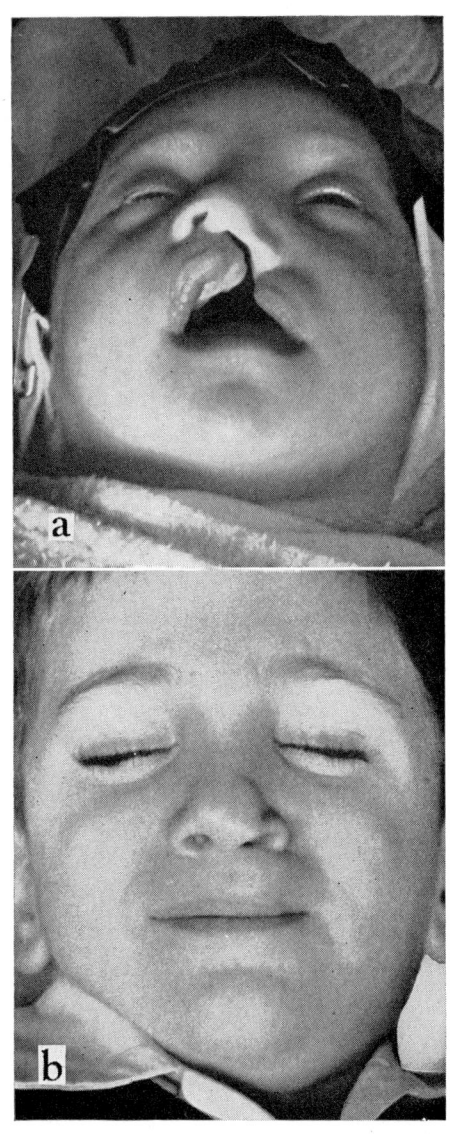

Case 35, *a:* Through-and-through left-sided cleft lip and palate. Closure of cleft of lip, formation of nostril, and bridging of the cleft in the alveolar process when child was five weeks of age. Axhausen-LeMesurier technique. Closure of cleft of palate at the age of two years.

b: Eight years later.

1040

CASE
36

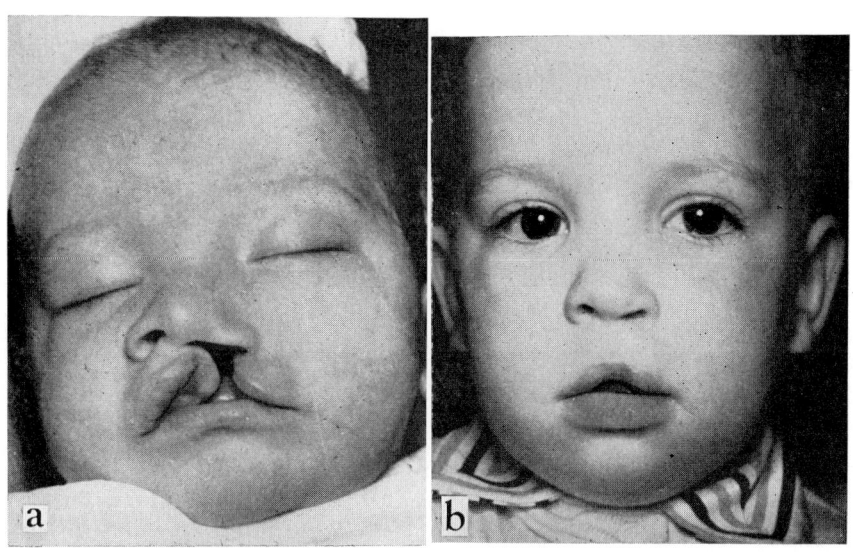

Case 36, *a:* Through-and-through cleft lip and palate. Closure of the cleft of lip, formation of nostril, and bridging of cleft in alveolar process when child was six weeks of age. Axhausen-LeMesurier technique. Closure of cleft of palate two years later.

b: Three years later.

CASE
37

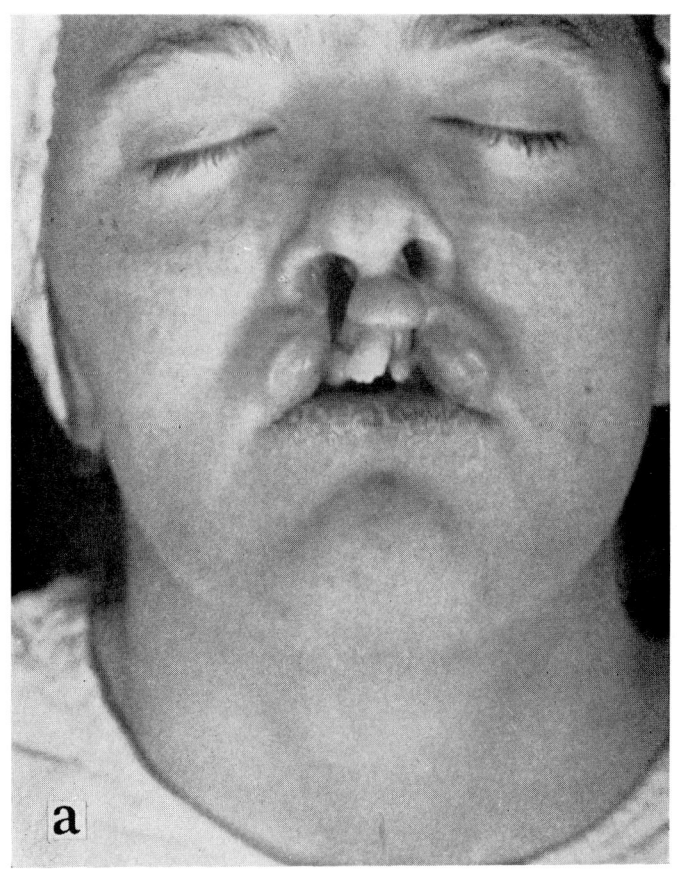

a

Case 37, *a:* Patient, aged seventeen, born with bilateral cleft lip and palate. Father would not give permission for operation in spite of numerous pleas from his family, friends, neighbors, and in spite of the fact he had to present his case once before court. At this age he reluctantly gave permission for surgical repair.

b, c: Closure of the bilateral lip defect in one stage.

d, e: Columella was elongated by use of skin of the prelabium (p. 318). Protruding premaxilla removed; missing teeth replaced with prosthesis which also had an appliance to hold the upper lip in normal protrusion.

1042

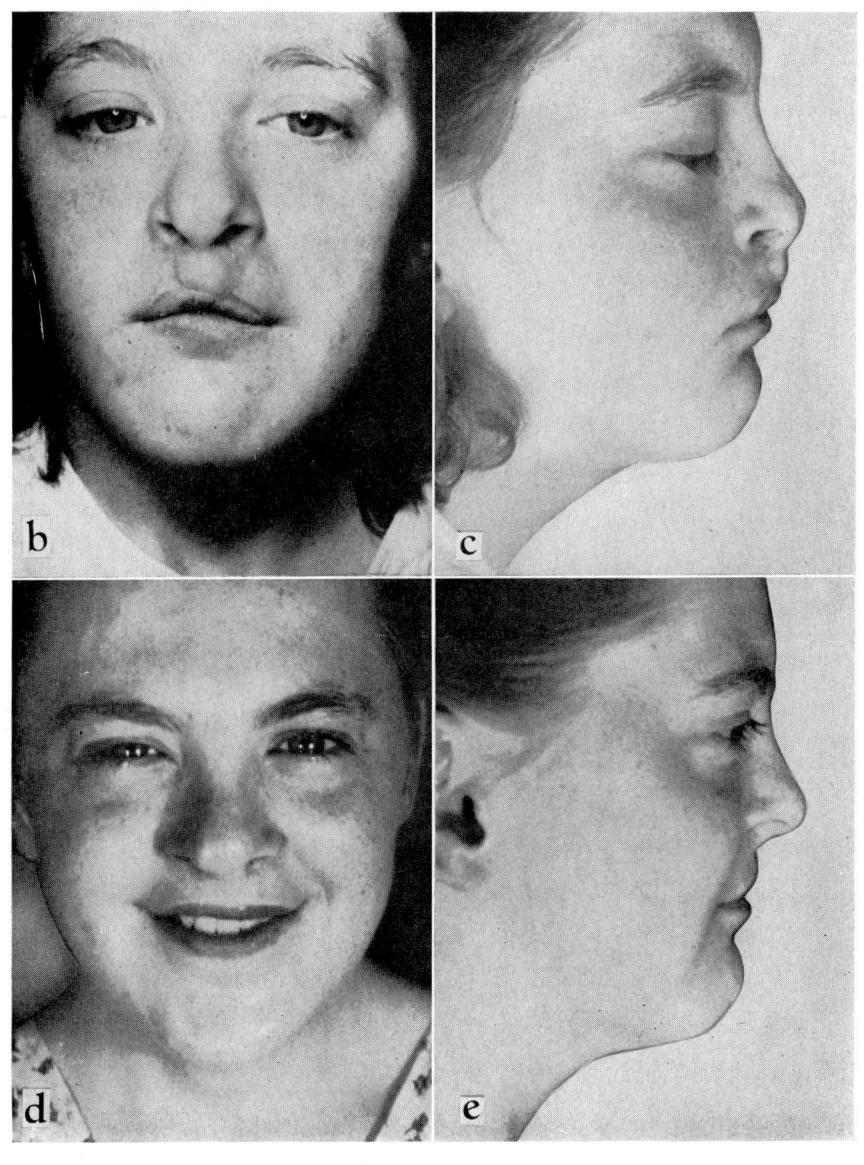

CASE
38

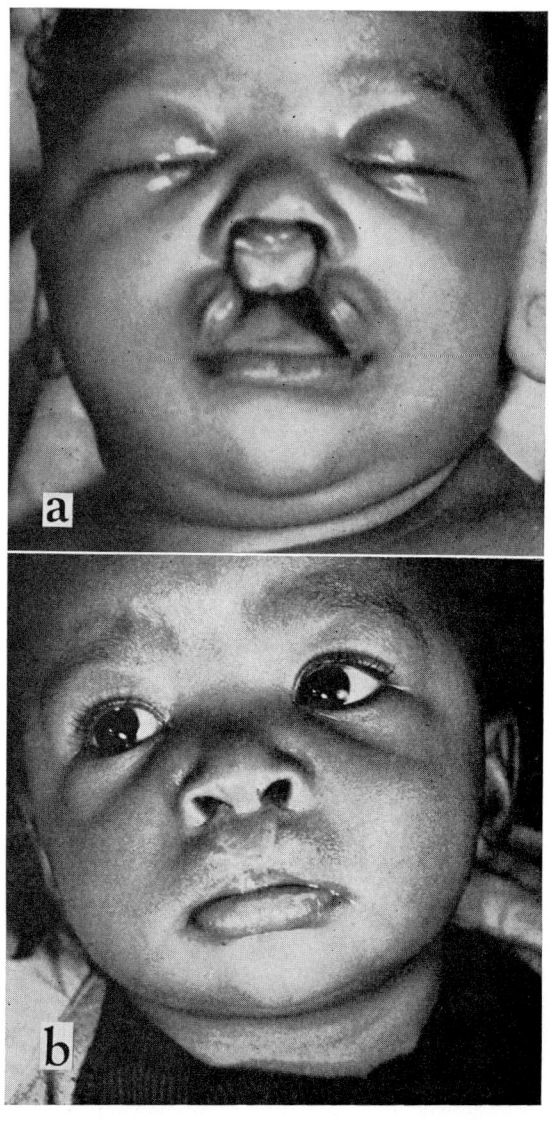

Case 38, *a, b:* Bilateral cleft lip and cleft in anterior part of palate. Both were closed when child was four weeks of age.

ILLUSTRATIVE CASES

CASE
39

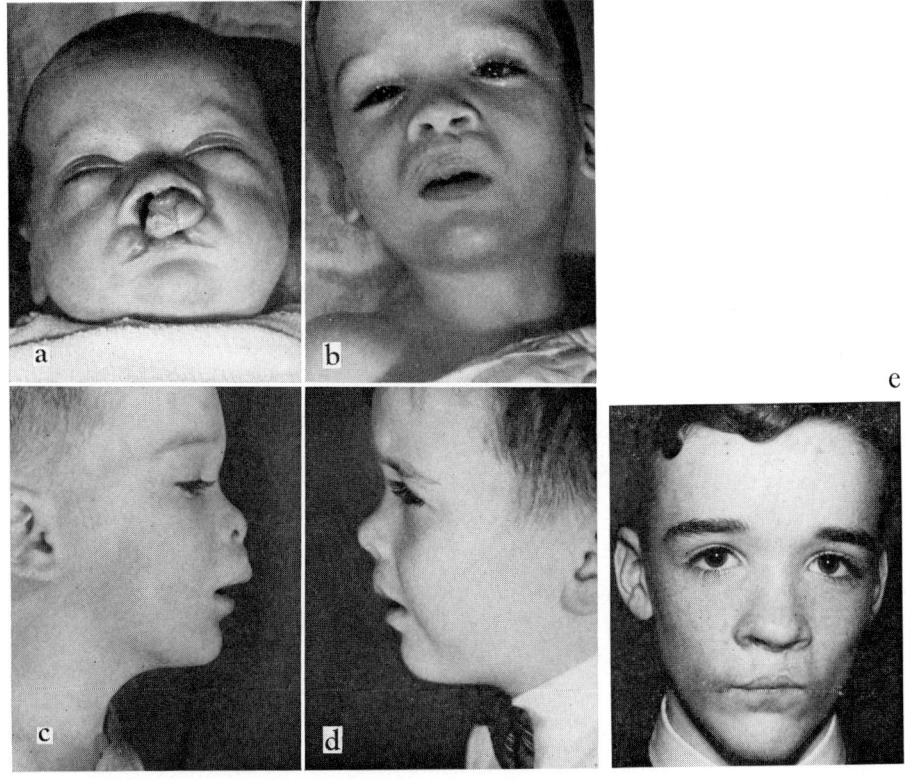

Case 39, *a:* Bilateral cleft lip and palate.

b: Closure of lip cleft and formation of nostrils and floor of nostrils in one stage. Closure of cleft of palate in two stages one and a half years later.

c: "Dogmouth" appearance from protrusion of premaxilla.

d: Removal of premaxilla (p. 320) at age four. Elevation of philtrum flap to lengthen columella. Four weeks later philtrum flap again elevated and folded to lengthen columella. Flap bed at philtrum skin grafted. Boy wears dentures with appliance to hold upper lip in normal protrusion.

e: At age fourteen, good cosmetic and functional results. Boy speaks with nearly normal voice, is on honor roll at school.

1045

ILLUSTRATIVE CASES

CASE
40

Case 40: Baby born with a left-sided transverse facial cleft (*a*). Familial history was negative. Cleft reached to the anterior border of the masseter muscle. Cleft edges were lined with vermilion tissue. In addition to the cleft the following deformities—all on the left side—were present: underdevelopment of left side of face, rudimentary ear cartilages situated in level of masseter muscle, no external auditory canal, absence of left Stensen's duct, no trace of parotid gland, underdevelopment of left side of mandible, absence of zygoma, notch in median third of upper lid, dermoid cyst and a rare lesion such as a chondroma of lateral half of conjunctiva, and coloboma of iris (*a* and *b*). X-ray examination demonstrated underdevelopment of the base of the skull, absence of malar arch, underdevelopment of mandible, possible absence of ascending ramus, no evidence of external ear or mastoid cells. Hence the deformity is comparable with the syndrome of the mandibular arch, a dysostosis mandibulo facialis (p. 355). At ten weeks of age the transverse cleft was repaired according to the method described on page 357 and the rudimentary ear cartilages were removed. Beneath the latter was found a cyst the size of a cherry filled with sebaceous matter and lined with epithelium; it represented the blind ending of the external auditory canal, and was removed. In a second operation, five months later, the vermilion-border junction between the Estlander flap and upper lip, which was bulging, was adjusted and the transverse scar, which had become hypertrophic, was excised and repaired. The scar again became hypertrophic and contracting (*c*). It was repaired by a Z-plasty (*d*). The hypertrophy did not recur and the cheek became fuller; hence, it is reasonable to assume that the tightness caused the hypertrophic changes.

e: Patient at age eleven after reconstruction of ear. Zygoma and ascending ramus—the latter to be replaced with fifth metatarsal bone—to be reconstructed at a later stage (at age fourteen or fifteen). (H. May: Plast. Reconstr. Surg.)

1046

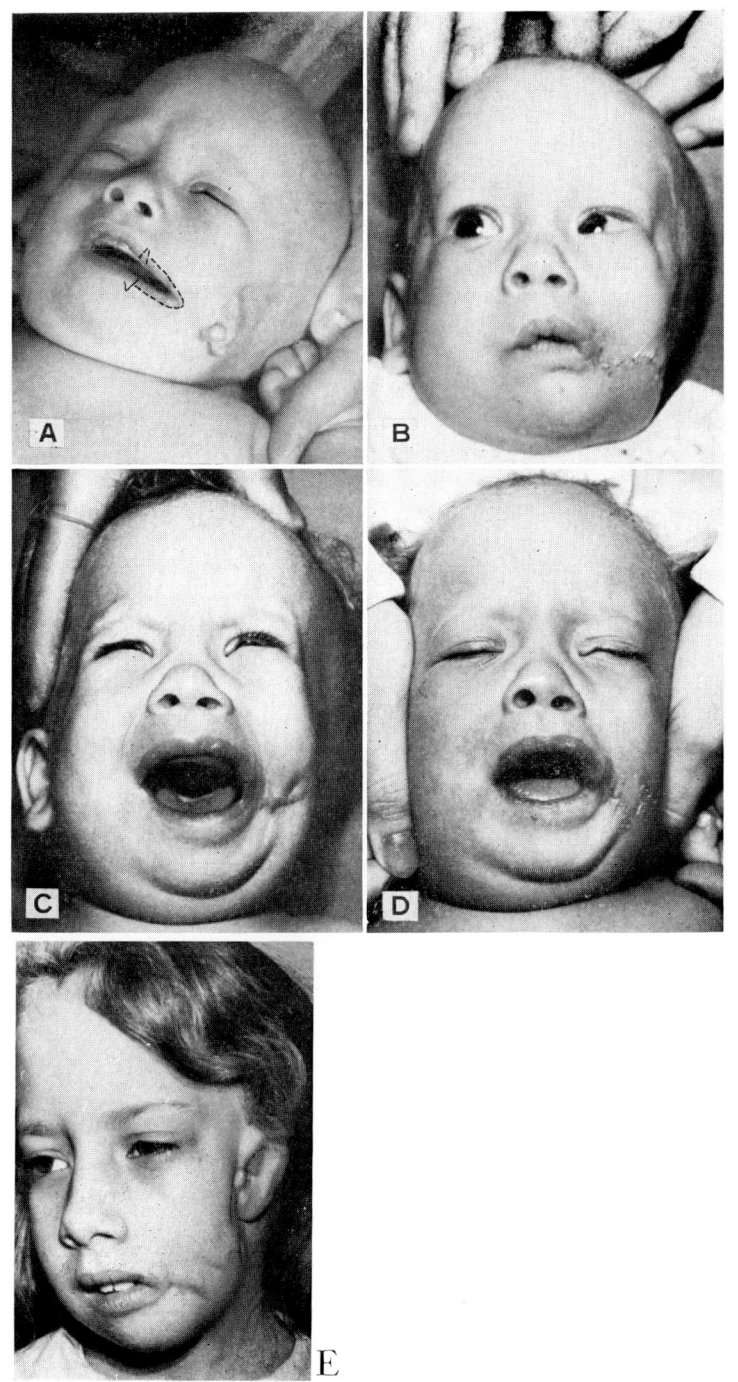

CASE
41

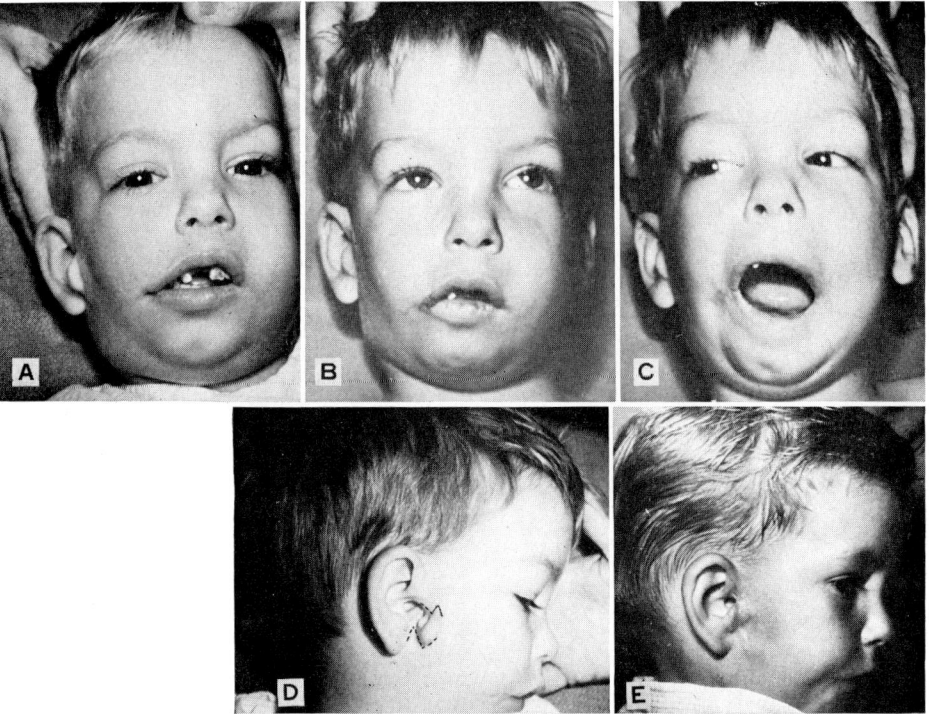

Case 41. This 2½-year-old boy was born with a right-side transverse facial cleft, underdevelopment of the right side of the mandible, and forward displacement of the tragus of the right ear (*A*). Familial history was negative. The cleft was about 2 cm. long, the cleft borders lined with skin. An oral commissure was absent because of lack of fusion of the orbicularis oris muscle; liquids drained from this opening. Due to underdevelopment of the mandible, the right side of the face seemed to be underdeveloped (*A*). The tragus was rather large and displaced forward without any connection with the auricle; back of it appeared to be a rudimentary tragus (*D*). The external auditory canal was present. *B, C:* The transverse cleft was closed according to the method described on page 357. The tragus was moved back by means of a two-stage Z-plasty (*D* and *E*). Later, the right side of the mandible could be lengthened. (H. May: Plast. Reconstr. Surg.)

CASE
42

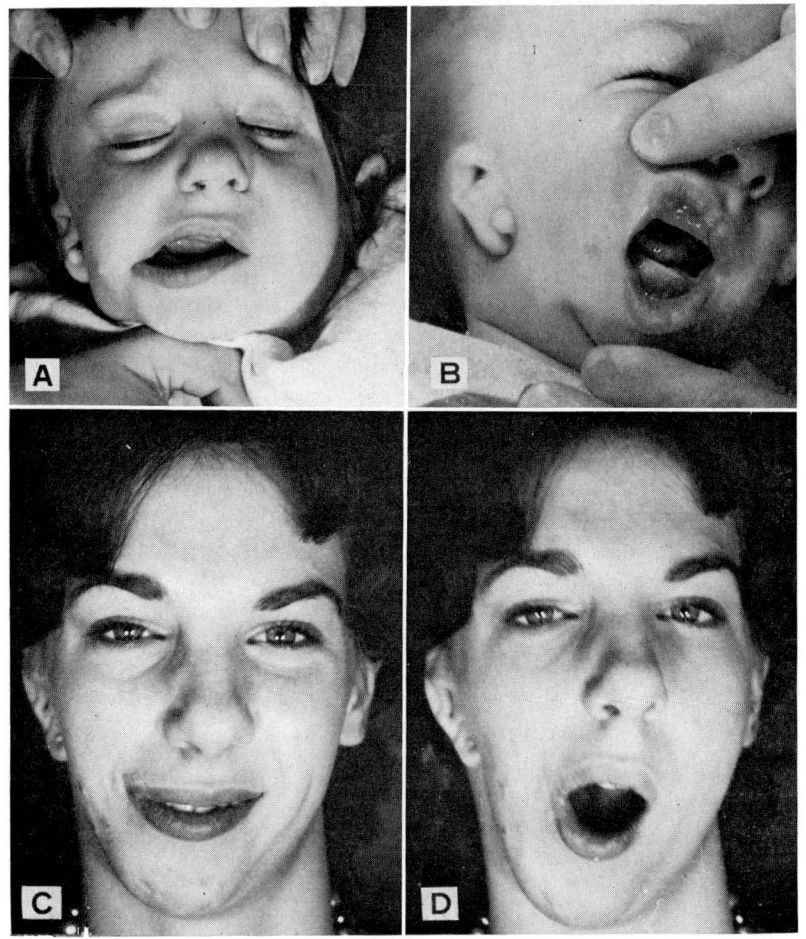

Case 42, *A* and *B:* Transverse facial cleft. Lower cleft border is vermilion lined and contains orbicularis muscle; upper border is shorter and skin lined, and has no orbicularis muscle (*B*); right side of mandible and right ear are underdeveloped (*B*).

C and *D:* After reconstruction of commissure, lengthening of right side of mandible and reconstruction of ear. (H. May: Plast. Reconstr. Surg.)

CASE
43

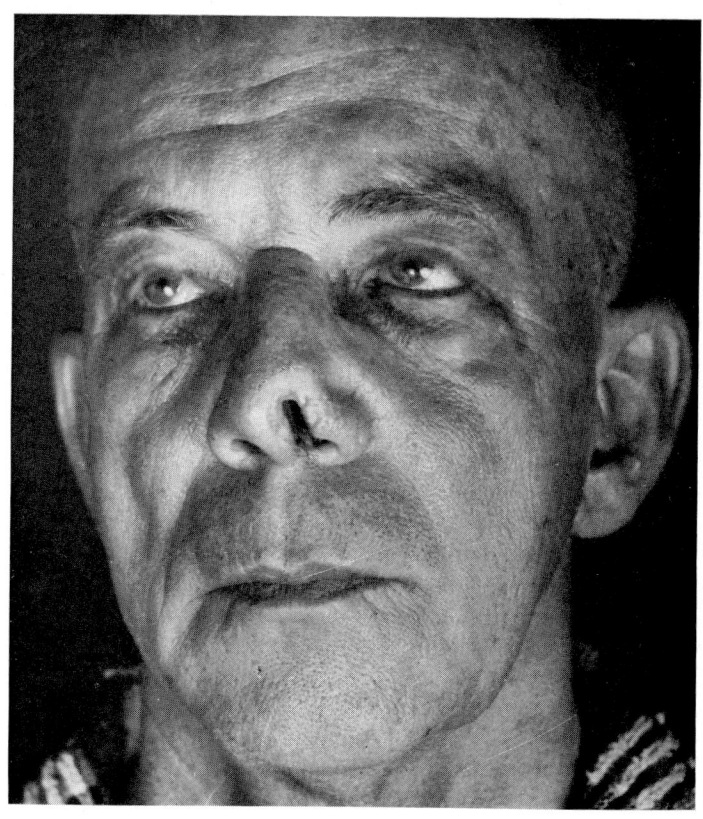

a

Case 43, *a:* Defect of left columella-alar angle five years after electrocoagulation of a basal cell carcinoma.

b: The defect at the columella-alar angle was closed with a composite skin cartilage graft (p. 388) which was taken from the rim of the
right ear. The defect at the ear was closed according to the method of
Figure 251 resulting in only slightly smaller ear. This picture depicts the
patient four weeks after the operation.

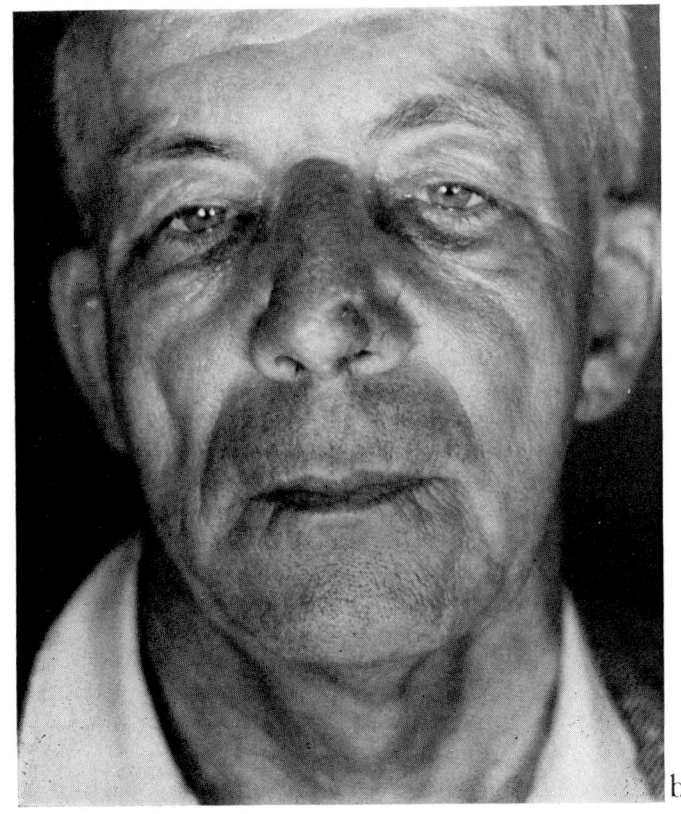

b

CASE
44

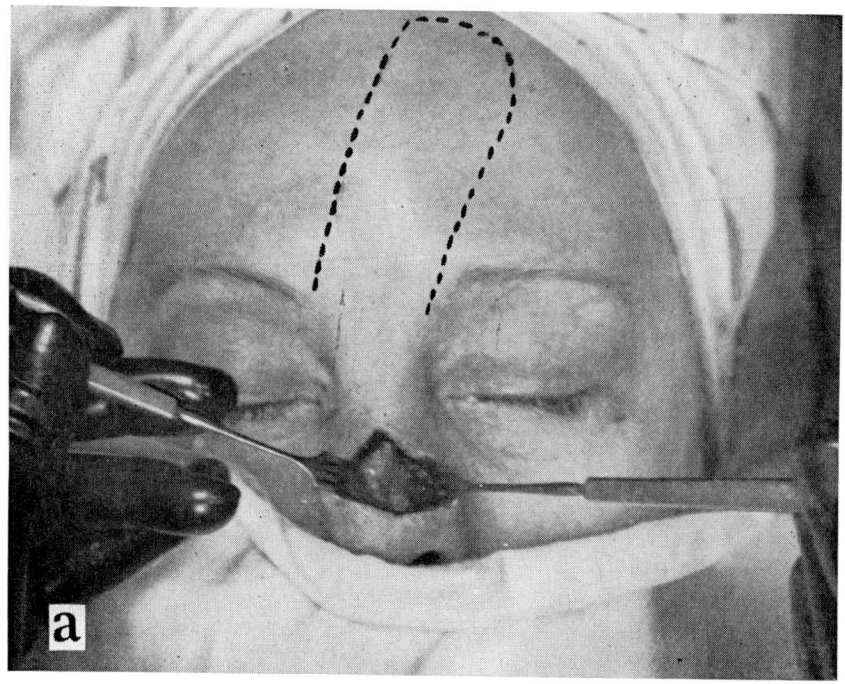

a

Case 44, *a:* Patient, aged sixty-two, was treated forty years ago with paraffin injection to elevate a traumatic flatness of the ridge of the nose. The cosmetic result was good and the patient had no symptoms until one summer when she exposed her nose to an extensive sunburn, the paraffin melted, the skin broke down and the cartilages were exposed. The entire damaged area was removed by excision leaving a full-thickness defect which was closed with a forehead flap.

b: Five weeks after transfer of forehead flap the pedicle was severed and flap and pedicle were adjusted.

c: Six months later the rather thick flap was defatted.

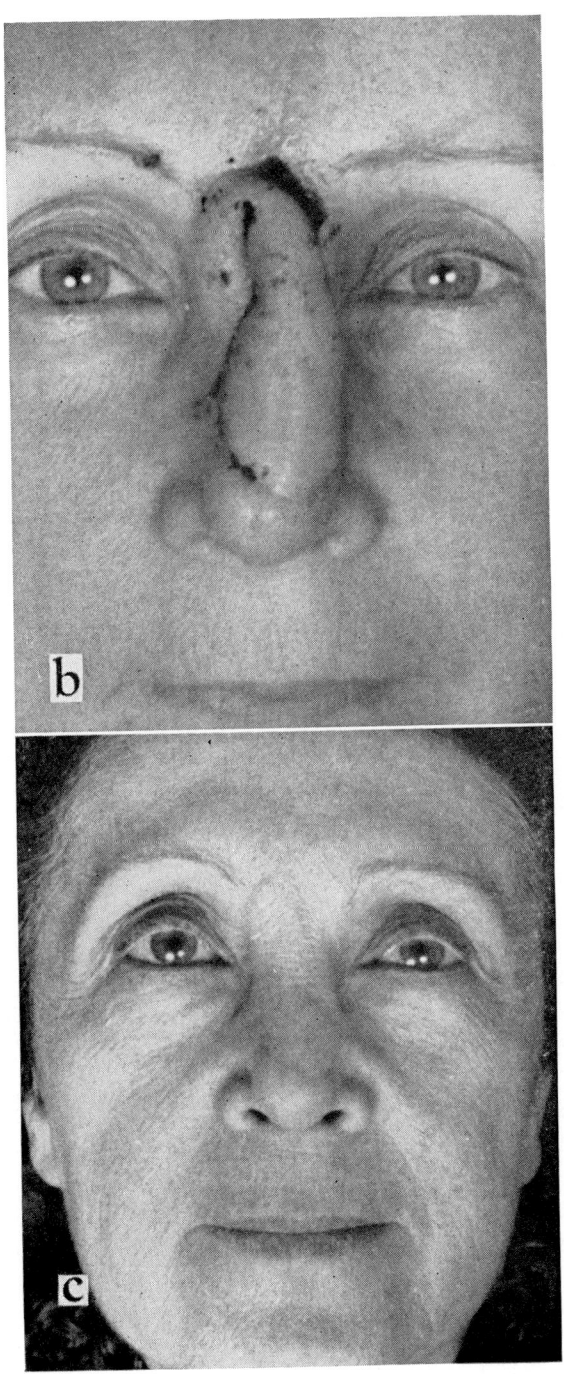

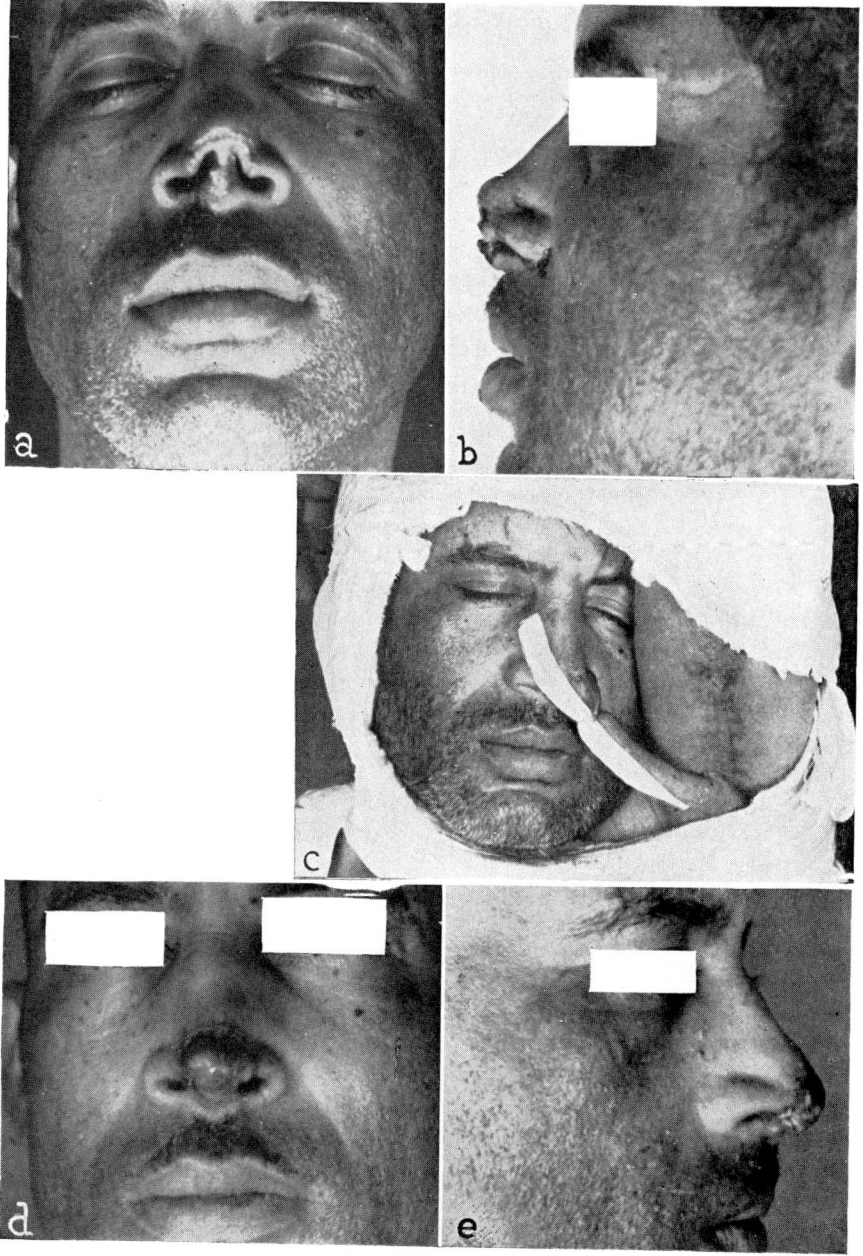

Case 45: Defect of tip of nose, nose, and parts of alae and columella from human bite; reconstructed with tube flap from arm.

CASE
46

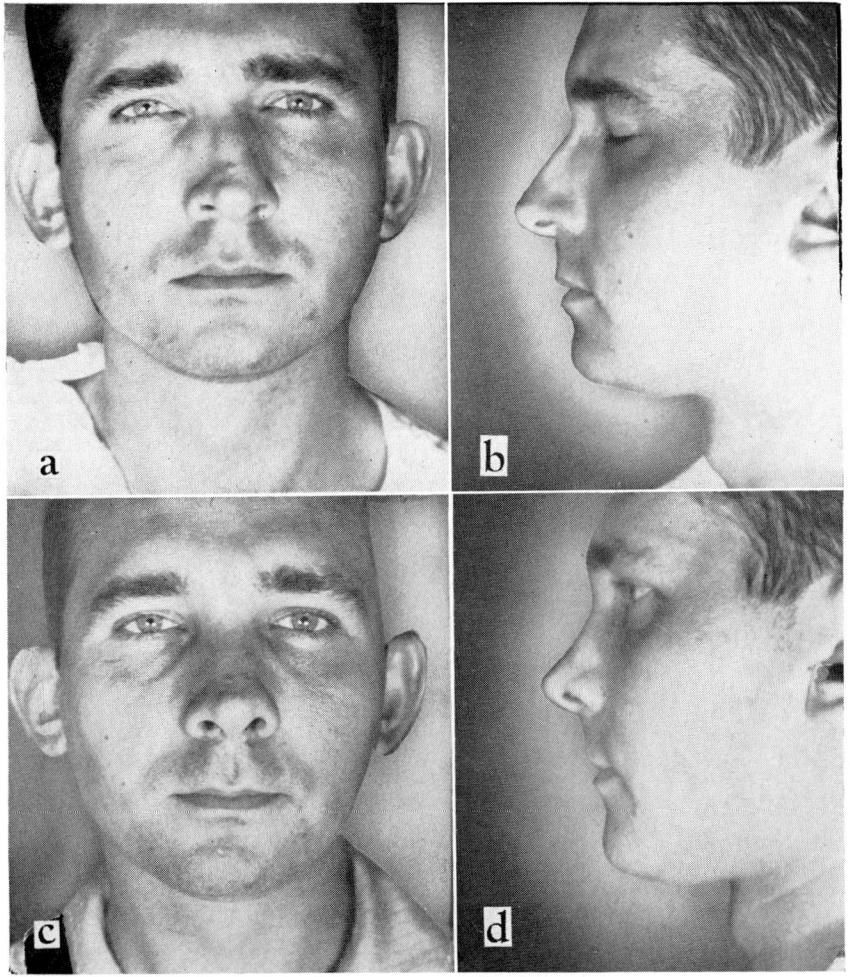

Case 46, *a, b:* Traumatic left-sided deviation of nose. Impairment of breathing from marked right-sided deviation of septum while the free edge of the septal cartilage was found deviated in the left nostril.

c, d: After rhinoplasty which consisted of slight reduction of the osseous ridge of the nose (greater reduction was made on elongated right side than on left side). Both anterior processes of maxilla were severed and both nasal bones shifted into midline. Removal of the deviated free end of the cartilaginous septum. The impairment of breathing remained. Patient may need submucous resection in the future.

CASE
47

Case 47: Patient, aged sixty-four, had had basal-cell cancer of the right side of the nose for sixteen years. He had had a full course of x-ray radiation (3000 R from sides, 3000 R from front, unfiltered). The lesion had continued to advance, and involved the tip of the nose. Radical excision of the right ala, parts of the tip of the nose, and parts of the right lateral wall of the nose was performed. There was no evidence of recurrence. The defect was closed with a lined sickel flap from the scalp, which was developed in several stages, according to the method of Figure 184, page 394. The first mobilization consisted of elevation of the scalp flap between temple and frontal pedicle.

a: Four weeks later, the flap was mobilized again between the two pedicles, and the frontal pedicle was severed. Four weeks later, the frontal part of the flap was elevated and lined with a composite graft consisting of skin and cartilage. The latter was taken from the anterior surface of the concha of the right ear. The raw surface of the concha was covered with a thick split graft. The pedicle was returned. Both grafts took completely.

b: Two weeks later, transplantation of the flap from the forehead to the nasal defect was effected. The borders of the defect were circumscribed with an incision and hinged inward, to increase the raw surface and to provide a broader base for the flap. Forehead area was covered with a full-thickness graft taken from the right supraclavicular region. The wound edges of the flap bed were held together with mattress sutures, which were tied over bismuth tribromophenate (xeroform) gauze. One week later, the pedicle was partially separated. Five days later, the pedicle was severed entirely, followed two days later by replacement of the pedicle to the flap bed on the skull and adjustment of the flap to the nasal defect edges.

c: Two months after the last stage.

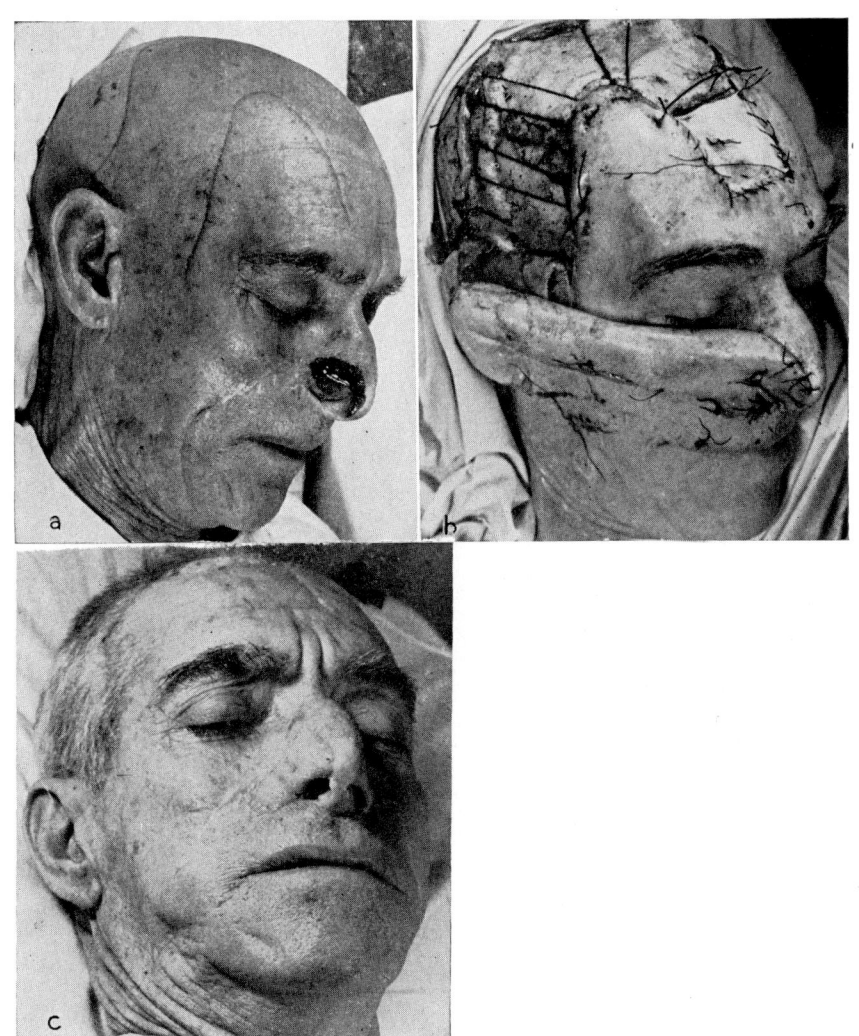

CASE
48

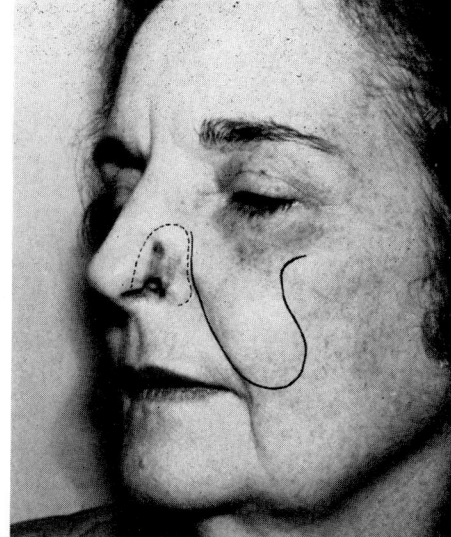

a

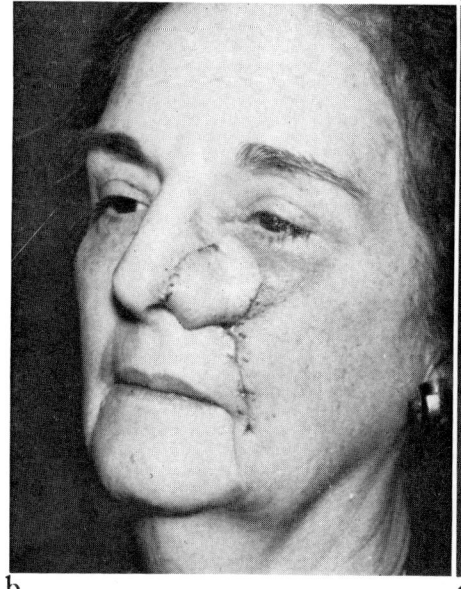

b   c

Case 48, *a:* Carcinoma of left ala. Part to be excised lined out with dotted lines; adjacent cheek flap lined out according to method described on page 392.

b: Distal end of flap doubled up to form lining and rim of ala; flap rotated. Scar from closure of flap bed comes to lie within nasolabial fold.

c: After configuration of base of ala was improved with Z-plasties, and flap was defatted and adjusted.

1058

CASE
49

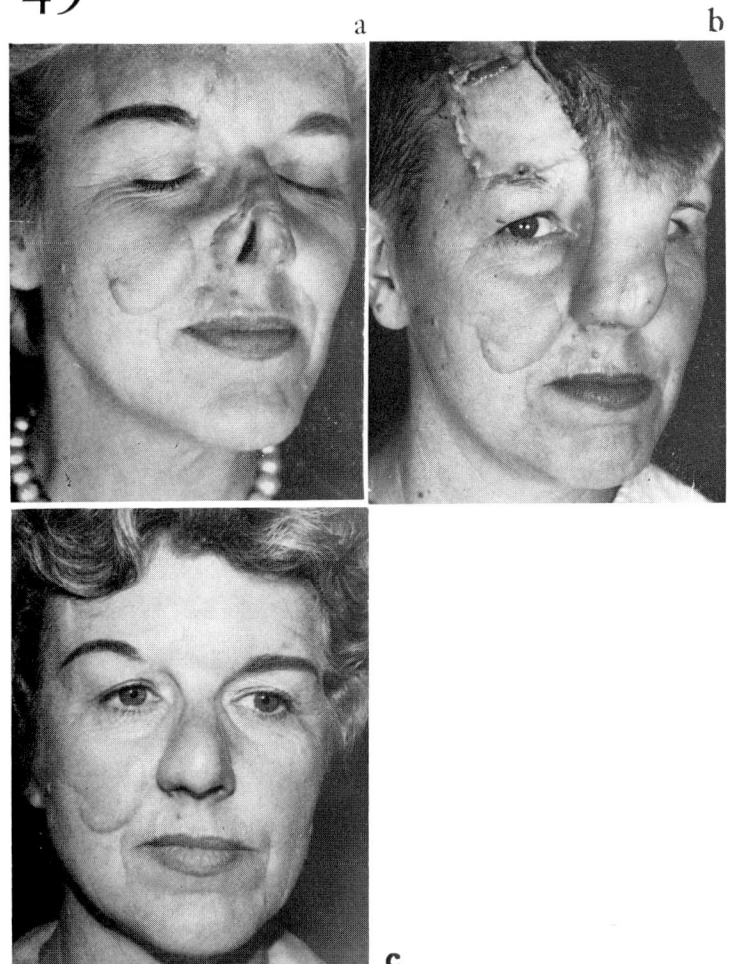

a   b

c

Case 49, *a:* Traumatic defect of most of right ala and lower ridge of nose and tip; surface defects of tip and lateral nasal walls replaced with skin grafts as emergency measure.

b: Replacement of defect and skin grafted areas with scalp-forehead flap after Converse (p. 402). Skin grafting of forehead defect. Pressure dressing of scalp defect. Three weeks later partial separation of pedicle, followed by complete separation of pedicle and return of scalp part of flap to scalp. Two weeks later adjustment of nasal flap after J. Penn. (p. 403).

c: After defatting and minor adjustments of nasal flap and improvement of cheek scar.

1059

CASE
50

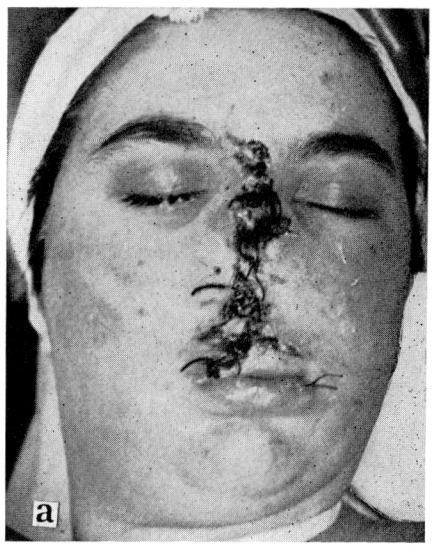

Case 50, *a:* Girl, aged nineteen, with partial loss of upper lip and nose from an automobile accident. The upper jaw was fractured in four places and severed through the sinuses. The mandible was fractured in two places. Emergency treatment was performed elsewhere, consisting of arresting hemorrhage mainly by pulling the facial wound edges together with thick silk sutures, tracheotomy, and shock treatment.

b: After transfer of the patient (ten days after the accident) the facial wounds were separated, and reduction and fixation of the maxillary fragments with the arch bar method and suspension of the maxilla were carried out (see p. 564 and Figure 264). The fractures of the mandible were stabilized with intramedullary Kirschner wires. Three weeks later the missing part of the right side of the upper lip was replaced with a flap from the lower lip by the Estlander-Abbé method. Six weeks later a forehead sickle flap, pedicled in the left temporal-mastoid area, was elevated in preparation for reconstruction of the nose. In the first stage the flap was elevated between two pedicles and returned. Two weeks later the peripheral pedicle over the eyebrows was severed; three weeks later the entire flap was elevated and returned.

c: After all edema in the flap had subsided, i.e. two months after the last stage, the flap was raised, the peripheral end folded to shape the nose and the remainder of the flap tubed. The donor area at the forehead was covered with a thick split skin graft. The scalp wound edges were held together with heavy mattress sutures. Three and one-half weeks later the flap was incised above the nose and a laboratory clamp applied for gradual crushing of the pedicle. Three days later the flap was severed and the pedicle returned to the skull. One week later the nose flap was adjusted.

1060

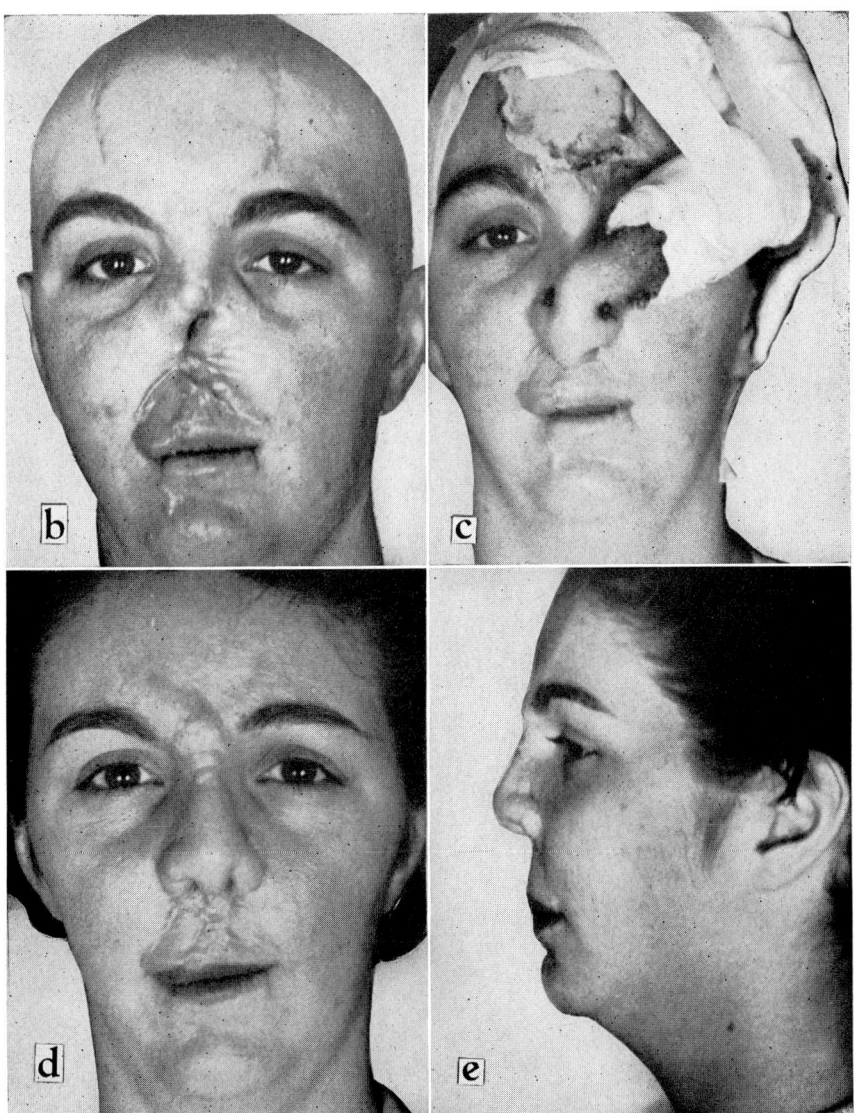

d, e: It took several readjustments of the nose flap to give the nose the final shape and to open the nostrils. Four months later an autogenous rib cartilage graft was inserted to hold the ridge of the nose elevated.

All of the patient's scars (face, arms, tracheotomy scars) became hypertrophic. Irradiation smoothed out all but those of upper lip which can be disguised to certain degree with makeup.

1061

CASE
51

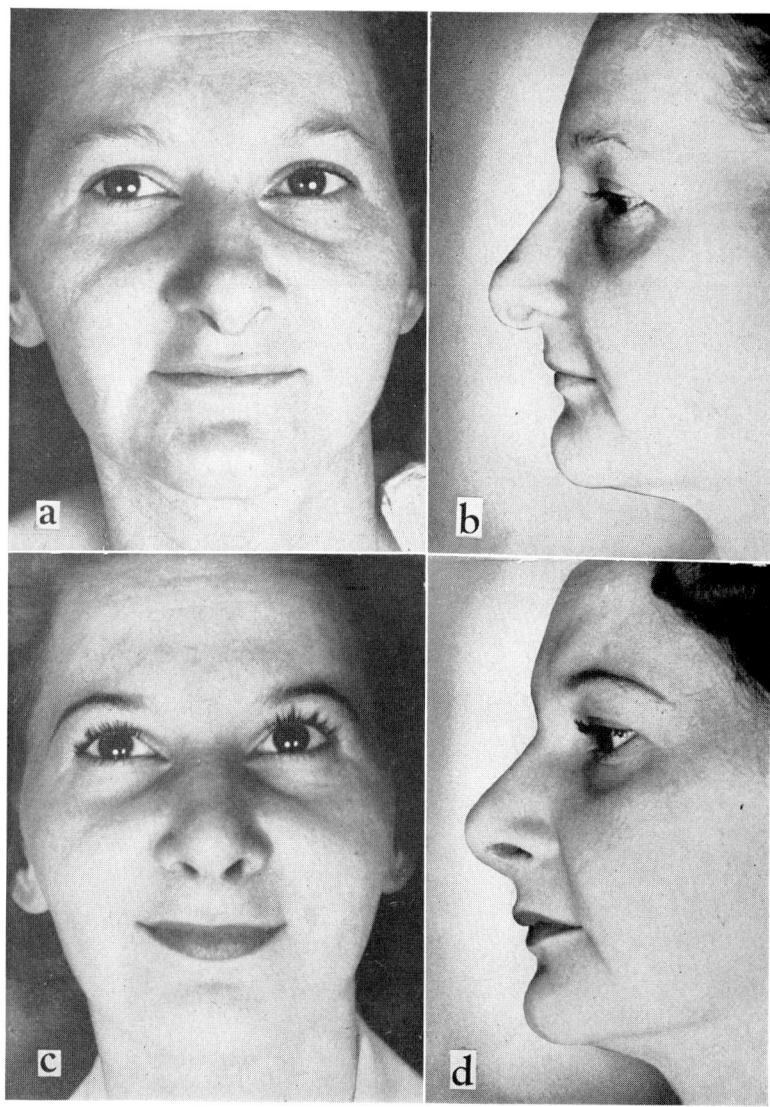

Case 51, *a, b:* Nasal deformity mainly consisting of bulbous tip, enlargement of the lower lateral cartilages, and hanging columella.

c, d: From a Réthi incision the lower lateral cartilages were reduced in height as well as in width. The columella cartilages were reduced in height. The upper lateral cartilages were reduced in width. The hanging of the columella was overcome by excision of a strip of free edge of the cartilaginous septum and reduction of the columellar cartilages.

CASE
52

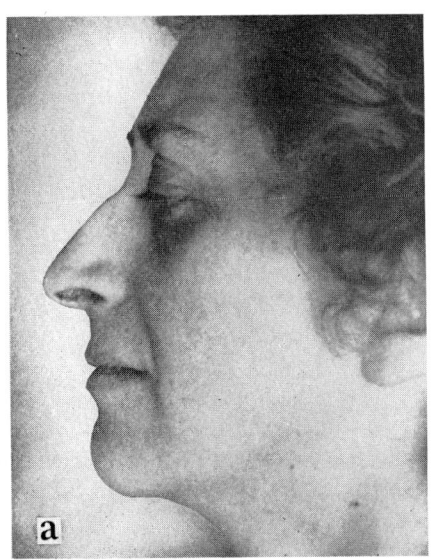 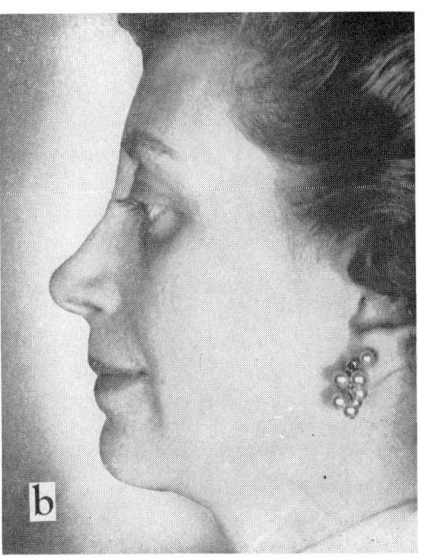

Case 52, *a:* Hump nose. Long nose.

   b: Rhinoplasty consisting of reduction of the nose in height as well
as in length.

CASE
53

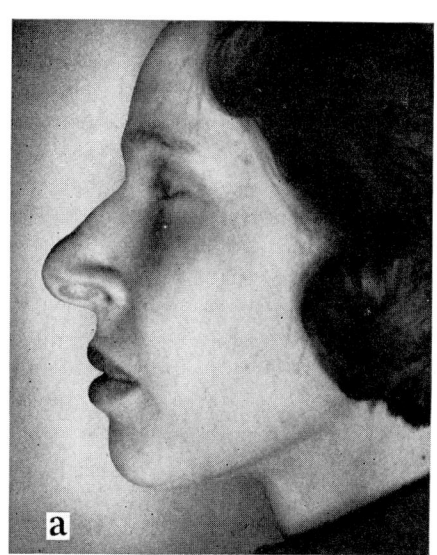 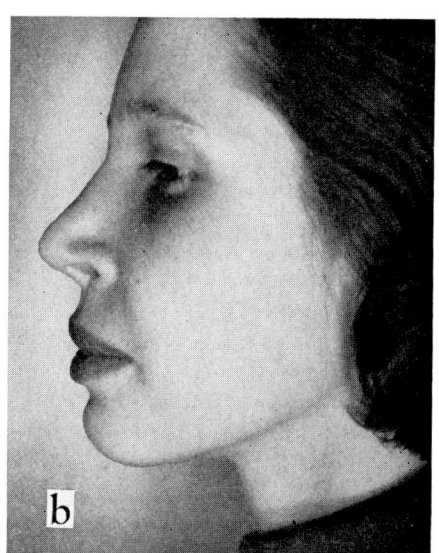

Case 53, *a:* Long, large nose. Drooping columella.

b: Correction of the nasal deformity by reduction of the nose in height and length. Hanging of columella overcome by reduction of width of columellar cartilages.

CASE
54

a

b

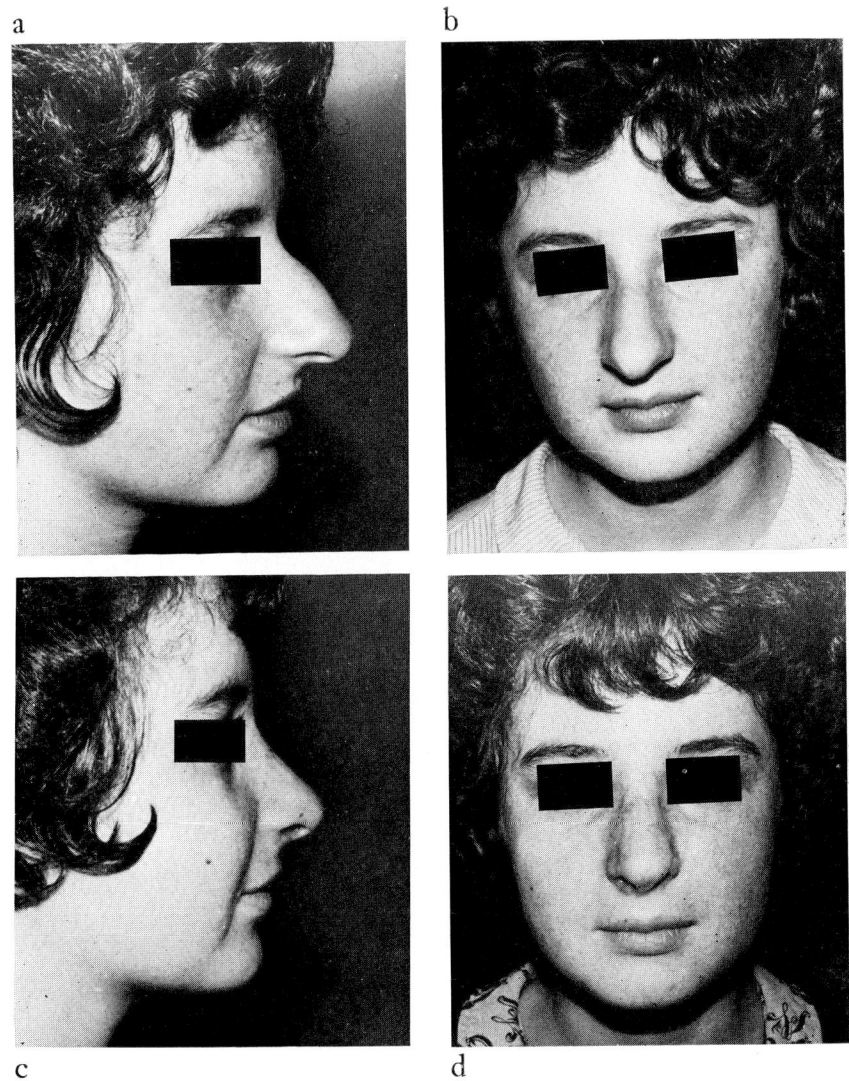

c

d

Case 54, *a* and *b:* Marked enlargement of nose in height as well as in length. Note narrow upper lip and retrusion of chin.

c and *d:* After rhinoplasty which consisted of marked reduction of all parts of the nose. Upper lip has become longer from shortening of nose and reduction of the crest of the tuberculum maxillae. Chin appears more prominent, although it was not built up.

a   b

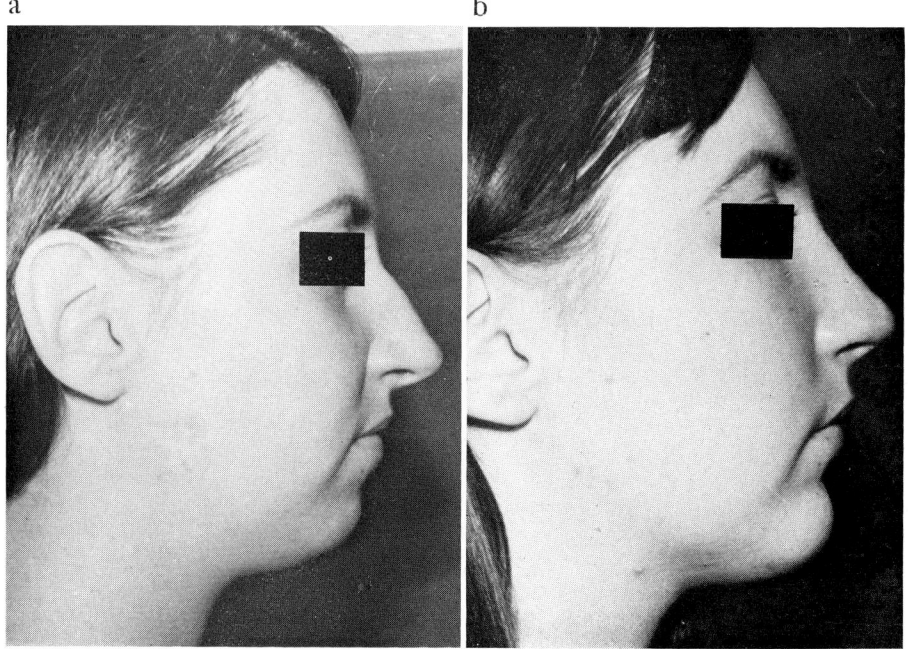

Case 55, *a:* The nose is slightly enlarged, elongated and humped. Upper lip is narrow. The deformity is accentuated by retrusion of the chin.

b: The chin is built up with a perforated silicon prosthesis and the nose properly shaped by a rhinoplasty; note increase in height of upper lip.

1066

CASE
56

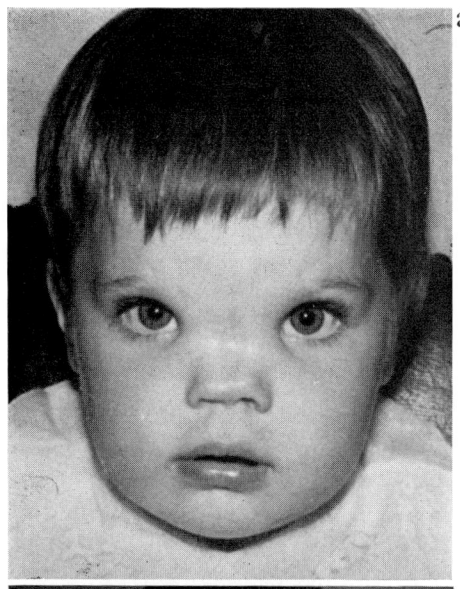

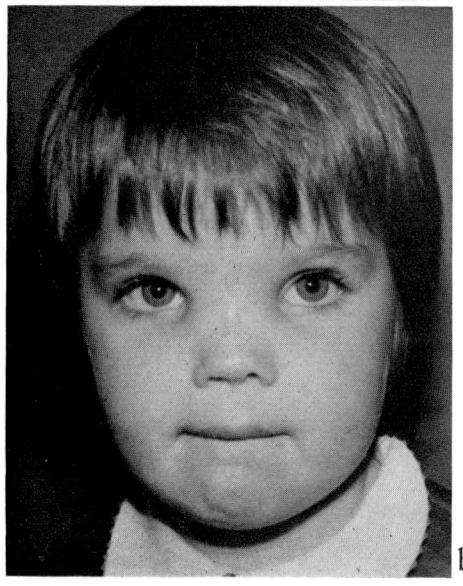

Case 56, *a:* 2½-year-old girl with cleft nose and seeming hypertheliorism of eyes.

b: Four years after repair of cleft nose (p. 435). Hypertheliorism appears less pronounced.

CASE
57

a   b

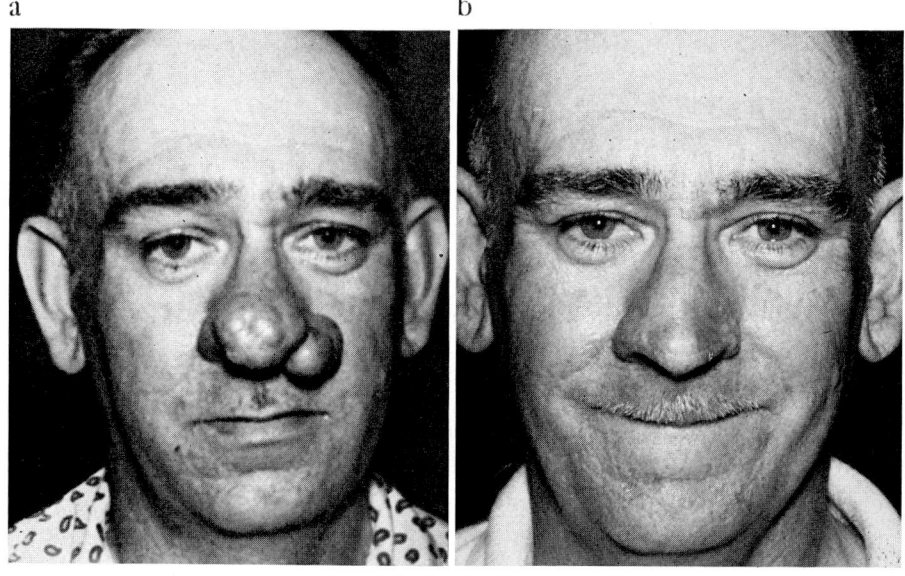

Case 57, *a:* Patient, aged forty-four, with a rhinophyma of many years' duration.

b: Entire skin of the nose containing the rhinophyma was removed and replaced with a thick split skin graft from the upper part of the chest.

1068

CASE
58

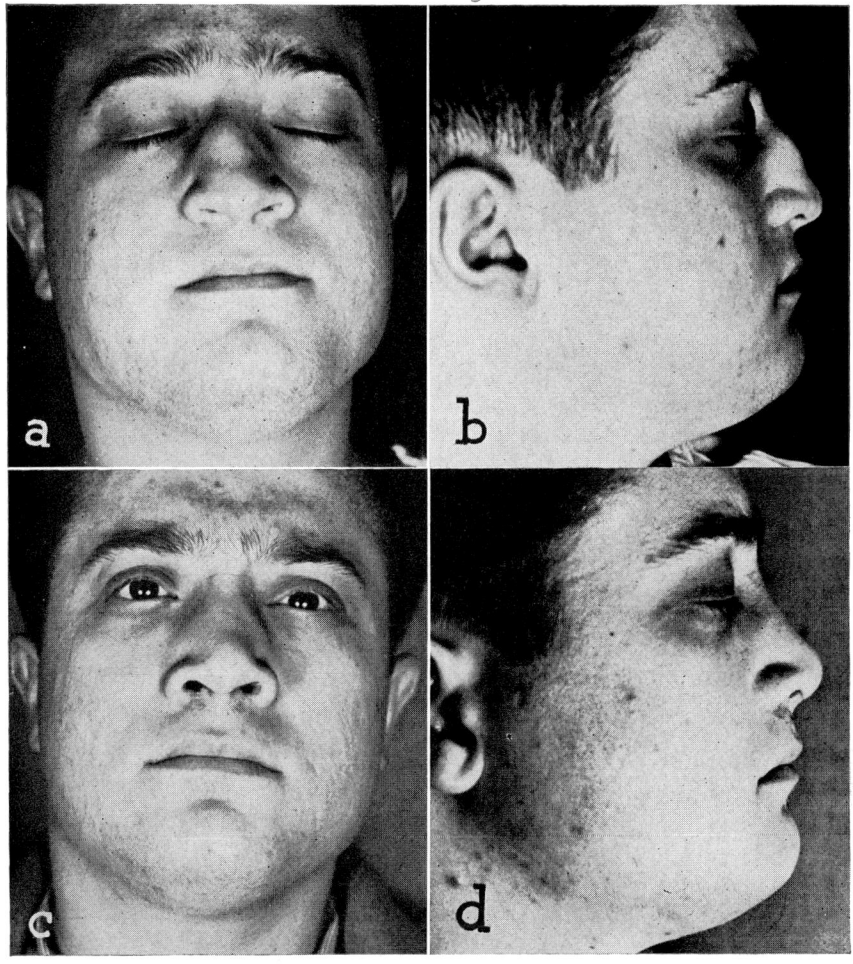

Case 58, *a, b:* Patient, aged twenty, with traumatic deformities of nose: deviation of nose, hump formation, shallow depression of cartilaginous ridge, wide nasal tip, wide nostrils, and marked deviation of septum causing impaired nasal breathing.

c, d: After removal of the hump, severance of the anterior process of the maxilla, shifting the nasal pyramid toward the left, reduction of width of tip, reflection of the median part of these cartilages toward the midline and suturing them back to back to fill out the slight depression of the cartilaginous ridge. Reduction of width of nostrils, submucous resection, severance of the septum from its base, and shifting of septum into the midline.

CASE
59

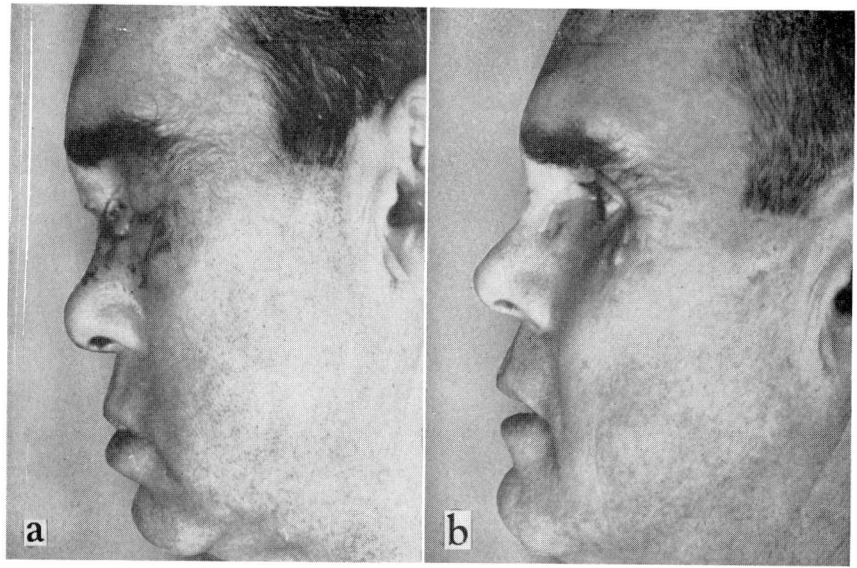

a   b

Case 59, *a:* Patient, aged forty-four, received multiple fractures of both orbits, zygomatic arch; entire maxilla was severed from base of skull; fracture of ridge of nose (Le Fort III type of fracture). After reduction and suspension of the maxillary fractures (p. 564) reconstruction of the ridge of the nose was carried out with an autogenous rib graft after healing of fractures.

b: Two years after the accident.

CASE
60

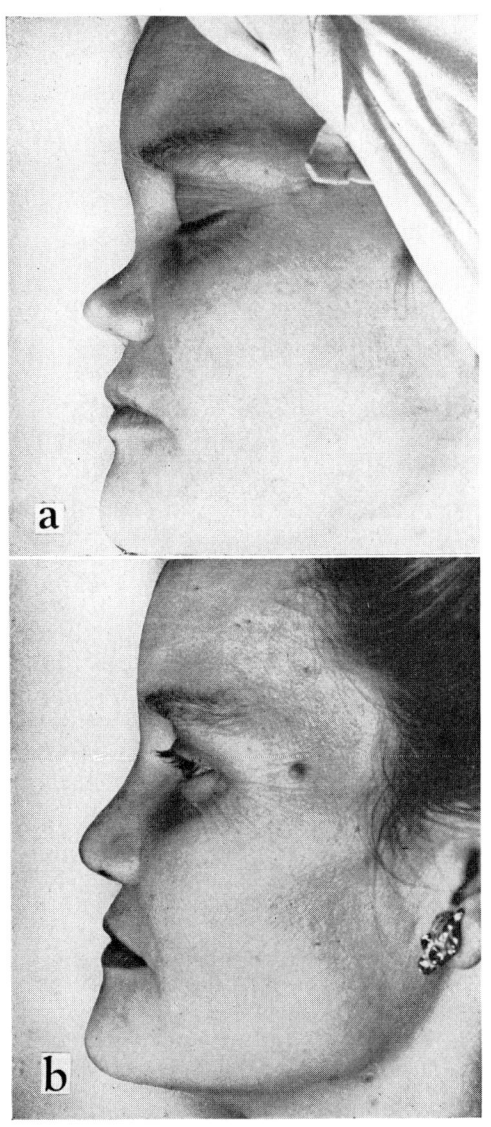

Case 60, *a:* Traumatic saddle nose.

b: After implantation of an autogenous rib cartilage graft from V-shaped inversion below tip of nose.

CASE
61

a   b

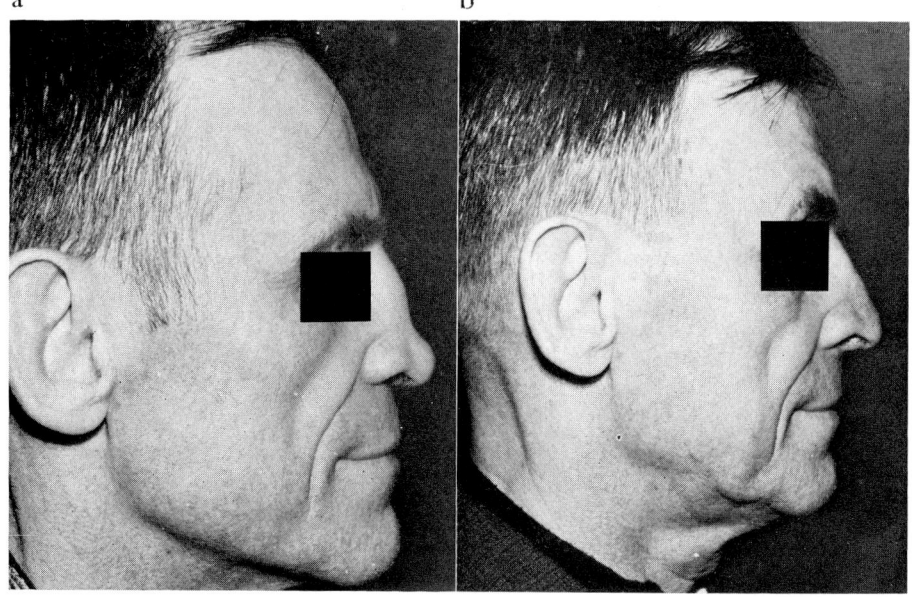

Case 61, *a:* Traumatic saddle nose after submucous resection of entire lower part of cartilaginous septum for severe traumatic deviation. Due to lack of support tip and columella are hanging.

b: After insertion of a piece of autogenous rib cartilage graft from a split columella incision to fill out depressed nasal ridge and the insertion of a second perpendicular narrow piece in a second stage to act as a strut to support the first graft (p. 431).

1072

CASE
62

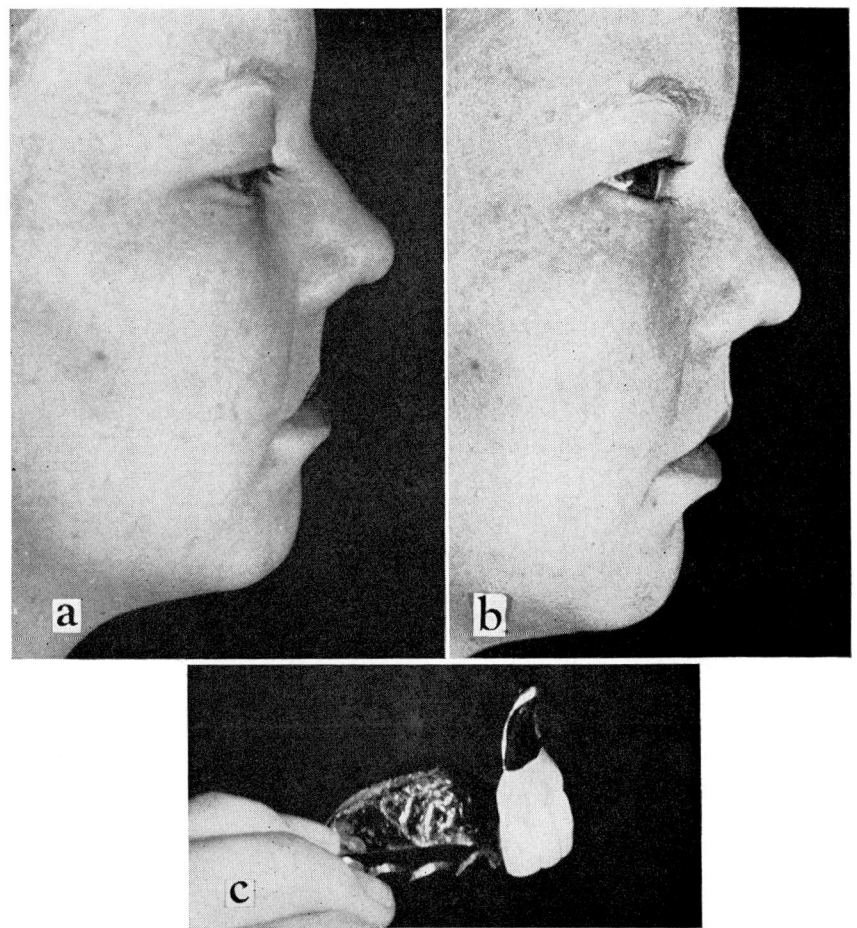

Case 62, *a:* Retrusion of upper lip from fracture of upper jaw after automobile accident. So-called "dishface" deformity.

b: After widening the upper labial sulcus with inlay skin graft.

c: Patient wears a prosthesis which is fastened to the upper teeth and has an appliance attached to it for forward displacement of upper lip.

CASE
63

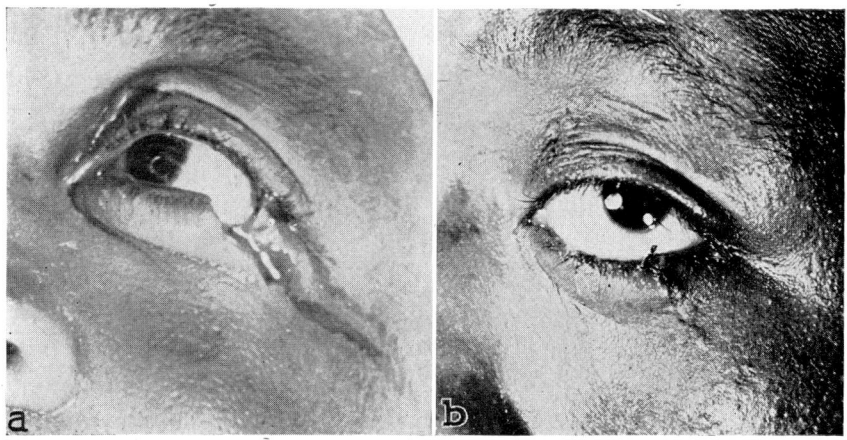

Case 63, *a:* Horizontal wound of upper eyelid; vertical wound of lower eyelid.

b: The latter repaired by the halving method to avoid later notching (Figure 223, page 463). The sutures were removed on the fourth day, with the exception of the marginal suture, which was left in place for ten days.

CASE
64

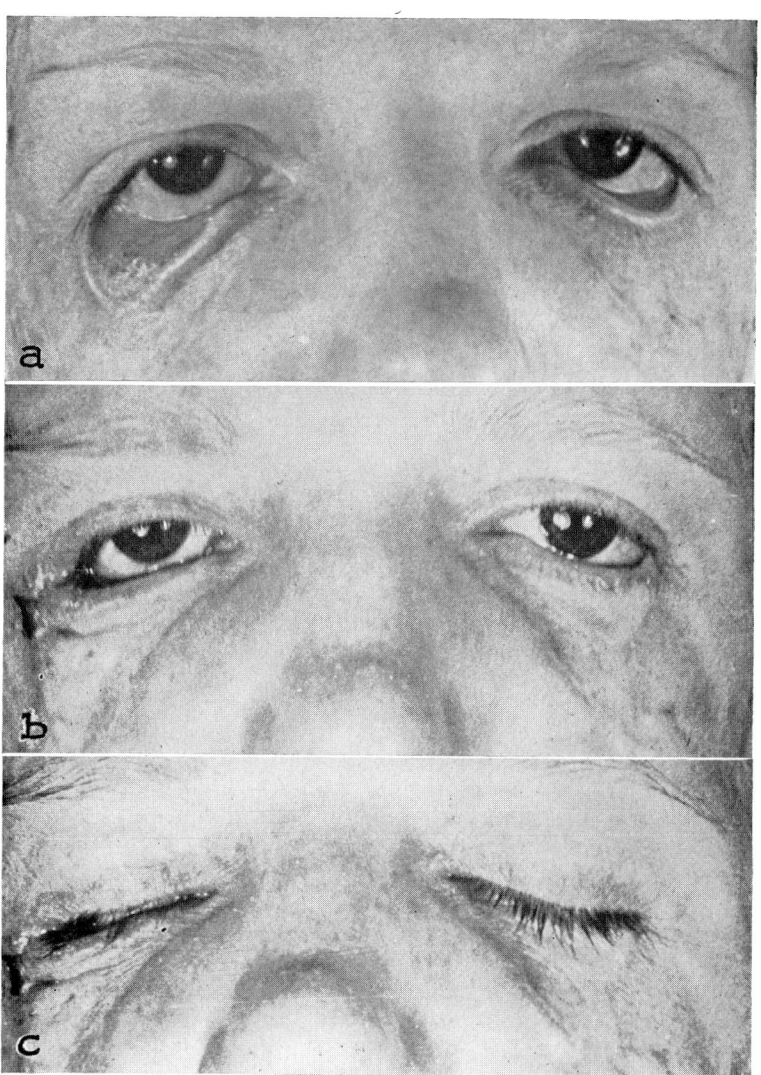

Case 64, *a:* Cicatricial ectropion of right and left lower lid after treatment for lupus vulgaris.

b, c: Repair of the deformity of the right eyelid by the use of two full-thickness grafts: one taken from the upper lid of the same eye to cover the upper half, one from the right postauricular region to cover the lower half of the defect (see Fig. 210, p. 452). Left-lid deformity repaired with a full-thickness graft from the upper lid of the same eye.

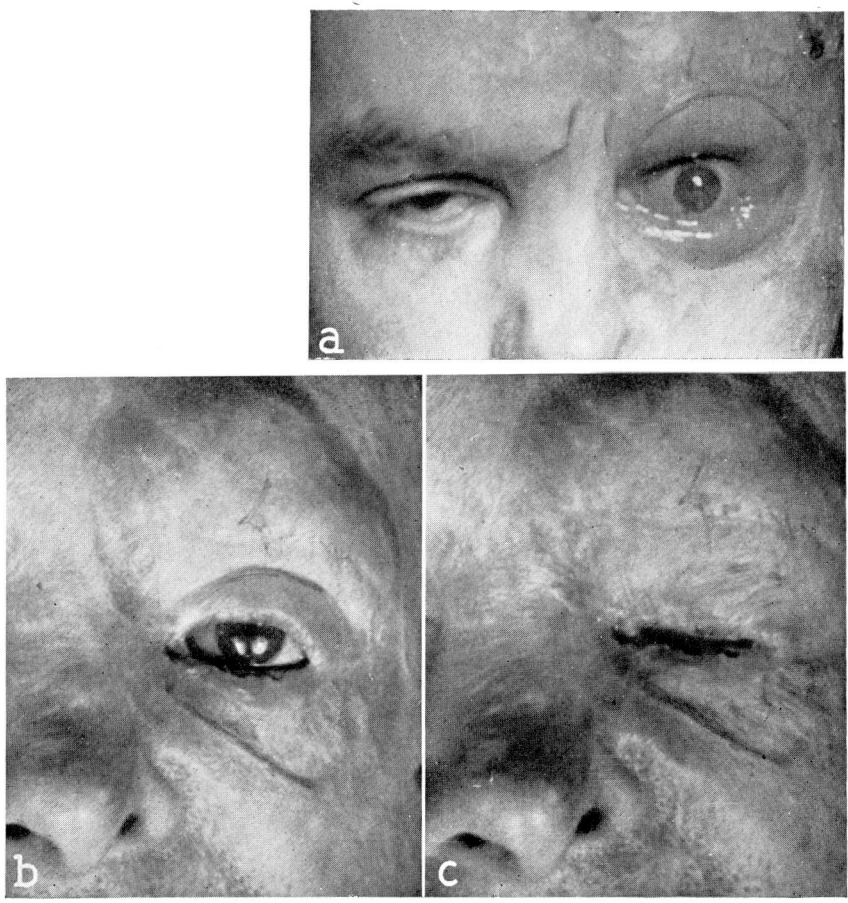

Case *65*, *a:* Cicatricial ectropion of upper and lower lid after third-degree burn. Note margin of upper lid retracted above level of site of former eyebrow. Vision almost completely absent, owing to corneal ulcers and extensive conjunctivitis.

b, c: Repair of both lids in one stage, according to the technique of Figure 210, page 452. Use of two full-thickness grafts from the hairless region of left upper arm. The intermarginal adhesions were not severed for three months. Vision almost completely restored.

1076

CASE
66

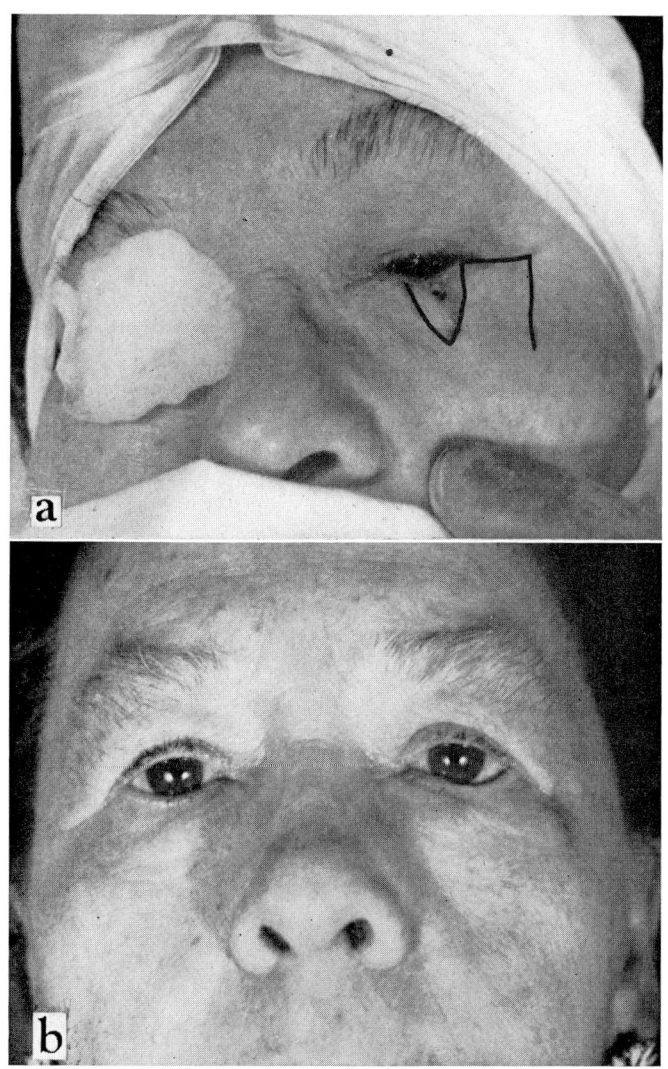

Case 66, *a:* Patient, aged fifty-eight, with cancer of left lower eye-lid. V-shaped excision and Dieffenbach flap for closure of defect (compare with Fig. 224, p. 465) are outlined. Since the tumor had only involved the skin it was not necessary to remove the conjunctiva.

b: Four months after the operation.

CASE
67

Case 67: Basal-cell cancer of lateral half of lower lid. The tumor involves the skin only. The width of the excision and the flap to close the defect are outlined. To facilitate rotation of the flap, a triangle of skin is excised at the extremity of the incision (after Imré) (see Fig. 213, p. 457). Since parts of the conjunctiva could be left behind, flap did not need to be lined.

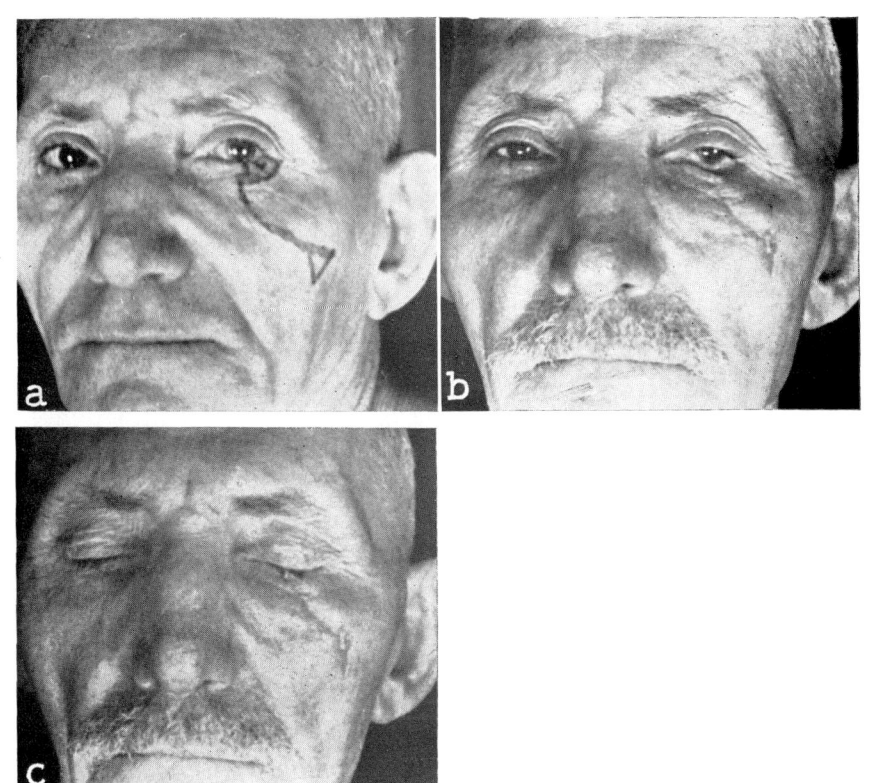

CASE
68

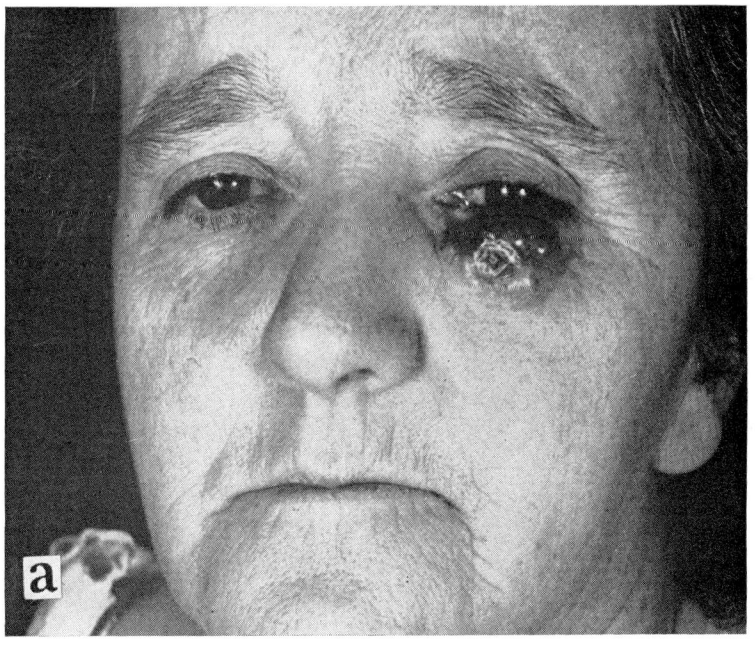

Case 68, *a:* Patient, aged fifty-one, with extensive basal cell carcinoma of left lower lid of one and one-half years' duration.

b: Tube flap constructed from mastoid to clavicular region. Five weeks later tube flap was lengthened. This part remained untubed. Four weeks later the lower pedicle was clamped as depicted. Four weeks later a mucous membrane graft, taken from the oral side of lower lip, was transplanted beneath flap (see dotted lines) for replacement of conjunctiva.

c: Three weeks later the entire lower lid was excised and the flap transplanted. Four weeks later flap was severed after clamp had been applied several days previously.

d, e: No evidence of reactivation four years after the last operation.

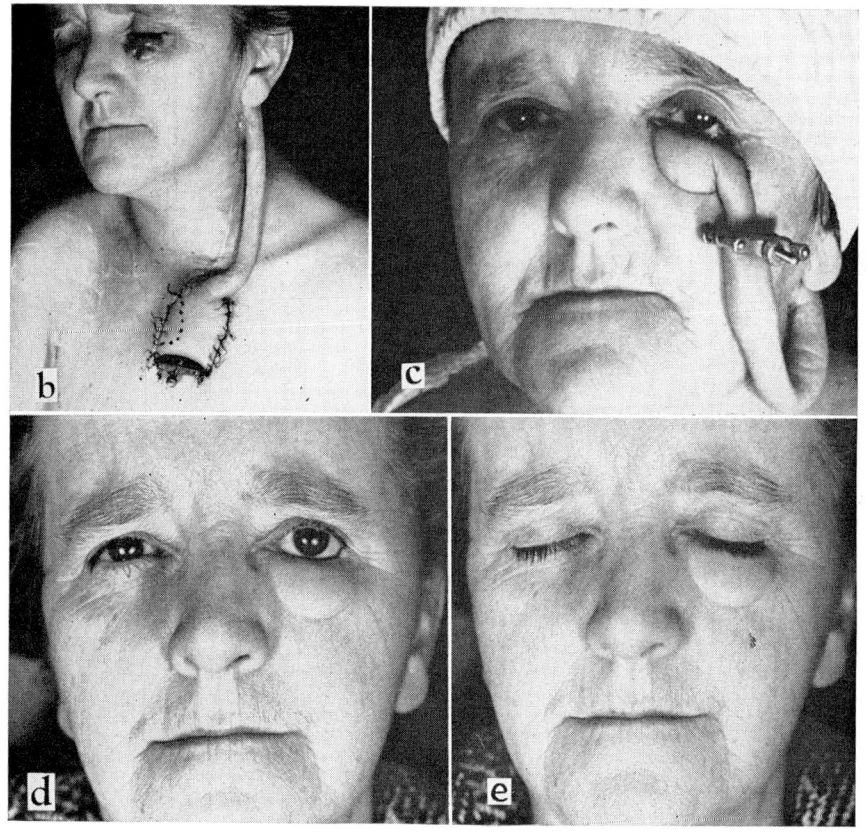

CASE
69

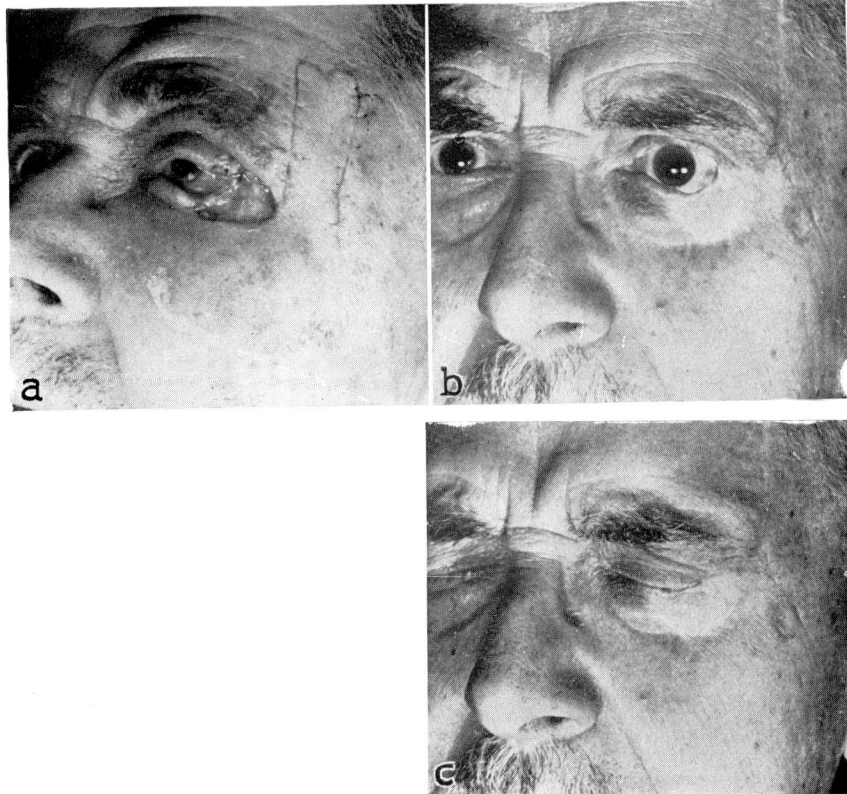

Case 69, *a:* Defect of lateral canthal angle, including lateral fourth of upper and lower lid after radiation for cancer. A temporal flap was raised, its peripheral end given the shape of the canthal angle. The flap was returned to its original site. After three weeks, it was raised again. Owing to blanching of the peripheral end, transfer was again delayed. After three more weeks, the defect was prepared. Two small turnover flaps were made from the median wound edges to replace the lining. The flap was rotated into the defect. The raw area of the flap bed was closed by undermining the wound edges and skin sliding. Six weeks later, the pedicle of the flap was severed and adjusted in place, as depicted in Figure 228, page 469.

b, c: Three years after operation.

1082

CASE
70

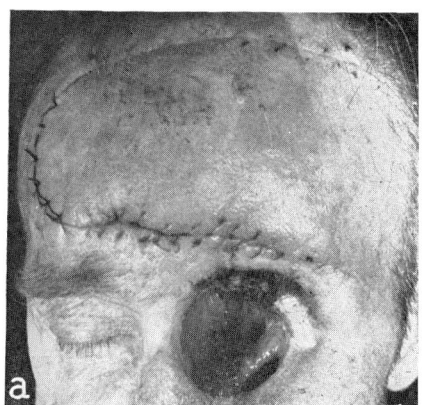

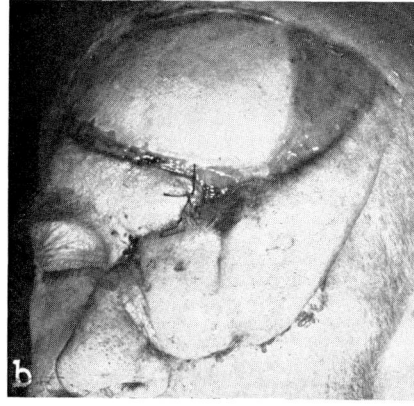

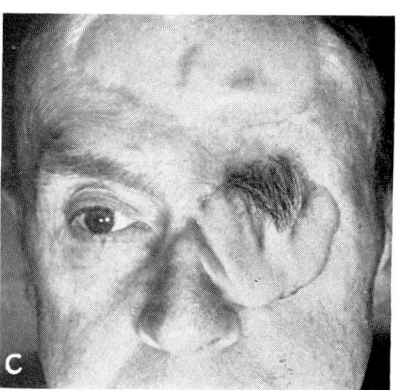

Case 70, *a:* Basal-cell cancer of eyelids, with invasion of the orbit, treated by removal of eyelids, exenteration of orbit, and removal of lateral bony wall of nose. No evidence of recurrence after four years. To close the big hole, a lined forehead flap, pedicled in left temporal region, was transplanted. The flap was mobilized between two parallel incisions, and returned and sutured. The upper incision includes a small part of the hair-bearing scalp to replace the eyebrow. Two weeks later, the right pedicle was severed and sutured; one week later, the peripheral end of the flap was elevated and lined with a split skin graft. Another week later, the entire flap was elevated, and the distal part of the flap bed covered with split skin graft. Blanching of the distal parts of the flap made another delay of transfer advisable.

b: Two weeks later, the flap was transplanted into the defect. The defect edges were denuded and split into two layers. The lining of the flap was sutured to the deep layer, the skin to the skin edges.

c: Six weeks later, the flap was severed from its pedicle, and the flap was adjusted in place. The patient wore spectacles, with ground glass on the left side, to conceal the deformity.

CASE
71

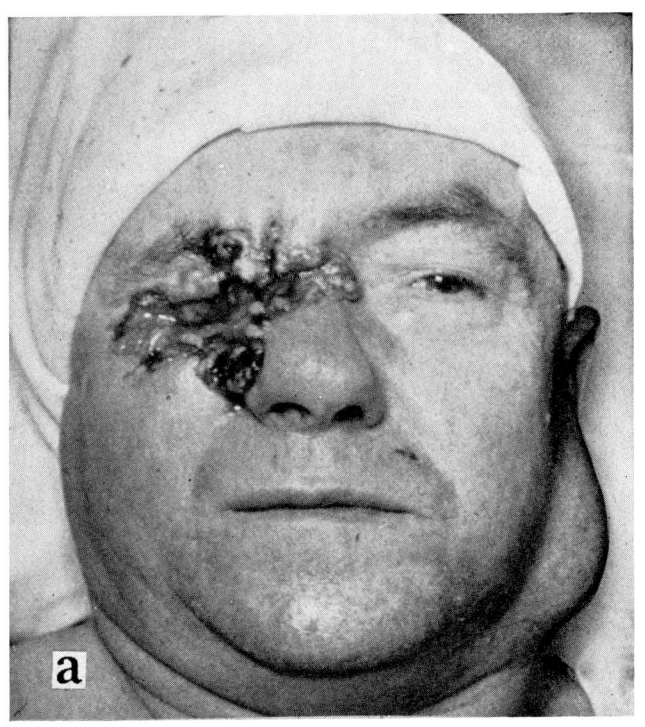

Case 71, *a:* Extensive basal cell carcinoma of right orbital region of ten years' duration. Mixed tumor of left parotid gland.

b: Radical operation consisting of removal of the right eye, right half of nose, wide excision of the tumor. Periosteum of the orbit could be preserved.

c: Two months later an inlay skin graft was transplanted to line the orbital cavity. Two years after the operation small recurrence at the nose which was electrocoagulated. No further reactivation four years after the first operation. Patient died from other causes.

1084

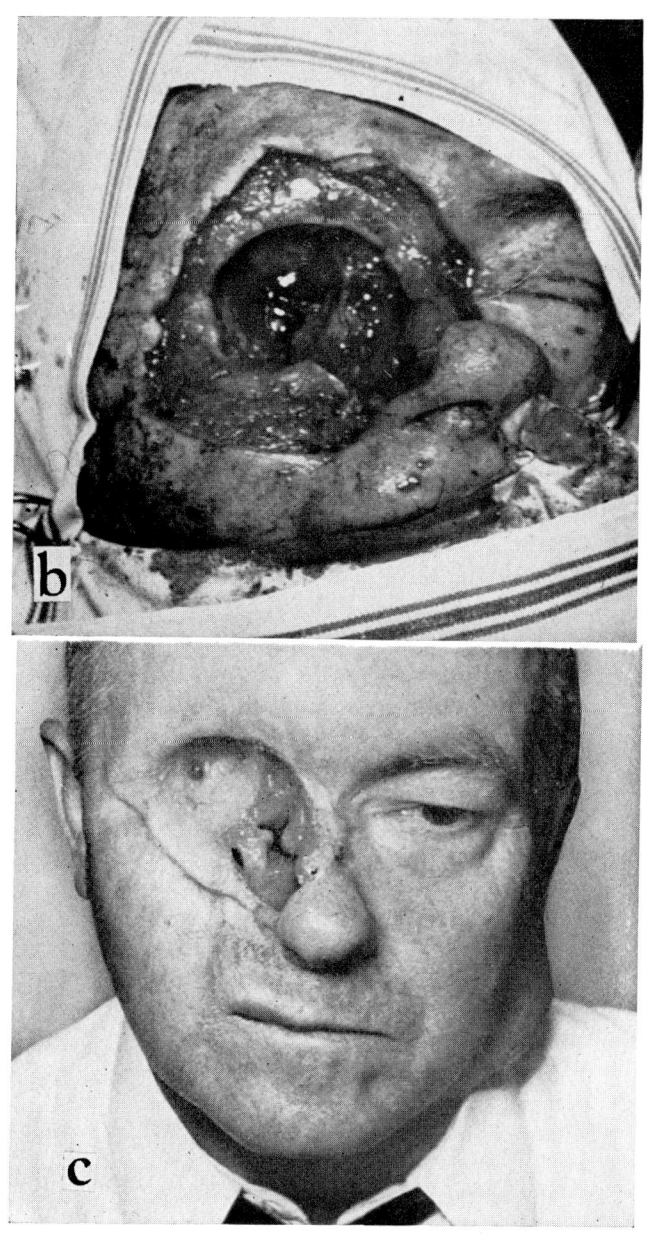

CASE

72

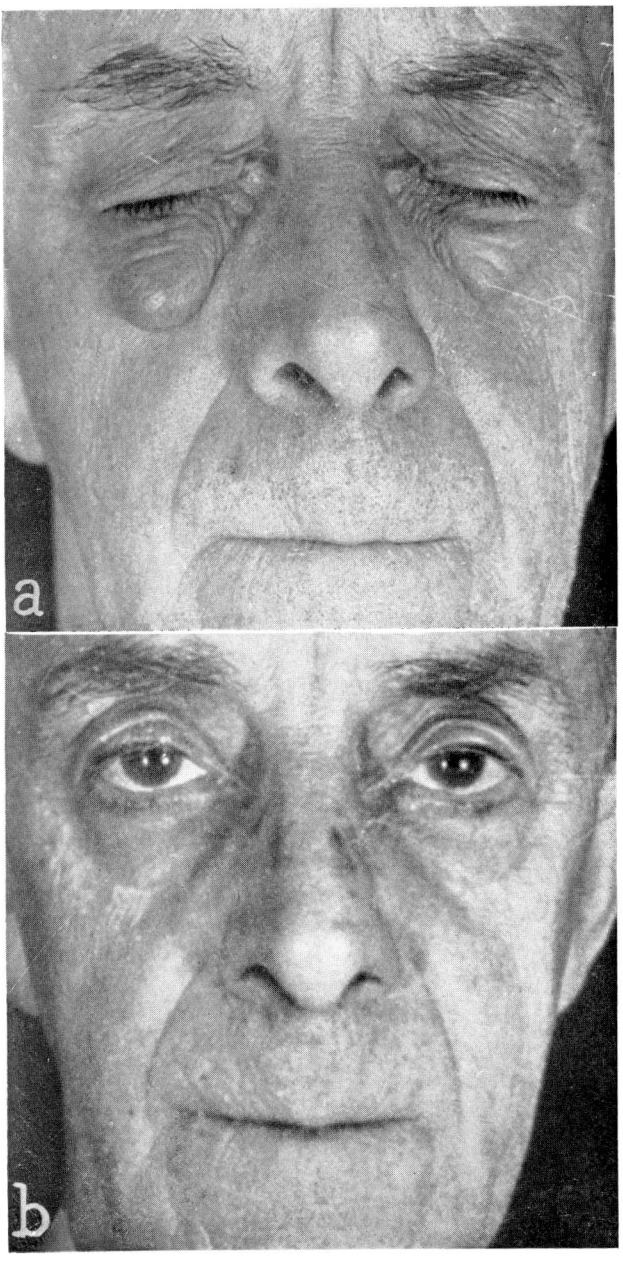

Case 72: Sagging pouches of lower lids, corrected by excision along the base. The lower incision runs along a natural fold. A triangular piece of skin was removed from the lateral end of the incision to avoid puckering (compare with Figure 240, p. 499).

CASE
73

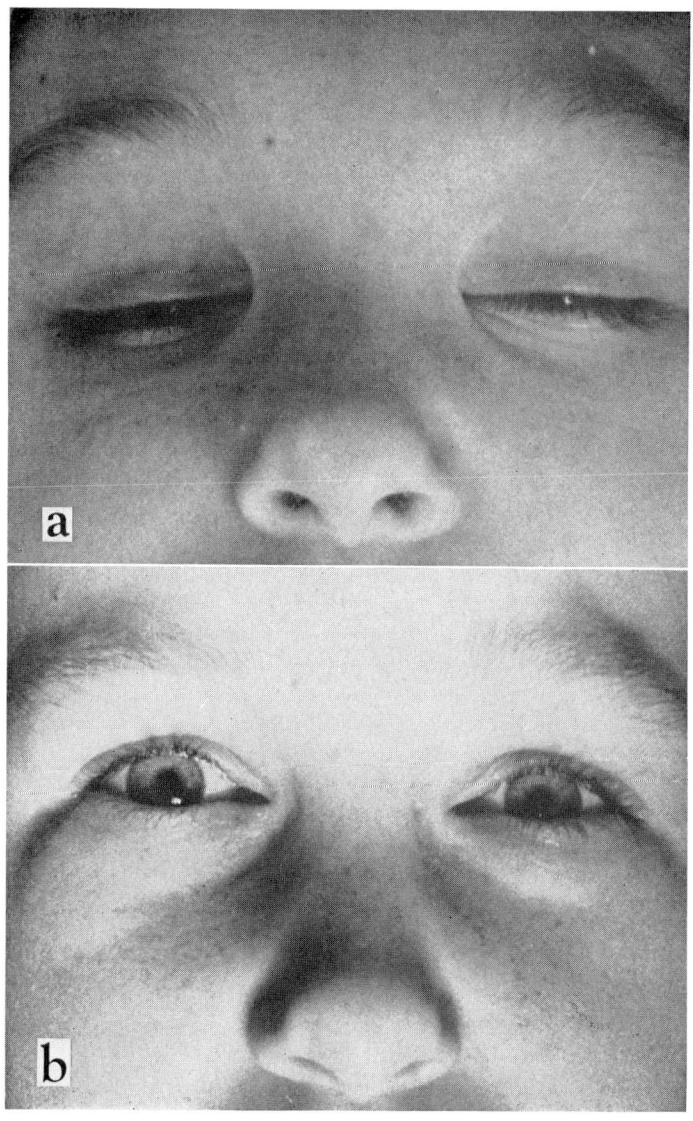

Case 73, *a:* Girl, aged nine, with bilateral epicanthus (Mongolian fold).

b: After bilateral epicanthus operation with double Z-plasty (Fig. 75, p. 253).

CASE

74

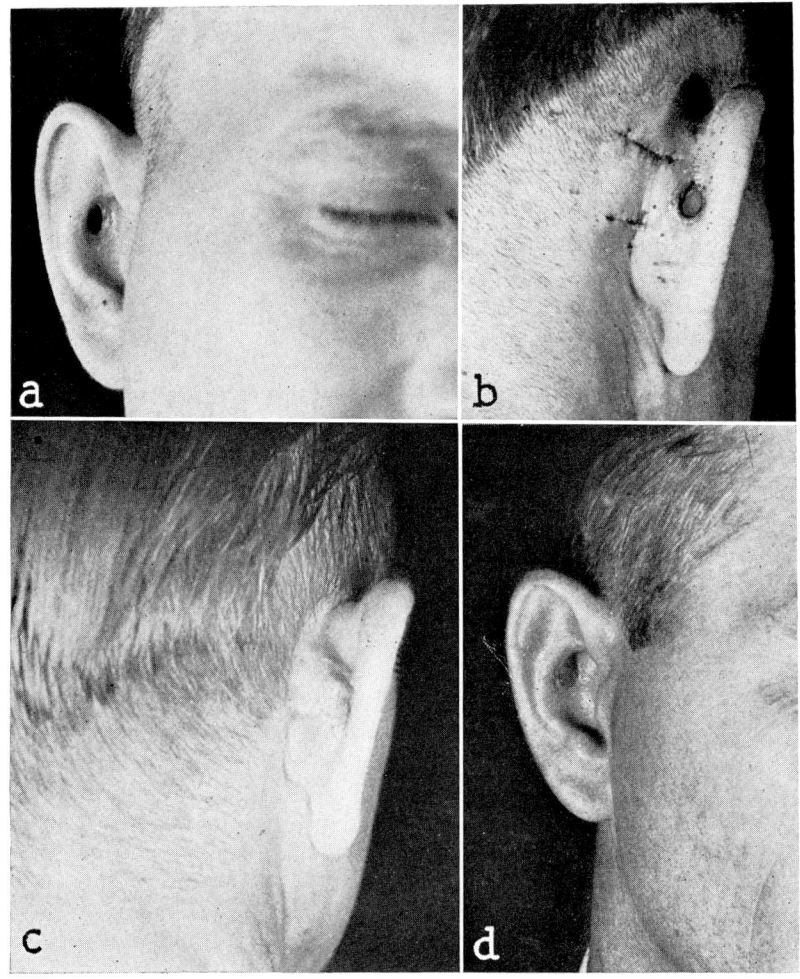

Case 74, *a:* Bullet wound through concha.

b: A double-pedicle flap in postauricular region, one third larger than required, was elevated and returned. A rim of skin surrounding the edge of the defect to be hinged forward later on was elevated and returned. After two weeks, the pedicle near the hole was severed and sutured.

c, d: After another two weeks, the whole flap was raised, the rim of skin surrounding the edge of the hole in the concha was hinged forward; the auricle was held back and the flap sutured into the defect. After three weeks, the backward tilt of the ear was overcome by severing the central pedicle in the mastoid region, undermining and advancing the flap. Resulting raw surface was skin grafted.

CASE
75

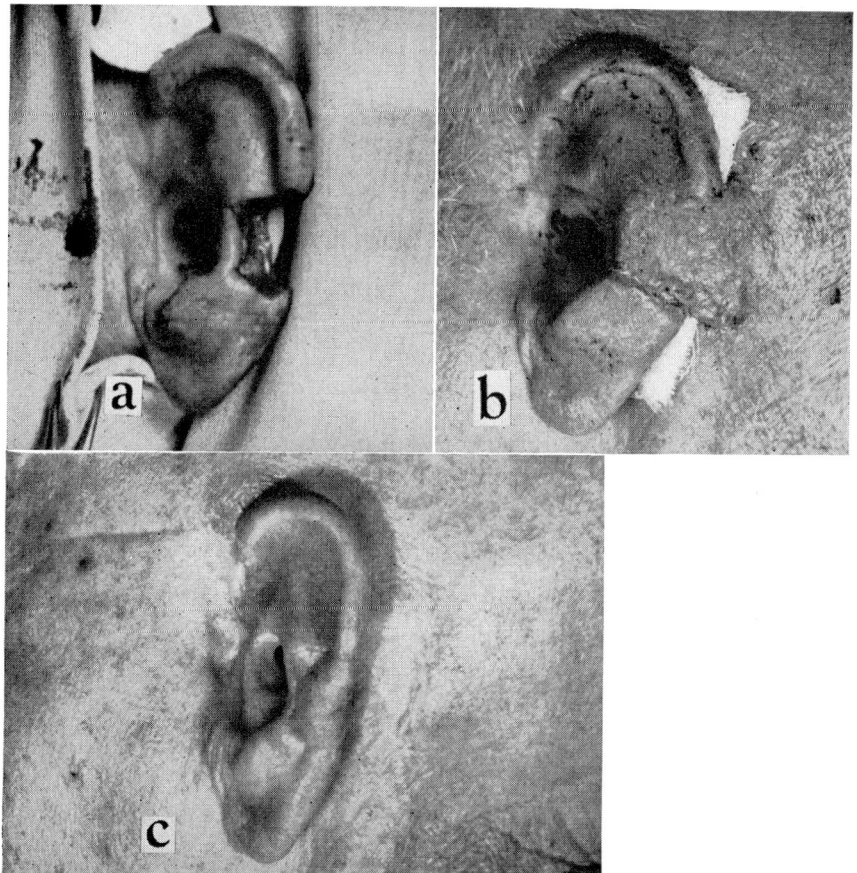

Case 75, *a:* Patient, aged sixty-two, after excision of helix and anthelix for removal of squamous cell carcinoma.

b: Transplantation of mastoid flap in same stage of operation. Donor
area of flap at mastoid region skin grafted.

c: Three weeks later partial separation of flap. Four days later separation of flap and adjustment of the same.

1089

CASE
76

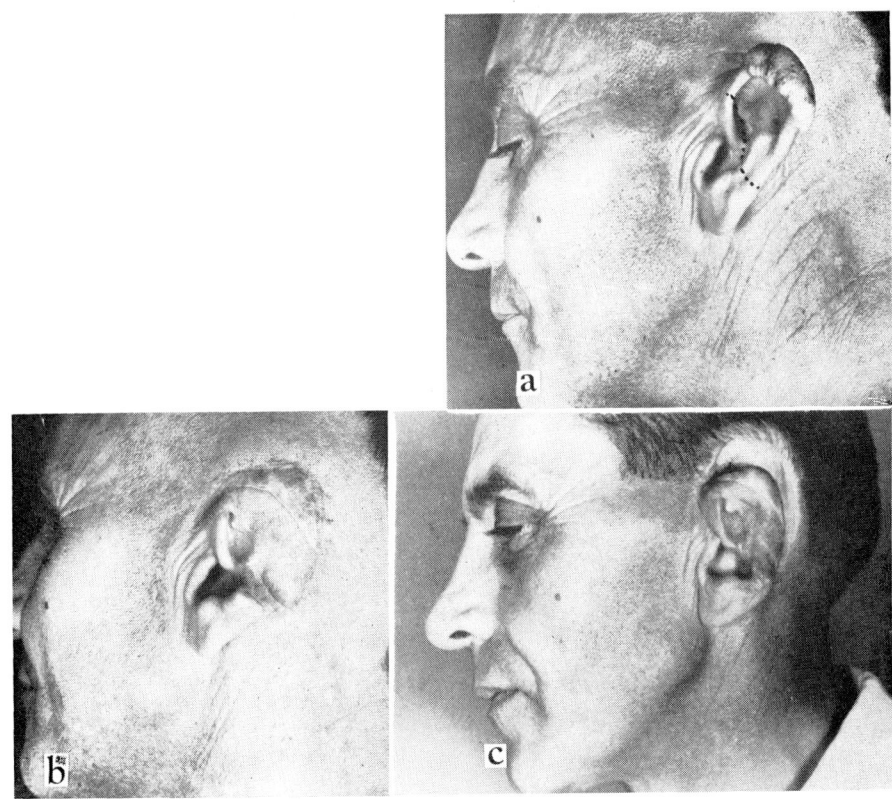

Case 76, *a:* Patient with squamous-cell carcinoma of ear, Grade I. (Line of excision marked with dotted lines.)

b: Subtotal removal of ear and mobilization of mastoid flap between an incision which outlined the upper helix rim and another in level of earlobe stump. Two weeks later rim incision completed, depilation of flap and transplantation of skin graft to depilated area. Three weeks later elevation of entire flap and transplantation of rib cartilage beneath the flap.

c: Six months later elevation of composite mastoid flap, flap attached to ear lobe, skin grafting of postauricular raw surface.

CASE
77

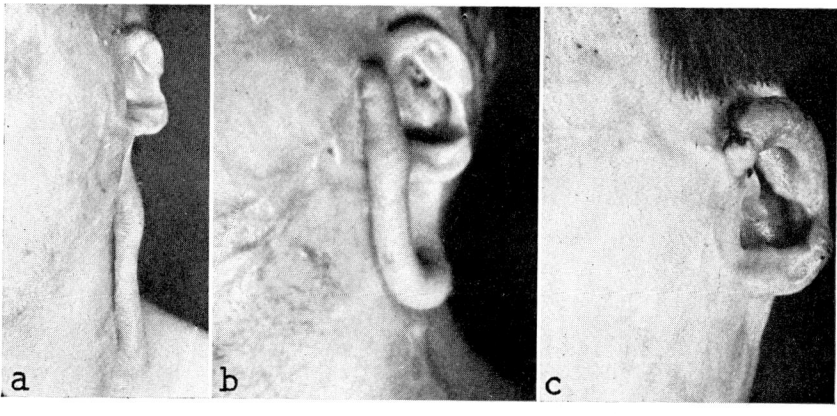

a   b   c

Case 77, *a:* Burn of face and ear. Helix absent. The concha was adherent to the mastoid region. The concha was moved forward by excision of the cicatricial tissue of the postauricular region, and the raw surface was skin grafted. A cervical tube flap was made to reconstruct the absent helix.

b: Four weeks later, the inferior pedicle of the flap was transferred to a place just above the tragus.

c: Three weeks later, the pedicle in the mastoid region was severed. One week later, the flap was opened along its seam, and draped around the auricle in such a way as to form the helix.

CASE
78

a   b

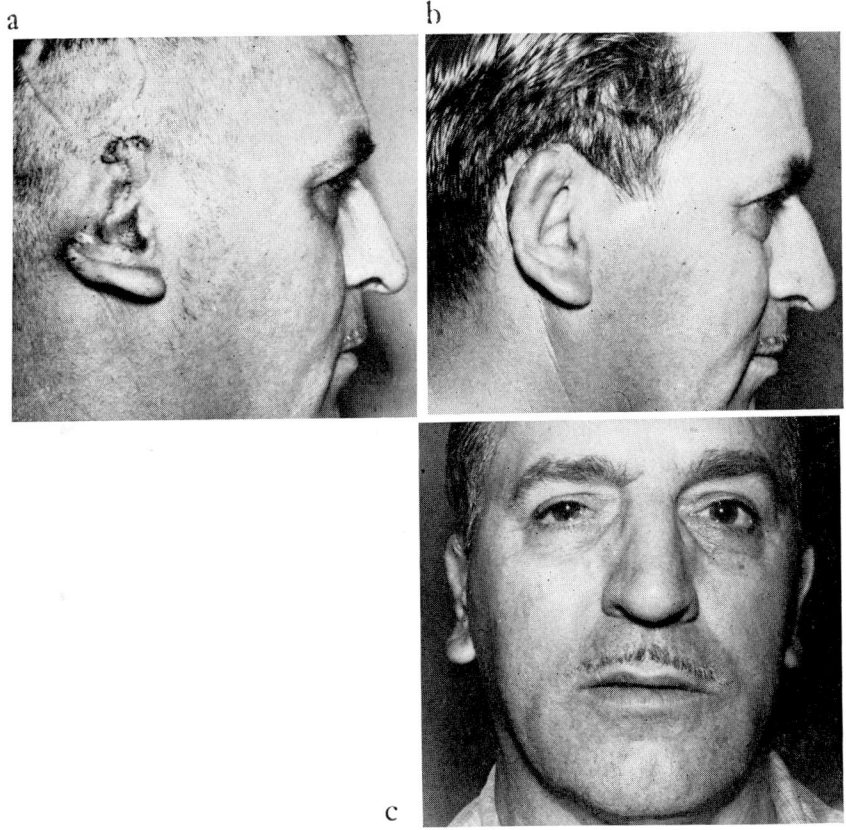

c

Case 78, *a:* Subtotal traumatic defect of right ear reconstructed according to technique described on page 510. First stage of reconstruction consisted of readjustment and attachment of the upper and lower ear remnants to the mastoid skin. Second stage (three weeks later), depilation of upper mastoid area (p. 204). Third stage (three weeks later), insertion of rib cartilage graft to form helix and anthelix. Fourth stage (three months later), elevation of compound mastoid flap and skin grafting of posterior ear surface and flap bed.

b, c: Six months after reconstruction.

1092

CASE
79

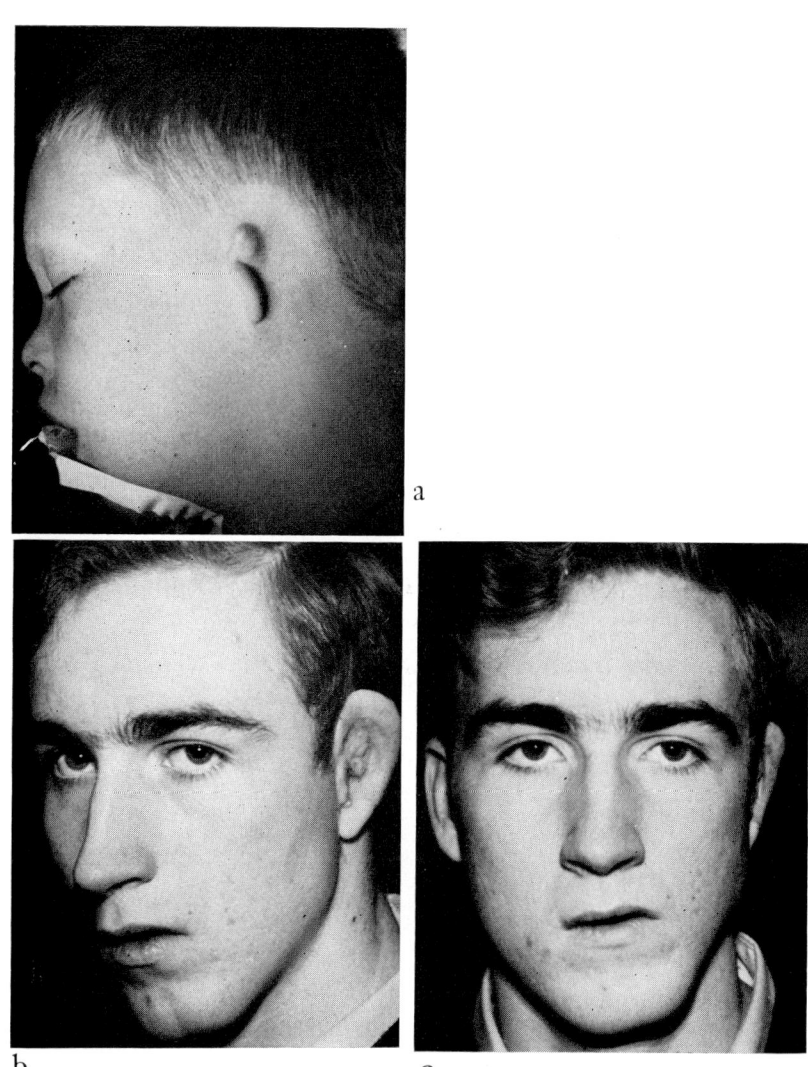

a

b   c

Case 79, *a-c:* Congenital absence of most parts of ear. Reconstructed according to method described on page 510. Reconstruction was
started at eight years of age. Ear was made larger to compensate for
possible retardation of growth.

   b-c: Eighteen years of age.

CASE
80

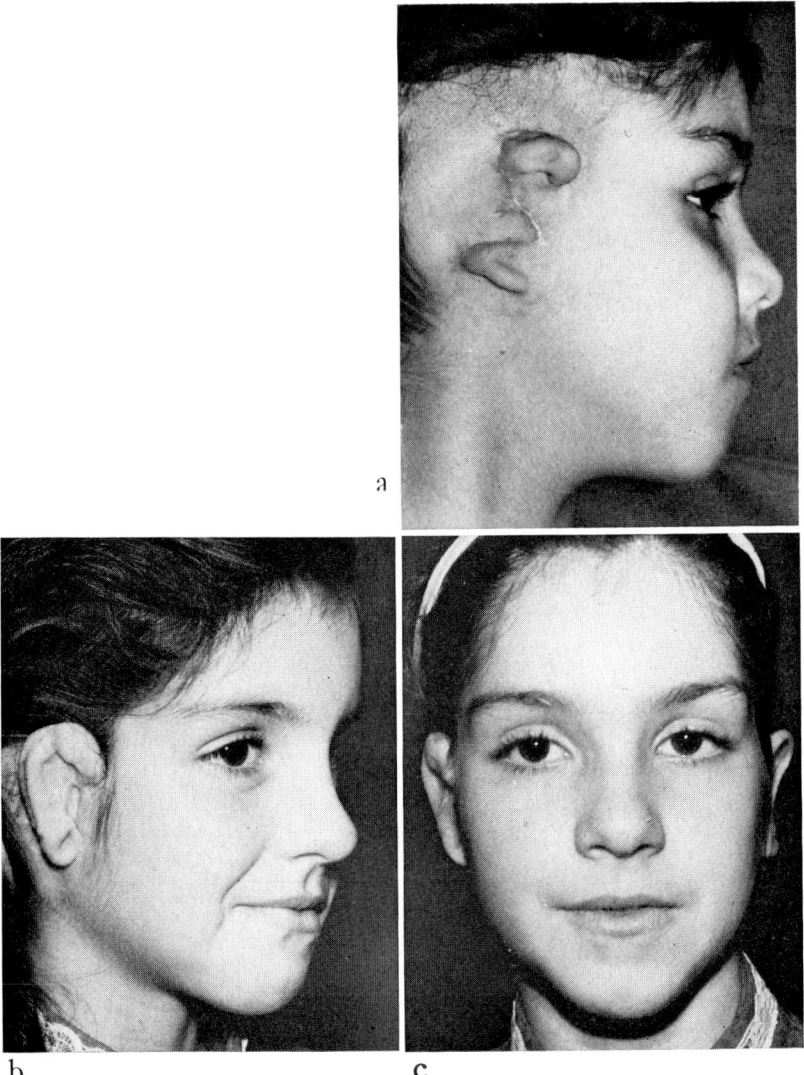

Case 80, *a:* Congenital absence of ear (age seven) except for remnants which have been switched upward and downward according to technique described on page 510. (For preoperative condition, see Fig. 244*A*, p. 514.)

b, c: Five years after reconstruction.

CASE
81

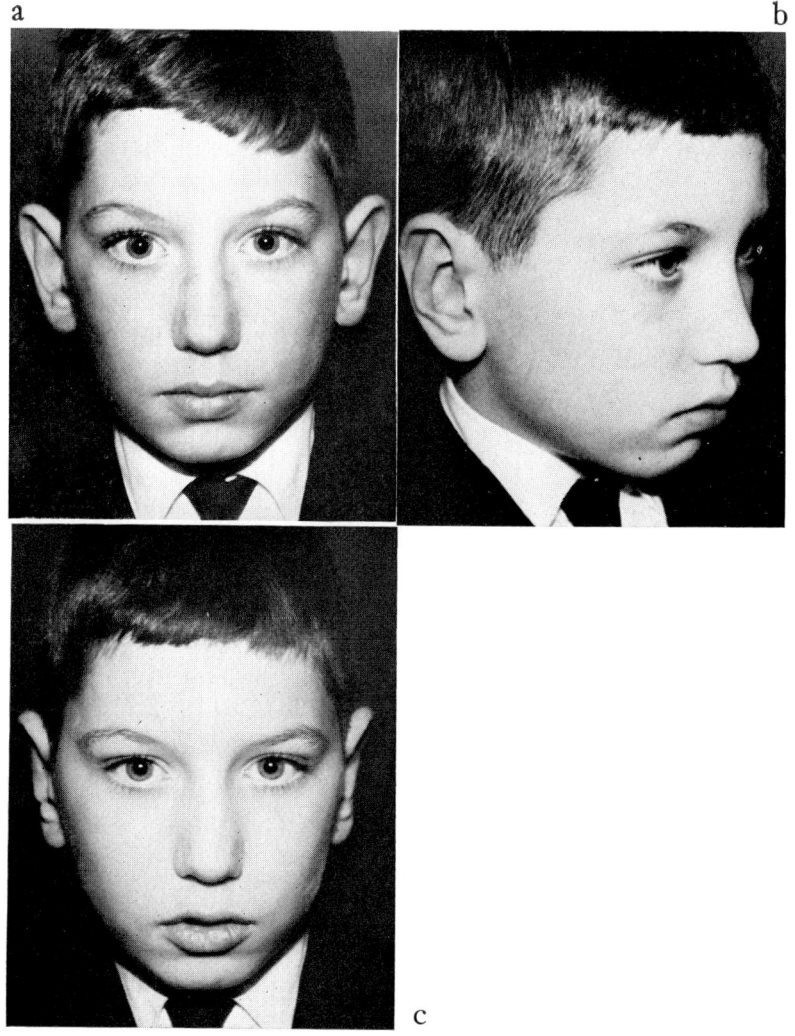

Case 81, *a:* Protrusion of ears from absence of anthelix.
b, c: Reconstruction of anthelix after Converse (p. 527).

CASE

82

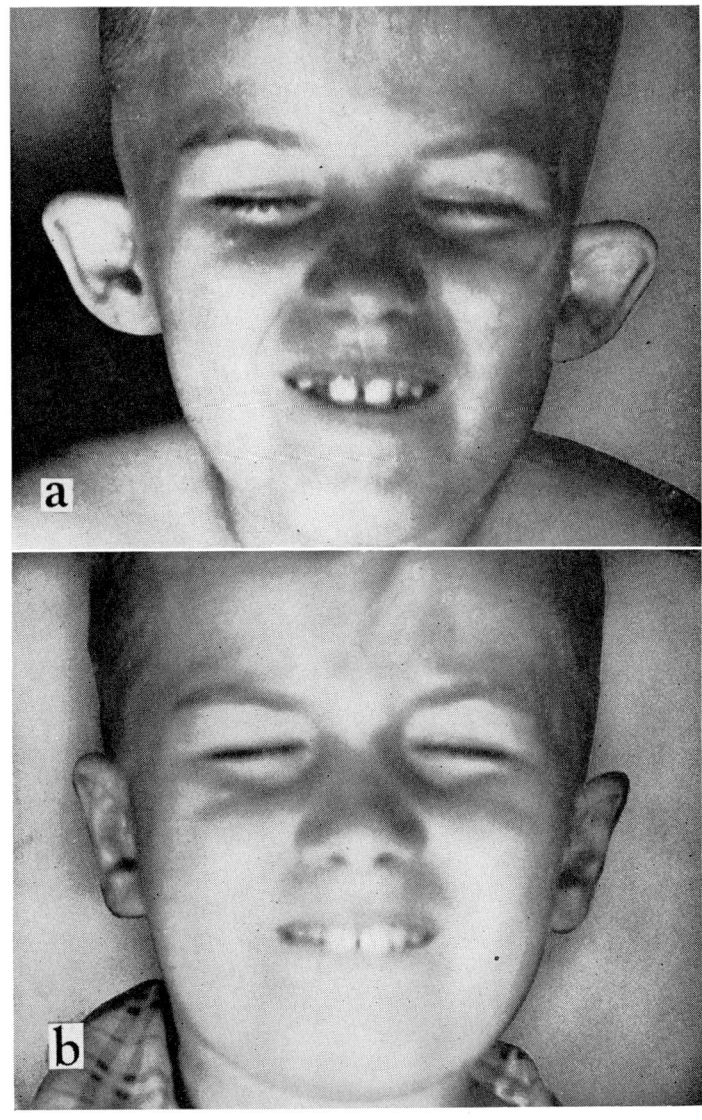

Case 82, *a:* Bilateral protrusion of ears from absence of anthelix.
b: After bilateral ear plasty consisting of construction of anthelix and excision of redundant skin.

CASE
83

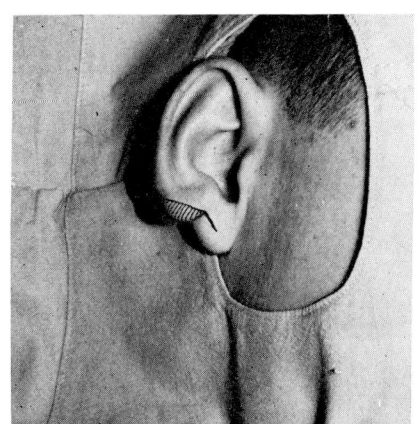 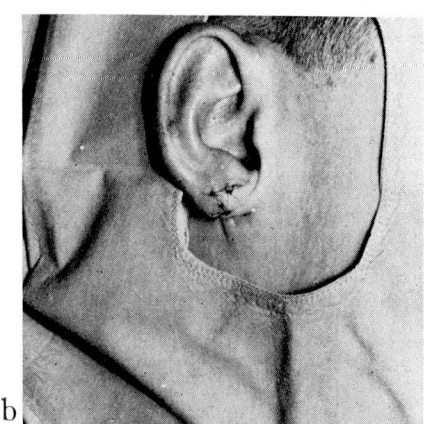

a   b

Case 83, *a:* Congenital split of earlobe. Line of excision (striped area) marked, quadrangular lobe flap lined out with solid line.
   b: After operation.

CASE

84

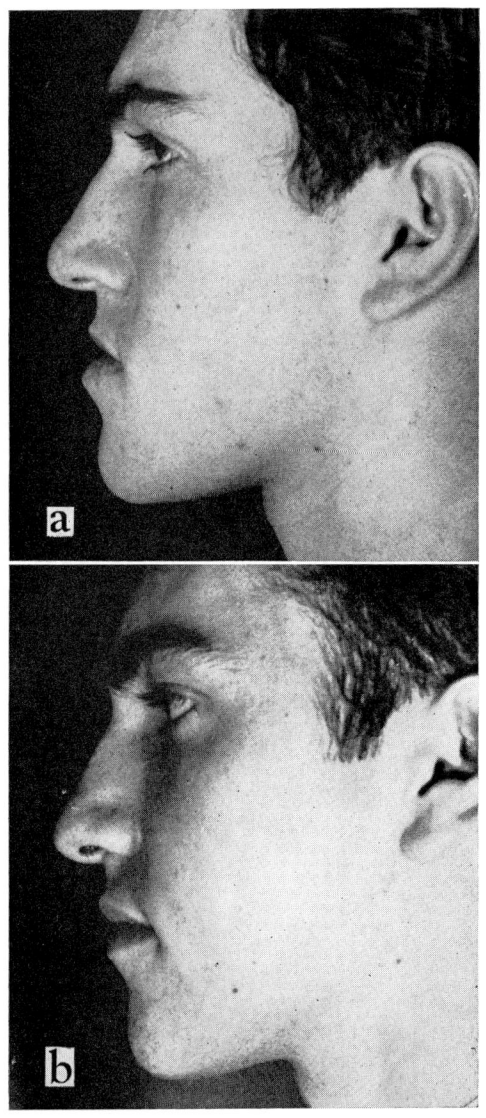

Case 84, *a:* Patient, aged nineteen, with mandibular prognathism and malocclusion of the teeth.

b: After correction of mandibular prognathism through osteotomy of the ascending ramus (p. 573). Teeth are in satisfactory occlusion.

CASE
85

a   b

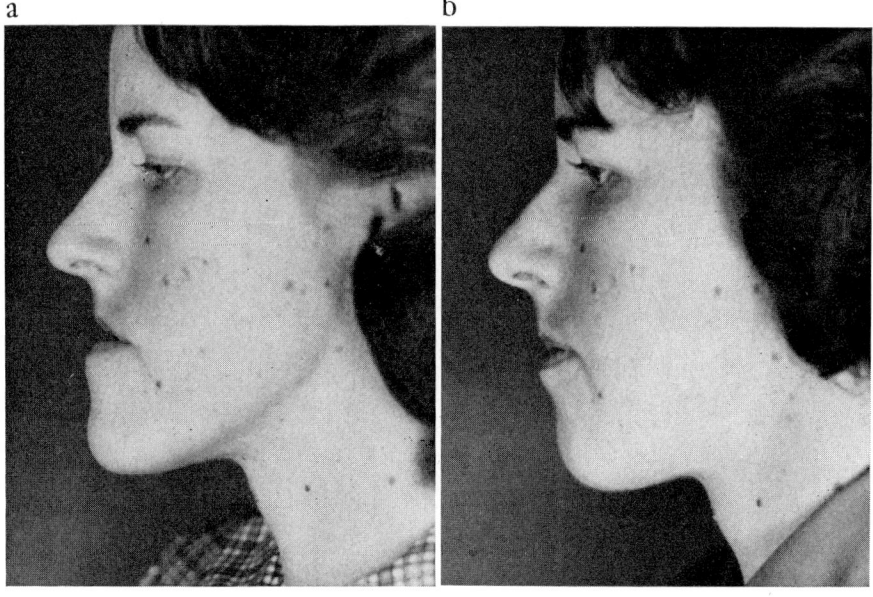

Case 85, *a:* Protrusion of mandible and malocclusion of teeth.
    b: After intraoral resection of horizontal ramus of mandible according to Converse (p. 576).

CASE
86

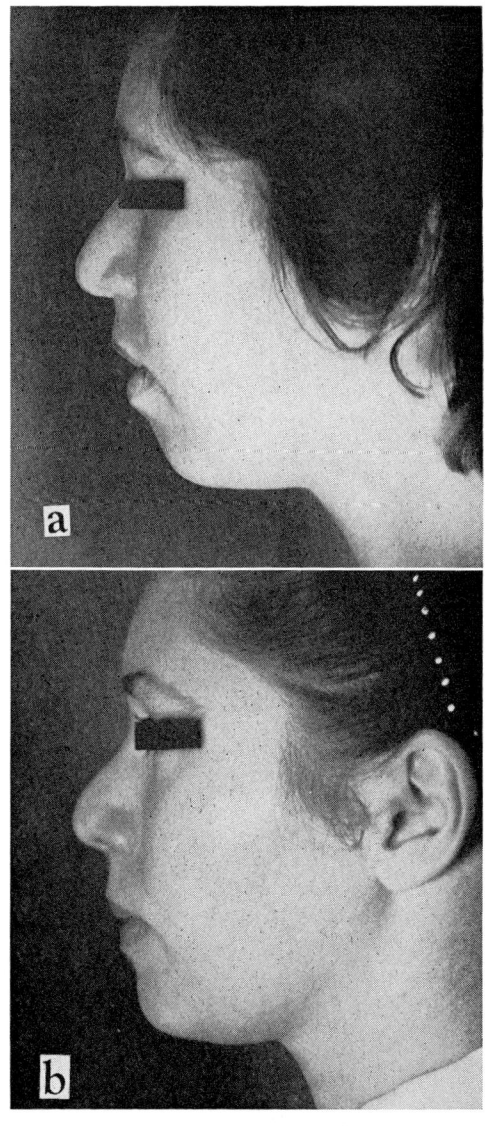

Case 86, *a:* Patient, aged twenty-four, with retrusion of chin. Teeth were in good occlusion.

b: After correction of retrusion of the chin with bone grafts from ilium which were inserted through an intraoral incision (see p. 580).

CASE
87

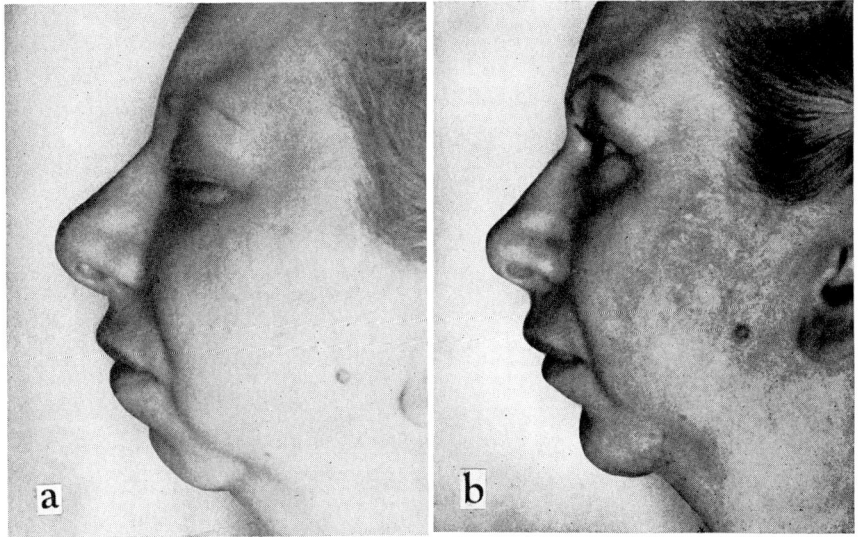

Case 87, *a:* Patient, aged thirty-nine, with marked retrusion of mandible. Teeth, however, were in perfect occlusion.

b: After correction of the retrusion of mandible through build-up of the chin with two superimposed autogenous rib cartilage grafts which were inserted from incision below the chin and held in position with two wire mattress sutures. Note that nose appears smaller after build-up of the chin.

CASE
88

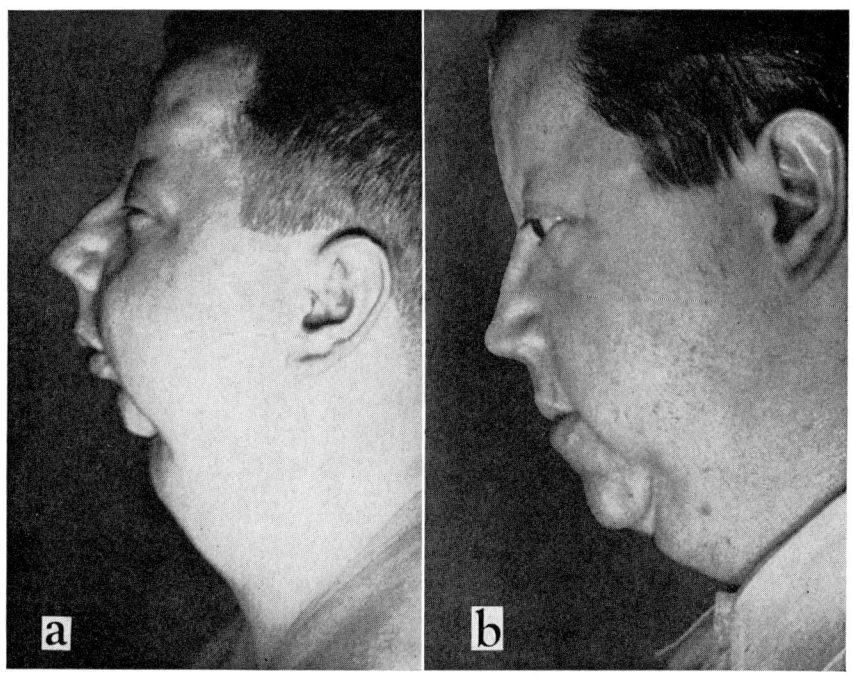

Case 88, *a:* Patient, aged twenty-five, with "bird face" from extensive retrusion and maldevelopment of mandible, open bit; teeth of lower jaw one inch behind teeth of upper jaw (compare with Figure 275*A*, p. 585).

b: Repair of micrognathia with bone graft from ilium which was fastened upon the anterior part of the mandible from an incision below the chin (compare with Figure 274, p. 584) (lengthening of mandibular bone was impossible owing to aplasia of the bone). Eight months later the lower gingival sulcus was enlarged and deepened with an inlay skin graft. A dental prosthesis was inserted into this pocket with artificial teeth. Good occlusion of these teeth with teeth of upper jaw (compare with Figure 275*B*, p. 585). Note that nose, which has not been operated upon, appears smaller after build-up of chin.

CASE
89

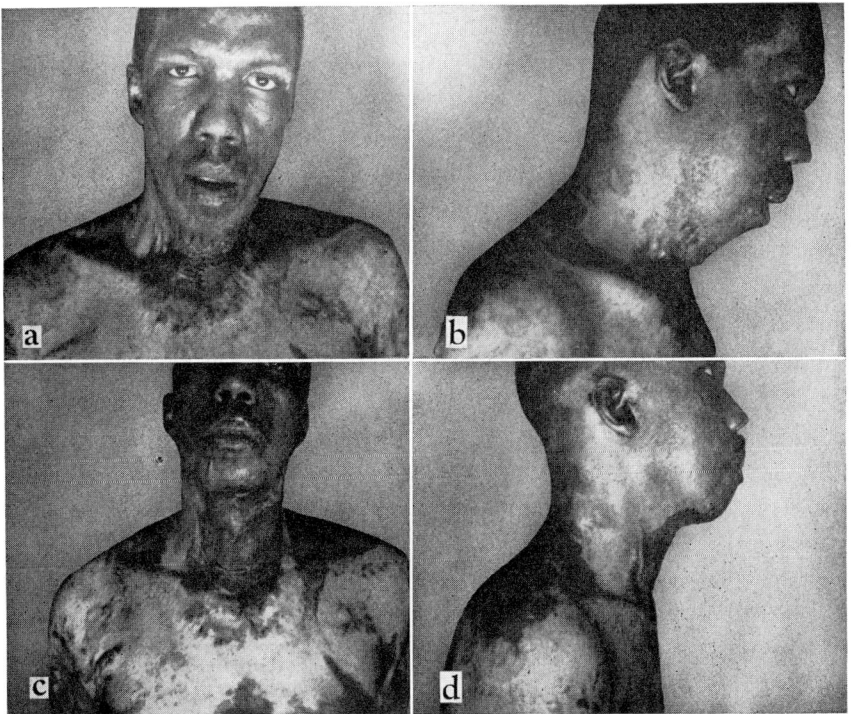

Case 89, *a, b:* Patient, aged thirty-four, with contracture of neck from extensive third-degree burn.

c, d: After excision of contracting scar and platysma and application of split skin grafts. Patient wore a brace (see Figure 276, p. 602) for three months day and night and for an additional three months overnight only.

CASE
90

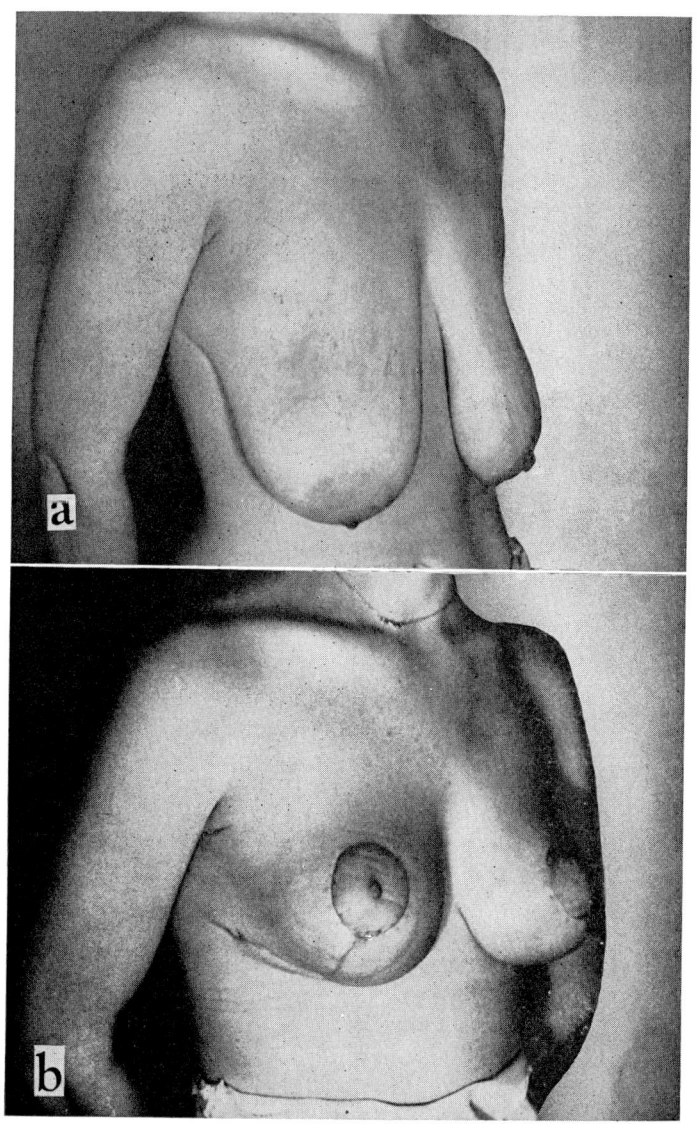

Case 90, *a:* Patient, aged twenty-five, with pendulous, hypertrophic breasts.

b: Six months after breast plasty with preservation of function of the glands.

CASE
91

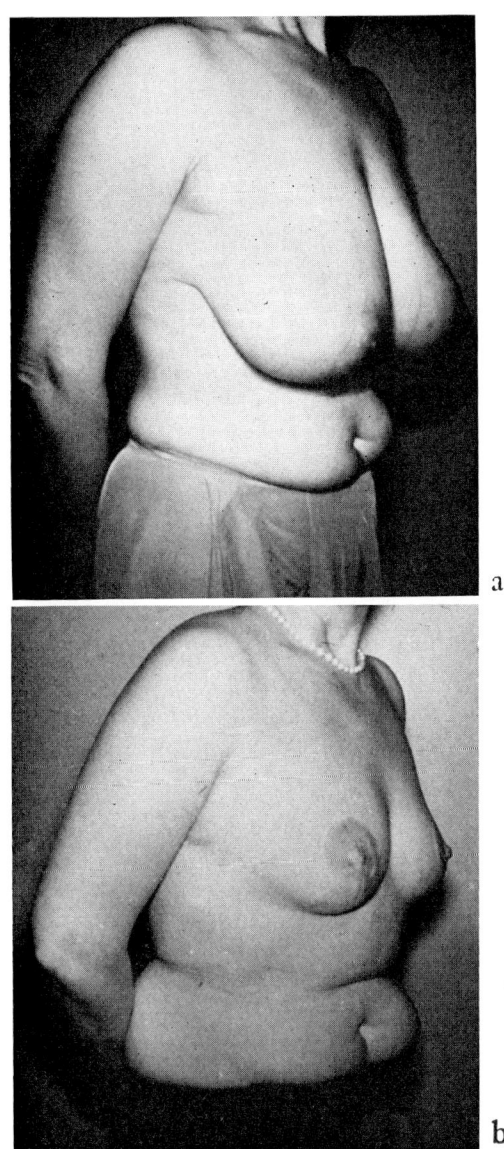

a

b

Case 91, *a, b:* Hypertrophic pendulous breasts. Breast plasty after Lexer-Biesenberger (p. 622).

CASE
92

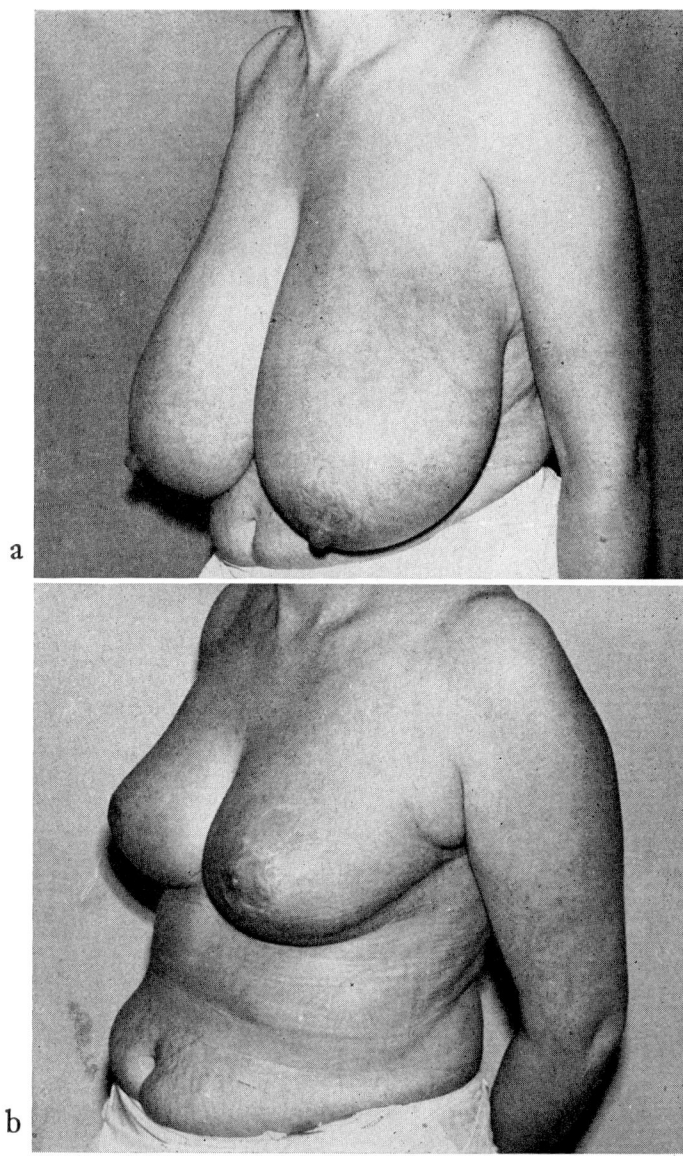

a

b

Case 92, *a:* Patient, aged forty-six, with marked hypertrophy of breasts.

b: After breast plasty with transplantation of areolae as free grafts.

CASE
93

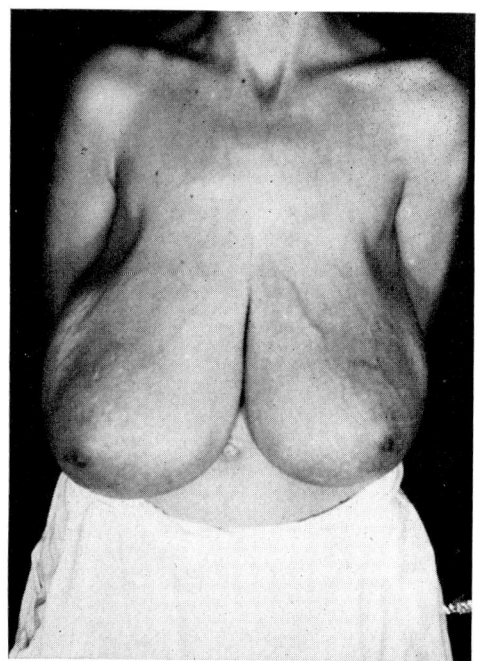

a

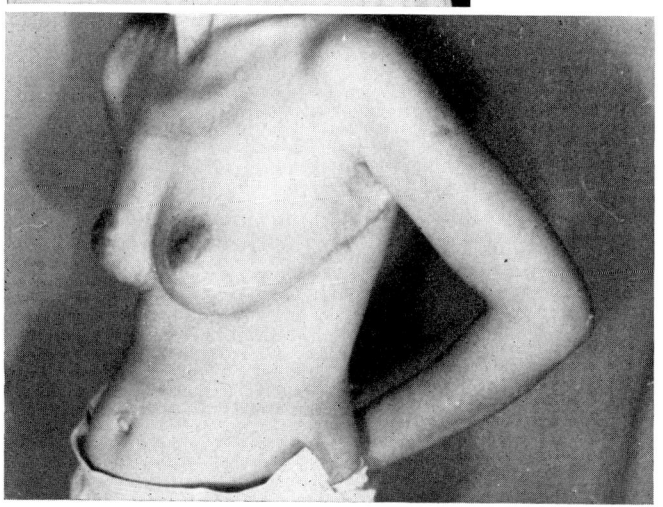

b

Case 93, *a:* Patient, aged forty-two, with marked hypertrophy of breasts, engorgement of subcutaneous veins. No lactation in two pregnancies.

b: Two years after breast plasty with free transplantation of areolae.

CASE
94

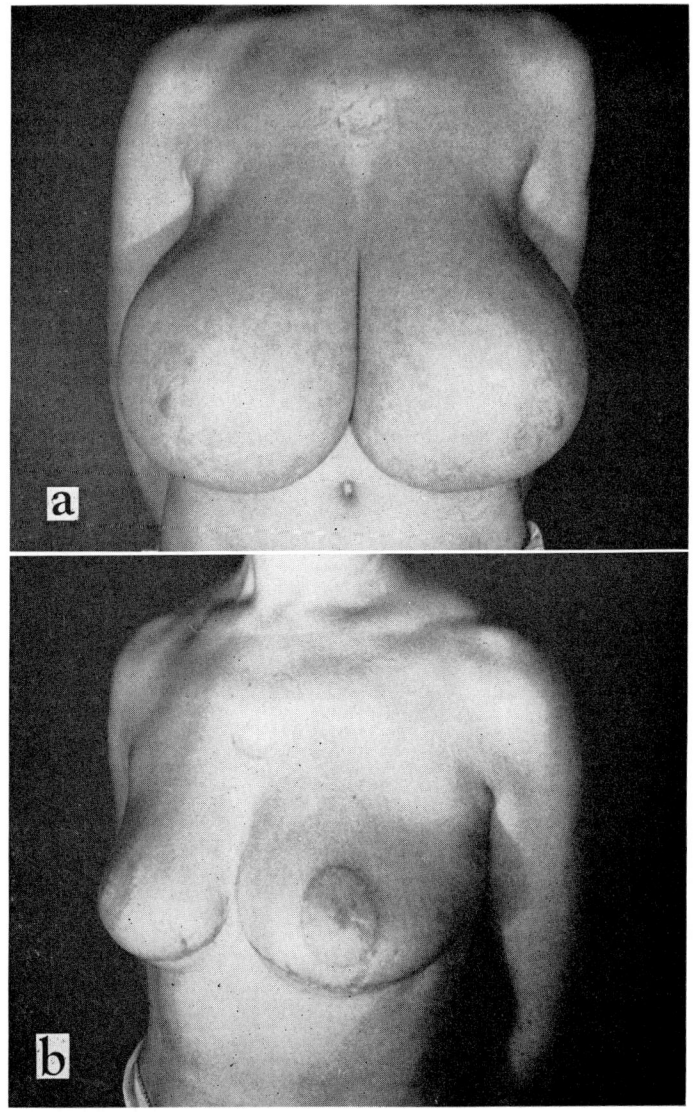

Case 94, *a:* Patient, aged twenty-seven, with marked hypertrophy of both breasts.

b: Seven months after breast plasty with transplantation of the nipples as free grafts. Patient went through two pregnancies; engorgement of breasts could promptly be overcome by injection of stilbestrol.

CASE
95

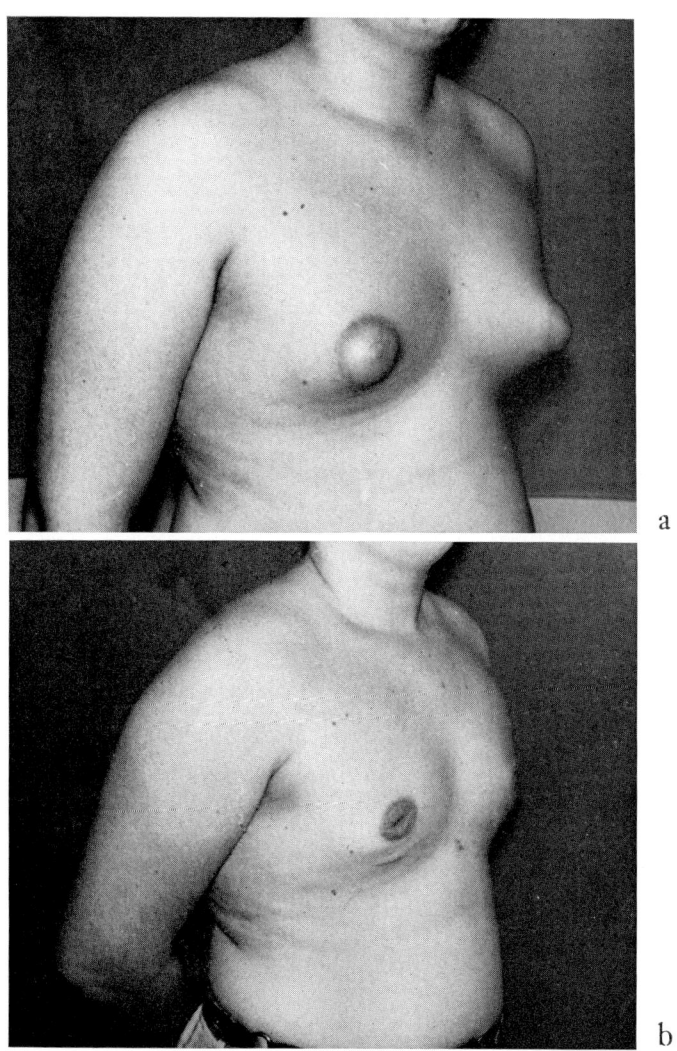

a

b

Case 95, *a:* Patient, aged twenty-nine, with gynecomastia.

b: Excision and repair of gynecomastia after the method of J. Webster (p. 635).

CASE
96

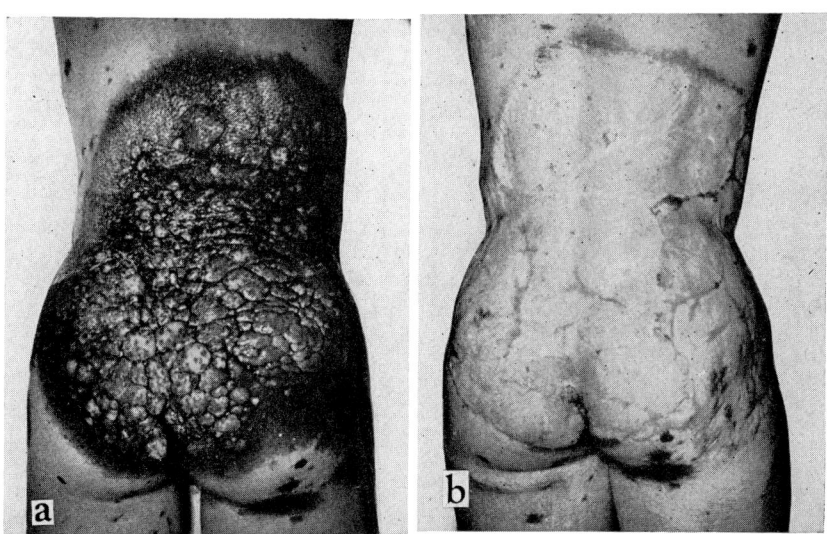

Case 96, *a:* Boy, aged seventeen, with large hairy birthmark (pigmented dermal nevus). In some places the nevus was 5 cm. (2 inches)
thick. It had crevices particularly around the anus with frequent infections.

b: The birthmark was excised in seven stages and skin grafted with
thick split skin grafts in each stage.

1110

CASE
97

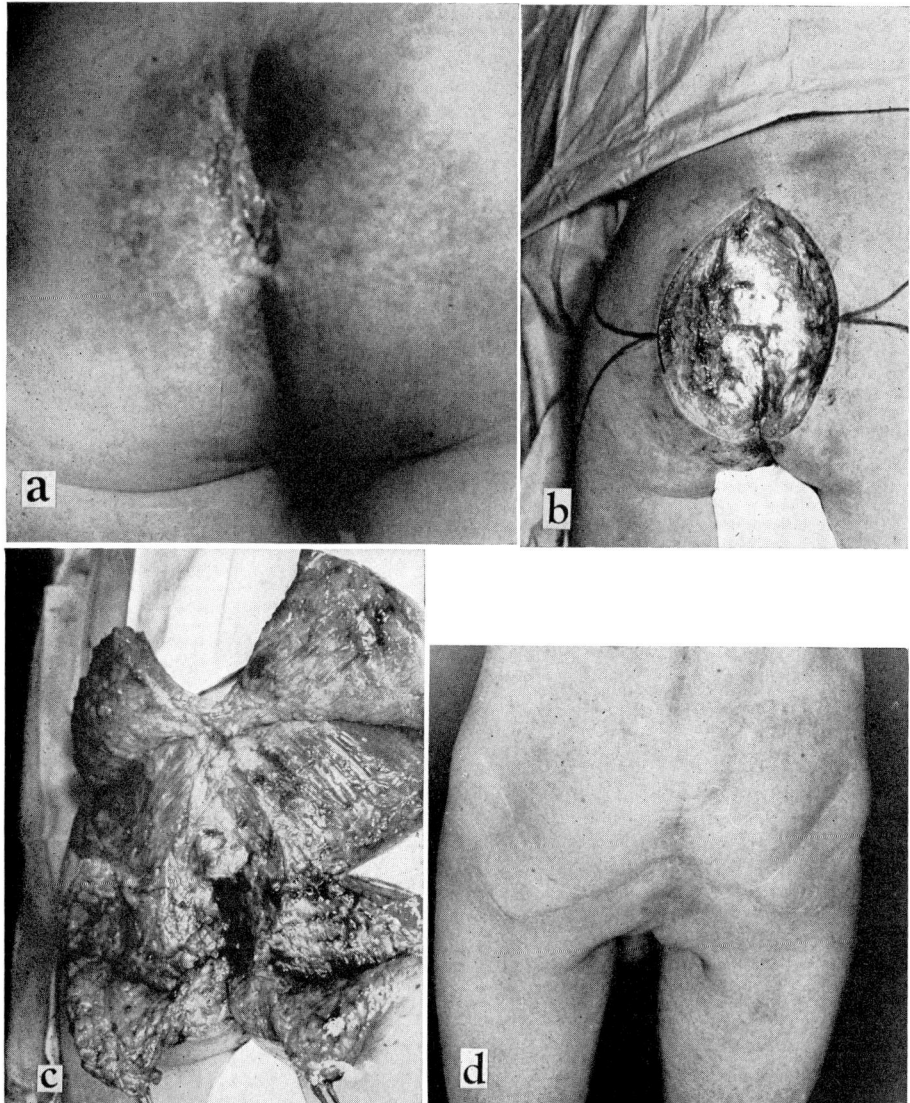

Case 97, *a:* Patient aged sixty-seven, with extensive x-ray burns of sacral region after irradiation of a carcinoma of the bladder.

b: Temporary colostomy performed. After excision of the x-ray damaged skin four local flaps were outlined.

c: After excision of necrotic sacrum and coccyx and elevation of flaps.

d: One year after flaps had been rotated into the defect.

CASE
98

a

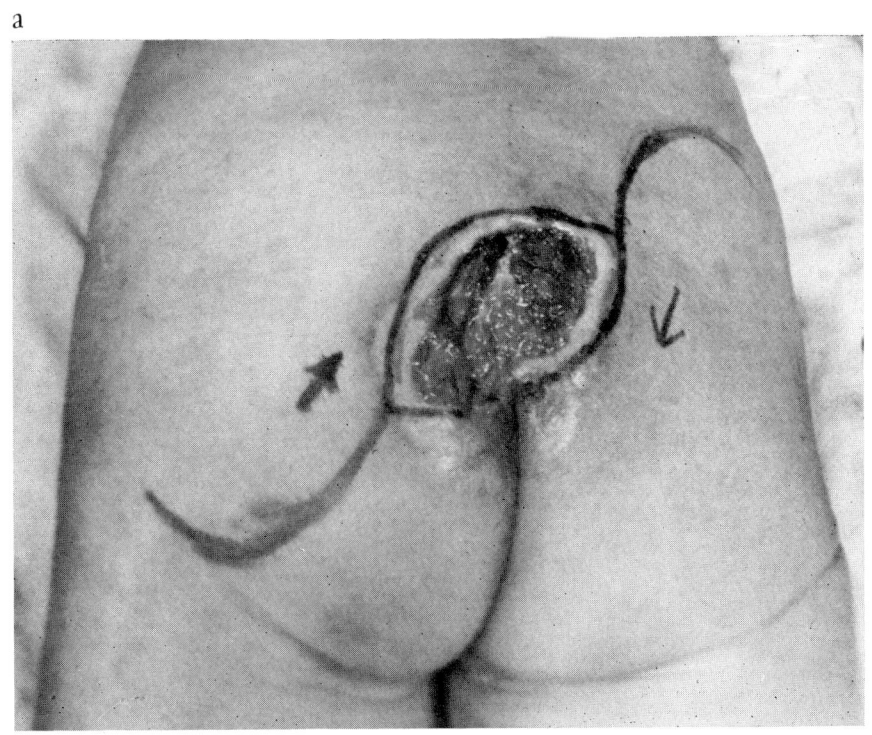

Case 98, *a:* Patient, aged seventy-two, with decubital ulcer. Local flaps for rotation are outlined.

b: Four weeks after operation.

b

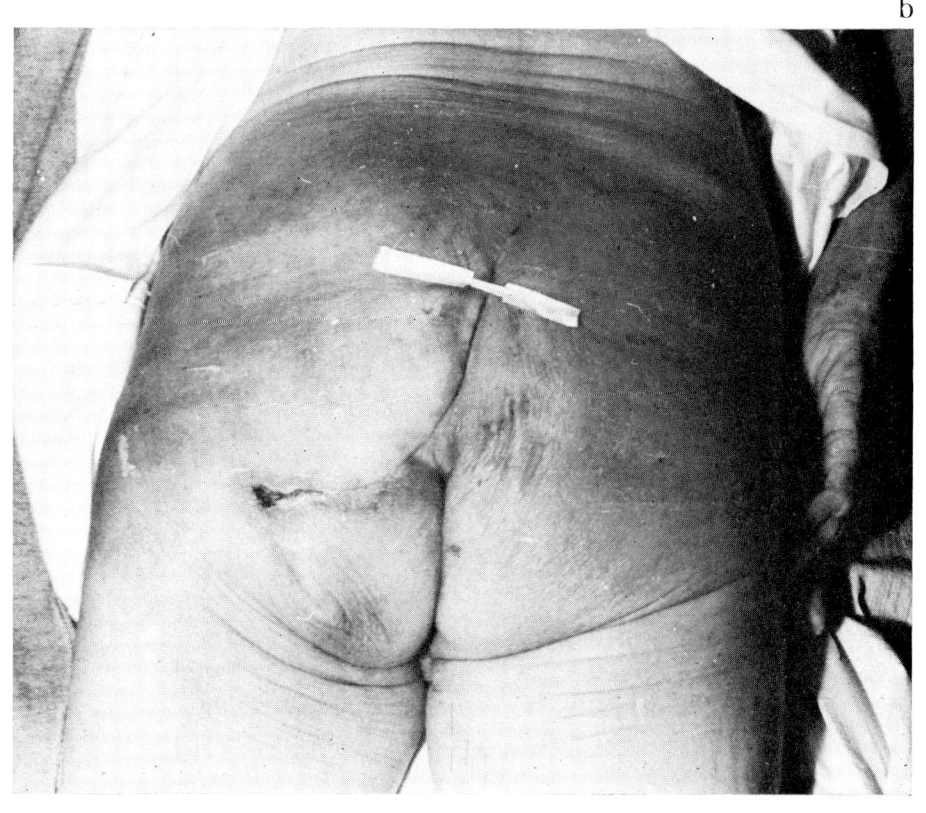

CASE
99

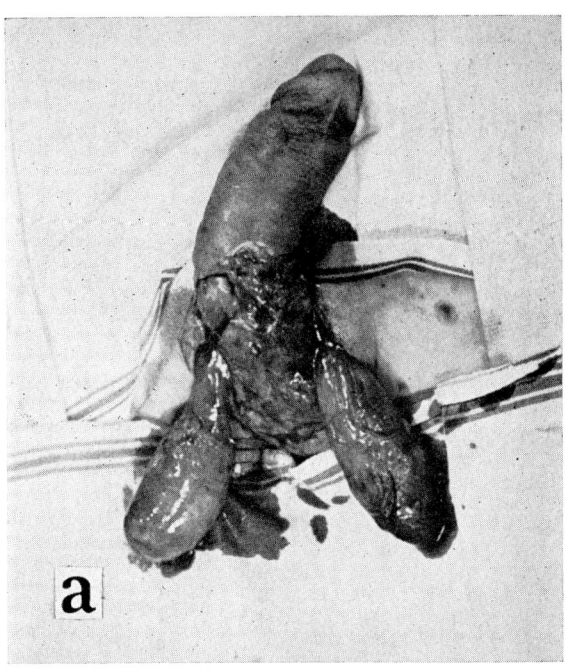

a

Case 99: A twenty-year-old patient was working on a printing machine. His trousers were caught between steel rollers just above the knees. They were pulled off along with the rest of his clothes, including the leather belt, which tore apart over his back. The accident resulted in complete denudation of the testicles and penis, and contusion of his back. The patient was in extreme shock for which he was treated immediately. About two hours after his admission the emergency dressings were changed; it was found that the scrotum, as well as the entire skin of the penis, was torn off. The skin of the penis was hanging on a narrow thin pedicle at

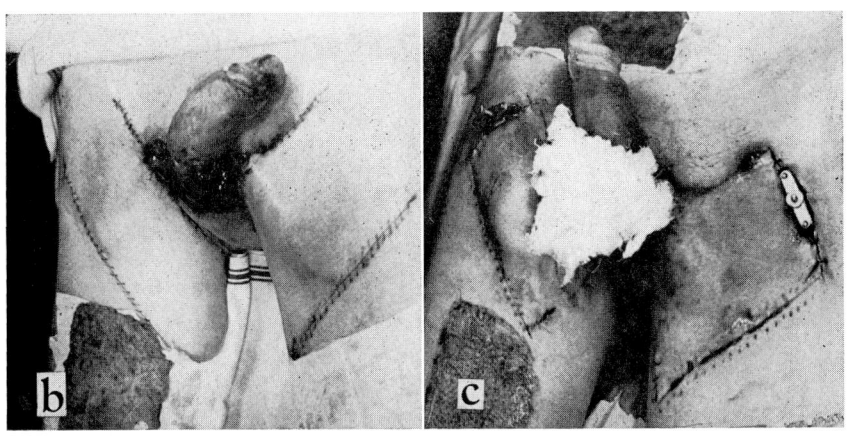

the corona of the glans; this was replaced and a pressure dressing applied. The scrotum, however, was not replaced immediately, since the patient's condition did not permit more repair work, but was placed in saline solution which contained 400,000 units of penicillin. It was replaced the next day and held in place with a light pressure dressing. The dressings were changed on the fifth day. The scrotum was found black and had to be removed. The distal two thirds of the skin of the penis had taken completely, the proximal third, however, was necrotic. After three weeks the

(Continued on next page)

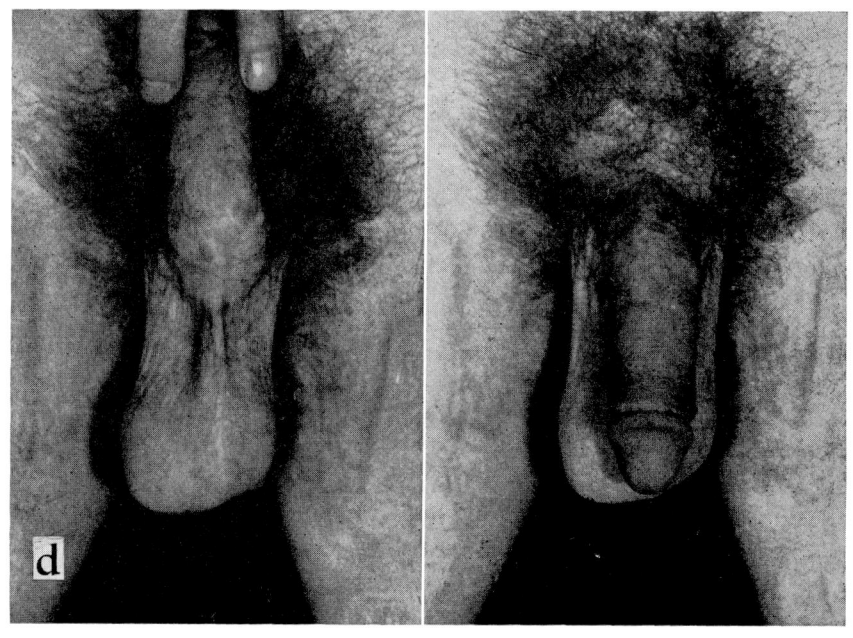

patient was referred for reconstruction of the scrotum. A double-pedicle oblique bridge flap was formed on the anteromedian surface of the thigh. The upper incision was made just below (about 2.5 cm. [one inch] distally) and parallel to the crease of the groin. The measurements of the flaps were 15 by 8 cm. Both flaps were elevated from the fascia lata. The testicle and spermatic cord were now buried beneath the flap. The proximal and posterior part of the plexus was resting upon the narrow strip of skin of the crease of the groin. The remainder of the posterior part of the plexus and the testicle would have come to lie upon the raw surface of the thigh. To prevent the testicle from growing to the donor area and also to prevent the flap from becoming reattached to its donor area, the donor area was skin grafted at this stage, using a nylon-backed thick split graft, cut with the dermatome from the median surface of the same thigh. The flap was now sutured to the wound edges of the donor area; in the region of the spermatic cord, it was sutured to the raw area *b*. A heavily padded pressure dressing was applied. Within the following weeks the pedicles of the flaps were gradually severed. The median pedicles were partially severed nine days after the first operation; five days later the lateral pedicle was severed one third from each side, and a laboratory clamp was applied to the median third (*c*), which within the following few days was gradually crushed. During the same stage the raw area of the proximal third of the shaft of the penis was skin grafted (*c*). One week after the third operation the flaps with the testicles closely attached were elevated. The skin grafts beneath them had taken well; the nylon backing was removed. The flaps, however, became cyanotic, hence were returned to their former site. One week later the flaps were again raised and were anastomosed to each other in the following manner: The lateral pedicles became the posterior and the median pedicles the anterior raphe; the lower oval openings of the flaps were sutured together, thus forming the bottom of the new scrotum. The posterior rim of the upper oval opening was sutured posteriorly to the perineal region, the anterior rim sutured to the pubic region (*d*).

Upon the request of a follow-up report, eight years after the accident, the patient wrote as follows: "I am happy to report to you I am feeling fine. My testicles do not bother me at all. I have not worn my suspensory to hold my testicles up for the last two years. I am also happy to tell you I have a fine young son . . . . He is two and one-half years old now. I have a job working as an airplane mechanic . . . . I have also been playing baseball for the past three years. So you can see I am feeling fine. In fact I don't think I have ever felt better." There was another boy born three years later.

1117

CASE
100

Case 100, *a:* Patient, aged forty-four, was circumcised. The operation resulted in loss of entire skin of penis. The corona glandis became adherent to the scrotum, and the shaft of the penis was buried in the scrotum, causing much distress upon erection.

b: The corona was freed from the scrotum; the shaft of the penis was dissected free, and covered with a skin graft and pressure dressing.

c: Two months after operation. Patient stated having no discomfort in any way. A similar follow-up report was received five years later.

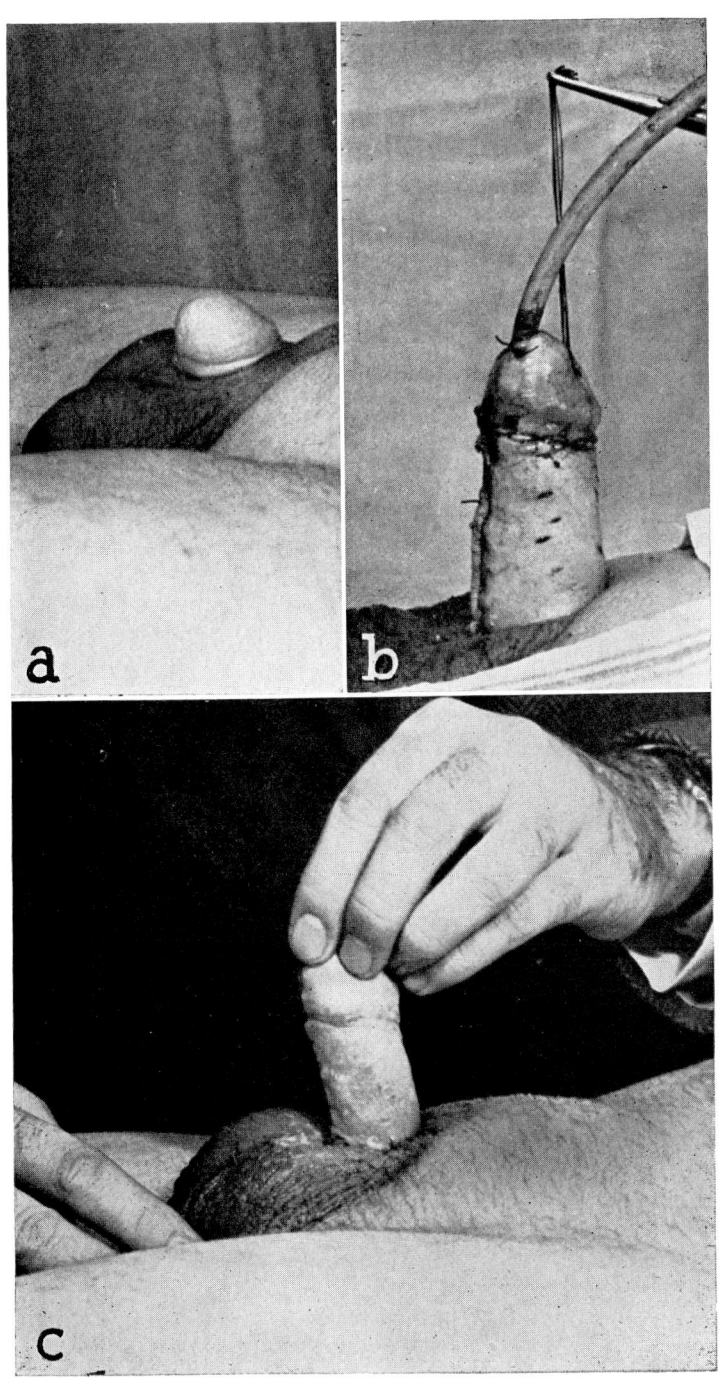

CASE
101

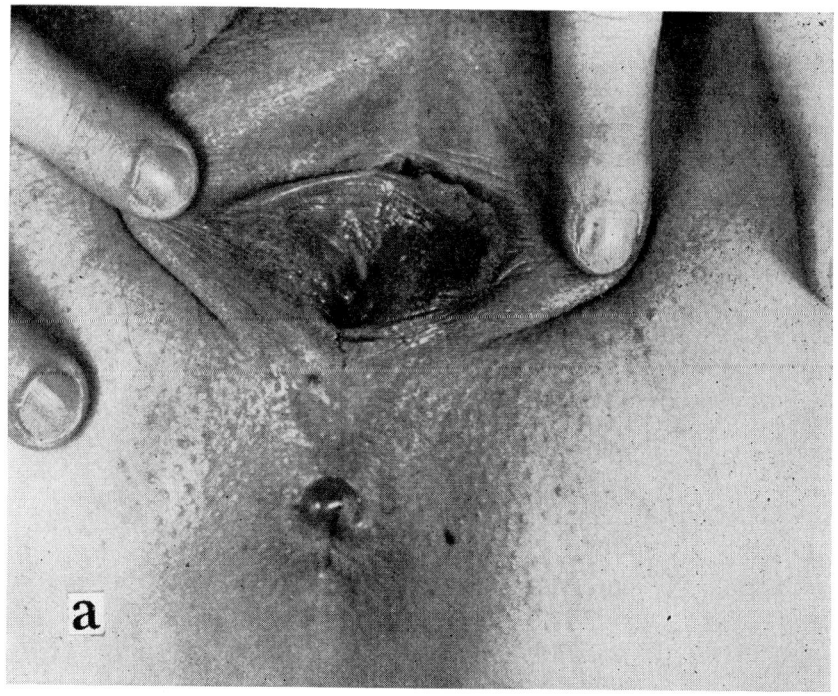

Case 101, *a:* Patient, aged eighteen, born with almost complete absence of the vagina. Since age seventeen she noticed a monthly pain in lower abdomen which repeated itself almost clocklike on the twenty-eighth day. From this time on the breasts started to develop. A gynecological examination under anesthesia revealed no uterus but both ovaries.

b: Reconstruction of vagina with inlay skin graft. Skin grafts were wrapped around a stent of plexiglass. Grafts were taken from the hairless region of the median surface of the thighs.

c: Rubber tubing fastened to a belt held the stent in place.

d: After stent was worn for three months day and night and after another three months only at night, vagina remained wide open. Patient has married; although some subsequent shrinkage occurred, intercourse is satisfactory. They adopted a child.

1120

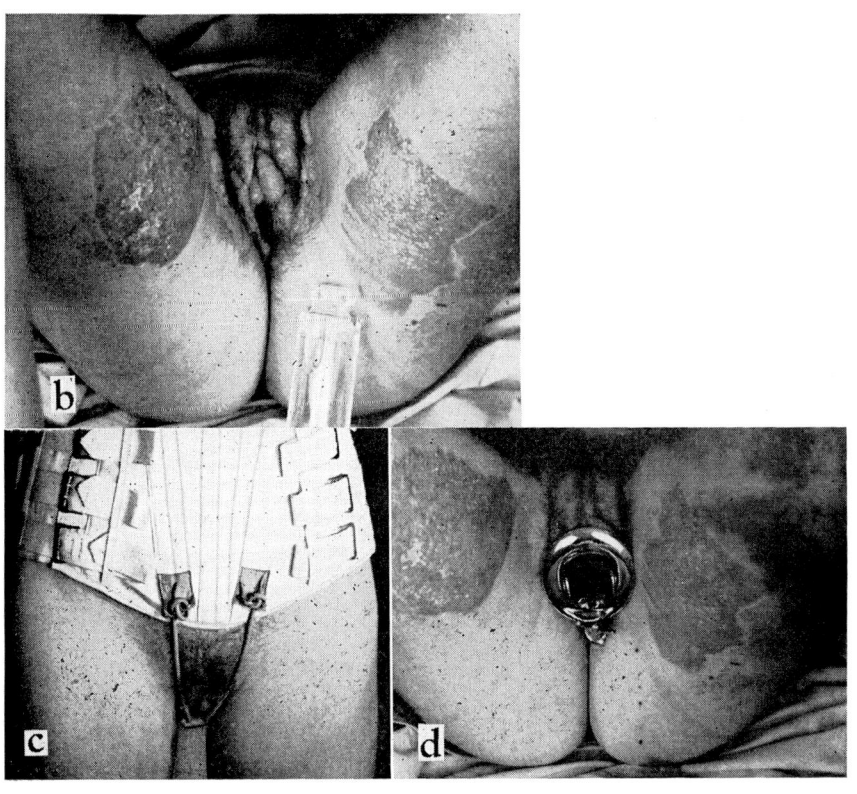

CASE
102

Case 102, *a:* Patient, aged twenty, was a pseudohermaphrodite who had been brought up as a female. At the age of twelve an exploratory laparotomy was performed elsewhere which did not establish the sex. The pelvis was found empty and gonads could not be found anywhere else. Endocrine studies failed also to clarify the sex pattern. Examination at the time of admission revealed an individual five feet seven inches tall, 163 pounds, large features, hands and feet, breasts small, voice only slightly low, female hair distribution, no facial hirsutism, and slightly broad hips. The inguinal regions were well padded with subcutaneous fat tissue and for this reason were difficult to palpate. There was no evidence of a hernia or a mass. The clitoris was about 5 cm. long and resembled a penis; it was held downward by a chordee and had complete hypospadia. The urethra opened into a vestibule surrounded by small labia minora. Behind it was a small fistulous opening representing the vaginal outlet. A probe could be passed through this opening for about 6 or 7 cm. Labia majora were present and of normal size; they were empty. These findings suggested that the individual was a pseudohermaphrodite and probably of male pattern. The psychosexual patterns were however female. At the age of nineteen she fell in love with a boy of her age. She requested reconstruction of the vagina and amputation of the phallus. *b:* The vagina was reconstructed with a free inlay skin graft. Amputation of the phallus was deferred. Subsequently she developed symptoms of a strangulated left-sided inguinal hernia. Operation revealed however a normal sized testicle with appendages and spermatic plexus surrounded by a hydrocele. A testicle was found in the right inguinal region. It was left behind. Subsequently the patient decided to remain female and castration and further estrogenization were carried out. Patient married a male and intercourse is satisfactory to both. Amputation of the phallus is indefinitely postponed since erection of the same upon sexual excitation provides a feeling of "pleasure" to her.

Conclusion: This individual proved to be a male pseudohermaphrodite. It must be assumed, although actual proof is lacking, that the testicle secreted a sufficient amount of female hormones to cause a gynecoid orientation. The psychosexual trauma inflicted later in life as the result of the discovery of the testicles would have increased had the patient been fitted to the gonadal sex. Through reconstruction of the vagina, castration, and estrogenization, the gynecoid pattern could be enhanced.

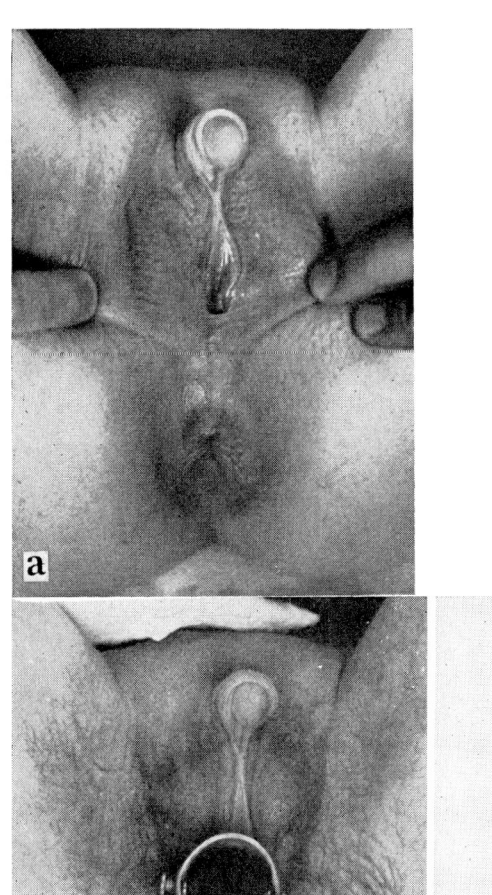

This case proves that the gonads, although primarily influencing the secondary sex characteristics of an individual and making the individual anatomically male or female, may not direct sex orientation and psychosexual behavior.

1123

CASE
103

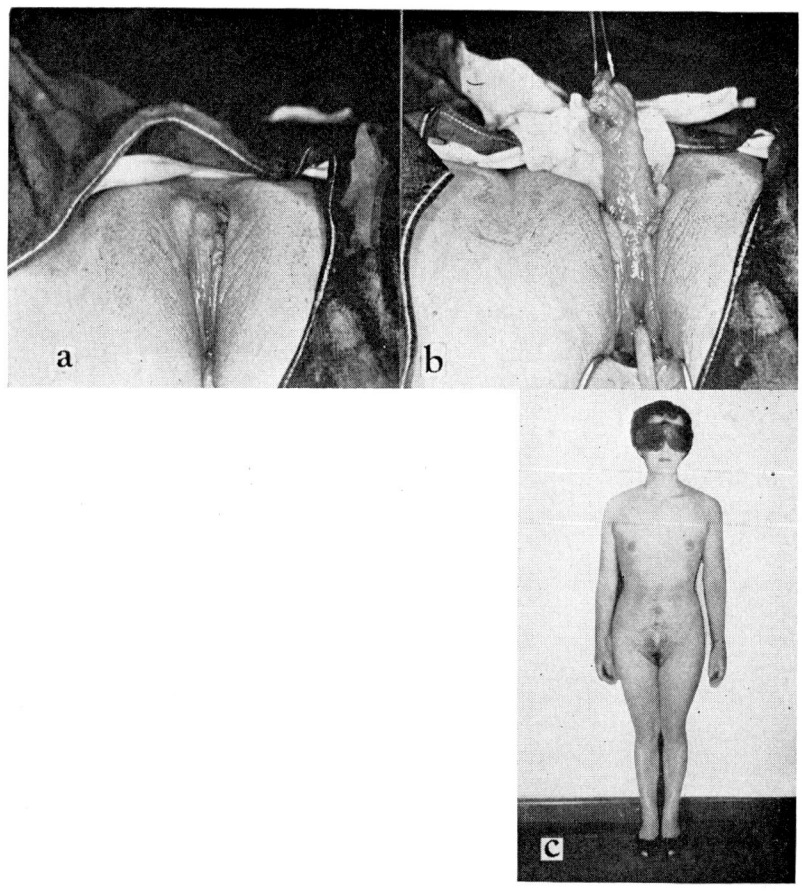

Case 103, *a:* This case had been formerly classified by the author as female pseudohermaphroditism (Plast. Reconst. Surg. 16:201, 1955), but from subsequent studies it became evident that the diagnosis must be corrected. The problem of female pseudohermaphroditism is complicated by the fact that the vast majority of "female hermaphrodites" actually have congenital adrenal hyperplasia, and this individual appears to be one of these cases.

Patient, aged nineteen, at birth was pronounced female. She has one brother. Family history is irrelevant. When one and one-half years old, mother noticed an enlargement of the child's clitoris. After consultation with several physicians, an exploratory laparotomy was carried out.

At operation a normal infantile uterus, tubes and ovaries were found. The urachus was persistent and quite definite and by palpation seemed to disappear as it passed laterally along the posterior wall of the abdomen toward the left kidney. The surgeon was unable to palpate any growths in the region of either kidney. A partial amputation of the clitoris, which was one and one-half inches long, was performed for symptomatic relief. An exploration of the adrenal glands was abandoned. It was hoped that as she grew older a possible tumor of the glands (adrenal) could be more easily dealt with. She was readmitted two years later for exploration of the adrenal glands; the right one was found normal, the left one could not be explored since operation had to be discontinued because of acceleration of the pulse. After she was four years old hair started to grow on the face and extremities. At six years of age she had a bloody discharge from the vagina for about two days. This occurred again for four days at age of fourteen years. Her voice grew deeper at age sixteen. Although early in youth she liked to play with girls, she became later attracted by boys as well as by girls. The clitoris after the partial amputation started to grow soon again. Ever since she can remember she experienced occasional erection of the clitoris, even at night; erection became more and more painful because the stump of the clitoris had been buried beneath the pubic skin at the first operation. Erections occurred upon excitation by men as well as women. In *a* (lithotomy position) the clitoris is seen bulging beneath the pubic skin.

She was referred for reconstruction of the vagina, which apparently was absent, and removal of the clitoris. The urinary hormone assays were reported as follows: June 22nd, 1947, 17 ketosteroids 53.6 mg. per 24 hours. September 22nd, 1953, 26.1 mg. and 32.3 mg. Urine volume 450 to 550 cc. per day.

(Continued on next page)

CASE

103 *(Continued)*

Operation was carried out under general anesthesia with the patient in lithotomy position (*b*). Between the underdeveloped labiae a wide urethral opening was disclosed, more posteriorly than normally situated. A catheter was passed into the urethral opening but failed to withdraw urine. Only after several more attempts could the Foley catheter be passed into the bladder. Thus it became obvious that the wide urethral opening was the urogenital sinus into which vagina and urethra opened. An incision was made from the posterior rim of this opening through the perineum toward the rectum. The incision was deepened for about an inch. When the vaginal cavity was reached, the vagina was of normal width but little shorter than normal. There was no cervix palpable or visible and no anterior enlargement simulating a prostate. A mobilization of the vagina was carried out to join it to the skin wound at the perineum. An incision was now made over the buried clitoris and a penis-like structure with two corpora cavernosa was dissected free. It measured 4 x 1 inch. A typical operation for amputation of the penis was carried out, leaving only a little stump where the corpora divided into a right and left branch. The mucous membrane was sutured over it. Recovery was uneventful.

She returned to her endocrinologist and estinyl was administered. This apparently caused intrauterine bleeding resulting in hematometra, since the cervix was absent. She consulted the gynecologist who upon operation found a blind vaginal pouch unconnected with the uterus; upon abdominal section the uterus was found markedly enlarged, tubes and ovaries appeared normal; the abdomen was closed and the operation continued by vaginal approach; the operative procedure consisted of connecting the vaginal vault to the presumed cervix, allowing drainage of the massive hematometra. Biopsies which had been taken from the ovaries showed immature structures with follicles in abundance. She then was placed on cortisone treatment. The hair of face and of extremities decreased almost immediately, and the breasts started to develop. She has irregular vaginal bleedings, or rather spottings, sometimes lasting about five days. The patient has now been happily married for four years.

Her endocrinologist, Dr. A. M. Bongiovanni, summarizes her and similar cases as follows: "The basic defect is an inability to synthesize cortisone. As a result of this the pituitary puts out very large amounts of ACTH in an attempt to force the synthesis of cortisone, but due to a congenital lack of the enzymes in the adrenal cortex necessary for the synthesis, the adrenal is unable to respond properly. However, instead of making cortisone, the gland does manufacture very large amounts of androgen since there is no defect in its ability to do so. Since the androgens do not satisfy the pituitary, the ACTH stimulation continues unabated. This whole disease begins in the uterus and the female fetus, whose organs are entirely normal otherwise, is under the influence of androgens which bring about changes only in the external genitalia but always leave the internal genitalia undisturbed. Therefore the ovaries and uterus are practically always normal. The surgical approach requires only correction of the external genitalia. However, for proper femininization to occur at the right age, cortisone must be administered continuously throughout life. The doses of cortisone employed are very small and approximate the amount that the normal adrenal would be making. These doses in no way resemble those used in rheumatoid arthritis or other such diseases. When the small dose of cortisone satisfies the pituitary, the adrenals no longer make androgens and the entire picture is reversed." Dr. Bongiovanni's outstanding work in this field is included in Wilkin's Endocrine Disorders in Childhood and Adolescence, published in 1960.

The diagnosis of congenital adrenal hyperplasia should be suspected in any infant born with ambiguous or abnormal external genitalia. It is important to make the diagnosis at a very early age to prevent the undesirable disturbances of metabolism which may occur. As has been emphasized by Jones et al., it is no longer necessary to subject a patient suspected of congenital adrenal hyperplasia to a laparotomy for purposes of diagnosis, or sex, or tumor of the adrenal. A female chromosomal sex arrangement (by means of buccal smear or some similar method) plus the presence of elevated urinary 17-ketosteroids which are suppressed by cortisone are sufficient to establish the diagnosis.

CASE
104

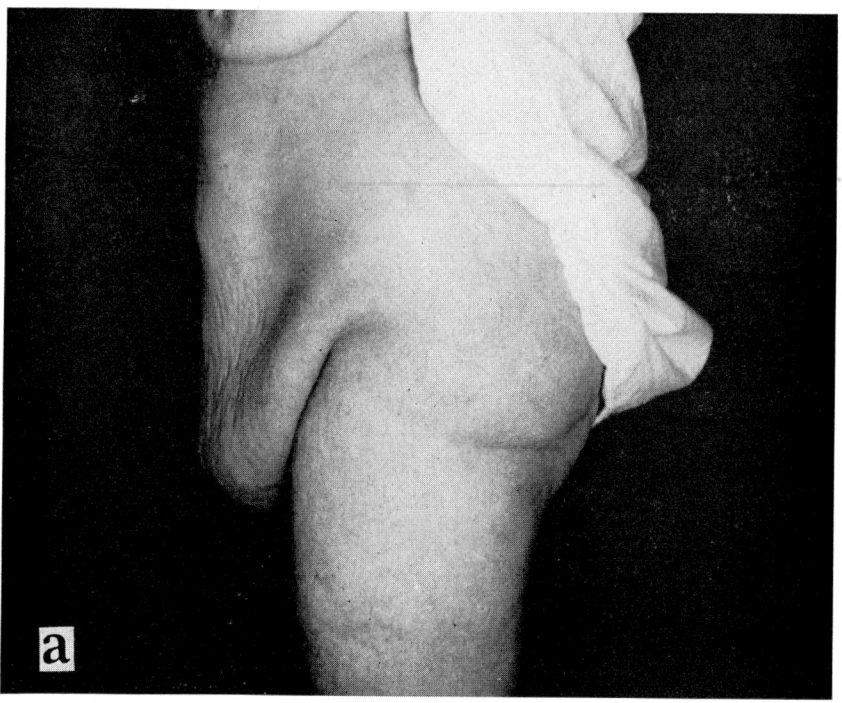

Case 104, *a:* Patient, aged sixty-one, had six children and with each pregnancy the adipose tissue of the abdomen enlarged and became flabby like an apron.

b, c: Three months after excision of the redundant skin and fat tissue and repair of a wide diastasis of the rectus muscle and transverse shortening of the fascia and muscle with a Mayo overlap technique. No symptoms or recurrence after fifteen months.

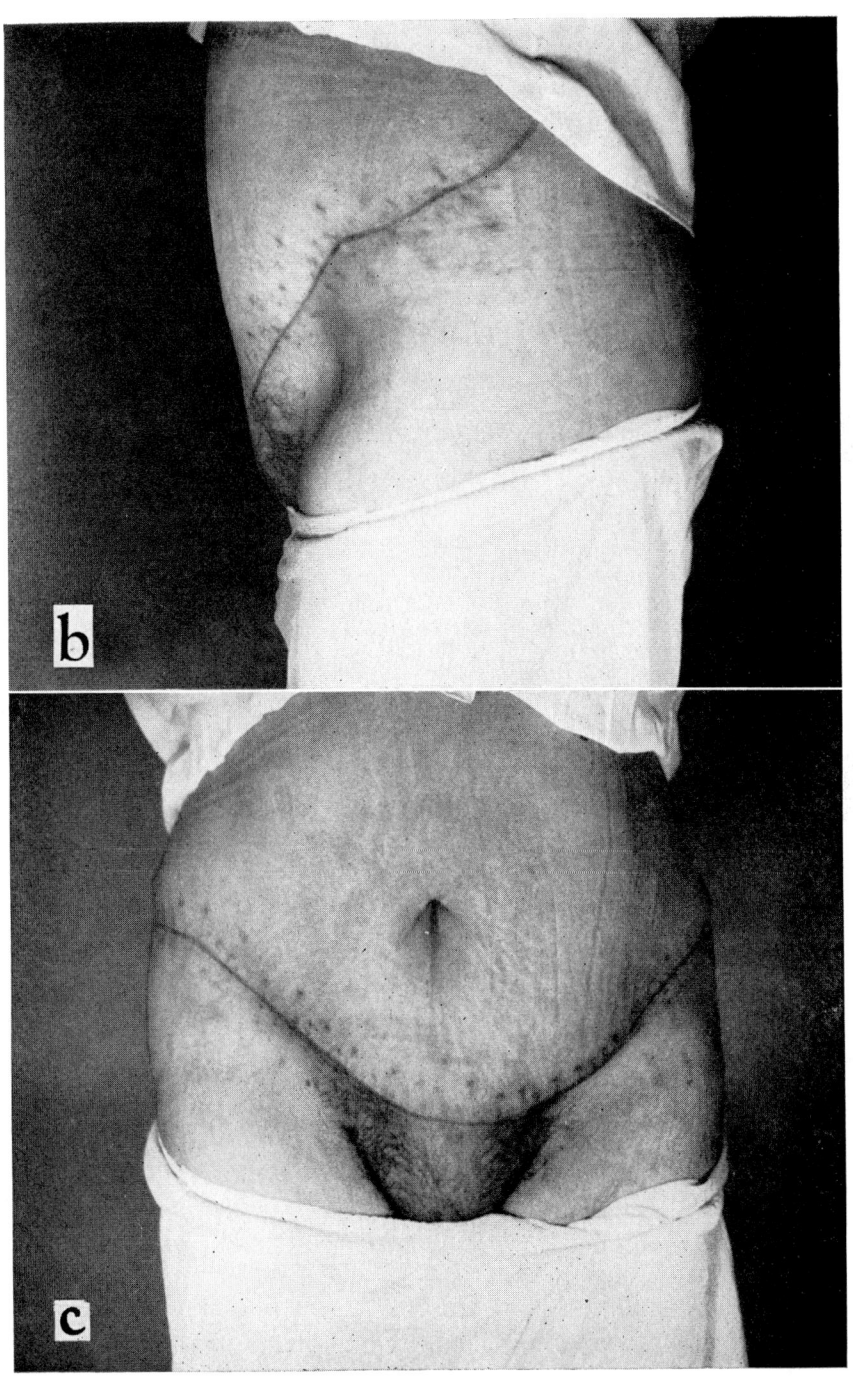

CASE
105

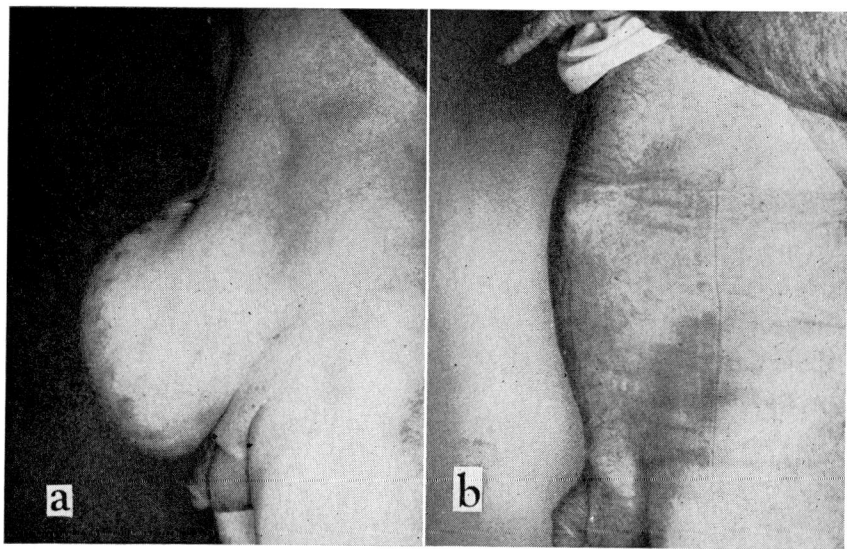

Case 105, *a:* Extensive incisional hernia of lower half of abdomen.
b: The operation consisted of the Mayo overlap method of closure. The flaps were made longitudinally of fascia and the rectus sheath. There was much tension on the whole area; hence a dermal graft was utilized which consisted of the excised redundant skin minus its epidermis. The patient wore an abdominal belt for six months. There is no evidence of recurrence thirteen months after operation. Patient works as a janitor of a school.

CASE
106

Case 106, *a:* The patient presented himself in the Metabolic Ward of the Lankenau Hospital weighing 691 pounds. He gave a history of excessive dietary intake of all sorts of foods. He required 5000 calories a day to sustain his weight. He was placed on an 800-calorie formula diet of varying constituency. Following 723 days of this, his weight reached a low point of 179 pounds—a total loss of 512 pounds.

b, c: Much redundancy of skin after weight loss.

d: After removal of the abdominal fat apron there was another, smaller, fat apron hanging over the genitalia; this was removed in another stage. The removal of redundant skin of thighs and arms followed, in successive stages.

a
b

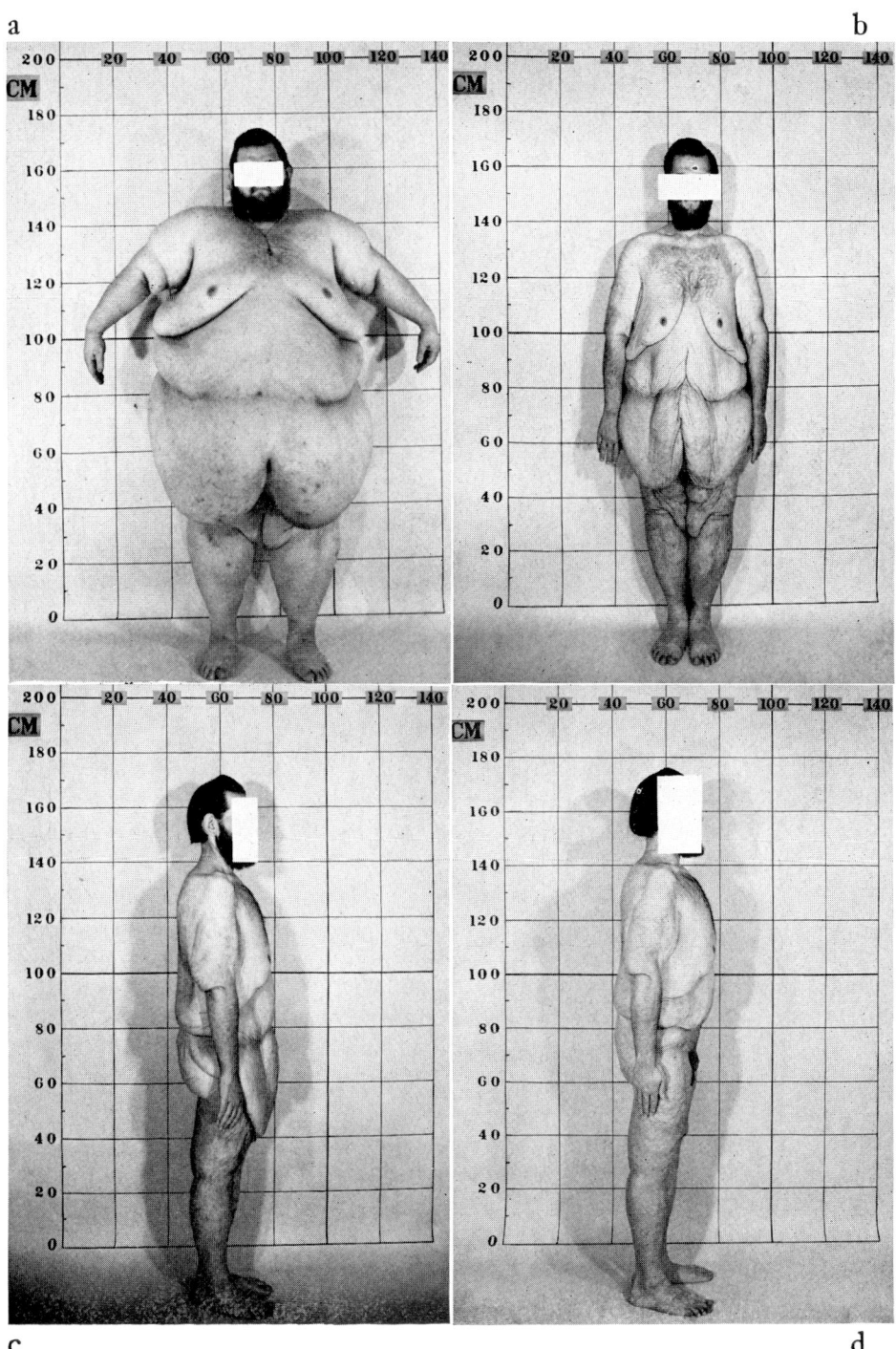

c
d

CASE
107

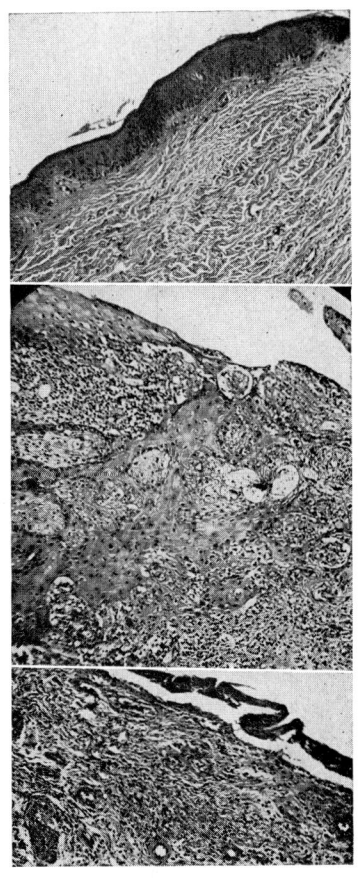

Case 107, *a:* Boy, aged four, with extensive burns of both legs. He was referred to the author's service three months after the burn. In three skin graft operations both legs and knee joints were covered with autogenous split grafts.

b: The general condition of the patient, however, deteriorated; hence homogenous split skin grafts (from his father) were used to close all raw surfaces. His general condition improved immediately.

c: The first homogenous graft started to disintegrate two months later. Four more operations were required to close the remaining raw surface with autogenous grafts.

d: One year later cicatricial adduction contractures of the groins and thighs were corrected with Z-plasty and skin grafts.

1132

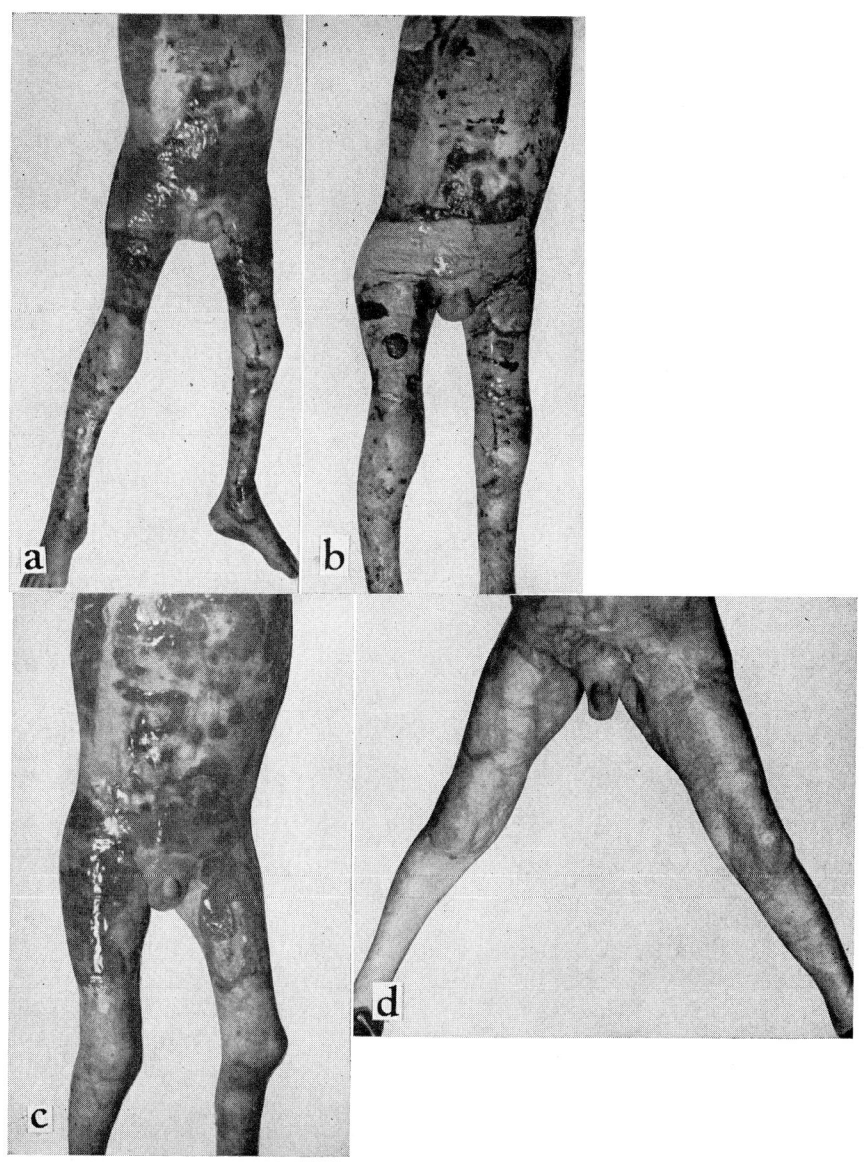

Microscopic picture depicts the homogenous skin graft five weeks after transplantation. Graft has "taken" well; note absence of any proliferative activity. Lower sections show homogenous skin graft in process of sloughing off. Extensive fibrous tissue reaction.

CASE
108

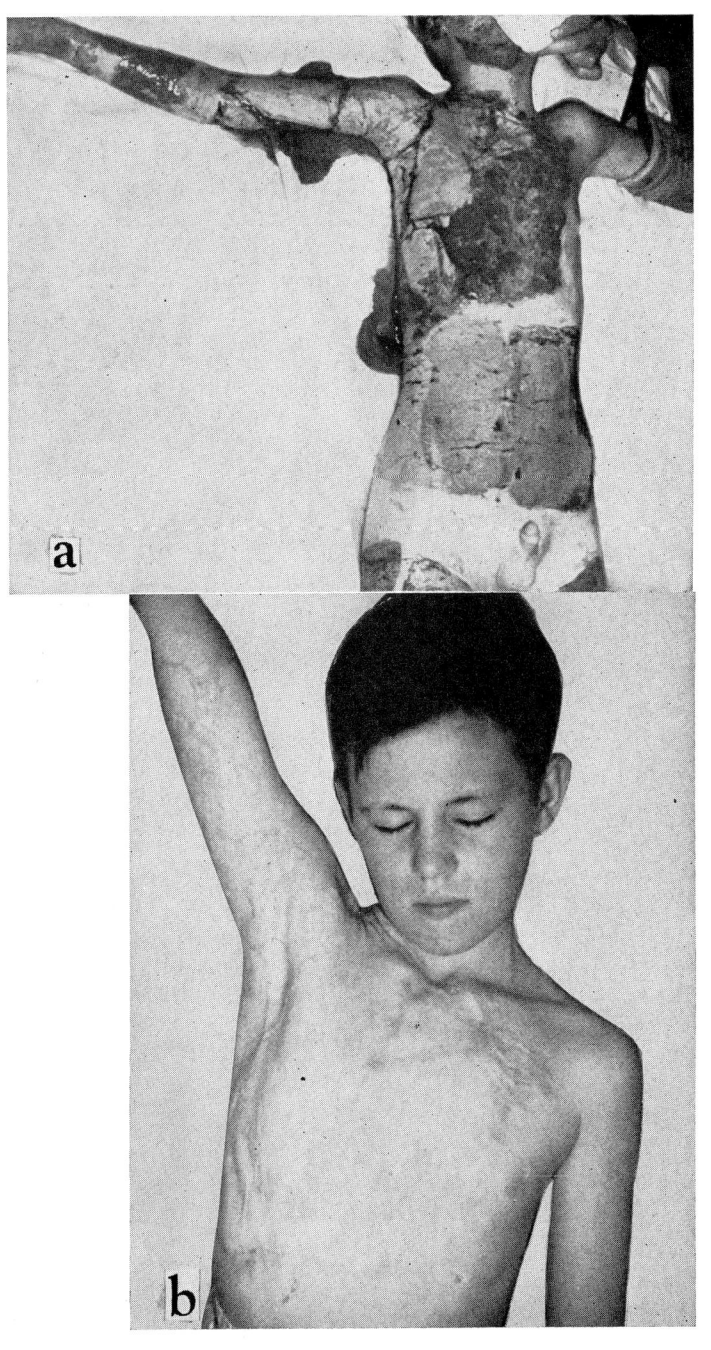

Case 108, *a:* Extensive burns of chest, right shoulder, right arm and neck. Shock treatment. Local treatment consisted of pressure dressings. The eschar started to come off on the twelfth day. It was completely excised on the eighteenth day. First skin graft operation on the twenty-fourth day. *b:* Three skin graft operations and later a Z-plasty were required to overcome a contracture of the right axilla.

CASE
109

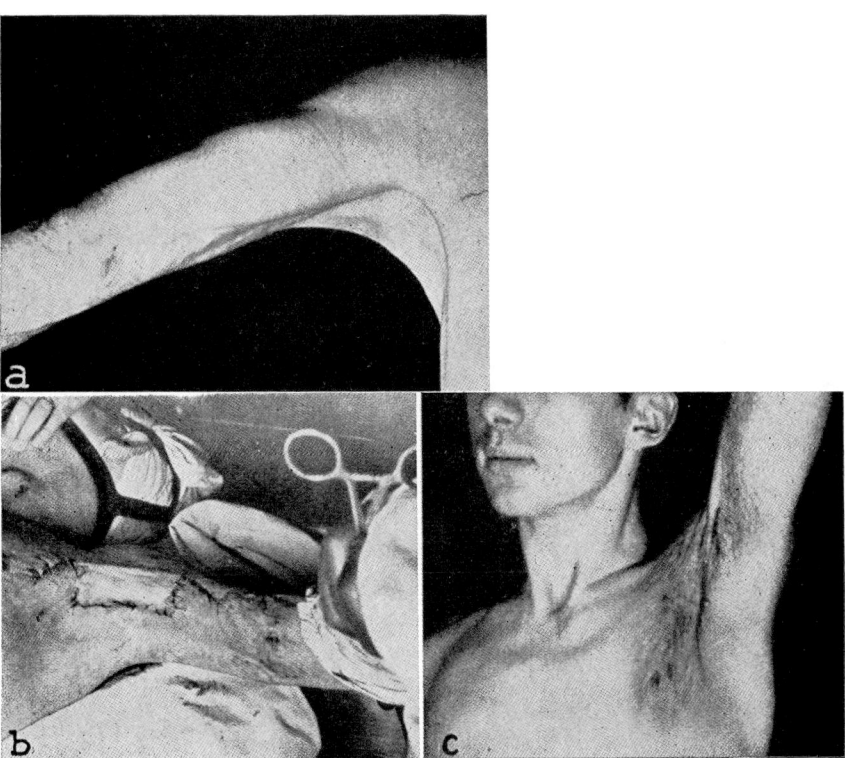

Case 109, *a:* Posterior view of patient with a binding web of anterior part of axilla after burn.

b: Condition corrected by double Z-operation, which broke up the binding web and released the contracture (Fig. 52, p. 186).

c: Patient three months after repair.

1135

CASE
110

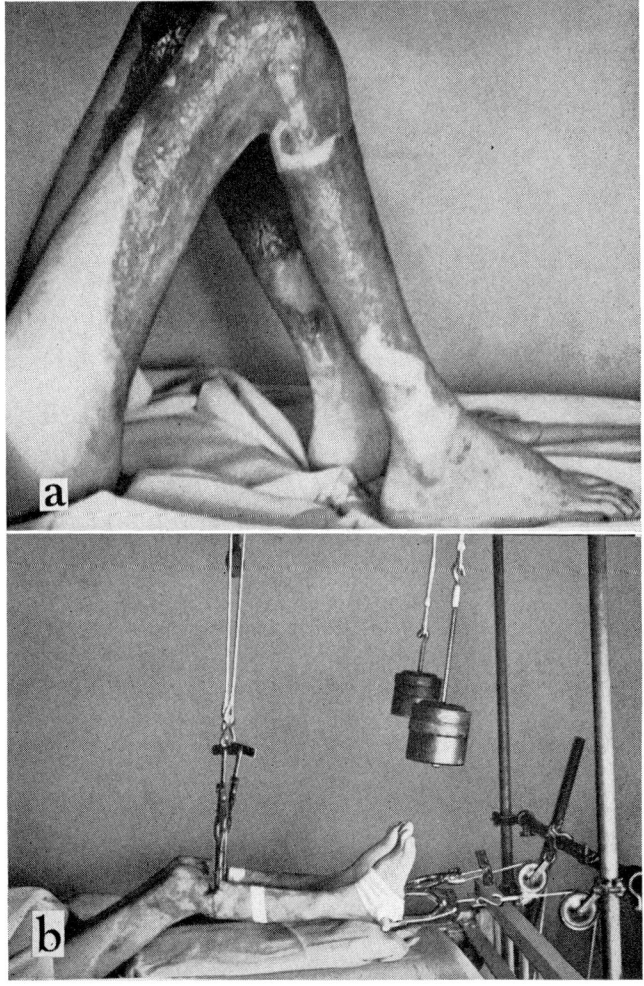

Case 110, *a:* Extensive burn of both legs, contracture of both knee joints (patient referred to author for repair six months after the accident).

b: The raw surfaces covered with skin grafts, the contracture partly reduced. Posterior subluxation of the tibia due to contracture of posterior ligaments and capsules, to be overcome by longitudinal and vertical traction.

c, d: X-ray pictures of same patient, showing on the left the posterior subluxation of the tibia, on the right the reduction of the subluxation by traction. Later, a plaster cast was applied in this position with incorporation of the wires.

e, f: One year after operation. (H. May: Surg. Clin. N. Amer.)

1136

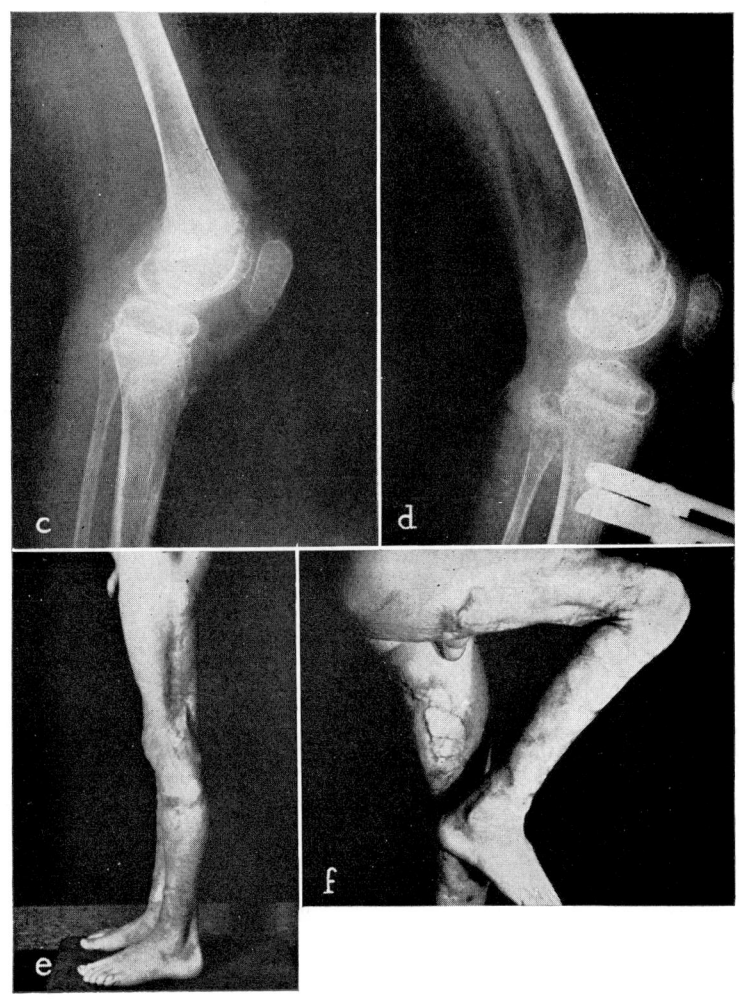

CASE
111

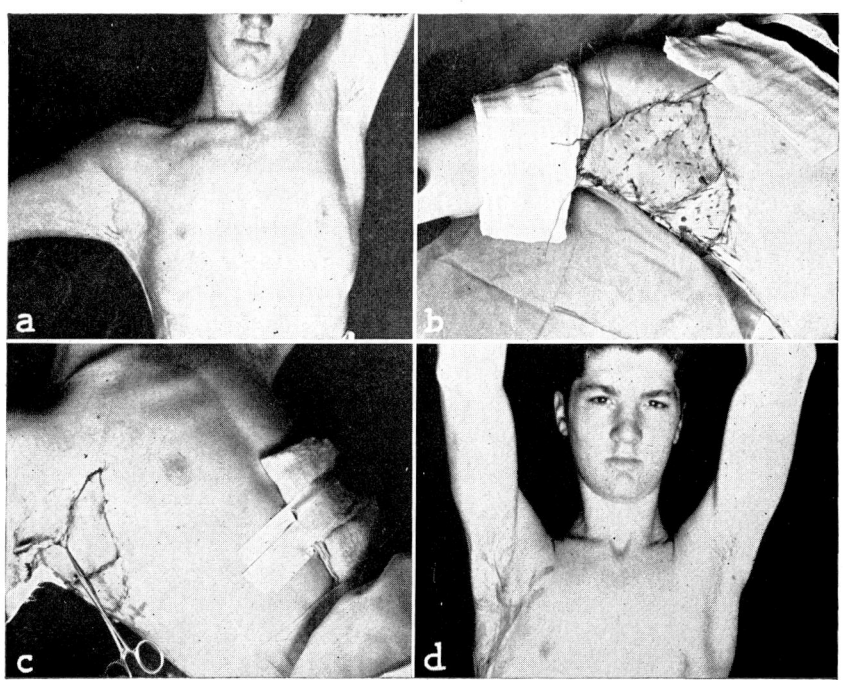

Case 111, *a:* Contracture of right axilla from old burn.

b: Repair similar to that of Case 112. Note probes behind the everted skin.

c: At the time of the first change of the dressing, the everted skin flap was released.

d: Result three months later. (H. May: Surg. Clin. N. Amer.)

CASE
112

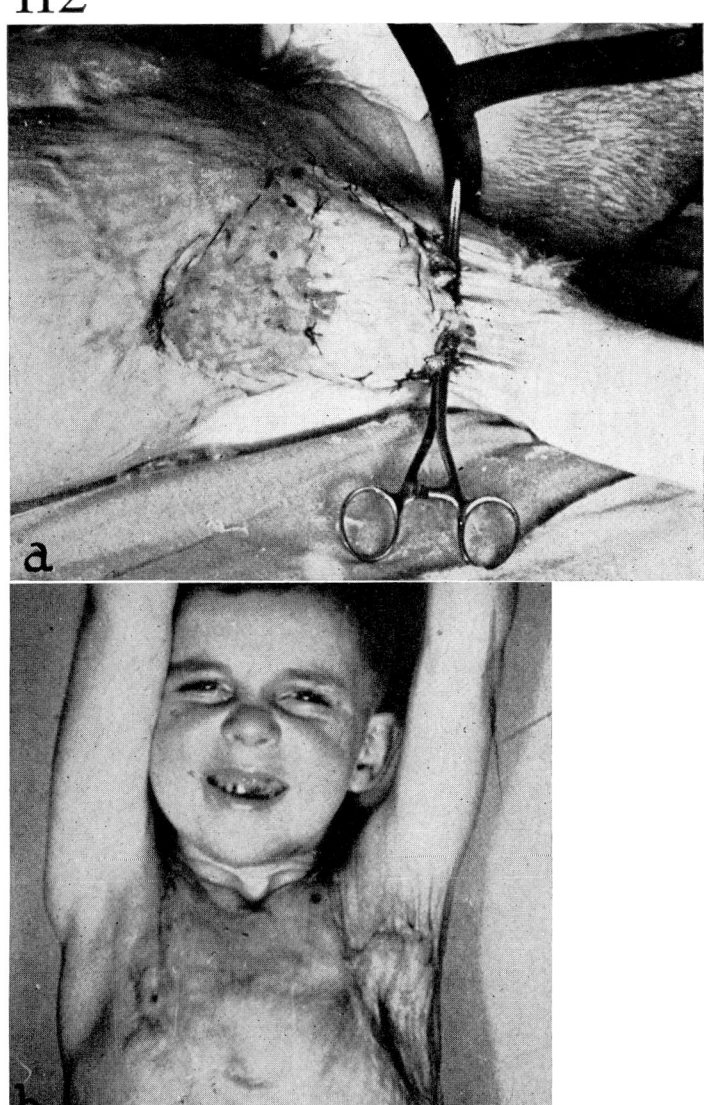

Case 112, *a:* Contracture of left axilla from old burn scar. Contracting scar was incised, the contracture reduced. The lateral wound edge
was everted and sutured to the skin of the arm so that skin came to lie on
skin (Kelly clamp behind the everted skin). This increased the raw surface
to counteract recontracture. The defect was covered with two skin grafts.

   b: After four months.

CASE
113

Case 113, *a:* Extensive contracture of left axilla from burn.

b: The scar was incised near the chest, the contracture reduced, and the defect covered with two skin grafts. Result six months after operation.

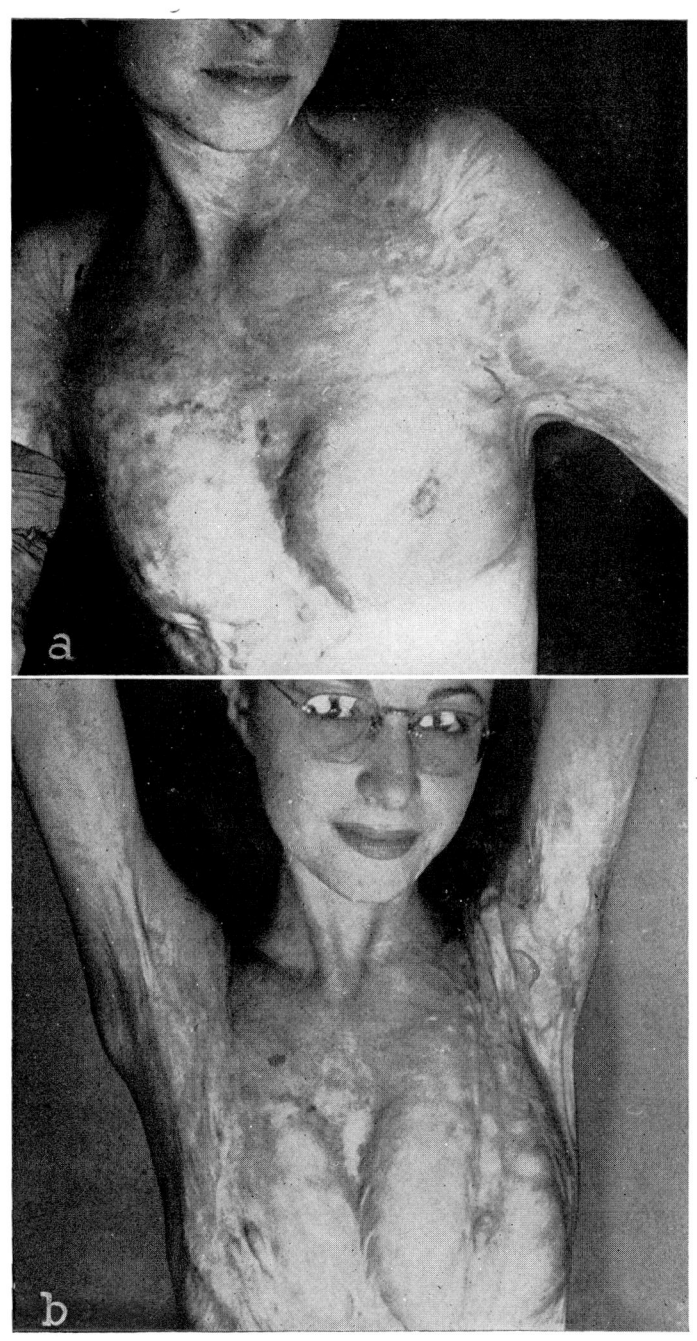

CASE
114

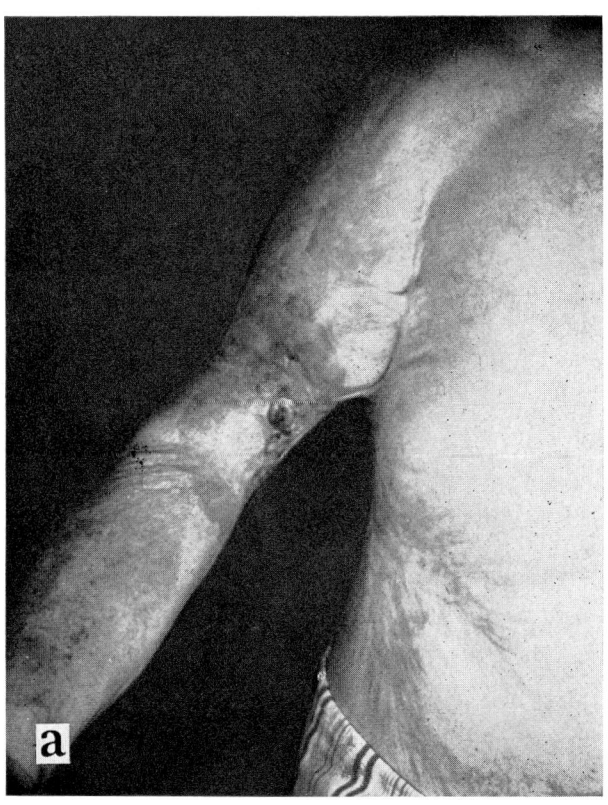

Case 114, *a:* Patient, aged sixty-one, with old burn contracture of right axilla. An ulcer developed in the scar. It was excised. The microscopic examination did not show any evidence of malignancy. The entire area of the ulcer was excised and skin grafted.

b: Eight months later a melanosarcoma developed on the other side of the arm within the burn scar. The entire scar and the tumor were excised, i.e., practically the entire surface of the right upper arm. The axilla was opened from a relaxation incision. All axillary glands were dissected. Vessels and nerves were covered with flaps from the neighborhood while the remaining raw surfaces were closed with a skin graft.

c: Six months after the operation. Patient died one and one-quarter years later from metastases.

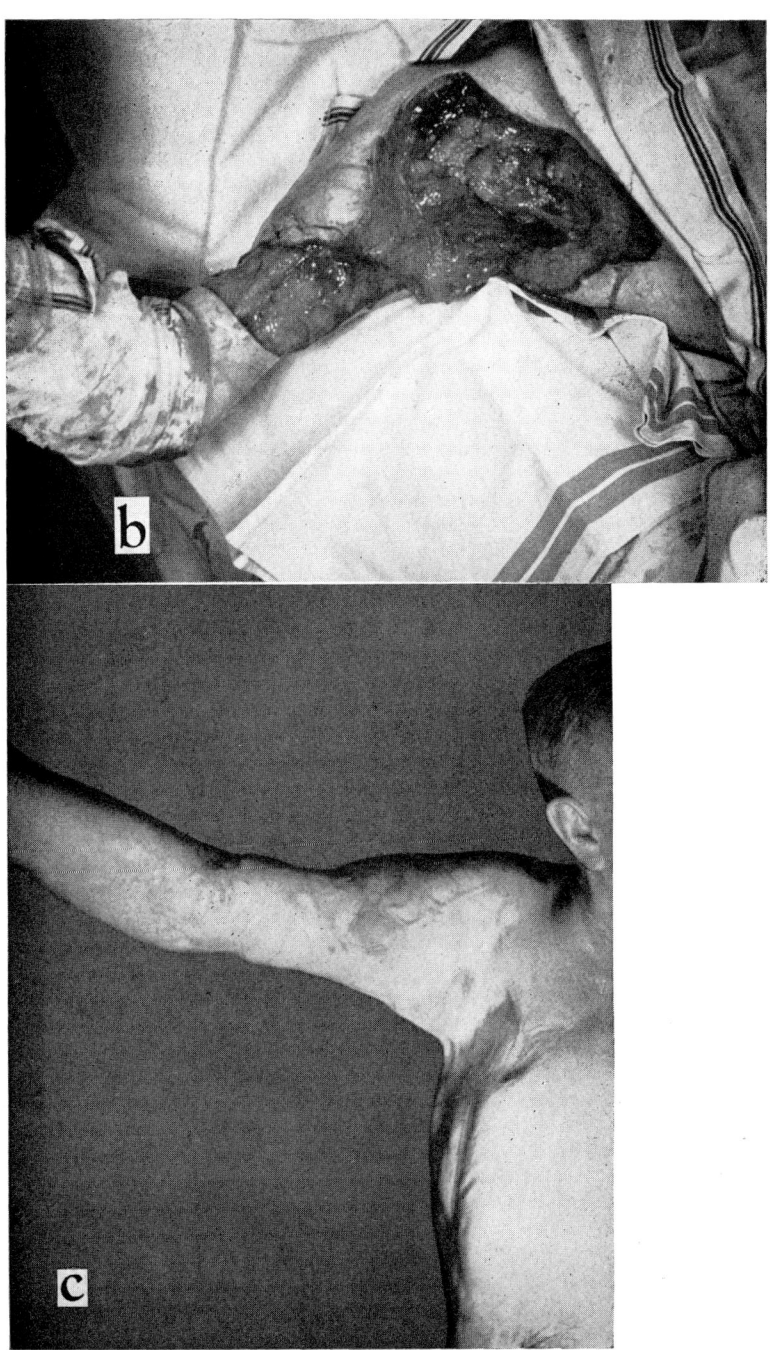

CASE
115

Case 115, *a:* Contracture of both axillae and right elbow joint from burn, normal skin in right axilla. An incision was made along the median border of the normal skin at the right side of chest (see dotted line). This part of the skin was undermined and the contracture reduced. The defect was covered with one large skin graft. A skin-graft repair to overcome the contracture of left axilla was unsuccessful; hence, a tube flap was made from the immediate neighborhood and transplanted in stages. The contracture of right elbow joint was repaired by a Z-plastic operation. *b:* Result four years after operation. (H. May: Surg. Clin. N. Amer.)

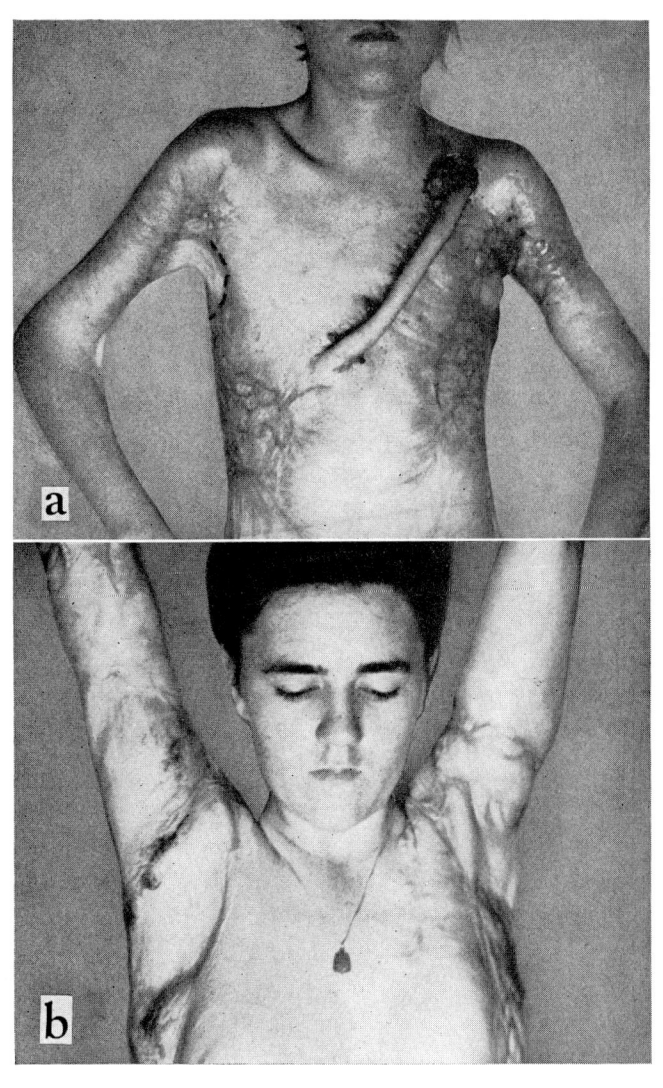

CASE
116

Case 116, *a:* Eight-year-old boy with contracted scar of right elbow joint and axilla from burns. Burned area included entire right half of chest and abdomen. Contracting scar of right elbow joint was thick and heavy. A tube flap was made from left thoracoepigastric region.

b: The lower end of the tube flap was severed after three months, and fastened to the left wrist. The upper pedicle was severed after seventeen days.

c: The contracting scar at elbow joint was incised, the contracture reduced, and the insertion of the biceps severed (no impairment of function resulted later from severance of biceps insertion). The tube flap was opened and sutured into the defect. Both arms were immobilized in a plaster cast.

d: The flap was severed from the wrist after two weeks. Condition three years after repair. Note length of flap (x–x). (H. May: Surg. Clin. N. Amer.)

1146

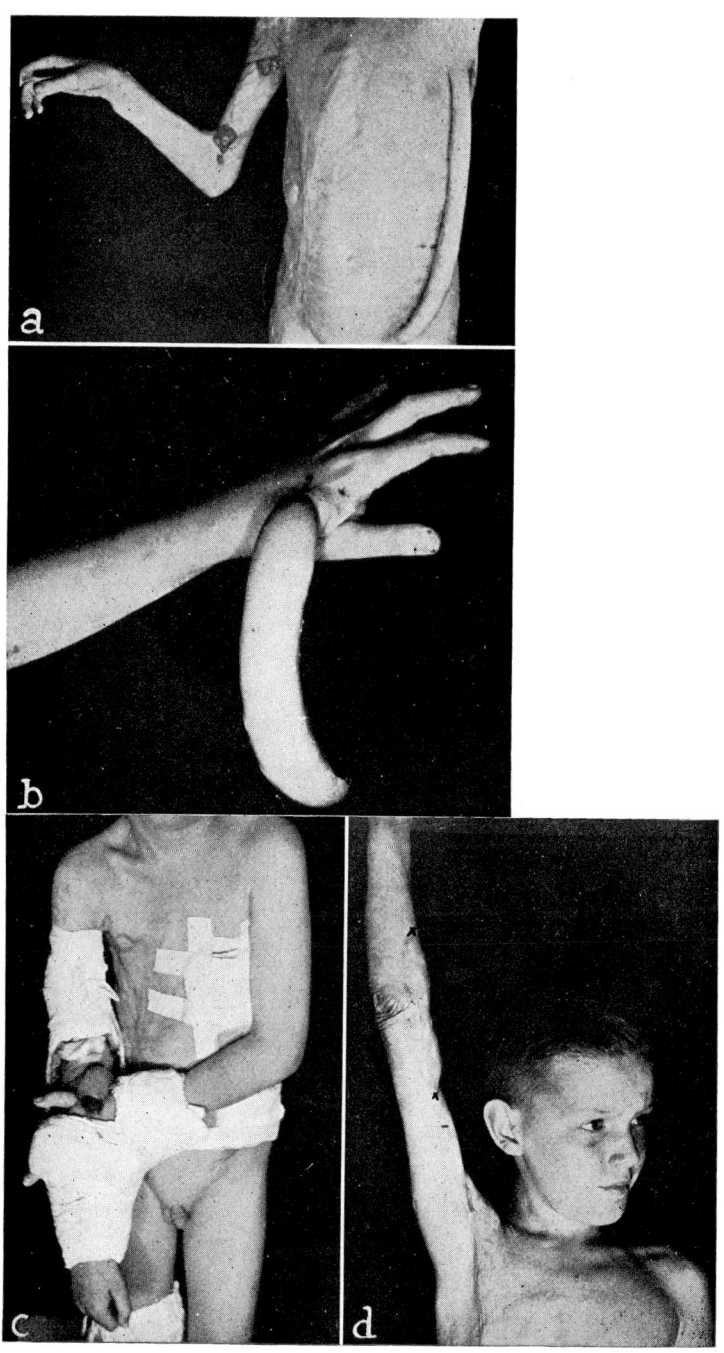

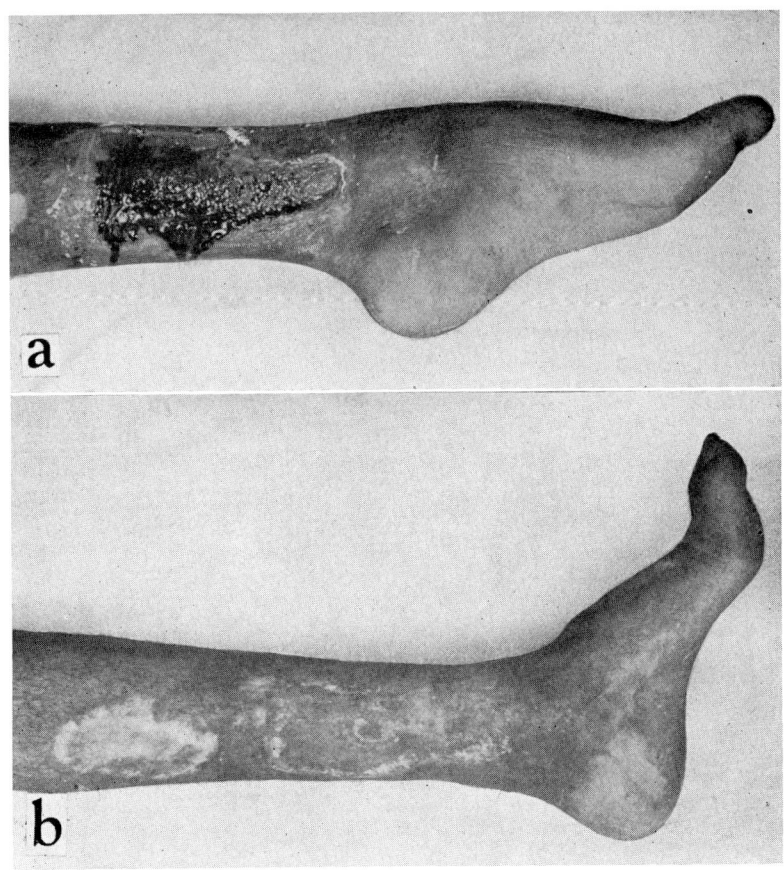

Case 117, *a:* Leg ulcer of long standing. Cultures revealed the anaerobic hemolytic streptococcus. Extensive contracture of the Achilles tendon. After zinc peroxide treatment for one week, cultures were negative.

b: The ulcer was excised, the defect skin grafted. The contracture of the Achilles tendon was overcome by gradual stretching under anesthesia and encasing the extremity in a plaster cast in four sittings, three weeks apart.

CASE
118

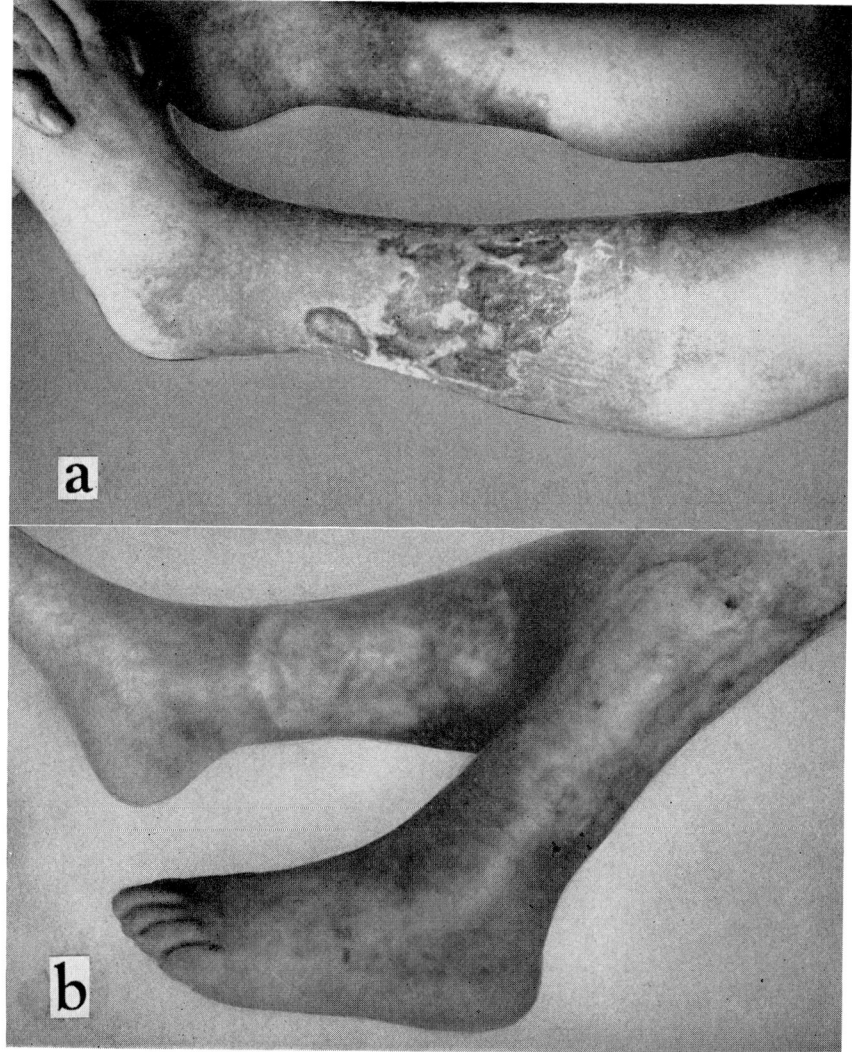

Case 118, *a:* Patient, aged sixty-three, with bilateral extensive vari-cose ulcers. After ligation and stripping of varicose veins the right ulcer was widely excised down to the deep fascia and split skin grafts were applied. In a subsequent operation six months later the left ulcer was treated the same way. Three years later there were small recurrences of both ulcers; hence both ulcers had to be excised again and skin grafted.

b: Since that time, four years later, no evidence of recurrence.

CASE
119

Case 119, *a:* Patient, aged sixty-seven, had a large cancer over his shoulder joint and scapula. Several attempts with radiation did not allay the growth. Wide excision of the area was performed, in which the spine of the scapula was partly removed (to be seen in the center of the wound); part of the deltoid muscle was also removed. This defect was to be covered with a tube flap from the abdomen, transferred by means of the left hand.

b: The tube flap was constructed in the right thoracoepigastric region. The diagram on the left side points out the way in which the tube flap was closed by staggering. Three and a half months later, the distal pedicle was gradually severed. This took seven days.

c: Two weeks later, the free end of the flap was fastened to the dorsum of the left hand. Two weeks later, the proximal pedicle was gradually severed. This took one week.

1150

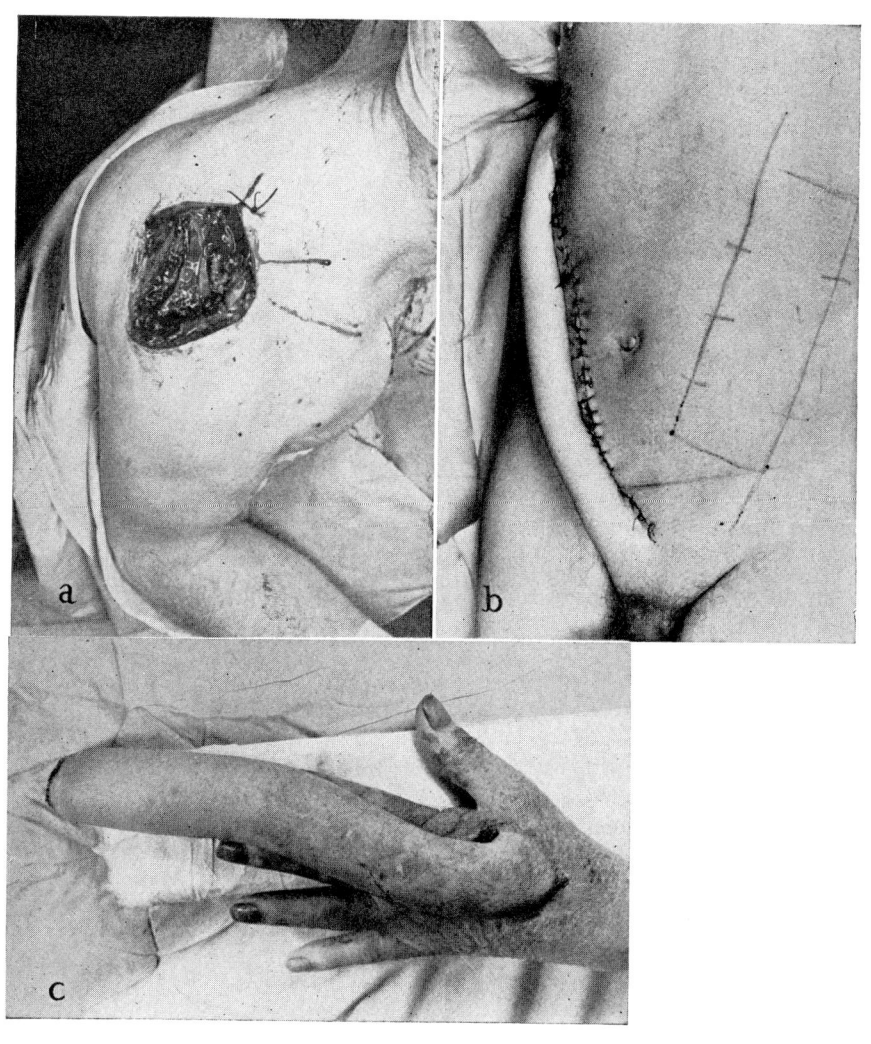

CASE
119 *(Continued)*

Case 119 *(continued)*, *d:* Three weeks later, the flap was transplanted and fastened to the defect. One week later, the flap was gradually severed from its pedicle. This took two days. The pedicle was then severed from the hand and discarded. One week later, the flap was adjusted in place.

e: Three years after the first operation. No evidence of recurrence. Full function of the shoulder joint.

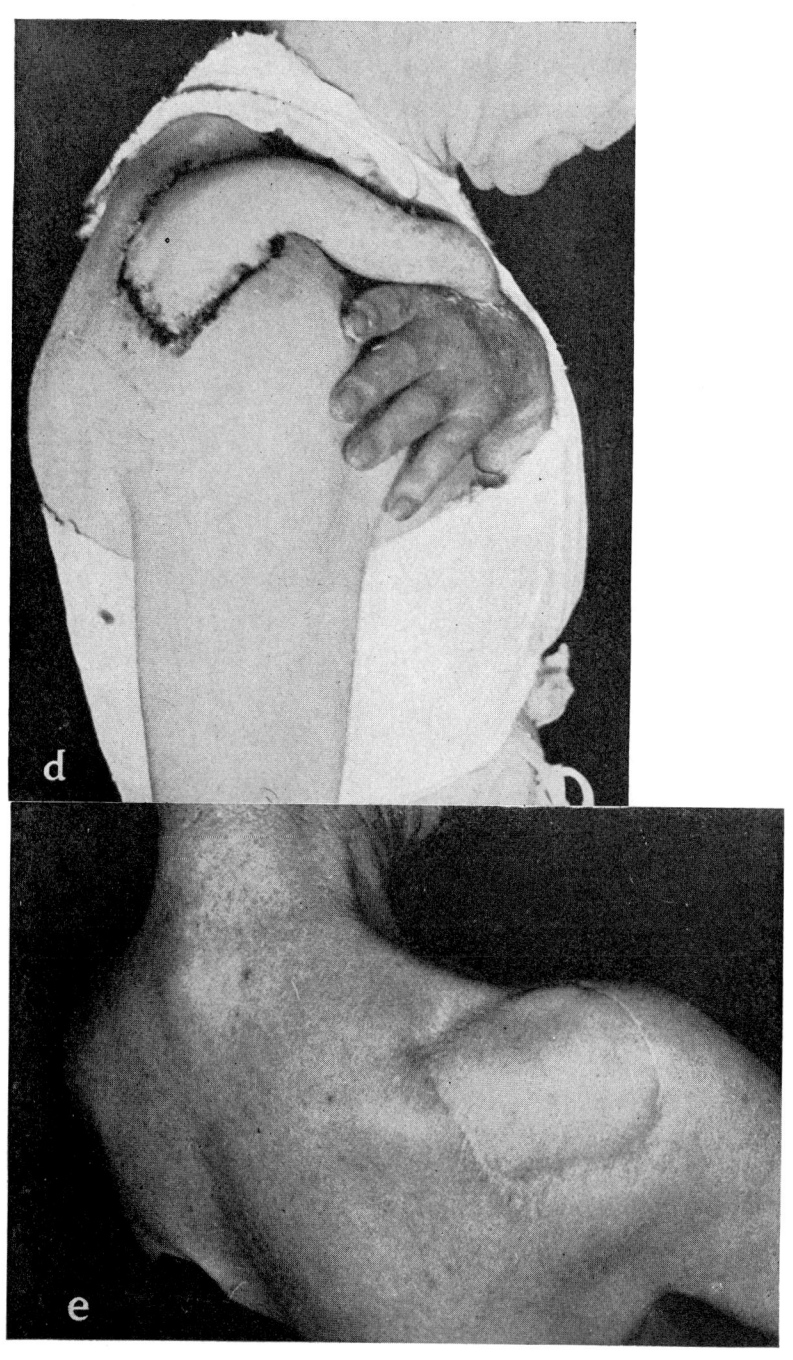

CASE
120

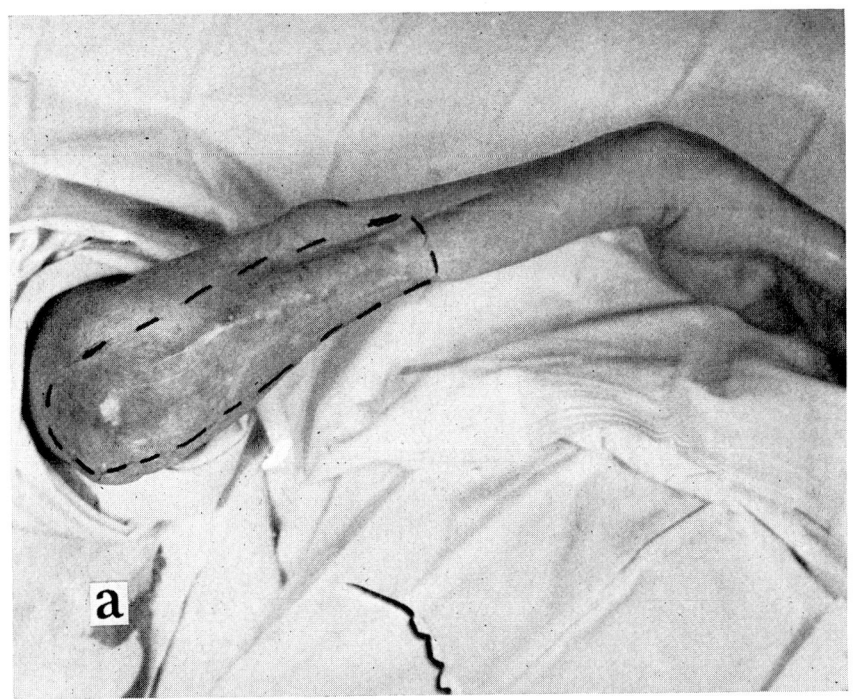

Case 120, *a:* Patient, aged forty-one, with atrophic traumatic scar formation over right elbow joint and upper half of lateral surface of forearm. Scar was unstable and broke down. Extent of the excision is outlined.

b: A large flap was developed from the adjacent chest region with a distal pedicle and transplanted in one stage. The raw area of the flap bed was skin grafted.

c: The flap was gradually severed on the twelfth day, complete severance on the twenty-first day with adjustment of flap and pedicle.

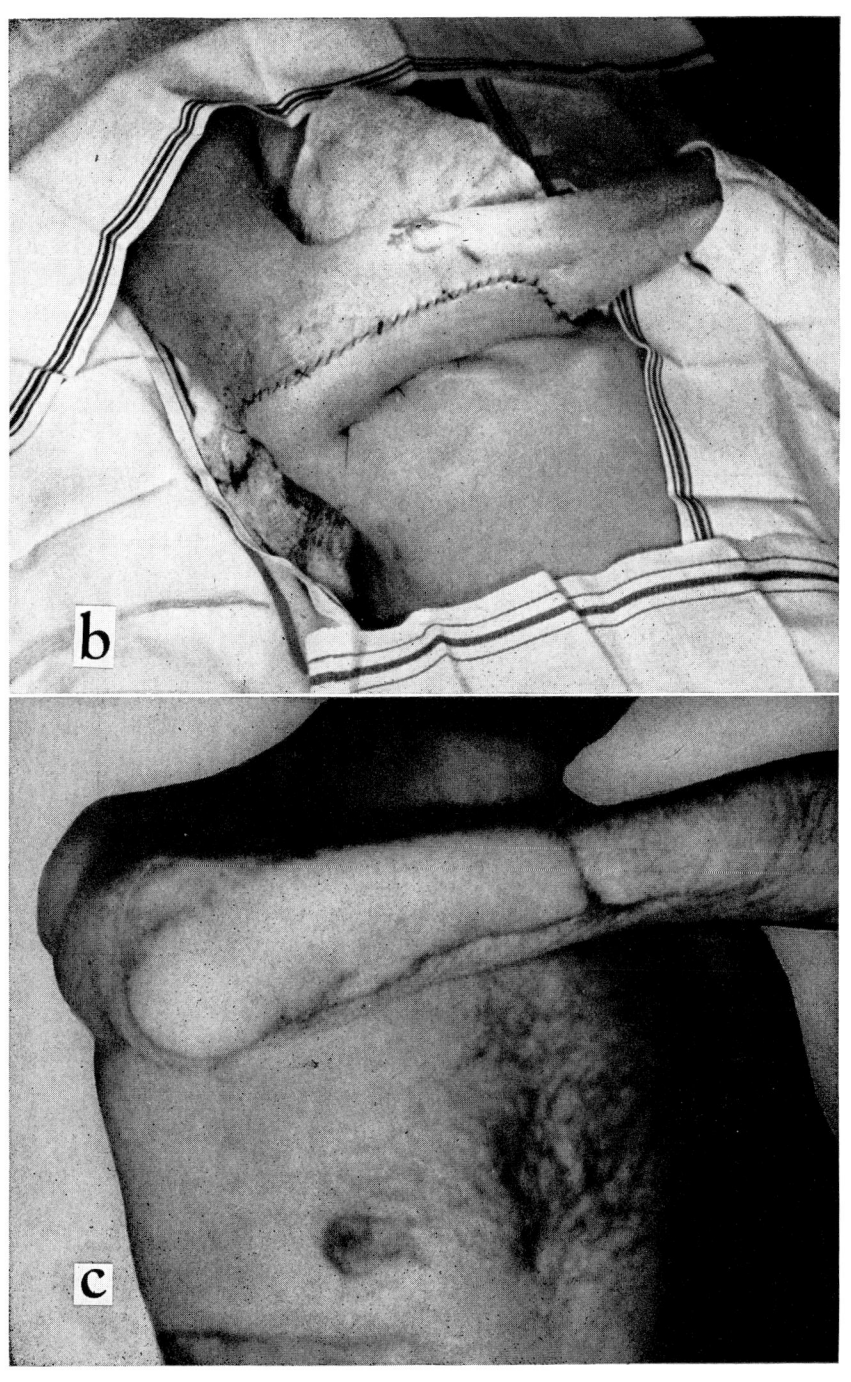

CASE
121

Case 121, *a:* Ulceration and cicatricial changes over tibia after compound fracture of leg followed by osteomyelitis.

b, c: After removal of sequestrum and scar tissue, the surface defect was closed by relaxation incisions and mobilization of the skin between the incisions and defect. Thus, double-pedicle flaps were formed which were shifted into the defect. The secondary defects were skin grafted.

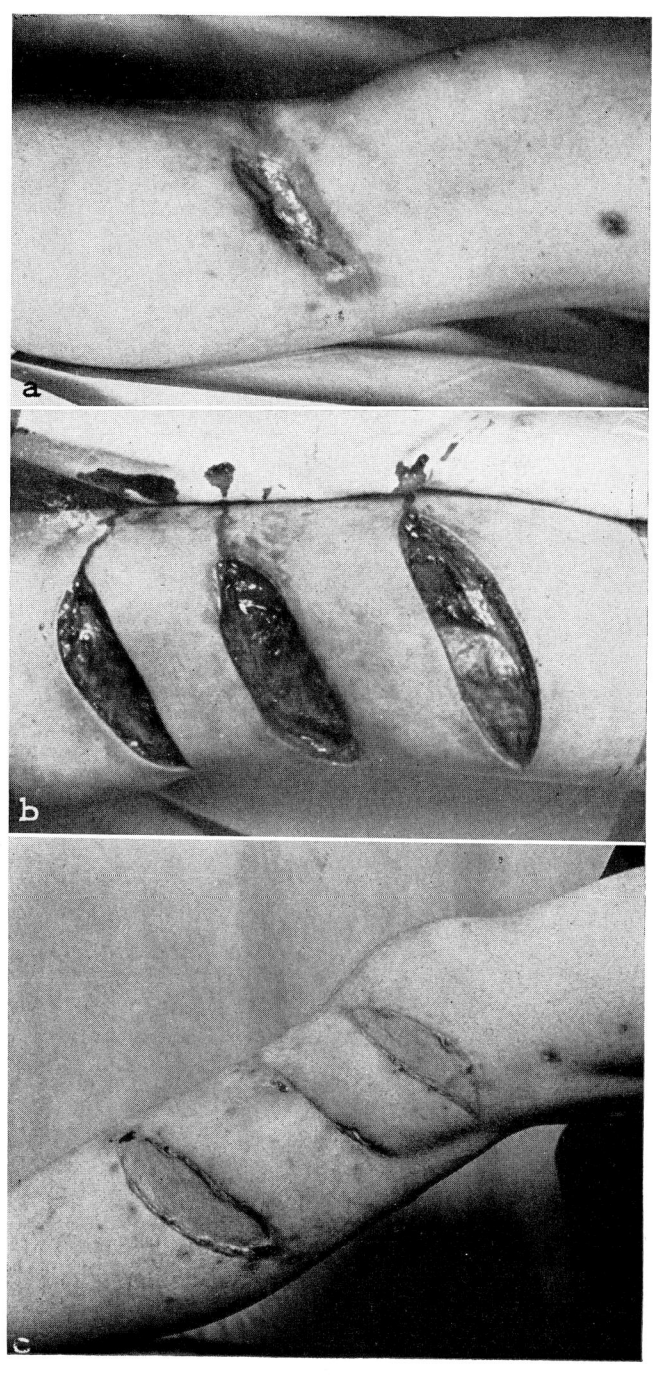

ILLUSTRATIVE CASES

CASE

122

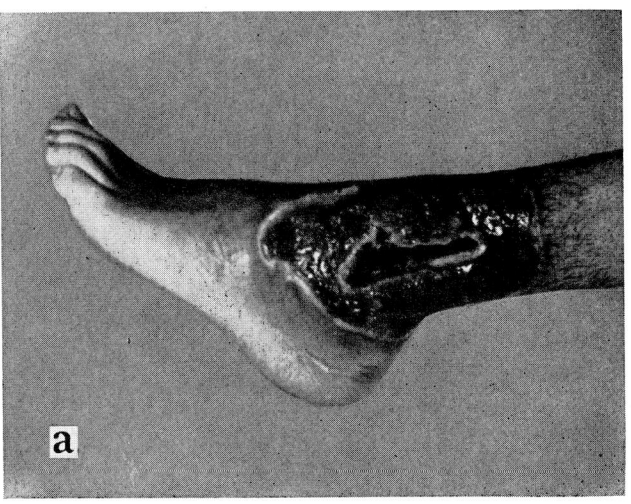

Case 122, *a:* Patient, aged twenty-two, with extensive third-degree burn of lateral surface of left ankle, with exposure of fibula and fracture of left humerus after automobile accident.

b: A cross-leg flap was developed from the right thigh in stages. First stage consisted of elevation of proximal half between two parallel incisions. Two weeks later the upper and lower half were elevated between two parallel incisions. Two weeks later the entire flap was elevated between the two pedicles, the proximal pedicle was incised from either side and a laboratory clamp was applied and gradually clamped to the middle portion of the pedicle. Clamp was removed two weeks later.

c: Six weeks later the flap was elevated and the flap bed covered with a split skin graft. The terminal portion of the flap became cyanotic and for this reason it seemed advisable to return the flap. It was laid upon the grafted flap bed and held in this position with a few sutures. Two weeks later the flap was elevated again. The ulcer of the left ankle was excised, the flap sutured to the raw area of ankle and both legs held in position with a plaster cast. One week later the pedicle of the flap was incised from either side and an elastic clamp applied to remainder of the pedicle. One week later the pedicle of the flap was severed completely, and the cast removed. Another week later flap at left ankle and pedicle at right thigh were adjusted in place.

d: Five months after the accident.

1158

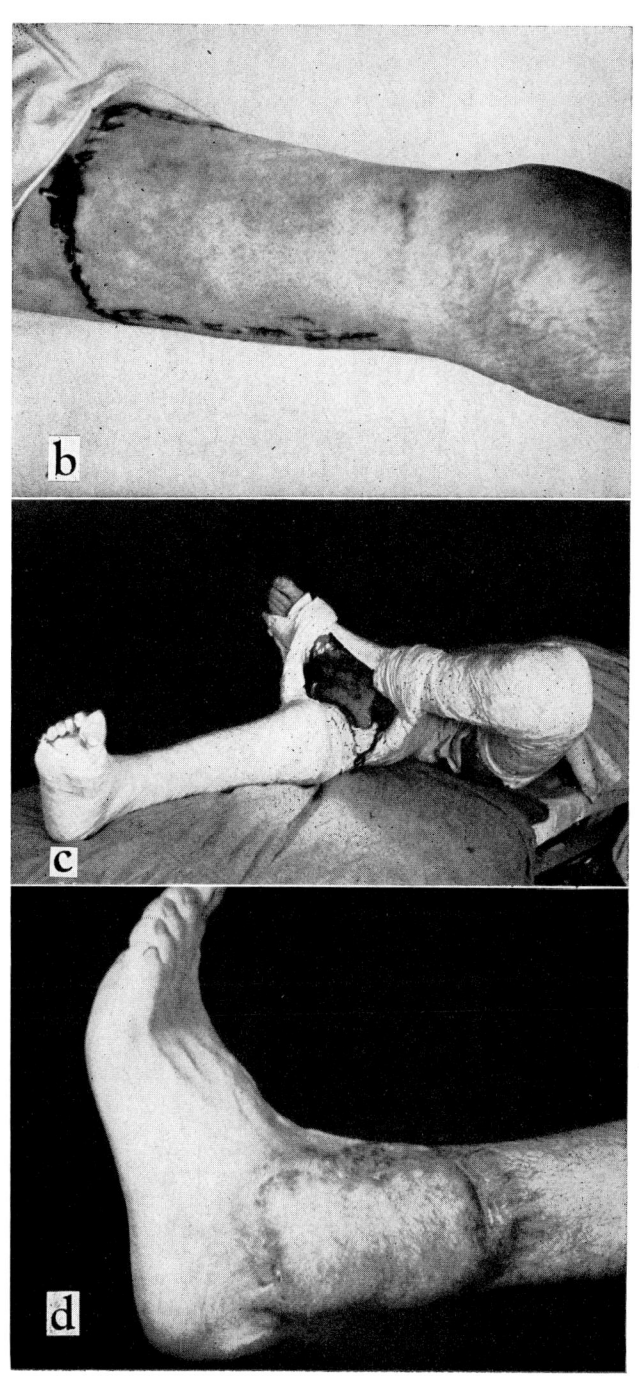

CASE
123

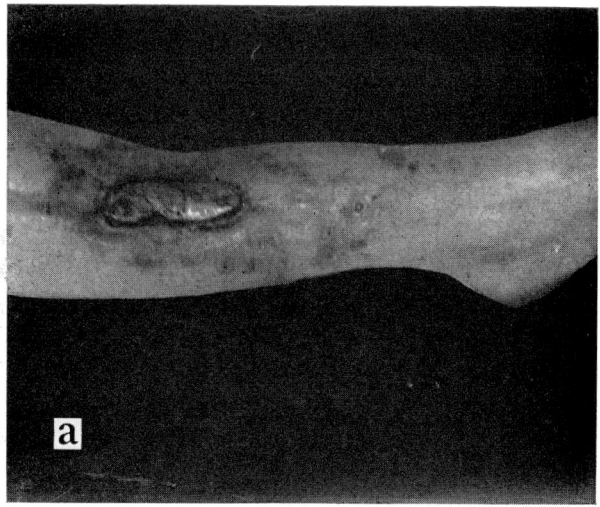

Case 123, *a:* Patient, aged nineteen, suffered from a compound fracture and extensive loss of skin over the left leg from a motorcycle accident. The fracture of the tibia was reduced and held stabilized with vitallium bone splint. After the fracture had healed patient was referred for closure of surface defect.

b: A flap from the calf of the right leg was elevated between two parallel incisions. Four weeks later the flap was elevated again and the distal pedicle was incised from either side, while a laboratory clamp was applied to the middle part of the pedicle. The clamp was gradually tightened, and could be removed four days later. Four weeks later the distal half of the flap was elevated and returned. The tibial bone plates were removed. Four weeks later the entire flap was elevated and returned. The circulation of the flap appeared adequate. The flap, however, became edematous and infiltrated during the following two weeks; hence it was advisable to wait another six weeks until all edema had subsided in the flap before it was transplanted.

c: After removal of a large sequestrum the flap from the right calf was elevated and transplanted to cover the raw surface on the left leg. The raw flap bed at the calf was covered with a skin graft. Ten days later the pedicle of the flap was incised from either side and a laboratory clamp was applied. The pedicle was gradually crushed so that four days later the pedicle could be severed. Five days later flap and pedicle were adjusted in place.

d: Subsequently several sequestra drained through the flap. All wounds have healed since that time and the leg is stable.

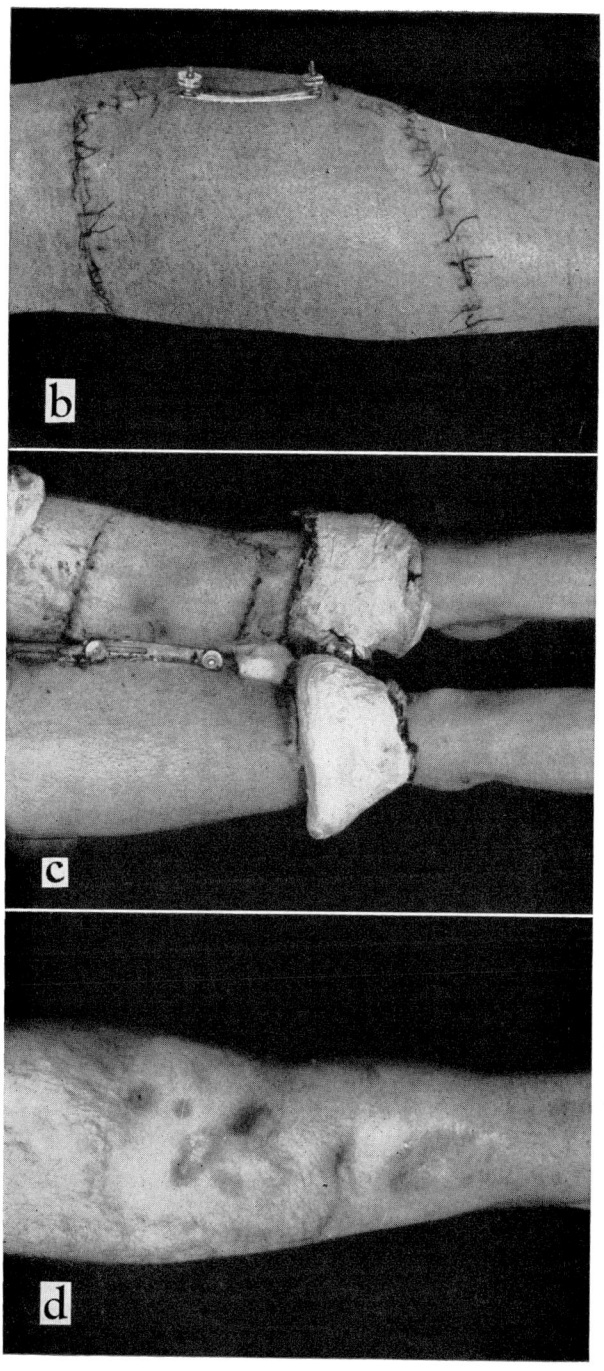

CASE

124

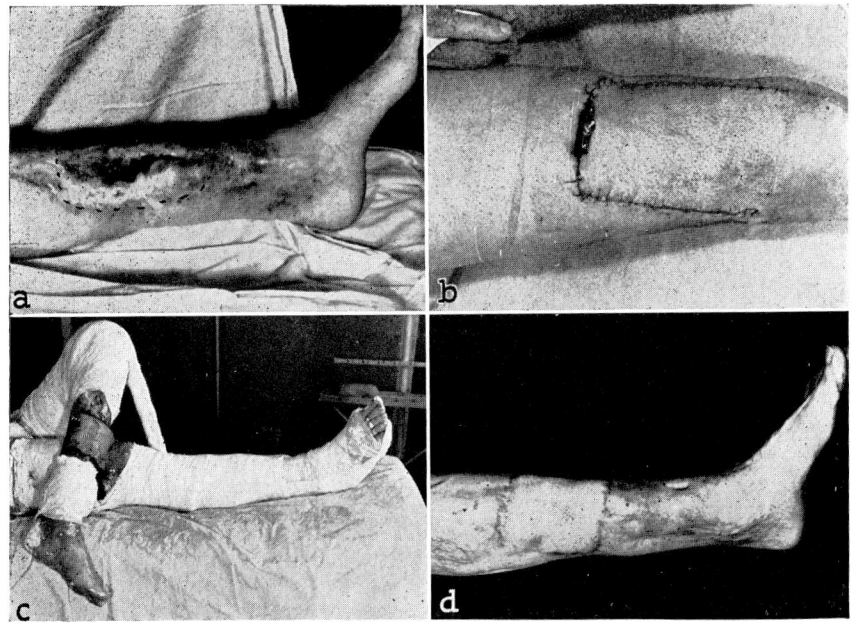

Case 124, *a:* A patient with extensive scarring, ulceration, and sequestration over the left tibia after osteomyelitis.

b: A double-pedicle flap was raised at the right thigh. First, the upper half was mobilized and returned to its original site. Two weeks later, the entire flap was mobilized and returned to its original site. Two weeks later, the flap was elevated again; the peripheral pedicle was incised from each side one third of its width, leaving a middle bridge attached to which a laboratory clamp was applied. The laboratory clamp was tightened every day, crushing the middle pedicle within one week. Three weeks later, the entire flap was raised. The flap was again returned to its original site.

c: Two weeks later, the flap was again raised; the scars over the tibia were removed. The tibia was "saucerized"; all sequestra were removed. The leg was crossed, and the flap was sutured in place after the flap bed had been skin grafted. The flap was severed gradually ten days later in the same way as the distal pedicle was severed. Separation was completed one week later; the cast was removed. Three weeks later, the flap was adjusted in place.

d: Three months after operation. (H. May: Surgery.)

CASE
125

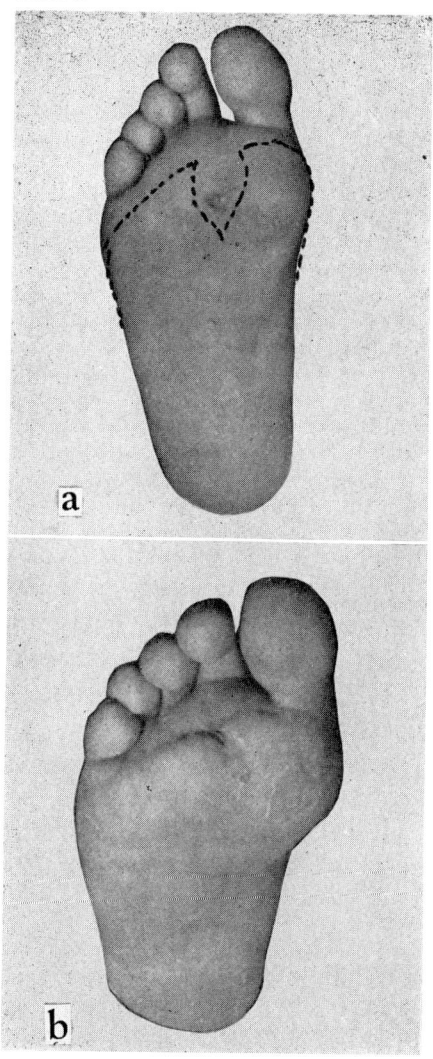

Case 125, *a:* Patient, aged thirty-five, with plantar wart of right foot, treated by irradiation. After two years the wart returned and the area became very painful. The involved area was excised and skin grafted. The skin graft, however, broke down after full weight bearing. The area was then excised and closed by sliding flaps—lines of excision as well as flaps are outlined.

b: Three months after operation. One year later patient notified author by letter that there were no symptoms and no evidence of recurrence of the plantar wart.

CASE

126

Case 126, *a:* Patient, aged thirty-three, had a plantar wart on left foot for fifteen years. Numerous conservative methods, such as radiation and cauterization, had failed to cure the lesion. Hence, radical excision and closure of the defect with a pedicle flap became advisable. The flap was prepared at the right thigh, as described on page 83. In the first stage, it was elevated between two parallel incisions. Clamping of the peripheral pedicle resulted in discoloration of the flap. Hence, the flap was returned to its original site. After three weeks, it was again elevated. The median pedicle was narrowed from each side, leaving a middle bridge to which a laboratory clamp was attached. By tightening the thumbscrew, the remainder of the pedicle was gradually crushed within five days. Two weeks later, the entire flap was raised. The peripheral parts changed color; hence, the flap was again returned.

b: One week later, the flap was again elevated, the flap bed at the thigh was skin grafted, and the flap was transplanted after excision of the plantar wart, which had reached the first metatarsophalangeal joint. (For technique of immobilization of the crossed legs, see p. 720.)

c: One week after the transfer of the flap, a laboratory clamp was applied to the pedicle, which was gradually crushed. It was severed eleven days after the transfer. The cast was removed. The free end of the pedicle at the thigh was adjusted in place, while the free end of the flap at the foot was sutured in place ten days later. The patient was not permitted weight bearing for four weeks. She was last seen seven years after the last operation. She had no pain and no limp.

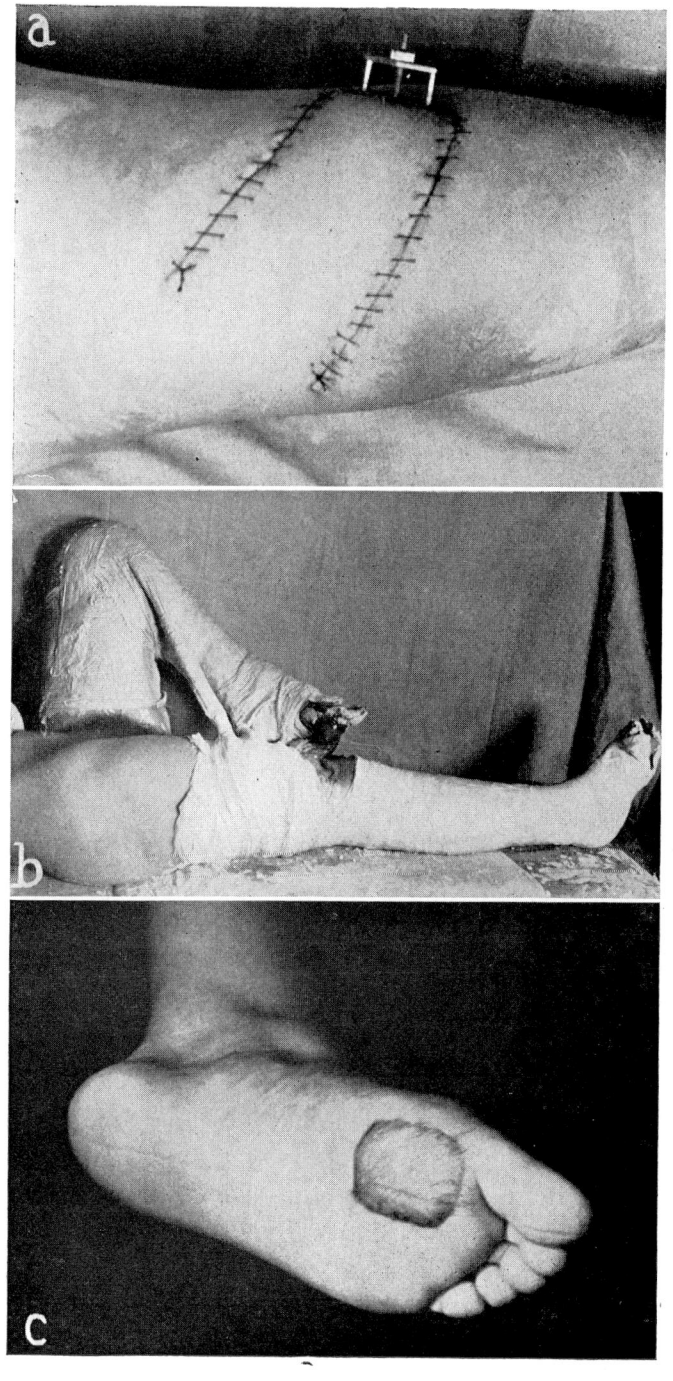

CASE
127

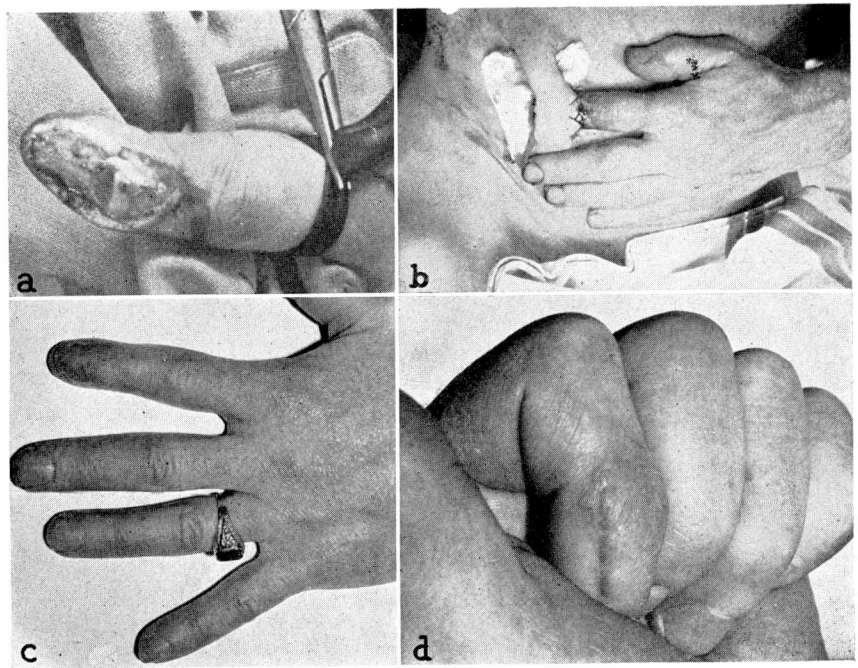

Case 127, *a:* Grinding injury of dorsum of left index finger. Note loss of dorsal half of bone of terminal phalanx and exposure of terminal joint. (Patient is left-handed.)

b: After excision of the wound, a pocket flap from opposite side of the abdomen was transferred immediately. The donor area was closed by skin sliding. The arm was immobilized in a plaster cast (for technique of application of cast, see p. 808).

c, d: Severance of the proximal pedicle after seven days, of the distal pedicle after ten days. Adjustment of the free ends of the flap and defect edges two weeks later.

1166

CASE
128

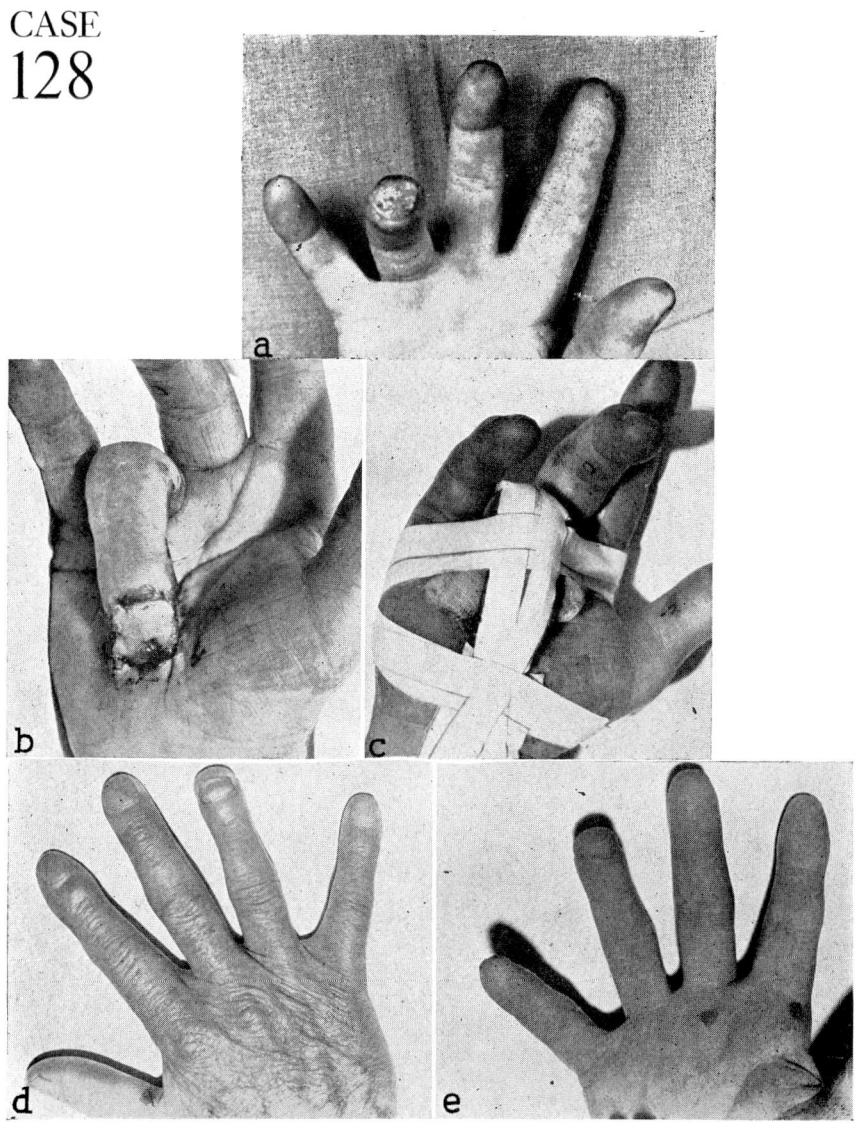

Case 128, *a:* Traumatic defect of tip of fourth finger. Exposure of bone. Conservative treatment for four weeks elsewhere was unsuccessful.

b: A flap with a proximal pedicle was raised from the palm and sutured to the defect.

c: Immobilization of finger with adhesive strips: one or two running over dorsum of hand and finger to palm; one or two running transversely over finger and just proximal to flap.

d, e: The pedicle of the flap was narrowed on the eighth postoperative day and severed on the eleventh day, followed by adjustment and approximation of the free edge of the flap and defect edge on the fourteenth day.

1167

CASE
129

Case 129, *a:* Traumatic defect of dorsum of terminal phalanx of left thumb. Note loss of dorsal half of bone of terminal phalanx and exposure of terminal interphalangeal joint.

b: After excision of the wound, immediate transfer of a single-pedicle flap from left upper abdominal wall. The donor area was closed by skin sliding. Immobilization in a plaster cast (for technique of application of cast, see p. 808).

c: Clamping of the pedicle was begun on the ninth postoperative day (see p. 85). The flap was severed on the twelfth day. Eleven days later, the free end of the flap was undercut and sutured to the defect edge.

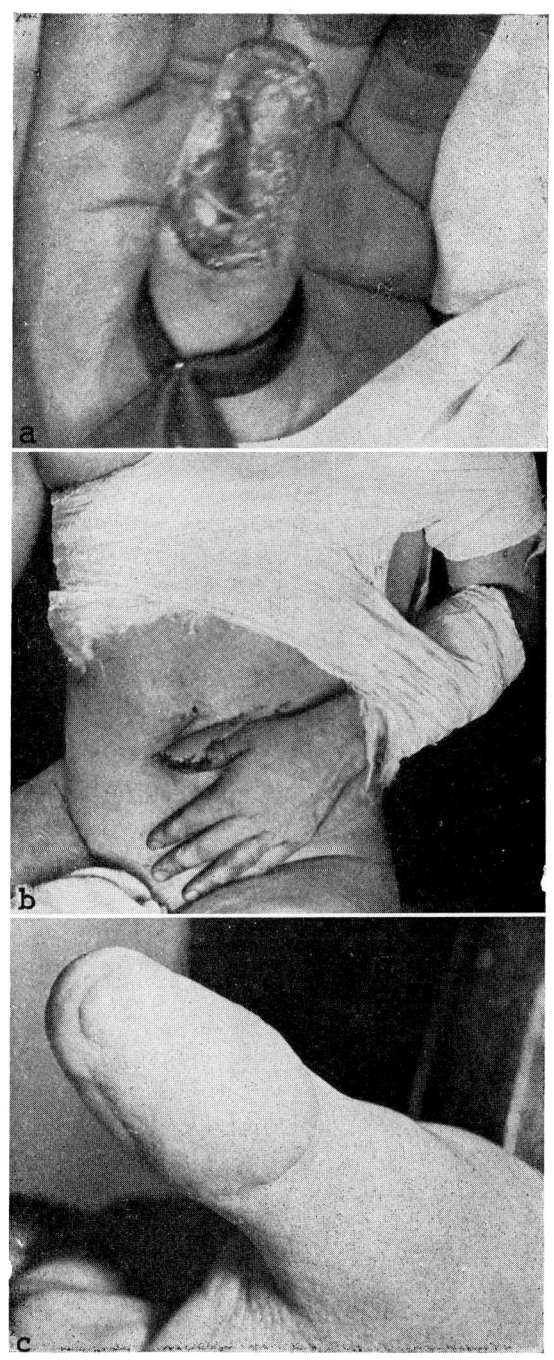

CASE
130

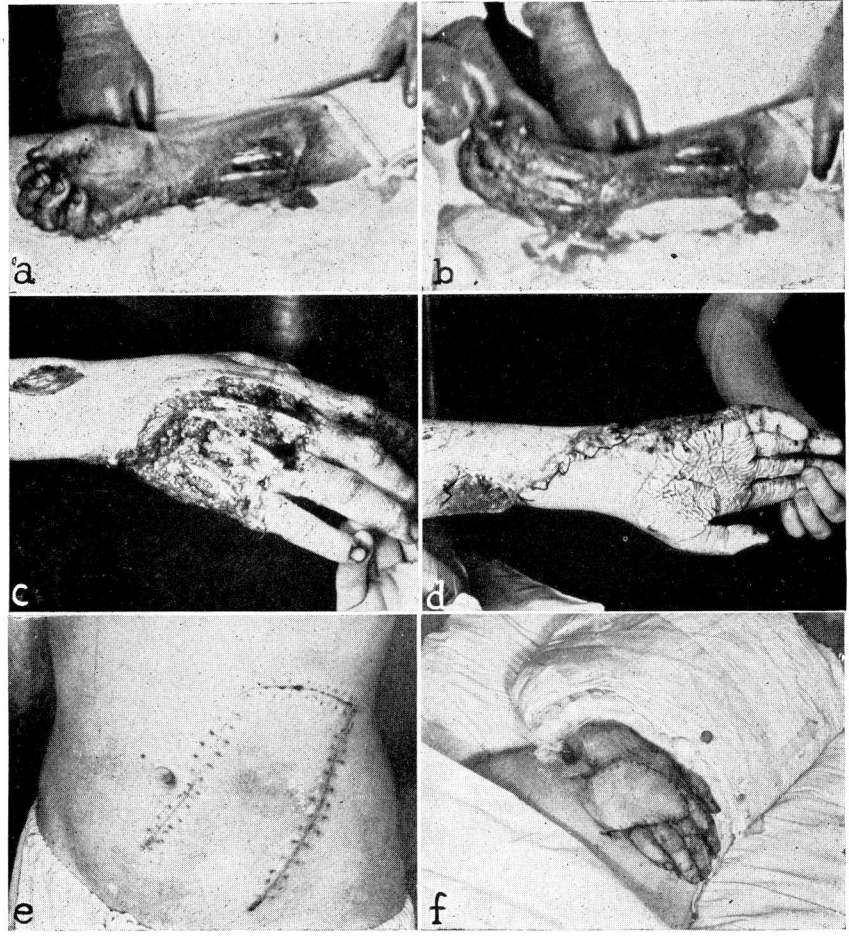

Case 130, *a, b, c:* Extensive loss of surface tissue on volar and dorsal side of forearm and hand. Exposure of tendons; loss of extensor tendon of fifth finger.

d: After excision of the wound, the defect was immediately closed at the forearm by wide undermining of the wound edges and skin sliding. A relaxation incision on the dorsum of the forearm facilitated skin sliding.

e: An open abdominal flap was raised from the opposite side of the abdomen in the same operation. The flap was raised between two parallel incisions. After one week, the proximal pedicle was incised and sutured.

f: The flap was raised on the fourteenth postoperative day; it did not change color. The flap bed was skin grafted. The flap was transferred to the right hand and accurately sutured in place. The arm was immobilized in a plaster cast.

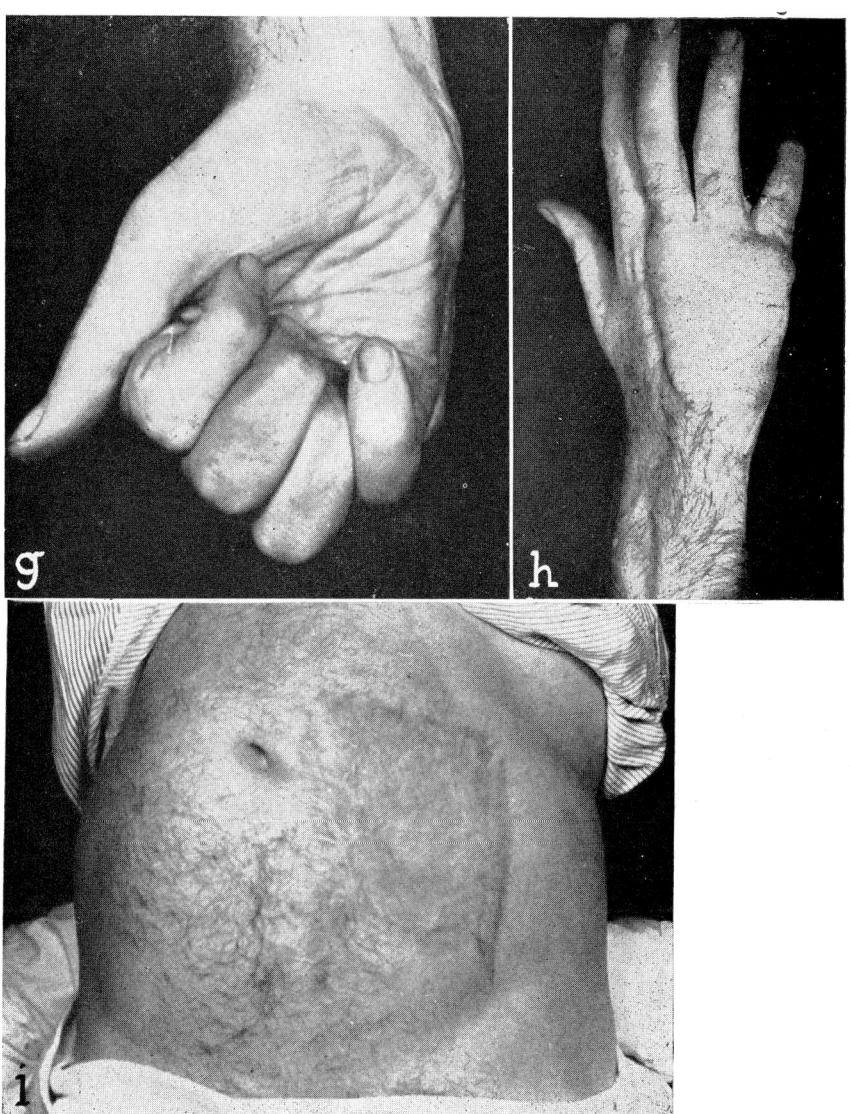

g, h: The pedicle of the flap was partly severed ten days after transfer of the flap, and was entirely separated on the fourteenth day. Adjustment and approximation of the free edge of flap and defect were performed two weeks later.

i: Donor area was skin grafted as soon as the flap was raised.

CASE
131

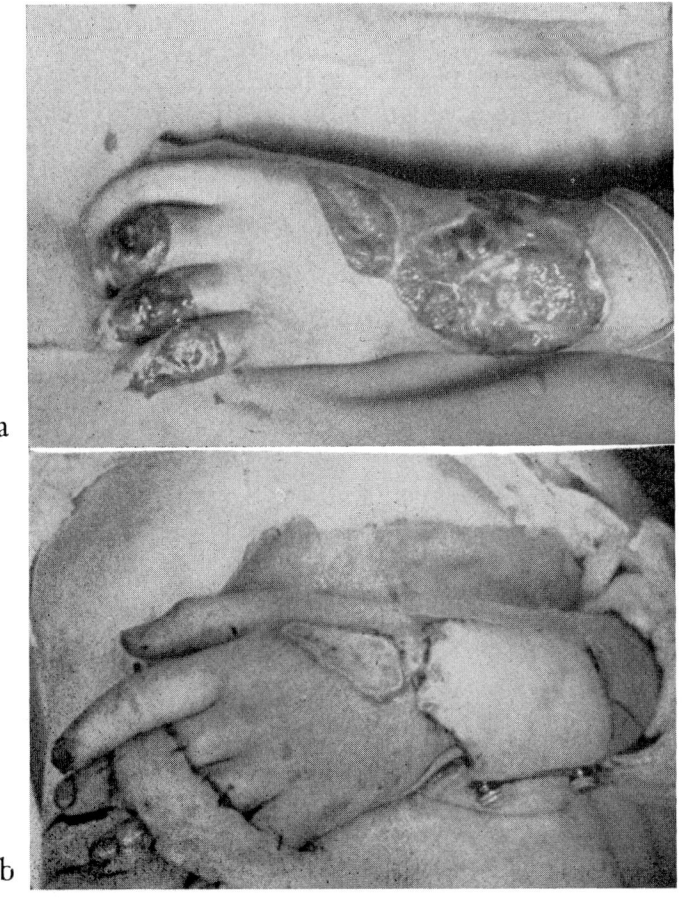

a

b

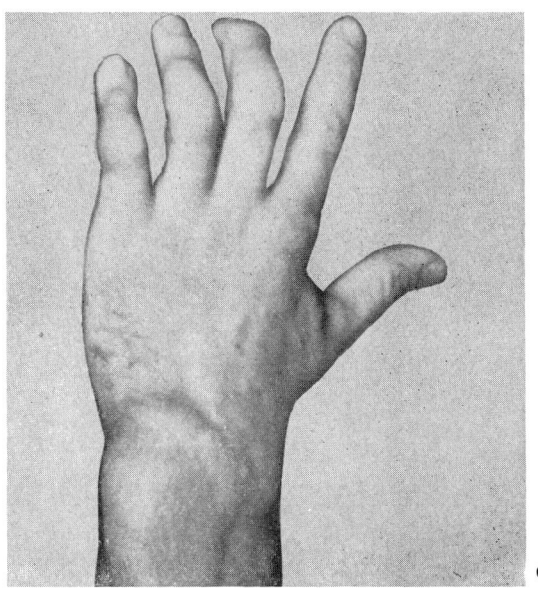

c

Case 131, *a:* Patient, aged twenty-six years, sustained severe crush and burn injury of left hand and forearm, after arm was caught in a hot press. There was a fracture in the lower third of ulna, and a hematoma and contusion of the median nerve. Emergency treatment consisted of decompression of the median nerve. Fifteen days after the injury the burn eschar was excised.

b: Six days later, skin graft was applied to one of the superficial surface defects of the dorsum of the wrist. An abdominal flap was elevated for closure of the other surface defects but the flap had to be returned, since the peripheral end became discolored. One week later three narrow pocket flaps were formed at the abdomen for coverage of the surface defects over the knuckles of the interphalangeal joints of third, fourth, and fifth fingers. The abdominal flap was elevated again. The flap bed was skin grafted and flap transplanted to the wrist. Seven days later the base of the main flap was incised on each side and a laboratory clamp was placed to the middle part. The bases of the finger flaps between two fingers were severed and a small laboratory clamp was applied to the lateral pedicles. All clamps were gradually tightened. Six days later all pedicles were severed. Twenty days later flaps and pedicles were adjusted in place. At the third and fifth fingers the adjustment consisted of excision of a wedge-shaped piece of tissue at each side of the flap and suturing of the edges of the flap to the wound edges of the fingers. At the fourth finger, however, no adjustment of flap edges was made since they were too short.

c: One year later all flaps were defatted in a two-stage operation. The median nerve in the meantime had regained full function.

CASE

132

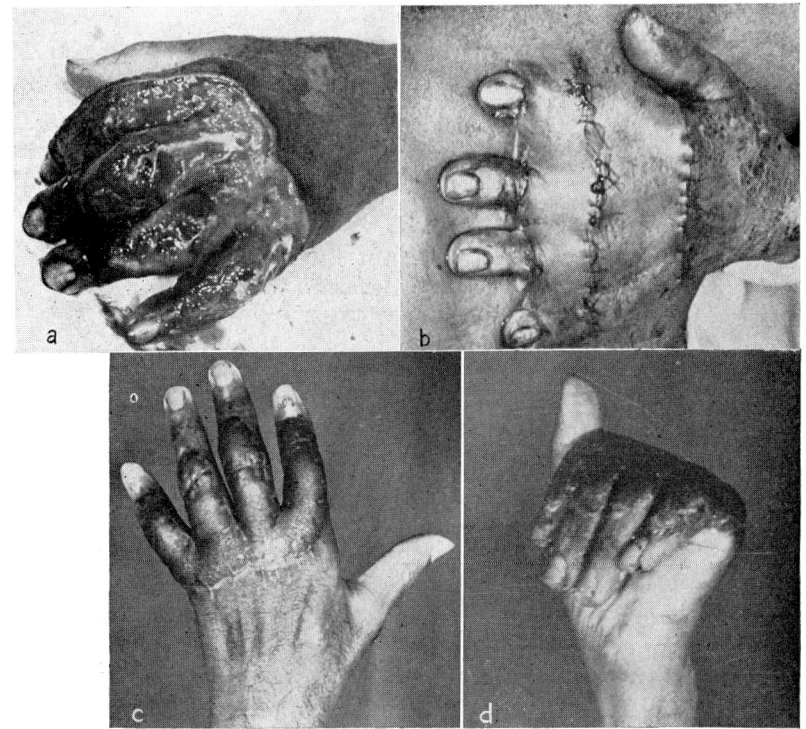

Case 132, *a:* Extensive wringer injury of distal half of dorsum of left hand, including a major part of the dorsum of the second to fifth fingers. After the necrotic skin had sloughed off, all tendons were found to be intact. Tendons, however, as well as joint capsules of the first interphalangeal joints, were exposed. Actually, the joint capsules of the first interphalangeal joints of the third and fourth fingers were necrotic so that the joint surfaces were exposed. Owing to the exposure of all these structures, skin grafting had to be abandoned in favor of flap transplantation.

b: A large pocket flap was formed on the left side of the abdomen, into which the fingers were fitted, as into a glove. Seven days after the operation, the proximal pedicle—that is, the pedicle running along the radial surface of the index finger—was severed. The flap edges were sutured to the wound edges of the index finger. Twelve days later, all pedicles were severed, with the exception of the one which ran along the ulnar surface of the fifth finger. Two days later, the last pedicle was severed. Four weeks later, the skin bridges between the fingers were severed down to the webs of the fingers, and each flap was attached to the respective wound edge of the fingers.

c, d: Functional result six weeks after the final operation. Patient has returned to former duties.

CASE
133

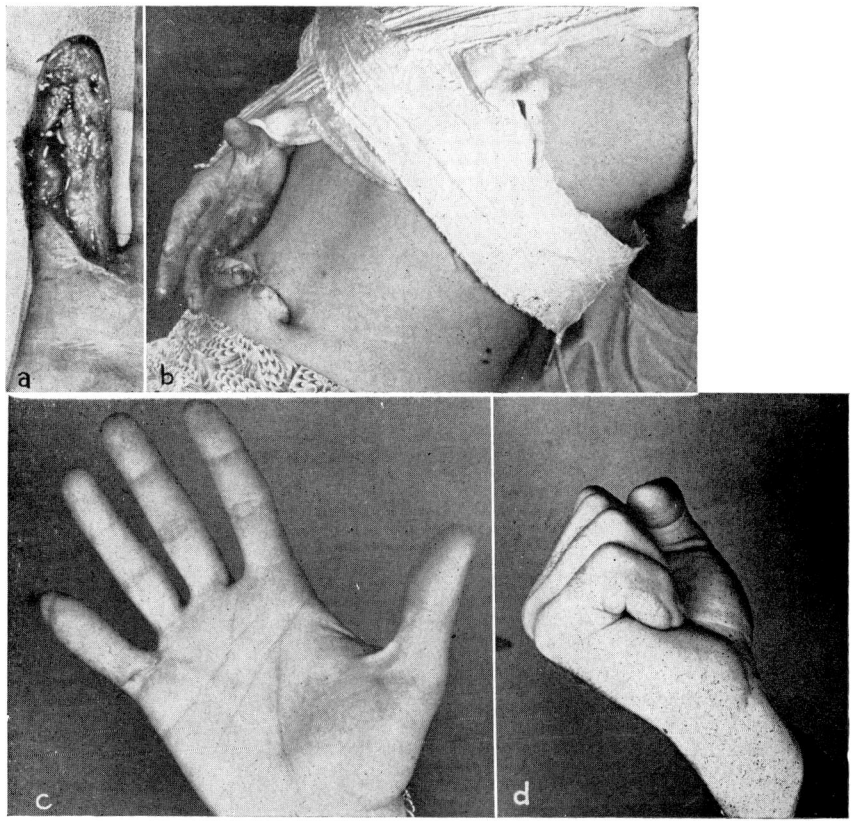

Case 133, *a:* Patient, aged twenty-nine, admitted with extensive laceration of the volar surface and part of the ulnar surface of the right fifth finger. Tendons were exposed, as well as all vessels and nerves on the volar side. In some parts, the tendon sheaths were missing.

b: A single-pedicle flap was prepared at the right side of the abdomen with a proximal pedicle. The flap was then transplanted to the raw surface of the finger, and the arm was immobilized in a plaster cast. The raw surface of the flap bed could be closed by skin sliding. Eight days later, partial separation of the flap was performed, with application of laboratory clamp according to the method described on page 85. Three days later, the pedicle was separated. One week later, flap and pedicle were adjusted.

c, d: Functional result one month after operation.

CASE
134

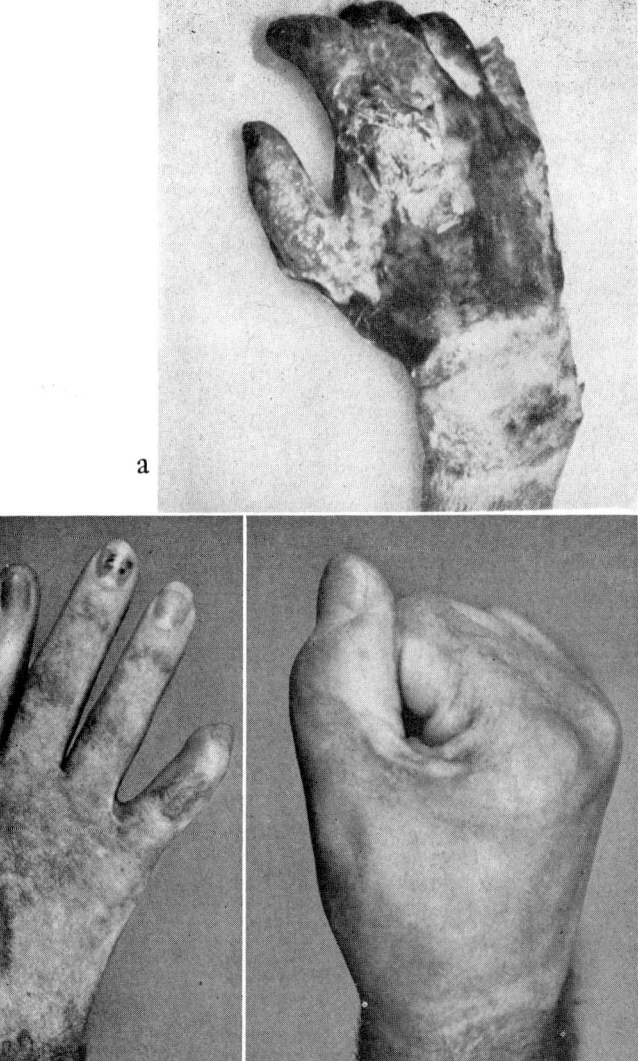

a

b   c

Case 134, *a:* Extensive third-degree burn treated locally with pressure dressings. Condition twelve days after accident. On the eighteenth day the necrotic skin was excised, followed daily by application of saline solution dressings. On the twenty-fourth day all raw surfaces were covered with split skin grafts.

b, c: Result one year after the operation.

CASE

135

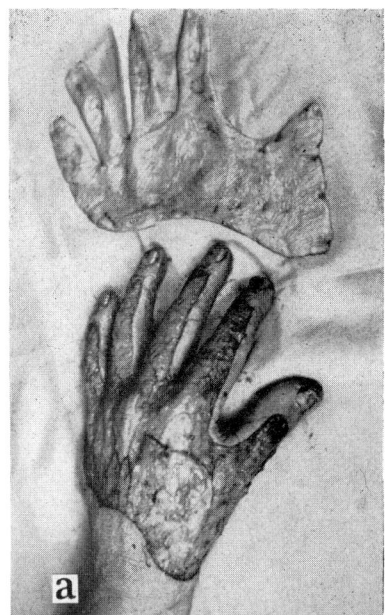

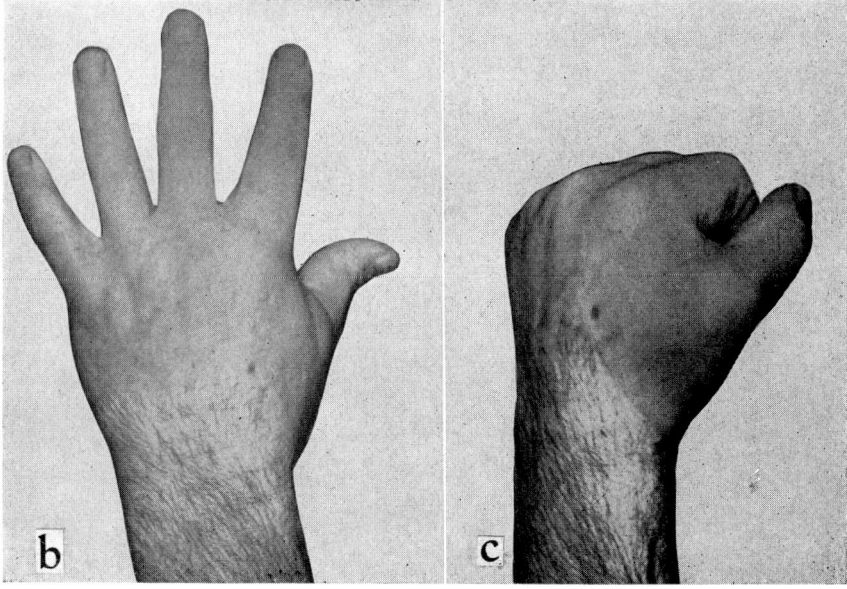

Case 135, *a:* Unstable and contracting scar of dorsum of hand and fingers from deep second-degree burn. The entire scar was excised in toto and the surface defect covered with a thick split skin graft.

b, c: Five months after operation.

CASE
136

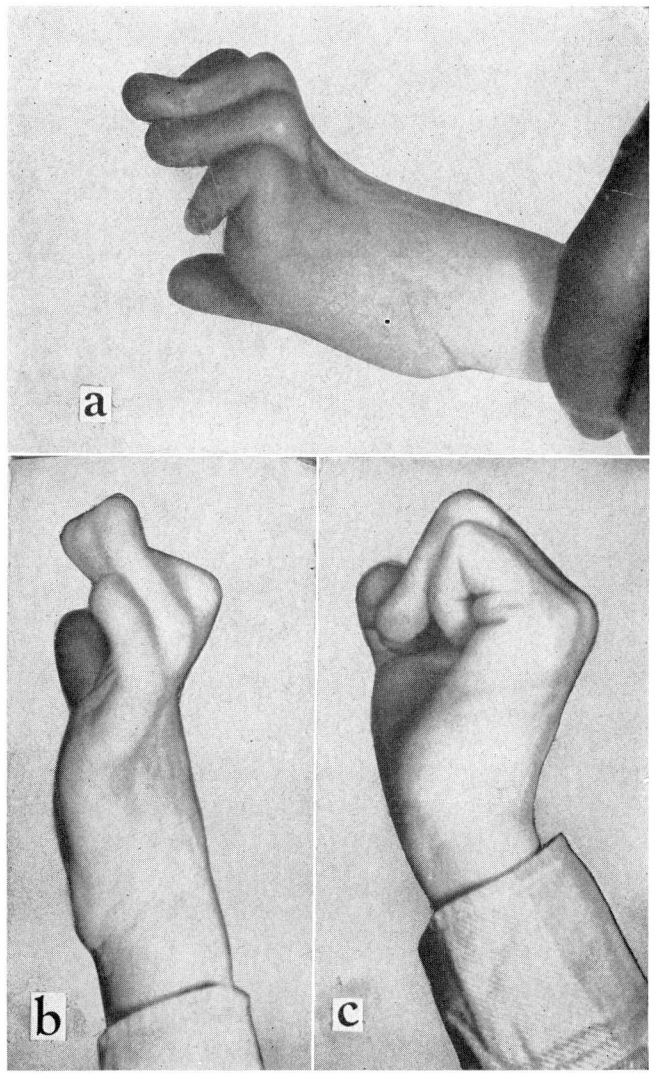

Case 136, *a:* Patient, aged five, had caught hand in a mangle. Skin graft had been applied but apparently did not take. Patient was referred three years later for repair of marked claw deformity of hand.

b, c: All the contracting scar tissue was excised. The collateral ligaments of the metacarpophalangeal joints were severed, the contractures reduced as much as possible and the raw surface covered with thick split skin graft. Five years after operation.

CASE
137

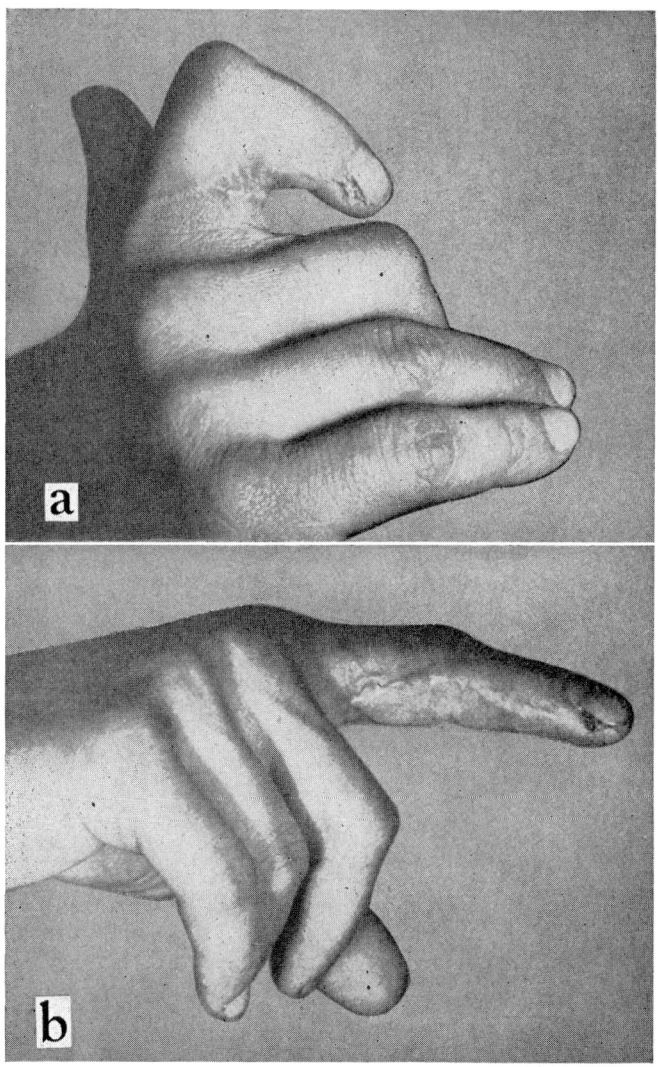

Case 137, *a:* Patient was treated in early youth for syndactylism of second and third finger. No skin grafts were employed. Local flaps were utilized for closure of the raw surfaces. A contracture developed in the index finger; web between index and third finger was obliterated.

b: After release of contracture and closure of the raw surface with a thick split skin graft.

1179

CASE
138

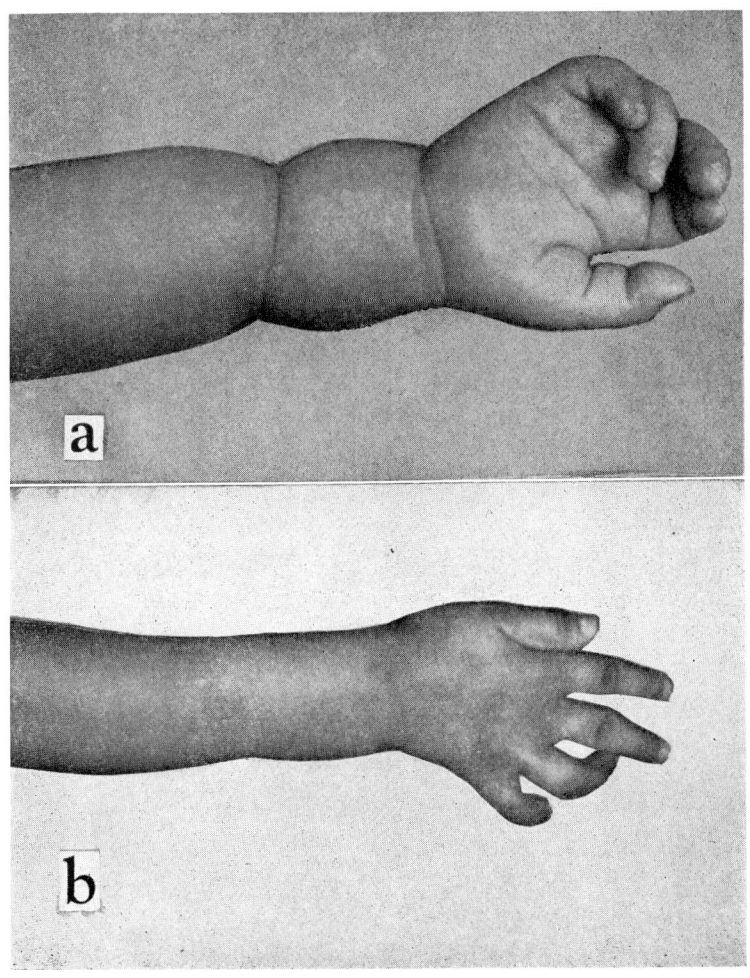

Case 138, *a:* Girl, aged two, with congenital constricting bands of right forearm.

b: Constricting bands were overcome in a two-stage operation consisting of multiple Z-plasties.

1180

CASE
139

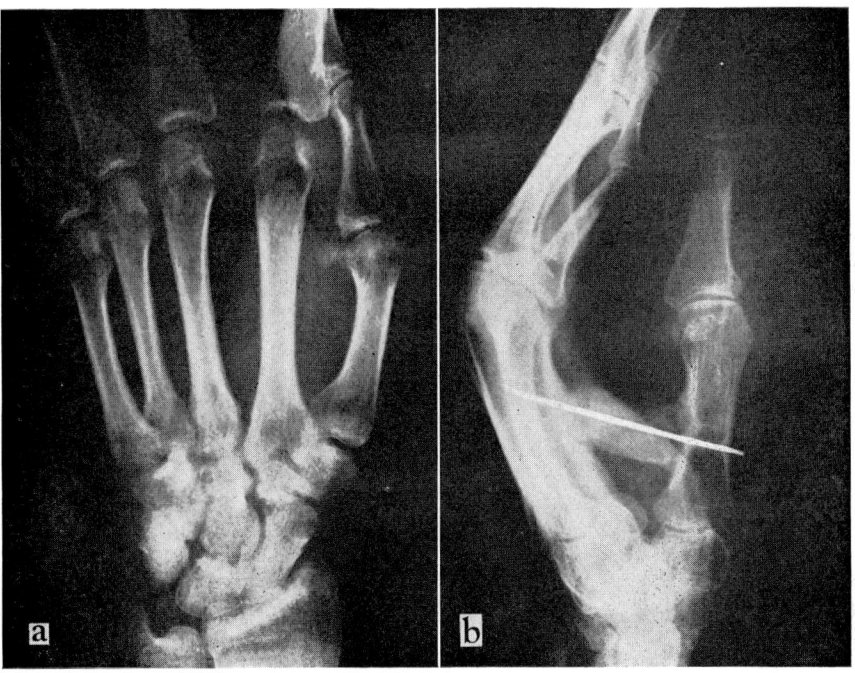

Case 139, *a:* Patient, aged twenty-three, received severe crush injury of the right arm and hand with extensive lacerations. There was much destruction of the muscles and other soft tissues in the thenar region and between first and second metacarpal bones. The injury resulted in obliteration of the web between the thumb and index finger and rigid adduction contracture of the thumb. The contracture was such that the thumb was in the way of the index finger when the index finger was flexed.

b: Operation consisted of removal of massive contracting scar tissue between the first and second metacarpal bones, lengthening of the web with a Z-plasty; to counteract recontracture a bone graft taken from the crest of the ilium was placed between the first two metacarpal bones with the thumb in abduction and opposition. A Kirschner wire was drilled through the metacarpals and bone graft for stabilization. There was no additional immobilization. This picture was taken seven months after operation.

CASE
140

Case 140: Patient, aged forty, received fourth-degree burns over the dorsum of the left hand at the level of the second and third metacarpal bones which were treated elsewhere. When first seen by the author, the patient had a thick, unstable scar over the dorsum of the hand, with loss of the extensor tendons of the second and third fingers.

a: The distal stumps of the tendons were adherent to the scar, preventing full flexion of the second and third fingers.

b: Abdominal flap was mobilized from the left side first, between two pedicles. The distal pedicle was partly severed and a laboratory clamp applied to it (see Fig. 36, p. 84). During the following week, the distal pedicle was crushed gradually by tightening the clamp. Three weeks later, the abdominal flap was mobilized. The peripheral part of the flap became cyanotic; hence, flap was returned to its original site. Six weeks later, the scar at the dorsum of the hand was excised. The abdominal flap was elevated, the flap bed skin grafted, and the flap transferred to the dorsum of the hand. Plaster cast was applied. One week later, the pedicle of the flap was partly incised and a laboratory clamp applied. Six days later, the flap was severed from its pedicle.

c: Three days later, the flap and pedicle were adjusted in place. Note the inability of patient to extend the second and third fingers. Two months later, the defects of the extensor tendons were bridged by transplanting a tendon graft, from the long extensor tendon of the fourth toe, to the second finger, and by reconstructing the junctura tendinum between the third and fourth fingers through utilization of a tendon graft from the proximal tendon stump of the third finger. Immobilization in extension for three weeks followed.

d, e: Patient regained almost full function of the second and third fingers. A recent examination revealed full return of function.

ILLUSTRATIVE CASES

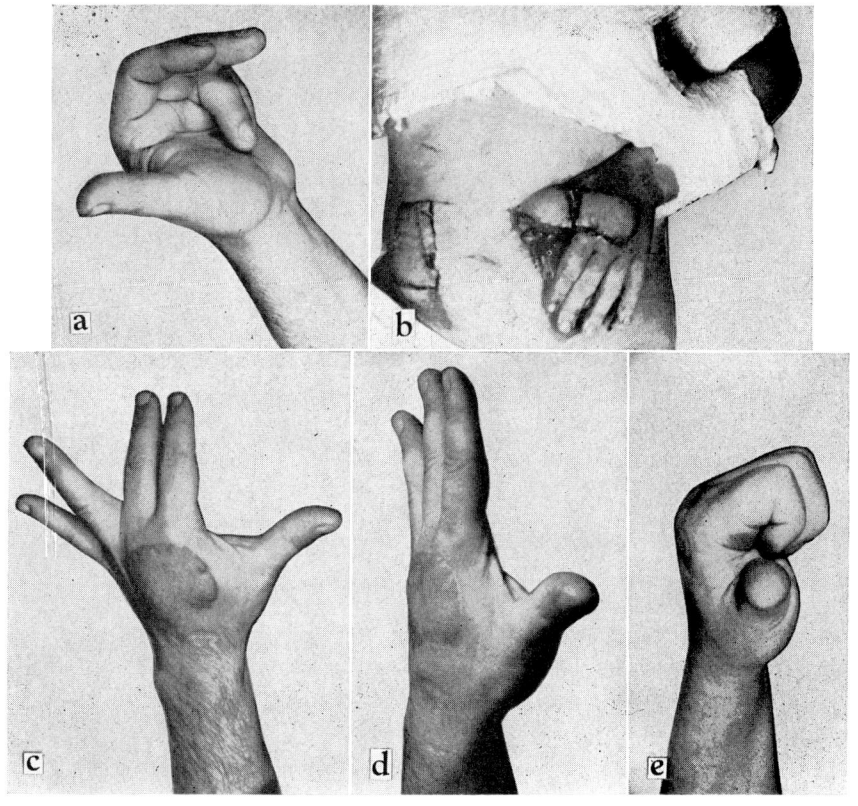

CASE

141

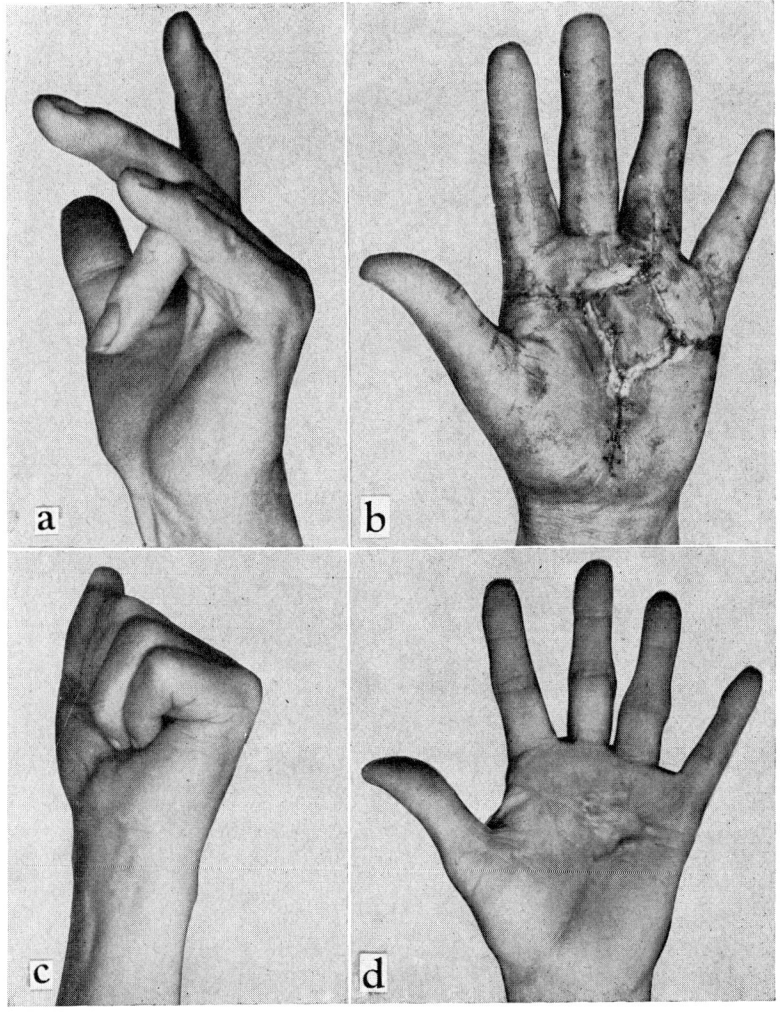

Case 141, *a:* Patient, aged forty-five, with Dupuytren's contracture of left hand of fifteen years' standing. The contracture primarily involved the third, fourth, and fifth fingers. There was, however, evidence of palmar nodules and contracting bands over the thenar region and the second finger.

b: The contracture was repaired, according to the method of Figure 344, page 827. The hand remained immobilized for two weeks. Active motility in hand bath was then permitted, but splint was reapplied for another week. The photograph depicts the condition three weeks after the operation. Thick split graft took completely.

c, d: The patient regained full motility of her hand within eight weeks after the operation.

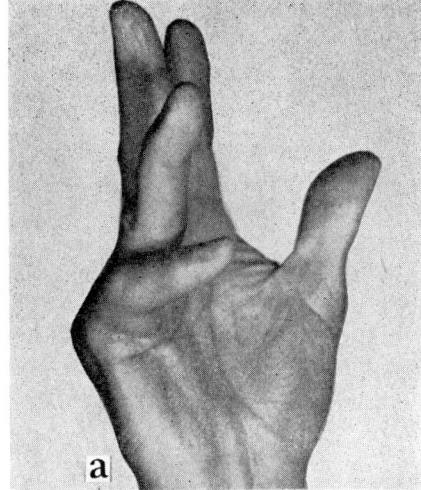

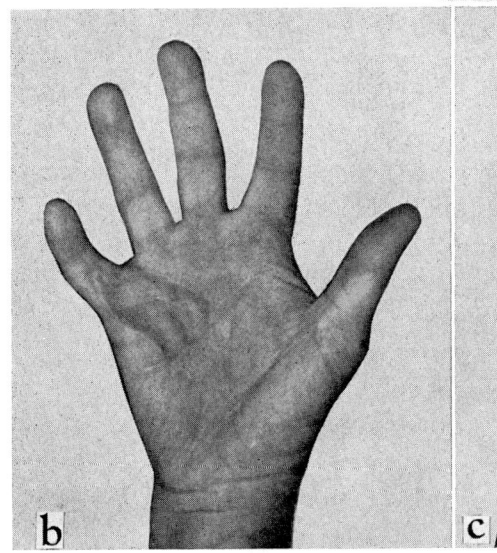

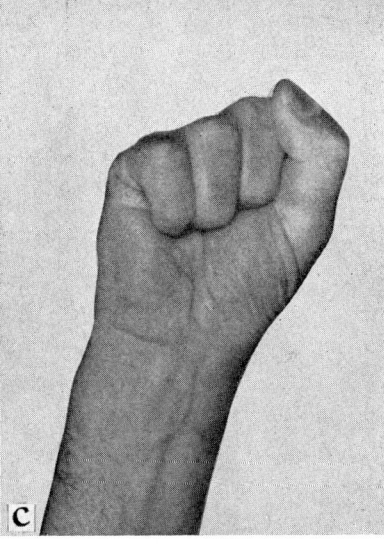

Case 142, *a:* Patient, aged fifty-eight, received a Colles fracture of the right wrist. Soon thereafter he noticed a gradual increasing contracture of the third, fourth and fifth fingers of right hand.

b, c: A typical Dupuytren's contracture developed which was operated on by excision of the entire palmar fascia and of the nodulous skin in the palm in the region of the fourth and fifth finger. Defect was replaced with a thick split skin graft. Two weeks after the operation the graft had taken well. Immobilization was continued until the twenty-first day. An Ace bandage was applied to prevent swelling and patient was urged to take active motion exercises and daily hand baths. One week later the bandage was left off temporarily but swelling of the knuckles and the dorsum of the hand occurred; the bandage was reapplied. Four weeks later much function of the hand was regained and the bandage could be left off. There was no swelling.

CASE
143

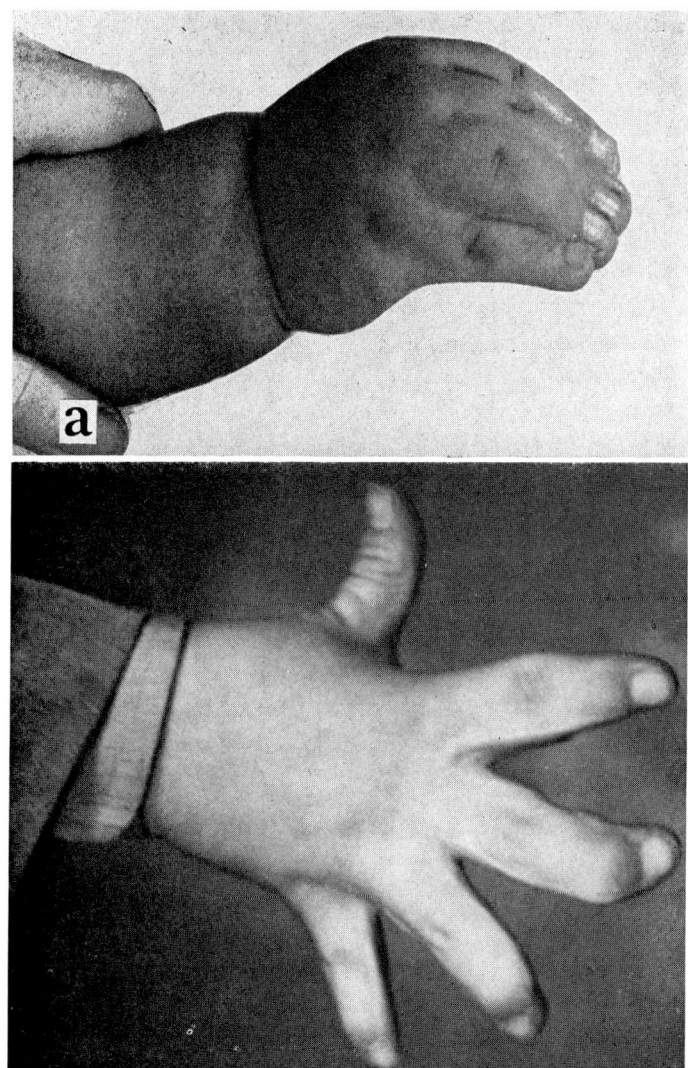

Case 143, *a:* Boy, aged two, with fusion of second to fifth finger of his right hand. Bony fusion was found between the terminal phalanges of the fourth and fifth fingers. The remainder of the fusion consisted of soft tissue. At birth the fingers were straight but subsequently became flexed because the shorter finger held the longer finger back in growth.

b: A two-stage operation was performed consisting of severance of fusion between the fourth and fifth fingers and third and second fingers, and application of a full-thickness graft to cover the raw surfaces in the first stage; five months later severance of the fusion between the third and fourth fingers with application of a full-thickness graft. Many of the scars along the grafted areas became hypertrophic. X-ray treatment softened the scars. Full function of all fingers was restored.

CASE
144

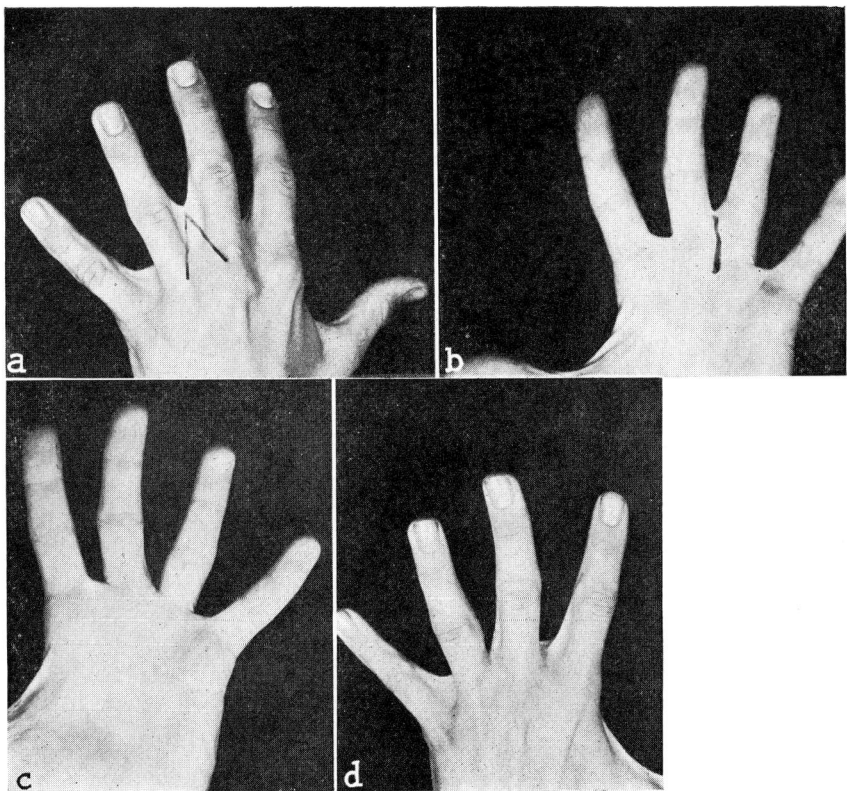

Case 144, *a:* Incomplete syndactylism between third and fourth fingers, repaired with a dorsal triangular skin flap (after Zeller). The base of the flap is at the level of the metacarpophalangeal joints, the tip at the level of the proximal interphalangeal joint. The flap is mobilized and reflected dorsally.

b: The fused volar portion is severed longitudinally.

c, d: In this case, the raw surfaces along the fingers could be covered with the redundant skin after severance of the volar fusion. The base of the web was covered by reflecting the dorsal triangular flap to the volar side.

CASE
145

Case 145: Patient, aged thirty-one, while window-cleaning fell through a window and lacerated the right wrist. Preoperative examination revealed separation of the tendons of the musculus flexor carpi radialis, flexor carpi ulnaris, flexor digitorum sublimis and musculus flexor digitorum profundus of the second, third, fourth, and fifth fingers, separation of the median and ulnar nerves and of the ulnar artery. Immediate repair of all structures, ligation of the ulnar artery and vein. Immobilization on a dorsal molded plaster-cast splint. The splint was temporarily removed on the fourteenth postoperative day, and physical therapy, including galvanization, was started. The patient received daily treatments. The splint was worn for three months until the neurological examination demonstrated return of sensory and motor function of the injured nerves. Physical therapy was continued every other day for another six months. At that time, the patient was discharged, with full functional return of the injured tendons and nerves.

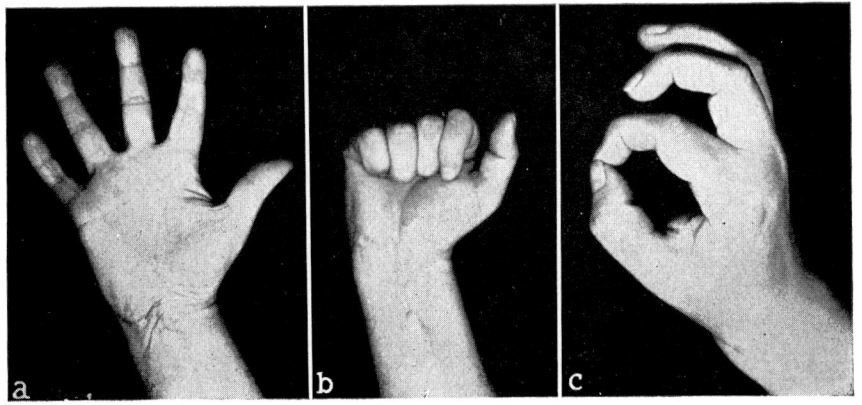

CASE
146

Case 146: Patient's left hand was caught in an electric saw. He had extensive lacerations of the dorsum of the hand over fourth and fifth fingers; severance of the two extensor tendons of the fifth finger; compound dislocation of the first interphalangeal joint of the fourth finger and of the terminal joint of the third finger; severance of the extensor tendons of the fourth and fifth fingers at the joint openings; and comminuted compound fracture of terminal phalanx of third finger. Immediate repair of the injured structures (one hour after the accident). Immobilization on a volar molded plaster-cast splint. The splint was removed after two weeks, and physical therapy was started. He returned to light work. Physical therapy was continued every other day for two months. Patient was then discharged with good function of the hand.

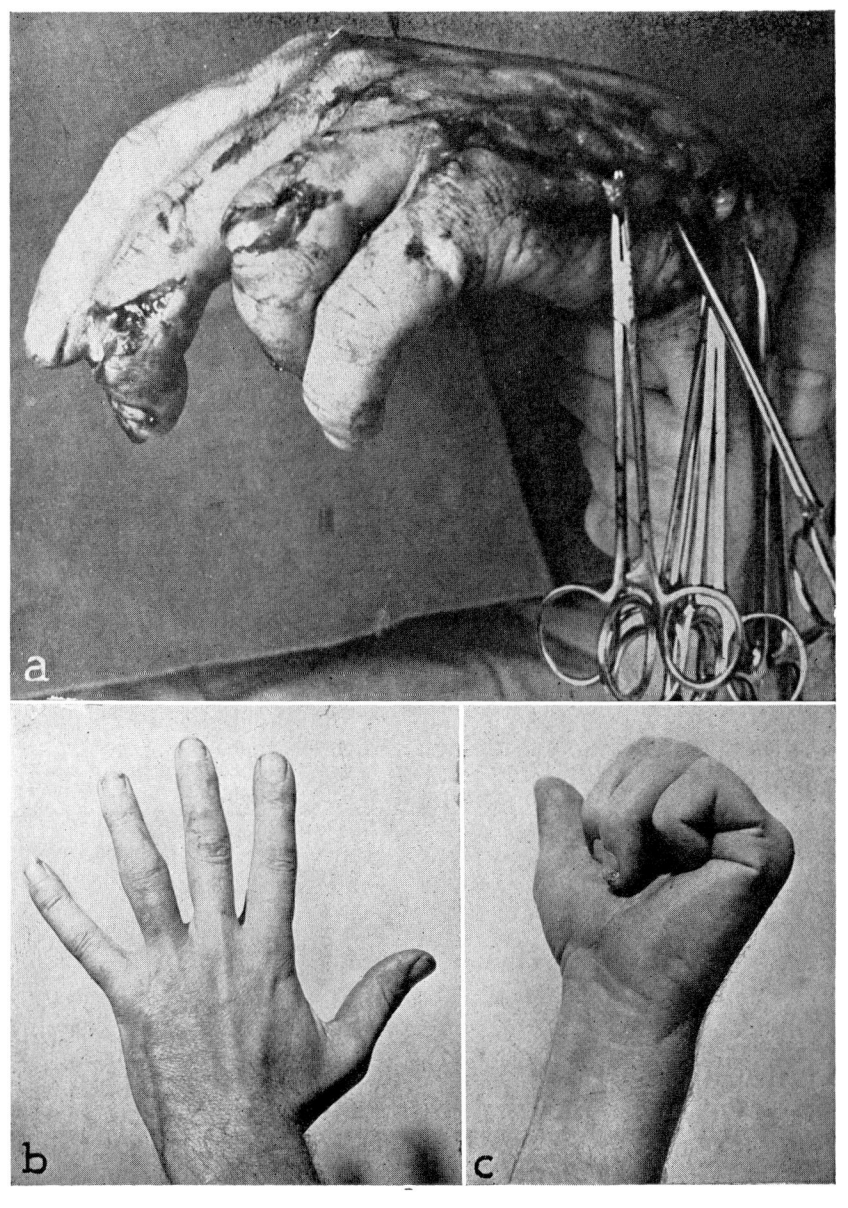

CASE
147

Case 147, *a:* Boy, aged eleven, had a laceration of the tendons of the musculus palmaris longus, flexor carpi radialis, flexor pollicis longus, flexor digitorum sublimis, and musculus flexor digitorum profundus, and of the median nerve and ulnar artery and vein (treated elsewhere). The severed tendons and nerves were repaired. The arm was immobilized for two weeks, and physical therapy instituted. After four months, it became evident that the sutured median nerve was not regenerating. Upon consultation, it was found that at the time of the accident an injury of the ulnar nerve must have been overlooked. The clinical picture was typical for paralysis of all intrinsic muscles of the hand (see p. 885). When he extended hand and fingers, the latter flexed as shown in *a.* Note wasting of thenar region. An exploratory operation was advised and carried out. The repaired tendons were found intact, but the proximal stump of the median nerve had been sutured to the distal stump of the ulnar nerve. Both nerves were severed from each other. The distal stump of the median nerve and the proximal stump of the ulnar nerve were located. All nerve ends were cicatricial, and had to be shortened for some distance until normal nerve fibers were encountered. Under extreme flexion of the wrist, the corresponding nerve stumps were sutured together. The arm was immobilized on a dorsal molded plaster-cast splint. The splint was temporarily removed three weeks after the operation, and physical therapy and occupational therapy were instituted. First return of nerve function was noticed two months later. The splint was removed.

b–d: Patient's hand had regained almost full function nine months after the second operation.

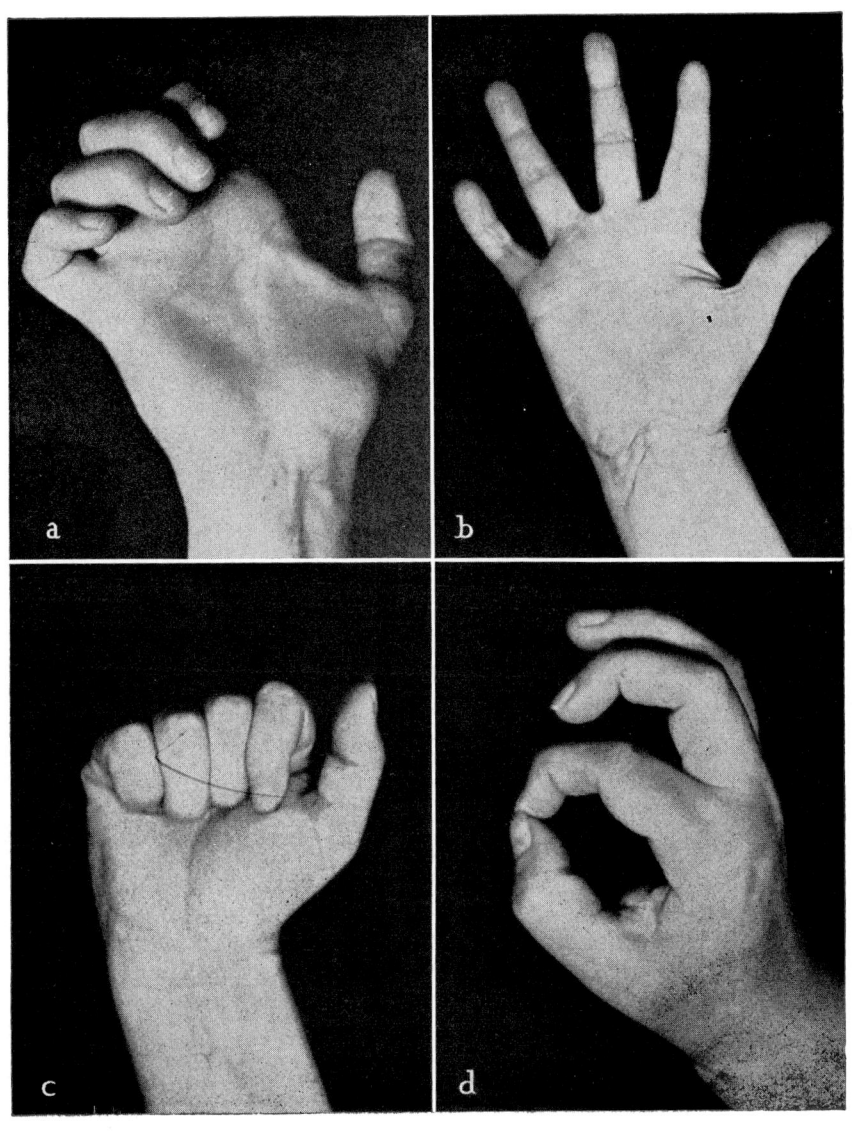

ILLUSTRATIVE CASES

CASE
148

Case 148, *a:* Combined median and ulnar palsy after unsuccessful nerve suture of both nerves following deep laceration of forearm. Note atrophy of thenar and hypothenar regions. Eight months after injury an exploratory operation revealed extensive neuroma formation at the site of nerve sutures. After resection of the neuromas the nerve gaps measured two inches. Nerve suture was impossible. A nerve graft was taken from proximal end of ulnar nerves to bridge gap in median nerve. One year later there was return of opposition of the thumb and some sensation along the distribution of the median nerve. A tendon transfer was now carried out to improve function of the fingers: sublimis of third finger to lumbricale muscles of second, third, fourth and fifth fingers and extensor pollicis brevis to first interosseous muscle of the index finger. Patient regained good function of metacarpophalangeal joints and abduction of index finger, but interphalangeal joints became stiff except in index finger. One year later all interphalangeal joints of third, fourth and fifth fingers were arthrodesed in position of function.

b, c: After completion of reconstruction. Note (*b*) that thenar region is no longer atrophied, but hypothenar region is. Return of opposition.

1194

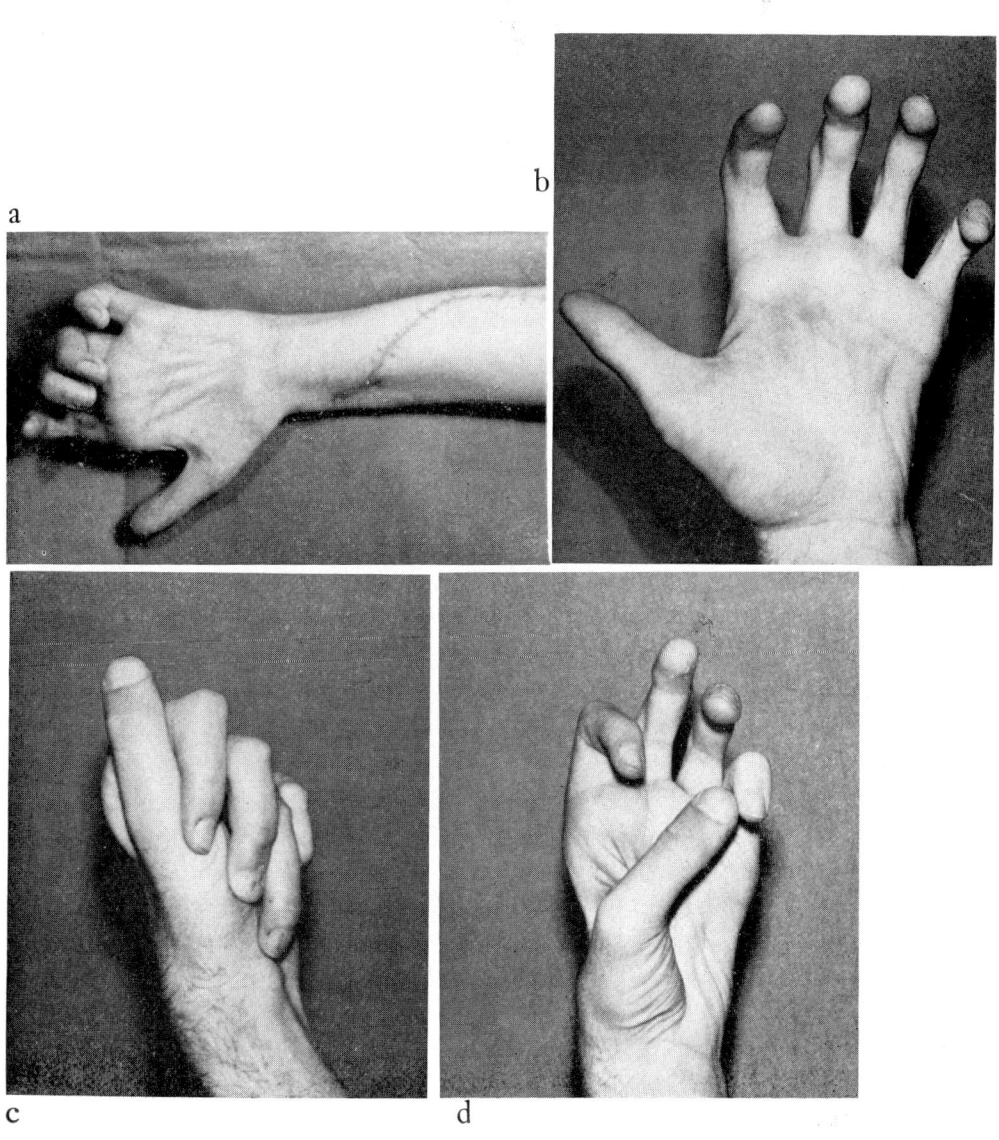

CASE
149

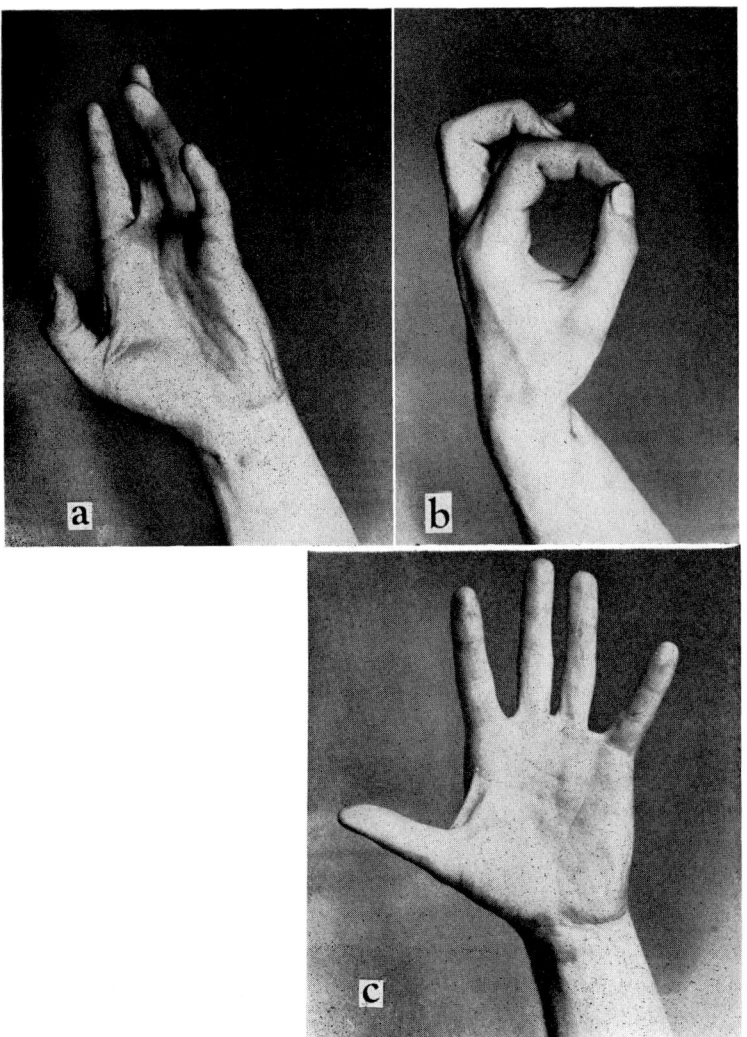

Case 149: Patient, aged nineteen, severed flexor pollicis longus of left thumb just distal to the flexor crease of the metacarpophalangeal joint. Only the skin wound was sutured.

a-c: Five months later the divided flexor pollicis longus was replaced with a tendon graft from the long extensor tendon of the fourth toe. The tendon was inserted to the terminal phalanx and to the flexor pollicis stump in the wrist.

CASE
150

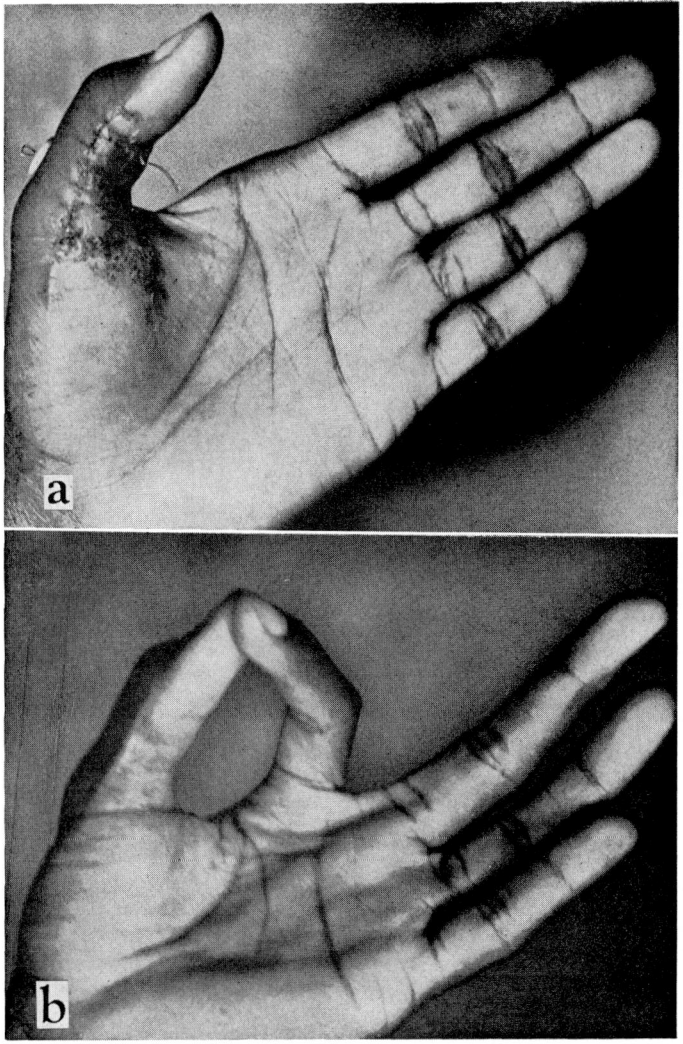

Case 150: Division of flexor pollicis longus. Primary repair had been attempted but had failed. The second operation revealed much scar tissue and for this reason a tendon grafting operation seemed to be contraindicated. A tenodesis was performed by incorporating the distal stump of the flexor pollicis longus into the first phalanx holding the terminal joint in 45-degree flexion. The pull-out wire method after Bunnell was used to hold the tendon in a canal which was drilled through the phalanx. Further immobilization of this joint was achieved by insertion of an intramedullary Kirschner wire (see Fig. 357, p. 863). The wire was removed later.

CASE
151

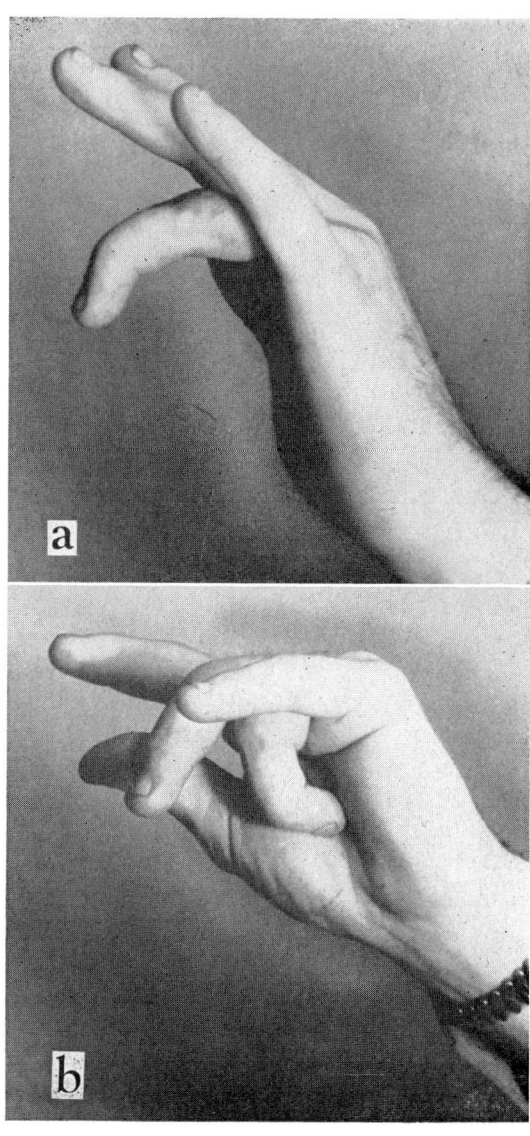

Case 151, *a*, *b:* Severance of the profundus tendon of fourth finger over the middle phalanx. Six weeks after tenodesis of distal stump of severed profundus tendon to bone of middle phalanx to hold terminal phalanx in 45-degree flexion permanently. (Compare with Case 150.)

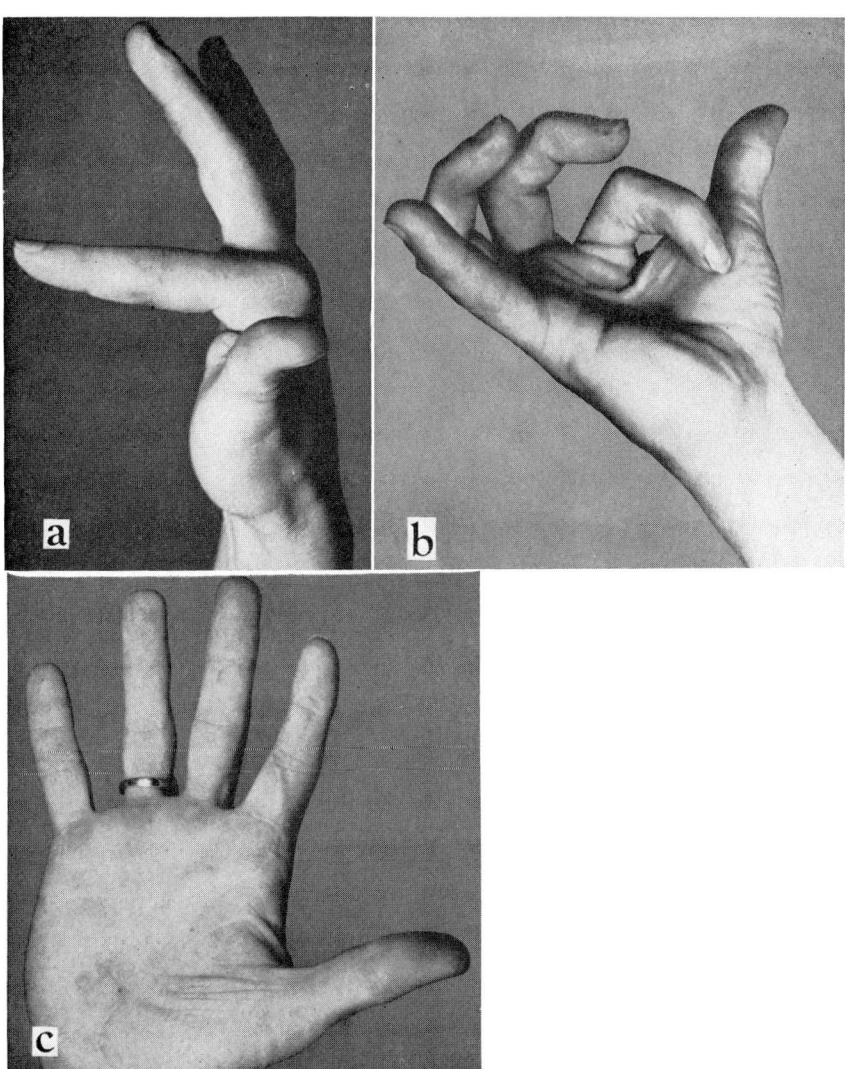

Case 152, *a:* Patient, aged twenty-seven, with severance of profundus and sublimis tendons of right index finger in level of the web.

b, c: After replacement of both tendons with a tendon graft from the sacrificed sublimis tendon.

CASE
153

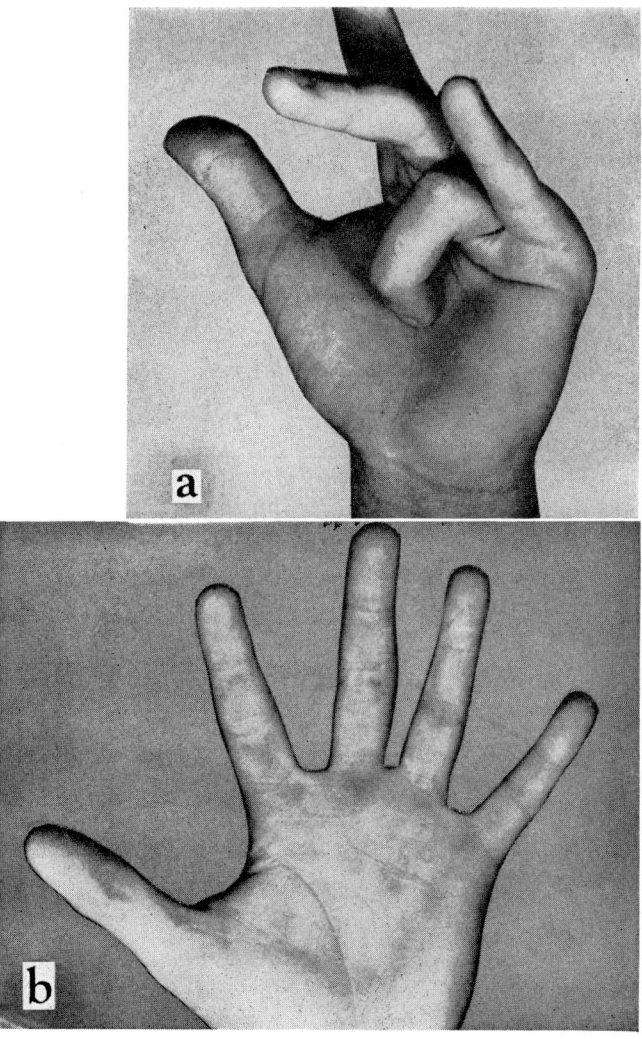

Case 153, *a, b:* Patient, aged thirteen, received a rupture of the profundus tendon of fourth finger while tackling during football. Two months later the sublimis tendon was sacrificed and the profundus tendon replaced with a tendon graft from the long extensor tendon of the fourth toe. Result five months after operation.

CASE
154

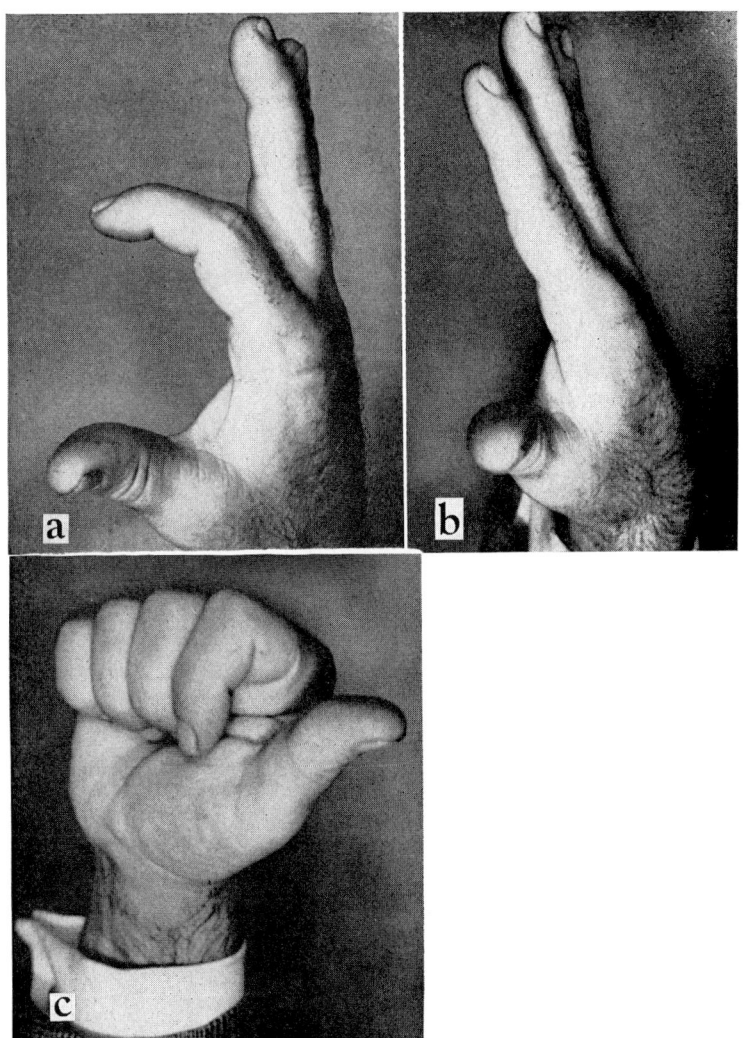

Case 154, *a:* Patient, aged thirty-nine, fell on a piece of glass and severed the extensor tendons of the second finger. The tendon became adherent and prevented flexion as well as extension of the finger.

b, c: After tenolysis and bridging the tendon defect with a tendon graft from the long extensor tendon of the fourth toe.

CASE
155

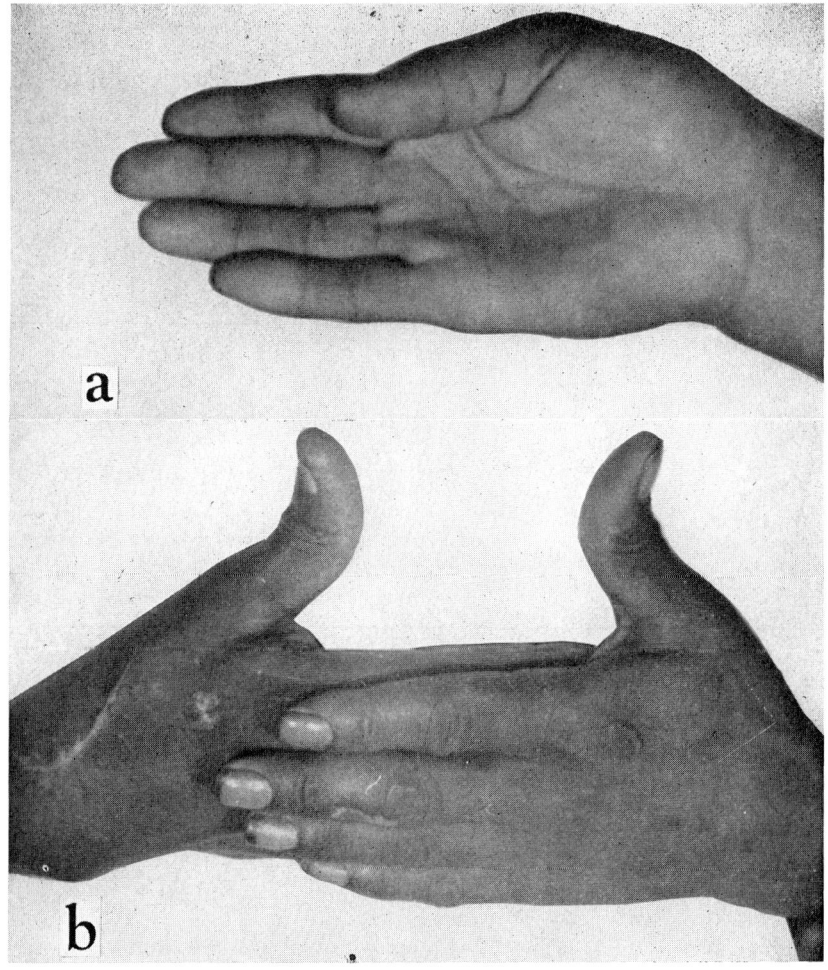

Case 155: Patient's long and short extensors and abductor of the right thumb were severed in an accident without attempt at repair. Upon operation several months later the six tendon stumps and the severed superficial radial nerve were identified. The tendon stumps were frayed and needed much shortening; end-to-end suture became impossible and tendon grafting had to be employed. The proximal end of the abductor pollicis was used as a graft. The distal ends of the extensor pollicis longus and brevis were sutured together and the gap between these combined tendons and the proximal stump of the extensor pollicis longus was bridged with the tendon graft. To increase the motor power the extensor pollicis brevis was sutured upon the extensor pollicis longus. The superficial radial nerve stumps were approximated. The hand was immobilized in cock-up position of the wrist with extension and opposition of the thumb for three weeks. Functional result (*a*) before, and (*b*) four months after the operation.

CASE
156

a

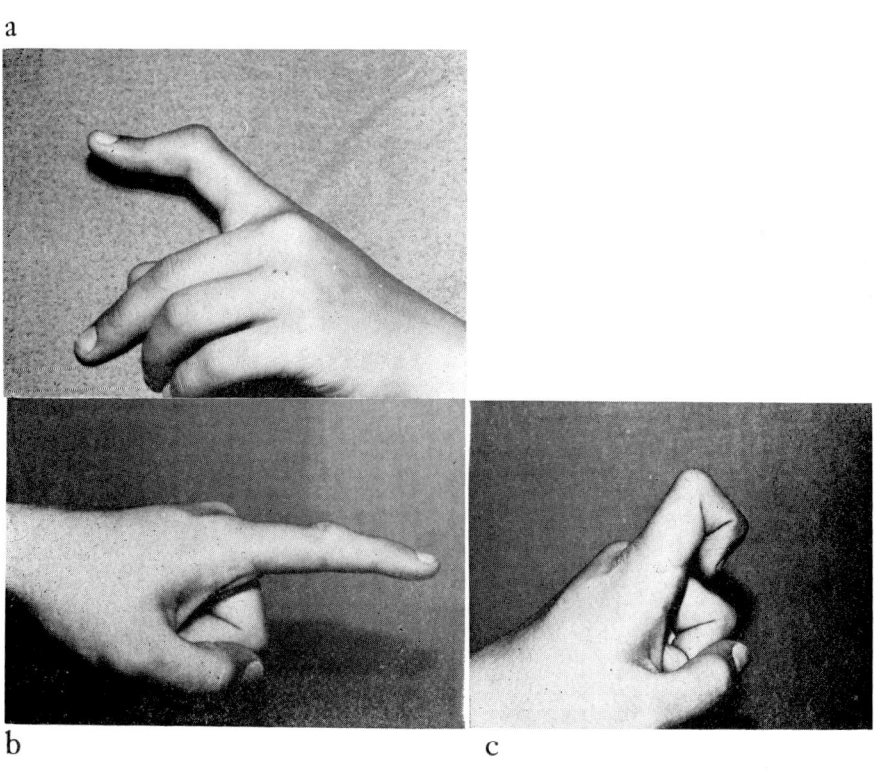

b   c

Case 156, *a:* Button-hole injury due to ruptured distal aponeurosis over first interphalangeal joint.

b, c: Repaired according to technique described on page 880.

Case 157, *a*, *b:* Patient, aged twenty-six, came in touch with a high tension wire and received deep extensive burns of the left hand. The soft tissues of the flexor surface of the forearm and the midpalmar space sloughed out and were débrided. This resulted in loss of the musculus flexor carpi radialis, flexor pollicis longus, the median nerve, and long flexors of second, third, and fourth fingers. The defect was closed with an abdominal flap.

c, *d:* Two months later tendon grafting was performed to replace the action of the profundus tendon of the second, third, and fourth fingers. The peroneus brevis tendon was used as a graft and was sutured to the distal end of the profundus muscle stump in the forearm. The other end was split into two strands; one strand was sutured to the profundus tendon of the second finger and the other one to the profundus of the fourth finger. The profundus of the third finger was sutured into the point of division of the graft. Two months later opposition of the thumb was restored by transferring the extensor pollicis brevis to the severed and rerouted extensor carpi ulnaris. The latter was rerouted just proximal to the ulnar epiphysis.

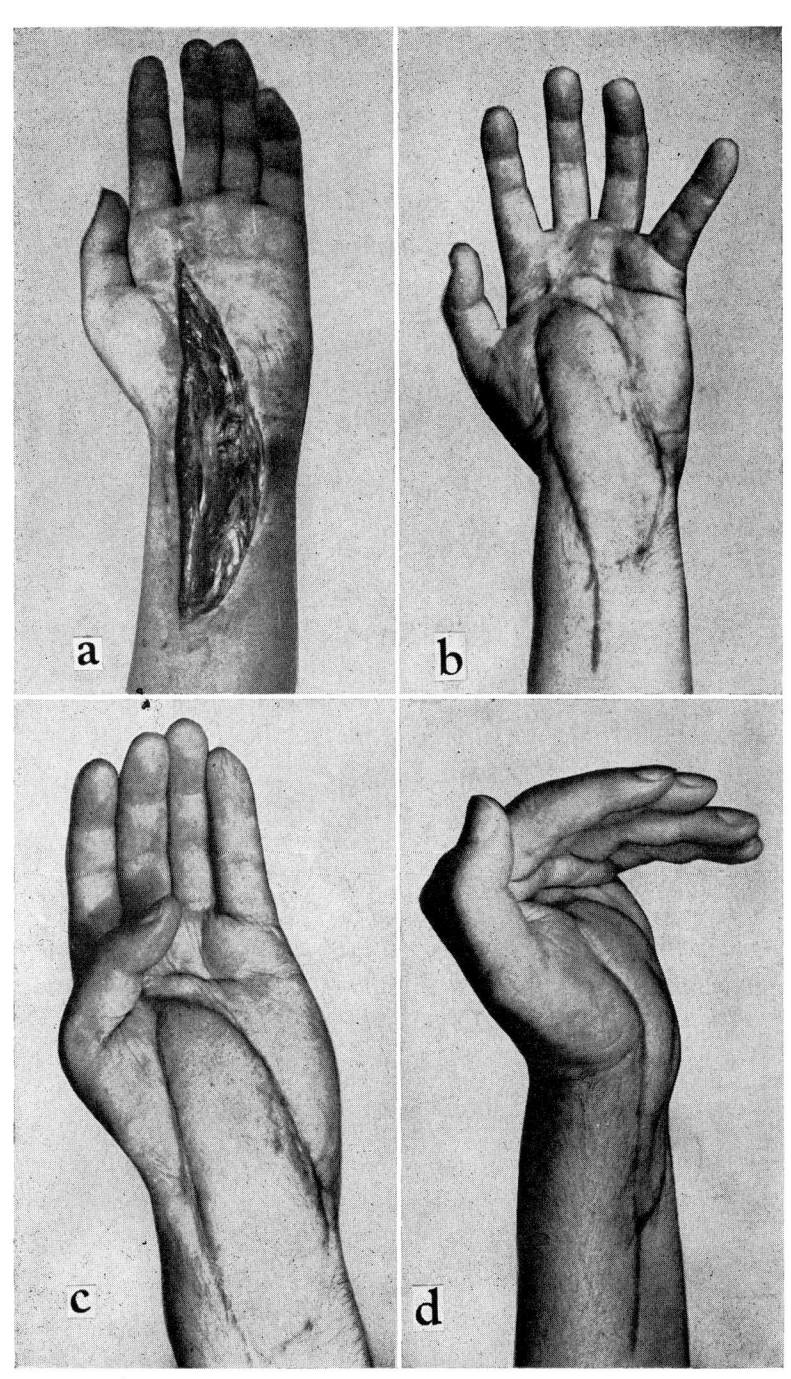

CASE
158

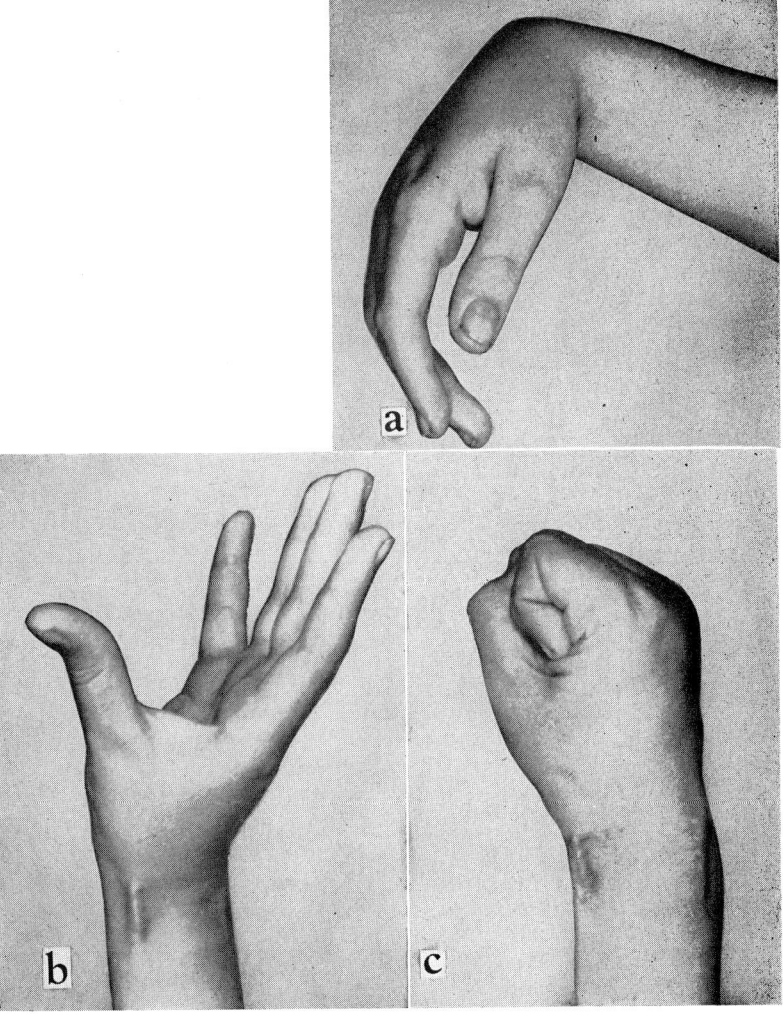

Case 158, *a:* Boy, aged twelve, with irreparable radial palsy from severance of the radial nerve in the right upper arm after a previous accident. The nerve ends had been sutured together but the nerve did not regenerate. Thirteen months later a tendon transfer was performed consisting of transfer of the flexor carpi ulnaris tendon to the extensor tendons of second to fifth fingers and transfer of the palmaris longus tendon to the severed extensor pollicis longus tendon.

b, c: Function of wrist and fingers was almost normal three months after the operation.

CASE
159

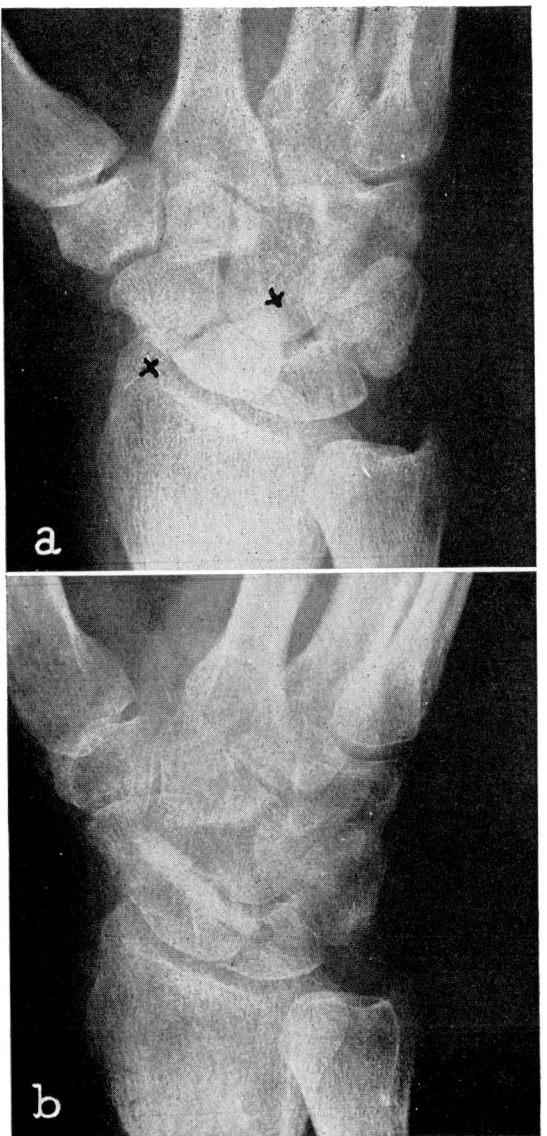

Case 159, *a:* Patient, aged twenty-eight, with nonunion of os navic-ulare of two months' duration. Fracture line x-x in roentgenogram. Both fragments revealed same density, hence appeared to be alive. The wrist was immobilized in a plaster cast in cock-up position for three months; no evi-dence of healing after that time.

b: A bone-pegging operation was performed (p. 929) and the wrist immobilized. After three months, the x-ray examination revealed complete union.

CASE
160

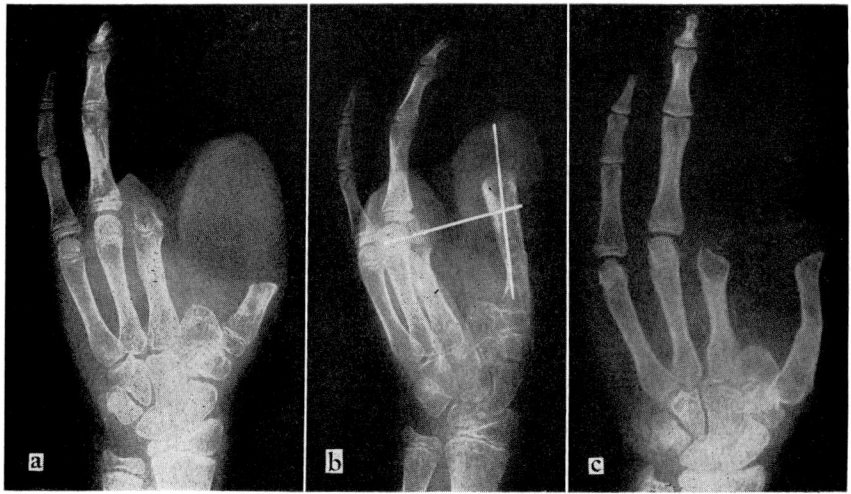

Case 160, *a-f:* Boy, eleven and one-half years of age, lost radial half of right hand as result of an explosion (*d*).

A rather large abdominal flap was transplanted in one stage to provide coverage of the raw surface and an extension later to receive a bone graft to lengthen the first metacarpal stump. Eight days later the flap was partially separated and a laboratory clamp was applied to the remaining pedicle to gradually crush the pedicle. Five days later the flap was severed. Four days later the flap was adjusted in place (*e*).

Roentgenograms: Metacarpal stumps over which the soft tissue flap is faintly outlined (*a*).

Five months after the flap transfer a metatarsal bone (the fifth) was placed upon the stump of the first metacarpal bone and transfixed with intramedullary wires (*b*).

Three months later the horizontal cross pin was removed and after another three months the vertical pin (*c*).

Demonstration of functional result (*f, g*).

1208

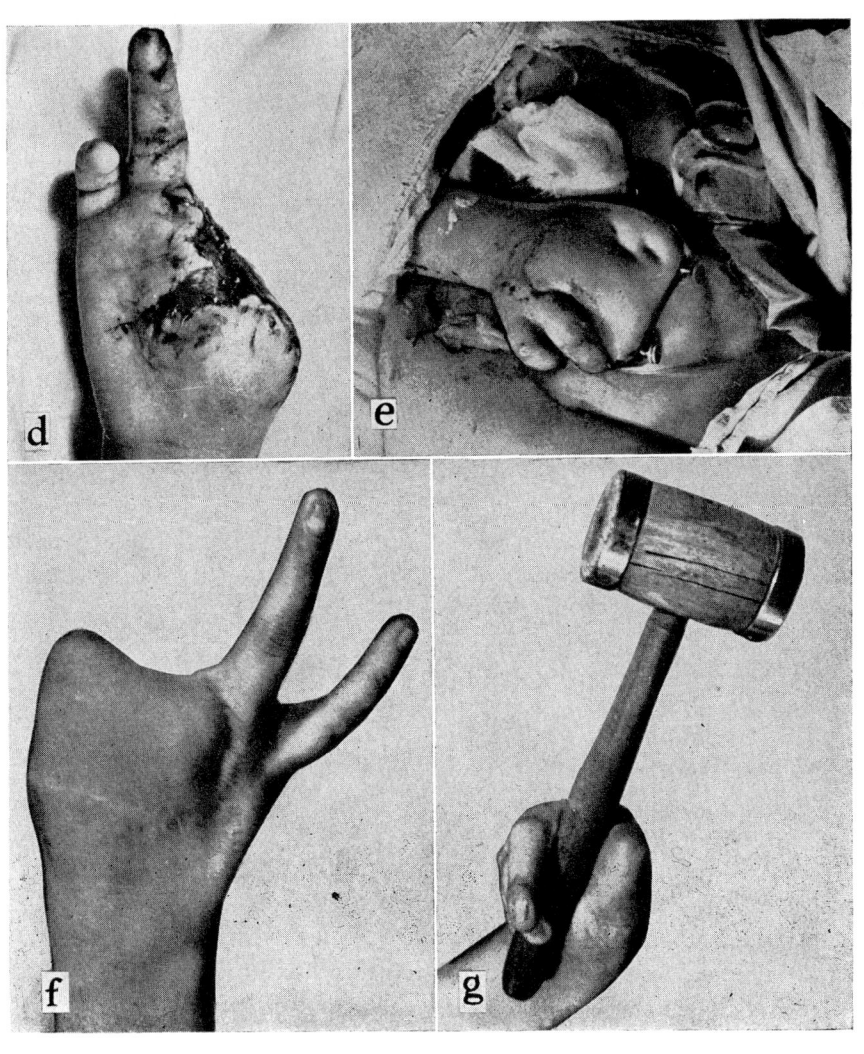

CASE
161

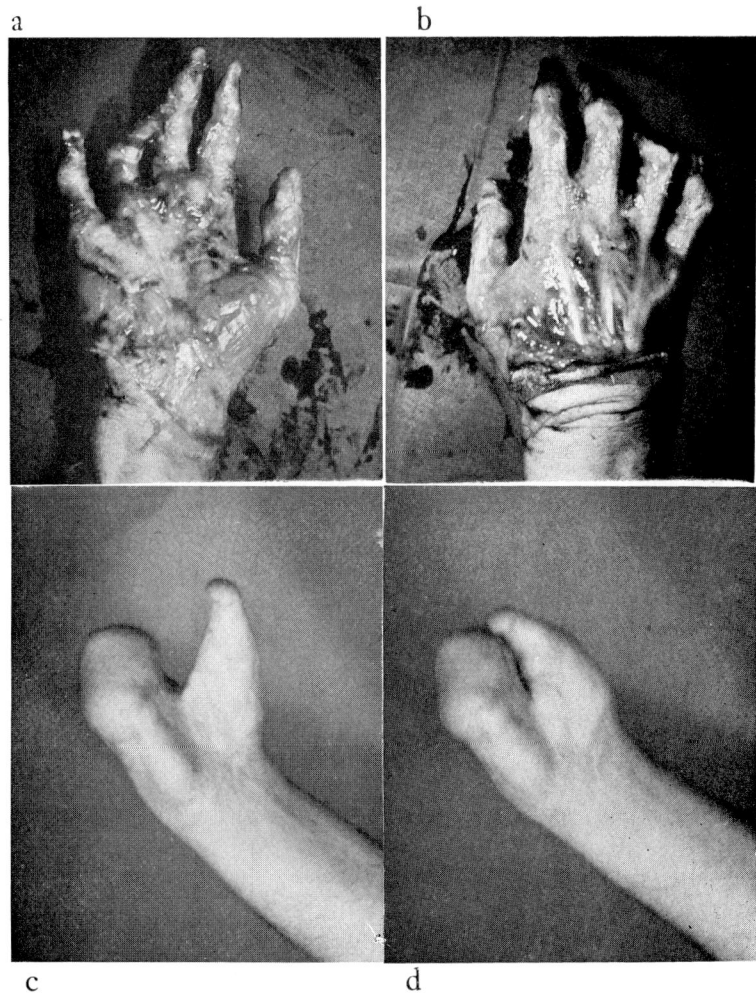

a   b

c   d

Case 161, *a, b:* "Degloving" of hand after latter was pulled between rollers. Immediate coverage with skin grafts. Second, third, fourth and fifth fingers became necrotic.

c, d: After disarticulation of second to fifth fingers through metacarpophalangeal joints, stumps were covered with an abdominal flap. Note that stump of thumb is covered with a flap which was transferred from the flap covering the finger stumps. Patient is now employed as a radio dispatcher at a police station.

1210

CASE
162

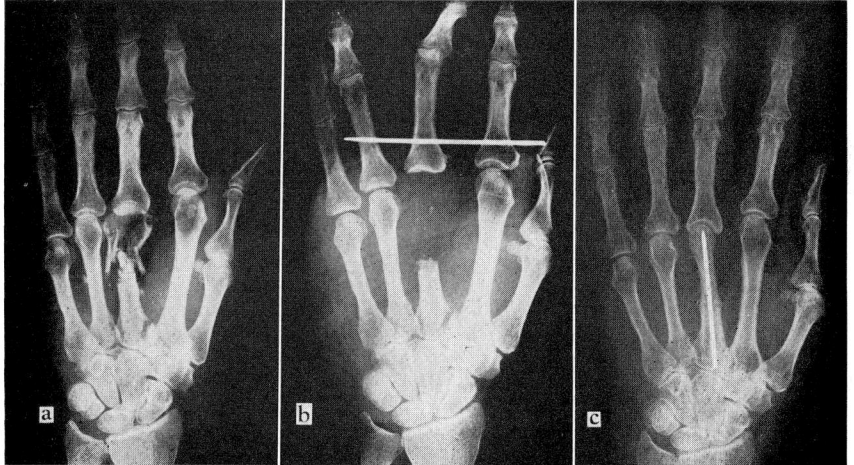

Case 162, *a:* Patient, aged sixty-two, was shot accidentally in the dorsum of the right hand. The injury resulted in extensive loss of surface tissue and a badly comminuted and compound fracture of the third metacarpal bone.

b: Distal two thirds of the third metacarpal bone was removed. The third finger was suspended upon the first phalanges of the second and third fingers by cross pinning. The pin was laid just beneath the webs of the finger and buried subcutaneously. A flap was transplanted from the abdomen in one stage. It was clamped ten days later and severed two days later, and adjusted in place five days later.

c: Three months later the third metacarpal bone was replaced with the fifth metatarsal bone and was stabilized with a longitudinal intramedullary wire and a cross pin through the sides of the metacarpals. This cross pin was removed five months later, while the vertical wire is still in place eight years after the accident.

d, e: Functional result.

(*Continued on next page*)

CASE
162 *(Continued)*

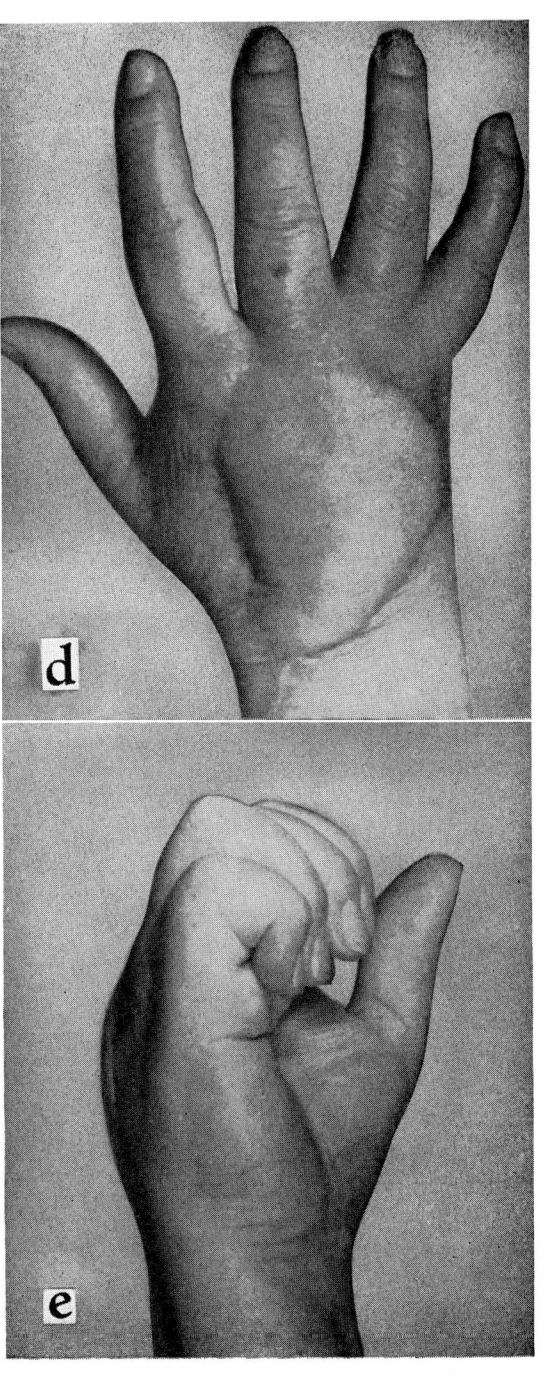

CASE
163

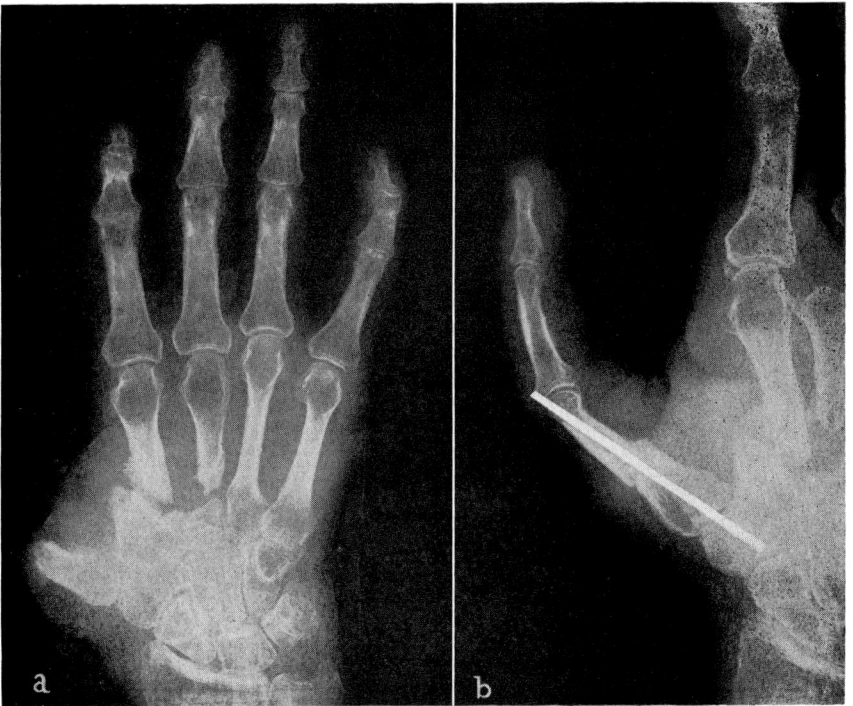

Case 163: Patient, aged forty-six, sustained a crushing injury to his left hand with loss of the thumb (*a*). The destroyed soft tissues of the thenar region and web were replaced with an abdominal flap (*c*). There was marked impairment of motility in all finger joints. To increase the function of this badly damaged hand, a thumb substitution operation was considered. Since the index finger showed distinct evidence of impairment of circulation (prolonged paleness after tourniquet test) the third finger was selected to replace the thumb with the Lucksch-Hilgenfeldt procedure. (*d*): Flap and incisions towards the thumb are outlined. (*e*): Exposure of the neurovascular bundle. (*f*): The finger is being moved to the stump of the thumb metacarpal. (*h*): Fixation of the transposed finger to the stump of the first metacarpal with an intramedullary wire. An additional cast was applied for five weeks. Then the profundus tendon of the third finger was shortened. It could not be joined with the flexor pollicis longus since the latter was frayed and adherent. The intramedullary wire was removed nine weeks after the finger transfer. (*g*), (*h*), and (*i*) depict the functional result six months after the transfer. In spite of a previous tenolysis adhesions recurred, preventing the fingers from fully functioning. The new thumb has sufficient sensitivity, although some of the sensitivity is projected along the radial side of the fourth finger.

(*Continued on next page*)

1213

CASE
163 *(Continued)*

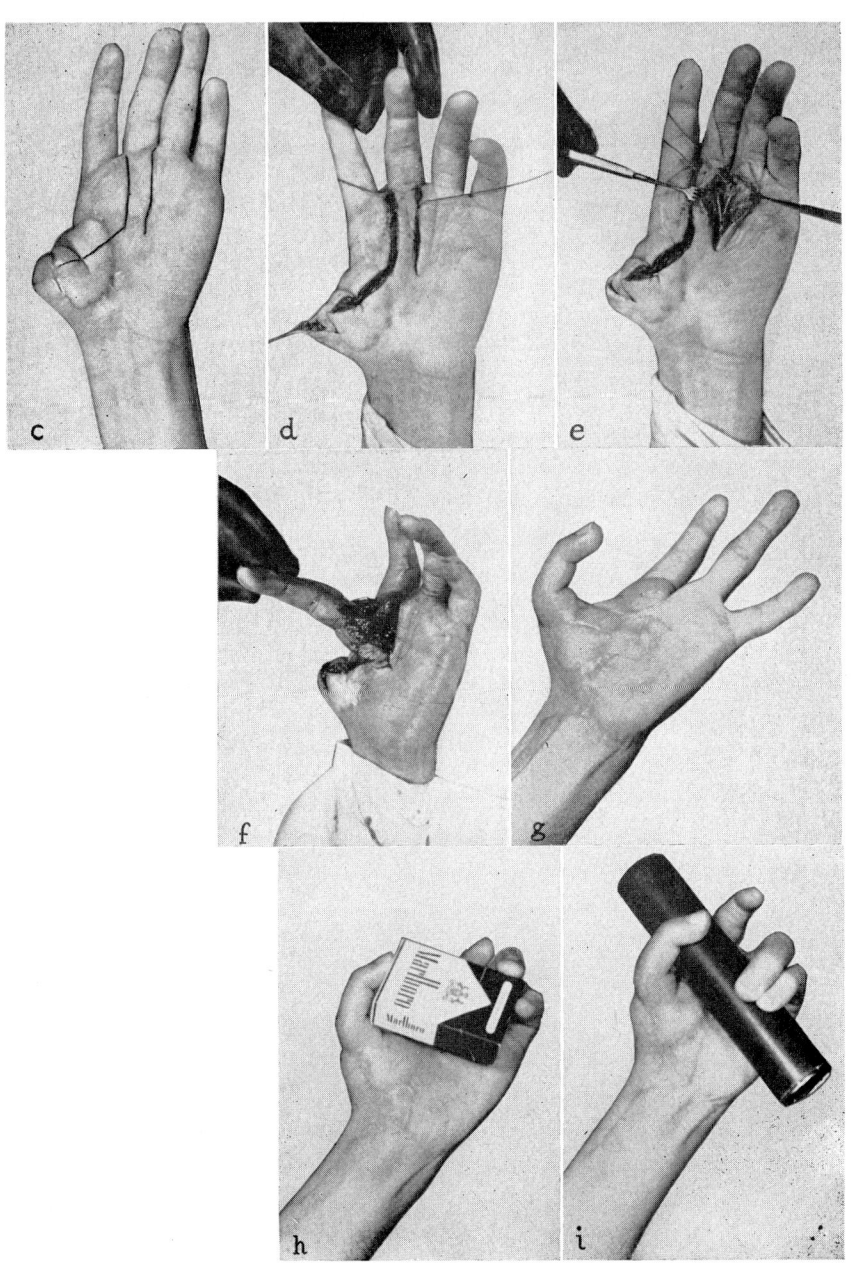

CASE
164

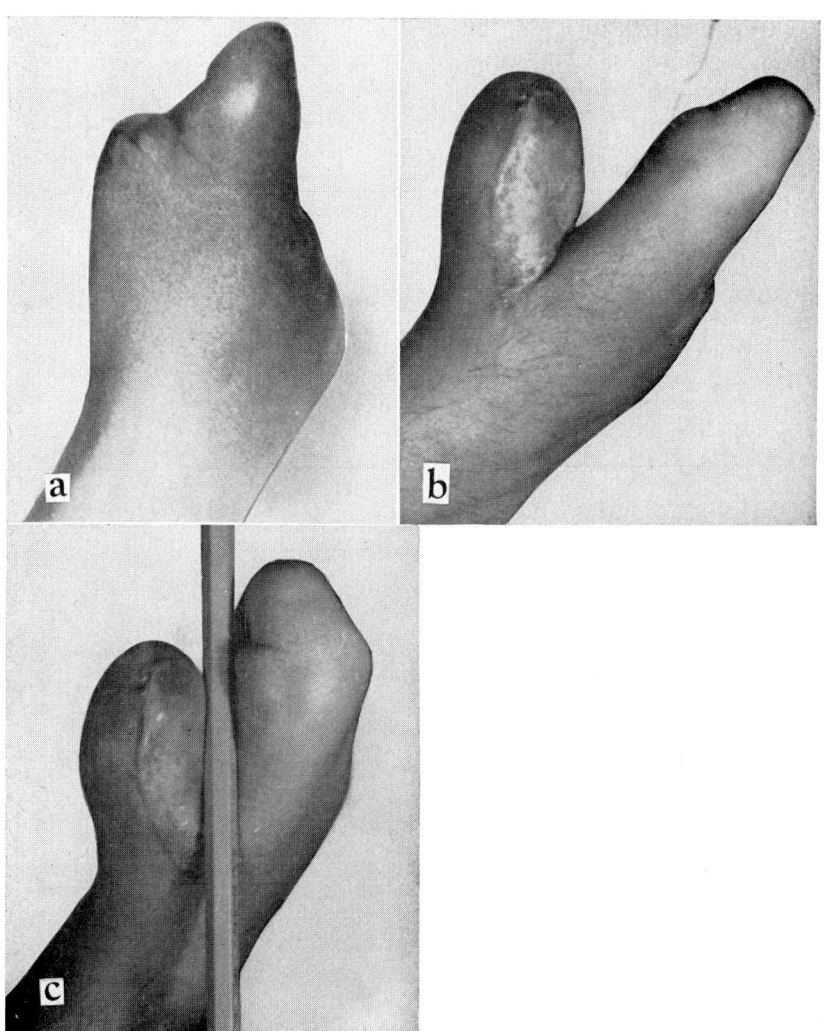

Case 164, *a:* Patient, aged thirty-five, with traumatic amputation of the right thumb through the proximal phalanx, traumatic amputation of index finger through the middle phalanx, and of third, fourth, and fifth fingers through the metacarpals.

b, c: An operation for phalangization was performed (p. 953) to create a cleft between the first and second metacarpal bones.

CASE
165

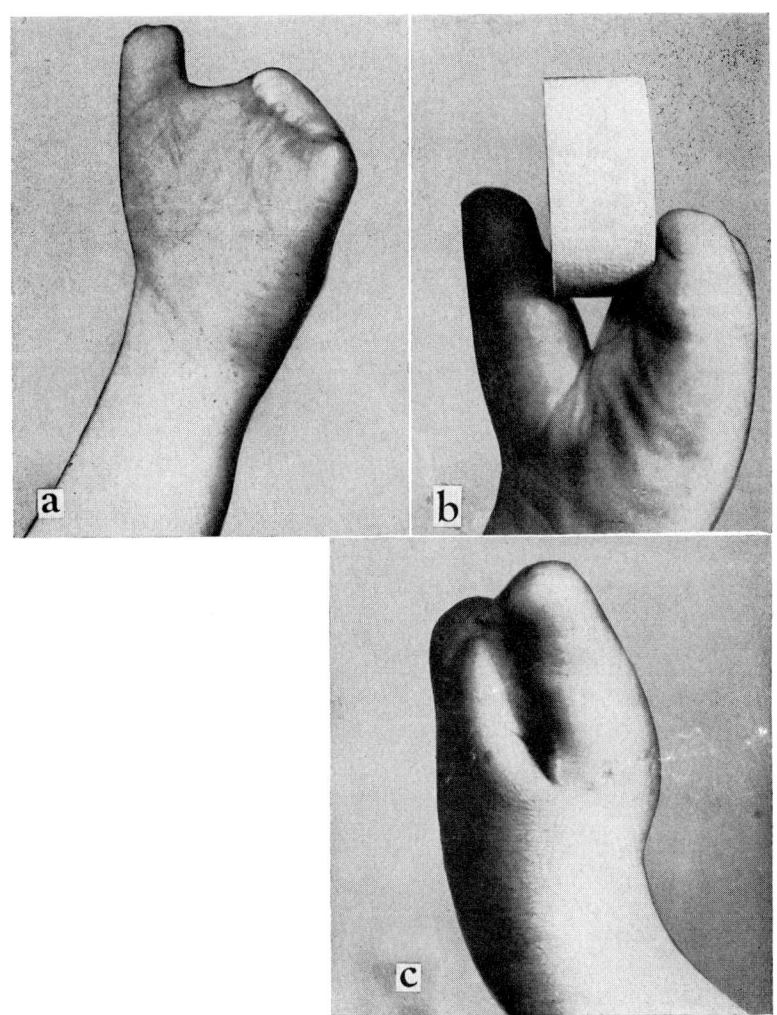

Case 165, *a:* Patient, aged thirty-one years, with traumatic amputation of second, third, fourth, and fifth fingers, and loss of thumb through the middle of the proximal phalanx of left hand. Heads of the metacarpals were immediately covered with an abdominal flap which was severed in stages.

b, c: Four months later an operation for phalangization was performed to create a cleft between the first and second metacarpal bones (p. 953). Too much of the adductor of the thumb had been sacrificed resulting in loss of power of adduction. To restore latter the stump of the extensor of the second finger was rerouted between the second and third metacarpal bone through the palm to the first metacarpal bone where it was fastened to the bone through a drill hole with a pull-out wire.

1216

CASE
166

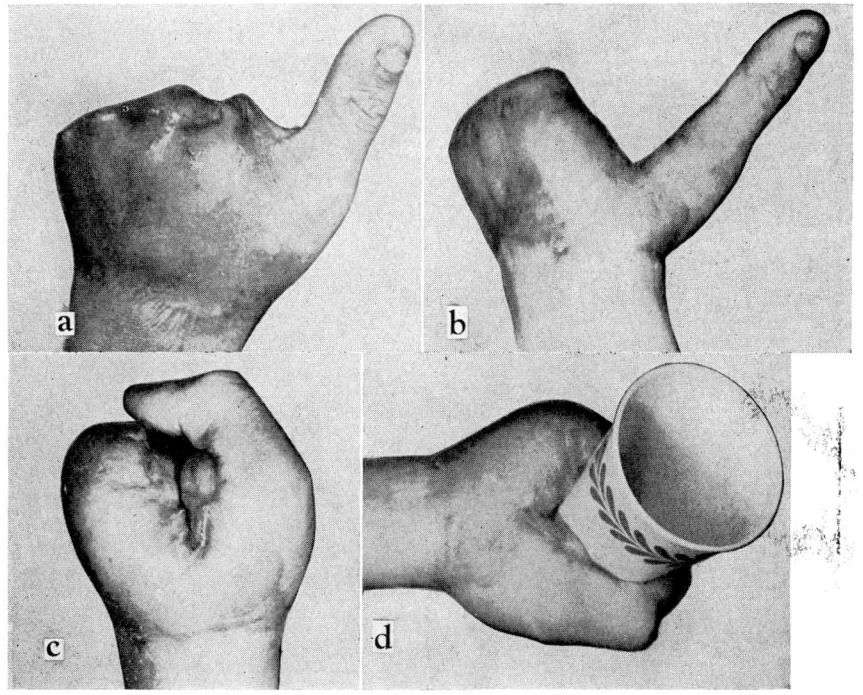

Case 166, *a:* Traumatic disarticulation of the second, third, fourth, and fifth fingers.

b: The second metacarpal was removed. An operation for phalangization was performed with removal of the first interosseous muscle and portion of the adductor muscle (p. 953). At the same time excision of the articular surface of the third, fourth, and fifth metacarpal and transplantation of an abdominal flap were carried out to close the raw surface over the metacarpal stumps. The flap was severed eleven days after transfer and three days later adjusted in place.

c, d: Functional result.

CASE
167

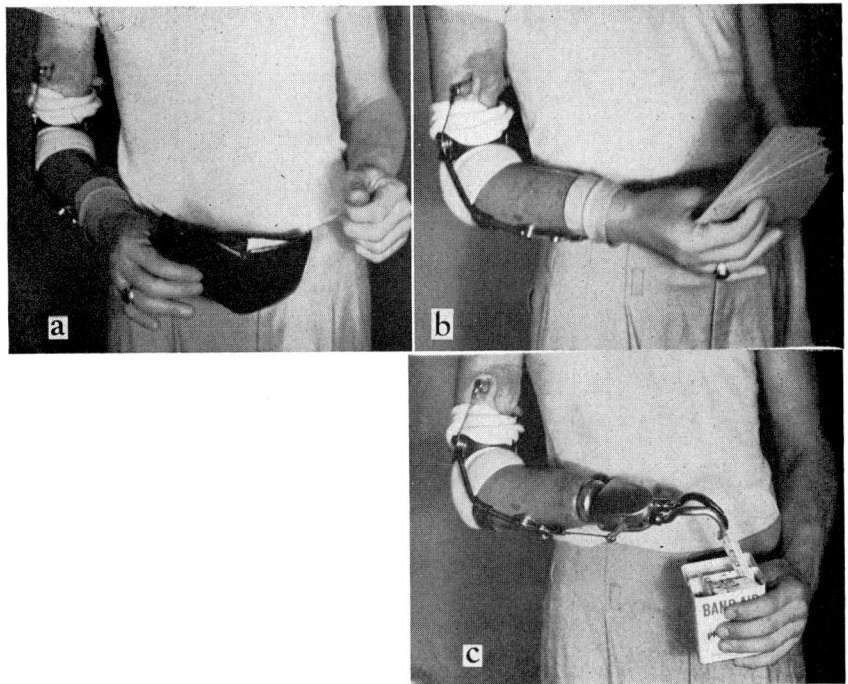

Case 167, *a-c:* Patient, aged eighteen years, who had right fore-arm amputated through the distal third after an extensive crushing injury. A cineplasty was performed through the biceps muscle. Demonstration of functional result. Hand and hook units are interchangeable.

CASE
168

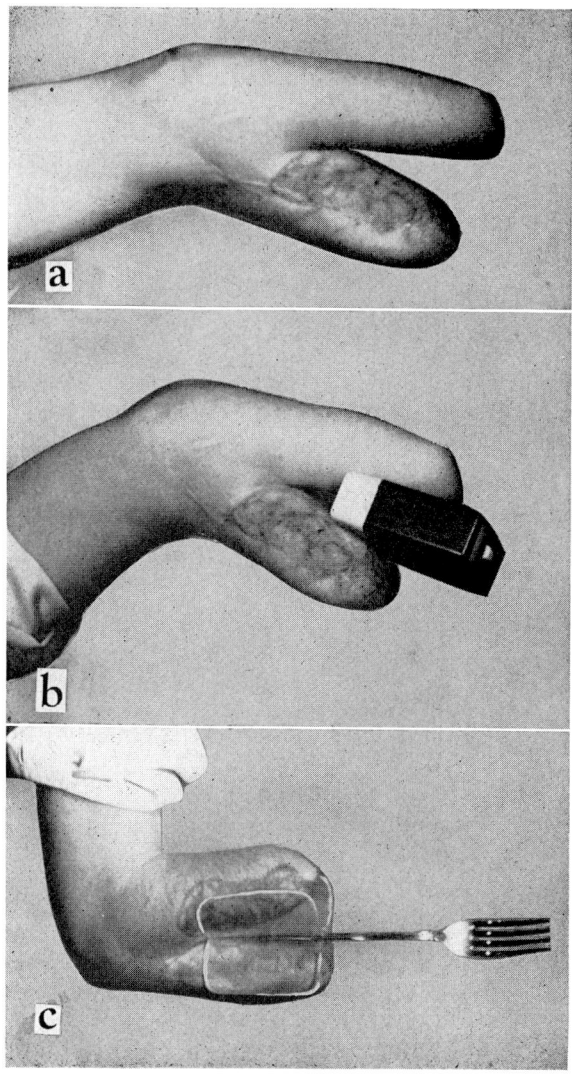

Case 168, *a-c:* Patient, aged sixty-three years, who had forearm amputated just above the wrist after severe crushing injury of the hand. A Krukenberg forcipication operation was carried out. Demonstration of functional result.

CASE
169

a

b

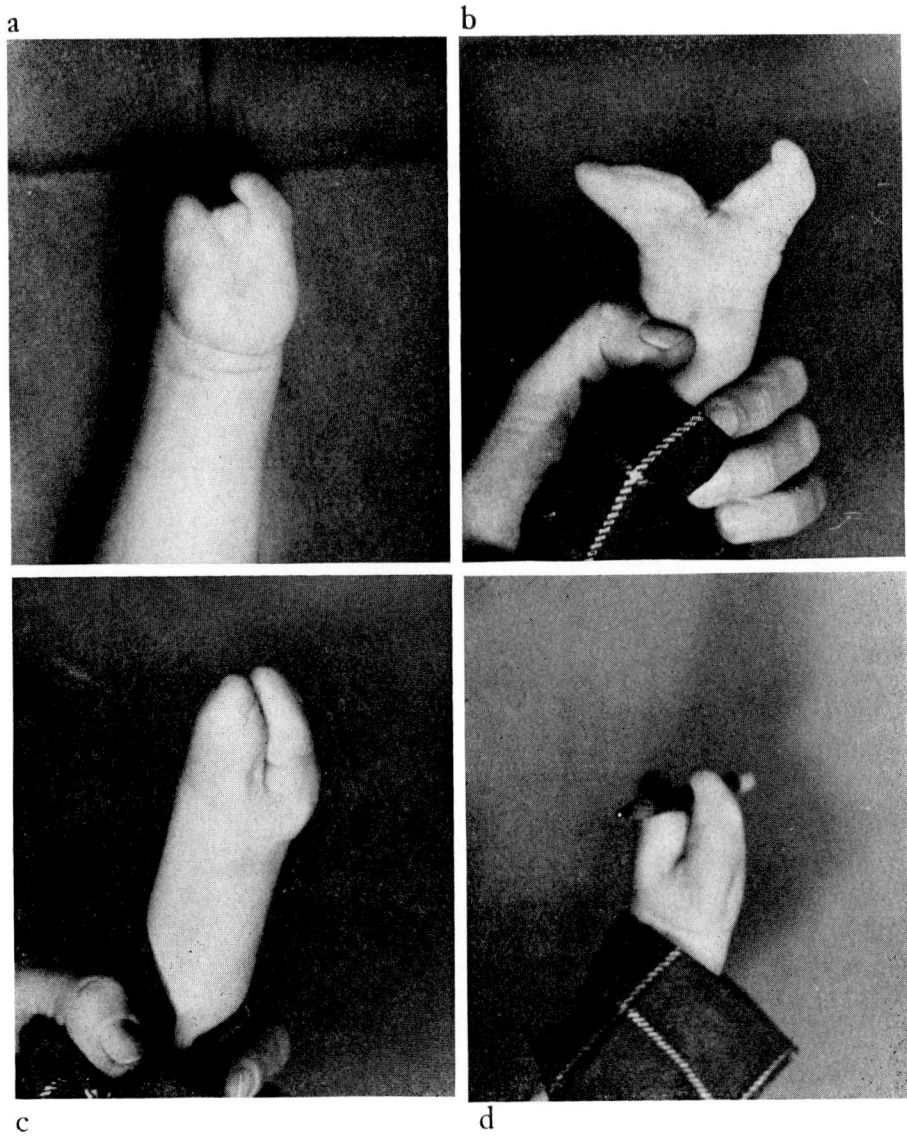

c

d

Case 169, *a:* Congenital "lobster-claw" formation of hand.
   b-d: Reconstruction consisting of resection of center section of hand, and skin grafting (see p. 980).

INDEX

INDEX

INDEX

INDEX

1224

INDEX

INDEX

INDEX

1230

INDEX

INDEX

1233

INDEX

INDEX

INDEX

INDEX

INDEX

1239

INDEX

1241

INDEX

INDEX

INDEX

INDEX

1248

INDEX

INDEX

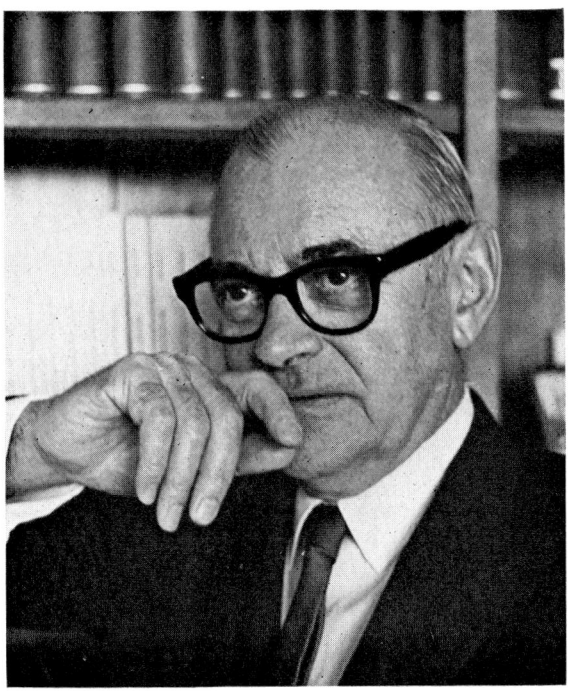

Following his graduation from the University of Freiburg, Germany, in 1926, Dr. May studied pathology under Ludwig Aschoff. In 1927 he joined the Surgical Clinic of the University of Munich, where he received training in general and in plastic and reconstructive surgery under the great teacher Dr. Erich Lexer. As Dr. Lexer's assistant, the author had the good fortune to participate in his chief's scientific pioneering and to work with him closely in writing and teaching. He left the Clinic in 1934 to make his home in Philadelphia.

Before his retirement in 1969, Dr. May was actively engaged in the practice of plastic and reconstructive surgery and in graduate teaching at the institutions with which he was affiliated. He was Associate Professor of Surgery at the Graduate School of Medicine, University of Pennsylvania, and Chief of the Department of Plastic and Reconstructive Surgery at Lankenau Hospital, Germantown Hospital, and St. Christopher's Hospital for Children.

The author is a diplomate of the American Board of Surgery and a member of the Founders' Group of the American Board of Plastic Surgery. He is affiliated with numerous national and international medical and surgical societies.